MW00653629

ADVANCED DRUG DELIVERY

ADVANCED DRUG DELIVERY

Edited by

ASHIM K. MITRA
Division of Pharmaceutical Sciences
University of Missouri—Kansas City
Kansas City, MO

CHI H. LEE
Division of Pharmaceutical Sciences
University of Missouri—Kansas City
Kansas City, MO

KUN CHENG
Division of Pharmaceutical Sciences
University of Missouri—Kansas City
Kansas City, MO

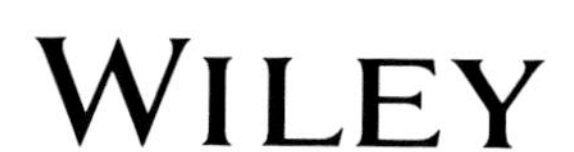

Published by John Wiley & Sons, Inc., Hoboken, New Jersey.
Published simultaneously in Canada.

Library of Congress Cataloging-in-Publication Data:

Advanced drug delivery/edited by Ashim K. Mitra, Chi H. Lee, Kun Cheng.
p.; cm.
Includes bibliographical references and index.
ISBN 978-1-118-02266-5 (cloth)
I. Mitra, Ashim K., 1954- II. Lee, Chi H. (Professor) III. Cheng, Kun (Professor)
[DNLM: 1. Drug Delivery Systems. QV 785]
RM301.12
615.1–dc23

2013014003

Printed in the United States of America

10 9 8 7 6 5 4 3 2 1

I would like to dedicate this book to the pharmaceutical industry.

Ashim K. Mitra

I owe my deepest gratitude to my wife, Dr. Yugyung Lee, for her love, devotion, and enormous support. I am pleased to mention my children, Eddie and Jason, who have given me encouragement and endless challenge.

Chi H. Lee

I dedicate this book to my parents, Mr. Guangxiong Cheng and Mrs. Pingqing Xu; my wife Lizhi Sun; my children Daniel and Jessica for their love and continuous support; and my mentors who have inspired me to pursue a career in science.

Kun Cheng

CONTENTS

PREFACE

During the past four decades, we have witnessed unprecedented breakthroughs in advanced delivery systems for efficient delivery of various therapeutic agents including small molecules as well as macromolecules. The development of advanced drug delivery systems for small-molecule drugs not only improves drug efficacy but also opens up new markets for the pharmaceutical industry. The global market for advanced drug delivery systems is expected to increase to $196.4 billion through 2014. On the other hand, remarkable progresses in molecular biology and biotechnology over the past two decades have not been matched by progresses in efficient delivery systems for the improvement of therapeutic efficacy. Therefore, it is integral to transform our knowledge in molecular biology and biotechnology into the development of effective delivery systems for macromolecular therapeutics.

Advanced Drug Delivery aims to provide up-to-date information of the basics, formulation strategies, and various therapeutic applications of advanced drug delivery. The goal of this book is to teach the philosophy of how to articulate practically the concepts of pharmaceutical sciences, chemistry, and molecular biology in such an integrated way that can ignite novel ideas to design and develop advanced delivery systems against various diseases.

This book is divided into four parts, starting with fundamentals related to physiological barriers, stability, transporters, and biomaterials in drug delivery. Then, it moves on to discuss different strategies that have been used for advanced delivery of small molecules as well as macromolecules. The third part focuses on regulatory considerations and translational applications of various advanced drug delivery systems in the treatment of critical and life-threatening diseases, such as cardiovascular diseases, cancer, sexually transmitted diseases, ophthalmic diseases, and brain diseases. The book ends with the applications of advance drug delivery in emerging research fields, such as stem cell research, cell-based therapeutics, tissue engineering, and molecular imaging. Each chapter provides objectives and assessment questions to facilitate student learning.

According to the report from the American Association of Pharmaceutical Scientists (AAPS), there is a critical shortage of well-trained pharmaceutical scientists in the areas of product development and related pharmaceutical technologies. We hope that this book will serve as a valuable tool not only for pharmacy graduate and undergraduate students but also for those healthcare professionals who have no pharmacy background but are engaged with drug development.

Finally, we would like to express our sincere appreciation and gratitude to all the contributors who spent enormous effort to share their knowledge and expertise in multiple aspects of advanced drug delivery.

Ashim K. Mitra
Chi H. Lee
Kun Cheng

ABOUT THE AUTHORS

Ashim K. Mitra received his Ph.D. in pharmaceutical chemistry in 1983 from the University of Kansas. He joined the University of Missouri—Kansas City (UMKC) in 1994 as chairman of the Pharmaceutical Sciences Department. He is currently the Vice Provost for Interdisciplinary Research, the UMKC Curators' Professor of Pharmacy, and a co-director of the Vision Research Center, UMKC School of Medicine. He has more than 30 years of experience in the field of ocular drug delivery and disposition. He has authored and co-authored over 280 refereed articles and 60 book chapters in the area of formulation development and ocular drug delivery; he has been awarded 9 patents and has presented (along with his research group) well over 500 presentations/abstracts at national and international scientific meetings. Prof. Mitra's work has attracted over US$6 million in funding from government agencies such as the National Institutes of Health (NIH), Department of Defense (DOD), and pharmaceutical companies. He is the recipient of numerous research awards from NIH, AAPS, AACP, ARVO, and pharmaceutical organizations.

Chi H. Lee received his B.S. degree in pharmacy from Seoul National University, South Korea. After getting his M.S. degree at the University of Washington, Seattle, he attended Rutgers University, North Brunswick, NJ, where he earned his Ph.D. degree. He completed his postdoctoral training at the University of Michigan Medical Center, Ann Arbor.

Prof. Lee was previously a member of the faculty at the University of Louisiana, Monroe, College of Pharmacy, before he moved to the University of Missouri—Kansas City, where his responsibilities include teaching undergraduate and graduate pharmacy students.

Prof. Lee has been actively involved in pharmaceutical research for more than three decades and has a special interest in the areas of formulation development and pathological mechanisms on microbicidal and cardiovascular devices and polymer-based systems. He has authored more than 55 articles and three book chapters on those subjects, and he has delivered more than 200 scientific presentations at local, national, and international symposia. Prof. Lee has received grants from various funding agencies including the National Institutes of Health (NIH) and the American Heart Association. He has served as a member of the American Association of Pharmaceutical Scientists, Society for Biomaterials, American Association of College of Pharmacy, Controlled Release Society, and American Heart Association.

Kun Cheng is an associate professor of pharmaceutical sciences at the University of Missouri—Kansas City (UMKC). He received his B.S. and M.S. degrees in pharmaceutical sciences from China Pharmaceutical University. He also received an M.S. degree in pharmacy from the National University of Singapore. He worked at the Bright Future Pharmaceutical Company in Hong Kong prior to joining the University of Tennessee Health Science Center, where he received his Ph.D. in pharmaceutical sciences. His current research focuses on the development of novel drug delivery systems for siRNA and small-molecule drugs.

Much of the effort from his laboratory has dealt with the therapeutic exploration of macromolecular agents, which have poor stability and inefficient cellular uptake.

Prof. Cheng has been actively engaged in extramural professional activities and in teaching graduate and PharmD students. He has edited one book titled *Advanced Delivery and Therapeutic Applications of RNAi* and two theme issues for the journals *Molecular Pharmaceutics* and *Pharmaceutical Research.* He is the recipient of the 2011 American Association of Pharmaceutical Scientists (AAPS) New Investigator Grant Award in Pharmaceutics and Pharmaceutical Technologies.

CONTRIBUTORS

Gayathri Acharya, University of Missouri—Kansas City, Kansas City, MO, USA

Vibhuti Agrahari, University of Missouri—Kansas City, Kansas City, MO, USA

Megha Barot, University of Missouri—Kansas City, Kansas City, MO, USA

Haibo Cai, East China University of Science and Technology, Shanghai, China

Mei-Ling Chen, Office of Pharmaceutical Science, Center for Drug Evaluation and Research, U.S. Food and Drug Administration, Silver Spring, MD, USA

Zhijin Chen, University of Missouri—Kansas City, Kansas City, MO, USA

Kun Cheng, Division of Pharmaceutical Sciences, School of Pharmacy, University of Missouri—Kansas City, Kansas City, MO, USA

Hoo-Kyun Choi, School of Pharmacy, Chosun University, Gwangju, South Korea

Kishore Cholkar, University of Missouri—Kansas City, Kansas City, MO, USA

Hari R. Desu, Department of Pharmaceutical Sciences, College of Pharmacy, University of Tennessee Health Science Center, Memphis, TN, USA

Omid C. Farokhzad, Laboratory of Nanomedicine and Biomaterials, Department of Anesthesiology, Brigham and Women's Hospital, Harvard Medical School, Boston, MA, USA

Weiwei Gao, Brigham and Women's Hospital, Harvard Medical School, Boston, MA, USA

Mitan R. Gokulgandhi, University of Missouri—Kansas City, Kansas City, MO, USA

Nazila Kamaly, Laboratory of Nanomedicine and Biomaterials, Department of Anesthesiology, Brigham and Women's Hospital, Harvard Medical School, Boston, MA, USA

Varun Khurana, University of Missouri—Kansas City, Kansas City, MO, USA

Deep Kwatra, Department of Molecular and Integrative Physiology, University of Kansas Medical Center, Kansas City, KS, USA

Chi H. Lee, Division of Pharmaceutical Sciences, School of Pharmacy, University of Missouri—Kansas City, Kansas City, MO, USA

Yugyung Lee, School of Interdisciplinary Computing and Engineering, University of Missouri—Kansas City, Kansas City, MO, USA

Zheng-Rong Lu, Department of Biomedical Engineering, Case Western Reserve University, Cleveland, OH, USA

Rubi Mahato, University of Missouri—Kansas City, Kansas City, MO, USA

Nanda K. Mandava, University of Missouri—Kansas City, Kansas City, MO, USA

Mukul Minocha, University of Missouri—Kansas City, Kansas City, MO, USA

Ashim K. Mitra, Division of Pharmaceutical Sciences, School of Pharmacy, University of Missouri—Kansas City, Kansas City, MO, USA

Mridul Mukherji, University of Missouri—Kansas City, Kansas City, MO, USA

D. Alexander Oh, Clinical Pharmacology Akros Pharma, Inc., Princeton, NJ

Dhananjay Pal, University of Missouri—Kansas City, Kansas City, MO, USA

Ashaben Patel, University of Missouri—Kansas City, Kansas City, MO, USA

Mitesh Patel, University of Missouri—Kansas City, Kansas City, MO, USA

Durga Paturi, University of Missouri—Kansas City, Kansas City, MO, USA

Bin Qin, University of Missouri—Kansas City, Kansas City, MO, USA

Animikh Ray, University of Missouri—Kansas City, Kansas City, MO, USA

Jwala Renukuntla, University of Missouri—Kansas City, Kansas City, MO, USA

Maxim G. Ryadnov, National Physical Laboratory, Teddington, Middlesex, UK

Sujay Shah, University of Missouri—Kansas City, Kansas City, MO, USA

Ravi S. Shukla, University of Missouri—Kansas City, Kansas City, MO, USA

Robhash K. Subedi, College of Pharmacy, Chosun University, Gwangju, South Korea

Wanyi Tai, University of Missouri—Kansas City, Kansas City, MO, USA

Wen-Song Tan, East China University of Science and Technology, Shanghai, China

Laura A. Thoma, Department of Pharmaceutical Sciences, College of Pharmacy, University of Tennessee Health Science Center, Memphis, TN, USA

Ramya Krishna Vadlapatla, University of Missouri—Kansas City, Kansas City, MO, USA

Aswani Dutt Vadlapudi, University of Missouri—Kansas City, Kansas City, MO, USA

Divya Teja Vavilala, University of Missouri—Kansas City, Kansas City, MO, USA

Shaoying Wang, University of Missouri—Kansas City, Kansas City, MO, USA

Wuchen Wang, University of Missouri—Kansas City, Kansas City, MO, USA

Xiaoyan Yang, University of Missouri—Kansas City, Kansas City, MO, USA

Zhaoyang Ye, The State Key Laboratory of Bioreactor Engineering, School of Bioengineering, East China University of Science and Technology, Shanghai, China

Yan Zhou, East China University of Science and Technology, Shanghai, China

PART I

INTRODUCTION AND BASICS OF ADVANCED DRUG DELIVERY

1

PHYSIOLOGICAL BARRIERS IN ADVANCED DRUG DELIVERY: GASTROINTESTINAL BARRIER

D. ALEXANDER OH AND CHI H. LEE

1.1 CHAPTER OBJECTIVES

- To outline gastrointestinal anatomy and physiology impacting advanced oral drug delivery systems.
- To review key physiological and physicochemical factors influencing drug absorption.
- To illustrate efficient strategies for overcoming gastrointestinal barriers in drug delivery.

1.2 INTRODUCTION

Drug delivery through oral administration is a complicated process: A drug must withstand the digestive processes and penetrate through the gastrointestinal (GI) barrier into the bloodstream. Drugs absorbed from the GI tract travel through portal veins to the liver, and then they are subjected to first-pass metabolism by the hepatic enzymes before entering the systemic circulation [1]. The oral route of drug administration is traditionally known as the most preferred route for systemic drug delivery, even though there are disadvantages, such as unpredictable and erratic absorption, gastrointestinal intolerance, incomplete absorption, degradation of drug in GI contents, and presystemic metabolism, mostly resulting in reduced bioavailability.

The primary functions of the GI tract are absorption and digestion of food, as well as secretion of various enzymes or fluids [2]. The gastrointestinal mucosa forms a barrier between the body and a luminal environment that contains not only nutrients but also potentially hostile microorganisms and toxins. The normal function of the GI barrier, which is referred to the properties of the gastric and intestinal mucosa, is essential for disease prevention and overall maintenance of health. The major challenge in drug delivery through the GI tract is to achieve efficient transport of nutrients and drugs across the epithelium while rigorously excluding passage of harmful molecules and organisms into the body.

The performance of GI barriers to drug transport may largely depend on the physicochemical characteristics of drugs. Water-soluble small molecules may not be easily absorbed unless a specific transporter to those molecules is present, while lipophilic drugs can be relatively well absorbed through GI barriers. Mucosal transporters include PEPT, OATP, OCT, MCT, ASBT, MDR1, MRP, and BCRP among others [3] as shown in Figure 1.1. Large-molecule drugs, such as antibodies and proteins, may suffer extensive enzymatic degradation in the GI tract [4].

In this chapter, gastrointestinal mucous membranes and gut physiology will be intensively covered from the perspective of physiological barriers, which will lead to thorough understanding of key obstacles to advanced oral drug delivery.

Advanced Drug Delivery, First Edition. Edited by Ashim K. Mitra, Chi H. Lee, and Kun Cheng.

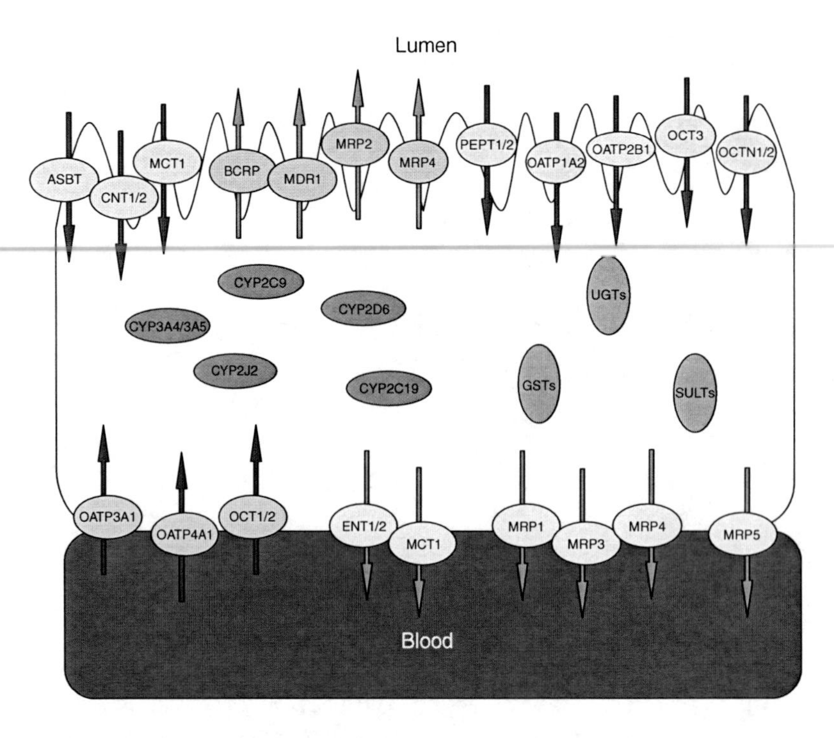

FIGURE 1.1 The intestinal metabolizing enzymes and uptake/efflux transporters [3].

1.2.1 Anatomy of Gastrointestinal Tract

1.2.1.1 Gastrointestinal Anatomy The major components of the gastrointestinal tract are the stomach, small intestine, and large intestine. The small intestine with a length of about 6 m includes the duodenum, jejunum, and ileum [5]. The stomach is a pouch-like structure lined with a relatively smooth epithelial surface. Extensive absorption of numerous weakly acidic or nonionized drugs and certain weakly basic drugs were demonstrated in the stomach under varying experimental conditions [2, 6, 7].

The small intestine is the most important site for drug absorption in the gastrointestinal tract. The epithelial surface area through which absorption of drug takes place in the small intestine is enormously large because of the presence of villi and microvilli, finger-like projections arising from and forming folds in the intestinal mucosa as shown in Figure 1.2 [8]. The surface area decreases sharply from proximal to distal small intestine and was estimated to range from 80-cm^2/cm serosal length just beyond the duodeno-jejunal flexure to about 20-cm^2/cm serosal length just before the ileo-cecal valve in humans [9]. The total surface area of the human small intestine is about 200 to 500 m^2 [6, 7]. The small intestine is made up of various types of epithelial cells, i.e., absorptive cells (enterocytes), undifferentiated crypt cells, goblet cells, endocrine cells, paneth cells, and M cells. There is also a progressive decrease in the average size of aqueous pores from proximal to distal small intestine and colon [10, 11].

The small intestine is the most involved region for carrier-mediated transport of endogenous and exogenous compounds. The proximal small intestine is the major area for absorption of dietary constituents including monosaccharides, amino acids, vitamins, and minerals. Both vitamin B_{12} and bile salts appear to have specific absorption sites in the ileum [2]. The large intestine has a considerably less irregular mucosa than the small intestine.

1.2.1.2 Pores The aqueous pores render the epithelial membranes freely permeable to water, monovalant ions and hydrophilic solutes with a smaller molecular size [2, 6, 7]. It was estimated that the hypothetical pores in the proximal intestine have an average radius of 7.5 Å, and those in distal intestine (ileum) have that of about 3.5 Å [10]. The pore sizes of the aqueous pathway for buccal and sublingual mucosa in pigs were estimated as 18–22 and 30–53 Å, respectively [12]. Since the molecular size of most drug molecules are larger than a pore size in the membrane, drug transport through pores seems to be of minor importance in drug absorption. However, some larger polar compounds with molecular weights up to several hundreds are still absorbed through active participation of the membrane components.

1.2.1.3 Tight Junctions Tight junctions are closely associated areas of two cells whose membranes join together, forming a virtually impermeable barrier to fluid. Tight

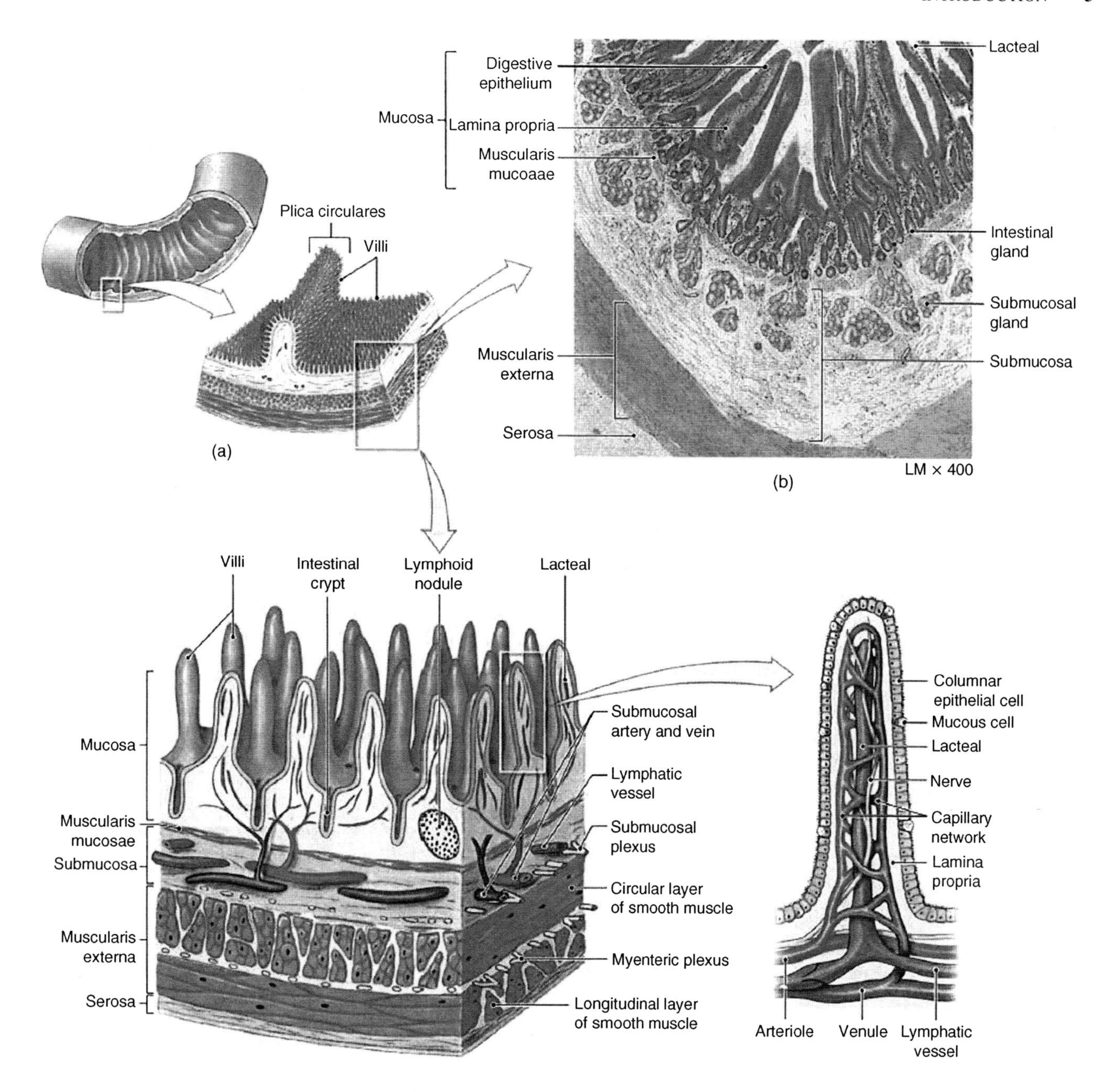

FIGURE 1.2 Gastrointestinal anatomy [8].

junctions are composed of the structural proteins (occludin and claudins), the scaffold proteins (ZO-1, ZO-2, fodrin, cingulin, symplekin, 7H6, and p130), and the actin cytoskeleton [13]. Paracellular transport of drugs mostly occurs via tight junctions (Figure 1.3). The permeability of intestinal epithelium to large molecules or ionized drugs depends on the combination of transcellular transport via adsorptive endocytosis and paracellular transport through tight junctions.

Tight junctions were conceptualized a century ago as secreted extracellular cement, forming an absolute and unregulated barrier within the paracellular space [2, 6, 7]. The contribution of the paracellular pathway of the gastrointestinal tract to the general correlation between environment and host molecular interaction was considered to be negligible. It is apparent that tight junctions have extremely dynamic structures engaged with developmental, physiological, and pathological situations.

To date, particular attention has been placed on the role of tight junction dysfunction in the pathogenesis of several diseases, particularly autoimmune diseases with viral etiology [2, 6, 7]. Pathophysiological regulation of tight junctions is influenced by various factors including secretory

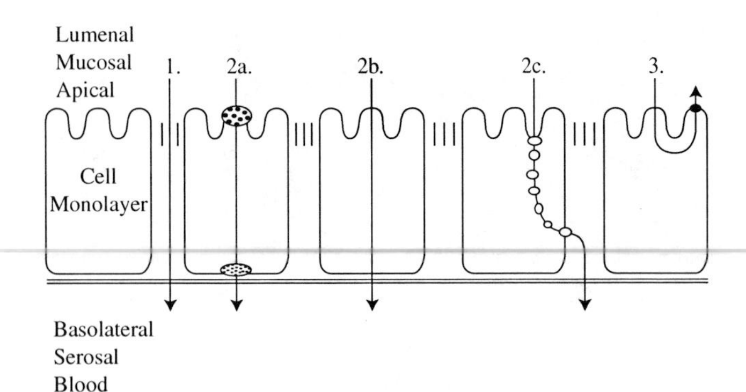

FIGURE 1.3 Mechanism of drug transport through epithelial membranes. 1. Paracellular; 2. Transcellular: 2a. Carrier-mediated; 2b. Passive diffusion; 2c. Receptor-mediated endocytosis; 3. Mediated efflux pathway. (See color figure in color plate section.)

IgA, enzymes, neuropeptides, neurotransmitters, dietary peptides and lectins, yeast, aerobic and anaerobic bacteria, parasites, proinflammatory cytokines, free radicals, and regulatory T-cell dysfunction [2].

1.2.2 Gastrointestinal Physiology

A comprehensive review of the physiological parameters that affect oral absorption in the context of formulation performance and drug dissolution was recently published [14]. This physiologically relevant information to oral human drug delivery could serve as a basis for the design of advanced drug delivery systems.

1.2.2.1 Gastrointestinal Components

(i) *Bile Salts.* Bile salts are known to enhance the absorption of hydrophobic drugs by enhancing their wettability. The absorption rates of such drugs as griseofulvin can be facilitated when they are taken after meals as a result of the increase of bile salts excretion that promotes their dissolution rates [2]. On the contrary, bile salts reduced the absorption of certain drugs, such as aminoglycosides, neomycin, and nystatin, through the formation of non-absorbable complexes with bile salts [15].

(ii) *Mucin.* Mucin is a viscous muco-polysaccharaide (glycoprotein) that lines the gastrointestinal mucosa for protection and lubrication purposes [16]. Mucin has a negative anionic charge, so it may form a nonabsorbable complex with some drugs, such as aminoglycosides and quaternary ammonium compounds, subsequently affecting their absorption.

(iii) *Enzymes.* Since GIT fluid contains high concentrations of enzymes needed for food digestion, some enzymes may act on drugs. For example, esterases secreted by pancreas affect the metabolic process of ester derivative drugs including aspirin and propoxyphene through the hydrolysis process in the intestine [17]. In epithelial cells, the partial location of the enzyme on the basolateral pole underlies the vectoral transport of salts, water, and organic solutes (e.g., bile salts) across the tissue, whereas in nonepithelial cells, such as fibroblasts, the enzyme is evenly distributed on the cell surface [4].

1.2.2.2 Gastrointestinal Blood Flow About 28% of cardiac output is supplied to the gastrointestinal tract by blood capillaries [2, 6, 7]. The blood perfusion of the gastrointestinal tract plays a critical role in drug absorption by continuously preserving the concentration gradient across the epithelial membrane. Polar molecules that are slowly absorbed exhibit no significant dependence on blood flow, but lipid-soluble molecules and molecules that are small enough to penetrate easily through the aqueous pores are greatly affected by the rate of blood flow. In general, the drug absorption rate is not significantly affected by physiological variability in mesenteric blood flow because blood flow is rarely a rate-limiting step in the drug absorption process through the gastrointestinal tract.

1.2.2.3 Luminal pH The pH of gastric fluid varies considerably according to the sites and contents. Gastric secretions have a pH of less than 1, but the pH of gastric contents is usually between 1 and 3 as a result of dilution and diet [2, 6, 7]. The pH of the stomach contents is briefly but distinctly elevated after a meal; thus, pH values of 5 or even greater are not unusual. Fasting tends to decrease the pH of gastric fluids and subsequently influences the pH of the stomach.

The luminal pH in the small intestine is about 6 to 7 [18], and large intestines have a similar luminal pH as described in Table 1.1. The acidic microclimate pH in the human jejunum was elevated in disease states and contributed to the deviation of the absorption profiles of weak electrolytes from the pH-partition hypothesis [19].

The pH at the absorption site is an integral factor in drug absorption because most drugs are either weak organic acids or bases [2, 6, 7]. Since the gastrointestinal barrier is highly permeable to uncharged and lipid-soluble solutes, a drug may be well absorbed from the segment of the gastrointestinal tract where a favorable pH exists but poorly absorbed from other segments where a less favorable pH exists. Weakly acidic drugs rapidly dissolve in alkaline pH, while basic drugs are more soluble in acidic pH. In addition, disintegration of certain pharmaceutical dosage forms is pH dependent; for example, enteric coated tablets dissolve only in alkaline pH. Luminal pH can influence the stability of some drugs including erythromycin, which is rapidly degraded in the acidic pH [20, 21].

TABLE 1.1 Gastrointestinal Physiology in Humans

GI Region	Length (cm)	Surface Area (cm^2)	Diameter (cm)	pH	Flow Rate (mL/min)	Average Residence Time
Entire GI tract	530–870	2×10^6		1.5–7		Up to 38 h
Mouth cavity	15–20	700				
Esophagus	20	200				
Stomach	25					
Fasted state		65		1.4–2.1		0.5–1.5 h
Fed state		660		2–5		2–6 h
Small intestine	370–630	$2.1–5.9 \times 10^6$		4.4–7.4		3 ± 1 h
Duodenum	20–30	$1.13–2.83 \times 10^5$	3.5–6	4.9–6.4		3–10 min
Jejunum	150–260	$2.70–7.50 \times 10^5$	2.5–4	4.4–6.4	0.73 (fasted); 3.0 (fed)	0.5–2 h
Ileum	200–350	$3.60–10.50 \times 10^5$	2.3–8	6.5–7.4	0.33 (fasted); 2.35 (fed)	0.5–2.5 h
Large intestine	150	15,000		5.5–7.4		Up to 27 h
Caecum	7	500		5.5–7		
Colon	90–150	15,000		5.5–7.4		
Rectum	11–16	150		7		

Source: Adapted from Refs. 1, 14, 82, and 90.

1.2.2.4 Gastric Emptying and Gastrointestinal Motility The volume of gastric contents greatly influences the concentration of a drug in the stomach. The rate of gastric emptying is governed by the volume of gastric contents and has a direct impact on the chemical and physical properties of chyme in the duodenum and jejunum [6]. Standard low bulk meals and liquids are transferred from the stomach to the duodenum in an apparent first-order fashion with a half-life of 20 to 60 minutes in healthy adults [6]. In addition, numerous factors as described in Table 1.2 can influence the rate of the gastric emptying process.

Gastric emptying is the major factor that greatly contributes to unusually large intersubject variability in the absorption of drugs released from enteric-coated tablets [22]. Gastric emptying is retarded by fats and fatty acids in the diet, high concentrations of electrolytes or hydrogen ion, high viscosity, mental depression, lying on the left side, and diseases, such as gastroenteritis and gastric ulcer [23]. Gastric emptying of liquids is much faster than that of solid food or solid dosage forms. Gastric emptying is promoted at low stomach pH and retarded at alkaline pH. Various drugs including atropine and narcotic analgesics, amitriptyline, propantheline, and imipramine can also retard gastric emptying [24, 25].

The gastrointestinal tract during the fasting state undergoes the characteristic sequences of motion (i.e., waves of activity) known as the interdigestive myoelectric complex or migrating motility complex [6]. The motility of the small intestine called the small bowel transit time also plays an integral role in drug absorption. The mean transit time of unabsorbed food residues or insoluble granules through the human small intestine is estimated to be about 4 hours [26].

Apart from dissolution of a drug and its permeation through the GI membrane, gastric emptying can also serve as a rate-limiting step in the drug absorption from the intestine. It is generally accepted that fast gastric emptying increases the bioavailability of most drugs. For example, a good correlation was found between stomach emptying time and peak plasma concentration for acetaminophen [27]. The rapid gastric emptying is desirable, when a fast onset of drug action is required (i.e., pain killers), when dissolution of a drug occurs in the intestine, when a drug is not stable in the gastric media, or when a drug is best absorbed from the distal part of the small intestine (e.g., vitamin B_{12}) [2]. Delayed gastric emptying may be preferred, if the food and/or gastric juice promote the disintegration and dissolution of a drug, if

TABLE 1.2 Factors Affecting Gastric Emptying

Gastric Emptying	Influencing Factors	Drugs
Increase	Higher temperature of food, volume of meal (initially), liquid meal, low pH, anxiety and stress, fasting, hyperthyroidism	Cisapride, domperidone, metoclopramide
Decrease	Lying on the left side, type of meal (fatty food > proteins > carbohydrates), solid food, volume of meal, bulky material, higher pH, vigorous exercise, depression	Antacids, anticholinergics (e.g., atropine), narcotic (e.g., morphine), analgesic (e.g., aspirin), tri-cyclic antidepressants, amitriptyline, propantheline, imipramine

a drug like griseofulvin dissolves slowly, if a drug irritates the gastric mucosa (e.g., aspirin), or if a drug is absorbed from the proximal part of the intestines and prolonged duration of action is needed (e.g., vitamin C) [21, 28]. Delayed intestinal transit time may be suitable for enteric coated formulations, sustained release dosage forms, and drugs with site-specific absorption in the intestines.

1.2.3 Gastrointestinal Barrier

1.2.3.1 Barrier to Bioavailability Bioavailability is traditionally defined as a ratio of drug amount at the systemic circulation to the amount taken into gut lumen, which is equivalent to an extent of absorption. The whole absorption process is a sequential event and includes dissolution and precipitation in the gut, enzymatic and chemical degradation, permeation through epithelial membrane, and metabolism at both the intestinal wall and the liver. It also includes other physiologic conditions, such as blood flow and transit time as described above, which are all together considered as barriers against complete absorption. The other element of the absorption process is the rate of absorption, which is governed by a series of time-dependent steps, such as dissolution, gastric emptying, intestinal transit time, and membrane permeability, at the brush border epithelial cells [28].

For a drug administered orally, the two most common reasons for its poor bioavailability are the decreased absorption and presystemic first-pass effects [28]. Low solubility and/or less optimal membrane permeability are key parameters for decreased absorption [29]. Before a drug reaches the blood circulation, it has to pass for the first time through organs of elimination, namely, the GI tract and the liver. The loss of drug through biotransformation by such eliminating organs during its passage to systemic circulation is called first-pass or presystemic metabolism. The low drug concentration or complete absence of the drug in plasma after oral administration is indicative of first-pass effects.

The presystemic metabolism of a drug is influenced by luminal, gut wall, bacterial, and hepatic enzymes [28]. Luminal enzymes are the enzymes present in the gut fluids as well as those from intestinal and pancreatic secretions. The enzymes from pancreatic secretions include hydrolases that metabolize ester drugs like choramphenicol and peptides, split the amide linkages through hydrolysis, and ultimately inactivate the protein and polypeptides drugs [2]. Gut wall enzymes also known as mucosal enzymes are mostly present in stomach mucosa. Intestinal mucosa has both phase I and phase II enzymes, e.g., CYP3A4/5, CYP2C9, CYP2C19, CYP2D6, UGT, GST, and SULT as shown in Figure 1.1 [3]. The activity of phase I enzymes in the gut wall is the highest at the duodenum and decreases distally. The highest expression of phase I enzymes was found between villous tips and midvilli. The GI microbes are rich in colon, whereas they are poorly present in stomach and small intestines [2]. Thus, many orally administered drugs remain unaffected by bacterial enzymes.

The colonic microbes generally render a drug more potent or toxic on biotransformation. For example, sulfasalazine, a drug used in ulcerative colitis, is hydrolyzed to sulfa pyridine and 5-amino-salicylic acid by the microbial enzymes of the colon. Hepatic enzymes play a major role in biotransformation of most drugs going through the first-pass effect before they reach the systemic circulation. Liver has both phase I (oxidation, reduction, hydrolysis) and phase II (glucuronidation, sulfation, methylation, acetylation) enzymes [2, 6]. Among them, cytochrome P450 enzymes are responsible for metabolism and bioactivation of about 75% of all drugs [30].

In the lumen of the small intestine, dietary fat is hydrolyzed to its components, monoacylglycerol (MG) and free fatty acids (FAs), and subsequently dispersed in bile acids. The pH in close proximity to the enterocyte surface is lower than other sites, causing protonation of the fatty acids. Free FAs then dissociate from the bile salt micelles and either passively diffuse or are transported across the brush border membrane by protein-mediated transporters like cluster determinant 36 (CD36), fatty acid binding protein (FABPpm), and fatty acid transport protein family members (FATPs) [31]. Both CD36 and FABPpm are found to reside in specialized microdomains known as lipid rafts [32].

Like dietary fat and cholesterol, lipid-soluble drugs are absorbed by the fat absorption pathways [2]. The oral absorption rates of griseofulvin and vitamin D were enhanced by certain oily formulations including the bile salt micelles that were transferred to blood circulation via the intestinal lymph system. The process of lipid absorption is classified into 3 steps: 1) the uptake, 2) assembled into lipoproteins, and 3) secretion of lipid into the lymphatic circulation. Each step in lipid absorption may be subjected to the pathway-involved regulation.

1.2.3.2 Barrier to Immunity The intestinal epithelium is the largest mucosal surface, providing an interface between the external environment and the mammalian host. The intestinal mucosa is continuously exposed to an immense load of antigens from ingested food, resident bacteria, and invading viruses [33]. The single-cell epithelial layer lining the gut lumen (Table 1.1, surface area $\sim$2.1 to 5.9×10^6 cm^2) has biphase functions, playing a major role in the digestion and absorption of nutrients and simultaneously constituting the organism's most important barrier between the internal and external environments. Epithelial permeability to nutrients depends on the regulation of intercellular tight junctions (TJs) as well as the activity of transcellular transport via endocytosis [13]. Epithelium has its ability to regulate the trafficking of macromolecules between the host organ and its environment through barrier properties. Intact macromolecules can be absorbed either via the transcellular or the paracellular pathway. For the transcellular pathway, the uptake of macromolecules occurs through the endocytosis process, followed by fusion with lysosomes (phagolysosomes) with potential degradation of the macromolecules before being delivered into the submucosa. In contrast, macromolecules penetrate the intestinal epithelium through the paracellular pathway, reaching the submucosa mostly in an intact form.

Paracellular passage of macromolecules under either physiological or pathological conditions is safeguarded by gut-associated lymphoid tissue (GALT) [34]. GALT serves as a containment system that prevents potentially harmful intestinal antigens from accessing the systemic circulation and induces systemic tolerance against luminal antigens through the processes involved with polymeric Ig A secretion and induction of T-regulatory-cell activity and immune tolerance [34]. Macrophages, leukocytes, and mucosal mast cells (MMCs) release numerous mediators that alter gut function. MMCs release various preformed mediators, such as histamine, serotonin, and mast-cell proteases, as well as newly synthesized mediators including leukotrienes, prostaglandins, platelet-activating factor, interleukin-4, and TNF-α· Most of these mediators affect epithelial permeability, which might explain, in part, enhanced intestinal permeability featured in both T helper 1 (Th1)-mediated and Th2-mediated pathologies [34].

In disease conditions including inflammatory bowel disease, excessive penetration of antigens through the epithelial layer may result in inappropriate immune stimulation, leading to chronic gastrointestinal inflammation [33]. The permeability of substrates through the intestinal epithelium depends on the regulation process of the mucosal immune system and intercellular tight junctions. Serum immunoglobulin to food antigen macromolecules were found in patients with inflammatory bowel disease and celiac disease, indicating that an enhanced amount of these proteins permeate through the intestinal epithelium, and trigger a systemic immune response. The permeability of substrates through the intestinal barrier increased in such disease conditions as food sensitivity, intestinal diseases [35], acute gastroenteritis, chronic intestinal infections, surgery, exercise, stress, extensive burns, malnutrition, secretory IgA deficiency, anti-inflammatory drugs, and viral infections [33].

1.2.3.3 Barrier to Microorganisms The acidic pH of the stomach and the antibacterial activity of pancreatic enzymes, bile, and intestinal secretions have also served as GI tract barriers [36]. Peristalsis and the natural loss of epithelial cells remove microorganisms. If peristalsis is slowed, the removal process of microorganisms is delayed, producing certain infections including symptomatic shigellosis. Compromised GI defense mechanisms may predispose patients to particular infections. Normal bowel microflora can inhibit pathogens; alteration of this flora with antibiotics allows for overgrowth of inherently pathogenic microorganisms or super infection with ordinarily commensal organisms such as *Candida albicans*.

1.2.4 Absorption Models

The barrier properties of the intestinal epithelium are generally investigated by assessing the permeability to various probe/marker molecules *in vivo* or *in vitro* with intestinal segments mounted in Ussing-type chambers. Although *in vivo* studies are more physiological, the *in vitro* approach makes it feasible to study epithelial permeability to a greater range of probes including proteins, and to determine the mechanisms and routes of passage involved. *In vitro* cell culture models, such as Caco-2, MDCK, or HT-29 cells, are used to measure drug permeability. The *in vivo* quantitative assessment models currently available are human jejunal perfusion technique, intravital microscopy of fluorescent bacteria, and *in vivo* fluorescence microscopic imaging for intestinal mucosa permeability [37, 38].

There are numerous *in vivo*, *in situ*, *in vitro*, and *in silico* models for assessment of absorption/transport-related mechanisms in addition to examining barrier properties [39, 40]. The absorption models and tools for *in silico, in vitro*, and *in vivo* experiments/methods used to get various parameters influencing human dosage regimen are shown in Figure 1.4. For example, an intestinal perfusion model allows for estimation of effective permeability (Peff), which enables estimation of bioavailability (F). Similarly, the Ussing chamber or Caco-2 model can provide apparent permeability [40], whereas the parallel artificial membrane permeability assay (PAMPA) enables estimation of passive permeability in a high throughput mode. Other *in vitro* models, such as everted gut sacs, brush border membrane vesicles (BBMVs), or intestinal rings, can serve as a means to investigate apparent absorption rates of drugs [40].

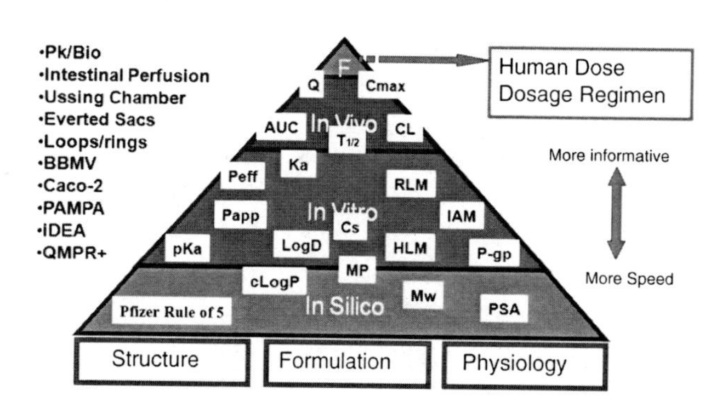

FIGURE 1.4 Absorption models and tools for *in silico, in vitro*, and *in vivo* experiments/methods to get various parameters influencing human dosage regimen.

It is also feasible to calculate various descriptors, such as Lipinski's Rule of Five, molecular weight (MW), polar surface area (PSA), clogP, solubility, and permeability, to a certain extent directly from the structure of a drug [40]. By taking the fundamental complexity of GI physiology and formulation characteristics into further consideration, the advanced absorption model could accurately estimate oral bioavailability and successfully predict an individual dosage regimen, which are crucial in the new drug development process.

Pharmacokinetics and biopharmaceutics are the fundamental areas for development of new drug formulations and evaluation of their clinical efficacy. Pharmacokinetics is divided into drug disposition features including the extent and rate of absorption, distribution, metabolism, and excretion. This is commonly referred to as the ADME scheme [41]. The kinetic approach using a compartment model has been frequently used, and the formation and ADME profiles of each metabolite have been broadly defined [42, 43]. Advanced evaluation and prediction tools for bioavailability/bioequivalence of drugs are also required in every stage of the drug assessment process. The drawbacks of biopharmaceutical estimation have mainly resulted from the physicochemical properties of drugs or the physiological factors of patients. Scientists have been enthusiastic to develop a theoretical model capable of predicting oral drug absorption in humans based on various mechanistic approaches, which can also address intrapatients' variances.

The mechanistic approaches are classified into three categories based on their dependence on spatial and temporal variables [44]: quasi-equilibrium models, steady-state models, and dynamic models. The quasi-equilibrium models are independent of spatial and temporal variables, and they include the pH-partition hypothesis and absorption potential concept. The steady-state models are independent of temporal variables, but they are dependent on spatial variables and include the film model, macroscopic mass balance approach, and microscopic balance approach [45]. The steady-state models are restricted to prediction of the extent rather than the rate of oral drug absorption [44]. The dynamic models deals with the relationship between spatial and temporal variables and include dispersion models and compartmental models [3]. The dynamic models can predict both the rate and extent of oral drug absorption, and thus, they are considered an improvement over the steady-state models.

1.3 PHYSIOLOGICAL FACTORS INFLUENCING DRUG ABSORPTION

Gastrointestinal absorption of orally administered drugs is influenced by various factors including physiological, physicochemical, and formulation factors [2, 7]. Physiological factors are age, blood flow to the GI tract, gastric empting and intestinal transit, disease state, first-pass effect, pH of luminal contents, a surface area of absorptive site, digestive enzymes, and microbial flora. Solubility, stability, buffers, complexation, particle size, crystal properties, pKa, and diffusion coefficient are classified as physicochemical factors that can affect drug absorption.

Formulation factors include dosage forms and pharmaceutical excipients that are needed to secure stability, acceptability, bioavailability, or functionality of the drug product [39]. Oral dosage forms, such as solution, suspension, tablet, or capsules, are influenced by these factors. Multiple excipients in a dosage form may cause poor absorption and low bioavailability of drugs [39]. Excipients commonly used are binders, buffers, coatings, diluents, disintegrants, lubricants, suspending agents, sweeteners, colorants, and surfactants [39]. Since drug absorption is concomitantly affected by various factors, it is quite difficult to determine which factors are mainly responsible for the poor bioavailability of specific drugs.

1.3.1 Epithelial Membranes

All cells are bound by membranes [46], which consist of the phospholipids bilayer with embedded proteins as described in Figure 1.5. Cell membranes are involved with a variety of cellular processes, such as cell adhesion, ion conductivity, and cell signaling. Cell membranes serve as the attachment surface for the extracellular glycocalyx, cell wall, and intracellular cytoskeleton. The lipid bilayer of cell membranes is impermeable to most water-soluble molecules.

Membrane transport processes in most biological events occur during the formation process of electrochemical potentials and the uptake process of nutrients, such as sugars and amino acids, removal of wastes, endocytotic internalization of macromolecules, and oxygen transport in respiration [4, 47]. The movement of many ions, nutrients, and metabolites across cellular membranes is catalyzed by specific transport proteins, i. e., transporters that show saturation and substrate specificity [48]. Thus, cell membrane is selectively permeable to ions and organic molecules. The epithelium lies on top of connective tissue, from which it is separated by a basement membrane. It is composed of tightly clustered cells connected by tight junctions and desmosomes. The gastrointestinal barrier that separates the lumen of the stomach and intestines from the systemic circulation has the properties similar to a semipermeable membrane with the complex structure composed of lipids, proteins, lipoproteins, and polysaccharides. Lipid-soluble molecules penetrate the barrier directly through the lipophilic portion of the membrane.

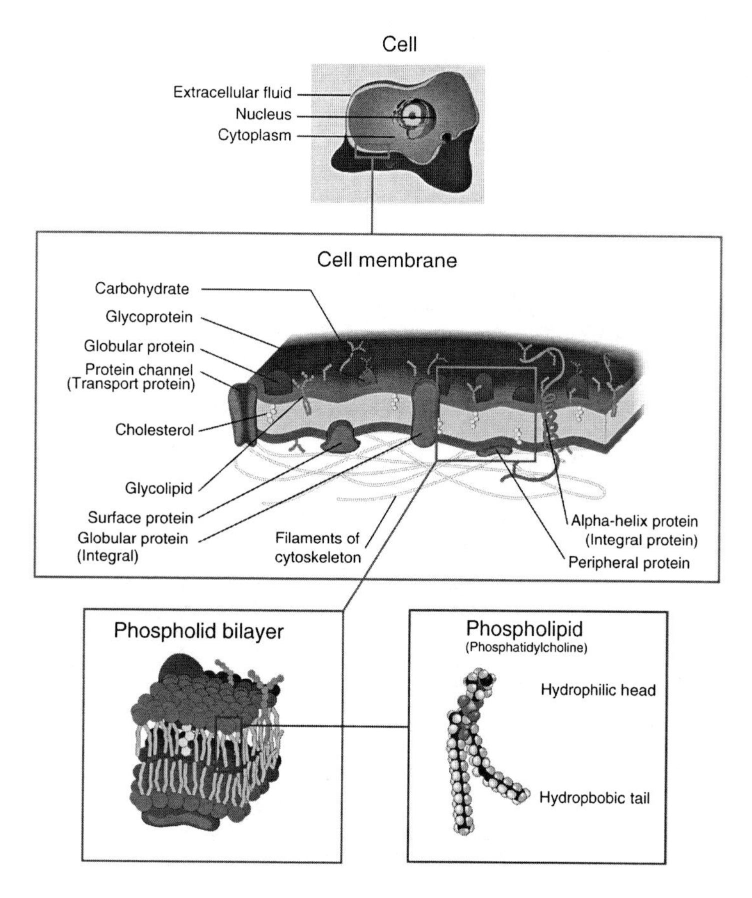

FIGURE 1.5 Illustration of a eukaryotic cell membrane. The cell membrane is a biological membrane that separates the interior of all cells from the outside environment [46].

1.3.2 Absorption Processes

Absorption processes include passive or facilitated diffusion, ion channels, primary and secondary active transporters, and macromolecular and bulk transporters [48]. The characteristics of the absorption processes were summarized in Table 1.3. The mechanisms involved with drug transport through epithelial membranes are shown in Figure 1.3.

*1.3.2.1 **Passive Diffusion*** Passive diffusion is the movement of a solute across the membrane down the electrochemical gradient in the absence of the assistance of a transport protein. It does not require any biological energy but follows Fick's law:

$$V = P \cdot A \cdot \Delta C = \left(\frac{D \cdot K}{\delta}\right) \cdot A \cdot \Delta C \qquad (1.1)$$

TABLE 1.3 Characteristics of Absorption Processes

Type	Transport Protein	Saturation	Concentration Gradient	Energy Dependence	Examples	Energy Source
Simple diffusion	No	No	No	No	Oxygen, water	
Ion channels	Yes	No	No	No	Na^{+} channel	
Facilitated diffusion	Yes	Yes	No	No	Glucose transporter	
Primary active transport	Yes	Yes	Yes	Yes	H^{+}-ATPase, Ca^{2+}-ATPase, $Na^{+}K^{+}$ ATPase, MDR1, BCRP, MRPs	ATP, light, substrate oxidation
Secondary active transport	Yes	Yes	Yes	Yes	Na^{+}/Ca^{2+} antiporter, Na^{+}/amino acid symporters, SGLT, H^{+}/ peptide transporter, OATP, MCT	Ion gradient

Source: Adapted from Ref. 48.

where V is a transport rate, A is the surface area, ΔC is a concentration difference across the membrane, D is the diffusivity of a solute, K is the partition coefficient between membrane and water, and δ is the membrane thickness. The general plot for a simple diffusion is shown in Figure 1.5. As expected from Equation (1.1), the transport rate is proportional to the substrate concentration, displaying a linear relationship (Pattern A). Numerous small lipid-soluble molecules, oxygen, N_2, CO_2, and NH_3, are transported through biological membranes via simple diffusion [4].

*1.3.2.2 **Ion Channels*** As ion fluxes are involved with regulation of inorganic ions, such as Na^+, K^+, Ca^{2+}, and Cl^-, ion transport across the cell membranes plays a critical role in numerous cell processes, such as cell growth and proliferation [4]. As previously reported, the high concentration of Na^+ ion outside the cell is balanced mainly by extracellular chloride ions [4]. On the other hand, the high concentration of K^+ ion inside the cell is balanced by a variety of negatively charged intracellular ions, such as Cl^-, HCO_3^-, and PO_4^{3-}, or negatively charged organic molecules [4].

Various enzymes and transport mechanisms regulate the pH and the concentrations of Na^+, K^+, Ca^{2+}, and Cl^- and other anions in cell, mitochondria, or organelle compartments [49]. Ionic gradients, established at the expense of metabolic energy, e.g., ATP hydrolysis, are used to transfer solutes across the membranes (e.g., amino acids and sugars) into the cell by multitransporters and protons out of the cell by antiporters [4]. The outward K^+ gradient generated across the plasma membrane is a major determinant of the inside negative transmembrane potential of cells [4]. In epithelial tissues, the polarized distribution of enzymes and ion carriers provides the driving force for movement of ions and molecules across the cell interior.

Ion channels have basically two conformations: open or closed. When they are open, ions flow through the channel and reproduce an electric current. For example, the rate of Na^+ movement through the acetylcholine receptor ion channel has a linear relationship with extracellular Na^+ concentration and the process is not saturable (Pattern A in Figure 1.6), which is similar to simple diffusion [48]. The ion channel of the acetylcholine receptor behaves as though it provides a hydrophilic pore within the lipid bilayer through which an ion of the right size, charge, and geometry can diffuse down its electrochemical gradient [48].

*1.3.2.3 **Facilitated Diffusion*** Molecules transport through cells according to their electrochemical potential gradient when an energy source is not required [4]. The facilitated diffusion process does not require energy and is accelerated by the specific binding process between a solute and membrane proteins [4].

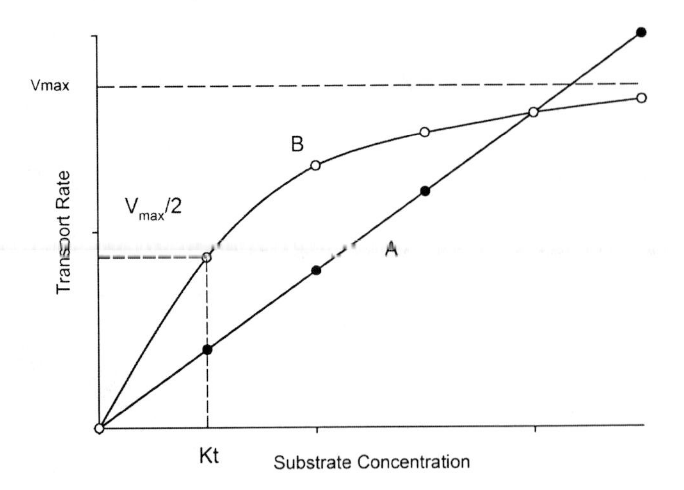

FIGURE 1.6 Concentration dependence of membrane transport: linear (A) and saturable (B) transport processes. Simple diffusion and ion channels obey the linear dependency on the substrate concentration. Facilitated transporter and active transporters follow a saturable pattern [48]. (See color figure in color plate section.)

Some essential features of the facilitated diffusion process can be summarized as follows [50]: 1) The facilitated diffusion process by a mobile transporter system operates such that solute flows from a higher to a lower electrochemical potential; 2) the solute flows at a rate greater than that predicted based on its size or hydrophilicity; 3) the penetration rate does not follow Fick's law except at very low concentrations (at higher concentrations, saturation kinetics are observed as seen in Figure 1.6 (Pattern B)); 4) competitive inhibition occurs between chemically and sterically similar substrates; 5) inhibitory action may be exerted by other compounds, especially those reacting with or ligating reactive groups in proteins; and 6) it is often feasible for the flow of substrate to propel temporarily in the opposite direction against the electrochemical potential gradient of analogs (an overshoot phenomenon) for the accumulation of an analog (or isotope). A well-known example of facilitated diffusion is displayed with erythrocyte glucose transport, in which glucose enters the erythrocyte via a specific transporter that allows for glucose entry into the cell at a rate about 50,000 times greater than its simple diffusion through a lipid bilayer [4].

*1.3.2.4 **Active Transporters*** Active transport results in the accumulation of a solute on one side of the membrane and often against its electrochemical gradient. It occurs only when solute accumulation is coupled with the exergonic process directly or indirectly [4]. During the transport process, energy sources, such as adenosine triiphosphate (ATP), electron transport, or an electrochemical gradient of another ion, are used to drive ions or molecules against their electrochemical potential gradients [4]. The active transport process maintains membrane potential and ion gradients, storage of energy for secondary transporters, and pH regulation inside the cell [4].

In primary active transport, solute accumulation is directly coupled with the exergonic reaction (conversion of ATP to adenosine triiphosphate (ADP) + Pi) [4]. Secondary active transport occurs when uphill transport of one solute is coupled with the downhill flow of another solute that was originally pumped uphill flow by primary active transport.

An example of the primary active transporter is the Na^+K^+ATPase in the mammalian cells that is energized by ATP [4]. Animal cells maintain a lower concentration of Na^+ and a higher concentration of K^+ intracellularly than are found in extracellular fluid. This concentration difference is established and maintained by primary active transport systems in the plasma membrane. The process is mediated by the enzyme Na^+K^+ATPase that couples the breakdown of ATP with the simultaneous and electrogenic movements of both Na^+ and K^+ against their concentration gradients (i.e., three Na^+ ions move outward for every two K^+ ions that move inward) [4].

In animal cells, the differences in cytosolic and extracellular concentrations of Na^+ and K^+ are maintained by active transport via Na^+K^+ATPase, and the generated Na^+ gradient is used as an energy source by a variety of symport and antiport systems [4]. The Na^+K^+ATPase shows specific distribution patterns on the animal cell surface. A few primary active transporters, such as MDR1, MRP2, MRP4, and BCRP in the epithelial membrane, and MRP1, MRP3, MRP4, and MRP5 in the basolateral membrane, are shown in Figure 1.1.

1.3.2.5 Secondary Active Transporters There are a few secondary active transport systems in which the free energy for translocation is not directly provided from metabolic changes but from the energy stored in ionic gradients. In secondary active transport, a single co-transporter couples the flow of one solute (such as H^+ or Na^+) down its concentration gradient with the pumping of a second solute (such as sugar and amino acid) against its concentration gradient [4]. In intestinal epithelial cells, glucose and certain amino acids are accumulated by symport with Na^+ [4]. Peptide transporters in the intestine and kidneys mediate small peptide transport via an inward-directed electrochemical H^+ gradient [51]. A few examples of the secondary active transporters, such as MCT1 and PEPT1 in the epithelial membrane, are shown in Figure 1.1.

Membrane transporters play an integral role in drug entrance and exit from the body. In addition, it is possible to use transporters for drug delivery, e.g., improving oral absorption via the peptide transporter. The identification of the membrane transporters and a better understanding of their regulation process will allow for development of an efficient drug delivery strategy.

Competition between two similar substances for the same transport system and subsequent reduced absorption of one or both compounds are additional functional properties of the carrier-mediated transport process [52]. The contribution quotient of a carrier-mediated process to the overall absorption rate decreases as the concentration increases, and it is negligibly low at sufficiently high concentrations. The capacity-limited characteristics of a carrier-mediated process indicate that the bioavailability of a drug absorbed through this manner decreases as its dose increases.

1.3.2.6 Macromolecular and Bulk Transport Macromolecules and inert particles are too big to transport across a lipid bilayer. Preformed proteins generally transport through membranes during fusion (secretion) or fission (e.g., pinocytosis) events. For example, during pinocytosis, macromolecules in the extracellular fluid phase are transferred into the cytoplasm via pinocytotic vesicles budding from the plasma membrane [4]. During exocytosis, however, storage vesicles fuse with the plasma membrane and thereby release loaded drugs into the extracellular environment [53]. Adsorptive pinocytosis during the transport process is engaged with transport receptors, such as the LDL receptor, which is a cell-surface integral membrane glycoprotein, recognizing LDL and regulating its endocytosis process [54].

1.3.3 Food

In general, gastrointestinal absorption is favored by an empty stomach. The absorption rate rather than the extent of absorption of drugs, such as sulfonamides and cephradine, is reduced in the presence of food [55, 56]. The effects of food on the absorption rate of drugs are mainly attributed to the delay in gastric emptying.

It has been frequently observed that administration of certain antibiotics, such as tetracyclines, penicillins [56, 57], lincomycin, captopril [58], and erythromycin [20, 59], right after a meal results in a significant decrease in both the rate and extent of their absorption. The absorption rate of some drugs including riboflavin, griseofulvin, and chlorothiazide is rather elevated when they are administered after a meal [28]. Interactions of drugs with specific food (e.g., grapefruit juice) or nutrients (e.g., calcium supplements) need to be investigated thoroughly to elucidate whether they generally follow theoretical predictions of physicochemical or physiological behaviors [60].

1.3.4 Age

Age is also known to affect the drug absorption through the GI tract. In infants, gastrointestinal pH is higher and intestinal surface and blood flow are lower than those in adults, resulting in poor drug absorption [2]. Drug absorption is also altered in elderly people as a result of changes in gastric emptying, achlorhydria, and bacterial overgrowth in the small intestine [2]. Accordingly, under current U.S. Food and Drug Administration (FDA) regulation after the Pediatric Research Equity Act enacted in 2003, pediatric assessment of drug products is strongly recommended.

1.3.5 Disease Status

The disease status may influence the rate and extent of drug absorption. It is highly likely that in those with clinical disorders, critical transport processes are either defective at the molecular level or not regulated properly in the physiological situation. The accumulative evidence suggests a role of modulated intestinal permeability in the early stage of the disease pathogenesis. Mutation can also produce defective transporters.

For example, an imbalance of gastric acid secretion causes gastric ulcers and diarrhea by cholera toxin, leading to solute loss and subsequent water loss [2]. Cystic fibrosis, an inherited disorder causing pancreatic, pulmonary, and sinus disease in children and young adults, is characterized with abnormal viscosity of mucous secretions caused by altered electrolyte transport across epithelial cell membranes [2]. The protein encoded by the gene defective in cystic fibrosis is the cystic fibrosis transmembrane conductance regulator (CFTR), which is a chloride channel regulated by cyclic adenosine monophosphate (AMP)-dependent protein kinase phosphorylation and requires binding of ATP for channel opening [61]. Abnormalities associated with celiac disease, which is characterized with loss of intestinal barrier functions [13], produce an increase in GI emptying rate and alteration of intestinal drug metabolism. Crohn's disease has a direct impact on intestinal transit time and lowers intestinal surface area [35]. Hepatic cirrhosis influences the bioavailability of drugs subjected to first-pass effects [62].

An enhanced mucosal permeability is engaged with pathogenesis and onset of pathological complications (e.g., viral and bacterial gastroenteritis, ulcerative colitis, and multiple organ dysfunction syndromes in patients with sepsis and trauma) [33]. The neuro-inflammation with alterations in the function of intestinal barriers is observed in various diseases including Alzheimer's disease, Parkinson's disease, Huntington's disease, multiple sclerosis, amyotrophic lateral sclerosis (ALS), and certain forms of depression [35, 63, 64].

1.4 PHYSICOCHEMICAL FACTORS INFLUENCING DRUG ABSORPTION

1.4.1 pH-Partition Theory

The dissociation constant and lipid solubility of a drug as well as the pH at the absorption site often define the absorption characteristics of a drug from the solution. The pH-partition theory of drug absorption is based on the assumption that the gastrointestinal tract is a simple lipid barrier to the transport of drugs and chemicals [65–67]. The nonionized form of an acid or basic drug is readily absorbed at the GI tract if it is sufficiently lipid soluble, whereas the ionized form is not. The fraction of drug in a nonionized form at the specific absorption site can be estimated by the oil–water partition coefficient of a drug; the more lipophilic the compound is, the faster its absorption is [67]. Organic anions or cations are likely absorbed in the small intestine, although they are absorbed at a much slower rate than the corresponding unionized form of the drug [68].

1.4.2 Drug pKa and Gastrointestinal pH

The relationship among pH, pKa, and the extent of ionization is described by the Henderson–Hasselbalch equation [28]:

for an acid

$$\mathrm{pKa} - \mathrm{pH} = \log(\mathrm{fu}/\mathrm{fi}) \tag{1.2}$$

for a base

$$\mathrm{pKa} - \mathrm{pH} = \log(\mathrm{fi}/\mathrm{fu}) \tag{1.3}$$

where fu and fi are the fractions of a drug present in the unionized and ionized forms, respectively.

Most acidic drugs are predominantly unionized at the low pH of gastric fluids and easily absorbed from the stomach as well as from the intestine. However, most weak acids are well absorbed in the small intestine. The major factors, such as a large surface area, a relatively long residence time, and the limited absorption of ionized forms of a drug (a factor not considered by the pH-partition theory), are contributed to the overall absorption rate of weak acids in the intestine. Most weak bases are poorly absorbed, if at all, in the stomach because they are largely ionized at low pH (Equation (1.3)). Strong bases with pKa values of 5 to 11 showed pH-dependent absorption. Stronger bases are ionized throughout the gastrointestinal tract and tend to be poorly absorbed [28].

1.4.3 Lipid Solubility

A basic principle of the lipophilic/hydrophilic nature of a drug is regulated by a property called the partition coefficient between a lipophilic solvent, such as chloroform, butanol, octanol, and water or aqueous buffer. Polar molecules like aminoglycosides and other antibiotics, quaternary ammonium compounds, or polypeptide drugs are poorly absorbed after oral administration as a result of a low partition coefficient [69]. On the other hand, lipid-soluble drugs, such as fentanyl and sufentanil with favorable partition coefficients, are generally well absorbed after oral administration.

Prodrugs designed to improve permeability and oral absorption of parent drugs are more lipid soluble than parent drugs and should be quickly converted to the parent compound during the absorption process in the gut wall or the liver. Ampicillin prodrugs, such as pivampicillin [70] and bacampicillin [71], are more lipid soluble, thus, being absorbed more than the parent compound after oral administration.

1.4.4 Unstirred Water Layer

Experimental evidences show that the pH-absorption profile is often shifted two or more pH units from the curve predicted by the pH-partition theory. This discrepancy can be explained by the experimental theory that an additional barrier to drug transport, called the unstirred or stagnant water layer, exists in parallel with the luminal surface of the intestinal membrane. The unstirred layer, whose thickness ranges from 0.01 to 1 mm [6], shifts the inflection point in the pH-absorption profile to the right for an acid and the left for a basic compound, reducing the absorption rate [72].

1.4.5 Dissolution

When a drug in a solid dosage form is given orally, the rate of its absorption is often controlled by its dissolution rate in the fluids. The solubility of numerous drugs increases as the environmental temperature of the solvent increases [28, 73]. Therefore, it is generally accepted that the dissolution rate is temperature dependent. The diffusion coefficient is inversely related to viscosity so that the dissolution rate could decrease as the viscosity of the solvent increases [73].

The degree of agitation or stirring of the solvent can affect the thickness of the diffusion layer. The greater the agitation is, the thinner the layer becomes and the faster the dissolution rate is. Changes in the solvent properties, such as pH, affect the solubility of the drug and, subsequently, the dissolution rate. Similarly, the use of different salts or other chemicals and physical forms (polymorphism) of a drug whose effective solubility is different from that of the parent drug usually affect the dissolution rate. An enhancement of the surface area of a drug exposed to various dissolution media generally increases the dissolution rate via reducing the particle size or attaining more effective wetting of the solid [28].

1.4.6 Hydrolysis in the Gastrointestinal Tract

The bioconversion through hydrolysis in the gastrointestinal tract is responsible for the poor bioavailability after oral administration [28]. The degradation rate of penicillin G decreases sharply as pH increases [74]. Some penicillins, notably amino-penicillins, are considerably more resistant to acid hydrolysis [73].

1.4.7 Complexation and Adsorption

Complexation of a drug in gastrointestinal fluids may alter the rate, and in some cases, the extent of absorption, because the drug complex usually differs from the free drug with respect to water solubility and lipid–water partition coefficient [28]. The complexing agent could be a substrate in the gastrointestinal tract, a dietary component, or a component of the dosage form. Some insoluble substances, such as charcoal, may adsorb co-administered drugs, often resulting in poor absorption of those drugs [28].

1.4.8 Deviation from pH-Partition Hypothesis

There are various reasons behind deviation of drug absorption from pH-partition hypothesis that is often observed in clinical situations: Some factors, such as variability in pH conditions in humans, unstirred water layer, and ion pair formation, may affect drug absorption through the GI tract.

The pH at membrane surfaces, i.e., microclimate pH, may alter the drug absorption rate based on pH-partition prediction. A more neutral pH in adult celiac disease would cause a smaller percentage of folic acid to be absorbed as a result of less ionized forms available, causing folate malabsorption [72, 75]. The negative charge on the membrane could attract the smaller number of cations toward the surface and subsequently repel the smaller number of anions.

In addition, the movement of water molecules into or out of the GI tract may affect the passage of small molecules across the membrane. The convective water flow can be produced as a result of the difference in osmotic pressure between blood and lumen contents, and the difference in hydrostatic pressure between lumen and perivascular tissues, for instance, derived from muscular contractions [73].

1.5 STRATEGIES TO OVERCOME GASTROINTESTINAL BARRIERS IN DRUG DELIVERY

1.5.1 Alternative Formulations

Various drug delivery strategies based on the physicodynamic characteristics of a drug can be opted to overcome the poor absorption/bioavailability. In improving the poor absorption/bioavailability, scientists need to deal with complex issues, such as stability in lumen or plasma, solubility, and permeability at the same time. Therefore, it is ideal to find which parameters are of particular importance in each strategy.

If solubility is an underlying problem, dissolution improvement may be a first priority. However, as this approach is not always successful, the chemical modification of a drug can be further considered for the enhancement of solubility. Depending on the lipophilicity of the compounds, either the water layer or the membrane becomes a limiting barrier to their absorption. For water-insoluble hydrophobic drugs, prodrugs have been synthesized to increase solubility, and later, they are converted back to the parent drugs by intestinal brush border membrane enzymes. For hydrophobic compounds, the diffusion water layer often serves as a barrier to the absorption rate [76]. For example, the solubility of hydrocortisone is only around 0.7 mM and above this concentration there was no significant increase in the uptake rate. The ester prodrugs of hydrocortisone enhanced their uptake rate by 20-fold [76]. Esterase and phosphatase in intestinal mucosal are responsible for reconverting of prodrugs back to parent hydrocortisone.

A popular approach for oral absorption enhancement of hydrophilic drugs is to use ester prodrugs which increase its hydrophobicity. Bacampicillin is a typical example of a prodrug for ampicillin [77]. Parent drugs containing –OH or –COOH groups can often be converted into esters from which the active drugs are regenerated by accountable esterases within the body.

Another strategy for oral absorption enhancement of hydrophilic drugs is to design suitable substrates subjected to a specific intestinal transporter [78]. Schematic representation of a general prodrug strategy to increase intestinal drug absorption is illustrated in Figure 1.7. Even though the parent drug is not a substrate of a particular transporter, when its prodrug becomes a substrate, then it can be taken up into the cells through a transporter-mediated process. Prodrugs need a metabolic process inside cells to be converted back to the parent drug and released into systemic circulation. Also, it would be highly desirable that any brush border or luminal enzymes are not directly involved with the metabolism of prodrugs. As the peptide transport system facilitates the absorption process of small peptides, peptide-like drugs and some β-lactam antibiotics and angiotensin converting enzyme inhibitors [52], a peptide transporter in

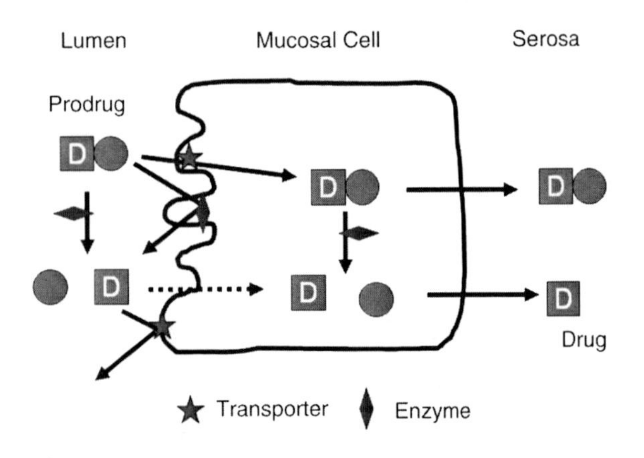

FIGURE 1.7 Schematic representation of transporter-targeted prodrug strategy.

the intestine could be used to enhance the bioavailability of poorly absorbed drugs. It has been retrospectively demonstrated that the peptide transporter improved oral absorption of valacyclovir [79] and valganciclovir (i.e., valyl ester of ganciclovir), both of which are a nonpeptidyl prodrug [80]. Ganciclovir has only 5–9% of bioavailability, and its dosing is about 100 mg 3 times daily taken with food. The prodrug valganciclovir has 10 times higher bioavailability than the parent drug, which is about 60%, and the dosing regimen can be improved once a day with a 450-mg dose.

Recently, the promising strategies that are commonly used in practice for long-term administration of drugs without interfering with human physiology have been reviewed [81]. One of the main goals is to replace injection formulations with various noninvasive technologies for simultaneously achieving improvement of safety and enhanced efficacy profiles. Other formulation objectives are modification of bioavailability, stability, permeability, solubility, dissolution rate, residence time, absorption area, and elimination [52]. Modulating barrier properties can be achieved by approaches involved with chemical enhancers, surfactants, iontophoresis, sonophoresis, micro needles, cell-penetrating peptides, ligand/vector-targeted delivery, and prodrugs [81]. Various controlled release formulations and noninvasive delivery technologies have been a main focus of product enhancement and life-cycle management for innovator biopharmaceuticals [82].

1.5.2 Alternative Routes of Administration

The most popular formulations for drug administration are oral dosage forms, such as tablets, capsules, powders, and granules. There are several advantages of oral dosage formulations: ease of accurate dosage, good physicochemical stability, good patient compliance, and cheaper manufacturing costs. However, one of the potential problems of oral medication is poor bioavailability, as the availability of the drug for absorption is affected by both disintegration and dissolution processes. Therefore, they should be stable chemically and/or enzymatically in the gastrointestinal tract during the absorption process.

Among various approaches available for enhancement of the bioavailability of the drug, targeted delivery to the colon via biodegradable polymers seems to be a potentially promising strategy. A wide range of the polysaccharides abundantly available in the market can be used solely for the purpose of colon-specific drug delivery [83]. This family of natural polymers has great appeal to the drug delivery community, as they comprise polymers having a large number of derivable groups, a wide range of molecular weights, varying chemical compositions, and for the most part, low toxicity and biodegradability with high stability [83].

In addition to oral medication, several alternative methods to the GI tract, such as buccal, sublingual, and rectal administrations, are available. The absorption of drugs through the oral mucosa provides an alternative route for systemic administration that bypasses the liver metabolism, even though the extent of absorption may be variable. In the oral mucosal cavity, the drug can be delivered by either the sublingual or the buccal route, which are well vascularized with venous blood draining the buccal mucosa, reaching the heart directly via the internal jugular vein [84, 85]. The drug absorption rate via the buccal route is less than that obtained via the sublingual mucosa as a result of the permeability barrier. The low mobility of the buccal musculature as compared with that of the sublingual route makes this site ideally suitable for sustained delivery of drugs [85]. Moreover, this route is convenient, accessible, and generally well complied by patients.

Significantly enhanced absorption through the oral mucosa has been achieved with compounds, such as glyceryl trinitrate, captopril, desoxycortisone acetate, isoprenaline, methacholine chloride, nifedipine, perphenazine, and morphine [85, 86]. The major mechanism of absorption through the sublingual route is simple diffusion. The optimal oil/water partition coefficient was within the range of 40 to 2000 for the sublingual route [73]

Additional routes of drug administration other than per the oral route are topical, inhalation, intramuscular, subcutaneous, intranasal, intraocular, rectal, or vaginal administration [87]. The alternative routes can serve as an efficient means to meet specific requirements in particular patient conditions. For example, rectal administration is an important route for children and old patients. The drugs can be administered as a solution or suppository and can bypass the presystemic hepatic metabolism. Drugs administered by this route include aspirin, acetaminophen [88], and few barbiturates [89].

1.6 SUMMARY

Physiological GI barriers are part of the protection mechanisms for the human body. The thorough understanding of GI barriers in drug delivery makes it possible to identify biopharmaceutical and pharmacokinetic problems on the new drug development process, to suggest alternative approaches to improve bioavailability, and further to predict the clinical efficacies of drugs. Physiological GI barriers include epithelial membrane, tight junctions, mucosa, gastrointestinal blood flow, luminal and microclimate pH, gastric emptying, GI motility, and age. Changes of GI barriers in disease states seem to have a direct impact on new drug development.

Depending on the lipophilicity of a drug, chemical modification, such as prodrug and bioconjugation, would be used for new formulation and drug development. Small-molecule solute or large-molecule transporters are potential targets, when the passive transmembrane transport is negligible as a result of its charge, size, or hydrophilicity. Prodrugs designed for solubility improvement, such as ester prodrugs, peptidyl drugs, or amino acid ester prodrugs, or designed as an efficient substrate to a specific transporter, are potentially powerful approaches to improving the absorption and intracellular delivery of drugs. Additional routes of drug administration other than per the oral route can serve as an efficient means to meet specific requirements in particular patients.

ASSESSMENT QUESTIONS

1.1. Which influencing factor does *not* increase gastric emptying of a drug?

- **a.** Higher temperature of food
- **b.** Lying on the left side
- **c.** Low pH
- **d.** Fasting

1.2. Which pharmacokinetic parameter will be optimized to develop a once-a-day extended release formulation of a short half-life drug? Explain why.

1.3. What are the key influencing factors on oral drug absorption of a drug "product?"

1.4. Which drug can be absorbed most from the intestinal tracts at pH 7?

- **a.** Quinine (pKa = 8.4)
- **b.** Benzoic acid (pKa = 4.2)
- **c.** Acetylsalicylic acid (pKa = 3.5)
- **d.** Salicylic acid (pKa = 3.0)

1.5. What are the biological barriers preventing oral delivery of protein drugs?

1.6. Which mechanism of drug transport through epithelial membranes will be the most feasible when nanoparticles are considered a potential delivery method of a vaccine? Which ones will contribute less?

1.7. Which mucosal solute transporters are present on the human gastrointestinal tract?

1.8. How would the maximal oral absorption be achieved for a drug? (Hint: Use Fick's law.)

1.9. Describe the following terms: (a) passive diffusion, (b) unstirred water layer, (c) tight junction, and (d) luminal pH.

1.10. What are the three key barrier functions of the gastrointestinal tract?

1.11. What is presystemic metabolism?

REFERENCES

1. Li, X., Jasti, B. *Design of Controlled Drug Delivery Systems*, McGraw-Hill, New York, NY, 2006.
2. Johnson, L.R. *Physiology of the Gastrointestinal Tract*, 2nd ed., Raven Press, New York, NY, 1987.
3. Huang, W., Lee, S.L., Yu, L.X. (2009). Mechanistic approaches to predicting oral drug absorption. *Journal of American Association of Pharmaceutical Scientists, 11*, 217–224.
4. Lehninger, A.L. *Principles of Biochemistry*, Worth, New York, NY, 1993.
5. Carr, K.E., Toner, P.G. Morphology of the intestinal mucosa, in T.Z. Csaky (ed.), *Pharmacology of Intestinal Permeability I*, Springer-Verlag, Berlin, Germany, 1984, pp. 1–50.
6. Davenport, H.W. *Physiology of the Digestive Tract*, 5th ed., Year Book Medical, Chicago, IL, 1982.
7. Guyton, A.C. *Textbook of Medical Physiology*, 6th ed., W.B. Saunders, Philadelphia, PA, 1981.
8. Wood, M.G. *Laboratory Manual for Anatomy & Physiology. Pig Version*, 4th ed., Pearson Education, San Francisco, CA, 2010, p. 659.
9. Wilson, J.P. (1967). Surface area of the small intestine in man. *Gut, 8*, 618–621.
10. Fordtran, J.S., Rector, F.C., Ewton, M.F. (1965). Permeability characteristics of the human small intestine. *Journal of Clinical Investigation, 44*, 1935–1944.
11. Chadwick, V.S., Phillips, S.F., Hofmann, A.F. (1977). Measurements of intestinal permeability using low molecular weight polyethylene glycols (PEG 400). II. Application to normal and abnormal permeability states in man and animals. *Gastroenterology, 73*, 247–251.
12. Goswami, T., Jasti, B.R., Li., X. (2009). Estimation of the theoretical pore sizes of the porcine oral mucosa for permeation of hydrophilic permeants. *Archives of Oral Biology, 54*, 577–582.
13. Fasanoa, A., Schulzke, J.D. The role of the intestinal barrier function in the pathogenesis of Celiac Disease, in A. Fasano, R. Troncone, and D. Branski (eds.), *Frontiers in Celiac Disease*, vol. 12, *Pediatric and Adolescent Medicine*, Basel, Karger AG, 2008, pp. 89–98.
14. Mudie, D.M., Amidon, G.L., Amidon, G.E. (2010). Physiological parameters for oral delivery and in vitro testing, *Molecular Pharmaceutics, 7*, 1388–1405.
15. Simon, G.L., Gorbach, S.L. (1986). The human intestinal microflora. *Digestive Diseases and Sciences, 3*, 147–162.
16. Jany, B.H., et al. (1991). Human bronchus and intestine express the same mucin gene. *Journal of Clinical Investigation, 87(1)*, 77–82.
17. Rainsford, K.D. (1975). The biochemical pathology of aspirin-induced gastric damage. *Inflammation Research, 5(4)*, 326–344.
18. Lui, C.Y., et al. (1986). Comparison of gastrointestinal pH in dogs and humans: Implications on the use of the beagle dog as a model for oral absorption in human. *Journal of Pharmacy and Pharmacology, 75(3)*, 271–274.
19. Lucas, M.L., et al. (1975). Direct measurement by pH-microelectrode of the pH microclimate in rat proximal jejunum. *Proceedings of the Royal Society of London—Series B: Biological Sciences, 192*, 39–48.
20. Welling, P.G., et al. (1978). Bioavailability of erythromycin stearate: Influence of food and fluid volume. *Journal of Pharmacy and Pharmacology, 67*, 764–766.
21. Shargel, L., Yu, A.B.C. *Biopharmaceutics, Encyclopedia of Pharmaceutical Technology*, Informa Healthcare USA, New York, NY, 2007, pp. 208–227.
22. Blythe, R.H., Grass, G.M., MacDonnell, D.R. (1959). The formulation and evaluation of enteric-coated aspirin tablets. *American Journal of Pharmacy, 131*, 206–216.
23. Nimmo, W.S., Prescott, L.F. (1978). The influence of posture on paracetamol absorption. *British Journal of Clinical Pharmacology, 5*, 348–349.
24. Hurwitz, A., Robinson, R.G., Herrin, W.F. (1977). Prolongation of gastric emptying by oral propantheline. *International Journal of Clinical Pharmacology, Therapy and Toxicology, 22*, 206–210.
25. Nimmo, J. (1973). The influence of metoclopramide on drug absorption. *Journal of Postgraduate Medicine, 49*, 25–28.
26. Eve, I.S. (1966). A review of the physiology of the gastrointestinal tract in relation to radiation doses of radioactive materials. *Health Physics, 12*, 131–161.
27. Heading, R.C., et al. (1973). The dependence of paracetamol absorption on the rate of gastric emptying. *British Journal of Pharmacology, 47*, 415–421.
28. Gibaldi, M. *Biopharmaceutics and Clinical Pharmacokinetics*, Lea & Febiger, Philadelphia, PA, 1984.
29. Amidon, G.L., et al. (1995). A theoretical basis for a biopharmaceutics drug classification: the correlation of in vitro drug product dissolution and in vivo bioavailability. *Research in Pharmacy, 12*, 413–420.
30. Guengerich, F.P. (2008). Cytochrome P450 and chemical toxicology. *Chemical Research in Toxicology, 21(1)*, 70.
31. Abumrad, N., Coburn, C., Ibrahimi, A. (1999). Membrane proteins implicated in long-chain fatty acid uptake by mammalian cells: CD36, FATP and FABPm. *Biochimica et Biophysica Acta, 1441*, 4–13.
32. Ehehalt, R., et al. (2006). Translocation of long chain fatty acids across the plasma membrane—lipid rafts and fatty acid transport proteins. *Molecular and Cellular Biochemistry, 284*, 135–140.
33. Söderholm, J.D., Perdue, M.H. (2001). Stress and the gastrointestinal tract II. Stress and intestinal barrier function. *American Journal of Physiology—Gastrointestinal and Liver Physiology, 280*, G7–G13.
34. Fasano, A., Shea-Donohue, T. (2005). Mechanisms of disease: The role of intestinal barrier function in the pathogenesis of gastrointestinal autoimmune diseases. *Nature Clinical Practice Gastroenterolgy & Hepatology, 2(9)*, 416–422.
35. Turner, J.R. (2009). Intestinal mucosal barrier function in health and disease. *Nature Reviews Immunology, 9*, 799–809.

36. Tunkel, A.R. Host defense mechanisms against infection, in *The Merck Manual for Health Care Professional*, 2009, section 15, chapter 178.
37. Olson, E.S., et al. (2010). Activatable cell penetrating peptides linked to nanoparticles as dual probes for in vivo fluorescence and MR imaging of proteases. *Proceedings of the National Academy of Sciences of the United States of America, 107(9)*, 4311–4316.
38. Sumen, C., et al. (2004). Intravital microscopy: Visualizing immunity in context. *Immunity, 21*, 315–329.
39. Dressman J.B., Lennernas, H. (eds.). *Oral Drug Absorption Prediction and Assessment*, Marcel Dekker, New York, NY, 2000.
40. Ehrhardt, C., Kim, K.J. (eds.). *Drug Absorption Studies: In Situ, In Vitro and In Silico Models (Biotechnology: Pharmaceutical Aspects)*, Springer, New York, NY, 2008.
41. Sheiner, L.B., Rosenberg, B., Marathe, V.V. (1977). Estimation of population characteristics of pharmacokinetic parameters from routine clinical data. *Journal of Pharmacokinetics and Biopharmaceutics, 5*, 445–479.
42. Sheiner, L.B., et al. (1979). Forecasting individual pharmacokinetics. *International Journal of Clinical Pharmacology, Therapy and Toxicology. 26(3)*, 294–305.
43. Bonate, P.L. (2005). Recommended reading in population pharmacokinetic pharmacodynamics (PDF). *Journal of American Association of Pharmaceutical Scientists, 7(2)*, E363–E373.
44. Yu, L.X., et al. (1996). Transport approaches to the biopharmaceutical design of oral drug delivery systems: Prediction of intestinal absorption. *Advanced Drug Delivery Reviews, 19*, 359–376.
45. Oh, D.M., Curl, R.L., Amidon, G.L. (1993). Estimating the fraction dose absorbed from suspensions of poorly soluble compounds in humans: A mathematical model. *Pharmaceutical Research, 10*, 264–270.
46. http://en.wikipedia.org/wiki/Cell_membrane. Accessed on January 28, 2012.
47. Lodish, H., et al., *Molecular Cell Biology*, Scientific American Books, New York, NY, 1995.
48. Oh, D.-M., Amidon, G.L. Overview of membrane transport. In G.L. Amidon and W. Sadee (eds.), *Membrane Transporters As Drug Targets*, Kluwer Academic/Plenum, New York, NY, 1999, pp. 1–27.
49. Hopfer, U., Liedtke, C.M. (1987). Proton and bicarbonate transport mechanisms in the intestine. *Annual Review of Physiology. 49*, 51–67.
50. West, I.C. *The Biochemistry of Membrane Transporter*, Chapman and Hall, London and New York, NY, 1983, p. 80.
51. Ganapathy, V., Leibach, F.H. (1996), Peptide transporters. *Current Opinion in Nephrology & Hypertension, 5*, 395–400.
52. Mahato, R.I., Narang, A.S., Thoma, L., Miller, D.D. (2003). Emerging trends in oral delivery of peptide and protein drugs. *Critical Reviews in Therapeutic Drug Carrier Systems, 20(2–3)*, 153–214.
53. Petty, H.R. *Molecular Biology of Membranes: Structure and Function*, Plenum, New York, NY, 1993, p. 404.
54. Yamamoto, T., et al. (1984). The human LDL receptor: A cysteine-rich protein with multiple Alu sequences in its mRNA, *Cell, 39*, 27–38.
55. Harvengt, C., et al. (1973). Cephradine absorption and excretion in fasting and nonfasting volunteers. *The Journal of Clinical Pharmacology, 13*, 36–40.
56. Welling, P.G. (1977). Influence of food and diet on gastrointestinal drug absorption: A review. *Journal of Pharmacokinetics and Biopharmaceutics, 5*, 291–334.
57. Klein, J.O., Finland, M.L. (1963). The new penicillins. *New England Journal of Medicine, 269*, 1019–1025.
58. Singhvi, S.M., et al. (1982). Effect of food on the bioavailability of captopril in healthy subjects. *The Journal of Clinical Pharmacology, 22*, 135–140.
59. Welling, P.G., Tse, F.L.S. (1982). The influence of food on the absorption of antimicrobial agents. *Journal of Antimicrobial Chemotherapy, 9*, 7–27.
60. Fleisher, D., Sweet, B.V., Parekh, A. Drug absorption with food, in J.I. Boullata and Vincent T. Armenti (eds.), *Handbook of Drug-Nutrient Interactions*, Humana Press, Totowa, NJ, 2004, pp. 129–154.
61. Schultz, S.G., et al. *Molecular Biology of Membrane Transport Disorders*, Plenum Press, New York, NY, 1996.
62. Regfirdh, C.G., et al. (1989). Pharmacokineties of felodipine in patients with liver disease, *European Journal of Clinical Pharmacology, 36*, 473–479.
63. Mhatre, M., Floyd, R.A., Hensley, K. (2004). Oxidative stress and neuroinflammation in Alzheimer's disease and amyotrophic lateral sclerosis: Common links and potential therapeutic targets. *Alzheimer's Disease Research Journal, 6(2)*, 147–157.
64. Tansey, M.G., Goldberg, M.S. (2010). Neuroinflammation in Parkinson's disease: its role in neuronal death and implications for therapeutic intervention. *Neurobiology of Disease, 37(3)*, 510–518.
65. Shore, P.A., Brodie, B.B., Hogben, C.A.M. (1957). The gastric secretion of drugs: A pH partition hypothesis. *Journal of Pharmacology and Experimental Therapeutics, 119*, 361–369.
66. Schanker, L.S., et al. (1958). Absorption of drugs from the rat small intestine. *Journal of Pharmacology and Experimental Therapeutics, 123*, 81–88.
67. Hogben, C.A.M., et al. (1959). On the mechanism of intestinal absorption of drugs. *Journal of Pharmacology and Experimental Therapeutics, 125*, 275–282.
68. Crouthamel, W.G., et al. (1971). Drug absorption IV. Influence of pH on absorption kinetics of weakly acidic drugs. *Journal of Pharmacy & Pharmaceutical Sciences, 60*, 1160–1163.
69. Lin, J.H. (1995). Species similarities and differences in pharmacokinetics. *Drug Metabolism and Disposition, 23*, 1008–1021.
70. Verbist, L. (1974). Triple crossover study on the absorption and excretion of ampicillin, pivampicillin, and amoxicillin. *Antimicrobial Agents and Chemotherapy, 6*, 588–593.
71. Bodin, N.-O., et al. (1975). Bacampicillin, a new orally well-absorbed derivative of ampicillin. *Antimicrobial Agents and Chemotherapy, 8*, 518–525.

72. Winne, D. (1978). Dependence of intestinal absorption *in vivo* on the unstirred layer. *Naunyn-Schmiedeberg's Archives of Pharmacology*, *304*, 175–181.
73. Florence, A.T., Attwood, D. *Physicochemical Principles of Pharmacy*, 2nd ed., Macmillan Press, London, 1988.
74. Lu, X.B., et al. (2008). Effect of buffer solution and temperature on the stability of penicillin G. *Journal of Chemical & Engineering Data*, *53*, 543–547.
75. Benn, A., et al. (1971). Effect of intraluminal pH on the absorption of pteroylglutamic acid. *British Medical Journal*, *1*, 148–150.
76. Amidon, G.L., Stewart, B.H., Pogany, S. (1985). Improving the intestinal mucosal cell uptake of water insoluble compounds, *Journal of Controlled Release*, *2*, 13–26.
77. Rautio, J., et al. (eds), *Prodrugs and Targeted Delivery: Towards Better ADME Properties*, Wiley-VCH Verlag GmbH, Weinheim, Germany, 2011.
78. Han, H.-K., Amidon, G.L. (2000). Targeted prodrug design to optimize drug delivery, *Journal of American Association of Pharmaceutical Scientists*, *2*(*1*), article 6.
79. Han, H., et al. (1998). 5′-Amino acid esters of antiviral nucleosides, acyclovir, and AZT are absorbed by the intestinal PEPT1 peptide transporter. *Research in Pharmacy*, *15*, 1154–1159.
80. Jung, D., Dorr, A. (1999). Single-dose pharmacokinetics of valganciclovir in HIV-and CMV- seropositive subjects. *The Journal of Clinical Pharmacology*, *39*, 800–804.
81. Pint, João F. (2010). Site-specific drug delivery systems within the gastro-intestinal tract: From the mouth to the colon. *International Journal of Pharmaceutics*, *395*(*1–2*), 44–52.
82. Zhang, H., Surian, J.M. Biopharmaceutic consideration and assessment for oral controlled release formulations, in Hong Wen and Kinam Park (eds), *Oral Controlled Release Formulation Design and Drug Delivery Theory to Practice*, Wiley, NJ, 2010, pp. 33–45.
83. Jain, A., Gupta, Y. Jain, S.K. (2007). Perspectives of biodegradable natural polysaccharides for site-specific drug delivery to the colon, *Journal of Pharmacy and Pharmacology*, *10*(*1*), 86–128.
84. McElany, J.C. Buccal Absorption of Drugs. In: *Encyclopedia of Pharmaceutical Technology*, vol. 2, J. Swarbick, and J.C. Boylan (eds.), Marcel Dekker, Inc., New York, NY, 1990.
85. Shojaei, A.H. (1998). Buccal Mucosa as a route for systemic drug delivery: A review. *Journal of Pharmacy & Pharmaceutical Sciences*, *1*(*1*), 15–30.
86. Turunen, E., et al. (2011). Fast-dissolving sublingual solid dispersion and cyclodextrin complex increase the absorption of perphenazine in rabbits. *Journal of Pharmacy and Pharmacology*, *63*(*1*), 19–25.
87. Lee, C.H., Chien, Y.W. *Drug delivery, Vaginal Route. Encyclopedia of Pharmaceutical Technology*, 3rd ed., Informa Healthcare2, New York, NY, 2011, pp. 961–985.
88. Owczarzak, V., Haddad, J. (2006). Comparison of oral versus rectal administration of acetaminophen with codeine in postoperative pediatric adenotonsillectomy patients. *The Laryngoscope*, *116*(*8*), 1485.
89. Larsson, L.E., et al. (1987). Effects of rectal thiopentone and methohexitone on carbon dioxide tension in infant anaesthesia with spontaneous ventilation. *Acta Anaesthesiologica Scandinavica*, *31*(*3*), 227–230.
90. Davies, B., Morris, T. (1993). Physiological parameters in laboratory animals and humans, *Research in Pharmacy*, *10*(*7*), 1093–1095.

2

SOLUBILITY AND STABILITY ASPECTS IN ADVANCED DRUG DELIVERY

Hoo-Kyun Choi, Robhash K. Subedi, and Chi H. Lee

2.1 CHAPTER OBJECTIVES

- To outline fundamental aspects of drug solubility and stability in advanced drug delivery.
- To update advancement in knowledge and technology related to solubility and stability of pharmaceuticals.

2.2 SOLUBILITY

2.2.1 Introduction

The combinatorial chemistry, high-throughput screening (HTS), and synchronization with other innovative processes have accelerated the discovery of new chemical entities (NCEs) as potential drug candidates [1–3]. Despite a vast number of novel drug molecules, only a few of them are successfully launched in the market. Discovering and developing a drug is a time-consuming and costly process with a recent estimation of about 13 years and US$900 million, respectively [4]. Major causes of attrition in clinic are lack of efficacy (accounting for approximately 30% of failures) and safety (toxicology and safety accounting for approximately 30%) [4]. Interestingly, adverse pharmacokinetic profiles and low bioavailability were the prime reason for attrition accounting for approximately 40% in 1991, which dropped to approximately 10% in 2000, indicating that significant progress has been made during the period of 1991–2000 in understanding pharmacokinetics and solving the problems related to it. These data give the glimpse of attrition on clinical evaluation; however, more drug candidate molecules are withdrawn before reaching clinical evaluation.

Although receptor affinity in high-throughput screening serves as the basic criterion for the selection of drug candidates, much attention is paid to biopharmaceutical characterization of lead substances for marketability assessment. The selection of the lead substances is considered part of the development process performed at various stages in drug discovery and clinical assessment. The major characteristics considered for the selection of the lead substances are listed in Table 2.1. Early assessment on various characteristics of drug substances from the chemical, pharmacological, toxicological, and biopharmaceutical points of view from the multidisciplinary team provides insight into the ability to develop drug substances transformed into effective and safe medicinal products [5]. The systemic approaches adapted for efficient drug discovery and development processes are outlined in Figure 2.1 [6].

General pharmacokinetic studies in the drug development process have focused on delineating the release profiles of drugs from dosage forms, which are determined by the absorption, distribution, metabolism, elimination, toxicity, and activity/response in the target site (LADMET-R) and considered gold standards [6]. Biopharmaceutical properties like solubility, permeability, and stability govern the bioavailability of the drug molecules, which in turn manifests

Advanced Drug Delivery, First Edition. Edited by Ashim K. Mitra, Chi H. Lee, and Kun Cheng.

TABLE 2.1 Potential Characteristics for Lead Substance Selection

Molecular weight	Charge
Functional groups	Solubility
H-bond donors	Polymorphism
H-bond acceptors	Salt formation
Clog P or M log P	Crystallinity
Conformation	Permeability
Lipophilicity	Metabolism
Stereochemistry	

Reproduced with permission from Ref. 5.

the efficacy and safety of the drug [7]. As the solubility and stability of drug molecules are the integral physicochemical properties [8], high-throughput screening for these parameters should be conducted beginning in the early stage of the drug development process [9]. Moreover, advancement in knowledge and technology has facilitated a better understanding of the issues related to solubility and stability. This chapter mainly covers the properties of and involved technologies for the solubility and stability of pharmaceuticals applied to advanced drug delivery.

2.2.2 General Concept

The official IUPAC definition of solubility (Section 9.1.8) [10] is as follows: "The solubility of a solute (solid, liquid or gas) is the analytical composition of a saturated solution expressed in terms of the proportion of the designated solute in a designated solvent." Solubility is an intrinsic material characteristic for a specific molecule and can be qualitatively defined as the spontaneous interaction of two or more substances to form a homogenous molecular dispersion [11]. Solubility depends on the physical and chemical properties of the solute and the solvent as well as on such factors as temperature, pressure, the pH of the solution, and to a lesser extent, the state of subdivision of the solute [12]. Solubility can be described concisely via the Gibbs phase rule [13]:

$$F = C - P + 2 \tag{2.1}$$

where F is the number of degrees of freedom, C is the smallest number of components that are adequate to describe the chemical composition of each phase, and P is the number of phases.

The equation derived from thermodynamic considerations for an ideal solution of a solid in a liquid is:

$$-\ln X_2^i = \frac{\Delta H_f}{R}\left(\frac{T_o - T}{TT_o}\right) \tag{2.2}$$

For a nonideal solution, the equation can be expressed as:

$$-\ln X_2 = \frac{\Delta H_f}{R}\left(\frac{T_o - T}{TT_o}\right) - \ln \gamma_2 \tag{2.3}$$

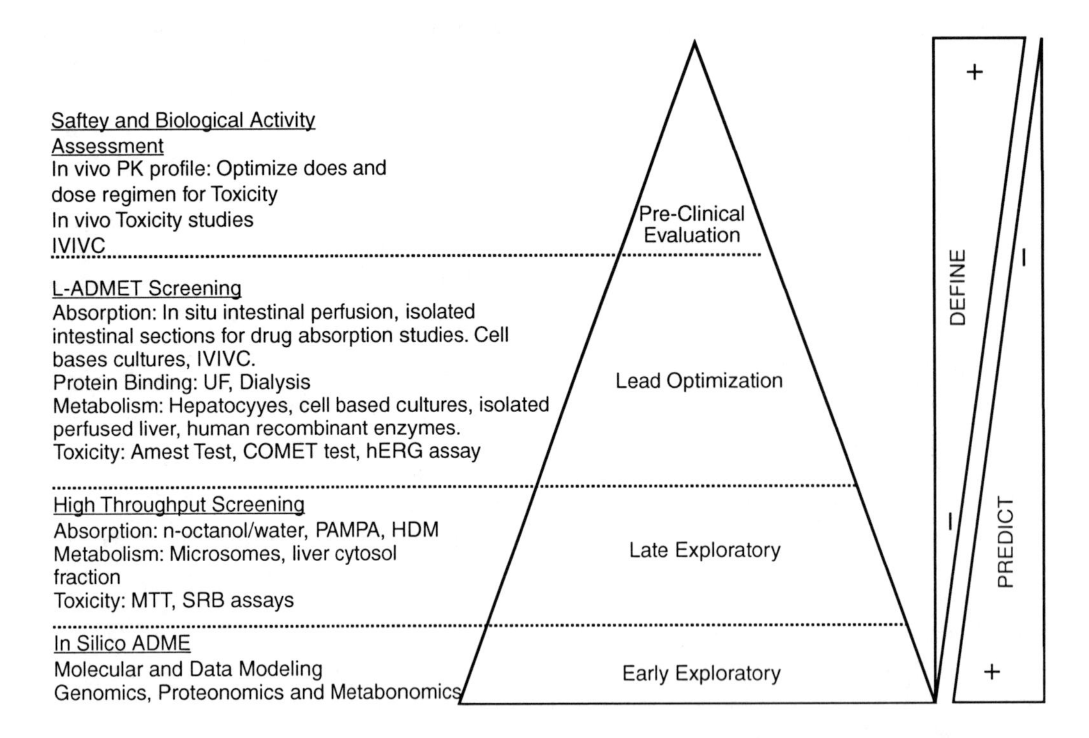

FIGURE 2.1 Systemic approach for drug discovery and development. Reproduced with permission from Ref. 6.

where X_2^i is the ideal solubility of solute expressed in mole fraction, R is the gas constant, ΔH_f is the molar heat of fusion, T_o is the melting point of the solute in absolute degrees, T is the temperature of the solution, and γ_2 is the rational activity coefficient [11].

Solubility is an important determinant in drug release and absorption, hence, playing an integral role in its bioavailability. For a drug to be absorbed, it must be present in the form of an aqueous solution at the site of absorption. This is true regardless of the mechanism of absorption, whether it be passive diffusion, convective transport, active transport, facilitated transport, or ion pair transport, except in the case of pinocytosis. If the drug is insoluble or very poorly soluble, it poses a problem of dissolution and/or absorption because the flux of the drug across an intestinal membrane is proportional to its concentration gradient between the apical side and the basolateral sides of the gastrointestinal tract. The Noyes–Whitney equation (modified) (Equation (2.4)) confers the significance of solubility in dissolution of a drug [14]:

$$DR = \frac{dX}{dt} = \frac{A \times D}{h} \times \frac{C_s - X_d}{V} \tag{2.4}$$

where DR is the dissolution rate, A is the surface area available for dissolution, D is the diffusion coefficient of the drug, h is the thickness of the boundary layer adjacent to the dissolving drug surface, C_s is the saturation solubility of the drug, X_d is the amount of dissolved drug, and V is the volume of dissolution media.

Poor solubility is caused by two main factors: 1) high lipophilicity and 2) strong intermolecular interactions [15]. The aqueous solubility of solid compounds is mostly governed by interactions between molecules in the crystal lattice, intermolecular interactions in the solution, and the entropy changes accompanying fusion and dissolution [3]. Equation (2.3) can be simplified as:

$$\ln X_w = \ln X_i - \ln \gamma_w \tag{2.5}$$

where X_w is the observed mole fraction solubility, X_i is related to its ideal mole fraction solubility, and γ_w is the activity coefficient in water. Equation (2.5) indicates that solubility can be regulated by changing the crystalline structure as well as the activity coefficient.

Drug solubility criteria are dependent on the required amount of a dose (i.e., drug potency). As a rule of thumb, a compound with an average potency of 1 mg/kg should have a solubility of at least 0.1 g/L to be adequately soluble [16]. If a compound with the same potency has a solubility of less than 0.01 g/L, it can be considered poorly soluble. The solubility estimation is based on the concept of maximum absorbable dose (MAD) [1], which is a conceptual tool estimating the maximum amount of drug that can be absorbed during the time the drug stays in the intestine as a solution. It is expressed as:

$$\begin{aligned} \text{MAD(mg)} = {} & S(\text{mg/mL}) \times K_a(\text{per min}) \\ & \times \text{SIWV(mL)} \times \text{SITT(min)} \end{aligned} \tag{2.6}$$

where S is the solubility at pH 6.5 reflecting a typical small intestine condition, K_a is the transintestinal absorption rate constant determined by a rat intestinal perfusion experiment, SIWV is the small intestinal water volume available for drug solubilization generally accepted as 250 mL, and SITT is the small intestine transit time, typically around 270 min. For a general description of "solubility," the United States Pharmacopoeia (USP) uses seven different solubility expressions as shown in Table 2.2 [17].

2.2.3 Biopharmaceutics Classification System (BCS)

The biopharmaceutics classification system provided by the U.S. Food and Drug Administration (FDA) is used as a practical guide for predicting the intestinal drug absorption. The FDA has issued a guide titled "Waiver of in vivo bioavailability and bioequivalence studies for immediate-release solid oral dosage forms based on biopharmaceutics classification system" [18]. Being combined with the dissolution rate of the drug, BCS takes into account three major factors that govern the rate and extent of drug absorption from immediate-release solid oral dosage forms: dissolution, solubility, and intestinal permeability [19]. According

TABLE 2.2 Solubility Definition in the USP

Solubility Definition	Parts of Solvent Required for One Part of Solute	Solubility Range (mg/mL)	Solubility Assigned (mg/mL)
Very soluble (VS)	<1	>1000	1000
Freely soluble (FS)	From 1 to 10	100–1000	100
Soluble	From 10 to 30	33–100	33
Sparingly soluble (SPS)	From 30 to 100	10–33	10
Slightly soluble (SS)	From 100 to 1000	1–10	1
Very slightly soluble (VSS)	From 1000 to 10,000	0.1–1	0.1
Practically insoluble (PI)	>10,000	<0.1	0.01

TABLE 2.3 BCS Classification of Drugs

Class	Solubility	Permeability
I	High	High
II	Low	High
III	High	Low
IV	Low	Low

to the BCS, drug substances are classified depending on their levels of solubility and permeability as given in Table 2.3.

Solubility that is based on a USP description and intestinal permeability is compared with the intravenous injection [20]. Since 85% of the drugs in the U.S. and European market are orally administered, all these factors should be primarily considered in the drug development process.

The importance of solubility and permeability on drug absorption can be illustrated by application of Fick's first law to membrane absorption across the mucosal surface [21]:

$$J_w = P_w \times C_w = \frac{dM}{dt} \times \frac{1}{A} \quad (2.7)$$

where J_w is the mass transport across the gut wall, P_w can be assumed as the effective permeability, C_w is the concentration of the drug at the membrane, and A is the surface area. As shown in Table 2.3, increasing the solubility of class II drugs can enhance the bioavailability of drugs significantly. Moreover, for class III drugs, the aqueous solubility of the drug should be modified to make it more lipophilic for higher permeability. Modification in both aqueous solubility and permeability will improve the bioavailability of class IV drugs. Hydrophilic–lipophilic balance is of utmost importance in achieving greater bioavailability of drugs.

2.3 BIOAVAILABILITY IMPROVEMENT

2.3.1 Enhancement of Solubility

Most new chemical entities discovered through combinatorial chemistry and HTS have higher molecular weight, enhanced lipophilicity, and decreased aqueous solubility [2, 22]. Out of 100 substances launched during the period of 1995–2000, 14 were considered class I, 12 were considered classified as class II, 28 were class III, and 46 were class IV substances [23]. About 30–40% of the lead substances available today have an aqueous solubility less than 10 μM or 5 mg/mL at pH 7 [5]. Hence, much effort is placed on enhancement of solubility of poorly soluble compounds. As discussed earlier, the candidate molecules with optimum solubility is crucial to achieving their target bioavailability and therapeutic responses. Moreover, solubility is of critical importance in pharmacological and toxicological profiling during the early stage of drug development. The candidate molecules are screened in nanomolar receptor assays that select the molecules with the best receptor binding for further preclinical studies [5]. Some common approaches frequently implemented for enhancing drug solubility are outlined below.

2.3.1.1 ***Prodrugs*** Prodrugs are compounds that are not biologically active by themselves but should be transformed into active products by chemical or enzymatic reactions [24–26]. Prodrugs can be classified into four major categories [27]: 1) carrier linked (active agent is linked to a carrier whose activation occurs by hydrolysis, oxidation, or reduction), 2) bioprecursors (which do not contain a premoiety yet are activated by hydration, oxidation, or reduction), 3) drug-polymer conjugates (where the carrier is a macromolecule such as a polyethylene glycol), and 4) drug-antibody conjugates (where the carrier is an antibody raised against tumor cells).

Solubility Enhancement Prodrug approaches are employed for various purposes, such as to increase solubility, increase stability, improve oral/local absorption, enhance brain penetration, reduce presystemic metabolism, reduce toxicity, reduce local irritation, and for patent line extension [25]. Several successful prodrugs are developed for enhancement of solubility, and the strategies applied as shown in Figure 2.2 will be covered in this section.

A common prodrug approach to enhancing water solubility is an addition of polar functionalities to the parent compound [26]. A phosphate prodrug represents one such successful approach. Highly water-soluble phosphate prodrugs can be obtained via preparation of phosphoric acid esters, phosphoric acid amides, or (phosphonooxy) methyl esters [25]. Phosphate esters are converted into a parent compound by brush-border enzyme, alkaline phosphatase in the gastrointestinal tract [28]. An example of a phosphate prodrug is fosamprenavir, a prodrug of HIV protease

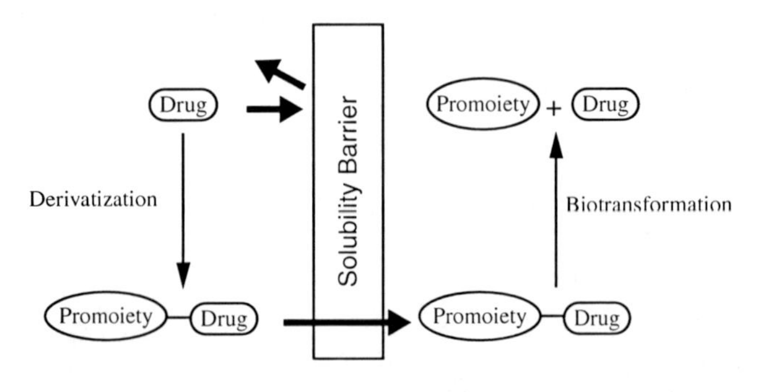

FIGURE 2.2 A schematic representation of the prodrug concept. Reproduced with permission from Ref. 26.

inhibitor amprenavir [29]. Fosamprenavir is applied orally as a calcium salt. As a result of its tenfold higher water solubility as compared with the parent drug, fosamprenavir exhibits increased peroral bioavailability as well. Another example is fosphenytoin, a prodrug of phenytoin, whose oral availability is greatly enhanced as compared with its parent drug [30]. In fosphenytoin, a phosphate group is attached via a spacer or linker. Clindamycin phosphate (parent drug: clindamycin), stachyflin phosphate (parent drug: stachyflin), etoposide disodium phosphate (parent drug: etoposide), miproxifene phosphate (parent drug: miproxifene), and estramustine phosphate (parent drug: estramustine) are also successful examples of phosphate prodrugs that showed enhanced oral delivery [26]. 20-phosphoryloxymethylcamptothecin (parent drug: camptothecin), aminodarone disodium phosphate (parent drug: aminodarone), prednisolone sodium phosphate (parent drug: prednisolone), fludarabine phosphate (parent drug: vidarabine), and entacapone phosphate (parent drug: entacapone) are other examples of phosphate prodrugs used in parenteral drug delivery.

Amino acid ester prodrugs represent another valid approach for enhancement of water solubility through esterification of the parent drug with amino acid [31]. The well-known examples are valacyclovir and valganciclovir, both of which are valine esters of the potent antiviral drugs acyclovir and ganciclovir, respectively. The enhanced peroral bioavailability of these prodrugs is not only a result of increased water solubility, but in addition, they are substrates of small peptide transporters (PEPT1) and, therefore, actively absorbed [25]. Both phosphate and amino acid ester prodrugs showed high chemical stability, efficient enzymatic cleavage, and greatly enhanced water solubility, and they are suitable for both oral and parenteral applications. In addition, amino acid ester prodrugs show significantly improved bioavailability, as they are a substrate of small peptide transporters (PEPT1). The hemisuccinate ester prodrug, another example of the prodrug approach for enhancement of solubility, however, is chemically metastable and a weak substrate for esterase cleavage [26]. Three of the earliest parenteral prodrugs are chloramphenicol, prednisolone, and methylprednisolone hemisuccinates.

Apart from the above-mentioned strategies, numerous alternative prodrug approaches have been performed for enhancement of water solubility. For example, paclitaxel has been attached to polymers, such as polyethylene glycol, albumin, and carboxymethyl dextran, for enhancement of water solubility [32], and the promising results have warranted further attempts with similar approaches.

Stability Enhancement The objective of prodrug design, as summarized in Figure 2.3, is not limited to improvement in solubility to facilitate oral absorption. The prodrug approach offers a wide range of property modulation covering from improvement in the chemical stability of an active ingredient to allowing tissue-selective delivery that can even lead to its *in situ* activation.

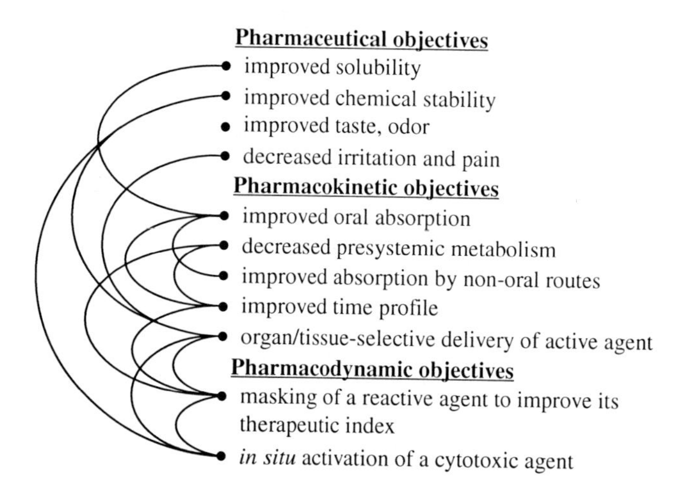

FIGURE 2.3 A schematic list of objectives in prodrug research, together with the overlaps. Reproduced with permission from Ref. 27.

In the case of etoposide, a chemically complex antitumor agent, the phenolic group was monophosphorylated to increase its water solubility and chemical stability [33]. After parenteral administration of prodrug to patients, rapid and quantitative conversion of prodrug to the parent drug was observed. An example of erythromycin also offers evidences for both organoleptic property and stability issues. To avoid its bad taste, which is the major excuse of rejection from children, erythromycin is normally administered to children as its 2′-ethyl succinate, a taste-free prodrug, which, however, undergoes slow but non-negligible hydrolysis in the medicine bottle. To resolve the stability issue, a far more stable pro-prodrug, which consists of 9-enol ether in erythromycin 2′-ethyl succinate [34], has been developed. This double prodrug is very poorly soluble in water and, thus, remains stable in solution, but in the acidic stomach, it rapidly converts into erythromycin 2′-ethyl succinate that eventually hydrolyzes to erythromycin.

L-Dopa is the drug of choice in the management of Parkinson's disease. However, as a result of its extensive metabolic decarboxylation process, oral bioavailability of L-Dopa is only 33% [35]. A tripeptide mimetic dopamine prodrug was developed and found to be sufficiently stable toward enzymatic degradation prior to absorption [36]. Subsequently, the addition of D-Asp-Ala as a suitable pro-moiety to enhance the intestinal permeability of small drug molecules was attempted and its high efficacy was successfully demonstrated [37]. The advantage of this pro-moiety over the di- or tri-peptides was to maintain stability in the gastrointestinal environment, thus, releasing the active compound in the blood and/or at its site of action [19, 38].

2.3.1.2 Salts A salt is formed from the reaction of an acid with a base, and this simple chemical reaction involves

TABLE 2.4 Potential Counterions Used in Preparation of Pharmaceutical Salts [39]

Cation	Anion
Bismuth	Hydrochloride
Potassium	Hydrobromide
Sodium	Sulfate
Lithium	Nitrate
Calcium	Tosylate
Magnesium	Mesylate
Ethanolamine	Napsylate
Zinc	Beylate
Choline	Maleate
Aluminum	Phosphate
TRIS	Salicylate
Ammonia	Tartrate
Diethylamine	Lactate
Procaine	Citrate
Benzathine	Benzoate
Meglumine	Succinate
	Acetate
	Fumarate

either protonation or a neutralizing reaction. Numerous drugs are either weak acids or weak bases and may form a wide range of salts with appropriate bases or acids, respectively. Salt formation could be used to alter the physicochemical, biopharmaceutical, and processing properties of a drug substance without modifying its fundamental chemical structure [39]. Acidic and basic drugs in their salt forms have higher solubility than their corresponding acid or base forms, leading to improved bioavailability or ease of formulation [40]. Typical counterions, anions, and cations used for preparation of salts of acidic and basic drugs are summarized in Table 2.4.

The principle of salt formation for basic or acidic drugs can be explained in terms of pH-solubility interrelationships. The schematic representation of the pH-solubility profile of a basic drug is shown in Figure 2.4 [41]. As shown in Figure 2.4, solubility can be expressed by two independent curves and that the point where two curves convene is the pH_{max}, the pH of maximum solubility. At $pH > pH_{max}$, the solid phase that is in equilibrium with a solution is free base and the solubility decreases as pH increases. The region of steepest slope in the curve represents an ionizing portion of the curve and begins around the pK_a value [42]. As pH is lowered further, pH_{max} is obtained where the maximum solubility of the drug is observed. This is the only point where theoretically both the free base and the salt can coexist as solids [40]. At $pH < pH_{max}$, a plateau region of the curve is obtained where the salt solubility of a drug prevails and is almost constant.

The schematic diagram for the pH-solubility interrelationship of free acid and its salt form is shown in Figure 2.5. The equilibrium species at pHs below pH_{max} are the free acid, which will convert into a salt at pHs above pH_{max}. The pH_{max} is the point where the acidic drug has the highest solubility and a point where theoretically both free acid and its salt forms coexist. Salt formation will be favored for the basic drug having a high pH_{max} (with higher pK_a), higher intrinsic solubility, and a lower salt solubility [40]. Salt formation will be favored for acidic drugs having low pH_{max} (i.e., lower pK_a), higher intrinsic solubility, and lower salt solubility.

The presence of a counterion in solution decreases the aqueous solubility of salt as a result of a common ion effect, which will be less pronounced for a salt form of drugs with higher K_{sp} (i.e., higher solubility).

$$\text{drug} \cdot \text{salt} \leftrightarrow \text{drug ion} + \text{salt counterion} \quad (2.8)$$

$$K_{sp} = [\text{drug ion}][\text{salt counterion}] \quad (2.9)$$

$$S = \sqrt{K_{sp}} \quad (2.10)$$

As most drugs newly synthesized or discovered have low aqueous solubility, their respective salts also have relatively

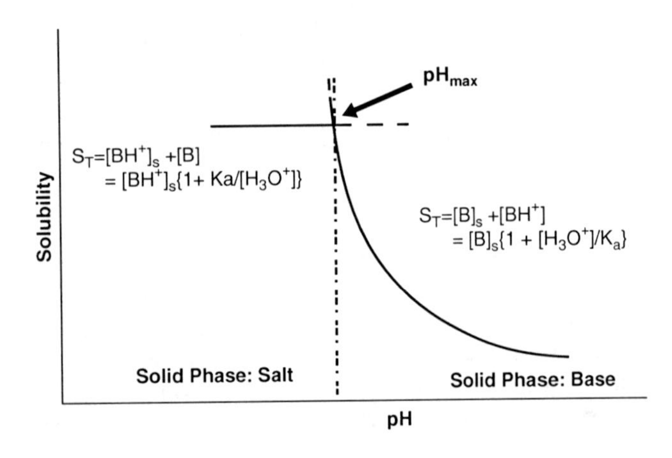

FIGURE 2.4 Schematic representation of the pH-solubility profile of a basic drug. Reproduced with permission from Ref. 41.

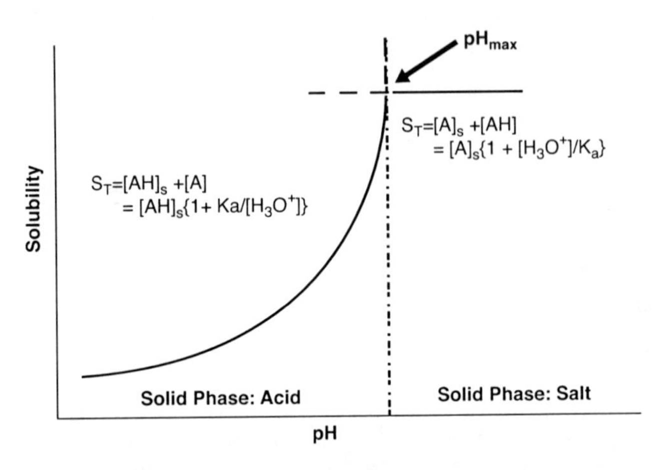

FIGURE 2.5 Schematic representation of the pH-solubility profile of an acidic drug. Reproduced with permission from Ref. 41.

low aqueous solubility. Hence, an impact of common ions is critical and precaution must be paid to the selection of cations or anions during the salt formation process as they may precipitate into their free acids or bases in gastrointestinal fluid after oral administration. It was reported that salt forms of numerous drug molecules undergo self-association in the solution, exhibiting nonideal pH-solubility behavior [41, 43, 44]. For example, the solubility of papaverine hydrochloride reached to >120 mg/mL at an almost constant pH of 4 ± 0.1 as a deviation from its normal solubility of 40 mg/mL [40]. The solubility of salts of specific drugs varies according to the salt-forming agents used. The overall effect of counterions on the solubility of salts depends on the difference in hydration energies or crystal lattice energies as a result of changes in salt structure [45]. Despite several problems related to salt formation, the salt formation approach will remain the primary means to improve solubility and the dissolution rate of poorly water-soluble acidic or basic drugs. Of approximately 300 NCEs approved by the FDA from 1995 to 2006, 120 in the market were in salt forms [40].

2.3.1.3 ***Crystal Engineering*** Crystal engineering approaches can be applied to a wide range of crystalline materials and offer an alternative and potentially fruitful means to improve solubility, dissolution rate, and subsequent bioavailability of poorly soluble drugs. Changes in operational conditions in the crystallization process, such as degree of saturation, temperature, solvent, pH, and impurity, can produce crystals with different properties [46].

Several examples in the literature demonstrate the effects of changing crystal morphology on *in vivo* dissolution rate with potential for improving bioavailability. The habit modification of dipyridamole by crystallization showed that dissolution of rod-shaped particles was faster than rectangular needle-shaped crystals [46]. Similarly, phenytoin can be crystallized into a needle-like rhombic shape with different dissolution properties [47], which is ascribed to changes in surface area rather than to improvements in the wetting of more polar surface moieties. However, it was also noted that the crystal habit of doped crystals played an integral role in the enhancement of the intrinsic dissolution rate of phenytoin as a result of increased abundance in polar groups [48]. The nature of a structure adopted by a given compound during the crystallization process would have a broad impact on the solid-state properties of the system [28].

It was reported that various polymorphs could have different solubility and dissolution rates, exhibiting nonequivalent bioavailability for polymorphs [46]. Polymorphism in crystalline solid is defined as materials with the same chemical composition but different lattice structures and/or different molecular composition [49], whereas pseudo-polymorphism is a term that refers to crystalline forms with solvent molecules as an integral part of the structure [49, 50]. Metastable polymorphs are characterized with a higher energy state, lower melting point, and higher aqueous solubility. Metastable crystalline forms of phenobarbital, spironolactone, and carbamazepine have shown a higher dissolution rate and enhanced bioavailability [46]. Similarly, two polymorphs of phenylbutazone showed differences in the dissolution rate and bioavailability in beagle dogs [51]. The metastable polymorph of etoposide provides a two times higher dissolution rate than a stable polymorph [52].

Even after a product is launched in the market, product recall becomes a necessity as a result of the biopharmaceutical issues, as was seen with Norvir (Abbott Laboratories, Abbott Park, IL). Two years after entry into the market, a previously unknown, but thermodynamically more stable, polymorph of the active ingredient (ritonavir) was discovered. This new form (form II) was approximately 50% less soluble in the hydroalcoholic formulation vehicle, resulting in poor dissolution behavior [53]. This eventually caused withdrawal of the original Norvir capsule from the market. It is, therefore, imperative that solubility and stability studies be integrated in guiding selection, development, and optimization of drug and dosage form. The additives or solvents (impurities) that can prevent the conversion of metastable form into the stable one could be used to exploit the superior solubility of the metastable form [46]. For example, trimesic acid was used to disrupt the conversion of the stable form of glutamic acid from the metastable form. Although the utilization of metastable polymorphs could offer a means to improve dissolution and oral bioavailability, there remain some concerns with respect to conversion of these materials into more stable crystalline forms during the processing and storage. In general, the range of solubility differences between two polymorphs is typically two- to threefold as a result of relatively small differences in free energy [54]. In addition, because of the higher potential risk of interconversion into more stable and less soluble forms in the gastrointestinal tract, the strategy involved with metastable polymorph development is less favored than other strategies.

Hydrates can stoichiometrically incorporate water at a definite position in the crystal lattice. The water present in these species forms hydrogen bond(s) and/or coordinate covalent bond(s) with the anhydrate molecule [55]. Incorporation of solvent molecules into the crystal lattice produces a molecule with different physicochemical properties. Generally, the anhydrous form of a drug has greater solubility than the hydrates. For example, the anhydrate form of naproxen sodium holds higher solubility than its hydrate [56]. However, the organic (nonaqueous) solvates have greater solubility than the nonsolvates. For instance, glibenclamide has been isolated as pentanol and toluene solvates, which exhibited higher solubility and dissolution rate than two nonsolvated polymorphs [57]. Similarly, the solvated form of spironolactone exhibited the enhanced dissolution rate [58]. Therefore, in the solvate formulation process, any property changes in stability and toxicity on interaction with mobile solvent and its components should be addressed.

The amorphous form of pharmacologically active materials has received considerable attention, as it represents the most energetic solid state of a material and offers higher solubility, dissolution, and bioavailability. An amorphous solid has a short-range molecular order [59]. However, unlike a crystalline solid, an amorphous solid having flexible constituent molecules does not have a long-range order of molecular packing or well-defined molecular conformation [60]. An amorphous solid can be produced by quenching of melts, prompt precipitation by antisolvent addition, freeze-drying, spray drying, and introduction of impurities. Amorphous solids can also be produced by solid dispersion processes that introduce mechanical or chemical stress (e. g., grinding, milling, and wet granulation) and dehydration of crystalline hydrates. Amorphous drug forms significantly enhance solubility as compared with its crystalline counterpart, displaying 1.4-fold for indomethacin, 2.0-fold for cefalexin, 2.5-fold for teteracycline, and approximately 10.0-fold for macrolide antibiotic and novobiocin acid [61]. The amorphous systems, however, pose a major challenge in achievement of proper physical and chemical stability.

An alternative approach for the enhancement of drug solubility, dissolution rate, and bioavailability uses the application of crystal engineering of co-crystals. A co-crystal is defined as a crystalline material that consists of two or mole molecular (and electrically neutral) species held together by noncovalent bonds [62]. Co-crystals can be prepared by evaporation of a heteromeric solution, grinding the components together, sublimation, growth from the melt, and slurry preparation [46]. The key benefits of a co-crystallization approach are the practical capacity of all types of drug molecules including weakly ionizable and nonionizable to form co-crystals and the existence of numerous potential counter-molecules including food additives, preservatives, pharmaceutical excipients, as well as other active pharmaceutical ingredients (APIs), for co-crystal synthesis [63, 64]. The dissolution of co-crystals of itraconazole with weak acids, such as succinic acid, malic acid, and tartaric acid, was 4- to 20-fold higher than the crystalline form [65]. The co-crystal of the API formed with glutaric acid increased its aqueous dissolution rate by 18 times over that of homomeric crystalline forms [66]. The co-crystals of carbamazepine, fluoxetine hydrochloride, ibuprofen, indomethacin, and norfloxacin have also achieved improved solubility and dissolution [67]. The major challenges in the co-crystal development are lack of efficient screening technologies and infamously difficult preparation procedures [68]. The co-crystallization approach is rapidly evolving and represents an emerging area of pharmaceutical investigation, which is still relatively unexplored and thus requires further profound studies.

2.3.1.4 ***Particle Size Reduction*** The relationship of curvature, interfacial free energy, and solubility of particles is described using a Gibbs–Thomson effect. The Gibbs–Thomson effect on the relative solubility of spherical particles of identical materials of varying size is expressed using an Ostwald–Freundlich equation as described below [69]:

$$\frac{RT\rho}{M}\ln\frac{S_1}{S_2} = 2\sigma\left(\frac{1}{r_1} - \frac{1}{r_2}\right) \tag{2.11}$$

where R is the gas constant, T is the absolute temperature, M is the molecular weight of the solid in solution, σ is the interfacial tension between the solid and the liquid, ρ is the density of the solid, and S_1 and S_2 are the solubilities of particle of radius r_1 and r_2, respectively. The Ostwald–Freundlich equation predicts that the equilibrium solubility of particles changes exponentially as a function of particle size [70]. Particle size reduction may lead to super saturation insolubility. Because intrinsic solubility remains almost unaffected, the most profound effect of particle size reduction is observed on increase in the dissolution rate through enhancement of the particle surface area (Fick's first law, Noyes–Whitey equation) [46]. Also, it was experimentally found that the thickness of the diffusion layer decreased as the particle size decreased, leading to faster transport of solvated molecules to bulk solution and, hence, faster dissolution [71].

Micronization produces a reduced particle size in the range of 2–5 μm and size distribution normally ranging from 0.1 to 25 μm [72]. Numerous new drugs developed recently exhibited such a low solubility that micronization did not guarantee sufficient bioavailability. Hence, the particle size reduction process has moved to the next level of nanonization with a particle size below 1 μm and a typical size distribution between 200 and 500 nm [73]. Nanosized particles showed significant enhancement in the dissolution rate and bioavailability as compared with micronized particles resulting from enormous enhancement of the surface area. Nanoparticles are obtained by top-down processes (i.e., comminuting of larger particles down to nanoparticles) or bottom-up processes (i.e., precipitation starting from molecular solution) [74]. Other alternative ways are the combination of both principles (NANOEDGE) and via chemical reaction. A size reduction of pharmaceuticals (micronization and nanonization) is achieved by techniques like milling [73, 75], precipitation [76], cryo vacuum [77], spray drying [75], sonocrystallization [64], high-pressure homogenization [72], and supercritical fluid technology [78].

2.3.1.5 ***Co-solvency*** Co-solvency, the addition of water-miscible solvents to an aqueous system, is one of the oldest and most frequently used solubilization techniques [79]. Co-solvent solubilization is particularly important for parenteral dosage forms in which it is desirable to incorporate the required dose as a true solution in the smallest volume of liquid. Most co-solvents have hydrogen bond donor and/or acceptor groups as well as small hydrocarbon regions [80]. Their hydrophilic bonding groups ensure water miscibility, while their hydrophobic hydrocarbon regions interfere with water's hydrogen bonding network, reducing the overall intermolecular attraction of water. By disrupting water's self-association, co-solvents reduce water's ability to squeeze out nonpolar, hydrophobic compounds, thus, increasing solubility. By adapting a different paradigm in which the polar water environment was changed to a more nonpolar environment like the solute, co-solvents facilitate the solubilization process. Commonly employed co-solvents include propylene glycol, ethanol, glycerin, and polyethylene glycol 400. Among several models for the prediction of co-solvent solubilization of nonpolar drugs, the log-linear model that is considered most useful, simple, and accurate [81], depicts an exponential increase in nonpolar drug solubility with a linear increase in co-solvent concentration:

$$\log S_{\mathrm{mix}} = \log S_{\mathrm{w}} + \sigma f \tag{2.12}$$

where S_{mix} and S_{w} are the total solute solubilities in the co-solvent/water mixture and in water, respectively; σ is the co-solvent solubilization power for the particular co-solvent-solute system, and f is the volume fraction of the co-solvent in the aqueous mixture. Several examples of commercial products employed co-solvency as a solubilization enhancement technique [82]. Lanoxin (Digoxin, GlaxoSmithKline, London, U.K.) is an elixir formulation for pediatric use containing 10% ethanol as co-solvent. VePesid (Etopside, Bristol-Myers-Squibb, New York, NY) is a soft gelatin capsule using glycerin and PEG 400 as co-solvents. Kaletra (Lopinavir and Ritonavir, Abbott) was formulated as an oral solution with alcohol (42.2% v/v) as co-solvent. Valium (Diazepam, Roche Laboratories, Nutley, NJ) was formulated as IM/IV using propylene glycol (40%) and ethanol (10%) as co-solvents. Robaxin (Methocarbamil, A.H. Robins, Richmond, VA) used PEG 300 (50%) as co-solvent for IM/IV preparation. Zemplar (Paricalcitol, Abbott) was formulated for IV bolus injection that contained propylene glycol (30%) and ethanol (20%) as co-solvent.

2.3.1.6 Use of Surfactants Surfactants are compounds that lower the surface tension between two liquids or between a liquid and a solid, allowing for easier spreading between them. The use of surfactants to improve the dissolution rate of poorly soluble drugs has been successfully demonstrated. The presence of surfactants increased the solubility of the drug by lowering the surface tension [83]. The capacity of surfactants in solubilizing drugs depends on numerous factors, such as chemical structures of surfactant and drug, temperature, pH, ionic strength, etc. [84]. In a previous study, acetyl-trimethyl-ammonium bromide, a cationic surfactant, enhanced the dissolution rate of poorly water-soluble acidic drugs through enhancement of solubility of drugs in the medium [85]. Tween 80 (Sigma-Aldrich, St. Louis, MO), a hydrophilic nonionic surfactant, enhanced the solubility of compounds, leading to enhanced absorption of digoxin [86] and paclitaxel [87]. Sodium lauryl sulphate (SLS), an anionic surfactant, enhanced the solubility of triclosan at concentrations above the critical micelle concentration (CMC) by several orders of magnitude [88]. SLS forms micellar aggregates with hydrophobic organic tails in the center and anionic polar groups at the outside. The lipophilic triclosan molecules are trapped in or between the hydrophobic cores of the micelle, which accounts for the increase in solubility.

As a result of the unique characteristics of surfactants, their low concentrations added to water will form a stable monolayer. As an amount of surfactant added increases, a monolayer becomes a bilayer. If the concentration of surfactant is sufficiently high, the bilayer becomes unstable and micelles are formed [89]. An important property of micelles particularly in pharmaceutical application is their ability to increase the aqueous solubility of sparingly soluble substances. At surfactant concentrations above the CMC, the solubility of the drug increases linearly with the concentration of the surfactant. As the solubilization is the partitioning process of the drug between micelle and aqueous phase, the standard free energy of solubilization ($\Delta G_{\mathrm{s}}^{\mathrm{o}}$) can be expressed by the following equation [90]:

$$\Delta G_{\mathrm{s}}^{\mathrm{o}} = -RT \ln P \tag{2.13}$$

where R is the universal gas constant, T is the absolute temperature, and P is the partition coefficient between the micelle and the aqueous phase.

Micelles formed with low-molecular-weight surfactants usually have relatively high CMC and are unstable upon dilution, whereas, micelles formed with amphiphilic block co-polymers have a high solubilization capacity and rather low CMC [84]. The compatibility between the loaded drug and core-forming components determines the efficacy of drug loading [91]. A Flory–Huggins interaction parameter (X_{sp}) could be used to assess such compatibility:

$$X_{\mathrm{sp}} = (\delta_{\mathrm{s}} - \delta_{\mathrm{p}})^2 \frac{V_{\mathrm{s}}}{RT} \tag{2.14}$$

where X_{sp} is the interaction parameter between solubilized drug and core-forming polymer block, δ is the Scatchard–Hildebrand solubility parameter of the core-forming polymer block, and V_{s} is the molar volume of the solubilized drug [92].

Some examples of polymeric micellar solubilization include Pluronic-based (BASF Corporation, Florham Park, NJ) micelles for drugs including diazepam [93], adriamycin [94], and anthracycline antibiotics [95].

*2.3.1.7 **Complexation*** The improvement of drug solubility and subsequent bioavailability remains one of the most challenging tasks in the drug development process. Among numerous approaches available and reported in the literature for enhancement of the solubility of a poorly water-soluble drug, complexation seems to be a promising technique. Cyclodextrins, dendrimers, and other complexation resources and techniques offer formulation scientists a profound way to overcome problems stemming from inadequate and variable bioavailability and gastrointestinal mucosal toxicity [96].

Cyclodextrins (CDs) are cyclic oligosaccharides capable of encapsulating lipophilic molecules into their interior cavity [97]. The pharmaceutical application of CDs is mostly observed in the area of enhancement of drug solubility in aqueous solutions [98]. For example, complexes of CDs with drugs including ibuprofen [99], nifedipine [100], prostaglandin E1 [101], and artimisinin [102] demonstrated significantly improved solubility properties. The first pharmaceutical product that contained a highly soluble CD derivative is Sporonax (itraconazole/hydroxypropyl β-CD, Johnson & Johnson, New Brunswick, NJ), followed by Clorocil (Chloramphenicol/methyl β-CD, Edol, Portugal), Brexin (piroxicam/β-CD, Chiesi Pharmaceuticals, Rockville, MD), Prostin (Alprostadil/α-CD, Pfizer, New York, NY), and Voltaren Ophthalmic (Diclofenac sodium/hydroxypropyl γ-CD, Novartis Pharmaceuticals, Basel, Switzerland), all of which exhibited greatly enhanced aqueous solubility.

Dendrimers are macromolecules characterized with their highly branched 3D structure that allows for a high degree of surface functionality and versatility [103]. Dendrimers having a hydrophobic core and a hydrophilic surface layer have been termed uni-molecular micelles. Unlike traditional micelles, dendrimers, however, do not have a critical micelle concentration, which offers them at an entire concentration range the opportunity to be used as nanostructures suitable for a drug solubilization enhancer. Drugs can physically interact with dendrimers through either encapsulation into void spaces (nanoscale container) or association with surface groups (nano-scaffolding) or a mixture of both. Driving forces for the interactions are hydrogen bonding, van der Waals interactions, and electrostatic interaction between opposite charges on dendrimers and drugs [104].

One example of a dendrimer-mediated interaction is observed with indomethacin, which is poorly soluble in water and sparingly soluble in alcohol. Indomethacin formulated with poly (amidoamine) dendrimers G4 containing amino, hydroxyl, and carboxylate surface groups achieved enhanced water solubility of the drug (~25 μg/mL) by 29-fold, 26-fold, and 10-fold, respectively [105]. The high efficiency of amino-surface dendrimers can be a result of the presence of the carboxylic acid functional group in indomethacin, allowing for strong electrostatic and hydrogen bond interactions between a drug and a carrier. Along with the enhancement of solubility, dendrimers are also reported to reduce the toxicity of solubilized drugs [106]. Methotrexate, an antimetabolite and antifolate, can often exert toxic effects to the rapidly dividing cells of bone marrow and gastrointestinal mucosa. In a previous study, a reduction of methotrexate toxicity by melamine-based dendrimers was reported [106, 107]. The chemical structure in which methotrexate was encapsulated into 1, 3, 5-triazene dendrimer by physical mixing of drug and dendrimer in saline solution was depicted in Figure 2.6.

Stacking complexation between drugs and certain compounds can enhance the solubility of drugs. Complexes are formed through the overlapping of the planar regions of aromatic molecules. For example, nicotinamide has been widely used as a solubilizing agent, and its working mechanism is involved with an outcome of stacking complexation with drugs [108, 109]. It was previously reported that the improvement in solubility of 11 structurally diverse drugs was mainly a result of complexation with nicotinamide [110]. Judging from its high solubilization efficiency, low toxicity, and low cost, nicotinamide is considered an integral solubility enhancer in the pharmaceutical field.

N-methyl pyrrolidone (NMP), a water-miscible aprotic solvent, was also reported to act as a solubilizing agent for enhancement of the uptake of poorly soluble drugs [111]. The presence of a substantially large and nearly planar nonpolar region in NMP may result in hydrophobic interactions with drug molecule, facilitating to form a complex. Such interactions will stabilize the drug in a dissolved form and subsequently increase its solubility [112]. Solubilizing efficiencies of NMP were investigated with drugs like phenobarbital, carbendazim, griseofulvin, phenytoin, ketoprofen, testosterone, and amiodarone.

The solubility of triclosan increased through complex formation with N-methyl glucamine (NMG) [88], which occurred between the electronegative nitrogen of NMG and the enolic hydrogen of triclosan. Similarly, electron-donating oxygen of polyethylene glycols can also form a complex with acidic hydrogen of drugs such as phenobarbital [113].

Other substances, like carrageenan, can also improve the solubility of a drug through complexation. Carrageenan, a naturally occurring anionic polysaccharide, consists of the sulfate esters of galactose and 3,6-anhydrogalactose copolymers [114]. As a result of the presence of anionic sulfate groups, carrageenan can strongly exert ionic interaction with oppositely charged drugs. During the interaction process, the polymer chains in carrageenan created irregular orders/structures in the complex, leading to the formation of an amorphous structure that accounts for the increased solubility of the drug [115].

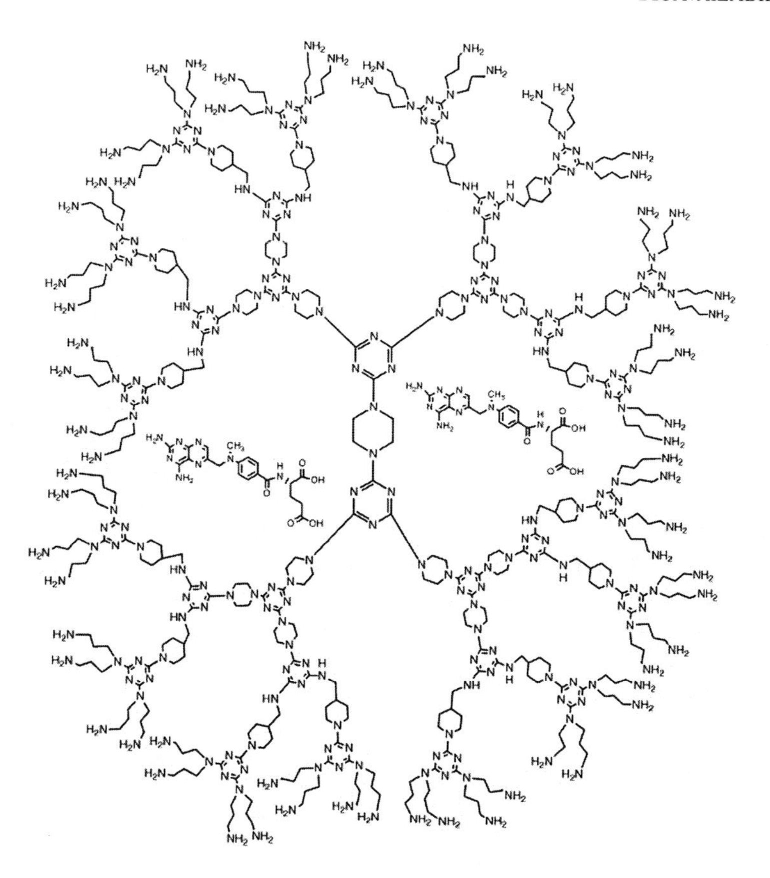

FIGURE 2.6 Structure of 1,3,5-triazene dendrimer encapsulating two molecules of methotrexate Reproduced with permission from Ref. 106.

2.3.1.8 Lipid-Based Formulations The capability of lipid-based formulations to facilitate gastrointestinal absorption of numerous poorly soluble drug candidates has been intensively studied [116]. The major advantages of the lipid based formulation approach are 1) improvement and reduction in the variability of gastrointestinal absorption of poorly water-soluble drugs and 2) possible reduction in or elimination of a number of development and processing steps (e.g., salt selection or identification of stable crystalline form of the drug, coating, and taste masking) [117]. The most frequently used excipients are dietary oils (e.g., coconut, palm seed, corn, olive, peanut, and sesame), lipid-soluble solvents (e.g., polyethylene glycol 400, ethanol, and glycerin), and various surfactants (e.g., Cremophor EL (BASF Corporation, Florham Park, NJ), Tween 80 (Uniqema, Paterson, NJ), Span 20 (Croda, Parsippany, NJ), Labrafil (Gattefosse, Paramus, NJ, USA), Labrasol (Gattefosse, Paramus, NJ, USA), and Gelucire (Gattefosse, Paramus, NJ, USA).

In the simplest case, such formulations could be the mixture of drug solubilized in a single lipid excipient. Digestion of the oily component(s) in the formulation will have a major impact on the fate of the drug in the gut [118]. In most cases, the digestion process has advantages over other methods in enhancement of drug solubility. For instance, the hydrophobic drugs can be highly solubilized within mixed micelles of bile components and the products of triglyceride lipolysis. Examples include Prometrium (Catalent Pharma Solutions, St. Petersburg, FL, USA) (progesterone in peanut oil), Teva-Valproic acid (Teva Pharmaceutical Ind., Petach Tikva, Israel) (valproic acid in corn oil), and Rocaltrol (Validus Pharmaceuticals LLC, Parsippany, NJ, USA) (calcitriol in medium-chain triglycerides), all of which in the market are sold in the form of soft gelatin capsules.

The conventional emulsion has limited applicability to the enhancement of the solubility of lipophilic drugs as a result of their instability. The thermodynamics of emulsion formation has been described using free energy associated with the emulsification process (ΔG) as expressed in the following equation [119]:

$$\Delta G = \sum N_i 4\Pi r_i^2 \sigma \qquad (2.15)$$

where N is number of droplets with radius r and σ is interfacial energy. The two phases tend to separate over a period of time to reduce the interfacial area between two phases and subsequently the free energy of the system. Surfactants form a layer around the emulsion particles, not only reducing the interfacial energy but also providing a barrier to coalescence.

Microemulsions are thermodynamically stable, isotropically clear dispersions of two immiscible liquids, such as oil and water, which are stabilized by an interfacial film of surfactant molecules [120]. As a result of their superior properties in solubilization and stability, microemulsions offer distinctive advantages over unstable dispersions like emulsions and suspensions. Oil-soluble drugs can be formulated in oil-in-water microemulsion, whereas water-soluble ones are better suited for water-in-oil systems. Cyclosporin A is formulated with corn oil and linoleoyl macrogolglycerides under the trade name Sandimmune (Novartis Pharmaceusticals) soft gel capsules.

Self-emulsifying drug delivery systems (SEDDSs) were used as an efficient means to improve the bioavailability of lipophilic drugs. SEEDSs are physically stable isotropic mixtures of oils, surfactants, or alternatively hydrophilic solvents and co-solvents [121, 122]. Furthermore, the formation of emulsion is thermodynamically spontaneous as a result of very low required free energy [123]. Upon mild agitation followed by dilution in aqueous media, SEDDSs form oil-in-water emulsions containing a drug in a solution state without necessitating the dissolution step, which frequently limits the rate of absorption of hydrophobic drugs from the crystalline state [124]. Itraconazole was formulated as SEEDS with tocopherol acetate used as the oil phase, Pluronic L 64 used as the surfactant, and Transcutol (Gattefosse, St. Priest, France) used as the co-solvent [125]. The formulation showed greatly enhanced bioavailability independent of the influence of food. Similarly, a higher bioavailability of simvastatin than a conventional tablet was observed from SEEDS formulation composed of Capryol 90 as oil phase, Cremophore EL as surfactant, and Carbitol as co-surfactant [126]. Formulations based on self-emulsification in the market are: Fortovase (Saquinavir, Hoffmann-La-Roche, Basel, Switzerland), Agenerase (Amrenavir, Glaxo SmithKline), and Lipirex (Fenofibrate, Genus Pharmaceuticals, Newbury Berkshire, U.K.).

2.3.1.9 Drug Dispersions in Formulation Carriers

Solid dispersion is one of the most promising techniques for enhancement of solubility and dissolution rate of poorly soluble drugs in carriers employed to produce drug dispersions [127, 128]. Solid dispersion refers to the dispersion of a group of solid products consisting of at least two different components, generally a hydrophilic matrix and a hydrophobic drug. The matrix can be either crystalline or amorphous, and the drug can be dispersed molecularly in amorphous particles (clusters) or in crystalline particles [129]. Solid dispersion can be prepared by two common methods: 1) fusion method and 2) solvent method [130].

1. *Fusion method:* This method is also referred as the melt method. In this method, a mixture of drug and carrier(s) is melted together under heat. The melt mass is then solidified by cooling. This method is especially suitable for low-melting-point drugs and carriers. Limitations of this method include incompatibility or phase separation of drug and carrier on the melt state, phase separation during cooling of melt mass, and degradation of drug at an elevated temperature [131]. There are numerous reported works, which used this method for improvement of solubility and dissolution of drugs. Solubility and dissolution of CoQ_{10} was improved by melting the drug with poloxamer 407 and Aerosil 200 at 70°C [132]. Nifedipine/mannitol solid dispersion was prepared by melting at 175°C with improvement in dissolution of nifedipine [133]. Hot-melt extrusion, which is used commercially, is an improved form of the fusion method for preparing solid dispersion. In this method, the drug/carrier mixture is simultaneously melted, homogenized, and then extruded and shaped as tablets, granules, pellets, sticks, or powder [127]. Another alternative method is hot-spin melting. In both methods, the drug exposure time to elevated temperature is significantly reduced as compared with the conventional hot-melt method. For example, solid dispersions of itraconazole [134] and hydrocortisone [135] were prepared using the hot-melt extrusion method, and solid dispersions of testosterone, progesterone, and dienogest [127] were prepared using hot-spin melting.
2. *Solvent method:* In this method, both drug and carrier(s) are dissolved in solvent(s). An important prerequisite for this method is both drug and carrier should have sufficient solubility in the solvent. The solvent from the solution can be removed by a number of methods, including vacuum drying, spray drying, freeze drying, and spray-freeze drying. Many drugs and polymers form solid dispersion using this technique. However, ecological and economical aspects of use of an organic solvent, toxicity related to the residual solvent in solid dispersion, and phase separation or crystallization during removal of solvent limit its application. Ternary solid dispersion of ofloxacin prepared by the solvent method showed significantly improved dissolution [136]. Solid dispersion of indomethacin with fine porous silica prepared by the solvent method and spray drying resulted in amorphous indomethacin with significantly improved dissolution of indomethacin [137]. Various modifications of the conventional solvent method including solvent-wetting method, melting solvent-method, and use of supercritical fluid technologies accomplished improvement in dissolution. Some reported works employing the aforementioned method include solid dispersion of felodipine using the solvent-wetting method [138] and solid dispersion

of carbamazepine [139] and felodipine [140] using supercritical fluid technologies.

Solid dispersion can be classified based on a molecular arrangement of drug and matrix in it as various types, namely, eutectics, amorphous precipitations in crystalline matrix, solid solution, glass suspension, and glass solution [131]. Enhancement in solubility and dissolution of hydrophobic drug from solid dispersion is brought by the following mechanisms [48, 141, 142]:

1. *Reduction in particle size:* Drug may exist molecularly or as amorphous clusters or as size-reduced crystals in the matrix in solid dispersion. When drug exists molecularly or in amorphous clusters, no energy is required to break the crystal lattice, thereby leading to enhancement in dissolution. Moreover, in the solid dispersion system, a supersaturated state is achieved during dissolution. If the drug precipitates, it remains in a metastable polymorphic form with higher solubility than the most stable crystal form [127]. An increase in surface area by reduction in drug crystal size leads to enhancement in both solubility and dissolution.
2. *Improved wettability of drug particles:* In a solid dispersion system, a drug is thoroughly dispersed in a hydrophilic carrier. Hence, drug wettability is enhanced in solid dispersions by the hydrophilic carriers even in the absence of surface-active agents. Furthermore, carriers can influence the drug dissolution profile through direct dissolution or co-solvent effects.
3. *Particles with higher porosity:* Particles in solid dispersions have been found to have a higher degree of porosity [143]. The increase in porosity also depends on the carrier properties; for example, solid dispersions with linear polymers produce larger and more porous particles than reticular polymers, therefore, leading to a higher dissolution rate [144]. The increased porosity of solid dispersion particles improves water penetration and, hence, causes rapid dissolution.

The carrier for solid dispersion is one of the most important factors for the dispersion process. As mentioned above, the variables including carrier/drug miscibility in melt state, ability to prevent recrystallization of drug, solvent solubility, and processing abilities should be considered for the selection of an optimum carrier. The most commonly used carriers and additives in solid dispersion are summarized in Table 2.5.

Solid dispersion has drawn an enormous amount of interest of drug delivery researchers for several years; however, its commercial utilization is still limited. Physical instability resulting from crystallization of drugs is one of the well-known problems of solid dispersion. Some marketed products of solid dispersion include Gris-PEG (griseofulvin in PEG, Novartis), Cesamet (nabilone in PVP, Lily) and Sporanox (itraconazole in HPMC and PEG 20,000 sprayed on sugar beads, Janseen Pharmaceuticals, Titusville, NJ/Johnson & Johnson) [131]. The major obstacles in the development of commercial products of solid dispersion are listed as follows [130, 145]:

1. Laborious and expensive methods of preparation
2. Reproducibility of physicochemical properties
3. Difficulty in development of dosage forms
4. Scale-up of manufacturing process
5. Stability of drug and vehicle

To date, various alternative strategies including hot-melt extrusion and electrostatic spinning method are applied to overcome the problems [145]. The solid dispersion approaches with advanced techniques to overcome the aforementioned problems may result in industrial-scale production.

TABLE 2.5 The Most Commonly Used Carriers and Additives in Solid Dispersion

S. No.	Chemical Class	Examples
1.	Acids	Citric acid, tartaric acid, succinic acid
2.	Sugars	Dextrose, sorbitol, sucrose, maltose, galactose, xylitol
3.	Polymeric materials	Polyvinylpyrrolidone, polyvinylalchohol, crospovidone, polyvinylpyrrolidone-polyvinylacetate copolymer, polyethylene glycol (M.W. 2000–20000), carboxymethylcellulose, hydroxypropyl cellulose, hydroxypropylmethyl cellulose, methylcellulose, hydroxypropylmethylcellulose phthalate, polyacrylates, polymethacrylates, guar gum, xanthan gum, sodium alginate, dextrin, cyclodextrins, galactomannan
4.	Surfactants	Polyoxyethyelene stearate, poloxamer, deoxycholic acid, tweens, spans, gelucire 44/14, vitamin E TPGS NF, sodium lauryl sulfate
5.	Miscellaneous	Pentaerythritol, phospholipids, Gelita® (hydrolysis product of collagen), urea, urethane, hydroxyalkyl xanthines

Reproduced with permission from Ref. 127.

2.3.2 Polarity Modification of Drugs

The very high polarity of drugs limits lipid solubility and subsequently their absorption through the gastrointestinal tract. Several prodrug approaches have been successfully pursued to enhance the lipid solubility of the polar compounds, such as carboxylates, phosphonates, and phosphates, via transformation to ester prodrugs [25]. Another type of highly polar compounds is sulfonates, whose low pK_a value (<1) causes them to be charged at physiologic pH values and, therefore, neither perorally bioavailable nor penetrate through the blood-brain barrier. The first lipophilic prodrug of sulfonates, converting them into chemically stable nitrophenyl esters (i.e., sulfophenylxanthine nitrophenyl esters), demonstrated its potential as perorally bioavailable compounds [146].

The presence of hydroxyl groups on peptides tends to promote hydrogen bonding with solvating water, leading to a concomitant decrease in the lipophilicity and subsequently membrane permeability [147]. The overall balance of polar to nonpolar groups within a drug molecule can be reduced either by removal of a polar group or addition of a nonpolar group [148]. The removal of two polar hydroxyl groups from dopamine, resulting in formation of phenethylamine, which increased lipid solubility approximately 50-fold with subsequent enhancement of brain permeability [149]. Masking of polar functional groups in drug molecules results in a reduction of hydrogen bonds and enhanced lipophilicity. Hydroxyl groups in drug molecules can be blocked irreversibly by methylation or reversibly by esterification. When one hydroxyl group in morphine is methylated, it becomes codeine whose membrane permeability increases approximately 10-folds, whereas when both hydroxyl groups are acetylated, it becomes heroin whose membrane permeability increases approximately 100-fold [150]. Also, halogenation of peptides or modification of the N-terminal of peptides with acylation or alkylation is an efficient means to enhance lipophilicity and membrane permeability [151].

Pharmaceutical salts are used for lowering the dissolution rate. For certain pharmaceutical applications, such as inhalation products and parenteral depot systems, drug substances are converted into less soluble forms through salt formation with long-chain fatty acids like stearic acid and palmitic acid [40]. For instance, abuterol stearate dissolved at pH 7.4 much more slowly than its free base and other salt forms, exhibiting the potential application in an aerosol system for sustained drug release in lungs [152]. Relatively slow dissolving salts using long-chain fatty acids including lauric acid are also investigated for the slow-release oral dosage forms containing candidate drugs like an antihypertensive agent [153, 154].

2.4 STABILITY

2.4.1 Stability of Pharmaceuticals

With the advancement of medicinal chemistry, numerous tools have been developed for the discovery of better compounds. Stability plays a major role in selecting high-quality HITS and steers drug discovery programs [155]. Chemical and physical degradation of drug compounds may change their pharmacological activities, resulting in altered efficacy as well as toxicological consequences. Pharmaceuticals should be stable and maintain their efficacy and safety until the time of usage or until their expiration date. Therefore, understanding the factors that influence the stability of pharmaceuticals and identifying methods to maintain their stability are critical [156]. Subsequently, shelf-life estimation, which is the essential part of stability study, should be based on the clear understanding of the multifaceted aspects of stability and proper optimality criteria [157].

2.4.1.1 Stability Assessment Methods Establishment and validation of the stability indicating assay method (SIAM) is critical for the analysis of drugs and their metabolites. With the advent of International Council of Harmonization (ICH) guidelines, it is integral to establish the SIAM that explicitly requires conduct of forced decomposition studies under a variety of conditions, such as pH, light, oxidation, dry heat, etc., and separation of drug from degradation products. As multiple components need to be separated during the analysis of stability samples, SIAM is expected to be efficient for analysis of individual degradation products. Among various analysis methods, chromatographic methods have taken precedence over the conventional analysis methods. High-performance liquid chromatography (HPLC) has gained popularity in stability studies as a result of its high-resolution capacity, sensitivity, and specificity. Nonvolatile, thermally unstable, or polar/ionic compounds can also be analyzed using this technique. Therefore, most SIAMs have been established using HPLC [158].

However, there might be numerous situations in which the mass balance may not be feasible as a result of the following situations: 1) formation of multiple degradation products, involving complex reaction pathways and drug excipient interaction products; 2) incomplete detection as a result of loss of ultraviolet (UV) chromophore or lack of universal detection; 3) loss of drug/degradation products as volatiles; 4) diffusive losses into or through containers; 5) elution/resolution problems; 6) in appropriate or unknown response factors as a result of lack of standards; and 7) errors and variability in the drug content assay.

In these cases, other analytical methods that can reduce the duration of SIAM performance and seem to be suitable for routine determination of the loaded compounds in pharmaceutical formulation should be selected for economy and time-saving purposes.

2.4.1.2 Modes of Chemical Degradation Instability may result in influencing various aspects, such as loss of APIs, alteration in bioavailability, loss of content uniformity, decline of microbial status, loss of pharmaceutical elegance and patient acceptability, formation of toxic degradation products, loss of package integrity, reduction of label quality, and modification of any factor of functional relevance [159]. The most common degradation pathways involve hydrolysis, dehydration, oxidation, intramolecular cyclization, photolysis, and racemization [155]. Multiple degradation pathways could be observed in some cases, which is highly subjected to the molecular states. For example, hydrolysis was the predominant degradation pathway of parthenolide, a major ingredient in feverfew extract, in solution, whereas the degradation pathway in a solid state was much more complicated [160].

According to the ICH guidelines, the amount of impurities allowed for the product during storage is between 0.05% and 1%, which is dependent on its dosage forms [161]. Chemical stability is generally expressed with a rate constant, k, representing the speed of either product formation or drug degradation. The rate equations are derived for zero- and first-order reactions based on the formation of product (D_0 is initial drug concentration, P_t is the degradation product concentration at time t; P_0, the initial product concentration is assumed to be zero):

$$\text{zero order}: P_t = kt \tag{2.16}$$

$$\text{first order}: \ln\left(1 - \frac{P_t}{D_0}\right) = -kt \tag{2.17}$$

For zero-order reactions (i.e., zero-order formation of product), the reaction rate is independent of the drug concentration, while for first-order reactions, the rate linearly depends on drug concentration [162].

Hydrolysis Hydrolyis is one of the most common reactions observed with pharmaceuticals. Numerous drug substances contain an ester bond, which is primarily hydrolyzed through nucleophilic attack of hydroxide ion or water. Carboxylic acid esters like benzocaine [163], aspirin [164], and methylphenidate [165] undergo hydrolysis. Lactones or cyclic esters like pilocarpine [166] and warfarin [167] exhibit ring opening as a result of hydrolysis. Carbamic acid esters, such as chlorphenesin carbamate [168], undergo hydrolysis in strongly acidic solutions. Cyclodisone [169], a sulfonic acid ester, was reported to be hydrolyzed in the neutral-to-alkaline pH range.

Amide bonds are less susceptible to hydrolysis than ester bonds because the carbonyl carbon of the amide bond is less electrophilic. However, drugs like lincomycin [170] are known to produce an amine and an acid through the hydrolysis process of its amide bonds. ß-Lactam antibiotics, such as penicillins and cephalosporins, which are cyclic amides or lactams, undergo rapid hydrolysis-induced ring opening [171, 172]. Recent study also demonstrated that the length of polysaccharide chain, the N- or O-sulfo groups are critical to the hydrolysis of 4,4′-(imidocarbonyl)-bis(N,N-dimethylaniline) monohydrochloride in addition to pH and ionic strength [173]. The findings from hydrolysis studies provide new insights into the catalytic phenomenon of pharmaceutical compounds.

Oxidation Oxidation is a well-known chemical degradation pathway for certain pharmaceuticals. Oxygen, which participates in most oxidation reactions, is abundant in the environment to which pharmaceuticals are exposed during either processing or long-term storage. Oxidation mechanisms for drug substances depend on the chemical structure of the drug and on the presence of reactive oxygen species or other oxidants [174]. Ascorbic acid is an example for the oxidation process which is well characterized in the numerous literatures [175, 176].

Protein molecules, widely used as pharmaceuticals for treating diseases including various types of tumors resulting from their great potency and specificity, are intrinsically unstable in aqueous solutions because of the physical and chemical degradation pathways including oxidation [177]. Comparative oxidation studies were performed to elucidate how the kinetics of oxidation of methionine residues in a model protein granulocyte-colony stimulating factor (G-CSF) by hydrogen peroxide (H_2O_2) affects its reactivity [178]. An understanding of the underlying mechanisms of oxidation pathways can serve as a better means to stabilize protein pharmaceuticals, enhance their efficacies, and avoid any side effects.

Photodegradation Photodecomposition usually leads to a loss of potency of the product. Even a trace amount of photodecomposition products formed during storage and administration may produce adverse effects [179]. For light-sensitive materials, sunlight or artificial light could lead to photodegradation of the active principle as well as change the physicochemical properties of the product. For example, as the product becomes discolored or cloudy in appearance, a loss in viscosity or a change in dissolution rate or a precipitation is observed [180]. The drug molecule may be affected directly or indirectly by irradiation, depending on how the radiant energy is transferred to the substance. Direct photochemical reactions occur when the drug molecule itself absorbs energy. In an indirect reaction, the energy may be absorbed by nondrug molecules (e.g., excipient, impurity, and degradation product) in the formulation. The energy is shared by the active ingredient, which is subjected to subsequent degradation [181]. The presence of pH-modifying substrates can affect the stability. Various types of buffer salts exert diverse effects on the photodegradation process as demonstrated by drugs such as daunorubicin and mefloquinine [182, 183]. A mixture of colors or pigments can cause catalytic fading or induce degradation of other components in the formulations by radical formation [184].

2.4.1.3 Factors Affecting Stability

Temperature Temperature is one of the primary factors affecting drug stability. The rate constant/temperature relationship has been described by Arrhenius equation:

$$\ln k = \ln A - \frac{E_a}{RT} \tag{2.18}$$

where R is a gas constant, E_a is the activation energy, and A is the frequency factor, an indication of the entropy of activation for the process. Arrhenius kinetics is a linear dependence of the natural logarithm of the reaction rate, k, versus the reciprocal of the absolute temperature, T. A prerequisite for the application of Equation (2.18) is that the degradation mechanism remains the same in the temperature range of interest. The systems involved with phase transitions, pH shifts, uncontrolled relative humidity, and complex reaction mechanisms can be described by the following equation:

$$k = AT^n e^{-Ea/RT} \tag{2.19}$$

where n is determined using nonlinear fitting programs ($0 < n < 1$).

The Arrhenius equation has been successfully applied to the prediction of the stability of various pharmaceuticals including the degradation of vitamin A dosage forms [185] and the degradation of multivitamin tablets [186].

pH The degradation rates of drug molecules are generally affected by pH because most degradation pathways are catalyzed by hydronium and/or hydroxyl ions [187]. As the rate law for decomposition contains a term involved with the concentration of hydrogen ion or hydroxyl ion, the reaction is said to be subject to specific acid–base catalysis. The effects of hydrogen ion on the acid-catalyzed hydrolysis of esters can be expressed as:

$$\log k_{obs} = -\text{pH} + \log k_1 \tag{2.20}$$

where log k_{obs} is the observed first-order reaction rate constant and k_I is the acid-catalyzed reaction rate constant. Thus, a plot of k_{obs} against pH should be linear with a slope equal to -1. The hydroxyl ion-catalyzed decomposition of an ester can be expressed as:

$$\log k_{obs} = -\text{pH} + \log k_2 \tag{2.21}$$

where k_2 is the base-catalyzed reaction rate constant. Thus, a plot of k_{obs} against pH should be linear with a slope equal to $+1$. Hydrolysis of methyl-dl-o-phenyl-2-piperidylacetate follows specific acid–base-catalysis. An increase in pH from 1 to 3 results in a linear decrease in hydrolysis rate (for specific hydrogen ion catalysis), whereas a further increase in pH from 3 to 7 results in a linear increase in hydrolysis rate (for specific hydroxide ion catalysis) [165]. Catalysis may occur in the buffer solution as a result of the involvement of one or more species of the buffer component. The reaction is then said to be subject to general acid or general base catalysis. In general acid or general base catalysis, a plot of k_{obs} against pH would not yield the slope of ± 1.

Verification of a general acid or general base catalysis may be made by determining the rates of degradation of a drug in a series of buffers. These buffers are maintained at the same pH (i.e., the ratio of salt to acid is constant) but are prepared with an increasing concentration of buffer species. For example, it was found that thiamine is stable at pH 3.90, where principal buffer component is acetic acid [188]. However, at higher pH values, the rate increases proportionally with the concentration of acetate that is used as a general base catalyst. In addition to possible general acid–base catalysis where a buffer can act as either a proton donor or an acceptor (Brönsted acid or base), the buffer species can also act as a Lewis acid or base through nucleophilic or electrophilic mechanisms. It has been reported that various phosphate species present in different buffer media enhance the degradation rate of numerous drug substances, such as cefadroxil [189] and carbenicillin [190].

When a drug has at least two ionizable groups, bell-shaped pH-rate profiles can be seen with the pH of maximum degradation occurring at pH corresponding to the isoelectric point, $(pK_{a1} + pK_{a2})/2$ [191]. At this pH, the concentration of the intermediate species is maximum. As shown in Figure 2.7, the decarboxylation of 4-aminosalicylic acid, an amphoteric electrolyte having a carboxylic group and an amino group, shows a bell-shaped pH-rate profile with a maximum at the isoelectric point.

Stability in GI fluids is essential for orally administered drugs. Compounds that are unstable in the GI tract will have poor oral bioavailability and low systemic exposure. Simulated gastric fluid (SGF; pH 1.2 with pepsin) and simulated intestinal fluid (SIF; pH 6.8 with pancreatin) have been developed to mimic GI conditions and to assist the assessment of the BCS of drugs for immediate-release solid dosage forms. The FDA has recommended stability studies of 1 h in SGF and 3 h in SIF at 37°C. Significant degradation (>5%) of a drug could be indicative of potential instability in the GI tract [192].

2.4.2 Preformulation Considerations in Stability

Preformulation studies, such as choice of crystalline form of the drug and excipients to be used in the dosage form, are an

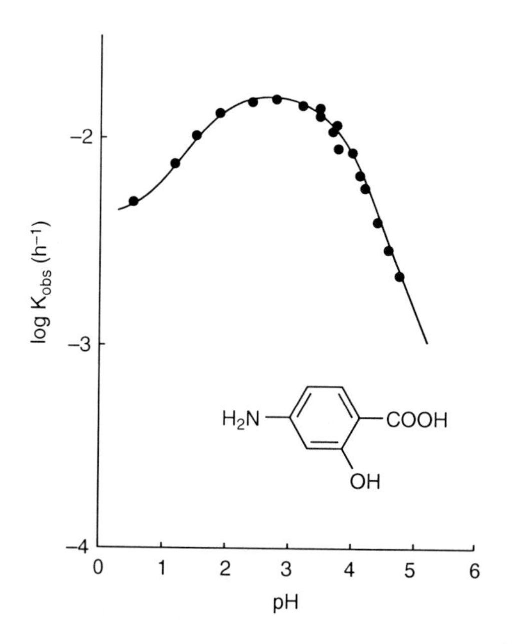

FIGURE 2.7 The pH-rate profile for decarboxylation of 4-aminosalicylic acid at 25°C [191].

integral step in developing stable pharmaceutical products [193]. Preformulation studies provide the initial data that help the formulator to select the best dosage-form strategy.

2.4.2.1 Analytical Tools Thermal analytical tools including differential scanning calorimetry (DSC), differential thermal analysis (DTA), and differential thermogravimetry (DTG) are indispensible in formulation screening because calorimetric changes and weight changes caused by chemical and physical degradation of pharmaceuticals can be readily detected [194]. For example, DSC was employed in the preformulation study of a poorly water-soluble drug substance, α-pentyl-3-(2-quinolinyl-methoxy) benzenemethanol [195]. The free base had an endothermic peak upon melting that was observed at the same position regardless of storage and measurement conditions. On the other hand, the anhydrous and monohydrate hydrochloride salt forms exhibited different behaviors depending on the measurement conditions. As the free base was found to be physically more stable than the hydrochloride salt, the free base of benzenemethanol was selected for formulation development. Thermal analysis often allows for detecting drug–excipient interactions; the interaction of ibuprofen with magnesium oxide was recognized based on changes in DSC thermograms [196].

2.4.2.2 Salt Formation Salt formation may be used to alter the physicochemical, biopharmaceutical, and formulation processing properties of a drug without modifying its fundamental structure. Both the physical and chemical stability of a drug may be altered by salt formation [197]. Studies have been carried out to investigate quantitative relationships between counterion characteristics and properties of the salt form [198]. The selection of an optimal salt form for the most stability requires consideration of counterion-related factors, such as crystal lattice energy, pH of the liquid microenvironment, and the possibility of counterion participation in the degradation of the drug [199]. Stronger crystal lattice forces generally result in superior solid-state stability, whereas the pH of the microenvironment is the function of counterion pK_a. Various studies have been conducted to identify the most stable salt form of drugs. For example, enalapril sodium was developed to resolve the instability status with enalapril maleate [200].

Similarly, in the case of lansoprazole, which exists as two optical isomers, a superior stability of amine salt of R-(+)-lansoprazole was reported [201]. Tris(hydroxymethyl) aminomethane salts of naproxen, ketorolac, 7′-oxo-7-thiomethoxy-xanthone-2-carboxylic acid, and 7-4(methylthibenzoyl)benzofuran-5-yl-acetic acid were significantly less hygroscopic as compared with either free acid or sodium salt forms [202]. Tosylate salt of the anti-neoplastic drug elsamitrucin resulted in stable parenteral solutions [203], whereas the stable amorphous calcium salt form of (6S)-N (5)-methyl-5,6,7,8-tetrahydrofolic acid was proposed for an injectable tumor agent [204].

2.4.2.3 Crystal Engineering APIs can exist in a variety of distinct solid forms, including polymorphs, solvates, hydrates, salts, co-crystals, and amorphous solids. Each form displays unique physicochemical properties that can profoundly influence the bioavailability, manufacturability/purification, stability, and other performance characteristics of the drug [205].

A good example of this crystalline complexity was observed with Sertraline hydrochloride, which has 27 purported crystal forms, including 17 polymorphs, 4 solvates, 6 hydrates, and the amorphous solid. As another example, the presence of crystals of nimodipine in a series of solid dispersions using polyethylene glycol as carrier was detected [206]. The crystal sizes were between one and several micrometers and seemed to increase with overall drug content. In samples examined 6 months after preparation, the crystals existed mainly as the racemic compound, whereas after 18 months of storage, mainly crystal conglomerates were present. Therefore, it is ideal for the pharmaceutical manufacturers to discover the most thermodynamically stable solid form to ensure the adequate bioavailability of the product over its shelf life.

Polymorphism It is generally accepted that the lowest energy crystalline polymorph should be identified and selected during the course of development of drug [54]. For some drugs, there is a potential danger that bioavailability could be reduced if the metastable form converts into the more stable form during the shelf life of the product. As an example, after storage at 40°C for 12 months, 60% of Phenylbutazone Form C was converted into Form A. Phenylbutazone Form C has a dissolution rate and solubility that are 1.5- and 1.2-fold, respectively, higher than those of Form A [207].

As another example, various marketed tablet formulations of glibenclamide exhibited different *in vitro* dissolution rates [208]. Glibenclamide displays polymorphs forms that differ by more than 10-fold in solubility assessed in simulated gastric fluid. The polymorphs (or pseudopolymorphs) of some drugs also exhibited different chemical stability. For example, the photodecay of form II of carbamazepine was 5.0- and 1.5-fold faster than forms I and III, respectively [209]. In addition to a change in the rate of decay, difference was also observed in the reactivity of different polymorphs of cinnamic acid derivatives [210]. In comparison with crystalline polymorphs, the amorphous form of a drug is generally expected to be less chemically stable as a result of various factors including the lack of a three-dimensional crystalline lattice, higher free volume, and greater molecular mobility.

Co-crystals Co-crystals incorporate acceptable guest molecules into a crystal lattice along with the APIs. The primary difference between solvates and co-crystals is the physical state of the isolated pure components: If one component is liquid at room temperature, the crystals are designated as solvates; if both components are solids at room temperature, the crystals are designated as co-crystals [211]. Pharmaceutical co-crystals have been used to resolve physical property issues in drug development, such as solubility, stability, and bioavailability, as opposed to changing the chemical composition of the API.

Co-crystal formation involves complexation of neutral molecules rather than of ions and, thus, has been potentially employed with all APIs, including acidic, basic, and nonionizable molecules [68]. Also, a large number of nontoxic "countermolecules" may be considered to be potential co-crystal candidates, possibly broadening the scope of pharmaceutical co-crystallization [212]. A pharmaceutical co-crystal formed between an inorganic acid and the phosphate salt of a drug candidate paved the way to develop a stable crystalline and bioavailable solid dosage form for pharmaceutical entities, where otherwise only unstable amorphous free form or salts could have been used [213]. It was also reported that Norfloxacin formed a stable salt with saccharin and that this salt formed a solid co-crystal with neutral saccharin, a norfloxacin saccharinate-saccharin dihydrate co-crystal [214].

2.4.3 Formulation Considerations in Stability

2.4.3.1 Excipients Pharmaceutical dosage forms are a complex system composed of not only drug substances but also various excipients, which may affect drug stability mediated through various mechanisms. The most obvious examples are those in which the excipients may participate directly in degradation as reactants. The impurities present in the excipient can promote oxidation reactions, such as nucleophilic/electrophilic addition with drugs [174]. Excipients may also exert catalyzing effects toward drug degradation. The nucleophilic catalysis effect of sugars and amines on the degradation of ester or amide drugs was previously reported [215, 216].

Other mechanisms involved are the effect of moisture present in excipients and the effect of pH changes caused by excipients. Excipients can affect drug stability by providing moisture. As a result of the high moisture content of polyvinyl pyrrolidone and urea, they significantly enhanced the hydrolysis rate of aspirin in solid dispersions [217]. Decreased drug stability for aspirin and ascorbic acid tablets in the presence of excipients having higher moisture was also reported [218]. The stability of trichlormethiazide (TCM) was nonhygroscopic and was not degraded even under humid conditions [219]. However, the stability of products of TCM decreased with increasing humidity in the presence of excipients, such as lactose, microcrystalline cellulose, corn starch, hydroxypropylcellulose (HPC), low-substituted HPC (L-HPC), calcium stearate, and light anhydrous silicic acid, suggesting that the adsorbed moisture by excipients causes TCM degradation.

Excipients having strong water-entrapping abilities tend to lower the drug degradation rates, as shown in colloidal silica [220]. The hydrolysis rate of nitrazepam in the presence of various excipients, such as microcrystalline cellulose, was measured based on the Brunauer Emmett Teller equation and found to be inversely proportional to the nitrogen-adsorption energy of the excipients [221]. The excipients having a higher adsorption energy lower water reactivity and thereby decrease the relative hydrolysis rates. Excipients that can form hydrates may enhance the drug degradation by releasing their water of crystallization during the grinding process. Lactose hydrate was reported to enhance degradation of 4-methoxyphenylaminoacetate hydrochloride upon grinding [222].

Excipients can also affect drug stability by altering microclimate pH. The surface acidity of excipients as a result of the presence of carboxylic acid groups has been reported to be a factor contributing to drug degradation. Lomustine exhibited faster degradation in poly (*d,l*-lactide) microspheres than in its pure crystalline state [223] because of the terminal carboxylic acid groups of poly (*d,l*-lactide) that changed the microenvironmental pH. Dye excipients may enhance oxidation and photodegradation of drugs by producing singlet oxygen that participates in the chain reactions, as is the case with phenyl butazone [224].

2.4.3.2 Stabilization Techniques As drug degradation is affected by various factors, numerous approaches for stability enhancement have been studied. To improve drug stability, structural modifications are conducted for the discovery of more stable analogs. The design of drugs with optimal potency and proper stability is a challenging task given the opposing requirements for absorption and metabolism [225]. An example of the analog development to enhance stabilization of parent drug is observed with clarithromycin, the methoxy substituted product of erythromycin [226]. Degradation of erythromycin at reactive hydroxyl groups via 6, 9-hemiketal breakdown under acidic pH conditions is prevented by substituting a methoxy group for the C-6 hydroxyl. Complex formation between drugs and excipients often increases the stability of drugs. The forces involved in complex formation include van der Waals forces, dipole–dipole interactions, hydrogen bonding, Coulomb forces, and hydrophobic interactions. Stabilization of ester drugs, such as tetracaine, in the presence of caffeine could be a result of the formation of a "stacking" complex [227]. Thus, attack on the ester bonds of tetracaine by water or hydroxide ion is hindered when tetracaine molecules are sandwiched between caffeine molecules. However, because of the non-inert nature of caffeine, clinical application of this approach may not be feasible.

To date, inert compounds like cyclodextrins (CDs) have received considerable interest. CDs are nonreducing cyclic oligosaccharides consisting of six (α-CD), seven (β-CD), or eight (γ-CD) dextrose units. CDs have a "doughnut" shape, with the interior portion of the molecule being relatively hydrophobic and the exterior being relatively hydrophilic [228]. As a result of their unique chemical structure, CDs are capable of forming "inclusion" complexes with various drug molecules to protect them from the chemical degradation.

Hydrolysis of bencyclane fumarate is inhibited by α-, β-, and γ-CD [229]. Other examples include stabilization of doxorubicin by γ-CD [187], thalidomide by 2-hydroxypropyl-β-CD [230], and tauromustine by 2-hydroxypropy-α-CD [231].

Entrapment of drug molecules in liposome, emulsions, or micelles affects their stability and, thus, can be used as a method for stabilizing pharmaceuticals. Anesthetics such as procaine are stabilized in liposome [232]. Physostigmine salicylate in a phospholipid emulsion was stabilized through interaction with phospholipids at the oil–water interface and through incorporation into the internal phase of the emulsion [233].

2.5 SUMMARY

The research related to advanced drug delivery requires improving quality and extending the length of life. However, because of the presence of the numerous attributes to drug profiles in the body that must be simultaneously optimized, it is a challenging task to find an efficient screening process. Solubility and stability issues are two major formulation huddles, and thus, understanding them is a prerequisite for identifying and discovering high-quality candidates. The poor biopharmaceutical properties often lead to extended timelines and a higher cost of manufacturing procedures. To avoid these problems and choose the best lead compounds from the biopharmaceutical perspective, physicochemical parameters, such as solubility and stability, need to be evaluated at the early stage. Approaches for the enhancement of solubility and stability have numerous advantages and disadvantages and should be carefully highlighted to achieve an efficacious product applicable to advanced drug delivery.

ASSESSMENT QUESTIONS

2.1. Define solubility.

2.2. Why is solubility enhancement necessary?

2.3. Explain with examples how crystal engineering can be used to improve the bioavailability of poorly soluble drugs?

2.4. Give the mechanism for miceller solubilization.

2.5. What are microemulsions?

2.6. How can the solid dispersion technique improve solubility?

2.7. What are the common modes of chemical degradation?

2.8. Explain how photodegradation affects a pharmaceutical product?

2.9. How can the stability of pharmaceuticals be predicted?

2.10. Justify how co-crystal formation may be a superior technique than salt formation to improve the stability of drug molecules.

2.11. Explain how excipients can affect drug stability in a dosage form.

2.12. Explain how cyclodextrins improve drug stability.

REFERENCES

1. Huang, L.F., Tong, W.Q. (2004). Impact of solid state properties on developability assessment of drug candidates. *Advanced Drug Delivery Reviews*, *56*, 321–334.
2. Lipinski, C.A. (2000). Drug-like properties and the causes of poor solubility and poor permeability. *Journal of Pharmacological and Toxicological Methods*, *44*, 235–249.

3. Panchangnula, R., Thomas, N.S. (2000). Biopharmaceutics and pharmacokinetics in drug research. *International Journal of Pharmaceutics*, *201*, 131–150.
4. Kola, I., Landis, J. (2004). Can the pharmaceutical industry reduce attrition rates? *Nature Reviews Drug Discovery*, *3*, 711–715.
5. Stegemann, S., et al. (2007). When poor solubility becomes an issue: From early stage to proof of concept. *European Journal of Pharmaceutical Sciences*, *31*, 249–261.
6. Garcia, A.G., et al. (2008). Pharmacokinetics in drug discovery. *Journal of Pharmaceutical Sciences*, *97*, 654–690.
7. Kaushal, A., Gupta, P., Bansal, A. (2004). Amorphous drug delivery systems: Molecular aspects, design, and performance. *Critical Reviews in Therapeutic Drug Carrier Systems*, *21*, 133–193.
8. Fernando, A., Alvarez-Núñez, Leonard, M.R. (2004). Formulation of a poorly soluble drug using hot melt extrusion: The amorphous state as an alternative. *American Pharmaceutical Rewiew*, *7*, 88–92.
9. Wolf, N.M., et al. (2006). Development of a high-throughput screen for soluble epoxide hydrolase inhibition. *Analytical Biochemistry*, *355*, 71–80.
10. Freiser, H., Nancollas, G.H. *Compendium of Analytical Nomenclature*, Blackwell Scientific, Oxford, Oxfordshire, and Boston, 1987, p. 279.
11. Sinko, P.J. *Martin's Physical Pharmacy and Pharmaceutical Sciences*, Lippincott Williams & Wilkins, Philadelphia, PA, 2006, p. 795.
12. Ain, S., Ain, Q., Parveen, S. (2009). An overview on various approaches used for solubilization of poorly soluble drugs. *The Pharma Research*, *2*, 84–104.
13. Gibbs, J.W. *The Collected Works of J. Williard Gibbs: Vol. I Thermodynamics*, Longmans Green, New York, London, and Toronto, 1928, p. 434.
14. Horter, D., Dressman, J.B. (2001). Influence of physicochemical properties on dissolution of drugs in the gastrointestinal tract. *Advanced Drug Delivery Reviews*, *46*, 75–87.
15. Horspool, K.R., Lipinski, C.A. (2003). Advancing new drug delivery concepts to gain the lead. *Drug Delivery Technology*, *3*, 34–44.
16. Faller, B., Ertl, P. (2007). Computational approaches to determine drug solubility. *Advanced Drug Delivery Reviews*, *59*, 533–545.
17. United States Pharmacopeia: The National Formulary. *The United States Pharmacopeia Convention*, Rockville MD, USP 31-NF 26, 2009.
18. F.D.A and U.S. Department of Health and Human Services. Guidance for industry-waiver of in vivo bioavailability and bioequivalence studies for immediate-release solid oral dosage forms based on biopharmaceutics classification system. Center for Drug Evaluation and Research, Washington, DC, 2000.
19. Amidon, G.L., et al. (1995). A theoretical basis for a biopharmaceutic drug classification: the correlation of in vitro drug product dissolution and in vivo bioavailability. *Pharmaceutical Research*, *12*, 413–420.
20. Wikipedia. *Biopharmaceutics Classification system*. 2011.
21. Lobenberg, R., Amidon, G.L. (2000). Modern bioavailability, bioequivalence and biopharmaceutics classification system. New scientific approaches to international regulatory standards. *European Journal of Pharmaceutics and Biopharmaceutics*, *50*, 3–12.
22. Lipinski, C.A., et al. (1997). Experimental and computational approaches to estimate solubility and permeability in drug discovery and development settings. *Advanced Drug Delivery Reviews*, *23*, 3–26.
23. Mehta, M. (2002). AAPS/FDA workshop on biopharmaceutics and classification system.
24. Albert, A. (1958). Chemical aspects of selective toxicity. *Nature*, *182*, 421–422.
25. Muller, C.E. (2009). Prodrug approaches for enhancing the bioavailability of drugs with low solubility. *Chemistry & Biodiversity*, *6*, 2071–2083.
26. Stella, V.J., Nti-Addae, K.W. (2007). Prodrug strategies to overcome poor water solubility. *Advanced Drug Delivery Reviews*, *59*, 677–694.
27. Testa, B. (2004). Prodrug research: Futile or fertile? *Biochemical Pharmacology*, *68*, 2097–2106.
28. Heimbach, T., et al. (2003). Absorption rate limit considerations for oral phosphate prodrugs. *Pharmaceutical Research*, *20*, 848–856.
29. Wire, M.B., Shelton, M.J., Studenberg, S. (2006). Fosamprenavir: clinical pharmacokinetics and drug interactions of the amprenavir prodrug. *Clinical Pharmacokinetics*, *45*, 137–168.
30. Varia, S.A., Stella, V.J. (1984). Phenytoin prodrugs VI: In vivo evaluation of a phosphate ester prodrug of phenytoin after parenteral administration to rats. *Journal of Pharmaceutical Sciences*, *73*, 1087–1090.
31. Song, X., et al. (2005). Amino acid ester prodrugs of the anticancer agent gemcitabine: Synthesis, bioconversion, metabolic bioevasion, and hPEPT1-mediated transport. *Molecular Pharmaceutics*, *2*, 157–167.
32. Dhanikula, A.B., Panchagnula, R. (2005). Preparation and characterization of water-soluble prodrug, liposomes and micelles of paclitaxel. *Current Drug Delivery*, *2*, 75–91.
33. Witterland, A.H.I., Koks, C.H.W., Beijnen, J.H. (1996). Etoposide phosphate, the water soluble prodrug of etoposide. *Pharmacy World & Science*, *18*, 163–170.
34. Bhadra, P.K., Morris, G.A., Barber, J. (2005). Design, synthesis, and evaluation of stable and taste-free erythromycin proprodrugs. *Journal of Medicinal Chemistry*, *48*, 3878–3884.
35. Bredberg, E., Lennernas, H., Paalzow, L. (1994). Pharmacokinetics of levodopa and carbidopa in rats following different routes of administration. *Pharmaceutical Research*, *11*, 549–555.
36. Wang, H.-P., et al. (1995). Synthesis and pharmacological activities of a novel tripeptide mimetic dopamine prodrug. *Bioorganic & Medicinal Chemistry Letters*, *5*, 2195–2198.
37. Steffansen, B., et al. (1999). Stability, metabolism and transport of-Asp (OBzl)-Ala—a model prodrug with affinity for

the oligopeptide transporter. *European Journal of Pharmaceutical Sciences, 8*, 67–73.

38. Smith, P.L., et al. (1993). Exploitation of the intestinal oligopeptide transporter to enhance drug absorption(review). *Drug Delivery, 1*, 103–111.
39. Corrigan, O.I., *Encyclopedia of Pharmaceutical Technology-Salt Forms: Pharmaceutical Aspects*, Informa Healthcare USA, New York, NY, 2006, pp. 3177–3186.
40. Serajuddin, A. (2007). Salt formation to improve drug solubility. *Advanced Drug Delivery Reviews, 59*, 603–616.
41. Stahl, P.H., Wermuth, C.G. *Handbook of Pharmaceutical Salts: Properties, Selection and Use*, Wiley-VCH, Weinheim, Germany, 2011, pp. 19–41.
42. Bhattachar, S.N., Deschenes, L.A., Wesley, J.A. (2006). Solubility: It's not just for physical chemists. *Drug Discovery Today, 11*, 1012–1018.
43. Rades, T., Muller-Goymann, C.C. (1997). Investigations on the micellisation behaviour of fenoprofen sodium. *International Journal of Pharmaceutics, 159*, 215–222.
44. Fini, A., et al. (1999). Formation of ion-pairs in aqueous solutions of diclofenac salts. *International Journal of Pharmaceutics, 187*, 163–173.
45. Nakashima, T., Fujiwara, T. (2001). Effects of surfactant counter-ions and added salts on reverse micelle formation of cetyltrimethylammonium surfactant studied by using (5, 10, 15, 20-tetraphenylporphyrinato) zinc (ii) as a probe. *Analytical Sciences, 17*, i1241–i1244.
46. Blagden, N., et al. (2007). Crystal engineering of active pharmaceutical ingredients to improve solubility and dissolution rates. *Advanced Drug Delivery Reviews, 59*, 617–630.
47. Nokhodchi, A., Bolourtchian, N., Dinarvand, R. (2003). Crystal modification of phenytoin using different solvents and crystallization conditions. *International Journal of Pharmaceutics, 250*, 85–97.
48. Chow, A.H.L., et al. (1995). Assessment of wettability and its relationship to the intrinsic dissolution rate of doped phenytoin crystals. *International Journal of Pharmaceutics, 126*, 21–28.
49. Saifee, M., et al. (2009). Drug polymorphism: A review. *International Journal of Health Research, 2*, 291–306.
50. Nangja, A., Desiraju, G.R. (1999). Pseudopolymorphism: Occurrences of hydrogen bonding organic solvents in molecular crystals. *Chemical Communications*, 605–606.
51. Pandit, J.K., et al. (1984). Effect of crystal form on the oral absorption of phenylbutazone. *International Journal of Pharmaceutics, 21*, 129–132.
52. Shah, J.C., Chen, J.R., Chow, D. (1999). Metastable polymorph of etoposide with higher dissolution rate. *Drug Development and Industrial Pharmacy, 25*, 63–67.
53. Bauer, J., et al. (2001). Ritonavir: An extraordinary example of conformational polymorphism. *Pharmaceutical Research, 18*, 859–866.
54. Singhal, D., Curatolo, W. (2004). Drug polymorphism and dosage form design: A practical perspective. *Advanced Drug Delivery Reviews, 56*, 335–347.
55. Zografi, G. (1988). States of water associated with solids. *Drug Development and Industrial Pharmacy, 14*, 1905–1926.
56. Martino, P.D., et al. (2001). Physical characterization of naproxen sodium hydrate and anhydrate forms. *European Journal of Pharmaceutical Sciences, 14*, 293–300.
57. Suleiman, M.S., Najib, N.M. (1989). Isolation and physicochemical characterization of solid forms of glibenclamide. *International Journal of Pharmaceutics, 50*, 103–109.
58. Salole, E.G., Al-Sarraj, F.A. (1985). Spironolactone crystal forms. *Drug Development and Industrial Pharmacy, 11*, 855–864.
59. Bansal, A. (2008). Amorphous pharmaceutical solids. *Sci. Topics*, http://www.scitopics.com/Amorphous_Pharmaceutical_Solids.html.
60. Yu, L. (2001). Amorphous pharmaceutical solids: Preparation, characterization and stabilization. *Advanced Drug Delivery Reviews, 48*, 27–42.
61. Hancock, B.C., Parks, M. (2000). What is the true solubility advantage for amorphous pharmaceuticals? *Pharmaceutical Research, 17*, 397–404.
62. Aakeroy, C.B. (1997). Crystal engineering: Strategies and architectures. *Acta Crystallographica Section B-Structural Science, 53*, 569–586.
63. Vishweshwar, P., et al. (2006). Pharmaceutical co-crystals. *Journal of Pharmaceutical Sciences, 95*, 499–516.
64. Dhumal, R.S., et al. (2009). Particle engineering using sonocrystallization: Salbutamol sulphate for pulmonary delivery. *International Journal of Pharmaceutics, 368*, 129–137.
65. Remenar, J., et al. (2003). Crystal engineering of novel cocrystals of a triazole drug with 1, 4-dicarboxylic acids. *Journal of the American Chemical Society, 125*, 8456–8457.
66. McNamara, D.P., et al. (2006). Use of a glutaric acid cocrystal to improve oral bioavailability of a low solubility API. *Pharmaceutical Research, 23*, 1888–1897.
67. Mirza, S., et al. (2008). Co-crystals: An emerging approach for enhancing properties of pharmaceutical solids. *DOSIS, 24*, 90–96.
68. Almarsson, O., Zaworotko, M.J. (2004). Crystal engineering of the composition of pharmaceutical phases. Do pharmaceutical co-crystals represent a new path to improved medicines? *Chemical Communications*, 1889–1896.
69. Born, P., et al. (2005). Research strategies for safety evaluation of nanomaterials, part V: Role of dissolution in biological fate and effects of nanoscale particles. *Toxicological Sciences, 90*, 23–32.
70. Florence, A.T., Attwood, D., *Physicochemical Principles of Pharmacy*, Chapman and Hall, London, 2006, pp. 139–176.
71. Tinke, A.P., et al. (2005). A new approach in the prediction of the dissolution behavior of suspended particles by means of their particle size distribution. *Journal of Pharmaceutical and Biomedical Analysis, 39*, 900–907.
72. Keck, C.M., Muller, R.H. (2006). Drug nanocrystals of poorly soluble drugs produced by high pressure homogenisation. *European Journal of Pharmaceutics and Biopharmaceutics, 62*, 3–16.

73. Jinno, J.J., et al. (2008). In vitro-in vivo correlation for wet-milled tablet of poorly water-soluble cilostazol. *Journal of Controlled Release*, *130*, 29–37.
74. Mijatovic, D.T., Eijkel, J.C., van den Berg, A. (2005). Technologies for nanofluidic systems: Top-down vs. bottom-up. A review. *Lab on a Chip*, *5*, 492–500.
75. Vogt, M., Kunath, K., Dressman, J.B. (2008). Dissolution enhancement of fenofibrate by micronization, cogrinding and spray-drying: Comparison with commercial preparations. *European Journal of Pharmaceutics and Biopharmaceutics*, *68*, 283–288.
76. Rasenack, N., Muller, B.W. (2002). Dissolution rate enhancement by in situ micronization of poorly water-soluble drugs. *Pharmaceutical Research*, *19*, 1894–1900.
77. Salvadori, B., et al. (2006). A novel method to prepare inorganic water-soluble nanocrystals. *Journal of Colloid and Interface Science*, *298*, 487–490.
78. Yasuji, T., Takeuchi, H., Kawashima, Y. (2008). Particle design of poorly water-soluble drug substances using supercritical fluid technologies. *Advanced Drug Delivery Reviews*, *60*, 388–398.
79. Millard, J.W., Alvarez-Nunez, F.A., Yalkowsky, S.H. (2002). Solubilization by cosolvents: Establishing useful constants for the log-linear model. *International Journal of Pharmaceutics*, *245*, 153–166.
80. Rubino, J.T., Yalkowsky, S.H. (1987). Cosolvency and cosolvent polarity. *Pharmaceutical Research*, *04*, 220–230.
81. Jain, P., Yalkowsky, S.H. (2007). Solubilization of poorly soluble compounds using 2-pyrrolidone. *International Journal of Pharmaceutics*, *342*, 1–5.
82. Strickley, R.G. (2004). Solubilizing excipients in oral and injectable formulations. *Pharmaceutical Research*, *21*, 201–230.
83. Patil, S., et al. (2011). Strategies for solubility enhancement of poorly soluble drugs. *International Journal of Pharmaceutical Sciences Review and Research*, *8*, 74–80.
84. Torchilin, V.P. (2001). Structure and design of polymeric surfactant-based drug delivery systems. *Journal of Controlled Release*, *73*, 137–172.
85. Park, S.H., Choi, H.K. (2006). The effects of surfactants on the dissolution profiles of poorly water-soluble acidic drugs. *International Journal of Pharmaceutics*, *321*, 35–41.
86. Zhang, H., et al. (2003). Commonly used surfactant, Tween 80, improves absorption of P-glycoprotein substrate, digoxin, in rats. *Archives of Pharmacal Research*, *26*, 768–772.
87. Malingre, M.M., et al. (2001). The co-solvent Cremophor EL limits absorption of orally administered paclitaxel in cancer patients. *British Journal of Cancer*, *85*, 1472–1477.
88. Grove, C., et al. (2003). Improving the aqueous solubility of triclosan by solubilization, complexation, and in situ salt formation. *Journal of Cosmetic Science*, *54*, 537–550.
89. Tanford, C. *The Hydrophobic Effect: Formation Of Micelles And Biological Membranes*, Wiley, New York, NY, 1980, p. 233.
90. Kadam, Y., Yerramilli, U., Bahadur, A. (2009). Solubilization of poorly water-soluble drug carbamezapine in Pluronic® micelles: Effect of molecular characteristics, temperature and added salt on the solubilizing capacity. *Colloids and Surfaces B: Biointerfaces*, *72*, 141–147.
91. Allen, C., Maysinger, D., Eisenberg, A. (1999). Nano-engineering block copolymer aggregates for drug delivery. *Colloids and Surfaces B: Biointerfaces*, *16*, 3–27.
92. Gadelle, F., Koros, W.J., Schechter, R.S. (1995). Solubilization of aromatic solutes in block copolymers. *Macromolecules*, *22*, 2403–2409.
93. Lin, S.Y., Kawashima, Y. (1987). Pluronic surfactants affecting diazepam solubility, compatibility, and adsorption from iv admixture solutions. *Journal of Parenteral Science and Technology*, *41*, 83–87.
94. Yokoyama, M., et al. (1998). Characterization of physical entrapment and chemical conjugation of adriamycin in polymeric micelles and their design for in vivo delivery to a solid tumor. *Journal of Controlled Release*, *50*, 79–92.
95. Batrakova, E.V., et al. (1996). Anthracycline antibiotics non-covalently incorporated into the block copolymer micelles: In vivo evaluation of anti-cancer activity. *British Journal of Cancer*, *74*, 1545–1552.
96. Rinaki, E., Valsami, G., Macheras, P. (2003). Quantitative biopharmaceutics classification system: The central role of dose/solubility ratio. *Pharmaceutical Research*, *20*, 1917–1925.
97. Rajewski, R.A., Stella, V.J. (1996). Pharmaceutical applications of cyclodextrins. 2. In vivo drug delivery. *Journal of Pharmaceutical Sciences*, *85*, 1142–1169.
98. Taraszewska, J., Migut, K., Kozbial, M. (2003). Complexation of flutamide by native and modified cyclodextrins. *Journal of Physical Organic Chemistry*, *16*, 121–126.
99. Charoenchaitrakool, M., Dehghani, F., Foster, N.R. (2002). Utilization of supercritical carbon dioxide for complex formation of ibuprofen and methyl-[beta]-cyclodextrin. *International Journal of Pharmaceutics*, *239*, 103–112.
100. Peeters, J., et al. (2002). Characterization of the interaction of 2-hydroxypropyl-beta-cyclodextrin with itraconazole at pH 2, 4, and 7. *Journal of Pharmaceutical Sciences*, *91*, 1414–1422.
101. Uekama, K., et al. (2001). Stabilizing and solubilizing effects of sulfobutyl ether beta-cyclodextrin on prostaglandin E1 analogue. *Pharmaceutical Research*, *18*, 1578–1585.
102. Usuda, M., et al. (2000). Interaction of antimalarial agent artemisinin with cyclodextrins. *Drug Development and Industrial Pharmacy*, *26*, 613–619.
103. Buhleier, E., Wehner, W., Vogtle, F. (1978). Cascade and nonskid-chain-like synthesis of molecular cavity topologies. *Synthesis*, *1978*, 155–158.
104. D'Emanuele, A., Attwood, D. (2005). Dendrimer-drug interactions. *Advanced Drug Delivery Reviews*, *57*, 2147–2162.
105. Chauhan, A.S., et al. (2004). Solubility enhancement of indomethacin with poly (amidoamine) dendrimers and targeting to inflammatory regions of arthritic rats. *Journal of Drug Targeting*, *12*, 575–583.

106. Neerman, M.F., et al. (2004). Reduction of drug toxicity using dendrimers based on melamine. *Molecular Pharmaceutics*, *1*, 390–393.
107. Agarwal, A., et al. (2008). Tumour and dendrimers: A review on drug delivery aspects. *Journal of Pharmacy and Pharmacology*, *60*, 671–688.
108. Rasool, A.A., Hussain, A.A., Dittert, L.W. (1991). Solubility enhancement of some waterâ insoluble drugs in the presence of nicotinamide and related compounds. *Journal of Pharmaceutical Sciences*, *80*, 387–393.
109. Agrawal, S., et al. (2004). Hydrotropic solubilization of nimesulide for parenteral administration. *International Journal of Pharmaceutics*, *274*, 149.
110. Sanghvi, R., Evans, D., Yalkowsky, S.H. (2007). Stacking complexation by nicotinamide: A useful way of enhancing drug solubility. *International Journal of Pharmaceutics*, *336*, 35–41.
111. Uch, A.S., Hesse, U., Dressman, J.B. (1999). Use of 1-methyl-pyrrolidone as a solubilizing agent for determining the uptake of poorly soluble drugs. *Pharmaceutical Research*, *16*, 968–971.
112. Sanghvi, R., et al. (2008). Solubility improvement of drugs using N-methyl pyrrolidone. *AAPS PharmSciTech*, *9*, 366–376.
113. Lim, J.K., Thompson, H.O., Piantadosi, C. (1964). Solubilization and stability of phenobarbital by some aminoalcohols. *Journal of Pharmaceutical Sciences*, *53*, 1161–1165.
114. Guiseley, K.B., Stanley, N.F., Whitehouse, P.A. *Handbook of Water-Soluble Gums And Resins: Carrageenan*, McGraw-Hill, New York, NY, 1980, p. 700.
115. Dai, W.G., Dong, L.C., Song, Y.Q. (2007). Nanosizing of a drug/carrageenan complex to increase solubility and dissolution rate. *International Journal of Pharmaceutics*, *342*, 201–207.
116. Strickley, R.G., *Oral Lipid-Based Formulations Enhancing the Bioavailability of Poorly Water-Soluble Drugs*, Informa Healthcare, New York, NY, 2007, pp. 1–32.
117. Hauss, D.J. (2007). Oral lipid-based formulations. *Advanced Drug Delivery Reviews*, *59*, 667–676.
118. MacGregor, K.J., et al. (1997). Influence of lipolysis on drug absorption from the gastro-intestinal tract. *Advanced Drug Delivery Reviews*, *25*, 33–46.
119. Reiss, H. (1975). Entropy-induced dispersion of bulk liquids. *Journal of Colloid and Interface Science*, *53*, 61–70.
120. Eccleston, G.M. *Encyclopedia of Pharmaceutical Technology: Microemulsions*, Marcel Dekker, New York, NY, 1992, pp. 31–71.
121. Craig, D.Q.M., et al. (1993). An investigation into the physico-chemical properties of self-emulsifying systems using low frequency dielectric spectroscopy, surface tension measurements and particle size analysis. *International Journal of Pharmaceutics*, *96*, 147–155.
122. Shah, N.H., et al. (1994). Self-emulsifying drug delivery systems (SEDDS) with polyglycolyzed glycerides for improving in vitro dissolution and oral absorption of lipophilic drugs. *International Journal of Pharmaceutics*, *106*, 15–23.
123. Wakerly, M.G., et al. (1986). Self-emulsification of vegetable oil-nonionic surfactant mixtures: A proposed mechanism of action. *ACS Symposium Series*, *311*, 242–255.
124. Charman, S.A., et al. (1992). Self-emulsifying drug delivery systems: formulation and biopharmaceutic evaluation of an investigational lipophilic compound. *Pharmaceutical Research*, *09*, 87–93.
125. Hong, J.Y., et al. (2006). A new self-emulsifying formulation of itraconazole with improved dissolution and oral absorption. *Journal of Controlled Release*, *110*, 332–338.
126. Kang, B.K., et al. (2004). Development of self-microemulsifying drug delivery systems (SMEDDS) for oral bioavailability enhancement of simvastatin in beagle dogs. *International Journal of Pharmaceutics*, *274*, 65–73.
127. Leunar, C., Dressman, J. (2000). Improving drug solubility for oral delivery using solid dispersions. *European Journal of Pharmaceutics and Biopharmaceutics*, *50*, 47–60.
128. Vasconcelos, T., Sarmento, B., Costa, P. (2007). Solid dispersions as strategy to improve oral bioavailability of poor water soluble drugs. *Drug Discovery Today*, *12*, 1068–1075.
129. Chiou, W.L., Riegelman, S. (1971). Pharmaceutical applications of solid dispersion systems. *Journal of Pharmaceutical Sciences*, *60*, 1281–1302.
130. Serajuddin, A. (1999). Solid dispersion of poorly water soluble drugs: early promises, subsequent problems, and recent breakthroughs. *Journal of Pharmaceutical Sciences*, *88*, 1058–1066.
131. Dhirendra, K., Lewis, S., Udupa, N., and Atin, K. (2009). Solid dispersions: A review. *Pakistan Journal of Pharmaceutical Sciences*, *22*, 234–246.
132. Nepal, P.R., Han, H.K., Choi, H.K. (2010). Enhancement of solubility and dissolution of Coenzyme Q10 using solid dispersion formulation. *International Journal of Pharmaceutics*, *383*, 147–153.
133. Zajc, N., et al. (2005). Physical properties and dissolution behaviour of nifedipine/mannitol solid dispersions prepared by hot melt method. *International Journal of Pharmaceutics*, *291*, 51–58.
134. Verreck, G., et al. (2003). Characterization of solid dispersions of itraconazole and hydroxypropylmethylcellulose prepared by melt extrusion—Part I. *International Journal of Pharmaceutics*, *251*, 165–174.
135. DiNunzio, J.C., et al. (2010). Fusion production of solid dispersions containing a heat-sensitive active ingredient by hot melt extrusion and Kinetisol® dispersing. *European Journal of Pharmaceutics and Biopharmaceutics*, *74*, 340–351.
136. Okonogi, S., Puttipipakhachorn, S. (2006). Dissolution improvement of high drug-loaded solid dispersion. *AAPS PharmSciTech*, *7*, E148–E153.
137. Takeuchi, H., et al. (2005). Solid dispersion particles of amorphous indomethacin with fine porous silica particles by using spray-drying method. *International Journal of Pharmaceutics*, *293*, 155–164.

138. Kim, E.J., et al. (2006). Preparation of a solid dispersion of felodipine using a solvent wetting method. *European Journal of Pharmaceutics and Biopharmaceutics*, *64*, 200–205.
139. Sethia, S., Squillante, E. (2004). Solid dispersion of carbamazepine in PVP K30 by conventional solvent evaporation and supercritical methods. *International Journal of Pharmaceutics*, *272*, 1–10.
140. Won, D.H., et al. (2005). Improved physicochemical characteristics of felodipine solid dispersion particles by supercritical anti-solvent precipitation process. *International Journal of Pharmaceutics*, *301*, 199–208.
141. Yonemochi, E., et al. (1997). Evaluation of amorphous ursodeoxycholic acid by thermal methods. *Pharmaceutical Research*, *14*, 798–803.
142. Yonemochi, E., et al. (1999). Physicochemical properties of amorphous clarithromycin obtained by grinding and spray drying. *European Journal of Pharmaceutical Sciences*, *7*, 331–338.
143. Vasconcelos, T., Costa, P. (2007). Development of a rapid dissolving ibuprofen solid dispersion. *Pharmaceutical Sciences World Conference*, DD-W-103.
144. Ghaderi, R., Artursson, P., Carifors, J. (1999). Preparation of biodegradable microparticles using solution-enhanced dispersion by supercritical fluids (SEDS). *Pharmaceutical Research*, *16*, 676–681.
145. Karanth, H., Shenoy, V.S., Murthy, R.R. (2006). Industrially feasible alternative approaches in the manufacture of solid dispersions: A technical report. *AAPS PharmSciTech*, *7*, E31–E38.
146. Yan, L., Müller, C.E. (2004). Preparation, properties, reactions, and adenosine receptor affinities of sulfophenylxanthine nitrophenyl esters: Toward the development of sulfonic acid prodrugs with peroral bioavailability. *Journal of Medicinal Chemistry*, *47*, 1031–1043.
147. Chikhale, E.G., et al. (1994). Hydrogen bonding potential as a determinant of the in vitro and in situ bloodâ "brain barrier permeability of peptides. *Pharmaceutical Research*, *11*, 412–419.
148. Habgood, M.D., Begley, D.J., Abott, N.J. (2000). Determinants of passive drug entry into the central nervous system. *Cellular and Molecular Neurobiology*, *20*, 231–253.
149. Fischer, E., et al. (1972). Phenethylamine content of human urine and rat brain, its alterations in pathological conditions and after drug administration. *Experientia*, *28*, 307–308.
150. Oldendorf, W.H., et al. (1972). Blood-brain barrier: Penetration of morphine, codeine, heroin, and methadone after carotid injection. *Science*, *178*, 984–986.
151. Witt, K.A., et al. (2001). Peptide drug modifications to enhance bioavailability and blood-brain barrier permeability. *Peptides*, *22*, 2329–2343.
152. Jashnani, R.N., Dalby, R.N., Byron, P.R. (1993). Preparation, characterization, and dissolution kinetics of two novel albuterol salts. *Journal of Pharmaceutical Sciences*, *82*, 613–616.
153. Benjamin, E.J., L.H., L. (1985). Preparation and in vitro evaluation of salts of an antihypertensive agent to obtain slow release. *Drug Development and Industrial Pharmacy*, *11*, 771–790.
154. Smith, S.W., Anderson, B.D. (1993). Salt and mesophase formation in aqueous suspensions of lauric acid. *Pharmaceutical Research*, *10*, 1533–1543.
155. Di, L., Kerns, E.H. (2009). Stability challenges in drug discovery. *Chemistry & Biodiversity*, *6*, 1875–1886.
156. Yoshioka, S., Stella, V.J. *Stability of Drugs and Dosage Forms*, Kluwer Academic/Plenum, New York, NY, 2000, p. 268.
157. Hedayat, A.S., Yan, X., Lin, L. (2006). Optimal designs in stability studies. *Journal of Biopharmaceutical Statistics*, *16*, 35–59.
158. Bakshi, M. (2002). Development of validated stability-indicating assay methods—critical review. *Journal of Pharmaceutical and Biomedical Analysis*, *28*, 1011–1040.
159. Carstensen, J.T., Rhodes, C.T. *Drug Stabilty, Principles and Practices*, Marcel Dekker, NewYork, NY, 2000, p. 520.
160. Jin, P., Madieh, S., Augsburger, L. (2007). The solution and solid state stability and excipient compatibility of parthenolide in feverfew. *AAPS PharmSciTech*, *8*, 200–205.
161. I.C.H (2003). Impurities in new drug products: Revised guideline on Q3B(R). *International Conference of Harmonization*, *68*, 64628–64629.
162. Waterman, K.C., Adami, R.C. (2005). Accelerated aging: Prediction of chemical stability of pharmaceuticals. *International Journal of Pharmaceutics*, *293*, 101–125.
163. Marcus, A.D., Baron, S. (2006). A comparison of the kinetics of the acid catalyzed hydrolyses of procainamide, procaine, and benzocaine. *Journal of the American Pharmaceutical Association*, *48*, 85–90.
164. Edwards, L.J. (1950). The hydrolysis of aspirin. A determination of the thermodynamic dissociation constant and a study of the reaction kinetics by ultra-violet spectrophotometry. *Transactions of the Faraday Society*, *46*, 723–735.
165. Siegel, S., Lachman, L., Malspeis, L. (1959). A kinetic study of the hydrolysis of methyl DL-alpha-phenyl-2-piperidylacetate. *Journal of the American Pharmaceutical Association*, *48*, 431–439.
166. Chung, P.T., Chin, Lach, J.L. (1970). Kinetics of the hydrolysis of pilocarpine in aqueous solution. *Journal of Pharmaceutical Sciences*, *59*, 1300–1306.
167. Garrett, E.R., Lippold, B.C., Mielck, J.B. (1971). Kinetics and mechanisms of lactonization of coumarinic acids and hydrolysis of coumarins I. *Journal of Pharmaceutical Sciences*, *60*, 396–405.
168. Hara, M., Hayashi, H., Yoshida, T. (1986). Kinetics and mechanism of degradation of chlorphenesin carbamate in strongly acidic aqueous solutions. *Chemical & Pharmaceutical Bulletin*, *34*, 3481–3484.
169. Umprayn, K., Waugh, W., Stella, V.J. (1990). Mechanism of degradation of the investigational cytotoxic agent, cyclodisone (NSC-348948). *International Journal of Pharmaceutics*, *66*, 253–262.

170. Forist, A.A., Brown, L.W., Royer, M.E. (1965). Acid stability of lincomycin. *Journal of Pharmaceutical Sciences, 54*, 476–477.
171. Blaha, J.M., et al. (1976). Kinetic analysis of penicillin degradation in acidic media. *Journal of Pharmaceutical Sciences, 65*, 1165–1170.
172. Yamana, T., Tsuji, A. (1976). Comparative stability of cephalosporins in aqueous solution: Kinetics and mechanisms of degradation. *Journal of Pharmaceutical Sciences, 65*, 1563–1574.
173. He, Y., Li, J., Chen, Y. (2011). Catalytic effects of different heparin analogs on the hydrolysis of auramine O. *Journal of Biopharmaceutical Science. Polymer Edition, 22*, 253–261.
174. Waterman, K.C., et al. (2002). Stabilization of pharmaceuticals to oxidative degradation. *Pharmaceutical Development and Technology, 7*, 1–32.
175. Dekker, A.O., Dickinson, R.G. (1940). Oxidation of ascorbic acid by oxygen with cupric ion as catalyst. *Journal of the American Chemical Society, 62*, 2165–2171.
176. Blaug, S.M., Hajrahvala, B. (1972). Kinetics of aerobic oxidation of ascorbic acid. *Journal of Pharmaceutical Sciences, 61*, 556–562.
177. Manning, M.C., et al. (2010). Stability of protein pharmaceuticals: an update. *Pharmaceutical Research, 27*, 544–575.
178. Pan, B. (2009). Mechanistic studies on chemical instabilities of recombinant proteins. *Massachusetts Institute of Technology.*
179. De Vries, H., et al. (1984). Photochemical decomposition of chloramphenicol in a 0.25% eyedrop and in a therapeutic intraocular concentration. *International Journal of Pharmaceutics, 20*, 265–271.
180. Tonnesen, H.H. (2001). Formulation and stability testing of photolabile drugs. *International Journal of Pharmaceutics, 225*, 1–14.
181. Thoma, K. *Photodecomposition and Stabilization of Compounds in Dosage Forms*, Taylor & Francis, London, 1996, pp. 111–140.
182. Islam, M.S., Asker, A.F. (1995). Photoprotection of daunorubicin hydrochloride with sodium sulfite. *Journal of Parenteral Science and Technology, 49*, 122–126.
183. Tønnesen, H.H. (1999). Photoreactivity of biologically active compounds. XV. Photochemical behaviour of mefloquine in aqueous solution. *Pharmazie, 54*, 590–594.
184. Konaka, R., et al. (1999). Irradiation of titanium dioxide generates both singlet oxygen and superoxide anion. *Free Radical Biology and Medicine, 27*, 294–300.
185. Carstensen, J.T. (1964). Stability patterns of vitamin A in various pharmaceutical dosage forms. *Journal of Pharmaceutical Sciences, 53*, 839–840.
186. Tardif, R. (1965). Reliability of accelerated storage tests to predict stability of vitamins (A, B1, C) in tablets. *Journal of Pharmaceutical Sciences, 54*, 281–284.
187. Loftsson, T., Brewster, M.E. (1996). Pharmaceutical applications of cyclodextrins. 1. Drug solubilization and stabilization. *Journal of Pharmaceutical Sciences, 85*, 1017–1025.
188. Windheuser, J.J., Higuchi, T. (1962). Kinetics of thiamine hydrolysis. *Journal of Pharmaceutical Sciences, 51*, 354–364.
189. Tsuji, A., et al. (1981). Degradation kinetics and mechanism of aminocephalosporins in aqueous solution: Cefadroxil. *Journal of Pharmaceutical Sciences, 70*, 1120–1128.
190. Zia, H., Tcharan, M., Zargarbashi, R. (1974). Kinetics of carbenicillin degradation in aqueous solutions. *Canadian Journal of Pharmaceutical Sciences, 9*, 112–117.
191. Jivani, S.G., Stella, V.J. (1985). Mechanism of decarboxylation of p-aminosalicylic acid. *Journal of Pharmaceutical Sciences, 74*, 1274–1282.
192. Asafu-Adjaye, E.B., et al. (2007). Validation and application of a stability-indicating HPLC method for the in vitro determination of gastric and intestinal stability of venlafaxine. *Journal of Pharmaceutical and Biomedical Analysis, 43*, 1854–1859.
193. Bharate, S.S., Bharate, S.B., Bajaj, A.N. (2010). Interactions and incompatibilities of pharmaceutical excipients with active pharmaceutical ingredients: A comprehensive review. *Journal of Excipients and Food Chemicals, 1*, 3–36.
194. El-Ries, M.A., et al. (2011). Thermal characterization of leflunomide. *Insight Pharmaceutical Sciences, 1*, 18–23.
195. Serajuddin, A.T., et al. (1986). Preformulation study of a poorly water-soluble drug, α-pentyl-3-(2-quinolinylmethoxy) benzenemethanol: Selection of the base for dosage form design. *Journal of Pharmaceutical Sciences, 75*, 492–496.
196. Kararli, T.T., et al. (1989). Solid-state interaction of magnesium oxide and ibuprofen to form a salt. *Pharmaceutical Research, 06*, 804–808.
197. Berge, S.M., Bighley, L.D., Monkhouse, D.C. (1977). Pharmaceutical salts. *Journal of Pharmaceutical Sciences, 66*, 1–19.
198. Anderson, B.D., and Conrady, R.A. (1985). Predictive relationships in the water solubility of salts of a nonsteroidal anti-inflammatory drug. *Journal of Pharmaceutical Sciences, 74*, 815.
199. Anderson, B.D., Flora, K.P. (1996). Preparation of water-soluble compounds through salt formation. *The Practice of Medicinal Chemistry*, 739–754.
200. Charles, S.B. (1999). Stable solid formulation of enalapril salt and process for preparation thereof. U.S. Patent 5690962.
201. Bhanu, M.N., Naik, S., Bodkhe, A. (2009). Stable R(+)-lansoprazole amine salt and a process of preparing the same. WO Patent 2010079504 A2.
202. Gu, L., Strickley, R.G. (1987). Preformulation salt selection. Physical property comparisons of the tris (hydroxymethyl) aminomethane (THAM) salts of four analgesic/antiinflammatory agents with the sodium salts and the free acids. *Pharmaceutical Research, 04*, 255–257.
203. Gore, A., et al. (2007). Stable elsamitrucin salts suitable for pharmaceutical formulations. U.S. Patent 20070293445.
204. Manzotti, R.I.P., Moreno, M. (2010). A process for the preparation of the stable, amorphous calcium salt of (6S)-N(5)-methyl-5,6,7,8-tetrahydrofolic acid. U.S. Patent20100168117.

205. Byrn, S.R., Pfeiffer, R.R., Stowell, J.G. *Solid State Chemistry of Drugs*, SSCI, West Lafayette, IN, 1999, p. 574.

206. Docoslis A, et al. (2007). Characterization of the distribution, polymorphism, and stability of nimodipine in its solid dispersions in polyethylene glycol by micro-Raman spectroscopy and powder X-ray diffraction. *The AAPS Journal*, *9*, E361–E370.

207. Tuladhar, M.D., Carless, J.E., Summers, M.P. (1983). Thermal behaviour and dissolution properties of phenylbutazone polymorphs. *Journal of Pharmacy and Pharmacology*, *35*, 208–214.

208. Blume, H., Ali, S.L., Siewert, M. (1993). Pharmaceutical quality of glibenclamide products a multinational postmarket comparative study. *Drug Development and Industrial Pharmacy*, *19*, 2713–2741.

209. Matsuda, Y., et al. (1993). pharmaceutical evaluation of carbamazepine modifications: comparative study for photostability of carbamazepine polymorphs by using Fourier-transformed reflection absorption infrared spectroscopy and colorimetric measurement. *Journal of Pharmacy and Pharmacology*, *46*, 162–167.

210. Cohen, M.D., Green, B.S. (1973). Organic chemistry in the solid state. *Chemistry in Britain*, *9*, 490–497.

211. Morissette, S., et al. (2004). High-throughput crystallization: Polymorphs, salts, co-crystals and solvates of pharmaceutical solids. *Advanced Drug Delivery Reviews*, *56*, 275–300.

212. Trask, A.V., Motherwell, W.D.S., and Jones, W. (2006). Physical stability enhancement of theophylline via cocrystallization. *International Journal of Pharmaceutics*, *320*, 114–123.

213. Chen, A.M., et al. (2007). Development of a pharmaceutical cocrystal of a monophosphate salt with phosphoric acid. *Chemical Communications*, 419–421.

214. Velaga, S.P., Basavoju, S., Bostrom, D. (2008). Norfloxacin saccharinate-saccharin dihydrate cocrystal—A new pharmaceutical cocrystal with an organic counter ion. *Journal of Molecular Structure*, *889*, 150–153.

215. Killion, R.B., Stella, V.J. (1990). The nucleophilicity of dextrose, sucrose, sorbitol, and mannitol with p-nitrophenyl esters in aqueous solution. *International Journal of Pharmaceutics*, *66*, 149–155.

216. Fujita, T., Harima, Y., Koshiro, A. (1983). Kinetic study of the degradation of cefotiam dihydrochloride in aqueous solution and of the reaction with aminoglycosides. *Chemical & Pharmaceutical Bulletin*, *31*, 2103–2109.

217. El-Banna, H.M., Daabis, N.A., El-Fattah, S.A. (1978). Aspirin stability in solid dispersion binary systems. *Journal of Pharmaceutical Sciences*, *67*, 1631–1633.

218. Lee, S.H., Dekay, G., Banker, G.S. (1965). Effect of water vapor pressure on moisture sorption and the stability of aspirin and ascorbic acid in tablet matrices. *Journal of Pharmaceutical Sciences*, *54*, 1153–1158.

219. Teraoka, R., et al. (2009). Effect of pharmaceutical excipients on the stability of trichlormethiazide tablets under humid conditions. *Chemical & Pharmaceutical Bulletin*, *57*, 1343–1347.

220. Gore, A.Y., Banker, G.S. (1979). Surface chemistry of colloidal silica and a possible application to stabilize aspirin in solid matrixes. *Journal of Pharmaceutical Sciences*, *68*, 197–202.

221. Pemer, P.R., Kesselring, U.W. (1983). Quantitative assessment of the effect of some excipients on nitrazepam stability in binary powder mixtures. *Journal of Pharmaceutical Sciences*, *72*, 1072–1074.

222. Irwin, W.J., Iqbal, M. (1991). Solid-state stability: The effect of grinding solvated excipients. *International Journal of Pharmaceutics*, *75*, 211–218.

223. Benita, S., et al. (1984). Characterization of drug-loaded poly (d,l-lactide) microspheres. *Journal of Pharmaceutical Sciences*, *73*, 1721.

224. Baugh, R., Calvert, R.T., Fell, J.T. (1977). Stability of phenylbutazone in presence of pharmaceutical colors. *Journal of Pharmaceutical Sciences*, *66*, 733.

225. Nassar, A.F. *Structural Modifications of Drug Candidates: How Useful Are They in Improving Metabolic Stability of New Drugs? Part I: Enhancing Metabolic Stability Pharmaceutical Sciences Encyclopedia: Drug Discovery, Development, and Manufacturing*, Wiley, New York, NY, 2010, pp. 253–268.

226. Nakagawa, Y., et al. (1992). Physicochemical properties and stability in the acidic solution of a new macrolide antibiotic, clarithromycin, in comparison with erythromycin. *Chemical & Pharmaceutical Bulletin*, *40*, 725–728.

227. Lachman, L., Higuchi, T. (1957). Inhibition of hydrolysis of esters in solution by formation of complexes III. Stabilization of tetracaine with caffeine. *Journal of the American Pharmaceutical Association*, *46*, 32–36.

228. Connors, K.A. (1997). The stability of cyclodextrin complexes in solution. *Chemical Reviews*, *97*, 1325–1357.

229. Fujioka, K., et al. (1983). Biopharmaceutical study of inclusion complexes. I. Pharmaceutical advantages of cyclodextrin complexes of bencyclane fumarate. *Chemical and Pharmaceutical Bulletin*, 2416–2423.

230. Krenn, M., et al. (1992). Improvements in solubility and stability of thalidomide upon complexation with hydroxypropyl- β-cyclodextrin. *Journal of Pharmaceutical Sciences*, *81*, 685–689.

231. Loftsson, T., Baldvinsdttir, J. (1992). Degradation of tauromustine (TCNU) in aqueous solutions. *Acta Pharmaceutica*, *4*, 129–132.

232. Habib, M.J., Rogers, J.A. (1987). Stabilization of local anesthetics in liposomes. *Drug Development and Industrial Pharmacy*, *13*, 1947–1971.

233. Pathak, Y.V., Rubinstein, A., Benita, S. (1990). Enhanced stability of physostigmine salicylate in submicron o/w emulsion. *International Journal of Pharmaceutics*, *65*, 169.

3

THE ROLE OF TRANSPORTERS AND THE EFFLUX SYSTEM IN DRUG DELIVERY

VARUN KHURANA, DHANANJAY PAL, MUKUL MINOCHA, AND ASHIM K. MITRA

3.1 CHAPTER OBJECTIVES

- To outline the fundamental concepts of drug transporters and their current status in absorption, distribution, metabolism, and elimination (ADME).
- To provide an idea regarding the role of influx and efflux transporters and substrate and inhibitor selectivity in drug delivery.
- To overcome challenges of drug efflux in drug delivery by the application of selective inhibitors/modulators.
- To evade drug efflux by employing prodrug concept and nanotechnology.
- To examine the potential application of *in vitro* models for transporter-mediated drug delivery.
- To provide recent advances in drug transporter research.

3.2 INTRODUCTION

Transporters are membrane proteins and an integral part of the cell membrane. These proteins are broadly involved in selective absorption of endogenous substances (substances such as anions and cations, vitamins, sugars, nucleosides, amino acids, peptides, etc.) and in elimination of toxic substances. In fact, transporters direct the influx of essential nutrients and ions and the efflux of cellular metabolites and xenobiotics. These proteins also play a pivotal role in drug absorption, distribution, elimination, and drug–drug interactions. Although the occurrence of multidrug resistance of bacteria was noticed more than 50 years ago, the discovery of P-glycoprotein (P-gp), a major factor for efflux of xenobiotics out of cell took 20 years. It is clear now that apart from the intestinal absorption barrier and the blood-brain barrier, different tumor cells express the P-gp, which plays a major role in drug resistance in chemotherapy. In fact, these transporters take a considerable role in the process of drug absorption, distribution, metabolism, and elimination (ADME) of drugs. Almost 2000 genes have been identified for transporters or transporter-related proteins [1]. Approximately 400 membrane transporters, in two superfamilies, have been identified and characterized for specific tissue localization, and several of these transporters have been cloned [2]. From a pharmacological point of view, two major superfamilies, ABC (adenosine triiphosphate (ATP) binding cassette) and SLC (solute carrier) transporters, are focused. The ABCs, as active transporters, operate by ATP hydrolysis to expel their substrate out of cells across a lipid bilayer. The ABC proteins are encoded by 49 genes and are categorized

Advanced Drug Delivery, First Edition. Edited by Ashim K. Mitra, Chi H. Lee, and Kun Cheng.

into seven subclasses [3]. The P-gp is the most well-documented transporter in the ABC superfamily and is encoded by the MDR1 (ABCB1) gene. The SLC superfamily consists of 43 families [3] that participate in drug absorption. There are many well-known SLC transporters, including serotonin (*SLC6A4*) and dopamine (*SLC6A3*) transporters. Besides carrying nutrients or extruding cellular waste or toxins, the wide-ranging role of membrane transporters is drug absorption, distribution, and elimination. These transporters also participate in drug–drug interactions. The role of these transporters in multidrug resistance has been well recognized. In addition to drug delivery service, some of these transporter proteins also serve as a protective barrier to particular organs such as the brain. For example, the P-gp in the blood-brain barrier (BBB) or blood-retinal barrier protects the brain and eyes, respectively, from toxic influx of a variety of structurally diverse molecules through an efflux pump. The ABC transporters also work in concert with drug metabolizing enzymes by eliminating drugs and their metabolites. Molecular cloning of transporter genes reveals the association of multiple genes encoding subtypes with a similar function with different tissue distribution and specificity toward drugs. Studying these subtypes (e.g., glucose transporters and GLUT 1-4) can unravel the structure-activity correlation for drug transport that may allow modulation of its activity when considered necessary. Sometimes transporters can be present in the form of multiple alleles with functional defects resulting in defective drug binding or transport. Although the importance of drug transporters in the process of ADME and drug–drug interactions is well documented, our knowledge in this area is still emerging. The U.S. Food and Drug Administration (FDA) and International Transporter Consortium (ITC) recently selected a few transporters: the organic anion transporter (OAT), organic anion transporting polypeptide (OATP), organic cation transporter (OCT), peptide transporter (PEPT), P-gp, multidrug resistance associated protein (MRP), and breast cancer resistance protein (BCRP), which are decisive to xenobiotics absorption, and drug–drug interactions. From a pharmacokinetic point of view, localization and function of these transporters in the intestine, liver, and kidney receives major attention. However, current evidence suggests that some of these transporters, particularly ABC transporters in the BBB, also have drawn interest for delivering drugs to the brain. In this chapter, we will discuss mainly those transporters as well as vitamin transporters that seem to be significant for drug delivery.

3.3 ABC TRANSPORTERS

3.3.1 ABC Proteins

The ATP binding cassette (ABC) family is a superfamily of membrane proteins responsible for translocation of various substances comprising sugars, amino acids, sterols, peptides, proteins, antibiotics, toxins, and xenobiotics. These proteins use the energy derived from hydrolysis of ATP for translocations of various substances across a concentration gradient. Forty eight different ABC transporters have been found in the human genome. The ABC transporter genes stand for the largest family of transmembrane proteins. Based on sequence homology and domain structure, they are categorized into seven different classes (ABCA–ABCG). So far, 13 different transporters have been identified from classes A, B, C, and G. These transporters play a significant role in the development of multidrug resistance (MDR) [4, 5]. First, Biedler and Riehm in 1970 reported that Chinese hamster ovary (CHO) cells identified for resistance to Actinomycin D also demonstrated cross-resistance to many other drugs such as duramycin, democoline, mithramycin, mytomycin C, puromycin, vinblastine, and vincristine [6–9]. It is also accountable for the efflux of HIV-protease inhibitors, anticancer agents, and many other drugs. It seemed that after selection of a single cytotoxic drug, mammalian cells simultaneously developed cross-resistance to a variety of therapeutic agents with different chemical structures and functions. This phenomenon was referred to multidrug resistance. Although it was believed that this drug resistance was a result of permeation alteration of the cell membrane, Juliano and Ling in 1976 revealed that drug resistance in CHO cells was from the presence of P-glycoprotein [7]. Why are so many efflux transporters present in life forms? Many toxins are present in nature, and clinicians administer many toxins to treat life-threatening diseases (cancer, HIV, diabetes, etc). The amphiphilic drug molecules are hydrophobic enough to diffuse through the lipid bilayer, but they are hydrophilic enough to reach the target. Once inside cells, these drugs can be inactivated by oxidation or conjugation to become more hydrophilic and get trapped inside the cells. These efflux transporters help them get out. Although the P-gp becomes a warrior in effluxing a wide range of therapeutic agents, the MRP family deserves credit in extruding drugs conjugated to glutathione (GSH), glucuronate, or sulfate and many other organic anions such as Methotrexate.

These ABC transporters always function unidirectionally as opposed to several others transporters that function bidirectionally [10]. All these ABC proteins show a minimal requirement of two transmembrane domains (TMDs) and two nucleotide binding domains (NBDs). This structural requirement can be assured by a single polypeptide chain or gathered from two homo-dimeric (equal) to hetero-dimeric (unequal) chains [11, 12]. All ABC transporters include a conserved sequence in NBD for binding ATP. The hydrolysis of ATP is required as a standard power for translocation by these transporters [13]. All ABC transporters demonstrate 25% homology. The conserved regions of sequence motifs consist of the 1) Walker A region, 2) Walker B region,

3) signature C motif (90-120 amino acids linker between Walker A and B regions), 4) glutamine loop (Q-loop), 5) histidine loop (H-loop), and 6) D-loop [14–16]. The Walker A and B regions play a vital role in nucleotide binding. The signature motif is considered a hallmark of ABC transporters that aids in communicating TMDs and ATP hydrolysis [17]. The glutamate and histidine loops assist in ATP hydrolysis [18, 19]. The other trademark of ABC transporters is the D-loop that contributes a vital function in communicating the catalytic sites [20]. Three important ABC transporters, P-gp, MRP, and BCRP, will be discussed further from a drug delivery point of view.

3.3.2 Efflux Transporters

The efflux transporter proteins belong to the ATP-binding cassette family. In particular, we are interested in the efflux transporters that are expressed at physiological barriers (e.g. intestinal absorption barrier, BBB, placental barrier, corneal and retinal barriers), in the liver, cancer cells, and other tissues responsible for drug clearance or excretion of xenobiotics. In this chapter, we will focus on three efflux transporters: P-gp, MRP, and BCRP. These transporters significantly influence ADME of a number of drugs and their metabolites and cause drug resistance for many therapeutic agents. The tissue distribution of these transporters (Table 3.1) and their localizations in various tissues are illustrated in Figure 3.1. These proteins along with primary metabolizing enzyme–cytochrome P450 (CYP) together constitute a highly efficient barrier for oral drug absorption. The P-gp is the most extensively studied efflux transporter that functions as a biological barrier by extruding toxins and xenobiotics into extracellular fluid. MRP belongs to the same ABC superfamily. Human MRP-1, MRP-2, and MRP-3 are known to be involved in the efflux of anti-HIV agents and their conjugated metabolites [21–25]. Substrate specificity and tissue localization of MDR protein differs from MRP. As a consequence of efflux, drug absorption is reduced and the bioavailability of xenobiotics diminishes at the target organs [26, 27]. In recent reviews, we have elaborately discussed the role of these efflux transporters in drug–drug and drug–herbal interactions [28, 29].

3.3.3 P-Glycoprotein

The P-gp, a product of an MDR gene, was first characterized as the ATP-dependent transporter, responsible for the efflux of therapeutic agents from resistant cancer cells. In the early 1970s, Juliano and Ling demonstrated a 170-kDa protein in Chinese hamster ovary cells resistant to colchicines [7] and that protein was absent in drug-sensitive cells. The word "P" stands for permeability because this transporter caused marked alteration in the permeation of several drugs across cell membranes. The P-gp is an integral membrane protein having two homologous halves, each consisting of one hydrophobic domain with six transmembrane segments and one hydrophilic nucleotide-binding domain. Two halves are connected by a short flexible polypeptide linker to form the functionally active 1280 amino acid protein. P-gp encoding genes have been identified in hamster, mice, human, and other species. It is a transporter protein, encoded by a small multigene family, described by MDR I, II, and III. P-gps from all three classes are present in rodents, whereas human cells express the P-gp belonging to classes I and III. It is the first ATP-dependent transporter found in the liver, and it represents the most studied member of the ATP binding cassette family of transporters. MDR proteins in humans and other species play a central role in protecting the cells against cytotoxic agents [30]. These efflux proteins exhibit a broad range of substrate specificity, such as digoxin, loperamide, doxorubicin, vinblastine, paclitaxel, fexofenadine cyclosporine-A, taxol, dexamethasone, lidocaine, erythromycin,

TABLE 3.1 Tissue Distribution of the P-gp, MRP, and BCRP [3, 28, 29]

Tissue	P-gp	MRP-1	MRP-2	BCRP
Small intestine	Epithelium, apical side of lumen	Basolateral membrane of lumen	Epical membrane of the lumen	Apical side of lumen
Colon	Epithelium, apical side of lumen	Not present	Apical membrane of the lumen	Apical side of lumen
Liver	Bile canalicular face of hepatocytes	Basolateral membrane of hepatocytes	Apical bile Canalicular	Bile canalicular
Kidney	Brush border surface of proximal tubules (apical)	Basolateral membrane of tubules	Apical proximal tubules	Not present
Placenta	Trophoblasts	Trophoblasts	Trophoblasts	Trophoblasts (facing maternal blood)
BBB	Luminal side of brain endothelium	Luminal side of brain endothelial cells	Luminal side of brain endothelial cells	Brain endothelial cells
Other major organs	Abundant on adrenal cortex	Basolateral membrane of sertoli cells	None	Breast lobules, apical; stem cells

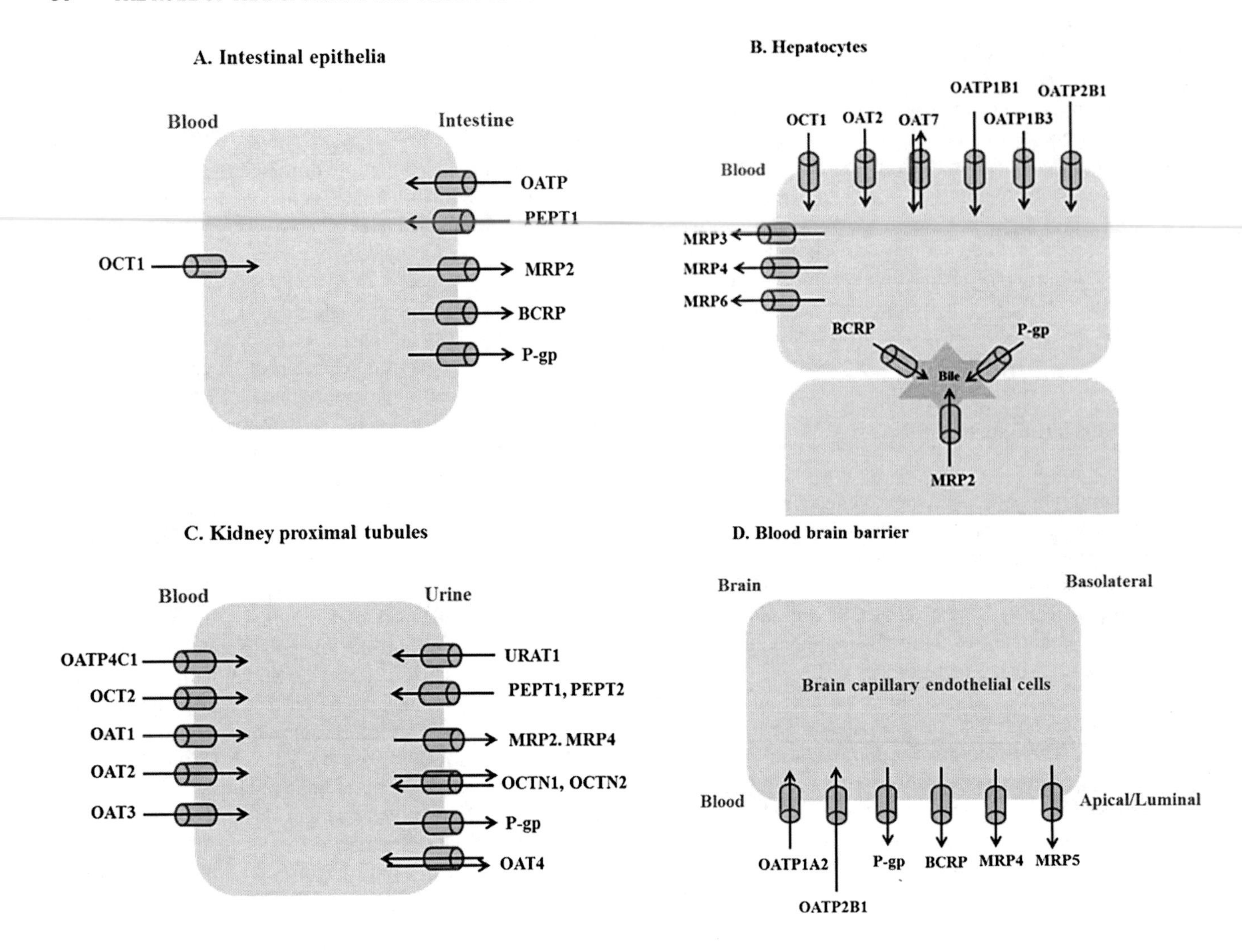

FIGURE 3.1 Localization of selected transporters in four tissues involved in ADME of drugs. Adapted from Ref. 2.

ketoconazole, rifampicin, protease inhibitors, and many anticancer agents [31–37]. Several P-gp substrates (including anticancer drugs, protease inhibitors, and a variety of other therapeutic agents from different classes) and its inhibitors are given in Table 3.2.

3.3.4 Multidrug Resistance Associated Proteins (MRPs)

The MRP family consists of at least nine members: MRP-1 and its eight isoforms, known as MRP2–9. MRP-2 has been recognized in the apical (luminal) membrane of rat brain capillary endothelium [39]. The transmembrane domains in this family vary among the members. MRP-4 (ABCC4), MRP-5 (ABCC5), and MRP-7 (ABCC7) have 12 transmembrane domains and two NBD-binding sites. Other members of the MRP family such as MRP-1 (ABCC1), MRP-2 (ABCC2), MRP-3 (ABCC3), and MRP-6 (ABCC6) have 17 transmembrane domains and two cytoplasmic NBD-binding sites. These membrane proteins (190 kD) mediate the ATP-dependent unidirectional efflux of glutathione, glucuronate, or sulfate conjugates of lipophilic drugs. In addition to many anionic conjugates, several unconjugated amphiphilic anions can serve as substrates for MRPs. There are numerous overlapping substrates among MRP, MATE (multidrug and toxin extrusion transporter), and MOAT (multispecific organic anion transporter) [2]. Gene symbol and other names used for the human MRP family have been shown in Figure 3.2. Recent reports have identified MRP in the brain capillary endothelium. A recent report revealed that MRPs play a significant role *in vivo* in the absorption of saquinavir across BBB [40]. Since the MRP family is capable of exporting GHS complexes such as cisplatin, their importance in drug resistance is gaining

TABLE 3.2 P-gp Substrates and Inhibitors [38]

Substrates	Inhibitors
Acebutolol, Acetaminophen, Actinomycin D, h-Acetyldigoxin, Amitriptyline, Amprenavir, Apafant, Asimadoline, Atenolol, Atorvastatin, Azidopine, Azidoprocainamide methoiodide, Azithromycin, Benzo(a)pyrene, Betamethasone, Bisantrene, Bromocriptine, Bunitrolol, Calcein-AM, Camptothecin, Carbamazepine, Carvedilol, Celiprolol, Cepharanthin, Cerivastatin, Chloroquine, Chlorpromazine, Chlorothiazide, Clarithromycin, Colchicine, Corticosterone, Cortisol, Cyclosporin A, Daunorubicin (Daunomycin), Debrisoquine, Desoxycorticosterone, Dexamethasone, Digitoxin, Digoxin, Diltiazem, Dipyridamole, Docetaxel, Dolastatin 10, Domperidone, Doxorubicin (Adriamycin), Eletriptan, Emetine, Endosulfan, Erythromycin, h-Estradiol, Estradiol-17h-d-glucuronide, Etoposide (VP-16), Fexofenadine, GF120918, Grepafloxacin, Hoechst 33342, Hydroxyrubicin, Imatinib, Indinavir, Ivermectin, Levofloxacin, Loperamide, Losartan, Lovastatin, Methadone, Methotrexate, Methylprednisolone, Metoprolol, Mitoxantrone, Monensin, Morphine, 99mTc-sestamibi, N-desmethyltamoxifen, Nadolol, Nelfinavir, Nicardipine, Nifedipine, Nitrendipine, Norverapamil, Olanzapine, Omeprazole, PSC-833 (Valspodar), Perphenazine, Prazosin, Prednisone, Pristinamycin IA, Puromycin, Quetiapine, Quinidine, Quinine, Ranitidine, Reserpine, Rhodamine 123, Risperidone, Ritonavir, Roxithromycin, Saquinavir, Sirolimus, Sparfloxacin, Sumatriptan, Tacrolimus, Talinolol, Tamoxifen, Taxol(Paclitaxel), Telithromycin, Terfenadine, Timolol, Toremifene, Tributylmethylammonium, Trimethoprim, Valinomycin, Vecuronium, Verapamil, Vinblastine,Vincristine, Vindoline, Vinorelbine	Amiodarone, Amitriptyline, Amlodipine, Astemizole, Atemoyacin-B, Atorvastatin, Aureobasidin A, Azelastine, Barnidipine, Benidipine, Bepridil, Bergamottin, Bergapten, Bergaptol, Biochanin A, Biricodar (VX-710), Bromocriptine, Buspirone, Caffeine, Carvedilol, Celiprolol, Cepharanthin, Chlorpyrifos, Cholesterol, Cimetidine, Clarithromycin, Clofazimine, Clomipramine, Clotrimazole, Colchicine, Cortisol, Cremophor EL, Cyclosporin, Cytochalasin E, Daunorubicin (Daunomycin), Desethylamiodarone, Desipramine, Desloratadine, Desmethylazelastine, Dexamethasone, Dexniguldipine, Digoxin, 6V,7V-Dihydroxybergamottin, Dihydrocytochalasin B, Diltiazem, Dipyridamole, Doxepin, Doxorubicin (Adriamycin), [d-Pen2, d-Pen5]-enkephalin, Efonidipine, Eletriptan, Emetine, Endosulfan, Epiabeodendroidin F, Ergometrine, Ergotamine, Erythromycin, Estramustine, Etoposide (VP-16), Fangchinoline, Felodipine, Fentanyl, Fluconazole, Fluoxetine, Fluphenazine, Fluvoxamine, Forskolin, Gallopamil, Genistein, GF120918, Haloperidol, Hydrocortisone, 1V-Hydroxymidazolam, Indinavir, Itraconazole, Ivermectin, Ketoconazole, Lansoprazole, Loperamide, Loratadine, Lovastatin, Manidipine, Methadone, Metoprolol, Mibefradil, Miconazole, Midazolam, Morin, Morphine, Naringenin, Nefazodone, Nelfinavir, Nicardipine, Nifedipine, Nilvadipine, Nisoldipine, Nitrendipine, Nobiletin, Norverapamil, Omeprazole, Pafenolol, Pantoprazole, Phenylhexyl isothiocyanate, Pimozide, Piperine, Pluronic block copolymer, Pristinamycin IA, Progesterone, Promethazine, PSC-833 (Valspodar), Quercetin, Quinacrine, Quinidine, Quinine, Ranitidine, Rapamycin, Reserpine, Ritonavir, Saquinavir, Silymarin, Simvastatin, Sirolimus, Mephenytoin, Spironolactone, Staurosporine, Sufentanil, Talinolol, Tamoxifen, Tangeretin, Taxol (Paclitaxel), Terfenadine, Tetrandine, Tetraphenylphosphonium, Trans-flupenthixol, Trifluoperazine, Triflupromazine, Trimethoxybenzoylyohimbine, Troleandomycin, Tween 80, Valinomycin, Verapamil, Vinblastine, Vincristine

attention. MRP4 and MRP5 can develop resistance to nucleotide analogs (PMEA) and purine base analogs (thioguanine and 6-mercaptopurine). Therefore, the role of MRPs in drug resistance cannot be ignored. A wide range of MRP substrates and inhibitors is provided in Table 3.3.

Gene Symbol	Protein	Other names used
ABCC1	MRP1	ABCC; MRP;GS-X;ABC29
ABCC2	MRP2	cMOAT, cMRP
ABCC3	MRP3	MOAT-D; cMOAT-2
ABCC4	MRP4	MOAT-B
ABCC5	MRP5	MOAT-C; pABC11
ABCC6	MRP6	MOAT-E; MLP-1;ARA
ABCC10	MRP7	
ABCC11	MRP8	

MOAT: multispecific organic anion transporter

FIGURE 3.2 Human MRP gene family.

3.3.5 Breast Cancer Resistant Protein (BCRP)

The BCRP belongs to a novel branch, subfamily G, of the large ABC transporter superfamily. The founding member of the ABCG subfamily, ABCG1, has been implicated in the regulation of cellular lipid homeostasis in macrophages through facilitating the efflux of cellular lipids including cholesterol and phospholipids. It is also known as a mitoxantrone-resistance protein. The BCRP is a 72-kD protein, described as a half transporter that contains only six transmembrane domains and one NBD-binding site. Predicted secondary structures of these drug efflux transporters of the ATP-binding cassette family are illustrated in Figure 3.3.

Two features that distinguish the subfamily G members from other ABC transporters are their unique domain organization. Functional characterization has demonstrated that the BCRP can transport a wide range of substrates ranging from chemotherapeutic agents to organic anion conjugates. P-gp substrates have a tendency to overlap the BCRP, but the latter includes acids or drug conjugates (mitoxantrone, methotrexate, topotecan, imatinib, irinotecan, statins,

TABLE 3.3 Substrates and Inhibitors for MRP2 [38]

Substrates	Inhibitors
N-Acetyl leukotriene E4, p-Aminohippurate, Arsenic, Azithromycin, Benzbromarone, Bilirubin bisglucuronide, Bilirubin monoglucuronide, Cadmium, Calcein, 5-Carboxyfluorescein, Cefodizime, Cisplatin, Copper, S-Decyl-glutathione, Dibromosulfophtalein, 2,4-Dinitrophenyl-S-glutathione (DNP-SG), Epicatechin-3-gallate, Epigallocatechin-3-gallate, Estradiol-17h-d-glucuronide, Etoposide (VP-16), N-Ethylmaleimide-glutathione, Ethinylestradiol-3-O-glucuronide, Ethinylestradiol-3-O-sulfate, Fluo-3, Glutathione, Glutathione-bimane, Glutathion-methylfluorescein, Glycyrrhizin, Grepafloxacin, Grepafloxacin glucuronide, Indinavir, Irinotecan, Leucovorin, Leukotriene C4, Leukotriene D4, Leukotriene E4, Methotrexate, 4_-OMethyl-epigallocatechin gallate, Ochratoxin A, Oxidized glutathione, Pravastatin, Probenecid, Ritonavir, Saquinavir, SN-38 carboxylate, SN-38 glucuronide, Sulfinpyrazone, Sulfobromophthalein, Sulfobromophthalein-S-glutathione, Taurochenodeoxycholate 3-sulfate, Taurolithocholate 3-sulfate, Temocaprilat, Vinblastine, Vincristine	Benzbromarone, Bergamottin, Bilirubin bisglucuronide, Bilirubin monoglucuronide, Cyclosporin, Daunorubicin, 6V,7V-Dihydroxybergamottin, Etoposide (VP-16), Furosemide, GF120918, Glibenclamide, Glutathione, LY335979, Leukotriene C4, MK571, Ochratoxin A, Oxidized glutathione, Pravastatin, Probenecid, Sulfinpyrazone, Tangeretin, Vincristine

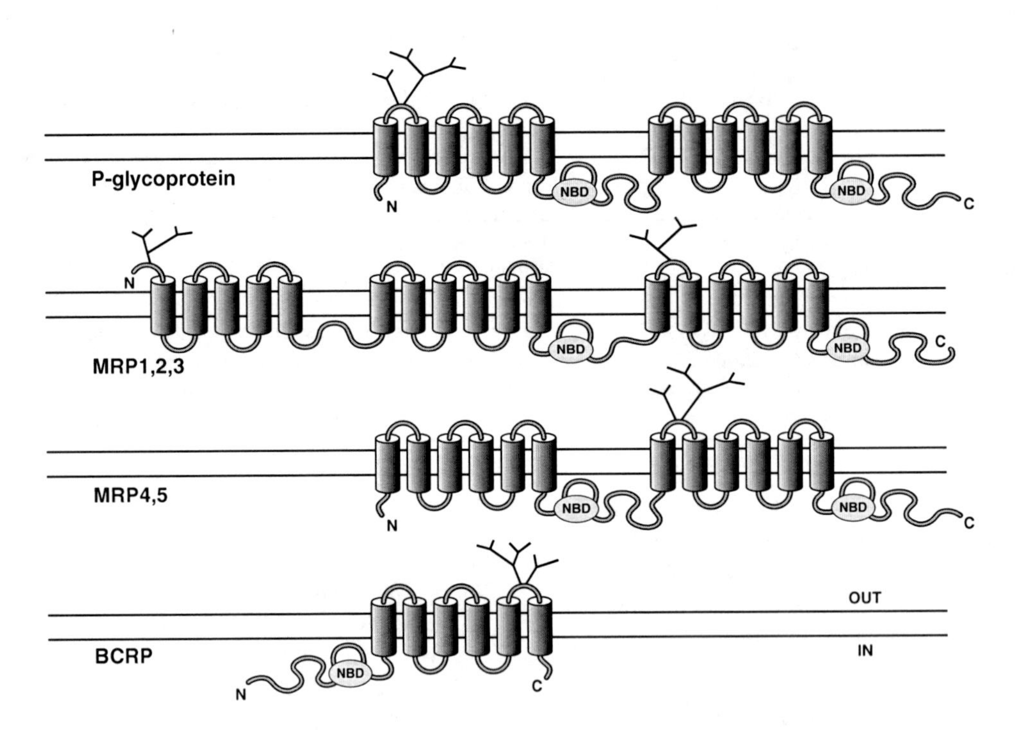

FIGURE 3.3 Predicted secondary structures of drug efflux transporters of the ATP-binding cassette family: Four classes are distinguished here, based on predicted structure and amino acid sequence homology. (1) P-glycoprotein consists of two transmembrane domains, each containing six transmembrane segments and two nucleotide-binding domains (NBDs). It is N-glycosylated (branches) at the first extracellular loop. (2) MRP1, 2, and 3 have an additional amino terminal extension containing five transmembrane segments, and they are N-glycosylated near the N-terminus and at the sixth extracellular loop. (3) MRP4 and 5 lack the amino terminal extension of MRP1–3 and are N-glycosylated at the fourth extracellular loop. (4) BCRP is a "half transporter" consisting of one NBD and six transmembrane segments, and it is most likely N-glycosylated at the third extracellular loop. Note that, in contrast to the other transporters, the NBD of BCRP is at the amino terminal end of the polypeptide. The BCRP almost certainly functions as a homodimer. N and C denote amino- and carboxy-terminal ends of the proteins, respectively. Cytoplasmic (IN) and extracellular (OUT) orientation indicated for BCRP applies to all transporters drawn here. Reproduced with permission from Ref. 41.

TABLE 3.4 Substrates and Inhibitors for BCRP [38]

Substrates	Inhibitors
Actinomycin D, 9-Aminocamptothecin, 2-Amino-1-methyl-6-phenylimidazole [4,5-b]pyridine (PhIP), Azidodeoxythymidine, Bodipy-FLPrazosin, C6-NBD-phosphatidylcholine, C6-NBD-phosphatidylserine, Cholesterol, Cimetidine, Daunorubicin, Dehydroepiandrosterone sulfate, Doxorubicin, Epirubicin, 17h-Estradiol, 17h-Estradiol-glucuronide, 17h-Estradiol-3-sulfate, Estrone, Estrone-3-sulfate, Etidium bromide, Etoposide, Flavopiridol, Fumitremorgin C, Genistein, Hoechst 33342, Indolocarbazole, Irinotecan, Lamivudine, Methotrexate, 4-Methylumbelliferone sulfate, Mitoxantrone, Progesterone, Pheophorbide, Protoporphyrin IX, Rhodamine 123, SN-38 (7-Ethyl-10-hydroxycamptothecin), SN-38 glucuronide, Tamoxifen, Testosterone, Topotecan, h-Sitosterol, Zidovudine	Acacetin, Apigenin, Beclomethasone, Biochanin A, Chrysin, Corticosterone, Cyclosporin A, Daidzein, Dehydroepiandrostrone sulfate, Diethylstilbestrol, Digoxin, Dexamethasone, Doxorubicin, 17h-Estradiol, 17h-Estradiol-3-sulfate, Estrone, Fumitremorgin C, Genistein, GF120918, Hesperetin, Imatinib mesylate, Kaempferol, Mitoxantrone, Naringenin, Naringenin-7-glucoside, Nelfinavir, Novobiocin, Omeprazole, Pantoprazole, Quercetin, Ritonavir, SN-38, Saquinavir, Silymarin, Stilbene resveratrol, Topotecan, Triamcinolone, Tryprost

sulphate conjugates, porphyrins, etc.). More evidence is emerging to suggest that the BCRP plays a significant role in drug disposition. Hence, it is important to examine its effect on pharmacokinetics and drug–drug interactions of therapeutic agents [42–48]. Information regarding various substrates and inhibitors of the BCRP has been depicted in Table 3.4.

3.3.6 Genetic Factors in Drug Response

Growing evidence suggests that genetic factors influence interindividual variation in drug response. Polymorphism has been indicated to vary with ethnicity. Mutations in genes may lead to genetic polymorphism. Several reports suggest that interindividual variability in drug response is linked to single nucleotide polymorphisms (SNPs). Polymorphism in a number of genes encoding for drug metabolizing enzymes and transporters has been reported. So far 28 SNPs have been detected at 27 positions on the MDR1 gene [49]. Mutations at exon 26 (C3435T) and 21(G2677T/A) of MDR are responsible for duodenal expression of the P-gp. A significantly reduced duodenal P-gp expression in homozygous (3435TT) individuals has been linked to a higher plasma digoxin level [23]. Also, C3435T has been reported to be a risk factor for HIV infection [50]. Chowbay et al. have described ethnic variability among Chinese, Malays, and Indians [51]. The pharmacogenetics of MDR1 in Asian populations are different from those in Caucasian and African populations. MDR1 is a well-conserved gene. But current evidence indicates that its polymorphism affects substrate specificity. Three SNPs frequently arise at positions 1236C > T, 2677G > T, and 3435C > T. In a recent review Fung and Gottesman have indicated that the frequency of synonymous 3435C > T polymorphism seems to vary significantly with ethnicity [52]. The *ABCB1* 3435C > T genotype was also found to alter the serum levels of cortisol and aldosterone during the postmenstrual phase of a normal cycle [53]. A common haplotype plays a significant role in drug response and efficacy. An evidence of high CYP3A4 expression in MDR1 2677T carriers was found in the human intestine [54]. The influence of MDR1 genotype on CYP3A4 expression adds additional complexity in drug–drug interactions.

3.3.7 Substrate Recognition by P-glycoprotein

The P-gp actively exports a wide range of chemically diverse compounds out of cells. TMDs 5–6 and 11–12 play a critical role in recognizing and binding its substrates. Seelig has reported on a general pattern of substrate recognition by the P-gp by analyzing more than 100 diverse compounds [55]. Well-defined two- or three-electron donor groups (recognition elements) are required for a substrate to bind the P-gp. These recognition elements are classified into two groups: type I and type II. Type I units compose of two electron donor groups with a spatial separation of 2.5 ± 0.3 Å, whereas type II units either consist of two or three electron donor groups with a spatial separation of 4.6 ± 0.6 Å. Accordingly, if a compound contains at least type I or type II units, then it is expected to be recognized by the P-gp. On the basis of the type and number of recognition elements, various compounds can be classified as nonsubstrate, weak substrate, or strong substrate. The structural elements responsible for a substrate–P-gp interaction reside in specific hydrogen bonding acceptor units. P-gp–substrate binding and its overexpression enhance the number and strength of hydrogen-bonding acceptor units [55].

3.3.8 Substrate and Inhibitor Selectivity

The P-gp-mediated efflux of substrates or therapeutic agents plays a major role in drug disposition across the biological barrier. Apart from cancer cells, the P-gp is expressed in many organs such as the intestine, liver, kidney, eye, and brain [56]. It has been proven that the oral absorption and brain penetration of P-gp substrates are significantly enhanced in MDR1 knockout mice compared with normal mice [57]. The oral bioavailability and brain permeability of

P-gp substrates can be significantly enhanced by co-administration of P-gp modulators [58, 59]. Both biliary excretion and renal clearance are significantly reduced in the presence of P-gp inhibitors [60, 61]. Now it is well accepted that appropriate P-gp inhibitors should be co-administered with P-gp substrates for therapeutic effectiveness. The activity of the P-gp-mediated efflux is a saturable process. This is a complex area of drug–drug or drug–inhibitor interactions. Such interactions can give rise to competitive inhibition, noncompetitive inhibition, and cooperative simulation [6]. These interactions can take place either at the P-gp binding site or at ATP binding domains. There is more than one P-gp binding location. The exact numbers of P-gp binding locations are yet to be confirmed. However, P-gp substrates and inhibitors can bind at different locations. In general, the substrate binding site and the two ATP-binding domains act together to operate the efflux pump. Therefore, inhibition of the P-gp-mediated drug efflux could potentially take place either as a result of the contest of the P-gp binding site and ATP-binding domains or as a result of blockage of ATP hydrolysis.

3.4 STRATEGIES TO OVERCOME ACTIVE EFFLUX

As we mentioned, MDR-mediated efflux poses a major impediment for successful drug delivery. Hence, strategies to overcome efflux proteins are warranted. We have briefly discussed the recent developments and research strategies to circumvent MDR-mediated efflux.

3.4.1 Pharmacological Inhibition of Efflux Proteins

Co-administration of chemical agents that can inhibit the activity of efflux proteins by either competitive or noncompetitive binding seems to be an attractive strategy for avoiding drug efflux. An ideal efflux modulator can inhibit the activity of efflux pumps at the apical membrane and subsequently enhance the permeability of the drug molecule in desired tissues. A schematic of this mechanism is depicted in Figure 3.4.

3.4.2 First-Generation MDR Modulators

Clinically approved Ca^{2+} channel blocker verapamil restored the cellular accumulation of vincristine in P-gp overexpressing cell lines. This finding stimulated development of several P-gp inhibitors [62, 63]. Antimalarial drugs quinine and quinidine and immunosuppressant cyclosporine A emerged as other first-generation inhibitors and were approved for therapeutic use in clinic [64–66]. Although these first-generation inhibitors were potent *in vitro*, very high doses required to block MDR-mediated efflux in humans led to potential life-threatening toxicity [67].

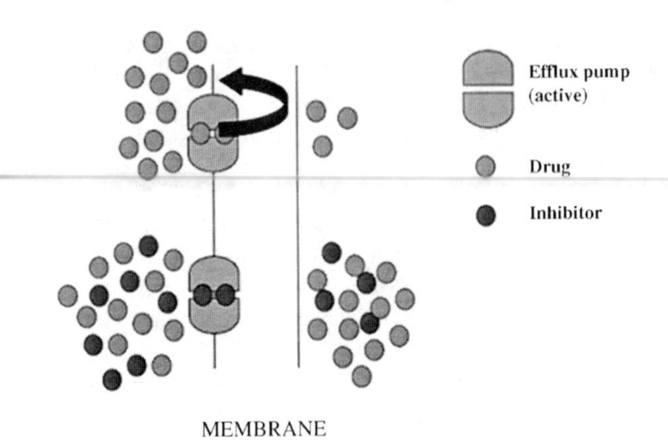

FIGURE 3.4 Combination therapy approach.

3.4.3 Second-Generation MDR Modulators

As a result of high toxicity with the first-generation modulators, the development of new MDR modulators with lower inherent toxicities was essential. Structural analogs of verapamil, including dexverapamil and an analog of Cyclosporin A, PSC-833 (Valspodar) were thus developed as second-generation modulators [68, 69]. However, these compounds seemed to alter the pharmacokinetic properties of co-administered anticancer drugs, such as paclitaxel, and doxorubicin, producing dose-dependent hematological side effects [70, 71]. This altered the pharmacokinetic profile of co-administered drugs and caused nonspecific interactions with CYP enzymes [72]. As a consequence, the dose adjustment of anticancer drugs seemed imminent to prevent an adverse outcome of the therapy.

3.4.4 Third-Generation MDR Modulators

These agents were designed to overcome the limitations of these previous modulators. This new set of efflux modulators is highly specific for MDR efflux pumps sparing any interaction with drug-metabolizing (CYP-450) enzymes that do not alter pharmacokinetic interaction with other therapeutic agents. For example, zosuquidar [73], tariquidar [74], and elacridar [75] are the MDR inhibitors that have shown promise in preclinical mouse model and more recently in the clinic. Zosuquidar and tariquidar are specific inhibitors of the P-gp. A noncompetitive inhibitory mechanism has been suggested because these are neither substrates for the P-gp nor transported by the ABC transporter [76]. Preclinical studies using such inhibitors with anticancer drugs showed significantly prolonged survival and reduction of MDR-bearing human tumors engrafted in mice [76]. No alterations in pharmacokinetic parameters of anticancer drugs such as doxorubicin, etoposide, daunorubicin, vincristine, and paclitaxel have been demonstrated during such co-administrations. Various phase I and phase II studies have been conducted during co-administration of zosuquidar with docetaxel and daunorubicin and doxorubicin for the treatment of breast cancer, leukemia, and non-Hodgkin's lymphoma [77–80]. Elacridar is a dual inhibitor of the P-gp and BCRP. Co-administration of elacridar has been reported to increase the oral bioavailability of topotecan in patients [81]. Preclinical studies suggest effective reversal of chemoresistance during co-administration of elacridar [82].

3.4.5 Herbal Modulation of MDR Efflux Proteins

Flavonoids such as chalcones, flavonols, flavones, procyanidins, flavan-3-ols (catechins), flavanones, and isoflavones are the major constituents among numerous other constituents of many naturally occurring herbal products on the market. There have been well-documented reports in the literature suggesting their interactions with efflux transporters, particularly P-gp [29]. To name a few, St. John's wort, garlic, ginseng, and grapefruit juice are well known as over-the-counter herbal products as dietary supplements and medications. In both preclinical and clinical settings, these products have been shown to interact with drugs that are substrates for P-gp. These herbal ingredients can either inhibit the ATPase activity of efflux pumps or act as competitive inhibitors for other drug molecules. Patel et al. demonstrated that the P-gp-mediated efflux of ritonavir was greatly reduced by quercetin in Caco-2 cells and MDCKII-MDR1 cells [83]. Similarly, intracellular accumulation of daunomycin was greatly enhanced in P-gp overexpressing K562 cells, with co-administration of various flavonoids [84]. Similar interactions of herbal products with other efflux transporters such as MRP2 and BCRP have also been reported in the literature. Flavonols such as myricetin and robinetin were shown to inhibit MRP2-mediated efflux of calcein in MRP2 overexpressing MDCKII cells [85]. Zhang et al. showed that chrysin, biochanin A, and 7,8-benzoflavone were the most potent flavonoids for inhibiting the efflux of mitoxantrone among 25 naturally occurring flavonoids tested in MCF-7 cells overexpressing BCRP [86, 87]. Likewise, genistein and naringenin were shown to reverse BCRP-mediated resistance [88].

Although the exact mechanism of the P-gp-mediated drug–drug interaction during co-administration of modulators and substrates has yet to be comprehended, it seems that substrate bioavailability does not follow simple kinetics. The competitive inhibition indicates two substrates operate at the same binding site of the P-gp where only one can bind on any one occasion, whereas noncompetitive inhibition suggests that two substrates are competent to translocate simultaneously at two distinct P-gp binding sites and may function independently. The situation may change when allosteric effects are engaged during interaction between substrate and modulator.

When a single drug is substrate for more than one efflux transporter, one specific inhibitor may not alter the pharmacokinetics profile. For example, vincristine is a substrate for both the P-gp and MRP2. In that case, co-administration of vincristine with either quinidine (inhibitor of the P-gp) or MK571 (inhibitor of the MRP) may not significantly change its brain absorption of vincristine. Because when one transporter is inhibited, another transporter overworks for pumping that drug out of the brain. In that case, selection of a dual inhibitor is critical. Recently we have shown that brain uptake of vandetanib (trade name Caprelsa; AstraZeneca, London, U.K.), an anticancer drug, was significantly enhanced in the presence of either GF120918 (elacridar) or everolimus (m-TOR inhibitor) compared with either Ko143 or LY335979. Vandetanib is a substrate for both the P-gp and BCRP. Although Ko143 and LY335979 are inhibitors of the P-gp and BCRP, respectively, GF120918 (elacridar) or everolimus can inhibit both the P-gp- and the BCRP-mediated efflux of vandetanib in a mouse brain [89].

3.4.6 Pharmaceutical Excipients as Inhibitors of MDR Efflux Proteins

A drug delivery system using novel Pluronic (BASF Corporation, Florham Park, NJ) block co-polymers has become popular for overcoming the efflux pump to overcome multidrug-resistant cancers. Improved oral drug absorption of topotecan, a model BCRP substrate, was observed after pretreatment of wild-type mice with Pluronic 85 (P85) and Tween 20 (BASF Corporation, Florham Park, NJ) [90]. In a separate study, the cellular accumulation of digoxin was increased by threefold in LLC-PK1 cells and by fivefold in the LLC-PK1-MDR1-transfected cells after addition of P85. Similar effects were observed for rhodamine-123 [91]. The co-administration of 1% P85 with radiolabeled digoxin in wild-type mice increased its brain permeation by threefold [91]. These data indicate that excipients such as P85 and Tween 20 can enhance the delivery of drug substrates through the inhibition of the P-gp- and the BCRP-mediated efflux mechanism.

3.4.7 Prodrug Strategy

Besides efflux transporters, such as the P-gp, MRP2, and BCRP, several nutrient (influx) transporters are also expressed on the cellular membranes. These nutrient transporters are responsible for the influx of various nutrients and drugs into various epithelial (enterocytes) and endothelial cells (e.g., blood-brain barrier). Recently, transporter-targeted prodrug derivatization has received great attention among drug delivery scientists. Prodrugs have been designed such that the modified compounds become substrates of nutrient transporters leading

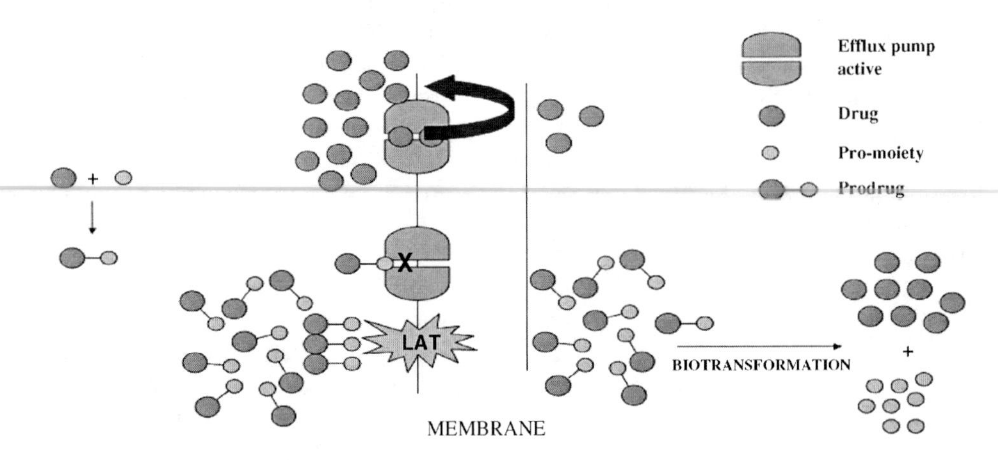

FIGURE 3.5 Transporter-targeted prodrug strategy: Improved permeability could be achieved by overcoming MDR efflux transporters during chemical modification of the parent drug molecule. (See color figure in color plate section.)

to enhanced absorption of these compounds across various physiological barriers, which upon crossing the membrane get biotransformed into parent drug and the promoiety (Figure 3.5). This strategy not only circumvents efflux pumps but can also reduce the toxic effects of the P-gp modulators. Jain et al. reported on evasion of the P-gp-mediated cellular efflux and enhanced permeability of HIV protease inhibitor saquinavir during prodrug modification. Di-peptide prodrugs, namely, valine-valine-saquinavir and glycine-valine-saquinavir showed enhanced absorption with reduced efflux relative to unmodified saquinavir across MDCKII-MDR1 cells [92]. In a similar study, parallel results were reported for evasion of the P-gp-mediated efflux of lopinavir [93] and quinidine [94] during peptide prodrug modifications.

3.4.8 Nanotechnology

Nanotechnology provides an alternative strategy for circumventing MDR by offering a means to encapsulate drugs to lipids, gelatins, and polymers producing nanoparticles that are resistant to drug efflux. These nanoparticles take advantage of the endocytosis process simultaneously evading MDR proteins on cell membranes. Moreover, these nanoparticles can be surface- decorated with folic acid, biotin, etc. for receptor-mediated targeted delivery. Figure 3.6 demonstrates the mechanism of efflux evasion via endocytosis after encapsulation of the drug molecules in nanoparticles. Inclusion of targeting ligands on the surface of nanoparticles has the potential of tumor-specific drug delivery and retention, thus, minimizing systemic toxicity [95].

Recently, numerous reports have been published showing encapsulation of chemotherapeutic agents such as doxorubicin and paclitaxel in liposomes or micelles. These encapsulated drugs exhibited high intracellular accumulations and 5–10-fold lower IC_{50} values in P-gp overexpressing cell lines in comparison with the free drugs [97]. Furthermore, accumulation DOX in the xenograft was approximately 20-fold higher when doxorubicin-loaded micelles with folate in their surface were administered in mice [98].

3.4.9 Antibodies Specific to the MDR1 Protein

To avoid the clinical side effects associated with a pharmacological chemosensitizer, monoclonal antibodies recognizing the P-gp have been explored as potential inhibitors of the P-gp. The studies using MRK-16, one of the P-gp monoclonal antibodies, suggested that their use, together with MDR-related cytotoxic drugs with or without a chemosensitizer, may have a potential effect as an anti-MDR therapy [99, 100]. Besides MRK-16, another monoclonal antibody UIC2 that targets the extracellular domain of the P-gp has been characterized [34]. However, an effective delivery of these large-molecular-weight monoclonal antibodies is a challenging task. To overcome this issue, recombinant DNA technology can be exercised to isolate new recombinant scFv antibodies that have a much smaller molecular weight with desired specificity and affinity directed toward a large array of antigens such as the MDR1 protein. Haus-Cohen et al. isolated and characterized such a recombinant scFv fragment capable of disrupting P-gp efflux activity, thereby reversing the MDR phenotype of drug-resistant human tumor cell lines [101].

3.5 INFLUX TRANSPORTERS

Influx transporters are integral plasma membrane proteins that control the influx of essential nutrients and ions. The presence of these transporters has been reported on various tissues and cell lines. These proteins play an important role in drug delivery. These influx transporters belong to the SLC

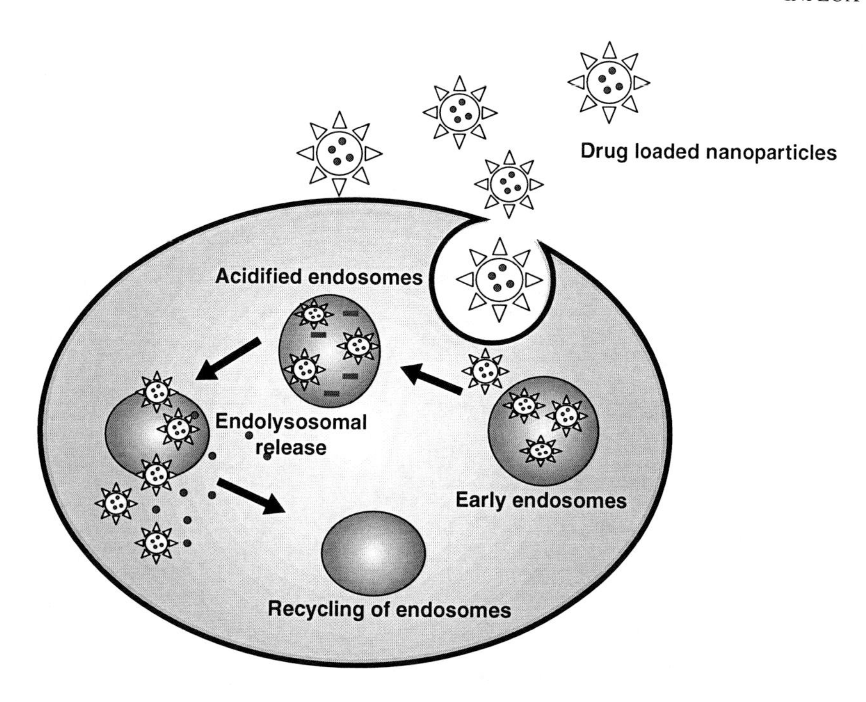

FIGURE 3.6 Evasion of MDR efflux proteins by surface-decorated nanoparticles: Substrate drug molecules encapsulated in the nanoparticles can evade MDR proteins during endocytosis. Adapted from Ref. 96.

(solute carrier) transporter family. These include carriers for peptides, vitamins, organic anions, organic cations, glucose, and other nutrients. These transporters are involved in pharmacokinetic and pharmacodynamic pathways of a drug molecule. Several drug molecules are modified chemically to achieve the desired lipophilicity and solubility, which will ultimately improve drug bioavailability. Designing a transporter targeted drug can be considered a rational approach for improving drug bioavailability. These modified drugs are often called "prodrugs" that are designed to target influx transporters. In this section, we will be discussing the influx transporters that can be exploited as molecular targets for tissue-selective drug delivery that may reduce systemic toxicity [102, 103]

3.5.1 Peptide Transporters

The cellular intake of dipeptides and tripeptides along with other peptidomimetics is mediated by peptide transporters. In mammals, two peptide transporters have been identified, peptide transporter 1 (PEPT1, SLC15A1) and peptide transporter 2 (PEPT2, SLC15A2). PEPT1 and PEPT2 share similar topology and consist of 708 and 709 amino acid residues, respectively. Apart from the intestine, PEPT is present in many tissues such as the colon, kidney, liver, lung, mammary gland, pancreas, eye, and central nervous system (CNS; Table 3.5) . Various drugs and prodrugs are substrates for peptide transporters like β-lactam antibiotics (cefadroxil, cefime, cefadrine, cycleacilin, and ceftibuten), angiotensin converting enzyme (ACE) inhibitors (captopril, enalapril, and fosinopril), aminopeptidase inhibitors (bestatin), and prodrug and nonpeptidic compounds (L-DOPA and valacyclovir; Table 3.6) [104]. Drug molecules can be chemically modified by introducing structural fragments (valyl, leucyl, isoleucyl, or glycine residues) for recognition by peptide transporters. Such a strategy has been successfully employed to nucleoside drugs such as acyclovir [105–107], ganciclovir [105, 108], azidothymidine [105, 109], floxuridine [105, 110], HIV protease inhibitors [93, 105], and L-DOPA [105, 111, 112] resulting in a significant improvement of oral absorption of these drugs by making use of the peptide transporter pathways [105]. To exert their pharmacological activity, these peptide prodrugs are metabolized by peptidase to release the free active drugs required for desired therapeutic effects.

Dipeptides, tripeptides, β-lactams, ACE inhibitors, and several prodrugs are taken up into cells by peptide transporter 1 (PEPT1) and PEPT2, against a concentration gradient. The acidic pH of the intestine generated by the brush-border Na^+/H^+ exchanger serves as the driving force for intestinal absorption of dipeptides and tripeptides and peptidomimetic drugs. The velocity of transport is determined by membrane voltage. By and large, the proton gradient is generated and maintained by NHE-3, the apical $Na^+–H^+$ antiporter with intracellular Na^+ removed by $Na^+–K^+$ ATPase in the basolateral membrane. Whereas dipeptides and tripeptides undergo rapid intracellular hydrolysis, free amino acids leave cells via basolateral transporters. Hydrolysis-resistant

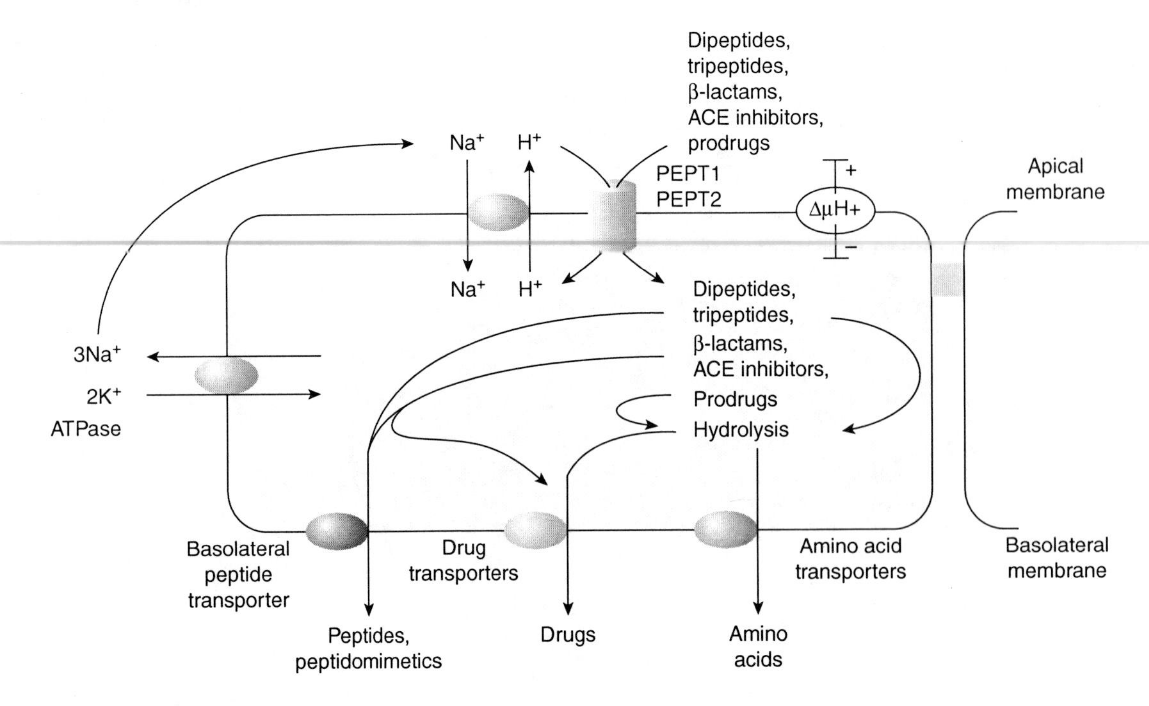

FIGURE 3.7 Model of peptide transport in epithelial cells from intestine and kidney. Reproduced with permission from Ref. 104.

substrates, such as most peptidomimetics, are released into the circulation by a basolateral peptide transporter that is yet to be identified or by other drug-transporting systems. A list of clinically relevant drugs or inhibitors of peptide transporter is presented in Table 3.6 and Figure 3.7.

3.5.2 Organic Anion Transporting Polypeptide (OATP)

OATPs are the members of the solute carrier organic anion transporter family (SLCO) classified within the SLC superfamily. The OATP protein encodes for 643–722 amino acids and has 9–12 transmembrane domains with intracellular amino and carboxy termini [138]. So far, 11 human isoforms (Table 3.7) and 14 rat isoforms have been identified in the OATP family. The OATP superfamily has been divided according to amino acid sequence identity, i.e., families (≥40% amino acid sequence identity) and subfamilies (≥60% amino acid sequence identity). OATP1B1, −1B3, and −2B1 are involved in the hepatic uptake of bulky and relatively hydrophobic organic anions. Several other OATPs are expressed in many tissues, such as the choroids

TABLE 3.5 Distribution of Peptide Transporters in Tissues, Cells, and Subcellular Compartments

Transporters	Tissue	Localization	References
PEPT1	Small intestine	Brush border membrane of enterocytes	[104, 113]
	Kidney	Brush border membrane of epithelial cells of the proximal tubule S1 segment	[104, 114]
	Bile duct	Apical membrane of cholangiocytes	[104, 115]
	Pancreas	Lysosomes of acinar cells	[104, 116]
	Cornea	Apical membrane	[117]
PEPT2	Kidney	Brush border membrane of epithelial cells of the proximal tubule (S2 and S3 segment)	[104, 114]
	Central nervous system	Epithelial cells of the choroid plexus, ependymal cells and astrocytes	[104, 118]
	Peripheral nervous system	Membrane and cytoplasm of glial cells	[104, 119]
	Lung	Apical membrane of bronchial and tracheal epithelial cells, membrane and cytoplasm pneumocytes type II	[104, 120]
	Mammary gland	Epithelial cells of the glands and ducts	[104, 121]
	Cornea	Apical membrane	[117]
	Iris ciliary body	—	[117]
	Retina/choroid	Basolateral membrane	[117]

Modified from Ref. 104.

TABLE 3.6 Example of Various Drugs/Prodrugs Acting as Substrates/Competitive Inhibitors of Peptide Transporters

Drug	Substrates/Competitive Inhibitors of		References
	PEPT1	PEPT2	
β-lactam antibiotics	+	+	[111, 122, 123]
Cephalexin	+	+	[111, 124]
Ceftibuten	+	+	[111, 125, 126]
Cefadroxil	+	+	[111, 127, 128]
Ciclacillin	+	+	[111, 124, 129]
Cefixime			
Photosensitizing agents	+	+	[111, 130]
5-Aminolevulinic acid			
Antitumor agents	+	+	[111, 131]
Bestatin	+	n.d.	[111, 132]
Floxuridine (prolyl and lysil prodrugs)			
Hypotensives	+	n.d.	[111, 133]
Midodrine			
Antivirals	+	+	[108, 111, 134]
Acyclovir	+	n.d.	[111, 134]
Zidovudine			
Dopamine receptor interactors	+	n.d.	[111, 135]
Sulpiride	+	n.d.	[111, 112]
Amino ester derivatives of L-DOPA			
Angiotensin-converting enzyme (ACE) inhibitors	+	+	[111, 136]
Fosinopril	+	+	[111, 137]
Captopril	+	+	[111, 137]
Enalapril			

+: Confirmed; n.d.: not determined.

plexus, brain, placenta, heart, intestine, lungs, kidneys, and testes [139]. Substrates for OATP include bile acids, eicosanoids, steroids, thyroid hormones, and their conjugates as well as xenobiotics such as anionic oligopeptides, organic dyes, several toxins, and numerous drugs (Table 3.7) [138, 140]. OATPs are ubiquitously expressed in the human body and mediate the Na^+-independent uptake of a wide range of amphipathic molecules (molecular weight > 300 kDa). The substrates of OATP are not limited to anions; they also transport cationic and neutral compounds. Altered expression levels of OATPs have been reported in different types of cancers (Table 3.8) [141].

3.5.3 Organic Anion Transporter (OAT)

OATs are another family of multispecific transporters, the major facilitator superfamily (MFS), and are encoded by the SLC22/Slc22 gene superfamily. OATs differ in their composition of amino acids. Human OAT1 and OAT3 consist of 563 and 542 amino acids, respectively. They have 12 α-helical transmembrane domains (TMDs) with intracellular amino and carboxy-termini [177, 178]. The main function of these transporters is to act as transmembrane uniporters, symporters, and antiporters and to translocate a diverse range of xenobiotics (drugs and toxins), endogenous metabolites (amino acids, sugars, neurotransmitters, etc.), and hydrophilic and amphiphilic substrates including inorganic ions (Na^+, Cl^-, HCO_3^-, etc.). They are responsible for the uptake of a wide range of low-molecular-weight substrates including steroid hormone conjugates, biogenic amines, various drugs, and toxins (Table 3.9) [177–181]. As a result of their expression on liver and kidneys, they might play a substantial role in maintaining endogenous homeostasis. They are capable of translocating a number of prescribed pharmaceuticals, such as loop and thiazide diuretics, methotrexate, ACE inhibitors, nonsteroidal anti-inflammatory drugs, and β-lactam antibiotics [182]. The presence of OATs on olfactory mucosa, choroid plexus, and retina corroborates their involvement in secretory processes [183]. The OAT family majorly represents the classic renal organic anion transport system. So far, eight isoforms (OAT 1–7 and URAT 1) of OAT have been identified (Table 3.9). Members of OAT belong to the SLC22A gene family and are structurally similar to organic cation transporters (OCTs) [139]. It is of clinical importance to understand the transport mechanism of OATs for critical elucidation related to drug handling and nephrotoxicity.

3.5.4 Organic Cation Transporter (OCT)

OCTs are also members of the SLC22A family of SLC transporters including novel organic cation transporters

TABLE 3.7 Characteristics and Selective Substrates of Human OATP Family Members

Protein Name	Amino Acids	Tissue Distribution	Substrates	Kinetic Parameter (K_m)	References
OATP1A2	670	Brain, kidney	Bromosulfophthalein	20 μM	[142–146]
			Estrone-3-sulfate	16 μM	
			Rosuvastatin	3 μM	
			Saquinavir	36 μM	
			Fexofenadine	6 μM	
OATP1B1	691	Liver	Atorvastatin	10 μM	[147–151]
			Bilirubin	0.01 μM	
			Estrone-3-sulfate	0.5 μM	
			Valsartan	1.4 μM	
			Enalapril	262 μM	
OATP1B3	702	Liver	Amanitin	4 μM	[151–157]
			Estradiol-17β-glucuronide	5–25 μM	
			Methotrexate	25–39 μM	
			Paciltaxel	7 μM	
			Rifampicin	2 μM	
OATP1C1	712	Brain, testis	Reverse triiodothyronine	0.12 μM	[158]
			Thyroxine	0.09 μM	
OATP2A1	643	Ubiquitous	Latanoprost	5.4 μM	[159]
OATP2B1	709	Ubiquitous	Fluvastatin	0.7 μM	[160–162]
			Bosentan	202 μM	
			Taurocholate	72 μM	
OATP3A1	710	Ubiquitous	Prostaglandin E1	0.05–0.1 μM	[163, 164]
			Prostagalndin E2	0.06–0.2 μM	
OATP4A1	722	Ubiquitous	Taurocholate	15 μM	[165]
			Triiodothyronine	1 μM	
OATP4C1	724	Kidney	Digoxin	8 μM	[166]
			Oubain	0.4 μM	
OATP5A1	848	—	—	—	—
OATP6A1	719	Testis	—	—	—

OCTN1 and OCTN2 (encoded by genes SLC22A4 and SLC22A5, respectively). They are responsible for the uptake of a wide range of low-molecular-weight, relatively hydrophilic organic cations such as prototypical cation TEA, neurotoxin MPP+, and endogenous compound N-methylnicotinamide (NMN) (Table 3.10) [201–203]. OCT consists of 543–557 amino acids. They have 12 TMDs with intracellular amino and carboxy-termini. Facilitated diffusion driven by the inside-negative membrane potential is the mechanism of uptake of organic cations via OCT [177, 201, 204–209]. The substrates of the OCTs are mostly cations with a rare exception for anionic or neutral compounds at physiological pH. Three isoforms of OCTs (OCT 1–3) have been cloned from humans, rabbits, rats, and mice. The paralogs of OCT1 and OCT2 share about 68–69% sequence homology for humans, rats, and mice, and 71% for rabbits [210]. Substrate specificity for orthologous OCT may vary as a result of difference in species. For example, the transport of tetrapropylammonium (TPA) or tetrabutylammonium (TBA) is mediated by human and rabbit OCT1 but not by rat and mouse Oct1. This example acts as a supporting statement for differences in recognition of OCT

TABLE 3.8 Expression of OATP in Various Cancer Tissues

	Cancer Tissue Expression		
OATP	Increased	Decreased	References
OATP1A2	In breast carcinoma cells and malignant breast tissue	In colon polyps and cancer	[167–169]
OATP1B1	—	In hepatocellular carcinoma	[170, 171]
OATP1B3	—	In hepatocellular carcinoma	[172]
OATP2A1	In malignant breast tissue and liver cancer	In tumors of bowel, stomach, ovary, lung, and kidney	[173–175]
OATP2B1	In bone cysts	—	[176]

TABLE 3.9 Tissue expression and Prototypical Substrates of OAT Family Members

	Tissue Expression				
OAT	Apical	Basolateral	Substrates	Inhibitors	References
OAT1	Mouse and rat choroid plexus	Renal proximal tubules and plasma membrane of skeletal muscles	p-Aminohippurate	Probenecid, novobiocin	[2, 177, 184–190]
OAT2	—	Renal proximal tubules and hepatocytes (rodents)	p-Aminohippurate	Bumetanide, chlorothiazide, cyclothiazide	[177, 191, 192]
OAT3	—	Renal proximal tubules	Estrone 3-sulfate	Probenecid, novobiocin	[2, 177, 193]
OAT4	Renal proximal tubules	Syncytiotrophoblasts in placenta	Estrone 3-sulfate	Olmesartan, telmisartan	[177, 191, 194–196]
OAT5	—	—	Ochratoxin A	Bumetanide, furosemide	[177, 191, 197]
OAT6	—	—	Estrone 3-sulfate	Benzylpenicillin, carbenicillin	[177, 191, 198]
OAT7	—	Hepatocytes	Estrone 3-sulfate	—	[177, 199]
URAT1	Renal proximal tubules	—	Urate	Losartan, telmisartan, furosemide	[177, 191, 200]

substrates across species [211]. Both the tissue expression and the localization of OCTs (Table 3.10) show that these transporters play a governing role in the excretion of toxic xenobiotic and endogenous organic cations. Their crucial involvement in drug disposition or drug response depicts tissue expression, substrate, and inhibitor specificity of the OCT family.

3.5.5 Sodium-Dependent Multivitamin Transporter (SMVT)

The SMVT is an important plasma membrane protein that facilitates the cellular uptake of vitamins and other essential co-factors such as biotin, pantothenic acid, and lipoic acid. The SMVT primarily facilitates the cellular uptake of biotin (vitamin B7) and is a highly sodium-dependent specific

TABLE 3.10 Tissue Expression and Substrates of OCT Family Members

	Tissue Expression				
OCT	Apical	Basolateral	Substrates	Inhibitors	References
OCT1	Lung epithelial cells	Hepatocytes, rodents, enterocytes, and proximal tubule epithelial cells (rodents)	Acyclovir, famotidine, metformin etc.	Quinine, quinidine, disopyramide	[2, 177, 201, 212–215]
OCT2	Lung epithelial cells	Distal convoluted tubules	Cimetidine, dopamine, metformin, etc.	Cimetidine, pilsicainide, cetirizine, testosterone, quinidine	[2, 177, 202, 203, 212, 214, 216]
OCT3	Lung epithelial cells and enterocytes	Hepatocytes and trophoblasts	Cimetidine, histamine, serotonin etc.	β-Estradiol, corticosterone, deoxycorticosterone, progesterone	[177, 202, 203, 214, 217–220]
OCTN1	Renal epithelial cells (rodents), intestinal epithelial cells, and lung epithelial cells	—	—	—	[177, 221]
OCTN2	Renal proximal tubules, syncytiotrophoblasts in placenta, and lung epithelial cells	—	—	—	[177, 222, 223]

vitamin carrier system. It has been referred to as the sodium-dependent multivitamin transporter because of its sodium and substrate specificity. The SMVT protein encodes for 635 amino acids and has 12 transmembrane domains. The expression of SMVT has been reported in various tissues such as placenta, intestine, brain, liver, lung, kidney, cornea, retina, and heart. Biotin has been used in drug delivery by covalently attaching or by surface modification of various therapeutic molecules [224]. Russell-Jones et al. reported on enhanced tumor accumulation of biotinylated fluorescently-labeled N-(2-hydroxypropyl) methacrylamide (HPMA) polymers after intravenous administration in mice [225]. Biotin has also been employed as a target moiety to deliver large peptides orally by varying the absorptive transport pathways and improving intestinal permeability. Ramanathan et al. demonstrated enhanced cellular accumulation of biotinylated PEG-based conjugates of Tat9 via the SMVT in Caco-2 and transfected CHO cells. The 29-kDa, peptide-loaded bioconjugate [PEG:(R.I-Cys-K(biotin)-Tat9)8] and biotin-PEG-3400 interact with human SMVTs to enhance the cellular accumulation of these large molecules. This strategy of conjugating high-molecular-weight compounds with targeting moiety enhances the intestinal absorption and oral bioavailability of macromolecules [224, 226]. Biotin-ganciclovir (B-GCV) uptake mediated by the SMVT was substantially higher compared with ganciclovir in both ARPE-19 cells and rabbit retina [227]. This study secularizes the intravitreal pharmacokinetics of GCV and B-GCV

TABLE 3.11 An Overview of Tissue Distribution and Kinetic Parameters of the SMVT on Cellular Accumulation

	Michaelis–Menten Kinetic Parameters		
Cells/Tissue	K_m	V_{max}	References
Bovine brain microvessel endothelial cells (BMECs)	49.1 μM	313.2 pmoles/mg protein/min	[229]
Human colonic epithelial cells (NCM460)	19.7 μM	38.8 pmoles/mg protein/3 min	[230]
Human-derived prostate cancer cells (PC-3)	19 μM	23 pmoles/min/mg protein	[231]
Human corneal epithelial (HCE) cells	296.23 μM	77.23 pmol/mgprotein/min	[232]
Human retinal pigmented epithelial cells (ARPE-19 and D407)	138.25 μM (ARPE-19) and 863.81 μM (D407)	38.85 pmoles/mg protein/min (ARPE-19) and 308.26 pmol/mgprotein/min (D407)	[228, 232]
Canine kidney cells (MDCK-MDR1) transfected with human *MDR1* gene	13 μM	21.5 pmoles/mg protein/min	[233]
Human retinoblastoma cells (Y-79)	8.53 μM	14.12 pmoles/mg protein/min	[234]
Human placental brush-border membrane	21 μM	4.5 nmoles/mg protein/min	[235]
Rabbit corneal epithelial cells (rPCECs)	32.52 μM	10.43 pmoles/mg protein/min	[227]
Rat retinal capillary endothelial cells (TR-iBRB2)	146 μM	0.223 nmoles/mg protein/min	[236]
Human proximal tubular epithelial cells (HK-2)	12.16 μM	14.4 pmoles/mg protein/7 min	[237]
Human intestinal cells (Caco-2)	9.5 μM	520 pmoles/mg protein/min	[238]
Human kidney cortex brush-border membrane	31 μM	82 nmoles/mg protein/30 sec	[239]
Human liver basolateral membrane vesicles	1.22 μM	4.76 pmoles/mg protein/10 sec	[240]
Human intestinal brush-border membrane (BBM)	5.26 μM	13.47 pmoles/mg protein/20 sec	[241]
Human rat kidney cortex brush-border membrane vesicles	55 μM	217 pmoles/mg protein/sec	[242]

by an ocular microdialysis technique. The AUC of Biotin-GCV (17.5 ± 1.38 mg*min*mL^{-1}) was significantly higher than GCV (10.6 ± 1.27 mg*min*mL^{-1}), and no statistically significant difference was observed between the half-lives of GCV and B-GCV [228]. The tissue distribution and kinetic parameters of the SMVT are presented in Table 3.11.

3.5.6 Sodium-Dependent Vitamin C Transporters (SVCT1 and SVCT2)

Ascorbic acid (AA or vitamin C) is an essential nutrient required for cellular function, wound healing, and immunity. Sodium-dependent vitamin C transporters (SVCT1 and SVCT2) were cloned recently from human and rat DNA libraries [243–245]. Both isoforms have a similar function and can mediate L-AA transport. This transporter is present in many tissues such as intestine [246, 247], kidney [248, 249], brain [250, 251], eye [252, 253], bone [254], and skin [255]. Luo et al. [256] reported on the presence of SVCT1 and SVCT2 in MDCK cells. Although SVCT1 expresses mainly on the apical membrane, SVCT2 is present on both the apical and the basolateral membrane. Uptake of ascorbic acid in MDCK-MDR1 cells seems to be a saturable and concentration-dependent process in a range with K_m of 83.2 μM and 7.27 μM for SVCT1 and SVCT2, respectively. Analysis of a deduced primary amino acid sequence of hSVCT1 and hSVCT2 suggests the presence of five putative PKC phosphorylation sites, while SVCT1 possesses an additional PKA site [257]. Various inter- and intracellular stimuli (hormones, paracrine factors, signaling molecules, etc.) are engaged in the expression of SVCT [258].

3.6 *IN VITRO* MODELS TO STUDY TRANSPORTERS

There are numerous cell-based models to study the function of these transporters. Kwatra et al. [259, 260] recently described the different models in detail. Although these cell-based models are easy-to-produce data, suitable for high-throughput screening, they also give some idea how these transporters operate. For example, colon carcinoma derived from the Caco2 cell and Madin–Darby canine kidney (MDCK) cells transfected with MDR1, MRP2, or BCRP are used for oral absorption studies. These efflux transporters in intestine work in conjunction with metabolizing enzyme cytochrome P-450 (CYP). Although both Caco2 cells and transfected MDCK cells express the efflux transporter, they do not contain CYP. Therefore, drug-transport data across these cell monolayers fail to produce equivalent *in vivo* kinetics data for oral absorption. We have developed the MDCK-MDR1-CYP3A4 cell line (MMC) as a model for oral absorption study [259]. This MMC along with the dual-chamber model containing hepatocytes or Hep-G2 transfected with CYP3A4 in the bottom chamber of transwell (Corning Costar Corp, Cambridge, MA) (Figure 3.8) may produce an equivalent *in vivo* kinetics data for oral absorption study. LS180 is another cell line that expresses both the efflux transporter and CYP but lacks sufficient tight junctions; therefore, it is unsuitable for drug transport studies. Several groups use CHO cells for transfection and functional characterization studies of a single transporter. This is a very good model for transporter characterization purposes. In our laboratory, we employ different corneal (SIRC, rPCC, and hCEC)

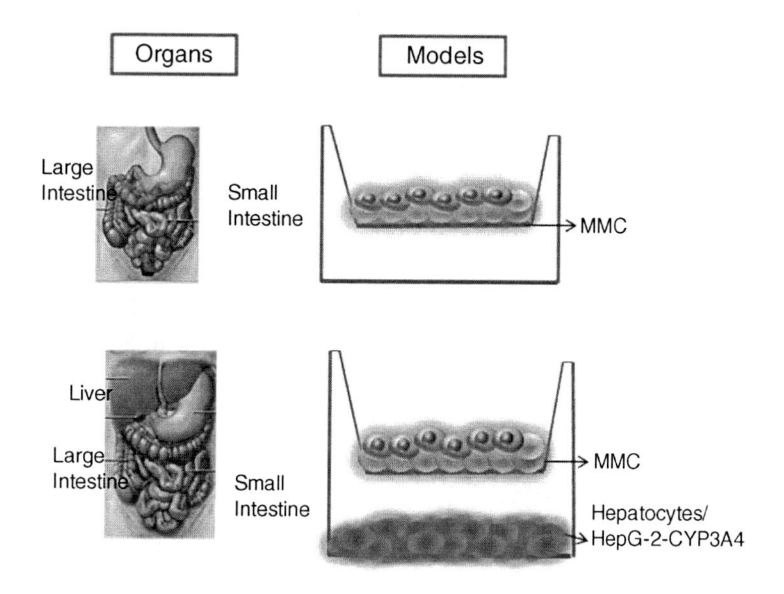

FIGURE 3.8 *In vitro* models for oral absorption studies of the MDCK-MDR1-CYP3A4 cell line (MMC) and the hepatic cell line transfected with CYP3A4 (HepG2-CYP3A4).

and retinal (ARPE19 and D407) cells for studying transporter-mediated drug delivery to the eye. These cell lines also lack sufficient tight junctions and cannot exactly generate equivalent *in vivo* kinetics data. Similarly, for BBB study, there are human, bovine, or rat brain microvessel endothelial cells, but none of these cell monolayers have sufficient tight junctions comparable with *in vivo* BBB. Therefore, it is not easy to select an *in vitro* model to investigate transporter-mediated drug delivery.

3.7 CONCLUSION

The new frontier of transporter research is forthcoming comprising transporter expression in normal cells versus cancer cells. In addition to increasing MDR, the tumor cells overexpress selected nutrient transporters. To meet an increased demand for nutrients for rapid proliferation, tumor cells upregulate glucose transporters (GLUT1/SLC2A1 and Na^+-coupled SGLT1) as well as amino acid transporters such as MCTs (monocarboxilates) [261]. Recently we have also shown that an enhanced uptake of folic acid, biotin, and arginine along with overexpression of FRα, SMVT, and $B^{(0,+)}$ (folate, multivitamin, and amino acid transporters, respectively) in retinoblastoma cells (Y79) compared with normal pigmented retinal epithelial cells (ARPE19) [262]. Overexpression of FRα has been reported in many cancer tissues such as breast ovarian cancer, mesothelioma, and breast, colon, renal, and lung tumors [263–268].

Numerous drug transporters are present, and several have been exploited for drug delivery, but the transport mechanisms of a few transporters have been only recently uncovered. Although it is important to identify all possible participants, their relative contributions in drug–drug interactions will give immediate benefit to determine the appropriate dose and target for the individual drug. Among numerous drug transporters, up to now, only P-gps, BCRPs, OATPs, OCTs, and OATs have been identified as critical players in clinical practice. To evaluate the ADME properties of drug molecules, transporter information is required by the FDA for drug labeling. Recently, the FDA has issued Drug Interaction Guidance to build up a strategy for addressing the transporter issue at the beginning of drug development [269–271].

The ITC has also provided guidance on using decision trees to delineate transporter-mediated drug–drug interactions [2]. The decision trees are subjected to modifications as transporter pharmacology advances. During development of new molecular entities (NMEs), the ITC has placed emphasis on the role of transporters, particularly the P-gp and BCRP in intestinal absorption and distribution across the blood-brain barrier. The other transporters such as OATP1B1, OATP 1B3, and OATP2B1 are also important for hepatocyte uptake and OATs and OCTs for renal excretion. It is imperative to consider that efflux transporters enhance the function of drug metabolizing in the intestine and liver. The subject becomes more complex when there may be superfluous influx and efflux in a given tissue and multiple transporters with overlapping substrate specificities control the drug concentration in that tissue. Another critical issue of selecting inhibitor(s) for delivering drugs is when one drug is a substrate for multiple transporters. For example, the concentration of vandetanib (a chemotherapeutic agent), a substrate for both the P-gp and BCRP, did not substantially enhance in the mouse brain in the presence of either specific P-gp (LY335979) or Bcrp1 (Ko143) inhibitors. Co-administration of elacridar, a dual P-gp/BCRP inhibitor, substantially enhanced the brain concentration of vandetanib. This suggests that appropriate selection of a drug combination is prudent to evade efflux for effective therapeutic success. As tumor cells overexpress, certain nutrient transporters such as folate or the biotin transporter can be used for tumor detection or for targeted drug delivery.

ASSESSMENT QUESTIONS

3.1. Write a brief note on membrane transporters, both influx and efflux transporters, that affect drug delivery.

3.2. MRP4 is localized on ___ side(s) of the intestine.

a. Apical
b. Basolateral
c. Apical and basolateral

3.3. Which of the efflux transporters is regarded as a "half transporter" because of its transmembrane domains?

a. P-glycoprotein
b. Multidrug resistance associated protein
c. Breast cancer resistant protein
d. None of the above

3.4. What are the strategies to overcome MDR-mediated efflux in drug delivery?

a. MDR modulators/inhibitors
b. Prodrug derivatization
c. Utilization of nanotechnology
d. Antibody targeted therapy
e. Both a and b
f. Both c and d
g. All of the above

3.5. How many isoform of peptide transporters have been identified in mammals?

a. 2
b. 4

c. 5
d. 7

3.6. Which OATP transporters are responsible for hepatic uptake of organic anions or amphipathic molecules?
a. OATP 1B1
b. OATP 1B3
c. OATP 2B1
d. OATP 1C1
e. OATP 4A1
f. A, B, and C

3.7. Which transporter(s) facilitates the cellular uptake of vitamins?

3.8. The SMVT protein encodes for __ amino acids and has __ transmembrane domains.
a. 635, 12
b. 557,12
c. 563, 12
d. 722, 9
e. 709, 12

3.9. Write a short explanation of sodium-dependent vitamin C transporters.

3.10. Describe the evasion of MDR efflux proteins by nanoparticles.

REFERENCES

1. Giacomini, K.M., Sugiyama, Y. *Membrane Transporters and Drug Response: Introduction*, Brunton, L.L., Chabner, B.A., Knollmann, B. C. (eds.), The McGraw-Hill Companies, New York, NY, 2011.
2. Giacomini, K.M., et al. (2010). Membrane transporters in drug development. *Nature Reviews Drug Discovery*, *9*, 215–236.
3. Borst, P., Elferink, R.O. (2002). Mammalian ABC transporters in health and disease. *Annual Review of Biochemistry*, *71*, 537–592.
4. Ambudkar, S.V., et al. (2003). P-glycoprotein: From genomics to mechanism. *Oncogene*, *22*, 7468–7485.
5. Gottesman, M.M. (2002). Mechanisms of cancer drug resistance. *Annual Review of Medicine*, *53*, 615–627.
6. Lin, J.H., Yamazaki, M. (2003). Clinical relevance of P-glycoprotein in drug therapy. *Drug Metabolism Reviews*, *35*, 417–454.
7. Juliano, R.L., Ling, V. (1976). A surface glycoprotein modulating drug permeability in Chinese hamster ovary cell mutants. *Biochimica et Biophysica Acta*, *455*, 152–162.
8. Kessel, D., Bosmann, H.B. (1970). Effects of L-asparaginase on protein and glycoprotein synthesis. *FEBS Letters*, *10*, 85–88.
9. Biedler, J.L., Riehm, H. (1970). Cellular resistance to actinomycin D in Chinese hamster cells in vitro: Cross-resistance, radioautographic, and cytogenetic studies. *Cancer Research*, *30*, 1174–1184.
10. Higgins, C.F. (1992). ABC transporters: From microorganisms to man. *Annual Review of Cell Biology*, *8*, 67–113.
11. Tusnady, G.E., et al. (1997). Membrane topology distinguishes a subfamily of the ATP-binding cassette (ABC) transporters. *FEBS Letters*, *402*, 1–3.
12. Kast, C., et al. (1995). Membrane topology of P-glycoprotein as determined by epitope insertion: Transmembrane organization of the N-terminal domain of mdr3. *Biochemistry*, *34*, 4402–4411.
13. Locher, K.P., Borths, E. (2004). ABC transporter architecture and mechanism: Implications from the crystal structures of BtuCD and BtuF. *FEBS Letters*, *564*, 264–268.
14. Kerr, I.D. (2002). Structure and association of ATP-binding cassette transporter nucleotide-binding domains. *Biochimica et Biophysica Acta*, *1561*, 47–64.
15. Dean, M., Rzhetsky, A., Allikmets, R. (2001). The human ATP-binding cassette (ABC) transporter superfamily. *Genome Research*, *11*, 1156–1166.
16. Linton, K.J., Higgins, C.F. (1998). The Escherichia coli ATP-binding cassette (ABC) proteins. *Molecular Microbiology*, *28*, 5–13.
17. Hrycyna, C.A., et al. (1998). Structural flexibility of the linker region of human P-glycoprotein permits ATP hydrolysis and drug transport. *Biochemistry*, *37*, 13660–13673.
18. Sauna, Z.E., Nandigama, K., Ambudkar, S.V. (2006). Exploiting reaction intermediates of the ATPase reaction to elucidate the mechanism of transport by P-glycoprotein (ABCB1). *Journal of Biological Chemistry*, *281*, 26501–26511.
19. Zaitseva, J., et al. (2005). A molecular understanding of the catalytic cycle of the nucleotide-binding domain of the ABC transporter HlyB. *Biochemical Society Transactions*, *33*, 990–995.
20. Jones, P.M., George, A.M. (2004). The ABC transporter structure and mechanism: Perspectives on recent research. *Cellular and Molecular Life Sciences*, *61*, 682–699.
21. Hulot, J.S., et al. (2005). A mutation in the drug transporter gene ABCC2 associated with impaired methotrexate elimination. *Pharmacogenet Genomics*, *15*, 277–285.
22. Letourneau, I.J., et al. (2005). Limited modulation of the transport activity of the human multidrug resistance proteins MRP1, MRP2 and MRP3 by nicotine glucuronide metabolites. *Toxicology Letters*, *157*, 9–19.
23. Huisman, M.T., et al. (2002). Multidrug resistance protein 2 (MRP2) transports HIV protease inhibitors, and transport can be enhanced by other drugs. *AIDS*, *16*, 2295–2301.
24. Naruhashi, K., et al. (2002). Involvement of multidrug resistance-associated protein 2 in intestinal secretion of grepafloxacin in rats. *Antimicrobial Agents and Chemotherapy*, *46*, 344–349.
25. Bakos, E., et al. (2000). Interactions of the human multidrug resistance proteins MRP1 and MRP2 with organic anions. *Molecular Pharmacology*, *57*, 760–768.

26. Wacher, V.J., et al. (1998). Role of P-glycoprotein and cytochrome P450 3A in limiting oral absorption of peptides and peptidomimetics. *Journal of Pharmacy & Pharmaceutical Sciences*, *87*, 1322–1330.
27. Sharom, F.J. (1997). The P-glycoprotein efflux pump: How does it transport drugs? *Journal of Membrane Biology*, *160*, 161–175.
28. Pal, D., et al. (2011). Efflux transporters- and cytochrome P-450-mediated interactions between drugs of abuse and antiretrovirals. *Life Science*, *88*, 959–971.
29. Pal, D., Mitra, A.K. (2006). MDR- and CYP3A4-mediated drug-herbal interactions. *Life Science*, *78*, 2131–2145.
30. Borst, P., et al. (2000). A family of drug transporters: The multidrug resistance-associated proteins. *Journal of the National Cancer Institute*, *92*, 1295–1302.
31. Borst, P., et al. (1993). Classical and novel forms of multidrug resistance and the physiological functions of P-glycoproteins in mammals. *Pharmacology Therapy*, *60*, 289–299.
32. Gottesman, M.M., Pastan, I. (1993). Biochemistry of multidrug resistance mediated by the multidrug transporter. *Annual Review of Biochemistry*, *62*, 385–427.
33. Ueda, K., et al. (1992). Human P-glycoprotein transports cortisol, aldosterone, and dexamethasone, but not progesterone. *Journal of Biological Chemistry*, *267*, 24248–24252.
34. Mechetner, E.B., Roninson, I.B. (1992). Efficient inhibition of P-glycoprotein-mediated multidrug resistance with a monoclonal antibody. *Proceedings of the National Academy of Sciences USA*, *89*, 5824–5828.
35. Hofsli, E., Nissen-Meyer, J. (1989). Reversal of drug resistance by erythromycin: Erythromycin increases the accumulation of actinomycin D and doxorubicin in multidrug-resistant cells. *International Journal of Cancer*, *44*, 149–154.
36. Roninson, I.B., et al. (1984). Amplification of specific DNA sequences correlates with multi-drug resistance in Chinese hamster cells. *Nature*, *309*, 626–628.
37. Bech-Hansen, N.T., Till, J.E., Ling, V. (1976). Pleiotropic phenotype of colchicine-resistant CHO cells: Cross-resistance and collateral sensitivity. *Journal of Cellular Physiology*, *88*, 23–31.
38. Takano, M., Yumoto, R., Murakami, T. (2006). Expression and function of efflux drug transporters in the intestine. *Pharmacology Therapy*, *109*, 137–161.
39. Miller, D.S., et al. (2000). Xenobiotic transport across isolated brain microvessels studied by confocal microscopy. *Molecular Pharmacology*, *58*, 1357–1367.
40. Park, S., Sinko, P.J. (2005). P-glycoprotein and mutlidrug resistance-associated proteins limit the brain uptake of saquinavir in mice. *Journal of Pharmacology and Experimental Therapeutics*, *312*, 1249–1256.
41. Schinkel, A.H., Jonker, J.W. (2003). Mammalian drug efflux transporters of the ATP binding cassette (ABC) family: An overview. *Advanced Drug Delivery Reviews*, *55*, 3–29.
42. Staud, F., Pavek, P. (2005). Breast cancer resistance protein (BCRP/ABCG2). *The International Journal of Biochemistry & Cell Biology*, *37*, 720–725.
43. Zhang, Z., et al. (2004). Regulation of the stability of P-glycoprotein by ubiquitination. *Molecular Pharmacology*, *66*, 395–403.
44. Sarkadi, B., et al. (2004). ABCG2—a transporter for all seasons. *FEBS Letters*, *567*, 116–120.
45. Haimeur, A., et al. (2004). The MRP-related and BCRP/ABCG2 multidrug resistance proteins: Biology, substrate specificity and regulation. *Current Drug Metabolism*, *5*, 21–53.
46. Abbott, B.L. (2003). ABCG2 (BCRP) expression in normal and malignant hematopoietic cells. *Hematology Oncology*, *21*, 115–130.
47. Doyle, L.A., Ross, D.D. (2003). Multidrug resistance mediated by the breast cancer resistance protein BCRP (ABCG2). *Oncogene*, *22*, 7340–7358.
48. Ejendal, K.F., Hrycyna, C.A. (2002). Multidrug resistance and cancer: The role of the human ABC transporter ABCG2. *Current Protein & Peptide Science*, *3*, 503–511.
49. Hoffmeyer, S., et al. (2000). Functional polymorphisms of the human multidrug-resistance gene: Multiple sequence variations and correlation of one allele with P-glycoprotein expression and activity in vivo. *Proceedings of the National Academy of Sciences USA*, *97*, 3473–2478.
50. Fellay, J., et al. (2002). Response to antiretroviral treatment in HIV-1-infected individuals with allelic variants of the multidrug resistance transporter 1: A pharmacogenetics study. *Lancet*, *359*, 30–36.
51. Chowbay, B., Zhou, S., Lee, E.J. (2005). An interethnic comparison of polymorphisms of the genes encoding drug-metabolizing enzymes and drug transporters: Experience in Singapore. *Drug Metabolism Reviews*, *37*, 327–378.
52. Fung, K.L., Gottesman, M.M. (2009). A synonymous polymorphism in a common MDR1 (ABCB1) haplotype shapes protein function. *Biochimica et Biophysica Acta*, *1794*, 860–871.
53. Nakamura, T., et al. (2009). Effects of ABCB1 3435C > T genotype on serum levels of cortisol and aldosterone in women with normal menstrual cycles. *Genetics and Molecular Research*, *8*, 397–403.
54. Lamba, J., et al. (2006). MDR1 genotype is associated with hepatic cytochrome P450 3A4 basal and induction phenotype. *International Journal of Clinical Pharmacology*, *79*, 325–338.
55. Seelig, A. (1998). A general pattern for substrate recognition by P-glycoprotein. *European Journal of Biochemistry*, *251*, 252–261.
56. Ambudkar, S.V., et al. (1999). Biochemical, cellular, and pharmacological aspects of the multidrug transporter. *Annual Review of Pharmacology and Toxicology*, *39*, 361–398.
57. Schinkel, A.H. (1998). Pharmacological insights from P-glycoprotein knockout mice. *International Journal of Clinical Pharmacology, Therapy and Toxicology*, *36*, 9–13.
58. Agarwal, S., et al. (2011). Breast cancer resistance protein and P-glycoprotein in brain cancer: Two gatekeepers team up. *Current Pharmaceutical Design*, *17*, 2793–2802.

59. Mayer, U., et al. (1997). Full blockade of intestinal P-glycoprotein and extensive inhibition of blood-brain barrier P-glycoprotein by oral treatment of mice with PSC833. *Journal of Clinical Investigation*, *100*, 2430–2436.
60. Kiso, S., et al. (2000). Inhibitory effect of erythromycin on P-glycoprotein-mediated biliary excretion of doxorubicin in rats. *Anticancer Research*, *20*, 2827–2834.
61. Song, S., et al. (1999). Effect of PSC 833, a P-glycoprotein modulator, on the disposition of vincristine and digoxin in rats. *Drug Metabolism and Disposition*, *27*, 689–694.
62. Harker, W.G., et al. (1986). Verapamil-mediated sensitization of doxorubicin-selected pleiotropic resistance in human sarcoma cells: Selectivity for drugs which produce DNA scission. *Cancer Research*, *46*, 2369–2373.
63. Inaba, M., et al. (1979). Active efflux of daunorubicin and adriamycin in sensitive and resistant sublines of P388 leukemia. *Cancer Research*, *39*, 2200–2203.
64. Kuhl, J.S., et al. (1992). Use of etoposide in combination with cyclosporin for purging multidrug-resistant leukemic cells from bone marrow in a mouse model. *Experimental Hematology*, *20*, 1048–1054.
65. Eliason, J.F., Ramuz, H., Kaufmann, F. (1990). Human multidrug-resistant cancer cells exhibit a high degree of selectivity for stereoisomers of verapamil and quinidine. *International Journal of Cancer*, *46*, 113–117.
66. Sehested, M., et al. (1989). Inhibition of vincristine binding to plasma membrane vesicles from daunorubicin-resistant Ehrlich ascites cells by multidrug resistance modulators. *British Journal of Cancer*, *60*, 809–814.
67. Ozols, R.F., et al. (1987). Verapamil and adriamycin in the treatment of drug-resistant ovarian cancer patients. *Journal of Clinical Oncology*, *5*, 641–647.
68. Jonsson, B., et al. (1992). SDZ PSC-833—a novel potent in vitro chemosensitizer in multiple myeloma. *Anticancer Drugs*, *3*, 641–646.
69. Pirker, R., et al. (1989). Enhancement of the activity of immunotoxins by analogues of verapamil. *Cancer Research*, *49*, 4791–4795.
70. Giaccone, G., et al. (1997). A dose-finding and pharmacokinetic study of reversal of multidrug resistance with SDZ PSC 833 in combination with doxorubicin in patients with solid tumors. *Clinical Cancer Research*, *3*, 2005–2015.
71. Wilson, W.H., et al. (1995). Phase I and pharmacokinetic study of the multidrug resistance modulator dexverapamil with EPOCH chemotherapy. *Journal of Clinical Oncology*, *13*, 1985–1994.
72. Lum, B.L., Gosland, M.P. (1995). MDR expression in normal tissues. Pharmacologic implications for the clinical use of P-glycoprotein inhibitors. *Hematology Oncology Clinics of North America*, *9*, 319–336.
73. Dantzig, A.H., et al. (1996). Reversal of P-glycoprotein-mediated multidrug resistance by a potent cyclopropyldibenzosuberane modulator, LY335979. *Cancer Research*, *56*, 4171–4179.
74. Dale, I.L., et al. (1998). Reversal of P-glycoprotein-mediated multidrug resistance by XR9051, a novel diketopiperazine derivative. *British Journal of Cancer*, *78*, 885–892.
75. Hyafil, F., et al. (1993). In vitro and in vivo reversal of multidrug resistance by GF120918, an acridonecarboxamide derivative. *Cancer Research*, *53*, 4595–4602.
76. Dantzig, A.H., et al. (2001). Reversal of multidrug resistance by the P-glycoprotein modulator, LY335979, from the bench to the clinic. *Current Medicinal Chemistry*, *8*, 39–50.
77. Ruff, P., et al. (2009). A randomized, placebo-controlled, double-blind phase 2 study of docetaxel compared to docetaxel plus zosuquidar (LY335979) in women with metastatic or locally recurrent breast cancer who have received one prior chemotherapy regimen. *Cancer Chemotherapy Pharmacology*, *64*, 763–768.
78. Lancet, J.E., et al. (2009). A phase I trial of continuous infusion of the multidrug resistance inhibitor zosuquidar with daunorubicin and cytarabine in acute myeloid leukemia. *Leukemia Research*, *33*, 1055–1061.
79. Morschhauser, F., et al. (2007). Phase I/II trial of a P-glycoprotein inhibitor, Zosuquidar.3HCl trihydrochloride (LY335979), given orally in combination with the CHOP regimen in patients with non-Hodgkin's lymphoma. *Leukemia Lymphoma*, *48*, 708–715.
80. Sandler, A., et al. (2004). A Phase I trial of a potent P-glycoprotein inhibitor, zosuquidar trihydrochloride (LY335979), administered intravenously in combination with doxorubicin in patients with advanced malignancy. *Clinical Cancer Research*, *10*, 3265–3272.
81. Kruijtzer, C.M., et al. (2002). Increased oral bioavailability of topotecan in combination with the breast cancer resistance protein and P-glycoprotein inhibitor GF120918. *Journal of Clinical Oncology*, *20*, 2943–2950.
82. Cisternino, S., et al. (2004). Expression, up-regulation, and transport activity of the multidrug-resistance protein Abcg2 at the mouse blood-brain barrier. *Cancer Research*, *64*, 3296–3301.
83. Patel, J., et al. (2004). In vitro interaction of the HIV protease inhibitor ritonavir with herbal constituents: changes in P-gp and CYP3A4 activity. *American Journal of Therapy*, *11*, 262–277.
84. Di Pietro, A., et al. (2002). Modulation by flavonoids of cell multidrug resistance mediated by P-glycoprotein and related ABC transporters. *Cellular and Molecular Life Sciences*, *59*, 307–322.
85. Zhang, L., et al. (2007). Mechanistic study on the intestinal absorption and disposition of baicalein. *European Journal of Pharmaceutical Science*, *31*, 221–231.
86. Zhang, S., et al. (2005). Structure activity relationships and quantitative structure activity relationships for the flavonoid-mediated inhibition of breast cancer resistance protein. *Biochemical Pharmacology*, *70*, 627–639.
87. Zhang, S., Yang, X., Morris, M.E. (2004). Combined effects of multiple flavonoids on breast cancer resistance protein (ABCG2)-mediated transport. *Research in Pharmacy*, *21*, 1263–1273.
88. Imai, Y., et al. (2004). Phytoestrogens/flavonoids reverse breast cancer resistance protein/ABCG2-mediated multidrug resistance. *Cancer Research*, *64*, 4346–4352.

89. Minocha, M., et al. (2012). Co-administration strategy to enhance brain accumulation of vandetanib by modulating P-glycoprotein (P-gp/Abcb1) and breast cancer resistance protein (Bcrp1/Abcg2) mediated efflux with m-TOR inhibitors. *International Journal of Pharmacology*, *434*, 306–314.
90. Yamagata, T., et al. (2007). Improvement of the oral drug absorption of topotecan through the inhibition of intestinal xenobiotic efflux transporter, breast cancer resistance protein, by excipients. *Drug Metabolism and Disposition*, *35*, 1142–1148.
91. Batrakova, E.V., et al. (2001). Pluronic P85 enhances the delivery of digoxin to the brain: In vitro and in vivo studies. *Journal of Pharmacology Experimental Therapeutics*, *296*, 551–557.
92. Jain, R., et al. (2005). Evasion of P-gp mediated cellular efflux and permeability enhancement of HIV-protease inhibitor saquinavir by prodrug modification. *International Journal of Pharmacology*, *303*, 8–19.
93. Agarwal, S., et al. (2008). Peptide prodrugs: Improved oral absorption of lopinavir, a HIV protease inhibitor. *International Journal of Pharmacology*, *359*, 7–14.
94. Jain, R., et al. (2004). Circumventing P-glycoprotein-mediated cellular efflux of quinidine by prodrug derivatization. *Molecular Pharmacology*, *1*, 290–299.
95. Fenske, D.B., Cullis, P.R. (2008). Liposomal nanomedicines. *Expert Opinion on Drug Delivery*, *5*, 25–44.
96. Acharya, S., Sahoo, S.K. (2011). PLGA nanoparticles containing various anticancer agents and tumour delivery by EPR effect. *Advanced Drug Delivery Reviews*, *63*, 170–183.
97. Dong, X., et al. (2009). Doxorubicin and paclitaxel-loaded lipid-based nanoparticles overcome multidrug resistance by inhibiting P-glycoprotein and depleting ATP. *Cancer Research*, *69*, 3918–3926.
98. Lee, E.S., Na, K., Bae, Y.H. (2005). Doxorubicin loaded pH-sensitive polymeric micelles for reversal of resistant MCF-7 tumor. *Journal of Control Release*, *103*, 405–418.
99. Naito, M., et al. (1996). Potentiation of the reversal activity of SDZ PSC833 on multi-drug resistance by an anti-P-glycoprotein monoclonal antibody MRK-16. *International Journal of Cancer*, *67*, 435–440.
100. Pearson, J.W., et al. (1991). Reversal of drug resistance in a human colon cancer xenograft expressing MDR1 complementary DNA by in vivo administration of MRK-16 monoclonal antibody. *Journal of National Cancer Institiute*, *83*, 1386–1391.
101. Haus-Cohen, M., et al. (2004). Disruption of P-glycoprotein anticancer drug efflux activity by a small recombinant single-chain Fv antibody fragment targeted to an extracellular epitope. *International Journal of Cancer*, *109*, 750–758.
102. Gaudana, R., et al. (2010). Ocular drug delivery. *Journal of American Association of Pharmaceutical Scientists*, *12*, 348–360.
103. Nakanishi, T. (2007). Drug transporters as targets for cancer chemotherapy. *Cancer Genomics Proteomics*, *4*, 241–254.
104. Rubio-Aliaga, I., Daniel, H. (2002). Mammalian peptide transporters as targets for drug delivery. *Trends in Pharmacological Sciences*, *23*, 434–440.
105. Kramer, W. (2011). Transporters, Trojan horses and therapeutics: Suitability of bile acid and peptide transporters for drug delivery. *Biological Chemistry*, *392*, 77–94.
106. Balimane, P.V., et al. (1998). Direct evidence for peptide transporter (PepT1)-mediated uptake of a nonpeptide prodrug, valacyclovir. *Biochemical and Biophysical Research Communications*, *250*, 246–251.
107. Ganapathy, M.E., et al. (1998). Valacyclovir: A substrate for the intestinal and renal peptide transporters PEPT1 and PEPT2. *Biochemical and Biophysical Research Communications*, *246*, 470–475.
108. Sugawara, M., et al. (2000). Transport of valganciclovir, a ganciclovir prodrug, via peptide transporters PEPT1 and PEPT2. *Journal of Pharmacy & Pharmaceutical Sciences*, *89*, 781–789.
109. Santos, C., et al. (2008). Dipeptide derivatives of AZT: Synthesis, chemical stability, activation in human plasma, hPEPT1 affinity, and antiviral activity. *ChemMedChem*, *3*, 970–978.
110. Tsume, Y., et al. (2008). Enhanced absorption and growth inhibition with amino acid monoester prodrugs of floxuridine by targeting hPEPT1 transporters. *Molecules*, *13*, 1441–1454.
111. Rubio-Aliaga, I., Daniel, H. (2008). Peptide transporters and their roles in physiological processes and drug disposition. *Xenobiotica*, *38*, 1022–1042.
112. Tamai, I., et al. (1998). Improvement of L-dopa absorption by dipeptidyl derivation, utilizing peptide transporter PepT1. *Journal of Pharmacy & Pharmaceutical Sciences*, *87*, 1542–1546.
113. Ogihara, H., et al. (1996). Immuno-localization of H+/peptide cotransporter in rat digestive tract. *Biochemical and Biophysical Research Communications*, *220*, 848–852.
114. Shen, H., et al. (1999). Localization of PEPT1 and PEPT2 proton-coupled oligopeptide transporter mRNA and protein in rat kidney. *American Journal of Physiology*, *276*, F658–F665.
115. Knutter, I., et al. (2002). H+-peptide cotransport in the human bile duct epithelium cell line SK-ChA-1. *American Journal of Physiology - Gastrointestinal and Liver Physiology*, *283*, G222–G229.
116. Bockman, D.E., et al. (1997). Localization of peptide transporter in nuclei and lysosomes of the pancreas. *International Journal of Pancreatology*, *22*, 221–225.
117. Zhang, T., et al. (2008). Drug transporter and cytochrome P450 mRNA expression in human ocular barriers: Implications for ocular drug disposition. *Drug Metabolism and Disposition*, *36*, 1300–1307.
118. Berger, U.V., Hediger, M.A. (1999). Distribution of peptide transporter PEPT2 mRNA in the rat nervous system. *Anatomy and Embryology (Berlin)*, *199*, 439–449.
119. Groneberg, D.A., et al. (2001). Expression of PEPT2 peptide transporter mRNA and protein in glial cells of rat dorsal root ganglia. *Neuroscience Letters*, *304*, 181–184.
120. Groneberg, D.A., et al. (2001). Localization of the peptide transporter PEPT2 in the lung: Implications for pulmonary oligopeptide uptake. *American Journal of Pathology*, *158*, 707–714.

121. Groneberg, D.A., et al. (2002). Peptide transport in the mammary gland: Expression and distribution of PEPT2 mRNA and protein. *American Journal of Physiology Endocrinology Metabolism*, *282*, E1172–E1179.

122. Bretschneider, B., Brandsch, M., Neubert, R. (1999). Intestinal transport of beta-lactam antibiotics: Analysis of the affinity at the H+/peptide symporter (PEPT1), the uptake into Caco-2 cell monolayers and the transepithelial flux. *Research in Pharmacy*, *16*, 55–61.

123. Daniel, H., Adibi, S.A. (1993). Transport of beta-lactam antibiotics in kidney brush border membrane. Determinants of their affinity for the oligopeptide/H+ symporter. *Journal of Clinical Investigation*, *92*, 2215–2223.

124. Ganapathy, M.E., et al. (1997). Interaction of anionic cephalosporins with the intestinal and renal peptide transporters PEPT 1 and PEPT 2. *Biochimica et Biophysica Acta*, *1324*, 296–308.

125. Ocheltree, S.M., et al. (2004). Mechanisms of cefadroxil uptake in the choroid plexus: Studies in wild-type and PEPT2 knockout mice. *Journal of Pharmacology and Experimental Therapeutics*, *308*, 462–467.

126. Boll, M., et al. (1994). Expression cloning of a cDNA from rabbit small intestine related to proton-coupled transport of peptides, beta-lactam antibiotics and ACE-inhibitors. *Pflügers Archiv/European Journal of Physiology*, *429*, 146–149.

127. Ganapathy, M.E., et al. (1995). Differential recognition of beta -lactam antibiotics by intestinal and renal peptide transporters, PEPT 1 and PEPT 2. *Journal of Biological Chemistry*, *270*, 25672–25677.

128. Fei, Y.J., et al. (1994). Expression cloning of a mammalian proton-coupled oligopeptide transporter. *Nature*, *368*, 563–566.

129. Wenzel, U., et al. (1996). Transport characteristics of differently charged cephalosporin antibiotics in oocytes expressing the cloned intestinal peptide transporter PepT1 and in human intestinal Caco-2 cells. *Journal of Pharmacology and Experimental Therapeutics*, *277*, 831–839.

130. Doring, F., et al. (1998). Delta-aminolevulinic acid transport by intestinal and renal peptide transporters and its physiological and clinical implications. *Journal of Clinical Investigations*, *101*, 2761–2767.

131. Saito, H., et al. (1996). Molecular cloning and tissue distribution of rat peptide transporter PEPT2. *Biochimica et Biophysica Acta*, *1280*, 173–177.

132. Landowski, C.P., et al. (2005). Targeted delivery to PEPT1-overexpressing cells: Acidic, basic, and secondary floxuridine amino acid ester prodrugs. *Molecular Cancer Therapy*, *4*, 659–667.

133. Tsuda, M., et al. (2006). Transport characteristics of a novel peptide transporter 1 substrate, antihypotensive drug midodrine, and its amino acid derivatives. *Journal of Pharmacology and Experimental Therapeutics*, *318*, 455–460.

134. Han, H., et al. (1998). 5′-Amino acid esters of antiviral nucleosides, acyclovir, and AZT are absorbed by the intestinal PEPT1 peptide transporter. *Research in Pharmacy*, *15*, 1154–1159.

135. Watanabe, C., et al. (2005). Na+/H+ exchanger 3 affects transport property of H+/oligopeptide transporter 1. *Drug Metabolism and Pharmacokinetics*, *20*, 443–451.

136. Shu, C., et al. (2001). Mechanism of intestinal absorption and renal reabsorption of an orally active ace inhibitor: Uptake and transport of fosinopril in cell cultures. *Drug Metabolism Reviews*, *29*, 1307–1315.

137. Zhu, T., et al. (2000). Differential recognition of ACE inhibitors in Xenopus laevis oocytes expressing rat PEPT1 and PEPT2. *Research in Pharmacy*, *17*, 526–532.

138. Hagenbuch, B., Gui, C. (2008). Xenobiotic transporters of the human organic anion transporting polypeptides (OATP) family. *Xenobiotica*, *38*, 778–801.

139. Sekinc, T., Miyazaki, H., Endou, H. (2006). Molecular physiology of renal organic anion transporters. *American Journal of Physiology - Renal Physiology*, *290*, F251–F261.

140. Konig, J., et al. (2006). Pharmacogenomics of human OATP transporters. *Naunyn-Schmiedeberg's Archives of Pharmacology*, *372*, 432–443.

141. Obaidat, A., Roth, M., Hagenbuch, B. (2012). The expression and function of organic anion transporting polypeptides in normal tissues and in cancer. *Annual Review of Pharmacology and Toxicology*, *52*, 135–151.

142. Ho, R.H., et al. (2006). Drug and bile acid transporters in rosuvastatin hepatic uptake: Function, expression, and pharmacogenetics. *Gastroenterology*, *130*, 1793–1806.

143. Su, Y., Zhang, X., Sinko, P.J. (2004). Human organic anion-transporting polypeptide OATP-A (SLC21A3) acts in concert with P-glycoprotein and multidrug resistance protein 2 in the vectorial transport of Saquinavir in Hep G2 cells. *Molecular Pharmacology*, *1*, 49–56.

144. Lee, W., et al. (2005). Polymorphisms in human organic anion-transporting polypeptide 1A2 (OATP1A2): Implications for altered drug disposition and central nervous system drug entry. *Journal of Biological Chemistry*, *280*, 9610–9617.

145. Cvetkovic, M., et al. (1999). OATP and P-glycoprotein transporters mediate the cellular uptake and excretion of fexofenadine. *Drug Metabolism and Disposition*, *27*, 866–871.

146. Kullak-Ublick, G.A., et al. (1995). Molecular and functional characterization of an organic anion transporting polypeptide cloned from human liver. *Gastroenterology*, *109*, 1274–1282.

147. Lau, Y.Y., et al. (2007). Effect of OATP1B transporter inhibition on the pharmacokinetics of atorvastatin in healthy volunteers. *Clinical Pharmacology Therapy*, *81*, 194–204.

148. Liu, L., et al. (2006). Vectorial transport of enalapril by Oatp1a1/Mrp2 and OATP1B1 and OATP1B3/MRP2 in rat and human livers. *Journal of Pharmacology and Experimental Therapeutics*, *318*, 395–402.

149. Yamashiro, W., et al. (2006). Involvement of transporters in the hepatic uptake and biliary excretion of valsartan, a selective antagonist of the angiotensin II AT1-receptor, in humans. *Drug Metabolism and Disposition*, *34*, 1247–1254.

150. Briz, O., et al. (2003). Role of organic anion-transporting polypeptides, OATP-A, OATP-C and OATP-8, in the human placenta-maternal liver tandem excretory pathway for foetal bilirubin. *Biochemical Journal*, *371*, 897–905.

151. Cui, Y., et al. (2001). Hepatic uptake of bilirubin and its conjugates by the human organic anion transporter SLC21A6. *Journal of Biological Chemistry*, *276*, 9626–9630.
152. Letschert, K., et al. (2006). Molecular characterization and inhibition of amanitin uptake into human hepatocytes. *Toxicological Sciences*, *91*, 140–149.
153. Smith, N.F., et al. (2005). Identification of OATP1B3 as a high-affinity hepatocellular transporter of paclitaxel. *Cancer Biology and Therapy*, *4*, 815–818.
154. Hirano, M., et al. (2004). Contribution of OATP2 (OATP1B1) and OATP8 (OATP1B3) to the hepatic uptake of pitavastatin in humans. *Journal of Pharmacology and Experimental Therapeutics*, *311*, 139–146.
155. Tirona, R.G., et al. (2003). Human organic anion transporting polypeptide-C (SLC21A6) is a major determinant of rifampin-mediated pregnane X receptor activation. *Journal of Pharmacology and Experimental Therapeutics*, *304*, 223–228.
156. Vavricka, S.R., et al. (2002). Interactions of rifamycin SV and rifampicin with organic anion uptake systems of human liver. *Hepatology*, *36*, 164–172.
157. Abe, T., et al. (2001). LST-2, a human liver-specific organic anion transporter, determines methotrexate sensitivity in gastrointestinal cancers. *Gastroenterology*, *120*, 1689–1699.
158. Pizzagalli, F., et al. (2002). Identification of a novel human organic anion transporting polypeptide as a high affinity thyroxine transporter. *Molecular Endocrinology*, *16*, 2283–2296.
159. Kraft, M.E., et al. (2010). The prostaglandin transporter OATP2A1 is expressed in human ocular tissues and transports the antiglaucoma prostanoid latanoprost. *Investigative Ophthalmology & Visual Science*, *51*, 2504–2511.
160. Treiber, A., et al. (2007). Bosentan is a substrate of human OATP1B1 and OATP1B3: Inhibition of hepatic uptake as the common mechanism of its interactions with cyclosporin A, rifampicin, and sildenafil. *Drug Metabolism and Disposition*, *35*, 1400–1407.
161. Noe, J., et al. (2007). Substrate-dependent drug-drug interactions between gemfibrozil, fluvastatin and other organic anion-transporting peptide (OATP) substrates on OATP1B1, OATP2B1, and OATP1B3. *Drug Metabolism and Disposition*, *35*, 1308–1314.
162. Nozawa, T., et al. (2004). Functional characterization of pH-sensitive organic anion transporting polypeptide OATP-B in human. *Journal of Pharmacology and Experimental Therapeutics*, *308*, 438–445.
163. Huber, R.D., et al. (2007). Characterization of two splice variants of human organic anion transporting polypeptide 3A1 isolated from human brain. *American Journal of Physiology—Cell Physiology*, *292*, C795–C806.
164. Adachi, H., et al. (2003). Molecular characterization of human and rat organic anion transporter OATP-D. *American Journal of Physiology - Renal Physiology*, *285*, F1188–F1197.
165. Fujiwara, K., et al. (2001). Identification of thyroid hormone transporters in humans: Different molecules are involved in a tissue-specific manner. *Endocrinology*, *142*, 2005–2012.
166. Mikkaichi, T., et al. (2004). Isolation and characterization of a digoxin transporter and its rat homologue expressed in the kidney. *Proceedings of the National Academy of Science USA*, *101*, 3569–3574.
167. Meyer zu Schwabedissen, H.E., et al. (2008). Interplay between the nuclear receptor pregnane X receptor and the uptake transporter organic anion transporter polypeptide 1A2 selectively enhances estrogen effects in breast cancer. *Cancer Research*, *68*, 9338–9347.
168. Ballestero, M.R., et al. (2006). Expression of transporters potentially involved in the targeting of cytostatic bile acid derivatives to colon cancer and polyps. *Biochemical Pharmacology*, *72*, 729–738.
169. Miki, Y., et al. (2006). Expression of the steroid and xenobiotic receptor and its possible target gene, organic anion transporting polypeptide-A, in human breast carcinoma. *Cancer Research*, *66*, 535–542.
170. Tsuboyama, T., et al. (2010). Hepatocellular carcinoma: Hepatocyte-selective enhancement at gadoxetic acid-enhanced MR imaging—correlation with expression of sinusoidal and canalicular transporters and bile accumulation. *Radiology*, *255*, 824–833.
171. Cui, Y., et al. (2003). Detection of the human organic anion transporters SLC21A6 (OATP2) and SLC21A8 (OATP8) in liver and hepatocellular carcinoma. *Laboratory Investigation*, *83*, 527–538.
172. Vavricka, S.R., et al. (2004). The human organic anion transporting polypeptide 8 (SLCO1B3) gene is transcriptionally repressed by hepatocyte nuclear factor 3beta in hepatocellular carcinoma. *Journal of Hepatology*, *40*, 212–218.
173. Wlcek, K., et al. (2011). The analysis of organic anion transporting polypeptide (OATP) mRNA and protein patterns in primary and metastatic liver cancer. *Cancer Biology and Therapy*, *11*, 801–811.
174. Holla, V.R., et al. (2008). Regulation of prostaglandin transporters in colorectal neoplasia. *Cancer Prevention Research (Philadelphia)*, *1*, 93–99.
175. Wlcek, K., et al. (2008). Altered expression of organic anion transporter polypeptide (OATP) genes in human breast carcinoma. *Cancer Biology and Therapy*, *7*, 1450–1455.
176. Liedauer, R., et al. (2009). Different expression patterns of organic anion transporting polypeptides in osteosarcomas, bone metastases and aneurysmal bone cysts. *Oncology Reports*, *22*, 1485–1492.
177. Roth, M., Obaidat, A., Hagenbuch, B. (2012). OATPs, OATs and OCTs: The organic anion and cation transporters of the SLCO and SLC22A gene superfamilies. *British Journal of Pharmacology*, *165*, 1260–1287.
178. Pao, S.S., Paulsen, I.T., Saier, M.H., Jr. (1998). Major facilitator superfamily. *Microbiology and Molecular Biology Reviews*, *62*, 1–34.
179. Ren, Q., Kang, K.H., Paulsen, I.T. (2004). TransportDB: A relational database of cellular membrane transport systems. *Nucleic Acids Research*, *32*, D284–D288.

180. Saier, M.H., Jr., et al. (1999). The major facilitator superfamily. *Journal of Molecular Microbiology and Biotechnology*, *1*, 257–279.
181. Reizer, J., et al. (1993). Mammalian integral membrane receptors are homologous to facilitators and antiporters of yeast, fungi, and eubacteria. *Protein Science*, *2*, 20–30.
182. Eraly, S.A., et al. (2004). The molecular pharmacology of organic anion transporters: From DNA to FDA? *Molecular Pharmacology*, *65*, 479–487.
183. Cha, S.H., et al. (2000). Molecular cloning and characterization of multispecific organic anion transporter 4 expressed in the placenta. *Journal of Biological Chemistry*, *275*, 4507–4512.
184. Ljubojevic, M., et al. (2007). Renal expression of organic anion transporter OAT2 in rats and mice is regulated by sex hormones. *American Journal of Physiology—Renal Physiology*, *292*, F361–F372.
185. Sykes, D., et al. (2004). Organic anion transport in choroid plexus from wild-type and organic anion transporter 3 (Slc22a8)-null mice. *American Journal of Physiology - Renal Physiology*, *286*, F972–F978.
186. Alebouyeh, M., et al. (2003). Expression of human organic anion transporters in the choroid plexus and their interactions with neurotransmitter metabolites. *Journal of Pharmacy & Pharmaceutical Sciences*, *93*, 430–436.
187. Takeda, M., et al. (2004). Evidence for a role of human organic anion transporters in the muscular side effects of HMG-CoA reductase inhibitors. *European Journal of Pharmacology*, *483*, 133–138.
188. Motohashi, H., et al. (2002). Gene expression levels and immunolocalization of organic ion transporters in the human kidney. *Journal of the American Society of Nephrology*, *13*, 866–874.
189. Pritchard, J.B., et al. (1999). Mechanism of organic anion transport across the apical membrane of choroid plexus. *Journal of Biological Chemistry*, *274*, 33382–33387.
190. Hosoyamada, M., et al. (1999). Molecular cloning and functional expression of a multispecific organic anion transporter from human kidney. *American Journal of Physiology*, *276*, F122–F128.
191. Burckhardt, G. (2012). Drug transport by organic anion transporters (OATs). *International Journal of Clinical Pharmacology, Therapy and Toxicology*, *136*, 106–130.
192. Enomoto, A., et al. (2002). Interaction of human organic anion transporters 2 and 4 with organic anion transport inhibitors. *Journal of Pharmacology and Experimental Therapeutics*, *301*, 797–802.
193. Cha, S.H., et al. (2001). Identification and characterization of human organic anion transporter 3 expressing predominantly in the kidney. *Molecular Pharmacology*, *59*, 1277–1286.
194. Ekaratanawong, S., et al. (2004). Human organic anion transporter 4 is a renal apical organic anion/dicarboxylate exchanger in the proximal tubules. *Journal of Pharmacology Science*, *94*, 297–304.
195. Ugele, B., et al. (2003). Characterization and identification of steroid sulfate transporters of human placenta. *American Journal of Physiology - Endocrinology and Metabolism*, *284*, E390–E398.
196. Babu, E., et al. (2002). Role of human organic anion transporter 4 in the transport of ochratoxin A. *Biochimica et Biophysica Acta*, *1590*, 64–75.
197. Asif, A.R., et al. (2005). Presence of organic anion transporters 3 (OAT3) and 4 (OAT4) in human adrenocortical cells. *Pflügers Archiv/European Journal of Physiology*, *450*, 88–95.
198. Sun, W., et al. (2001). Isolation of a family of organic anion transporters from human liver and kidney. *Biochemical and Biophysical Research Communications*, *283*, 417–422.
199. Shin, H.J., et al. (2007). Novel liver-specific organic anion transporter OAT7 that operates the exchange of sulfate conjugates for short chain fatty acid butyrate. *Hepatology*, *45*, 1046–1055.
200. Enomoto, A., et al. (2002). Molecular identification of a renal urate anion exchanger that regulates blood urate levels. *Nature*, *417*, 447–452.
201. Koepsell, H. (2004). Polyspecific organic cation transporters: their functions and interactions with drugs. *Trends in Pharmacological Sciences*, *25*, 375–381.
202. Jonker, J.W., Schinkel, A.H. (2004). Pharmacological and physiological functions of the polyspecific organic cation transporters: OCT1 2, and 3 (SLC22A1-3). *Journal of Pharmacology and Experimental Therapeutics*, *308*, 2–9.
203. Dresser, M.J., Leabman, M.K., Giacomini, K.M. (2001). Transporters involved in the elimination of drugs in the kidney: Organic anion transporters and organic cation transporters. *Journal of Pharmcology Science*, *90*, 397–421.
204. Wright, S.H. (2005). Role of organic cation transporters in the renal handling of therapeutic agents and xenobiotics. *Toxicology and Applied Pharmacology*, *204*, 309–319.
205. Wright, S.H., Dantzler, W.H. (2004). Molecular and cellular physiology of renal organic cation and anion transport. *Physiological Reviews*, *84*, 987–1049.
206. Koepsell, H., Endou, H. (2004). The SLC22 drug transporter family. *Pflügers Archiv/European Journal of Physiology*, *447*, 666–676.
207. Koepsell, H., Schmitt, B.M., Gorboulev, V. (2003). Organic cation transporters. *Reviews of Physiology, Biochemistry & Pharmacology*, *150*, 36–90.
208. Koepsell, H., Gorboulev, V., Arndt, P. (1999). Molecular pharmacology of organic cation transporters in kidney. *Journal of Membrane Biology*, *167*, 103–117.
209. Takeda, Y., Inoue, H. (1975). [Polyamines and cell multiplication]. *Horumon To Rinsho*, *23*, 111–119.
210. Choi, M.K., Song, I.S. (2008). Organic cation transporters and their pharmacokinetic and pharmacodynamic consequences. *Drug Metabolism and Pharmacokinetics*, *23*, 243–253.
211. Dresser, M.J., Gray, A.T., Giacomini, K.M. (2000). Kinetic and selectivity differences between rodent, rabbit, and human organic cation transporters (OCT1). *Journal of Pharmacology and Experimental Therapeutics*, *292*, 1146–1152.

212. Kimura, N., et al. (2005). Metformin is a superior substrate for renal organic cation transporter OCT2 rather than hepatic OCT1. *Drug Metabolism and Pharmacokinetics*, *20*, 379–386.

213. Bourdet, D.L., Pritchard, J.B., Thakker, D.R. (2005). Differential substrate and inhibitory activities of ranitidine and famotidine toward human organic cation transporter 1 (hOCT1; SLC22A1), hOCT2 (SLC22A2), and hOCT3 (SLC22A3). *Journal of Pharmacology and Experimental Therapeutics*, *315*, 1288–1297.

214. Lips, K.S., et al. (2005). Polyspecific cation transporters mediate luminal release of acetylcholine from bronchial epithelium. *American Journal of Respiratory Cell and Molecular Biology*, *33*, 79–88.

215. Karbach, U., et al. (2000). Localization of organic cation transporters OCT1 and OCT2 in rat kidney. *American Journal of Physiology - Renal Physiology*, *279*, F679–F687.

216. Gorboulev, V., et al. (1997). Cloning and characterization of two human polyspecific organic cation transporters. *DNA and Cell Biology*, *16*, 871–881.

217. Nies, A.T., et al. (2009). Expression of organic cation transporters OCT1 (SLC22A1) and OCT3 (SLC22A3) is affected by genetic factors and cholestasis in human liver. *Hepatology*, *50*, 1227–1240.

218. Muller, J., et al. (2005). Drug specificity and intestinal membrane localization of human organic cation transporters (OCT). *Biochemical Pharmacology*, *70*, 1851–1860.

219. Sata, R., et al. (2005). Functional analysis of organic cation transporter 3 expressed in human placenta. *Journal of Pharmacology and Experimental Therapeutics*, *315*, 888–895.

220. Wu, X., et al. (1998). Identity of the organic cation transporter OCT3 as the extraneuronal monoamine transporter (uptake2) and evidence for the expression of the transporter in the brain. *Journal of Biological Chemistry*, *273*, 32776–32786.

221. Tamai, I., et al. (1997). Cloning and characterization of a novel human pH-dependent organic cation transporter, *OCTN1*. *FEBS Letters*, *419*, 107–111.

222. Masuda, S., et al. (2006). Identification and functional characterization of a new human kidney-specific H+/organic cation antiporter, kidney-specific multidrug and toxin extrusion 2. *Journal of the American Society of Nephrology*, *17*, 2127–2135.

223. Wu, X., et al. (1998). cDNA sequence, transport function, and genomic organization of human OCTN2, a new member of the organic cation transporter family. *Biochemical and Biophysical Research Communications*, *246*, 589–595.

224. Vadlapudi, A.D., Vadlapatla, R.K., Mitra, A.K. (2012). Sodium dependent multivitamin transporter (SMVT): A potential target for drug delivery. *Current Drug Targets*, *13*, 994–1003.

225. Russell-Jones, G., et al. (2004). Vitamin-mediated targeting as a potential mechanism to increase drug uptake by tumours. *Journal of Inorganic Biochemistry*, *98*, 1625–1633.

226. Ramanathan, S., et al. (2001). Targeted PEG-based bioconjugates enhance the cellular uptake and transport of a HIV-1 TAT nonapeptide. *Journal of Control Release*, *77*, 199–212.

227. Janoria, K.G., et al. (2006). Biotin uptake by rabbit corneal epithelial cells: Role of sodium-dependent multivitamin transporter (SMVT). *Current Eye Research*, *31*, 797–809.

228. Janoria, K.G., et al. (2009). Vitreal pharmacokinetics of biotinylated ganciclovir: Role of sodium-dependent multivitamin transporter expressed on retina. *Journal of Ocular Pharmacology and Therapeutics*, *25*, 39–49.

229. Park, S., Sinko, P.J. (2005). The blood-brain barrier sodium-dependent multivitamin transporter: A molecular functional in vitro-in situ correlation. *Drug Metabolism and Disposition*, *33*, 1547–1554.

230. Said, H.M., et al. (1998). Biotin uptake by human colonic epithelial NCM460 cells: A carrier-mediated process shared with pantothenic acid. *American Journal of Physiology*, *275*, C1365–C1371.

231. Patel, M., et al. (2012). Molecular expression and functional activity of sodium dependent multivitamin transporter in human prostate cancer cells. *International Journal of Pharmacology*, *436*, 324–331.

232. Vadlapudi, A.D., et al. (2012). Functional and molecular aspects of biotin uptake via SMVT in human corneal epithelial (HCEC) and retinal pigment epithelial (D407) cells. *Journal of American Association of Pharmaceutical Scientists*, *14*, 832–842.

233. Luo, S., et al. (2006). Functional characterization of sodium-dependent multivitamin transporter in MDCK-MDR1 cells and its utilization as a target for drug delivery. *Molecular Pharmacology*, *3*, 329–339.

234. Kansara, V., et al. (2006). Biotin uptake and cellular translocation in human derived retinoblastoma cell line (Y-79): A role of hSMVT system. *International Journal of Pharmacology*, *312*, 43–52.

235. Grassl, S.M. (1992). Human placental brush-border membrane Na(+)-biotin cotransport. *Journal of Biological Chemistry*, *267*, 17760–17765.

236. Ohkura, Y., et al. (2010). Blood-to-retina transport of biotin via Na+-dependent multivitamin transporter (SMVT) at the inner blood-retinal barrier. *Experimental Eye Research*, *91*, 387–392.

237. Balamurugan, K., Vaziri, N.D., Said, H.M. (2005). Biotin uptake by human proximal tubular epithelial cells: Cellular and molecular aspects. *American Journal of Physiology - Renal Physiology*, *288*, F823–F831.

238. Ma, T.Y., Dyer, D.L., Said, H.M. (1994). Human intestinal cell line Caco-2: A useful model for studying cellular and molecular regulation of biotin uptake. *Biochimica et Biophysica Acta*, *1189*, 81–88.

239. Baur, B., Baumgartner, E.R. (1993). Na(+)-dependent biotin transport into brush-border membrane vesicles from human kidney cortex. *Pflügers Archiv/European Journal of Physiology*, *422*, 499–505.

240. Said, H.M., et al. (1992). Biotin transport in human liver basolateral membrane vesicles: A carrier-mediated, Na+ gradient-dependent process. *Gastroenterology*, *102*, 2120–2125.

241. Said, H.M., Redha, R., Nylander, W. (1987). A carrier-mediated, Na+ gradient-dependent transport for biotin in

human intestinal brush-border membrane vesicles. *American Journal of Physiology*, *253*, G631–G636.

242. Baur, B., Wick, H., Baumgartner, E.R. (1990). Na(+)-dependent biotin transport into brush-border membrane vesicles from rat kidney. *American Journal of Physiology*, *258*, F840–F847.
243. Daruwala, R., et al. (1999). Cloning and functional characterization of the human sodium-dependent vitamin C transporters hSVCT1 and hSVCT2. *FEBS Letters*, *460*, 480–484.
244. Wang, H., et al. (1999). Human Na(+)-dependent vitamin C transporter 1 (hSVCT1): Primary structure, functional characteristics and evidence for a non-functional splice variant. *Biochimica et Biophysica Acta*, *1461*, 1–9.
245. Tsukaguchi, H., et al. (1999). A family of mammalian Na+-dependent L-ascorbic acid transporters. *Nature*, *399*, 70–75.
246. Said, H.M., Mohammed, Z.M. (2006). Intestinal absorption of water-soluble vitamins: An update. *Current Opinion in Gastroenterology*, *22*, 140–146.
247. Maulen, N.P., et al. (2003). Up-regulation and polarized expression of the sodium-ascorbic acid transporter SVCT1 in post-confluent differentiated CaCo-2 cells. *Journal of Biological Chemistry*, *278*, 9035–9041.
248. Bowers-Komro, D.M., McCormick, D.B. (1991). Characterization of ascorbic acid uptake by isolated rat kidney cells. *Journal of Nutrition*, *121*, 57–64.
249. Rose, R.C. (1986). Ascorbic acid transport in mammalian kidney. *American Journal of Physiology*, *250*, F627–F632.
250. Astuya, A., et al. (2005). Vitamin C uptake and recycling among normal and tumor cells from the central nervous system. *Journal of Neuroscience Research*, *79*, 146–156.
251. Castro, M., et al. (2001). High-affinity sodium-vitamin C co-transporters (SVCT) expression in embryonic mouse neurons. *Journal of Neurochemistry*, *78*, 815–823.
252. Talluri, R.S., et al. (2006). Mechanism of L-ascorbic acid uptake by rabbit corneal epithelial cells: Evidence for the involvement of sodium-dependent vitamin C transporter 2. *Current Eye Research*, *31*, 481–489.
253. Garland, D.L. (1991). Ascorbic acid and the eye. *American Journal of Clinical Nutrition*, *54*, 1198S–1202S.
254. Dixon, S.J., et al. (1991). Ascorbate uptake by ROS 17/2.8 osteoblast-like cells: Substrate specificity and sensitivity to transport inhibitors. *Journal of Bone and Mineral Research*, *6*, 623–629.
255. Padh, H., Aleo, J.J. (1987). Characterization of the ascorbic acid transport by 3T6 fibroblasts. *Biochimica et Biophysica Acta*, *901*, 283–290.
256. Luo, S., et al. (2008). Activity of a sodium-dependent vitamin C transporter (SVCT) in MDCK-MDR1 cells and mechanism of ascorbate uptake. *International Journal of Pharmacology*, *358*, 168–176.
257. Liang, W.J., Johnson, D., Jarvis, S.M. (2001). Vitamin C transport systems of mammalian cells. *Molecular Membrane Biology*, *18*, 87–95.
258. Wilson, J.X. (2005). Regulation of vitamin C transport. *Annual Review of Nutrition*, *25*, 105–125.
259. Kwatra, D., Budda, B., Vadlapudi, A.D., Vadlapatla, R.K., Pal, D., Mitra, A.K. (2012). Transfected MDCK cell line with enhanced expression of CYP3A4 and P-glycoprotein as a model to study their role in drug transport and metabolism. *Molecular Pharmaceutics*, *9(7)*, 1877–1886.
260. Kwatra, D., Boddu, S.H.S., Mitra, A.K. *MDCK Cells and Other Cell-Culture Models of Oral Drug Absorption, Oral Bioavailability: Basic Principles, Advanced Concepts, and Applications*, vol. 28, Wiley, Hoboken, NJ, 2011.
261. Ganapathy, V., Thangaraju, M., Prasad, P.D. (2009). Nutrient transporters in cancer: Relevance to Warburg hypothesis and beyond. *International Journal of Clinical Pharmacology, Therapy and Toxicology*, *121*, 29–40.
262. Jwala, J., et al. (2012). Differential expression of folate receptor-alpha, sodium-dependent multivitamin transporter, and amino acid transporter (B (0, +)) in human retinoblastoma (Y-79) and retinal pigment epithelial (ARPE-19) cell lines. *Journal of Ocular Pharmacology and Therapeutics*, *28*, 237–244.
263. van Dam, G.M., et al. (2011). Intraoperative tumor-specific fluorescence imaging in ovarian cancer by folate receptor-alpha targeting: first in-human results. *Nature Medicine*, *17*, 1315–1319.
264. Allard, J.E., et al. (2007). Overexpression of folate binding protein is associated with shortened progression-free survival in uterine adenocarcinomas. *Gynecologic Oncology*, *107*, 52–57.
265. Dainty, L.A., et al. (2007). Overexpression of folate binding protein and mesothelin are associated with uterine serous carcinoma. *Gynecologic Oncology*, *105*, 563–570.
266. Parker, N., et al. (2005). Folate receptor expression in carcinomas and normal tissues determined by a quantitative radioligand binding assay. *Analytical Biochemistry*, *338*, 284–293.
267. Toffoli, G., et al. (1997). Overexpression of folate binding protein in ovarian cancers. *International Journal of Cancer*, *74*, 193–198.
268. Campbell, I.G., et al. (1991). Folate-binding protein is a marker for ovarian cancer. *Cancer Research*, *51*, 5329–5338.
269. Zhang, L., et al. (2008). A regulatory viewpoint on transporter-based drug interactions. *Xenobiotica*, *38*, 709–724.
270. U.S. Department of Health and Human Services, F.D.A., Center for Drug Evaluation and Research (CDER). *Drug Interaction Studies—Study Design, Data Analysis, Implications for Dosing, and Labeling Recommendations*, 2012.
271. U.S. Department of Health and Human Services, F.D.A., Center for Drug Evaluation and Research (CDER). *Drug Interaction Studies—Study Design, Data Analysis, and Implications for Dosing and Labeling*, 2004.

4

BIOMATERIAL IN ADVANCED DRUG DELIVERY

MEGHA BAROT, MITESH PATEL, XIAOYAN YANG, WUCHEN WANG, AND CHI H. LEE

"Biomaterial is a systemically and pharmacologically inert substance designed for implantation within or incorporation with living systems."

The Clemson University Advisory Board for Biomaterials [1]

4.1 CHAPTER OBJECTIVES

- To highlight the functional properties, categorization, and selection of biomaterials and mechanisms of tissue interactions with the material surface.
- To outline general requirements of biomaterials for biocompatibility and blood compatibility and enlist factors affecting interactions with tissue/blood.
- To provide applications of bioresorbable and biodegradable polymers, composite materials, and other materials in the field of biomedicines and drug delivery.
- To elucidate the potential usage and favorable design of biomaterials for other therapeutic applications.

4.2 CLASSIFICATION AND BIOCOMPATIBILITY OF BIOMATERIAL

4.2.1 Definition and Classification of Biomaterials

A *biomaterial* is a nonviable material used in a medical device intended to assess, treat, augment, or replace any nonfunctional part of a living system or to function in intimate contact with living tissues or biological systems. Biomaterials are of the human body [2–4]. The clinical success of biomaterial-based implants has been a critical step toward the medical needs of a rapidly aging population.

Biomaterials have been applied to heal or repair the human body for millennia, but human-made materials have been used only for four decades. Biomaterials can interact with tissues in various ways depending on the material type. Biomaterial has been categorized based on (A) the mechanism of tissue interaction to the material surface or (B) material selection, as shown in Table 4.1.

4.2.1.1 Mechanism of Tissue Interaction to the Material Surface It is vital to comprehend the structural and functional properties of biomaterials and their interactions with the physiological environment. Biomaterial has been classified based on the mechanism by which they were clinically effective in achieving suitable properties to match those of the replaced tissue with maximal biocompatible response and minimal toxicity in the host [4, 7, 8].

(i) **Bioinert biomaterials**, such as stainless steel and polyethylene, were classified as the first-generation biomaterials. Bioinert material upon placement within the biological system exhibits the least or no interaction with adjacent tissues [2]. This type of

Advanced Drug Delivery, First Edition. Edited by Ashim K. Mitra, Chi H. Lee, and Kun Cheng.

TABLE 4.1 Classification of Biomaterials [1,2,5,6]

Biomaterials	Examples
(A) Mechanism of tissue interaction to the material surface	
(i) Bioinert	Stainless steel, titanium, alumina, ultra-high molecular weight polyethylene
(ii) Bioactive (interactive)	Synthetic hydroxyapatite, glass ceramic, bioglass
(iii) Bioresorbable (viable)	Tricalciumphosphate,polylactic–polyglycolic acid co-polymers, calcium oxide, calcium carbonate, gypsum
(iv) Replant	Implantable materials consisting of native tissues, cultured *in vitro* from cells of patients
(B) Material selection	
(i) Composites	Carbon–carbon, wire- or fiber-reinforced, bone cement
(ii) Metals	Titanium, aluminum, cobalt chromium, gold, silver, stainless steels, iron, platinum, tungsten
(iii) Ceramics	
1. Nonabsorbable (relatively inert)	1. Alumina, zirconia, carbon
2. Bioactive or surface-reactive (semi-inert)	2. Glass, ceravital
3. Biodegradable or Resorbable (noninert)	3. Calcium phosphate, coralline, aluminum-calcium-phosphate, tricalcium phosphate
(iv) Biodegradable polymers	
(a) Natural polymers	(a)
1. Proteins	1. Collagen, elastin, fibrin, albumin
2. Polysaccharides (human origin)	2. Hyaluronic acid, chondroitin sulfate
3. Polysaccharides (non human origin)	3. Chitosan, alginic acid
(b) Synthetic polymers	(b) Polyglycolide, polylactides, polycaprolactone, polyphosphoester, poly(lactide-co-glycolide), polyanhydrides

material will not initiate any kind of adverse response toward the host system and, hence, will be widely used for hard tissue replacements and vascular surgery [9].

(ii) **Bioactive (interactive) biomaterial** upon placement within the biological system becomes bioactive as a result of interaction or recognition by the host system or of *in situ* phase transformations from liquid to solid or vice versa (in the presence of a biological system or external stimuli) [2]. Bioactive materials, such as hydroxyapatite-reinforced polyethylene (HAPEX) and bioglass that favorably interact with the body, were described as the second-generation biomaterials [57]. Bioactive materials are widely used for bone tissue engineering applications to elicit specific beneficial responses (ingrowth, adhesion) [10, 11].

(iii) **Bioresorbable (viable) biomaterials** were classified as the third-generation biomaterials as a result of their ability to heal the body [8]. The bioresorbable and bioactive material upon placement slowly starts to dissolve within the biological system. Viable biomaterial possibly incorporates live cells at implantation and is treated by the host as normal tissue matrices and is actively resorbed and/or remodeled [2]. As a result of its bioabsorptive nature, no further actions are required for removing bioresorbable material from the host system. This will also help in avoiding long-term complications associated with such synthetic materials. Bioresorbable materials are mostly used for short-term surgical applications, such as bone fixation, replacement, augmentation, and orthopedic devices [12, 13].

(iv) **Replant biomaterial** consist of native tissue, cultured *in vitro* from cells previously obtained from the specific patient. As a result of identical cellular markers as host, they should be the ultimate material for development of a harmonious interaction.

4.2.1.2 Material Selection The success of biomaterial relies on physicochemical properties (mechanical strength, stability) and biocompatibility (nontoxic, nonimmunogenic) of material being introduced into human tissue or organ [1]. Based on vital properties of biomaterial, four classes of synthetic material are extensively used for implantation within the human body.

(i) **Composites** are strong, tailor-made solids containing two or more distinct phases on a scale larger than the atomic. Elastic modulus property of composite can be modulated significantly relative to any other homogeneous material. Composites offer a substantial control over its material properties that opens up the possibility for the scientist to fabricate stiff, strong, or highly elastic and compliant materials [1, 14]. Composite biomaterials are mostly used in the field of bone tissue engineering as a dental filing composite (dental resin), bone cement, or orthopedic implants [14, 15].

(ii) **Metals** are inorganic and crystalline materials used as a biomaterial as a result of its strong and ductile nature. Titanium, cobalt-chromium, and stainless steel are three important metals used for implantation within human body as a result of their high strength, toughness, and biocompatible properties. Poor friction and susceptibility to corrode are common limitations associated with metal biomaterials. Metal biomaterials are frequently used for joint replacement, dental root implants, pacer and suture wires, bone plates, and screws [1, 16].

(iii) **Ceramics** are a refractory, polycrystalline, typically inorganic material. It is biocompatible and corrosion- and compression-resistant biomaterial with low electrical and thermal conductivities. The brittle and nonductile nature of ceramics is the major limitation as biomaterial. Based on biological reactivity, ceramics biomaterial can be classified as nonabsorbable (relatively inert), bioactive or surface reactive (semi-inert), and biodegradable or resorbable (noninert). Ceramics are mostly used for dental and orthopedic implants [5, 17].

(iv) **Polymers** are macromolecules built up by repeated bonding of smaller molecules called monomers. A wide range of biodegradable and natural and synthetic polymers has been investigated as a biomaterial for tissue engineering and controlled drug delivery. Biodegradable polymers are considered a versatile class of biomaterials as a result of its inherent flexibility and ability to match physical and mechanical properties of various tissues or organs of the body [17]. The limitation of polymeric biomaterials is its low mechanical resistance and easily degradable property. Polymeric biomaterials are used for sutures, arteries, veins, cements, artificial tendons, teeth, ears, noses, heart valves, lenses, testicles, and breasts implants [17, 18]. Based on structural properties, polymers have been classified into two major groups (Table 4.2): linear polymer and branched polymer.

a. *Linear polymers:* A homopolymer is the most basic and simplest linear polymer that has been widely used in production of nanoparticles as a result of its ability to form random coiled structures with a size of 5–15 nm and ease in introducing multiple functional groups in the polymeric backbone. Homopolymers have been extensively used for generating polymer drug conjugates. Principally, drug polymer conjugates consists of a polymer backbone that carries various exogenous compounds, such as solubilizing agent, therapeutic molecules, and targeting group along with a spacer [19]. Most frequently used linear polymers for drug delivery are vinyl polymers, polysaccharides, as well as poly(amino acids) and poly(ethylene glycols) (PEGs) [20, 21]. Factors including molecular weight, polydispersity, charge, and the hydrophilic–hydrophobic character of the polymer predominantly control drug-associated properties, such as biodistribution, clearance, biological activity, and toxicity [19].

Block co-polymers are another integral class of liner polymer that readily forms nanosized or microsized self-assemblies in the solvents. Block co-polymers are mostly amphiphilic in

TABLE 4.2 Classification of Polymers [19]

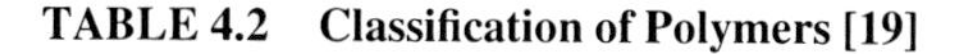

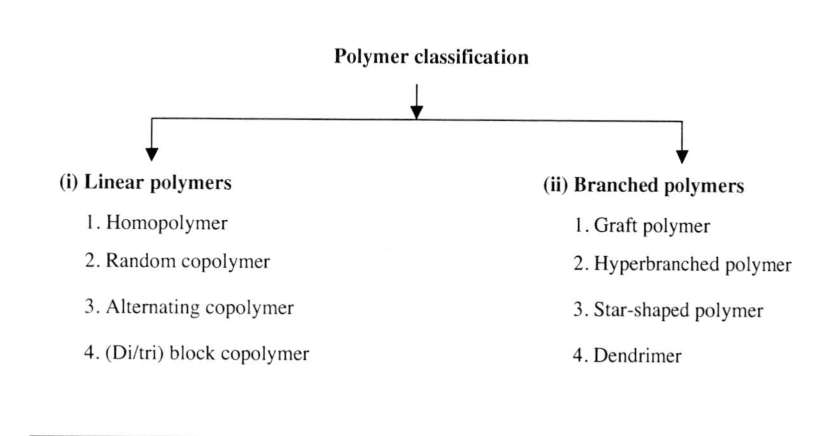

nature, and consist of both hydrophobic (A) and hydrophilic (B) blocks (AB-type diblock and ABA- or BAB-type triblock) in the same polymer chain [22, 23]. Block co-polymers are successful in developing micelles used for 1) drug targeting, 2) control drug delivery, or 3) enhancing drug solubility or stability [24]. The key regulating factors of block co-polymer as a drug delivery carrier include the molecular weight proportion of the A to B block, intrinsic affinity between the drug and hydrophobic block, and electrical charge [19].

b. *Branched polymers:* A branched polymer generates spheroid-shaped molecules holding primary, secondary, and tertiary charged amine groups. Polyethyleneimine (PEI) is the most typical branched polymer used for drug delivery. The cationic polyelectrolyte property of PEI attracts anionically charged organic and inorganic materials, thus, being extensively used for anionic DNA delivery [19, 25, 26]. A sequence of graft co-polymers based on hyper-branched PEI with a nonionic and hydrophilic block has been developed. The role of PEI in such a co-polymer was mostly to condense nucleic acids, while the hydrophilic block was used to increase the solubility and stability of the inter-polyelectrolyte complex against opsonization. Besides PEI-based graft polymers, most graft polymers are recognized as comb-type co-polymers because of their holding wide-ranging branching along with a linear polymer backbone [19, 27, 28].

A star polymer is another class of branched polymers, consisting of a three-dimensional hyper-branched structure produced by arm-first or core-first methods [29]. An application of the star polymer as a drug vector is limited as a result of the properties of a smaller hydrodynamic radius and lower solution viscosity as compared with linear polymers.

Dendrimers represent a new class of branched polymer. It consists of a unique three-dimensional structure, in which a series of layered branches regularly extend from a central core [30, 31]. The structural components of dendrimer include 1) a multifunctional central core, 2) branched units, and 3) surface groups. Dendrimers exhibit wide-ranging biomedical applications including drug delivery (gene, vaccines, and conventional drugs) and magnetic resonance imaging contrast agents [32–35]. A unique architecture of dendrimers offers several advantages over linear polymers. For instance, 1) an internal cavity of the dendrimer offers noncovalent encapsulation of a hydrophobic drug for successive controlled release; 2) a therapeutic drug, targeting and solubilizing groups, can be easily attached to the dendrimer periphery as a result of the multivalence nature of dendrimers; 3) the reproducible pharmacokinetic behavior of a drug can be achieved as a result of the low polydispersity of dendrimers; and 4) dendritic micelles offer superior stability over other polymeric micelles as a result of the presence of a strong unimolecular covalent bond [19].

4.2.2 Biocompatibility of Biomaterial

4.2.2.1 Biocompatibility Requirements The fundamental requirement to be qualified as a biomaterial is that material must be biocompatible, safe, cost-effective, and not generate any toxic, allergic, or carcinogenic responses [18]. Biocompatibility is the ability of a material to perform with an appropriate host response (local or systemic response of host to implanted material) in a specific application, and the success of biomaterials highly relies on its compatibility in biological system [1].

The biological compatibility or biocompatibility of biomaterial is a surface phenomenon, and material biocompatibility can be determined based on adverse host response intensity. The selection of material for biomedical application is mainly based on material compatibility within a biological system. Three important considerations in the selection of biocompatible material are as follows:

a. Biocompatibility may not be exclusively dependent on the material characteristics, but also it may depend on the location in which the material is used. It is highly likely that material response may vary from one application site to another.
b. It is sometimes required that material should interact rather than be inert in nature with the tissue to generate its effects (e.g., blood contacting materials designed to develop a neointima).
c. In some cases, it is required for material to degrade over time rather than remain intact for an indefinite period (e.g., resorbable materials, sutures, and biodegradable drug delivery systems) [36].

4.2.2.2 Types of Interactions Between Biomaterial and Host Tissues Biomaterial exhibits four different types of interactions within the biological system depending on the material properties.

(i) *Chemical interaction:* Metal biomaterials possess chemical interactions within the host system. The ultimate outcomes of metal interactions include corrosion, degradation, and protein deposition. Metal biomaterials in contact with host systems stimulate immune system by forming complexes with native proteins, and such complexes are considered candidate antigens in clinical applications. Dermal reactions (eczema, redness, and itching) are the most frequent outcome of the metal hypersensitivity. Although hypersensitivity has been categorized as an immediate humoral response (types I, II, or II) or delayed cell-mediated response (type IV), reactions associated with metal biomaterials are recognized as a type IV delayed hypersensitivity response. In addition to immunogenic responses, metal degradation products may also generate other responses, such as metabolic changes, initiation of lymphocyte toxins, variations in host–parasite interactions, and development of chemical carcinogenesis [1, 37–39].

(ii) *Mechanical interaction:* The development of a fibrous encapsulation, thrombus formation, and calcification are the ultimate outcomes of mechanical interaction between biomaterial and the host system. The biocompatibility of blood contacting biomaterial devices is mainly related to the thrombotic response induced by the materials. Biomaterial implants upon being implanted within the human body tend to adsorb protein biomolecules, the ultimate outcome of which would be blood coagulation, leukocyte recruitment and adhesion, foreign body reaction, and fibrous encapsulation. The outcomes of foreign body reaction and fibrous encapsulation serve as a biological restriction of integration and *in vivo* performance of biomaterial implants. Although no material has been found truly biocompatible, numerous cardiovascular devices function with small or tolerable risks of complications. Biomaterial-associated thrombotic complications can be arrested by actively blocking the pathway responsible for the intrinsic thrombogenicity of the materials [1, 40, 41].

(iii) *Pharmacological interaction:* Toxic leaching, embrittlement, and cell lysis are the major consequences of pharmacological biomaterial interactions. When a component of biomaterial dissolves in tissue, material becomes porous and creates large deformations that lead to toxic contaminants, such as residual monomers, stabilizers, emulsifiers, or sterilization by-products, mostly leaching from the implants. The mechanical properties of biomaterial may also be affected by leaching that, especially in the case of metal biomaterials, may lead to reduction in fracture strength as a result of formation of macroscopic voids [1, 42].

(iv) *Surface interaction:* Biomaterial-mediated surface interactions with the host system will trigger a series of host reactions including blood–material interactions (protein adsorption, and provisional matrix formation), complement activation on biomaterial surfaces, and macrophage adhesion followed by fusion (foreign body giant cell formation) or capsulation. The ultimate outcome of the above events would be acute or chronic inflammation, granulation, foreign body reaction, and fibrosis. Moreover, these events will initiate the release of degraded mediators, which are responsible for device failure [43].

Implantable devices or scaffolds are prone to various implant responses. In particular, the synthetic polymers, such as polylactic acid, poly-L-lactide acid, polyethylene glycol, and polyhydroxyl ethyl methacrylate, not only enhance the scaffold strength but also act as a bioactivity inducer. One of the major drawbacks of synthetic polymers is their faster degradation rates, which are much greater than that of a natural polymer, thus, producing rapid implant responses including capsule formation, tissue ingrowth, and tissue adhesion.

a. *Capsule formation:* The body reacts to the foreign materials by forming a fibrous capsule, isolating them in an enclosed space. Various types of cells, such as myocytes, macrophages, foreign body giant cells, myoblasts, and monocytes participate in this fibrotic reaction. Capsular contraction, which results from hardening and shrinkage of the preformed fibrous capsule, greatly affects the functionality and therapeutic efficacy of implantable devices [44].

In assessment of the biocompatibility of pectin/poly vinyl alcohol (PVA) composite hydrogel, it was found that inflammatory cell infiltration occurred in the muscular tissues around the PVA implants after a week, while fibrous capsulation around the implants was formed after four weeks [43]. In the study of biodegradable nerve guide conduit reinforced with genipin-cross-linked gelatin/β-tricalcium phosphate, a very thin fibrous capsule was formed surrounding the conduit upon being subcutaneously implanted on the dorsal side of a rat [45, 46]. Composite membrane containing polyvinyl alcohol (PVA) and porcine small intestinal submucosa (SIS) powder was developed as a novel coating material for coronary covered stents. In *in vivo* implantation tests, a thin capsule was formed by several layers of fibroblasts surrounding the implants, indicating the PVA-SIS composite membrane retained biomechanical and biological properties that can be used as a coating material for a coronary covered stent [47].

In the case of chitosan-hydroxyapatite composites, massive capsules consisting of dense connective tissue were formed, and the material showed signs of biodegradation in the form of fissures and cavities. The chitosan-hydroxyapatite-based implants exhibit a huge potential to generate a strong interaction with host cells [48].

b. *Tissue ingrowth:* Tissue ingrowth is a desired response for many implants. Good tissue ingrowth is dependent on the mechanical stability of the implant, and the nature of ingrowing tissue is dependent on the minimum size of the interconnections between pores. It was reported that the formation of a protein–protein composite scaffolds with desirable mechanical properties was obtained through silk fibroin microparticle reinforcements. These materials can enhance the compressive properties of porous silk fibroin sponges and closely simulate the mechanical features of native bone, producing significantly increased osteogenic differentiation [49].

A novel nanosize hydroxyapatite (HA) particles/poly(ester-urethane) composite scaffold for bone tissue engineering provided an osteoconductive surface to promote the ingrowth of new bone after implantation into bone defects. As compared with other groups, hydroxyapatite (HA) nanoparticles and polycaprolactone (PCL) particles induced the differentiation of primary human-bone–derived cells with significant upregulation of osteogenic gene expression and alkaline phosphatase activity, which are essential for bone ingrowth in load-bearing applications [50].

The porous bottom surface of polylactide/beta-tricalcium phosphate (PLA/beta-TCP) composite scaffolds displayed enhanced osteogenic differentiation potential, achieving a rapid growth of bone cells. An enhanced adhesion and proliferation of fibroblasts has been observed, when they are loaded onto a novel composite beta-tricalcium phosphate/silicone rubber (beta-TCP/SR) [51]. It was also noticed that the dense surface of the scaffold inhibited the ingrowth of osteoblasts and bone tissue, while simultaneously encouraging the ingrowth of chondrocytes [52].

c. *Tissue adhesion:* The cell adhesion to biomaterials, one of the major barriers to the extended use of biomaterial devices, causes the improper tissue integration or compatibility with biomaterial surfaces, leading to biomaterial-induced infection. These interactions are directed by numerous receptors and outer membrane molecules on the cell surface, as well as by the electronic state and geometry of the biomaterial surface. For instance, fibrovascular ingrowth into porous implants was greatly affected by implant porosity and composition rather than by angiogenic enhancing membrane molecules.

Nano-hydroxyapatite composite membranes in combinations with poly(vinyl alcohol) (*n*-HA/PVA) [53] or carboxyethylchitosan [54] revealed a reduced tensile strength and increase of Young's modulus of composite membranes, validating their potential as scaffold materials. Electrospun collagen/poly(ε-caprolactone) porous nerve conduits efficiently stimulated regenerated nerve fibers in the sciatic nerve gap, accomplishing similar electrophysiological and muscle renovation rates to autografts [55].

The adhesive chitosan/Pluronic (BASF Corporation, Florham Park, NJ) injectable hydrogels exhibited strong adhesiveness to soft tissues and mucous layer and demonstrated superior hemostatic properties. Hence, these hydrogels could be exploited for injectable drug delivery depots, tissue engineering hydrogels, tissue adhesives, and antibleeding materials [56]. An application of collagen-chitosan/fibrin glue asymmetric scaffolds has been explored in skin tissue engineering [57]. Shuttle-like fibroblasts adhering to the wall of the scaffold showed a gradual growth in the dermal layer of the scaffold, and constructed composite skin substitute with a histological structure similar to that of normal skin tissue.

4.2.3 Blood Compatibility

4.2.3.1 Mechanism In using biomaterials, it is important to monitor the biocompatibility and degradability of constituents of composite materials under a body environment, especially upon exposure to blood [58]. The blood compatibility of the implanted device depends on the properties of biomaterial, design of the device, and patient state. However, the biological properties of biomaterial are the only regulating factor to control blood compatibility. An implantation of biomaterial within a host system triggers a series of surface reactions including protein absorption followed by coagulation system activation that results in stimulation of the immune system.

Protein adsorption plays a crucial role in short-term and long-term blood compatibility of a biomaterial surface [59]. The most important consideration while selecting blood interfacing biomaterial implants is that it should not induce blood coagulation (clotting) or any blood cell damage (hemolysis). Blood coagulation occurs in response to intrinsic or extrinsic stimulations.

a. Intrinsic stimulations are initiated by blood contact with either a damaged portion of the blood vessel wall or another thrombogenic (clot causing) surface. It will take 7–12 minutes to form a soft clot.

b. Extrinsic stimulations are initiated as a result of the presence of a foreign body or tissue damage (other than blood vessel), and it will take 5–12 seconds to form a soft clot.

4.2.3.2 Factor Affecting Blood Compatibility

(i) **Surface roughness** is a crucial factor in defining blood compatibility as a rough surface has a greater exposure area for the blood component. Surface roughness will promote faster blood coagulation as compared with smooth surface material. Rough surfaces are sometimes used to promote initial clotting at porous interfaces to minimize the leakage of blood (e.g., polymer meshes used for vascular grafts).

(ii) **Surface wettability** of biomaterial corresponds to the hydrophilic or hydrophobic nature of the material surface. No consistent correlation was observed between the wettability parameter (the contact angle) and blood clotting time.

(iii) **Surface charge:** The intima of a normal blood vessel has a negative surface charge as a result of the presence of polysaccharides (chondroitin sulfate and heparin sulfate). The essential elements of blood (red cells, white cells, and platelets) also have a negative charge; hence, the natural repulsive force between intima and blood cells minimizes cell damage and coagulation.

The effect of the surface charge on the onset of clot formation has been demonstrated in the canine experiments using negatively charged and noncharged segments of vessel-simulating copper tubing [1]. Copper is normally thrombogenic (i.e., induce clot forming) material when they are implanted as an arterial replacement. When the tube was negatively charged, the onset of clot formation was delayed by a few days as compared to the control tube, which induced a clot within a few minutes. For synthetic biomaterials, surface charge occurs naturally only in polymers.

4.2.3.3 Approaches to Reduce Blood Coagulation Through Surface Modification

(i) *Generation of cell-membrane resembling surface:* Surface modification of parent material is an attractive approach for improving biomedical functionality of blood-contacting biomaterial. Surface modification may lead to generation of a material surface resembling a cell membrane that may be capable of altering or reducing protein adsorption. The self-monitoring polymeric coating can improve the performance of a biomaterial device by reducing protein adsorption on the blood–material interface. For instance, the modification of plasticized vinyl chloride (PVC) with the incorporation of cyclodextrin reduced fibrinogen adsorption, whose degree depends on the type and quantity of cyclodextrin used [59, 60].

(ii) *Generation of thrombo-resistant surfaces:* The generation of a thrombo-resistant biomaterial surface reduces coagulation, which can be achieved by several approaches, including:

a. *Fabrication of a negatively charged material surface:* An increase in negative charge could reduce the platelet response but enhance the contact activation phase of the intrinsic coagulation [60]. Anionic radicals can be included in the material structure to produce a negative surface charge.

b. *Lowering surface tension:* Surface tension is a complex, time-dependent phenomena resulting from the adhesion of other materials (i.e., circulating proteins) to the vessel surface. Blood cells are less likely to adhere to the surface with low surface tension. High surface tension materials tend to attract proteins that form a protective layer on the material, while low surface tension materials repel blood cells and minimize clotting. A theoretical range of surface tension that suppresses thrombosis should be specified for each device.

c. *Heparin conjugation:* Heparin is a polysaccharide with negative charges used to prevent clotting in general. An attempt was made to attach heparin chemically to the surface of the biomaterial implant [61]. Different categories of polysaccharide have been used for tissue-engineered scaffolds and drug-delivery applications, including 1) nonmammalian polysaccharides (alginate, chitin, and dextran), 2) mammalian polysaccharides (hyaluronan, chondroitin sulfate, and heparin), 3) multi-polysaccharide conjugates, and 4) polysaccharide mimetic.

(iii) *Composite application:* A biomimetic matrix composed of adhesive proteins and growth factors, for themselves or a combination with coating substrate for biomaterials, can be used for surface coating. Biomimetic composites have been suitable for tissue engineering not only to improve biological function but also to reduce cytotoxicity [58]. For instances, novel electro-spun polyurethane/gelatin composite meshes have been designed as a blood vessel substitute (i.e., vascular prosthesis), which previously has been lacking a functional synthetic small diameter [62].

The blood compatibility of composite membranes displayed its maximal value when they have the greatest hydrophilic property, simultaneously accomplishing fewer platelets adhered and spread, and showing a little distortion on the surface of materials [63]. In the platelet adhesion test for assessment of blood compatibility of surface coating, PLGA50/50 drug eluting film showed much enhanced blood compatibility as compared with anticorrosion micro-arc oxidation/poly-L-lactic acid (MAO/PLLA) coating film [64].

Chitosan has been widely used for biomaterial scaffolds in tissue engineering as a result of its superior mechanical properties and cytotoxic compatibility. However, biomedical utilization of chitosan, especially for blood-contacting tissue engineering, was limited as a result of its poor blood compatibility. Macroscopically homogeneous chitosan–heparin (Chi-Hep) blended suspension showed improved blood compatibility as well as good mechanical properties and endothelial cell compatibility [65]. Chi-Hep composite matrices could be a promising candidate for blood-contacting tissue engineering.

Chitosan was also used as a supplement substance for biomaterial scaffolds in tissue engineering to enhance their biocompatibility. The efficacy and blood compatibility of polyvinyl alcohol (PVA) hydrogels for artificial blood vessel applications were significantly improved by the addition of natural polymers including chitosan, gelatin, and starch [66]. *O*-butyryl chitosan (OBCS)-grafted polypyrrole (PPy) composite films have both excellent blood compatibility and high electrical conductivity, which warrant them to be suitable for biomaterials, such as electrically conducting blood vessels and functionally hemocompatible substrates of biosensors used directly in whole blood [67].

4.3 BIORESORBABLE AND BIOERODIBLE MATERIALS

Bioresorbable and bioerodible polymers are one class of biomaterials that has the unique ability of interacting with a biological system and therefore widely employed in tissue engineering. Bioresorbable polymers or bio-absorbable polymers are polymers that can be resorbed or metabolized in the human system without producing any side effects and are therefore advantageous over metallic systems [68]. This ability of bioresorbable and bioerodible materials made them suitable for their use as a drug delivery system, sutures, and implants, as it will avoid the requirement of a second surgical operation for their removal. Furthermore, the physical, chemical, and mechanical properties of these materials can be modified so as to improve their usability as medical devices.

Bioresorbable polymers are also commonly used in joint surgeries as they exhibit bone-like properties and aid in bone healing. Most of these polymers are naturally or synthetically derived and degrade into nontoxic products through hydrolysis [69]. Such advantages in addition to biocompatibility and biodegradability make bioresorbable and bioerodible polymers an interesting biomaterial for their use in tissue engineering. An ideal bioresorbable and bioerodible polymer should not produce an inflammatory response upon implantation, should have degradation time similar to the regeneration or healing of the targeted tissue, and should produce nontoxic products on degradation that can be easily excreted from the body [70]. The major advantages in applying bioresorbable polymers to the medical devices include:

I. Simultaneous replacement by soft tissues.
II. Elimination of corrosion, release of metallic particles, and a second surgery for the removal of an implanted device unlike metal implants.
III. Transfer of loads to the healing of soft tissue and bone fractures.
IV. Avoidance of difficulties in magnetic resonance imaging.
V. Accomplishment of enhanced drug release profiles by modifying the polymeric block ratio.

4.3.1 Application of Bioresorbable and Bioerodible Polymers

Bioresorbable and biodegradable polymers are versatile in various applications, as summarized in Table 4.3.

(i) *Replacement arthroplasty (joint replacement surgery):* Replacement arthroplasty or joint replacement surgery is a type of orthopedic surgery in which a severe arthritic joint surface is substituted with a prosthesis (an artificial medical device). It is usually used when the joint pain or joint dysfunction is not curable with noninvasive methods. Bioresorbable and bioerodible polymers are commonly used in orthopedic surgery as they eliminate the removal process of the implant with surgical operation [70].

(ii) *Soft contact lens:* A soft contact lens has been widely used for drug delivery in addition to its application in correcting vision difficulties such as hyperopia, myopia, and others. Soft contact lenses are usually prepared from hydrogels as they possess a water-absorbing capacity and are able to control the release rate of the loaded drugs. A soft contact lens has also been used as a drug delivery system for treating inflammation in the anterior segment of the eye (Table 4.3). Recently, a silicone hydrogels contact lens has been proposed to alleviate drying symptoms that are associated with a normal

TABLE 4.3 Application of Bioresorbable and Biodegradable Polymers

Polymer	Medical Devices/ Formulation	Inference	Reference
Poly-L/D-lactide 96/4	Scaffolds	Significant improvement in the function and structure of the joint without producing signs of osteolysis after implant resorption	[73]
Cholesterol bearing pullulan	Hydrogel	Highly efficient in delivering bone morphogenetic protein for inducing bone growth	[74]
Polylactate	Screws	Useful in the fixation of Pipkin fracture	[75]
Polylactide-co-glycolide	Microsphere	Symptoms of arthritis (limb swelling) were successfully relieved	[76]
Polyhydroxyl methyl methacrylate	Soft contact lens	Improved loading and sustained delivery of diclofenac in lacrimal fluid	[77]
Polyhydroxy ethyl methacrylate	Soft contact lens	Prolonged release of ciprofloxacin	[78]
Poly(w-pentadecalactone-co-*p*-dioxanone) copolyester	Suture material	Co-polymer was well tolerated and produced tissue responses similar to unmodified poly (*p*-dioxanone)	[79]
Polylactic acid-co-glycolic acid	Suture material	Cytosine-phosphorothioate-guanine oligonucleotides loaded suture exhibited greater suppression of neuroblastoma recurrence and improved survival rate	[80]
Poly(glycolide-co-ε-caprolactone)	Suture material	Suture possessed adequate tensile strength which facilitated wound healing and eventually degraded without causing irritation	[71]
Polylactide-polyglycolide acid	Bone plates	Significant enhancement in bone formation by inducing proliferation of osteoblasts	[81]
Poly-L/DL-lactic acid	Bone plates	Assisted healing and gradually transferred the physiological forces to the healing bone while gradually degraded over time	[72]
Polylactide-co-glycolide	Foamspheres, bone plates	Slow and sustained release of recombinant bone morphogenetic proteins. Excellent recovery of calvarial bone	[82]
Polylactide/D-lactide/ trimethylene carbonate	Bone mini plates	Found useful in fixing unilateral mandibular angle fractures without producing any serious complications	[83]
Poly(L-lactide-co-D/L-lactide)	Bone plates	Alternative to titanium plates in providing strong internal fixation of mandible fractures	[84]
Poly-L-lactide-polyglycolic acid	Screws	Could be utilized as a fixation implant in autogenous bone grafts	[85]
Polylactic-co-glycolic acid	Scaffolds	Significant growth and amount of axons were found in groups treated with implants carrying neural stem cells and Schwann cells	[86]
Poly-beta hydroxybutyrate	Scaffold	Significant improvement in the restoration of spinal cord injury	[87]
Chitosan	Solution	The conduction of nerve impulse in the spinal cord of guinea pigs were successfully restored	[88]
Collagen	Chitosan tubes	Tubes containing type I collagen showed significant production of new axons and recovery from the spinal cord injury	[89]

hydrogel contact lens, suggesting that the incorporation of silicone in a contact lens might be a viable approach for reducing dryness problems attributed by hydrogel contact lens [90].

(iii) *Sutures:* The use of sutures produced from bioabsorbable polymers is highly advantageous as the polymer will be slowly absorbed and degraded under physiological conditions unlike non-biodegradable polymers [71].

(iv) *Bone plates:* An ideal system intended to repair bone fractures should be able to provide adequate strength initially to facilitate bone healing followed by a decrease in strength so as to allow physiological force transfer to the healing bone. Biodegradable polymers are ideal biomaterials to fulfill these functions over metallic systems [72]. Several biodegradable polymers including polylactide, polyglycolide, and their co-polymers have been previously used for the fixation devices in maxillofacial, orthopedic, and craniofacial reconstructive surgical procedures (Table 4.2).

A polylactic acid–polyglycolic acid co-polymer plate and screw fixation system along with a resorbable collagen barrier have been recommended for clinical application in a guided bone regeneration procedure [91]. In this approach, the polylactic acid–polyglycolic acid co-polymer served as a scaffold that supported bone formation while the collagen barrier secured the graft material. Lately, novel poly(L-lactic acid) composite fibers carrying hydroxyapatite nanorods were recommended for load-bearing bone plate application [92].

(v) *Spinal rods:* A spinal rod is a type of spinal implants that is used so as to immobilize the spine in a right alignment [93]. These rods are usually strong but possess sufficient flexibility so that it can fit accurately in the alignment of the patient's spine. The study on the implantation effects of bioabsorbable polylactide rods and K-wire rods (rigid fixation) on the posterior interlaminar fusion investigated in rabbits displayed significant spinal fusion as compared with groups without implantation [94], suggesting that bioabsorbable polylactide rods and K-wire rods can serve as a potential implant for augmenting spinal fusion. Furthermore, the use of bioabsorbable polylactide rods would be convenient over K-wire rods as it will avoid the requirement of a surgical operation.

(vi) *Chin augmentation:* Chin augmentation is a surgical procedure where the implants are placed on the underlying part or structure of the face so as to provide balance and support to the facial structures [95]. It is one of the most commonly used techniques to generate significant correction, reshape chin size, and provide noticeable changes while fixating maxillofacial abnormalities. The implant placed at the target site provides a new surface for the growth of soft tissue thereby providing stronger support together [95]. It is usually used for balancing and restoring the facial structures of a person through enlarging and reshaping the chin as compared with the nose.

(vii) *Spinal cord injury:* Several biodegradable polymers such as polylactide-co-glycolide, chitosan, collagen, and others have been used for restoring function in traumatic conditions including spinal cord injury [96].

4.3.2 Implant Response to Tissue Ingrowth, Capsule Formation, and Tissue Adhesion

Artelon (Artimplant AB, Malmo, Sweden) Spacer CMC was a classic example of an implant inducing tissue ingrowth and capsule formation [97, 98]. It is a T-shaped device made from a biodegradable polymer, polycaprolactone-based polyurethane urea. It is used in the treatment of thumb base osteoarthritis also known as osteoarthritic trapeziometacarpal (CMC) joint or carpometacarpal joint that is a state where the base of the thumb is disabled as a result of osteoarthritis. The device is positioned in such a way that the trapezial bone is well separated from the metacarpal bone while forming an articular surface for cell adhesion. The capsular tissue on the dorsal surface grows thereby stabilizing the joint by strengthening the joint capsule. However, it has its own limitations as foreign body reactions associated with Artelon Spacer CMC were reported for the lack of its biocompatibility [99].

4.3.3 Biocompatibility Issues

Poly glycolic acid and polylactides/polyglycolides polymers have been widely used for producing bioabsorbable implants, sutures, and other biomedical devices. Previously, the rapid molecular weight loss of nine different bioabsorbable polymers has been reported to be the major factor responsible for producing strong tissue reactions. It was also reported that polylactide-co-glycolide polymer (25/75, 75/25) and poly-L-lactide polymer showed minimal inflammatory and fibrocellular response [100].

High-molecular-weight poly-L-lactic acid blended with a water-soluble amphiphilic phospholipid polymer containing phosphorylcholine groups (PMB30W) have been reported to minimize tissue responses as compared with poly-L-lactic acid implants. Furthermore, the thrombus formation and release of proinflammatory cytokines from human peripheral blood mononuclear cells were also significantly reduced with poly-L-lactic acid/PMB30W blended polymer [101].

Chitosan is an intensively studied biomaterial as scaffolds in the regeneration of bone, nerve, and cartilages. Recently, chitosan scaffolds have been found to provide an excellent environment for the growth of vascular, lung, and liver cells [102]. However, it has been reported that chitosan can cause blood coagulation, and therefore, its efficacy for blood-contacting tissue engineering should be carefully monitored [65].

Scaffolds prepared from a mixture of chitosan and heparin demonstrated excellent blood and endothelial cell compatibility [65]. *In vitro* studies showed that chitosan heparin films had lesser adsorption of albumin and fibrinogen than chitosan films. Furthermore, the formation of thrombus and adhesion of platelets on chitosan heparin films were significantly diminished as compared with chitosan films. This study demonstrates that heparin, a well-known anticoagulant, can be employed for providing a thrombo-resistant surface to chitosan.

The use of bioresorbable polymers has revolutionized the application of biomaterials in the field of biomedicines. Bioresorbable and bioerodible polymers are successfully used for not only drug delivery devices but also fixating fractures, chin augmentation, sutures, and in bone replacements. The biocompatibility, degradation rate, and strength of these polymers can be manipulated so as to improve their efficacy in application to the human body.

4.4 COMPOSITE MATERIALS

Composite materials are solids that contain two or more distinct constituent materials or phases. The properties of composite, including elastic modulus, are significantly altered as compared with those of a homogeneous material [103, 104]. Natural composites, such as foam with an empty space at one phase, are composed of bone, wood, dentin, cartilage, and skin [105, 106]. Hierarchical structures of natural composites exhibit particulate, porous, and fibrous features at different microscales.

Composite biomaterials have been broadly used as biomedical devices, such as dental filling composites, reinforced bone cement, orthopedic implants with porous surface, and bioactive glasses for healing [107–110]. Composite materials offer numerous advantages over homogeneous materials, motivating researchers and engineers to continuously exploit their detailed and small-scale material properties including stiffness, strength, lightweight, resilience, and compliance, over the larger scale structure [111].

Composite materials can be categorized into macro-filler composite (>10 μm), hybrid composite and homogenic micro-filler composite (0.01–0.1 μm), and inhomogenic micro-filler composite according to the filler size (0.01–0.1 μm) [112, 113]. Nanofillers and nanoclusters can enhance the long-term stability in hybrid composites, whereas microfiller composites additionally possess the polishing properties by the use of nanoparticles and nanoclusters. When superficial filler particles are disoriented as a result of abrasion, the nanoclusters of the nanocomposites are thereby broken down into nanoparticles.

Composite biomaterials are mostly made of synthetic polymers. Polyethylene remains a popular matrix source as nondegradable materials, while polymers, such as polylactic acid (PLA) and polyhydroxybutyrate (PHB), have been widely used as degradable matrix sources.

Hydroxyapatite-reinforced polyethylene (HAPE) was the first of the "second-generation" biomaterials that have been developed to be bioactive rather than bio-inert [114]. HAPE has steered to a range of other potentially bioactive composites, which can be degradable or nondegradable depending on the type and composition of the matrix polymer. The responses to most implantable composites have been safe, and no signs of macrophages and inflammation were observed until more than 30 months after implantation of composites [115].

4.4.1 Composite Materials for Biomedical Application

(i) *Composite materials for bone tissue engineering and joint replacement:* Biomaterials have been applied to bone implantation and replacement over four decades [116]. As the optimization of mechanical strength of the scaffold materials remain a big challenge in bone tissue engineering, composite materials are playing a prime role in enhancement of efficacy and strength of biomedical bone devices. The next generation of biomaterials seems to be a mixture of bioactive and bioresorbable materials that can achieve the proficiency of closely mimicking the natural function of bone and tissue regeneration.

Carbon nanotube is a promising material whose intrinsic adhesion properties can improve the mechanical strength of the biomedical devices, particularly those to be positioned in contact with bone, such as prostheses for arthroplasty, plates or screws for fracture fixation, drug delivery systems, and scaffolding for bone regeneration [117, 118]. Cell adhesion to a culture dish coated with multiwalled carbon nanotubes is much greater than those coated with other materials including collagen [119, 120].

Carbon nanotubes in a combination with recombinant human bone morphogenetic protein-2 exhibited excellent tissue compatibility and bone repair capability, thereby closely integrating with bone tissue and accelerating bone formation [121, 122]. It was also observed that the combination of carbon nanotubes with grafted chitosan enormously enhanced the mechanical strength of the composite [122], mimicking the organic portion as well as the inorganic portion of natural bone.

Calcium phosphatase bioceramics, such as hydroxyapatite (HA) and tricalcium phosphate, are promising materials for bone tissue engineering because these ceramic mixtures reflect the chemistry and structure of the native mineral components of the bone tissue [123]. The incorporation of HA nanoparticles into the polymer scaffold altered the pore surface morphology of the composite scaffolds whose properties were dependent on the ratio of HA and the polymer, rendering them to be more suitable for protein adsorption. The combination of HA and chitosan composite also exhibited an excellent biodegradability and biocompatibility in bone tissue engineering [124–128].

Recently, ceramics have been enormously used for orthopedics in the United States. Pure alumina was the first commercial implant for clinical use in the 1970s, and to date, applied components have been expanded to millions. A new ceramic composite, the alumina matrix composite, has been applied to the total joint replacement area, offering enhanced reliability and excellent performance [129]. The alumina matrix composites displayed the reinforcement of ceramics with tribological qualities and exhibited enhanced mechanical resistance as compared with pure alumina, pioneering new composite designs (i.e., new sizes for inserts and ceramic double mobility) for orthopedics.

(ii) *Composite materials for wound healing:* Biocomposites made of bioresorbable polymers and bioactive inorganic materials, such as bioactive glasses, are intensively explored for wound healing, bone reconstruction, and tissue engineering [130–132]. For instance, synthetic bioabsorbable biocomposites composed of polyglycolic acid (PGA), polylactic acid (PLA), and polyglycolide lactide (PGLA) co-polymers were developed as surgical sutures applied for wound healing [132].

Bioactive glasses have been used to coat surgical meshes and sutures using a novel textile technique [133, 134]. As compared with pure Bioglass (University of Florida, Gainesville, FL), the Bioglass-poly(D,L-lactide) (PDLLA) composite coatings exhibited improved microstructural homogeneity and uniformity along the suture length through an additional PDLLA coating [109].

In particular, the composite polyglactin 910, a synthetic absorbable monofilament surgical suture material, has exhibited excellent performance as sutures in wound healing applications with several integral advantages: good mechanical properties, minimal tissue reactions, and easy and reproducible fabrication [129]. This fibrous material is a promising precursor in fabrication of resorbable three-dimensional scaffolds made of bioactive ceramics or glasses for tissue engineering applications. As a moist environment promotes rapid wound healing, a hydrogel sheet composed of alginate, chitin/chitosan, and fucoidan composites has been used as a primary wound dressing to maintain an optimal moist environment [135].

(iii) *Composite materials for ophthalmic application:* Bioadhesives have limited usage in ophthalmic surgery, as they have inadequate tensile strength and are difficult to be retained at the tissue site. A scaffold of cyanoacrylate bioadhesive composite consisted of 2-octyl-cyanoacrylate and either a poly (L-lactic-co-glycolic acid) (PLGA) or a rehydrated porcine small intestine submucosa (SIS) accomplished enhanced adhesiveness and, thus, was used as an alternative to sutures in ophthalmic surgery [110].

It was demonstrated that the composite hydrogel was both nontoxic and biodegradable and that corneal endothelial cells transplanted by the composite hydrogel could survive and retain normal morphology, supporting corneal endothelium reconstruction. Hydrogels based on a water-soluble derivative of chitosan, hydroxypropyl chitosan (HPCTS), and sodium alginate dialdehyde (SAD) displayed their biocompatibilities and pharmacological efficacies as well as suitability in ophthalmic application [136].

A composite interpenetrating network of two biocompatible materials, poly(dimethyl siloxane) (PDMS) and Poly (*N*-isopropyl acrylamide) (PNIPAAM), was explored as artificial cornea and contact lens [137]. It generates polymers with preferred oxygen and glucose permeability and improved wettability as compared with PDMS homo-polymers. It also showed a greater mechanical strength as compared with PNIPAAM homopolymers, further demonstrating its potential as ophthalmic biomaterials for the controlled drug delivery.

(iv) *Electrically conducting composite materials for nerve tissue engineering:* The current clinical treatment strategy for peripheral nerve injuries with segmental nerve loss prefers the method of nerve autografts, which remain the only proven means of bridging lengthy gaps in the peripheral nerve [138–140]. A piece of noncritical nerve from a secondary site on the body has been used to replace the missing nerve section.

Electrically conductive polymer composites composed of polycaprolactone fumarate and polypyrrole (PCL-PPy) materials synthesized with five different anions have been developed for nerve regeneration [141]. *In vitro* studies showed that PCLF-PPy materials support cell attachment, proliferation, and neurite extension and that they are promising materials for future studies involving electrical stimulation. As this technique still has numerous drawbacks including donor site morbidity, insufficient donor nerve length, mismatch of diameter between donor nerve and recipient site, misaligned endoneurial tubes, and mismatched regenerating axons, further improvement in electrical conductivity is needed for the customary clinical application.

(v) *Composite for dental restorative materials:* Dental composites should be stable within the oral environment and relatively easy to handle [142–144]. Dental composites, however, still have several drawbacks including shrinkage during the polymerization process, potential failure of the resin–dentin interface leading to secondary caries, a high coefficient of thermal expansion, and a low wear resistance as compared with metal-based restorations [145, 146]. Several interesting developments and strong trends in the broader field of materials science that inspire future potential applications of dental composites to some extent include:

(a) *Nanoparticles for dental micro-filled substrate:* Nanoparticles, such as colloidal silica particles with a diameter around 40 nm, have been used as hybrid composites for a dental microfilled substrate for decades [147]. Nanoparticle composites for a dental microfilled substrate exhibited outstanding esthetics and enhanced wear resistance, fracture toughness, adhesion to tooth tissue, as well as ease of polishing [148]. However, the wear and fatigue properties of composites encapsulating nanoparticles were similar to or sometimes worse than a microfilled composite [149].

(b) *Antimicrobial activity materials:* Antimicrobial materials are used to fight bacteria and delay, reduce, or avoid the formation of biofilms on the materials [150]. Silver and titanium particles were incorporated into dental composites to introduce antimicrobial properties and enhance the biocompatibility of the composites [151].

    The antimicrobial activity of dental composites containing quaternary ammonium polyethylenimine (PEI) nanoparticles demonstrated a delay in biofilm formation as compared with conventional composites, indicating that quaternary ammonium PEI nanoparticles immobilized in resin-based materials have a strong antibacterial activity upon contact without leach-out of the nanoparticles and without compromise in mechanical properties [152]. Although the detailed mechanism of the antibacterial effect of these materials was not fully elucidated, it was speculated that PEI might cause lysis of the bacterial cells through binding to the cell wall components, causing leakage of the cytoplasmatic material.

(c) *Stimuli responsive materials:* Stimuli responsive materials, also known as smart materials, possess properties that are considerably altered by external stimuli, such as changes of temperature, mechanical stress, pH, moisture, or electric or magnetic fields [153, 154]. Smart dental composites seem to be relatively suitable for release-on-command of antimicrobial compounds or fluoride to fight microbes or secondary caries [155].

    Resin composites are used for a variety of applications in dentistry, including restorative materials, cavity liners, pit and fissure sealants, cores and buildups, inlays, onlays, crowns, provisional restorations, cements for single or multiple tooth prostheses and orthodontic devices, endodontic sealers, and root canal posts [156, 157]. It is likely that the use of resin will continue to grow and become smart dental material in both frequency and application as a result of their versatility.

    Stimuli responsive dental composites would demand more complicated structures and/or combined materials with adequate strength, high wear resistance, and polishability retention than normal dental composites [158, 159]. Subsequently, dental composites further necessitate new synthetic polymers with enhanced self-adhesive properties, leading to genuinely easy placement in the mouth [157].

(vi) *Self-repairing (self-healing) materials:* As dental materials have a limited lifetime and can self-degrade as a result of various physical, chemical, and/or biological stimuli, the renovation process in biological materials requires the integration of numerous factors related to the physiological nature [160, 161]. For example, the fact that natural bone is permanently remodeled and self-repaired (healed) even after a major fracture has occurred has motivated engineers and scientists worldwide to develop synthetic self-healing or self-repairing materials [162, 163].

    Dental tissues in the oral cavity, which are subjected to be regenerated, are dental enamel and dentin. During the last few years, numerous attempts have been made to create synthetic dental enamel or repair dental enamel modified from polymer–ceramic biomimetic composites [164]. It was demonstrated that a hydroxyapatite layer, which was obtained after the hydroxyapatite solution was deposited onto enamel, was very efficient in dental tissue regeneration [165].

    An epoxy system containing resin-filled microcapsules is one of the first self-repairing synthetic materials for dental application [166]. When a crack occurs in the epoxy composite material, the microcapsules near the creak are broken and release the resin. The resin subsequently fills the crack and reacts with a Grubbs catalyst dispersed in the epoxy composite, leading to the polymerization of the resin and repair of the crack. The efficacy of the healing action after a fracture event relies on the duration of healing time exerted by bulk polymer materials like dicyclopentadiene [167–169].

    As modern composite resins have not yet achieved the level of mechanical properties found in dental amalgam, leading to shorter and limited clinical service for composite resin materials as compared with amalgam, several advanced approaches with the new structural epoxy formulations were attempted. For instance, the self-repairing materials filled with glass filler and an acrylic-based system, as opposed to an epoxy-based system, efficiently recovered mechanical properties by the incorporation of embedded monomers and catalysts [170].

4.4.2 Composite Materials for Drug Delivery

Over the past few decades, composite materials have attracted significant research interest in the interdisciplinary field of material-related sciences with drug delivery systems. Four composite materials have been successfully designed as promising materials for drug delivery, which include:

(i) *Nanocomposite materials:* Nanoparticles have been incorporated into the nanostructured scaffolds to deliver biologically active molecules, such as growth and differentiation factors used for optimal tissue regeneration [171]. Composite materials, such as a polymeric scaffold blended with nano-sized material, could be a promising carrier for drug delivery. In particular, a stronger interaction between nanosize particles and the surrounding polymer material may result in improved mechanical strength in the composite scaffold, whereas enhanced surface roughness may increase osteoblastic functions.

The encapsulation or conjugation of the agents with biocompatible polymers, such as polyethylene glycol (PEG) and *N*-(2-hydroxypropyl)methacrylamide (HPMA), liposomes, and dendrimers, has been a successful approach for improving the water solubility of therapeutic agents, extending residency time in the body, and the uptake rate at tumor, in turn reducing required drug loads and associated toxic effects [172–174].

PEG, a U.S. Food and Drug Administration (FDA)-approved, nontoxic polymer exhibiting high resistance to protein adsorption, is a particularly popular candidate. PEG molecules are strongly hydrophilic and form a surface-bound hydrated layer around the nanoparticles [175–177]. The hydrated layer shields the nanoparticles from interactions with cell surface proteins, thereby limiting nanoparticles elimination by the immune system.

(ii) *Carbon nanotubes (CNTs):* CNTs have been exploited as a novel tool for the delivery of therapeutic molecules including peptides, RNA and DNA, and biomedical applications as sensors, actuators, and composites [122, 178–180]. The large inner volume of CNTs in contrast to their dimensions and easy immobilization process of the outer surface with biocompatible materials make them a superior nanomaterial for drug delivery [181, 182].

Studies reveal that CNTs are a versatile carrier for controlled and targeted drug delivery, especially for cancer cells, as a result of their cell membrane penetrability. Several studies on the fate of nanotubes in the body demonstrated that CNTs loaded with drug molecules could easily pass into cells and enter the cell nucleus, thus, accomplishing both cellular and nuclear levels of targeted delivery [183].

In recent years, a new generation of nanomaterials known as "smart bio-nanotubes" was introduced [184, 185]. The smart bio-nanotubes have a trilayered structure consisting of a microtubular protein called tubulin coated with a bilayer of lipid followed by coating of tubulin protein in the form of rings or spirals where proteins had either open ends (negatively overcharged) or closed ends (positively overcharged with lipid caps). The integral variable for smart bio-nanotubes that regulates the release profile of loaded drug is the comparative thickness of protein lipid versus protein coats, which can be competently optimized based on pharmacological efficacy.

(iii) *Electro-conductive composites:* Electro-conductive hydrogels (ECHs) are polymeric blends or co-networks that combine inherently conductive electroactive polymers with highly hydrated hydrogels [186, 187]. ECHs are used for the delivery of biological molecules, such as peptide sequences, enzymes antibodies, and DNA. ECHs offer a new class of devices with low interfacial impedances, which are suitable for neural prosthetic tools, such as deep brain stimulation electrodes; low-voltage actuation, which is suitable for electrically stimulated drug release devices; and *in vivo* biocompatibility, which is suitable for implantable biosensors [188].

Intrinsically conductive polymer composites (ICPCs) include both the mechanical properties of conventional polymers and the electrical properties of conducting polymers [189]. They can possess relatively high conductivities and dielectric constants, which can be easily transformed from insulating into conducting states through chemical processes, making ICPCs a very promising material for electromagnetic interference shielding (EMI) and other applications, such as organic solar cells, flexible transparent displays, and super-capacitors [190]. Polypyrrole-poly(acrylonitrile-co-vinyl acetate) composites were well suited to electromagnetic interference shielding applications, antistatic materials, and decoupling capacitors [191].

(iv) *Drug-loaded fibers and threads:* To incorporate a model drug, tetracycline hydrochloride (TCH), into poly(L-lactic acid) (PLLA) fibers, drug-loadable fibers and threads were developed via combining electrospinning with aligned fibers collection under either blend or coaxial electrospinning [192]. The blend TCH/PLLA fibers showed the smallest fiber diameter, whereas neat PLLA fibers and core-shell TCH-PLLA fibers showed a larger proximal average diameter, suggesting that the electrospinning technique provides a novel way to fabricate medical agent-loaded fibrous threads for tissue suturing and tissue regeneration applications. Drug-loadable fibers and threads can also be designed for stent coating against coronary diseases [193].

4.5 OTHER MATERIALS

The employment of metals and ceramics as biomaterials, exclusively or in combination with others, has been intensively explored, and thus, so far related research areas have been continuously expanding. The biomedical application of these metals highlights their distinct properties that either mimic physiological functions or provide additional support for bodily function [194].

4.5.1 Hydroxyapatite (HA)

(i) *HA scaffold designed for bone substitutes:* The scaffolds support cell/tissue attachment, determining the ultimate shape of the regenerated functional tissue, and leading to tissue growth [195]. Hydroxyapatite (HA), a major inorganic compound of human hard tissue, and its derivatives or composites have received enormous attention for their porogenecity and are considered superb candidates for enhancing mechanical strength and osteoconductive properties. As particulate HA was found to be incompetent to generate sufficient toughness when compared with natural bone, an infiltration of polymers, such as polycaprolactone (PCL), polycaprolactoneitaconate (PCLI), and poly(propylene fumarate) (PPF), was applied for improvement of compressive toughness of HA scaffold designed for bone substitutes [196, 197]. The thermal linking approach has resulted in huge reinforcement of mechanical strength and no adverse toxicity to osteo-cell lines, which has made it a promising bone regenerative candidate.

As it is of paramount concern that the cell adhered or attached, as well as penetrated through the HA scaffold surface into its body, the design of the macro-porosity of HA has been considered a criterion for examining its regenerative potential. Nano-crystalline generated via nonionic surfactant incorporation had a similar crystal size to that of natural apatites and a macroporous structure that stretches down to the micrometer scale [198]. The three-dimensional (3D) network compiled by nano-crystalline HA and coated with biopolymer having the pore size below 100 μm has been very effective for cell anchorage and colonization [199].

Numerous methods, such as foaming, leaching, and sintering out salt crystals, have been evaluated to achieve desirable bioresorbability and porosity of HA, and simultaneously enhance its structural merit for bone regeneration [200]. By adjusting manufacturing parameters, HA granules could have a controllable pore size, exhibiting a suitable pore structure and high porosity, as well as good mechanical properties [201]. With higher pore sizes, HA granules could obtain the ability to incorporate macromolecules, such as bone generating growth factors or antibodies, as a result, enhancing the therapeutic efficacy of HA and serving as an excellent substrate for bone tissue engineering.

(ii) *HA as bioactive surface coating materials:* HA is also used as bioactive surface coating materials for prevention or treatment of various physiological defects. The deposition of HA is highly effective in enhancing the biocompatibility of metal implants in the body. Early attempts of HA coating through various methods yield a layer that has a weak interaction with a metallic surface, significantly affecting the bonding strength between HA and the metal surface as well as the original bone tissue [202]. Variables, such as the enlargement of the metallic surface area and the structural interconnection among the surface array and HA morphology, are mainly considered solutions to the overall coating improvement [203].

Several new methods have been proposed to produce a smoother HA granule surface to avoid intrinsic inflammatory response and simultaneously promote natural osteo-integration. The control over the pore size and porosity, as well as smoothness, could be achieved by monitoring micro-channel structures through advanced instrumentations and different processing conditions. Recently, it was found that the osteogenic capacity of HA was enhanced through thermal spraying technology, in which silver (Ag) particles containing HA were used to coat titanium implants applied for joint replacement [204]. The optimal concentration of Ag particles containing HA was further determined to provide a good osteo-conductivity profile while maintaining low toxicity.

(iii) *HA particles designed as delivery vehicles:* Aside from being employed as bone substitutes or scaffolds in tissue engineering, spherical HA fabricated by various methods, such as interconnected pore channels generated through porogen introduction, liquid nitrogen, and freeze-drying, showed its effectiveness as a drug carrier [205]. Due to the bone integrative property of porous HA particles, they are primarily used as localized bone-inducing delivery vehicles [206]. Most compounds loaded in HA applications that fall under this category are anti-inflammatory drugs or antibacterial agents, such as dexamethasone, triamcinolone acetonide, and gentamicin [207].

HA in combination with the human demineralized bone matrix (hDBM) has offered an alternative means to promoting regenerative efficacy [208]. In contrast to lyophilized chips and uncombined HA products, hDBM has helped HA nanoparticles to achieve a significantly enhanced osteo-integration rate due to the demineralized property [209]. Bone morphogenetic protein-2 (BMP-2), which induces osteogenic differentiation, has been intensively used for local bone regeneration for the past decades. To mimic the biological condition that BMP-2s are continuously being produced and delivered into the bone formation site, HA nanoparticles were efficiently used as the BMP-2 carrier [210].

Injectable HA solution or gel has been widely used in soft-tissue augmentation [211]. Applications of an injectable HA system extend to not only bone regeneration but also to bone metastasis inhibition and anti-inflammation [212]. The chemical resorbability and structural similarity to bone tissue make HA carriers even more advantageous in fixing bone-related clinical cases, such as metastasized cancer that affects bone tissue. The chemotherapeutical adjuvants have been synergistically added to form rheologically competent HA ceramics, which served as a very efficient carrier for chemotherapies [213].

4.5.2 Titanium (Ti)

Being used as individual metal or alloy, titanium was broadly applied to numerous biomedical research areas Owing to its biocompatibility, anticorrosive properties, resistance to wear, and adequate mechanical strength [214]. Although its cost is relatively high as compared with other metal material, such as steel and cobalt alloys, the excellent performance makes it the first choice to patients seeking optimal care.

Clinical implantation of titanium and its alloys requires surface bonding with bone tissues to achieve long-term integration in them. Consequently, surface modification of such metals is often carried out before implantation. For instance, the titanium surface was modified with acid-alkali treatment, whose bioactivation plays a major role in enhancing the deposition performance of coated films, such as hydroxyapatite film, proving superior bonding between films with surface-activated metals to those with non-modified materials [215].

The employment of titanium particles in impaction grafting as the bone substitute has also been one of its clinical usages, especially for the purpose of osteoconduction. The insertion of titanium particles into a bone conduction chamber used as a model for evaluating bone ingrowth behavior enhanced fibrous armoring, although small particles are not so effective as larger sized particles in its osteoconduction capability [216]. Another advantage of this titanium-based grafting material over allograft is the resistance against the resorbability; while the allograft undergoes constant resorption into osteoblasts, titanium never does.

4.5.3 Nitinol

Nitinol has become major material for construction of the medical device, providing mechanical properties during the self-expanding procedure of the surgery and maintaining strong support against restenosis [217]. It is also advocated by its excellence in super-elasticity and shape memory, which serve as a foundation for most of its biomedical applications [218]. Nitinol, as a modified titanium alloy, is also employed in intravascular intervention technology including stents [219]. However, in some cases, a corrosive environment inside the lumen has triggered the release of nickel ions that have a potential to produce adverse inflammation, thus, necessitating a polymeric coating protection against thrombus formation [220].

The high adhesion strength of non-biodegradable polyhedral oligomeric silsesquioxanes (POSS) and poly(carbonate-urea)urethane (PCU) to the Nitinol stent surface proved to be a critical factor for enhancement of resistance to bare Nitinol peeling [221]. A nitinol wire is tested for its unique mechanical properties in biomaterial application in which the fatigue factor poses as a major challenge in evading clinical failure. Nitinol alloy containing 55.6 wt% is superelastic and exerts a strain-stress response under the testing cycle that simulates a real-life application [222]. There have been numerous attempts of chemical modification including forming the TiO_2 film to enhance the surface properties of nitinol medical devices, which mostly resulted in great enhancement of a corrosive resistance property [223].

4.5.4 Platinum (Pt)

Conducting metals like platinum and platinum-indium alloys are used for electrical medical devices including chronic electrode implants, which recorded electrical impulses in the brain [224].

Endovascular coils made of platinum have been developed for the alleviation of an intracranial aneurysm. The surface coating strategy using polymers is also involved in the bioactivation of the surface of the metal coils. Although there is no substantial mechanistic evidence to support the clinical merit of the coating technique, a review on the clinical examination of several trials using hydrogel-coated coils showed that major recurrence was significantly lowered with hydrogel-coated coils as compared with bare-platinum coils [225].

4.5.5 Magnesium (Mg)-Containing Alloys

Magnesium (Mg)-containing alloys were brought into the biomedical horizon because of their desirable biodegradability, which makes them suitable for an exclusively stenting stenotic vessel. The conventional stent implantation procedure suffers from a high risk of restenosis, whereas the gradual dissolution of the stent body mass could serve as an intermediate transmission that shifts the mechanical load toward tissues around the vessel implant site [226]. Although magnesium alloys are undergoing prompt corrosion in contact with the physiological fluid, they could be structurally modified so as to alter its susceptibility to both corrosion and mechanical strength. With proper compositional and surface modification, Mg alloys were found extremely instrumental as materials for stents and orthopedic implants [227].

Magnesium has been useful in orthopedic implants for its solubility enhancement to phosphates and in substituting calcium to form self-setting cement, which exhibited excellent biocompatibility in rabbit femoral condyle [228]. Recently, the progress in fabricating magnesium doped apatite cement (md-AC) containing magnesium oxide and calcium dihydrogen phosphate (MO-CDP) has opened a new era for biomedical application of magnesium [229]. The newly formed biocement containing md-AC readily increased compression strength and improved osteoconductivity of this biocement as compared with hydroxyapatite cement. As a result of its potential osteoconductivity and mechanical strength, md-AC proved to be very efficient in being translated into the clinical application for bone repair and regeneration.

4.5.6 Silver (Ag)

The element silver (Ag) is ubiquitous in nature and serves as an antibacterial agent in newly formed wounds. Several applications of silver products demonstrated its oxidative activity and potential in forming nanoscale composites, such as bactericidal sponge formulations in combination with natural polymers. The formation of Ag nanoparticles out of silver nitrate solution could produce homogenously scattered particles around the surface of composite sponge made of chitosan-based material [230]. The Ag nanoparticles as a bactericidal means also showed its potential in the treatment of postsurgery infection stemmed from titanium implants. TiO_2-nanotubes coated with Ag exhibited a controlled release rate of Ag that quickly reached an effective concentration range for exerting bactericidal activity, thus, prohibiting further surgery-induced infection [231].

4.5.7 Stainless Steel

Stainless steel has been mainly used in implanting surgery, in which it serves as supporting scaffold to counteract the adverse effect caused by the abnormality of tissue constriction [232]. Most biomedical devices made of stainless steel are vascular implantation devices, exploiting their malleability as well as the mechanical strength. Similar to other intrinsic problems associated with metal materials used in implantation, stainless steel is subjected to substantial corrosion in the presence of electrolytes in these fluids. Although various metal alloys undergo a great loss of the fundamental property in corrosion, stainless steel stands out as having a low release rate of corroded composites and a relatively low cost.

The surface properties of devices made of stainless steels still need to be altered to achieve sufficient biocompatibility. Numerous coating methods on functionalizing the stainless steel scaffold surface have been developed. Three major techniques, dip coating, electrodeposition, and atomic layer deposition, have been applied on a myriad of coating materials, such as silica, polymer film, amines, and thiols. For example, a new approach of shielding the stainless steel surface with a silica layer using the atomic layer deposition method and thereafter functionalized by moieties that contain trialkoxysilane derivatives for surface linking was proposed to maintain biocompatibility as well as biological activities [233].

4.5.8 Cobalt Chrome (CoCr)

CoCr is distinctive in its resistance to corrosion under the physiological condition and surface strength that counteract the abrasive wear after implantation. Among the most desirable attributes of CoCr to orthopedic implants, the ability to integrate gradually into bone tissue and a tendency of bone growth near the implants determine the long-term efficacy of the surgery [234]. One approach to addressing this issue is to incorporate osteogenic factors within the implant device. The incorporation of bone-morphogenetic protein 2 (BMP-2), which is considered a factor that stimulates cell-implant interface adherence, yielded highly differentiated osteoblasts and a bone matrix [235].

The CoCr alloy is found especially useful as posterior arthrodesis constructs, in contrast to titanium and stainless steel, which have different sensitivities to intraoperative contouring. It was reported that CoCr constructs have a greater fatigue life than Ti constructs at all of the tested loading levels, 700N, 400N, and 250N [236]. Therefore, the CoCr is considered to be more appropriate as lumbar screw–rod arthrodesis constructs. In cardiovascular intervention, a CoCr alloy stent could provide thinner struts that have the potential of lowering intravascular inflammation and facilitate re-endovascularization, demonstrating its superb efficacy with an enhanced success rate of 98.8% [237].

4.5.9 Bioceramics

As a family of inorganic materials, bioceramics have been frequently used to accommodate various bone imperfections, such as osteoporotic fractures and damaged hard tissue. Among the several clinically relevant qualities that bioceramics should possess, osteoconductivity is the most highly pursued attribute. The ability of the implant to induce further bone regeneration has become the focus of artificial bone engineering.

(i) *Bioceramics to deliver therapeutic ions/drugs:* Several bioceramics that are able to deliver therapeutic ions have been introduced into biomedical society. Stronium-doped zinc silicate glass ceramics were evaluated for an implant scaffold, which serves as an osteogenic template to provide structural support as well as conductive vascularization [238]. In a series of experiments, it was shown that the crystal phase of the ceramic structure underwent degradation and maintained the levels of Zn^{2+} and Sr^{2+} of around 600 ppm for each, which is identical to the clinical level in achieving osteogenesis, osteoclastic restoration, and antibacterial potency.

The bone resorption needs to be prevented in various cases including osteoporosis, in which bioceramic systems could deliver anti-osteoporotic drugs that reverse the resorption process. Bioceramics, such as mesoporous SBA 15, were used to incorporate the model drug, Zoledronate, whose release rate was optimized for its kinetics, potency, and interaction with ceramic scaffold pores [239].

(ii) *Bioceramics made of calcium phosphate derivatives:* Beta-tricalcium phosphate bioceramics have been examined for its osteoconductivity and osteostimulation for various purposes, such as bone defects, trauma, and injury. An artificial implant has provided good osteo-conductivity with an ideal surface area contributed by porosity; however, it lacks such stimulation power as those exhibited in natural osteoblasts. Scaffolds with the different weight ratio of beta-calcium silicate *in vivo* have dramatically improved osteogenesis and have lowered the degradation rate [240].

Ion-substitution of composition elements is a conventional approach to modifying bioceramics applied to bone tissue engineering. A novel discovery of the gallium (Ga) precursor has led to the successful formation of Ga-doped β-tricalcium phosphate (TCP) ceramics through substitution of one of the five calcium (Ca) sites [241]. As the Ga content increases, the substitution of Ga over calcium yields a more desirable unit-cell volume, accomplishing enhanced mechanical properties with higher compressive strength.

The incorporation of alkali metal elements like potassium, sodium, and strontium in calcium polyphosphate (CPP) is a promising attempt to promote its degradability for reinforcing the bone density and mechanical strength [242]. Calcium phosphate is rigid in conformation, thus, requiring the degradation process for P-O-P bond breakage, for which metal doping was previously used to enhance biodegradability [243]. Calcium polyphosphate replaced with alkali metals through a calcining-sintering technique provides a readily degradable structure of bioceramics through the hydrolysis process, achieving an enhanced osteoinduction and osteoconduction capability [244].

4.6 FUTURE DIRECTIONS

Upon introduction of the concept decades ago, biomaterials have demonstrated highly versatile capabilities in fixing a myriad of aspects of bodily ailments. As the need for artificial tissue or organs steadily grows and thrives in clinical settings, the potential of biomaterials in fixing tissue defects or replacing a failed organ becomes more intriguing and complicated and, hence, leans toward a more advanced stage [245]. The usage of biomaterials has since then bonded with the term "tissue engineering." However, the most recent advances in biomaterials encompass a broader spectrum of biomedical applications related with their enhanced bioconductivity, increasing control over topographical design and controlled delivery of therapeutics through nanotechnology

[246, 247]. Biomaterials designed in a cost-effective screening methodology could yield a mathematically favorable topography that discovers the previously unfathomable interaction between tissue cell and material surface or triggers specific cellular surface responses [248].

The design of biomaterials is already in an era of nano-level, embracing an endless potential that spans from diagnosis to prevention to cure of diseases. As the investigation of these potentials of biomaterials prospers, unprecedented circumstances could be reached and mechanisms revealed. Numerous ideas, such as remote triggering of drug release from stimulus sensing material, a magnetic field oriented collapse of sensitive membrane built up by a variety of macroscale polymers, and the extension of a conventional delivery route of drugs through the unique bio-mimic nature of materials, have surely led to the sustainable flourishing of therapeutic applications of biomaterial [249, 250].

ASSESSMENT QUESTIONS

4.1. What are biomaterials? Define the classification of biomaterial.

4.2. What are the fundamental requirements of biomaterials to be qualified for biomedical applications?

4.3. What are three important considerations when selecting biocompatible material?

4.4. Define the various types of interactions between biomaterial and host.

4.5. What are the factors affecting blood compatibility?

4.6. Which approach reduces blood coagulation through surface modification?

a. Fabrication of a negatively charged material surface
b. Heparin conjugation
c. Lowering the surface tension
d. All of the above

4.7. A synthetic polymer mediated implant response is/are:

a. Capsule formation
b. Tissue ingrowth
c. Tissue adhesion
d. All of the above

4.8. Which one of the items below is NOT a linear polymer?

a. Graft polymer
b. Homopolymer
c. Random co-polymer
d. Diblock polymer

4.9. What are biodegradable polymers? Give a few examples of biodegradable–bioresorbable polymers that are commonly used in tissue engineering.

4.10. How are biodegradable polymers advantageous over non-biodegradable and metallic systems in tissue engineering?

4.11. What basic properties should a biodegradable polymer possess for its utilization in producing implants for tissue engineering?

4.12. List a few biocompatibility issues that are associated with biodegradable polymers.

4.13. Which methods are not employed in generating hydroxyapatite (HA) with desirable bioresorbability and porosity?

4.14. What is the major concern in manufacturing hydroxyapatite that is suitable for macromolecules?

4.15. Apart from being used in bone tissue engineering and in coating the bioactive surface, what could possibly be an alternative for hydroxyapatite as biomaterials?

4.16. What are the major advantages of Titanium (Ti) as a bio-implant?

a. Anticorrosive property
b. Mechanical strength
c. Resistance to wear
d. All of the above

4.17. What's the major potential risk of using Nitinol alloy in constructing intravascular devices? How can the risk be reduced?

4.18. Which of the following properties is considered the main reason for choosing Magnesium (Mg)-containing alloys as biomaterials?

a. Mechanical strength
b. Biodegradability
c. Anticorrosive property
d. Ductility

4.19. In contrast to titanium and stainless steel, Cobalt-Chrome (CoCr) stands out as a posterior arthrodesis construct. Why?

4.20. Which one of the following properties should be most highly pursued for bioceramics while being used for accommodating bone imperfections?

a. Osteoconductivity
b. Biodegradability
c. Resorptivity
d. Density

4.21. What are the most commonly used approaches for functionalizing the stainless steel scaffold surface?

a. Electro-deposition
b. Atomic layer deposition
c. Dip coating
d. All of the above

4.22. Define the term "composite materials."

4.23. Explain the advantages of using composite materials as biomedical devices over homogeneous materials.

4.24. Give examples of natural composites.

4.25. What is the categorization of composite materials according to the filler size? Discuss the advantage and mechanism of microfiller composite materials composed of nanofillers and nanoclusters.

4.26. According to the filler types, the composites can be classified into which of the following?

a. Particulate
b. Short fiber
c. Long fiber
d. Laminate
e. All of the above

4.27. Explain the mechanism by which smart bio-nanotubes are the new generation of nanomaterial delivery regulating the release profile of the loaded drug.

4.28. Explain the differences among the three generations of bicomposites.

4.29. Give examples of co-polymers used in wound healing. Give some examples of a composite coated with these co-polymers.

4.30. Define the term "stimuli responsive material" (smart material).

4.31. Define the term "electro-conductive hydrogel composite."

4.32. Discuss the mechanism by which the self-repairing, resin-filled microcapsules act when a crack occurs in a dental application.

4.33. How can biocompatible polymer polyethylene glycol (PEG) extend the residency time of PEG-conjugated nanoparticulates in the body?

4.34. Which composite has been explored as an artificial cornea and contact lens?

a. Composite composed of polyethylene glycol and poly(L-lactic-co-glycolic acid)
b. Composite interpenetrating network of poly (dimethyl siloxane) and poly(*N*-isopropyl acrylamide)
c. Composites composed of polycaprolactone fumarate and polypyrrole (PCL-PPy)
d. Composites composed of polylactic acid and polyhydroxybutyrate

REFERENCES

1. Park, J., Lakes, R.S. *Biomaterials an Introduction*, 3rd ed., Springer Science, New York, NY, 2007, pp. 2–5.
2. Heness, G., Ben-Nissa, B. (2004). Innovative bioceramics. *Materials Forum*, *27*, 104–114.
3. Black, J. (1982). The education of the biomaterialist: Report of a survey, 1980–81. *Journal of Biomedical Materials Research*, *16*(2), 159–167.
4. Williams, D.F. *Definitions in Biomaterials, Proceedings of a Consensus Conference of the European Society for Biomaterials*, Vol. 4, Chester, U.K., March 3–5, 1986, Elsevier, New York, NY.
5. Billotte, W.G. Ceramic biomaterials, in Joseph D.Bronzino (ed.), *The Biomedical Engineering Handbook*, 2nd ed., CRC Press, Boca Raton, FL, 2000.
6. Nair, L.S., Laurenci, C.T. (2007). Biodegradable polymers as biomaterials. *Progress in Polymer Science*, *32*, 762–798.
7. Bonfield, W. (1988). Hydroxyapatite-reinforced polyethylene as an analogous material for bone replacement. *Annals of the New York Academy of Sciences*, *523*, 173–177.
8. Hench, L.L., Polak, J.M. (2002). Third-generation biomedical materials. *Science*, *295(5557)*, 1014–1017.
9. Allan, B. (1999). Closer to nature: New biomaterials and tissue engineering in ophthalmology. *The British Journal of Ophthalmology*, *83(11)*, 1235–1240.
10. Hoppe, A., Guldal, N.S., Boccaccini, A.R. (2011). A review of the biological response to ionic dissolution products from bioactive glasses and glass-ceramics. *Biomaterials*, *32*, 2757–2774.
11. Hubbell, J.A. (1999). Bioactive biomaterials. *Current Opinion in Biotechnology*, *10*(2), 123–129.
12. Berry, M. (2008). Bioresorbable composite materials for orthopaedic devices. *Medical Device Technology*, *19*(5), 69–70, 72.
13. Tormala, P., Pohjonen, T., Rokkanen, P. (1998). Bioabsorbable polymers: Materials technology and surgical applications. *Proceedings of the Institution of Mechanical Engineers. Part H, Journal of Engineering in Medicine*, *212*(2), 101–111.
14. Lakes, R. Composite biomaterials, in Joseph D.Bronzino (ed.), *The Biomedical Engineering Handbook*, 2nd ed., CRC Press, Boca Raton, FL, 2000.
15. Tanner, K.E. (2010). Bioactive composites for bone tissue engineering. *Proceedings of the Institution of Mechanical*

Engineers. Part H, Journal of Engineering in Medicine, *224(12)*, 1359–1372.

16. Ratner, B.D., Hoffman, A.S., Schoen, F.J., Lemons, J.E., Scheon, F.J. *Biomaterials Science, An Introduction to Materials in Medicine*, Academic Press, San Diego, CA, 1996.
17. Sáenz, A., et al. (1999). Ceramic biomaterials: An introductory overview. *Journal of Materials Education*, *21(5–6)*, 297–306.
18. Nair, L.S., Laurencin., C.T. (2006). Polymers as biomaterials for tissue engineering and controlled drug delivery. *Advances in Biochemical Engineering/Biotechnology*, *102*, 47–90.
19. Qiu, L.Y., Bae, Y.H. (2006). Polymer architecture and drug delivery. *Pharmaceutical Research*, *23(1)*, 1–30.
20. Hoste, K., Winne, K. De., Schacht, E. (2004). Polymeric prodrugs. *International Journal of Pharmaceutics*, *277(1–2)*, 119–131.
21. Okana, T., et al. *Advances in Polymeric Systems for Drug Delivery*, Gordon and Breach Science, Tokyo, Japan, 1994.
22. Kumar, N., Ravikumar, M.N., Domb, A.J. (2001). Biodegradable block copolymers. *Advanced Drug Delivery Reviews*, *53(1)*, 23–44.
23. Bae, Y., Kataoka. K. Polymer assemblies: Intelligent block copolymer micelles for the programmed delivery of drugs and genes, in G.S. Kwon (ed.), *Drug and the Pharmaceutical Sciences, Volume 148, Polymeric Drug Delivery Systems*, Taylor & Francis, Boca Raton, FL, 2005, pp. 491–532.
24. Yokoyama, M. Polymeric micelles for the targeting of hydrophobic drugs, in G.S. Kwon (ed.), *Drug and the Pharmaceutical Sciences, Volume 148, Polymeric Drug Delivery Systems*, Taylor & Francis, Boca Raton, FL, 2005, pp. 533–575.
25. Petersen, H., et al. (2002). Synthesis, characterization and biocompatibility of polyethylenimine-graft-poly(ethylene glycol) block copolymers. *Macromolecules*, *35*, 6867–6874.
26. Shuai, X.T., et al. (2003). Novel biodegradable ternary copolymers hy-PEIYg-PCLYb-PEG: Synthesis, characterization, and potential as efficient nonviral gene delivery vectors. *Macromolecules*, *36*, 5751–5759.
27. Xie, H.Q., Xie, D. (1999). Molecular design, synthesis and properties of block and graft copolymers containing polyoxyethylene segments. *Progress in Polymer Science*, *24*, 275–313.
28. Li, Y.X., Nothnagel, J., Kissel. T. (1997). Biodegradable brush like graft polymers from poly(D,L-lactide) or poly (D,L-lactide-coglycolide) and charge-modified, hydrophilic dextrans as backbone-synthesis, characterization and in vitro degradation properties. *Polymer*, *38(25)*, 6197–6206.
29. Jones, M.C., Ranger, M., Leroux, J.C. (2003). pH-sensitive unimolecular polymeric micelles: Synthesis of a novel drug carrier. *Bioconjugate Chemistry*, *14(4)*, 774–781.
30. Aulenta, F., Hayes, W., Rannard, S. (2003). Dendrimers: A new class of nanoscopic containers and delivery devices. *European Polymer Journal*, *39*, 1741–1771.
31. Gillies, E.R., Frechet, J.M. (2005). Dendrimers and dendritic polymers in drug delivery. *Drug Discovery Today*, *10(1)*, 35–43.
32. Vandamme, T.F., Brobeck, L. (2005). Poly(amidoamine) dendrimers as ophthalmic vehicles for ocular delivery of pilocarpine nitrate and tropicamide. *Journal of Controlled Release*, *102*, 23–38.
33. D'Emanuele, A., et al. (2004). The use of a dendrimer-propranolol prodrug to bypass efflux transporters and enhance oral bioavailability. *Journal of Controlled Release*, *95(3)*, 447–453.
34. Chauhan, A.S., et al. (2003). Dendrimer-mediated transdermal delivery: Enhanced bioavailability of indomethacin. *Journal of Controlled Release*, *90(3)*, 335–343.
35. Wiwattanapatapee, R., Lomlim, L., Saramunee, K. (2003). Dendrimers conjugates for colonic delivery of 5-aminosalicylic acid. *Journal of Controlled Release*, *88(1)*, 1–9.
36. Williams, D.F. (2008). On the mechanisms of biocompatibility. *Biomaterials*, *29(20)*, 2941–2953.
37. Hallab, N., Jacobs, J.J., Jonathan, B. Hypersensitivity associated with metallic biomaterials, in D.L. Wise (ed.), *Biomaterials Engineering and Devices: Human Application*, Vol. 1, Humana Press, New York, NY, 2000, pp. 15–17.
38. Wang, J.Y., et al. (1997). Prosthetic metals impair murine immune response and cytokine release in vivo and in vitro. *Journal of Orthopaedic Research*, *15(5)*, 688–699.
39. Bravo, I., et al. (1990). Differential effects of eight metal ions on lymphocyte differentiation antigens in vitro. *Journal of Biomedical Materials Research*, *24(8)*, 1059–1068.
40. Keselowsky, B.G., et al. (2007). Role of plasma fibronectin in the foreign body response to biomaterials. *Biomaterials*, *28(25)*, 3626–3631.
41. Gorbet, M.B., Sefton, M.V. (2004). Biomaterial-associated thrombosis: Roles of coagulation factors, complement, platelets and leukocytes. *Biomaterials*, *25(26)*, 5681–5703.
42. Zhang, M. Biocompatibility of material, in D. Shi (ed.), *Biomaterials and Tissue Engineering*, Qinghua da xue chu ban she, China, 2004, pp. 83–99.
43. Anderson, J.M., Rodriguez, A., Chang, D.T. (2008). Foreign body reaction to biomaterials. *Seminars in Immunology*, *20(2)*, 86–100.
44. Huang, C., Jin, D.D., Zhang, Z.M., Qu, D.B. (2008). Evaluation of the biocompatibility of pectin/poly vinyl alcohol composite hydrogel as a prosthetic nucleus pulposus material. *Journal of Southern Medical University*, *28(3)*, 453–456.
45. Yang, X., et al. (2010). Preparation and characterization of trace elements-multidoped injectable biomimetic materials for minimally invasive treatment of osteoporotic bone trauma. *Journal of Biomedical Materials Research. Part A*, *95(4)*, 1170–1181.
46. Yang, Y.C., et al. (2010). Characteristics and biocompatibility of a biodegradable genipin-cross-linked gelatin/beta-tricalcium phosphate reinforced nerve guide conduit. *Journal of Biomedical Materials Research. Part B, Applied Biomaterials*, *95(1)*, 207–217.
47. Jiang, T., et al. (2009). Heparinized poly(vinyl alcohol)—small intestinal submucosa composite membrane for coronary covered stents. *Biomedical Materials*, *4*(2), 025012.

48. Vogt, J.C., et al. (2008). A comparison of different nanostructured biomaterials in subcutaneous tissue. *Materials in Medicine*, *19*(*7*), 2629–2636.

49. Rockwood, D.N., et al. (2011). Ingrowth of human mesenchymal stem cells into porous silk particle reinforced silk composite scaffolds: An in vitro study. *Acta Biomaterialia*, *7*(*1*), 144–151.

50. Roohani-Esfahani, S.I., et al. (2010). The influence hydroxyapatite nanoparticle shape and size on the properties of biphasic calcium phosphate scaffolds coated with hydroxyapatite-PCL composites. *Biomaterials*, *31*(*21*), 5498–5509.

51. Zhang, Y.M., et al. (2009). Mechanical and biological evaluations of beta-tricalcium phosphate/silicone rubber composite as a novel soft-tissue implant. *Aesthetic Plastic Surgery*, *33*(*5*), 760–769.

52. Haaparanta, A.M., et al. (2010). Porous polylactide/beta-tricalcium phosphate composite scaffolds for tissue engineering applications. *Journal of Tissue Engineering and Regenerative Medicine*, *4*(*5*), 366–373.

53. Zeng, S., et al. (2011). Preparation and characterization of nano-hydroxyapatite/poly(vinyl alcohol) composite membranes for guided bone regeneration. *Journal of Biomedical Nanotechnology*, *7*(*4*), 549–557.

54. Shi, H., et al. (2011). Cellular biocompatibility and biomechanical properties of N-carboxyethylchitosan/nanohydroxyapatite composites for tissue-engineered trachea. *Artificial Cells, Blood Substitutes, and Immobilization Biotechnology*, *40*, 120.

55. Yu, W., et al. (2011). Sciatic nerve regeneration in rats by a promising electrospun collagen/poly(epsilon-caprolactone) nerve conduit with tailored degradation rate. *BMC Neuroscience*, *12*, 68.

56. Ryu, J.H., et al. (2011). Catechol-functionalized chitosan/pluronic hydrogels for tissue adhesives and hemostatic materials. *Biomacromolecules*, *12*(*7*), 2653–2659.

57. Han, C.M., et al. (2010). Application of collagen-chitosan/fibrin glue asymmetric scaffolds in skin tissue engineering. *Journal of Zhejiang University. Science. B*, *11*(*7*), 524–530.

58. Prasad, C.K., Krishnan, L.K. (2008). Regulation of endothelial cell phenotype by biomimetic matrix coated on biomaterials for cardiovascular tissue engineering. *Acta Biomaterialia*, *4*(*1*), 182–191.

59. Sevastianov, V.I. (2002). Blood compatible biomaterials: current status and future perspectives. *Trends in Biomaterials and Artificial Organs*, *15*(2), 20–30.

60. Courtney, J.M., et al. (2003). Modification of polymer surfaces: Optimization of approaches. *Perfusion*, *18*, 33–39.

61. Baldwin, A.D., Kiick, K.L. (2010). Polysaccharide-modified synthetic polymeric biomaterials. *Biopolymers*, *94*, 128–140.

62. Detta, N., et al. (2010). Novel electrospun polyurethane/gelatin composite meshes for vascular grafts. *Materials in Medicine*, *21*(*5*), 1761–1769.

63. Tu, M., Cha, Z.G., Feng, B.H., Zhou, C.R. (2006). Synthesis of novel liquid crystal compounds and their blood compatibility as anticoagulative materials. *Biomedical Materials*, *1*(*4*), 202–205.

64. Lu, P., et al. (2011). Controllable biodegradability, drug release behavior and hemocompatibility of PTX-eluting magnesium stents. *Colloids and Surfaces. B, Biointerfaces*, *83*(*1*), 23–28.

65. He, Q., et al. (2010). Preparation and characterization of chitosan-heparin composite matrices for blood contacting tissue engineering. *Biomedical Materials*, *5*(*5*), 055001.

66. Liu, Y., et al. (2009). Physically crosslinked composite hydrogels of PVA with natural macromolecules: Structure, mechanical properties, and endothelial cell compatibility. *Journal of Biomedical Materials Research. Part B, Applied Biomaterials*, *90*(2), 492–502.

67. Mao, C., et al. (2008). New biocompatible polypyrrole-based films with good blood compatibility and high electrical conductivity. *Colloids and Surfaces. B, Biointerfaces*, *67*(*1*), 41–45.

68. Gogolewski, S. (2000). Bioresorbable polymers in trauma and bone surgery. *Injury, 31 Suppl 4*, 28–32.

69. Gunatillake, P.A., Adhikari, R. (2003). Biodegradable synthetic polymers for tissue engineering. *European Cells & Materials*, *5*, 1–16.

70. Middleton, J.C., Tipton, A.J. (2000). Synthetic biodegradable polymers as orthopedic devices. *Biomaterials*, *21*(*23*), 2335–2346.

71. Huang, T.W., et al. (2010). Clinical and biomechanical analyses to select a suture material for uvulopalatopharyngeal surgery. *Otolaryngology—Head and Neck Surgery*, *143*(*5*), 655–661.

72. Turvey, T.A., Proffit, W.P., Phillips, C. (2011). Biodegradable fixation for craniomaxillofacial surgery: A 10-year experience involving 761 operations and 745 patients. *International Journal of Oral and Maxillofacial Surgery*, *40*(*3*), 244–249.

73. Honkanen, P.B., et al. (2009). A midterm follow-up study of bioreconstructive polylactide scaffold implants in metacarpophalangeal joint arthroplasty in rheumatoid arthritis patients. *The Journal of Hand Surgery, European*, *34*(2), 179–185.

74. Hayashi, C., et al. (2009). Osteoblastic bone formation is induced by using nanogel-crosslinking hydrogel as novel scaffold for bone growth factor. *Journal of Cellular Physiology*, *220*(*1*), 1–7.

75. Hermus, J.P., et al. (2005). Fixation of a Pipkin fracture with bio-absorbable screws. Case report and a review of the literature. *Injury*, *36*(*3*), 458–461.

76. Khaled, K.A., et al. (2010). Prednisolone-loaded PLGA microspheres. In vitro characterization and in vivo application in adjuvant-induced arthritis in mice. *AAPS PharmSciTech*, *11*(2), 859–869.

77. Dos Santos, J.F., et al. (2009). Soft contact lenses functionalized with pendant cyclodextrins for controlled drug delivery. *Biomaterials*, *30*(*7*), 1348–1355.

78. Ciolino, J.B., et al. (2009). A drug-eluting contact lens. *Investigative Ophthalmology & Visual Science*, *50*(*7*), 3346–3352.

79. Liu, J., et al. (2011). Biodegradation, biocompatibility, and drug delivery in poly(omega-pentadecalactone-co-p-dioxanone) copolyesters. *Biomaterials*, *32(27)*, 6646–6654.
80. Intra, J., et al. (2011). Immunostimulatory sutures that treat local disease recurrence following primary tumor resection. *Biomedical Materials*, *6(1)*, 011001.
81. Palmieri, A., et al. (2011). Biological effect of resorbable plates on normal osteoblasts and osteoblasts derived from Pfeiffer syndrome. *The Journal of Craniofacial Surgery*, *22(3)*, 860–863.
82. Weber, F.E., et al. (2002). Slow and continuous application of human recombinant bone morphogenetic protein via biodegradable poly(lactide-co-glycolide) foamspheres. *International Journal of Oral and Maxillofacial Surgery*, *31(1)*, 60–65.
83. Bayat, M., et al. (2010). Treatment of mandibular angle fractures using a single bioresorbable miniplate. *Journal of Oral and Maxillofacial Surgery*, *68(7)*, 1573–1577.
84. Gaball, C., et al. (2011). Minimally invasive bioabsorbable bone plates for rigid internal fixation of mandible fractures. *Archives of Facial Plastic Surgery*, *13(1)*, 31–35.
85. Matsumoto, M.A., et al. (2005). Tissue response to poly-L-lactide acid-polyglycolic acid absorbable screws in autogenous bone grafts: A histologic morphological analysis. *Clinical Oral Implants Research*, *16(1)*, 112–118.
86. Olson, H.E., et al. (2009). Neural stem cell- and Schwann cell-loaded biodegradable polymer scaffolds support axonal regeneration in the transected spinal cord. *Tissue Engineering. Part A*, *15(7)*, 1797–1805.
87. Novikova, L.N., et al. (2008). Biodegradable poly-beta-hydroxybutyrate scaffold seeded with Schwann cells to promote spinal cord repair. *Biomaterials*, *29(9)*, 1198–1206.
88. Cho, Y., Shi, R., Borgens, R.B. (2010). Chitosan produces potent neuroprotection and physiological recovery following traumatic spinal cord injury. *The Journal of Experimental Biology*, *213*, 1513–1520.
89. Li, X., et al. (2009). Repair of thoracic spinal cord injury by chitosan tube implantation in adult rats. *Biomaterials*, *30(6)*, 1121–1132.
90. Chalmers, R., et al. (2008). Improving contact-lens related dryness symptoms with silicone hydrogel lenses. *Optometry and Vision Science*, *85(8)*, 778–784.
91. Fabbri, G., et al. (2009). Guided bone regeneration technique in the esthetic zone: A novel approach using resorbable PLLA-PGA plates and screw fixation. A case report. *The International Journal of Periodontics & Restorative Dentistry*, *29(5)*, 543–547.
92. Aydin, E., Planell, J.A., Hasirci, V. (2011). Hydroxyapatite nanorod-reinforced biodegradable poly(L-lactic acid) composites for bone plate applications. *Materials in Medicine*, *22(11)*, 2413–2427.
93. Slone, R.M., MacMillan, M., Montgomery, W.J. (1993). Spinal fixation. Part 1. Principles, basic hardware, and fixation techniques for the cervical spine. *Radiographics*, *13(2)*, 341–356.
94. Bezer, M., et al. (2005). Absorbable self-reinforced polylactide (SR-PLLA) rods vs rigid rods (K-wire) in spinal fusion: An experimental study in rabbits. *European Spine Journal*, *14(3)*, 227–233.
95. Beekhuis, G.J. (1984). Augmentation mentoplasty with polyamide mesh. Update. *Archives of Otolaryngology*, *110(6)*, 364–367.
96. Nomura, H., Tator, C.H., Shoichet, M.S. (2006). Bioengineered strategies for spinal cord repair. *Journal of Neurotrauma*, *23(3–4)*, 496–507.
97. Nilsson, A., et al. (2010). The Artelon CMC spacer compared with tendon interposition arthroplasty. *Acta Orthopaedica*, *81(2)*, 237–244.
98. Nilsson, A., et al. (2005). Results from a degradable TMC joint spacer (Artelon) compared with tendon arthroplasty. *The Journal of Hand Surgery*, *30(2)*, 380–389.
99. Robinson, P.M., Muir, L.T. (2011). Foreign body reaction associated with Artelon: Report of three cases. *The Journal of Hand Surgery*, *36(1)*, 116–120.
100. Yuki, I., et al. (2010). Intravascular tissue reactions induced by various types of bioabsorbable polymeric materials: Correlation between the degradation profiles and corresponding tissue reactions. *Neuroradiology*, *52(11)*, 1017–1024.
101. Kim, H.I., et al. (2011). Tissue response to poly(L-lactic acid)-based blend with phospholipid polymer for biodegradable cardiovascular stents. *Biomaterials*, *32(9)*, 2241–2247.
102. Hirano, S., Noishiki, Y. (1985). The blood compatibility of chitosan and N-acylchitosans. *Journal of Biomedical Materials Research*, *19(4)*, 413–417.
103. Park, J.B., Lakes, R.S., *Biomaterials—An Introduction*, Plenum, New York, NY, 1992, pp. 169–183.
104. Lakes, R. Composite biomaterials, in Joseph D.Bronzino (ed.), *The Biomedical Engineering Handbook*, 2nd ed., CRC Press, Boca Raton, FL, 2000.
105. Katz, J.L. (1980). Anisotropy of Young's modulus of bone. *Nature*, *283(5742)*, 106–107.
106. Lakes, R, (1993). Materials with structural hierarchy. *Nature*, *361*, 511–515.
107. Simchi, A., et al. (2011). Recent progress in inorganic and composite coatings with bactericidal capability for orthopaedic applications. *Nanomedicine: Nanotechnology, Biology, and Medicine*, *7(1)*, 22–39.
108. Ko, H.F., Sfeir, C., Kumta, P.N. (2010). Novel synthesis strategies for natural polymer and composite biomaterials as potential scaffolds for tissue engineering. *Philosophical Transactions. Series A, Mathematical, Physical, and Engineering Sciences*, *368(1917)*, 1981–1997.
109. Chen, Q.Z., Blaker, J.J., Boccaccini, A.R. (2006). Bioactive and mechanically strong bioglass-poly(D,L-lactic acid) composite coatings on surgical sutures. *Journal of Biomedical Materials Research. Part B, Applied Biomaterials*, *76(2)*, 354–363.
110. Duffy, M.T., et al. (2005). Sutureless ophthalmic surgery: A scaffold-enhanced bioadhesive technique. *Journal of AAPOS*, *9(4)*, 315–320.
111. Gibson, R.F., (2011). Multifunctional composite materials and structures: A brief review. *Audio, Transactions of the IRE Professional Group on*, *130(4)*, 2325.

112. Zimmerli, B., et al. (2010). Composite materials: Composition, properties and clinical applications. *A literature review. Schweiz Monatsschr Zahnmed, 120(11)*, 972–986.
113. Lutz, F., Phillips, R.W. (1983). A classification and evaluation of composite resin systems. *The Journal of Prosthetic Dentistry, 50(4)*, 480–488.
114. Suwanprateeb, J., et al. (1997). Influence of Ringer's solution on creep resistance of hydroxyapatite reinforced polyethylene composites. *Materials in Medicine, 8(8)*, 469–472.
115. Tanner, K.E. (2010). Bioactive ceramic-reinforced composites for bone augmentation. *Journal of the Royal Society, Interface/the Royal Society, 7 Suppl 5*, S541–S557.
116. Wang, M. (2003). Developing bioactive composite materials for tissue replacement. *Biomaterials, 24(13)*, 2133–2151.
117. Rahmat, M., Das, K., Hubert, P. (2011). Interaction stresses in carbon nanotube-polymer nanocomposites. *ACS Applied Materials & Interfaces, 3(9)*, 3425–3431.
118. Samsonidze, G.G., Yakobson, B.I. (2002). Kinetic theory of symmetry-dependent strength in carbon nanotubes. *Physical Review Letters, 88(6)*, 065501.
119. Byrne, M.T., Gun'ko, Y.K. (2010). Recent advances in research on carbon nanotube-polymer composites. *Advanced Materials, 22(15)*, 1672–1688.
120. Terada, M., et al. (2009). Development of a multiwalled carbon nanotube coated collagen dish. *Dental Materials Journal, 28(1)*, 82–88.
121. Usui, Y., et al. (2008). Carbon nanotubes with high bone-tissue compatibility and bone-formation acceleration effects. *Small, 4(2)*, 240–246.
122. Wang, S.F., et al. (2005). Preparation and mechanical properties of chitosan/carbon nanotubes composites. *Biomacromolecules, 6(6)*, 3067–3072.
123. Teng, S.H., et al. (2009). Chitosan/nanohydroxyapatite composite membranes via dynamic filtration for guided bone regeneration. *Journal of Biomedical Materials Research. Part A, 88(3)*, 569–580.
124. Liuyun, J., Yubao, L., Chengdong, X. (2009). A novel composite membrane of chitosan-carboxymethyl cellulose polyelectrolyte complex membrane filled with nano-hydroxyapatite I. Preparation and properties. *Materials in Medicine, 20(8)*, 1645–1652.
125. Zhang, Y., et al. (2008). Electrospun biomimetic nanocomposite nanofibers of hydroxyapatite/chitosan for bone tissue engineering. *Biomaterials, 29(32)*, 4314–4322.
126. Kim, K., Fisher, J.P. (2007). Nanoparticle technology in bone tissue engineering. *Journal of Drug Targeting, 15(4)*, 241–252.
127. Manjubala, I., et al. (2008). Growth of osteoblast-like cells on biomimetic apatite-coated chitosan scaffolds. *Journal of Biomedical Materials Research. Part B, Applied Biomaterials, 84(1)*, 7–16.
128. Di Martino, A., Sittinger, M., Risbud, M.V. (2005). Chitosan: A versatile biopolymer for orthopaedic tissue-engineering. *Biomaterials, 26(30)*, 5983–5990.
129. Masson, B. (2009). Emergence of the alumina matrix composite in total hip arthroplasty. *International Orthopaedics, 33(2)*, 359–363.
130. Boccaccini, A.R., et al. (2003). Bioresorbable and bioactive composite materials based on polylactide foams filled with and coated by bioglass particles for tissue engineering applications. *Materials in Medicine, 14(5)*, 443–450.
131. Roether, J.A., et al. (2002). Development and in vitro characterisation of novel bioresorbable and bioactive composite materials based on polylactide foams and bioglass for tissue engineering applications. *Biomaterials, 23(18)*, 3871–3878.
132. Deng, X., Hao, J., Wang, C. (2001). Preparation and mechanical properties of nanocomposites of poly(D,L-lactide) with Ca-deficient hydroxyapatite nanocrystals. *Biomaterials, 22(21)*, 2867–2873.
133. Blaker, J.J., Nazhat, S.N., Boccaccini, A.R. (2004). Development and characterisation of silver-doped bioactive glass-coated sutures for tissue engineering and wound healing applications. *Biomaterials, 25(7–8)*, 1319–1329.
134. Boccaccini, A.R., et al. (2003). Composite surgical sutures with bioactive glass coating. *Journal of Biomedical Materials Research. Part B, Applied Biomaterials, 67(1)*, 618–626.
135. Murakami, K., et al. (2010). Hydrogel blends of chitin/chitosan, fucoidan and alginate as healing-impaired wound dressings. *Biomaterials, 31(1)*, 83–90.
136. Liang, Y., et al. (2011). An in situ formed biodegradable hydrogel for reconstruction of the corneal endothelium. *Colloids and Surfaces. B, Biointerfaces, 82(1)*, 1–7.
137. Liu, L., Sheardown, H. (2005). Glucose permeable poly (dimethyl siloxane) poly (N-isopropyl acrylamide) interpenetrating networks as ophthalmic biomaterials. *Biomaterials, 26(3)*, 233–244.
138. Shi, G., et al. (2004). A novel electrically conductive and biodegradable composite made of polypyrrole nanoparticles and polylactide. *Biomaterials, 25(13)*, 2477–2488.
139. Chen, S.J., et al. (2000). Template synthesis of the polypyrrole tube and its bridging in vivo sciatic nerve regeneration. *Journal of Materials Science Letters, 19*, 2157–2159.
140. Shustak, G., et al. (2007). A novel electrochemically synthesized biodegradable thin film of polypyrrole-poly- ethylene-glycol-polylactic acid nanoparticles. *New Journal of Chemistry, 31*, 163–168.
141. Runge, M.B., et al. (2010). The development of electrically conductive polycaprolactone fumarate-polypyrrole composite materials for nerve regeneration. *Biomaterials, 31(23)*, 5916–5926.
142. Jeong, T.S., et al. (2009). The effect of resin shades on microhardness, polymerization shrinkage, and color change of dental composite resins. *Dental Materials Journal, 28(4)*, 438–445.
143. Condon, J.R., Ferracane, J.L. (1997). Factors effecting dental composite wear in vitro. *Journal of Biomedical Materials Research, 38(4)*, 303–313.
144. Cook, W.D., Chong, M.P. (1985). Colour stability and visual perception of dimethacrylate based dental composite resins. *Biomaterials, 6(4)*, 257–264.

145. Okamura, H., Miyasaka, T., Hagiwara, T. (2006). Development of dental composite resin utilizing low-shrinking and low-viscous monomers. *Dental Materials Journal, 25(3)*, 437–444.

146. Ensaff, H., O'Doherty, D.M., Jacobsen, P.H. (2001). Polymerization shrinkage of dental composite resins. *Proceedings of the Institution of Mechanical Engineers. Part H, Journal of Engineering in Medicine, 215(4)*, 367–375.

147. Chen, M.H. (2010). Update on dental nanocomposites. *Journal of Dental Research, 89(6)*, 549–560.

148. Manhart, J., et al. (2000). Mechanical properties and wear behavior of light-cured packable composite resins. *Dental Materials, 16(1)*, 33–40.

149. Turssi, C.P., Ferracane, J.L., Ferracane, L.L. (2006). Wear and fatigue behavior of nano-structured dental resin composites. *Journal of Biomedical Materials Research. Part B, Applied Biomaterials, 78(1)*, 196–203.

150. Aydin Sevinc, B., Hanley, L. (2010). Antibacterial activity of dental composites containing zinc oxide nanoparticles. *Journal of Biomedical Materials Research. Part B, Applied Biomaterials, 94(1)*, 22–31.

151. Mitra, S.B., Wu, D., Holmes, B.N. (2003). An application of nanotechnology in advanced dental materials. *Journal of the American Dental Association, 134(10)*, 1382–1390.

152. Beyth, N., et al. (2006). Antibacterial activity of dental composites containing quaternary ammonium polyethylenimine nanoparticles against Streptococcus mutans. *Biomaterials, 27(21)*, 3995–4002.

153. Zhang, K., et al. (2004). Characterization of nanostructure of stimuli-responsive polymeric composite membranes. *Biomacromolecules, 5(4)*, 1248–1255.

154. Hamada, K., Kawano, F., Asaoka, K. (2003). Shape recovery of shape memory alloy fiber embedded resin matrix smart composite after crack repair. *Dental Materials Journal, 22(2)*, 160–167.

155. Endo, T., et al. (2008). Stimuli-responsive hydrogel-silver nanoparticles composite for development of localized surface plasmon resonance-based optical biosensor. *Analytica Chimica Acta, 611(2)*, 205–211.

156. Ferracane, J.L. (2011). Resin composite—state of the art. *Dental Materials Journal, 27(1)*, 29–38.

157. Jandt, K.D., Sigusch, B.W. (2009). Future perspectives of resin-based dental materials. *Dental Materials Journal, 25(8)*, 1001–1006.

158. Hahnel, S., et al. (2010). Investigation of mechanical properties of modern dental composites after artificial aging for one year. *Operative Dentistry, 35(4)*, 412–419.

159. Endo, T., et al. (2010). Surface texture and roughness of polished nanofill and nanohybrid resin composites. *Dental Materials Journal, 29(2)*, 213–223.

160. Bouillaguet, S., et al. (2006). Hydrothermal and mechanical stresses degrade fiber-matrix interfacial bond strength in dental fiber-reinforced composites. *Journal of Biomedical Materials Research. Part B, Applied Biomaterials, 76(1)*, 98–105.

161. Titley, K.C., et al. (1998). The effect of various storage methods and media on shear-bond strengths of dental composite resin to bovine dentine. *Archives of Oral Biology, 43(4)*, 305–311.

162. Fratzl, P. (2007). Biomimetic materials research: What can we really learn from nature's structural materials? *Journal of the Royal Society, Interface/the Royal Society, 4(15)*, 637–642.

163. Womer, R.B., Raney, Jr., R.B., D'Angio, G.J. (1985). Healing rates of treated and untreated bone lesions in histiocytosis X. *Pediatrics, 76(2)*, 286–288.

164. Yamagishi, K., et al. (2005). Materials chemistry: A synthetic enamel for rapid tooth repair. *Nature, 433(7028)*, 819.

165. Lippert, F., Parker, D.M., Jandt, K.D. (2004). In vitro demineralization/remineralization cycles at human tooth enamel surfaces investigated by AFM and nanoindentation. *Journal of Colloid and Interface Science, 280(2)*, 442–448.

166. White, S.R., et al. (2001). Autonomic healing of polymer composites. *Nature, 409(6822)*, 794–797.

167. Pyhalto, T., et al. (2005). Fixation of distal femoral osteotomies with self-reinforced poly(L/DL)lactide 70:30 and self-reinforced poly(L/DL)lactide 70:30/bioactive glass composite rods. An experimental study on rabbits. *Journal of Biomaterials Science, Polymer Edition, 16(6)*, 725–744.

168. Kessler, White, S.R. (2001). Self-activated healing of delamination damage in woven composites. *Composites, 32*, 683–699.

169. Kessler, M.R., White, S.R., Sottos, N.R. *Self-healing of Composites Using Embedded Microcapsules: Repair of Delamination Damage in Woven Composites*, 10th European Conference on Composite Materials, 2002.

170. Wertzberger, B.E., et al. (2010). Physical characterization of a self-healing dental restorative material. *Journal of Applied Polymer Sciences, 118*, 428–434.

171. Smith, I.O., et al. (2009). Nanostructured polymer scaffolds for tissue engineering and regenerative medicine. *Wiley Interdisciplinary Reviews. Nanomedicine and Nanobiotechnology, 1(2)*, 226–236.

172. Chandrawati, R., et al. (2009). Cholesterol-mediated anchoring of enzyme-loaded liposomes within disulfide-stabilized polymer carrier capsules. *Biomaterials, 30(30)*, 5988–5998.

173. Yellepeddi, V.K., Kumar, A., Palakurthi, S. (2009). Biotinylated poly(amido)amine (PAMAM) dendrimers as carriers for drug delivery to ovarian cancer cells in vitro. *Anticancer Research, 29(8)*, 2933–2943.

174. Wang, D., et al. (2003). Synthesis and evaluation of water-soluble polymeric bone-targeted drug delivery systems. *Bioconjugate Chemistry, 14(5)*, 853–859.

175. Minelli, C., Lowe, S.B., Stevens, M.M. (2010). Engineering nanocomposite materials for cancer therapy. *Small, 6(21)*, 2336–2357.

176. Pirollo, K.F., Chang, E.H. (2008). Does a targeting ligand influence nanoparticle tumor localization or uptake? *Trends in Biotechnology, 26(10)*, 552–558.

177. Veronese, F.M., Pasut, G. (2005). PEGylation, successful approach to drug delivery. *Drug Discovery Today, 10(21)*, 1451–1458.

178. Inigo, A.R., Henley, S.J., Silva, S.R. (2011). Dispersive hole transport in polymer: Carbon nanotube composites. *Nanotechnology, 22(26)*, 265711.

179. Heller, D.A., et al. (2011). Peptide secondary structure modulates single-walled carbon nanotube fluorescence as a chaperone sensor for nitroaromatics. *Proceedings of the National Academy of Sciences of the United States of America, 108(21)*, 8544–8549.

180. Cheung, W., et al. (2010). DNA and carbon nanotubes as medicine. *Advanced Drug Delivery Reviews, 62(6)*, 633–649.

181. Khripin, C.Y., Arnold-Medabalimi, N., Zheng, M. (2011). Molecular-crowding-induced clustering of DNA-wrapped carbon nanotubes for facile length fractionation. *ACS Nano, 5(10)*, 8258–8266.

182. Tessonnier, J.P., et al. (2009). Selective deposition of metal nanoparticles inside or outside multiwalled carbon nanotubes. *ACS Nano, 3(8)*, 2081–2089.

183. Pantarotto, D., et al. (2004). Functionalized carbon nanotubes for plasmid DNA gene delivery. *Angewandte Chemie, 43(39)*, 5242–5246.

184. Dinu, C.Z., Bale, S.S., Dordick, J.S. (2011). Kinesin I ATPase manipulates biohybrids formed from tubulin and carbon nanotubes. *Methods in Molecular Biology, 743*, 77–93.

185. Dinu, C.Z., et al. (2009). Tubulin encapsulation of carbon nanotubes into functional hybrid assemblies. *Small, 5(3)*, 310–315.

186. Guiseppi-Elie, A., et al. (1997). Electroconductive hydrogels: Novel materials for the controlled electrorelease of bioactive peptides. *Polymer Preprint, 38*, 608.

187. Guiseppi-Elie, A. (2010). Electroconductive hydrogels: Synthesis, characterization and biomedical applications. *Biomaterials, 31(10)*, 2701–2716.

188. Kumar, S., Gangopadhyay, R. (2005). Conducting polymer gel: Formation of a novel semi-IPN from polyaniline and crosslinked poly(2-acrylamido-2-methyl propanesulphonic acid). *Polymer, 46*, 2993–3000.

189. Murugendrappa, M.V., Khasim, S., Prasad, M.V.N.A. (2005). Synthesis, characterization, and conductivity studies of polypyrrole-fly ash composites. *Bulletin of Materials Science, 28*, 565–569.

190. Wojkiewicz, J.L., Fauveaux, S., Miane, J.L. (2003). Electromagnetic shielding properties of polyaniline composites. *Synthetic Metals, 135–136*, 127–128.

191. Sarac, A.S., et al. (2011). Morphology and electrical properties of intrinsically conducting polymer composites. *Plastic Research Online, June* 28th.

192. He, C.L., Huang, Z.M., Han, X.J. (2009). Fabrication of drug-loaded electrospun aligned fibrous threads for suture applications. *Journal of Biomedical Materials Research. Part A, 89(1)*, 80–95.

193. Perkins, L.E. (2010). Preclinical models of restenosis and their application in the evaluation of drug-eluting stent systems. *Veterinary Pathology, 47(1)*, 58–76.

194. Variola, F., et al. (2011). Nanoscale surface modifications of medically relevant metals: State-of-the art and perspectives. *Nanoscale, 3(2)*, 335–353.

195. Hutmacher, D.W. (2000). Scaffolds in tissue engineering bone and cartilage. *Biomaterials, 21(24)*, 2529–2543.

196. Sharifi, S., et al. (2011). Hydroxyapatite scaffolds infiltrated with thermally crosslinked polycaprolactone fumarate and polycaprolactone itaconate. *Journal of Biomedical Materials Research. Part A, 98(2)*, 257–267.

197. Lee, K.W., et al. (2010). Enhanced cell ingrowth and proliferation through three-dimensional nanocomposite scaffolds with controlled pore structures. *Biomacromolecules, 11(3)*, 682–689.

198. Chen, C.W., et al. (2004). Mechanochemical-hydrothermal synthesis of hydroxyapatite from nonionic surfactant emulsion precursors. *Journl of Crystal Growth. 270*, 615–623.

199. Cicuendez, M., et al. (2012). Biological performance of hydroxyapatite-biopolymer foams: In vitro cell response. *Acta Biomaterialia, 8(2)*, 802–810.

200. Chung, E.J., et al. (2011). Low-pressure foaming: A novel method for the fabrication of porous scaffolds for tissue engineering. *Tissue Engineering. Part C, Methods.*

201. Tan, Q., et al. (2011). Fabrication of porous scaffolds with a controllable microstructure and mechanical properties by porogen fusion technique. *International Journal of Molecular Sciences, 12(2)*, 890–904.

202. Piao, Z., et al. (2011). Effects of the nano-tubular anodic TiO2 buffer layer on bioactive hydroxyapatite coating. *Journal of Nanoscience and Nanotechnology, 11(1)*, 286–290.

203. Wang, L.N., Adams, A., Luo, J.L. (2011). Enhancement of the capability of hydroxyapatite formation on Zr with anodic ZrO nanotubular arrays via an effective dipping pretreatment. *Journal of Biomedical Materials Research. Part B, Applied Biomaterials, 99(2)*, 291–301.

204. Yonekura, Y., et al. (2011). Osteoconductivity of thermal-sprayed silver-containing hydroxyapatite coating in the rat tibia. *The Journal of Bone and Joint Surgery British, 93(5)*, 644–649.

205. Yang, J.H., et al. (2011). Synthesis of spherical hydroxyapatite granules with interconnected pore channels using camphene emulsion. *Journal of Biomedical Materials Research. Part B, Applied Biomaterials, 99(1)*, 150–157.

206. Cai, L., et al. (2011). Vascular and micro-environmental influences on MSC-coral hydroxyapatite construct-based bone tissue engineering. *Biomaterials, 32(33)*, 8497–8505.

207. Hong, M.H., et al. (2011). Drug-loaded porous spherical hydroxyapatite granules for bone regeneration. *Materials in Medicine, 22(2)*, 349–355.

208. Acarturk, T.O., Hollinger, J.O. (2006). Commercially available demineralized bone matrix compositions to regenerate calvarial critical-sized bone defects. *Plastic and Reconstructive Surgery, 118(4)*, 862–873.

209. Dallari, D., et al. (2012). A prospective, randomised, controlled trial using a Mg-hydroxyapatite—demineralized bone matrix nanocomposite in tibial osteotomy. *Biomaterials, 33(1)*, 72–79.

210. Xie, G., et al. (2010). Hydroxyapatite nanoparticles as a controlled-release carrier of BMP-2: Absorption and release kinetics in vitro. *Materials in Medicine, 21(6)*, 1875–1880.
211. Montufar, E.B., et al. (2010). Foamed surfactant solution as a template for self-setting injectable hydroxyapatite scaffolds for bone regeneration. *Acta Biomaterialia, 6(3)*, 876–885.
212. Koocheki, S., Madaeni, S.S., Niroomandi, P. (2011). Application of hydroxyapatite nanoparticles in development of an enhanced formulation for delivering sustained release of triamcinolone acetonide. *International Journal of Nanomedicine, 6*, 825–833.
213. Lopez-Heredia, M.A., et al. (2011). An injectable calcium phosphate cement for the local delivery of paclitaxel to bone. *Biomaterials, 32(23)*, 5411–5416.
214. Geetha, M., et al. (2009). Ti based biomaterials, the ultimate choice for orthopaedic implants—A review. *Progress in Materials Science, 54*, 397–425.
215. Wang, Q.Q., et al. (2011). Preparation of a HA/collagen film on a bioactive titanium surface by the electrochemical deposition method. *Biomedical Materials, 6(5)*, 055009.
216. Walschot, L.H., et al. (2011). The effect of impaction and a bioceramic coating on bone ingrowth in porous titanium particles. *Acta Orthopaedica, 82(3)*, 372–377.
217. Szold, A. (2006). Nitinol: Shape-memory and super-elastic materials in surgery. *Surgical Endoscopy, 20(9)*, 1493–1496.
218. Singh, D., et al. (2011). Use of nitinol shape memory alloy staples (NiTi clips) after cervical discoidectomy: Minimally invasive instrumentation and long-term results. *Minimally Invasive Neurosurgery: MIN, 54(4)*, 172–178.
219. Laird, J.R., et al. (2010). Nitinol stent implantation versus balloon angioplasty for lesions in the superficial femoral artery and proximal popliteal artery: Twelve-month results from the RESILIENT randomized trial. Circulation. *Cardiovascular Interventions, 3(3)*, 267–276.
220. Dake, M.D., et al. (2011). Nitinol stents with polymer-free paclitaxel coating for lesions in the superficial femoral and popliteal arteries above the knee: Twelve-month safety and effectiveness results from the Zilver PTX single-arm clinical study. *Journal of Endovascular Therapy, 18(5)*, 613–623.
221. Bakhshi, R., et al. (2011). Polymeric coating of surface modified nitinol stent with POSS-nanocomposite polymer. *Colloids and Surfaces. B, Biointerfaces, 86(1)*, 93–105.
222. Henderson, E., Nash, D.H., Dempster, W.M. (2011). On the experimental testing of fine Nitinol wires for medical devices. *Journal of the Mechanical Behavior of Biomedical Materials, 4(3)*, 261–268.
223. Perez, L.M., et al. (2009). Effect of Nitinol surface treatments on its physico-chemical properties. *Journal of Biomedical Materials Research. Part B, Applied Biomaterials, 91(1)*, 337–347.
224. Griffith, R.W., Humphrey, D.R. (2006). Long-term gliosis around chronically implanted platinum electrodes in the Rhesus macaque motor cortex. *Neuroscience Letters, 406 (1–2)*, 81–86.
225. White, P.M., et al. (2011). Hydrogel-coated coils versus bare platinum coils for the endovascular treatment of intracranial aneurysms (HELPS): A randomised controlled trial. *Lancet, 377(9778)*, 1655–1662.
226. Yang, J., Cui, F., Lee, I.S. (2011). Surface modifications of magnesium alloys for biomedical applications. *Annals of Biomedical Engineering, 39(7)*, 1857–1871.
227. Gastaldi, D., et al. (2011). Continuum damage model for bioresorbable magnesium alloy devices—Application to coronary stents. *Journal of the Mechanical Behavior of Biomedical Materials, 4(3)*, 352–365.
228. Wu, Z.Z., et al. (2005). Experimental study of a new type of cement on tibia plateau fractures treatment. *Clinical Medical Journal of China, 12*, 261–264.
229. Lu, J., et al. (2011). Preparation and preliminary cytocompatibility of magnesium doped apatite cement with degradability for bone regeneration. *Materials in Medicine, 22(3)*, 607–615.
230. Li, D., et al. (2011). Fabrication of new chitosan-based composite sponge containing silver nanoparticles and its antibacterial properties for wound dressing. *Journal of Nanoscience and Nanotechnology, 11(6)*, 4733–4738.
231. Zhao, L., et al. (2011). Antibacterial nano-structured titania coating incorporated with silver nanoparticles. *Biomaterials, 32(24)*, 5706–5716.
232. Hayes, J.S., Richards, R.G. (2010). The use of titanium and stainless steel in fracture fixation. *Expert Review of Medical Devices, 7(6)*, 843–853.
233. Slaney, A.M., et al. (2011). Biocompatible carbohydrate-functionalized stainless steel surfaces: A new method for passivating biomedical implants. *ACS Applied Materials & Interfaces, 3(5)*, 1601–1612.
234. Yarlagadda, P.K., Chandrasekharan, M., Shyan, J.Y. (2005). Recent advances and current developments in tissue scaffolding. *Bio-medical Materials and Engineering, 15(3)*, 159–177.
235. Poh, C.K., et al. (2011). Cobalt chromium alloy with immobilized BMP peptide for enhanced bone growth. *Journal of Orthopaedic Research, 29(9)*, 1424–1430.
236. Nguyen, T.Q., et al. (2011). The fatigue life of contoured cobalt chrome posterior spinal fusion rods. *Proceedings of the Institution of Mechanical Engineers. Part H, Journal of Engineering in Medicine, 225(2)*, 194–198.
237. Belardi, J.A. (2011). Cobalt-chromium stenting in patients with acute myocardial infarction: Thinner is better. *Catheterization and Cardiovascular Interventions, 77(5)*, 615–616.
238. Looney, M., O'Shea, H., Boyd, D. (2011). Preliminary evaluation of therapeutic ion release from Sr-doped zinc-silicate glass ceramics. *Journal of Biomaterials Applications.*
239. Manzano, M., et al. (2011). Anti-osteoporotic drug release from ordered mesoporous bioceramics: Experiments and modeling. *AAPS PharmSciTech, 12(4)*, 1193–1199.
240. Wang, C., et al. (2012). The enhancement of bone regeneration by a combination of osteoconductivity and osteostimulation

using beta-CaSiO3/beta-Ca3(PO4)2 composite bioceramics. *Acta Biomaterialia*, *8(1)*, 350–360.

241. Mellier, C., et al. (2011). Characterization and properties of novel gallium-doped calcium phosphate ceramics. *Inorganic Chemistry*, *50(17)*, 8252–8260.
242. Bruyere, O., et al. (2007). Relationship between change in femoral neck bone mineral density and hip fracture incidence during treatment with strontium ranelate. *Current Medical Research and Opinion*, *23(12)*, 3041–3045.
243. Song, W., et al. (2009). The study on the degradation and mineralization mechanism of ion-doped calcium polyphosphate in vitro. *Journal of Biomedical Materials Research, Part B, Applied Biomaterials*, *89*(2), 430–438.
244. Song, W., et al. (2011). A novel alkali metals/strontium co-substituted calcium polyphosphate scaffolds in bone tissue engineering. *Journal of Biomedical Materials research, Part B, Applied Biomaterials*, *98B*(2), 255–262.
245. Vallet-Regí, M., Ruiz-Hernández, E. (2011). Bioceramics: From bone regeneration to cancer nanomedicine. *Advanced Materials*, *23(44)*, 5177–5218.
246. Langer, R. (2009). The evolution of biomaterials. Interview by Alison Stoddart and Victoria Cleave. *Nature Materials*, *8(6)* 444–445.
247. Engelmayr, G.C.Jr, et al. (2008). Accordion-like honeycombs for tissue engineering of cardiac anisotropy. *Nature Materials*, *7(12)*, 1003–1010.
248. Unadkat, H.V., et al. (2011). An algorithm-based topographical biomaterials library to instruct cell fate. *Proceedings of the National Academy of Sciences of the United States of America*, *108*(*40*), 16565–70.
249. Yang, L., Zhang, L., Thomas, J.W. (2011). Nanobiomaterials: State of the art and future trends. *Advanced Engineering Materials*, *13*(*6*), B197–B217.
250. Timko, B.P., et al. (2011). Advances in drug delivery. *Annual Review of Materials Research*, *41*(*1*), 1–20.

PART II

STRATEGIES FOR ADVANCED DRUG DELIVERY

5

STRATEGIES OF DRUG TARGETING

Ravi S. Shukla, Zhijin Chen, and Kun Cheng

5.1 CHAPTER OBJECTIVES

- To enlist the fundamental concepts and principals needed for the development of targeted drug delivery systems.
- To understand different drug targeting strategies.
- To enlist and discuss numerous delivery systems used for targeting therapeutic agents to the distant diseased tissues.
- To learn the fundamental concepts and chemistry along with applications of ligands in developing a targeted drug delivery system.

5.2 INTRODUCTION

Targeted drug delivery refers to the specific accumulation of drug in a certain body region. Depending on the location of diseases, a targeted drug delivery system can specifically deliver drugs to a certain organ, a certain type of cell, or even a certain subcellular compartment. The primary advantage of using a targeted drug delivery system is that it has high therapeutic efficacy at diseased sites without inducing undesirable side effects in other healthy tissues. The recent rapid progress in identifying druggable targets and developing new medicines has not been matched by the development of efficient delivery systems to achieve the anticipated therapeutic effect for human patients. This is particularly true for macromolecular drugs that face more challenges in overcoming numerous biological barriers during systemic administration. Therefore, the development of targeted drug delivery systems is becoming a crucial step in transforming our knowledge and understanding of diseases to successful therapeutics.

The idea of drug targeting originates from the revolutionary "magic bullet" concept proposed by Paul Ehrlich, the founder of chemotherapy, almost 100 years ago. In this hypothetical concept, Ehrlich theorized that by targeting the receptors of pathogens, targeted medicines could selectively attack pathogens while leaving healthy tissues unaffected [1]. Since then, many scientists have dedicated their research to developing ideal targeting strategies to treat life-threatening diseases, and several these strategies have been marketed. Theoretically, any ideal targeted delivery system should have two characteristics: 1) increased efficacy of the drugs in diseased tissues; and 2) reduced toxicity of the drugs in other healthy tissues. In the new era of drug delivery, knowledge and expertise from different areas, such as nanotechnology, polymer chemistry, and molecular biology are being combined to develop targeted drug delivery systems. In general, a targeted drug delivery system contains a therapeutic drug, a carrier, and a targeting ligand. The behavior of the carrier and ligand determines the absorption, distribution, metabolism, and cellular uptake of the cargo. Consequently, the successful construction of a carrier and a targeting ligand can selectively deliver a drug to the target cells (Figure 5.1).

With the advancement of molecular biology and biotechnology techniques, the regulatory pathways of a variety

Advanced Drug Delivery, First Edition. Edited by Ashim K. Mitra, Chi H. Lee, and Kun Cheng.

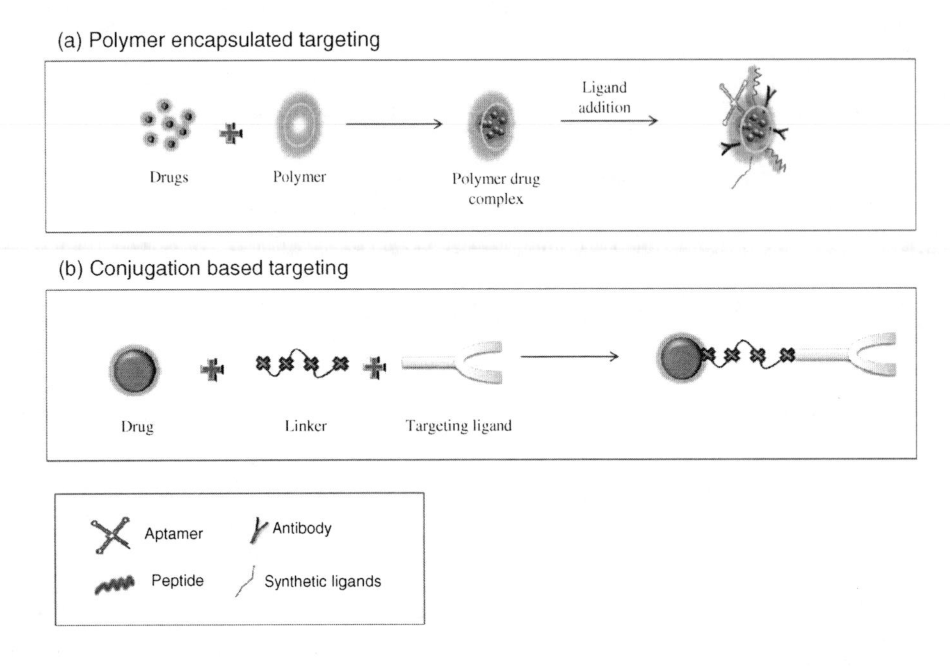

FIGURE 5.1 Schematic illustration depicting numerous drug targeting strategies: (a) encapsulation of therapeutic drugs in polymers and (b) conjugation of therapeutic drugs with targeting ligands via a liker.

of diseases have been elucidated. At the same time, scientists have unraveled several transporters and receptors that could be used to develop novel drug targeting strategies. As a result, many novel delivery systems have been developed that can, in principal, exert a better therapeutic effect than traditional therapies. In the past, many potent lead compounds were not marketed as a result of their toxicity to healthy tissues. To translate a drug molecule from the laboratory bench to market, it is necessary to either develop a potent chemical entity that can meet Lipinski's rule of five or incorporate the compound in a carrier system that can efficiently deliver the cargo to its target cells. Lipinski's rule of five is a universal rule that guides scientists in the development of a safe and conventional oral formulation [2, 3]. According to this rule, an active lead compound could become a drug if it has 1) no more than 5 hydrogen bond donors (expressed as the sum of amine groups and hydroxyl groups), 2) no more than 10 hydrogen bond acceptors (expressed as the sum of Ns and Os), 3) a molecular weight of less than 500 Da, and 4) partition coefficient log P less than five. However, most drug candidates developed in recent years cannot meet Lipinski's rule of five because of certain unfavorable characteristics, such as low solubility, poor stability, and poor cellular uptake. Consequently, a critical need remains in the pharmaceutical sciences to formulate new chemical entities in targeted drug delivery systems.

The aim of this chapter is to introduce the basic targeting mechanisms and various strategies used to achieve targeted drug delivery. Different approaches that have been employed to target a cargo to its site of action are presented. Subcellular targeting strategies are also described in this chapter.

5.3 DRUG TARGETING MECHANISMS

Targeted drug delivery can be achieved using various approaches from a simple, local administration to a sophisticated drug carrier that is modified with targeting ligands. In general, targeting mechanisms can be classified into physical targeting, passive targeting, and active targeting (Table 5.1 and Figure 5.2).

5.3.1 Physical Targeting

Physical targeting uses various external physical forces such as magnetic fields [13], ultrasound [14], light [15], temperature [5], and electric fields [16], to accumulate or release therapeutic agents at their target sites. The most common types of physical targeting include magnetic field-mediated targeting, ultrasound-mediated targeting, and light-mediated targeting (Figure 5.2a).

A magnetically targeted delivery system allows the accumulation of magnetic particles at a local site with the aid of external magnetic steering. Although magnetic particulate carriers have been employed in drug delivery since

TABLE 5.1 Different Types of Targeted Drug Delivery Systems

Method	Technology	Targeting Mechanism	Carrier	Advantage
Physical targeting	Heat sensitive	Temperature-mediated drug release	Temperature-sensitive biomaterials	Controlled and efficient drug release from the nanocarriers
	Ultrasound triggered	Ultrasound energy increases the permeability in the cells and degrade the carriers	Microbubbles	Accumulation and penetration into the deeper tissues
	Light induced	Light triggered irreversible structural change that allows for delivery of the entire dose regimen	Biomaterials containing photocleavable bonds [4]	Spatial and temporal control of compound release
	Magnetic nanocarriers	Accumulates the magnetic carrier in the tissues near the magnetic environment	Ferric oxide and other iron containing carriers [5]	Accumulation occurs in the presence of the external magnetic force that decreases the side effects
Passive targeting	Temperature	The carriers undergo a phase transition at different temperatures	Thermosenstive polymers	Drug carriers respond with the environmental condition
	EPR effect	The difference in the anatomy and pathology of solid tumors and normal tissues is used for drug targeting	Nanocarriers with size no larger than 200 nm [6]	Reduce the toxicity to the normal tissues
	pH sensitive	Drugs releases from pH-sensitive carriers under variations of pH	pH-sensitive biomaterials [7]	pH of tumor microenvironment is different from the normal tissues that allow higher drug accumulation
Active targeting	Folic acid	Folic acid could bind with folate receptors overexpressed on tumor cells	Folic acid as ligand on the biomaterials encapsulating drug	Higher therapeutic action at low drug concentration
	Mannan	Mannose receptors	Solid lipid nanoparticles [8]	Carriers decorated with mannan, anchored on the surface receptors of the macrophages and dendritic cells.
	Peptide	Peptide-receptor mediated targeting	Nanoparticles [9], micelle [10], liposomes [11]	Improve the cell uptake
	antibody	Antibodies bind to receptor overexpressed on tumor cells	Nanocomplex [12]	Increased targeted delivery

the 1970s [17], they did not attract much attention for drug targeting until the late 1980s [18]. Magnetic nanoparticles have gained a great deal of attention in recent years as a result of nanotechnology development. Specific properties of the magnetic nanoparticles make them an attractive platform for drug targeting. The advantages of magnetic nanoparticles include 1) magnetic dipole interactions lead to the accumulation of the magnetic nanoparticles in the desired sites under an external magnetic field; 2) the materials used for the preparation of the magnetic nanoparticles

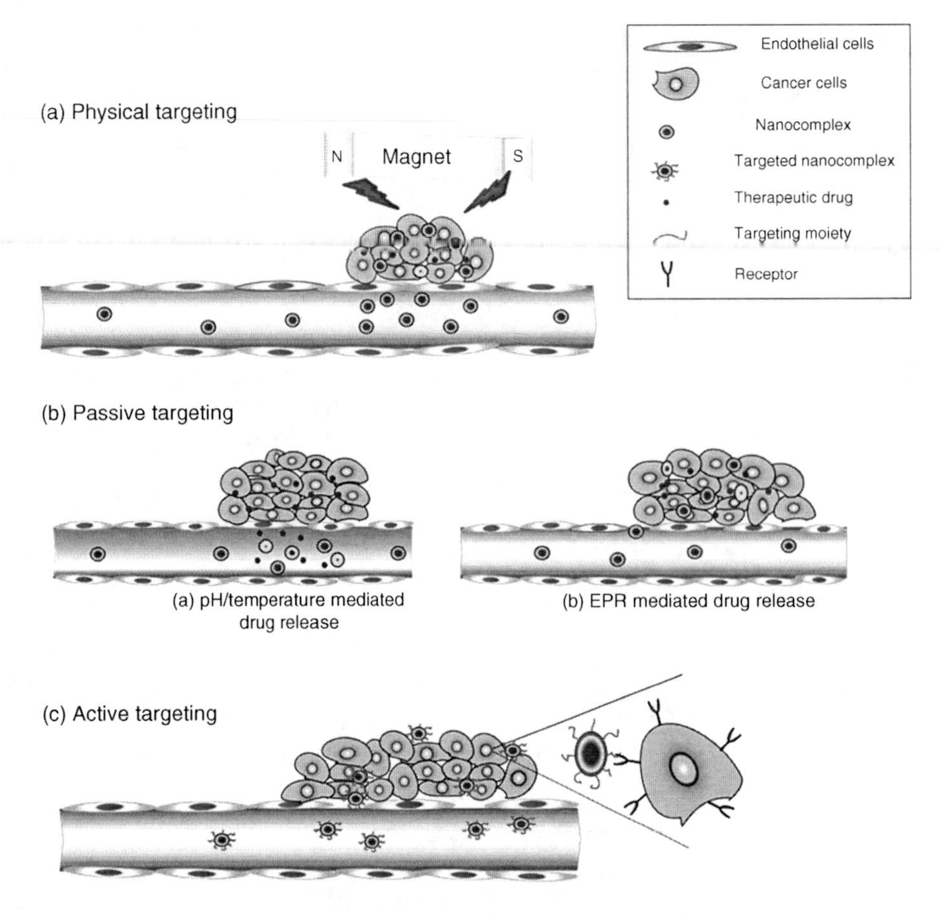

FIGURE 5.2 Schematic representation of different drug targeting methods. (a) physical targeting: requires external force such as magnetic field to accumulate the drug at the target site; (b) passive targeting: release the drug in the presence of unusual pH/temperature or large fenestration in capillaries; and (c) active targeting; requires ligands such as antibody/fragments, peptides, or small molecules on the surface of cargo to target the diseased tissues.

can be modified to improve biocompatibility; and 3) the magnetic nanoparticles can also be tailored with targeting ligands to further enhance cell-type specificity. The most successful magnetic nanoparticle is the super-paramagnetic iron oxide nanoparticle that has been approved by the U.S. Food and Drug Administration (FDA) as a magnetic resonance imaging contrast agent. For example, ferumoxides is a dextran-coated iron oxide nanoparticle in the 48–56-nm range [19]. The 5-nm monocrystalline magnetite (Fe_3O_4) cores of ferumoxides are coated with low-molecular-weight dextran, resulting in a hydrodynamic diameter of approximately 50 nm. Ferumoxides can be used in the detection and evaluation of liver lesions that are associated with alterations in the reticuloendothelial system (RES). Other studies have revealed that super-paramagnetic iron oxide nanoparticles show great potential in the evaluation of diseases in the RES, including changes in the liver, spleen, lymph nodes, and bone marrow [20]. In addition, the magnetic nanoparticles can be used as gene delivery systems [21].

Ultrasound-mediated delivery is a novel drug delivery system that combines ultrasound technology with microbubbles and therapeutic agents to facilitate cellular uptake using an external ultrasound field [22]. The strategy uses the acoustic energy of ultrasound to insonate the drug-carrying microbubbles at the desired sites, leading to the breakdown of these bubbles and drug release, thus, minimizing systemic side effects [23]. The ultrasound-mediated systems can achieve 1) local drug release, 2) enhanced permeability of the carriers and drugs, and 3) enhanced drug diffusion [23, 24]. Therefore, this system shows great promise in the targeted delivery of various therapeutic agents. The entrapped drugs can be released from the complexes by a short medical ultrasound treatment that destroys the bubbles. However, the drug-loading capacity of the carriers must be improved to meet the clinical requirements.

Light-triggered nanocarriers are designed to release drugs locally when exposed to light. They are modified with photosensitive materials such as photosensitive polymers and lipids that can absorb light energy [25], and they convert the light energy into heat to disrupt the carrier and subsequently release the encapsulated drug. This system allows for the release of encapsulated drugs at a specific time and location [26, 27]. Drug release is triggered by exposure to visible light or a laser. Furthermore, the light-sensitive system can be used to optimize the efficacy and safety of theranostics, the integration of therapy and diagnostics [26, 28].

5.3.2 Passive Targeting

Passive targeting refers to the selective accumulation of a drug in a target site that has unique physiological characteristics relative to other tissues in the body (Figure 5.2b). The most common example of passive targeting is tumor targeting by the enhanced permeation and retention (EPR) effect. In principal, drug carriers administered intravenously are restricted to the circulation system until they cross capillaries with large fenestrations. Cancer tissues grow rapidly and form new blood vessels to fill their nutritional demand by a process known as angiogenesis. The angiogenic blood vessels formed in tumor tissues are not as compact as normal blood vessels and have large gaps (600–800 nm) between their vascular endothelium. This leaky structure enhances the permeability and retention (EPR) of nanoscale particles (20–200 nm) in cancer tissues [29–32]. EPR-mediated targeting is a gold-standard targeting strategy in almost all cancers with the exception of prostate and pancreatic cancers that are less vascularized [33]. Injured or inflamed tissues also have increased permeability to enable leukocytes extravasation. This increased permeability also allows for the accumulation of nanocarriers at the desired sites of action. This approach has been successfully exploited for targeted drug delivery to inflammatory colonic mucosa in bowel disease [34].

The physico-chemical properties of nanocarriers, such as size, charge, and surface hydrophobicity, can affect the passive targeting efficiency. Although nanocarriers in the size range of 20–200 nm are preferred for passive targeting, a significant amount of them are rapidly entrapped in the RES after systemic administration. Nanocarriers tend to bind to the serum opsonins via a process called opsonization [35], and these opsonized nanoparticles are recognized by phagocytes as a result of the interaction between opsonins and the scavenger receptors present in the phagocytes. As part of the immune defense system in the body, the RES consists of various phagocytic cells including macrophages and monocytes. Phagocytic cells present in the spleen and liver recognize the opsonized particles and engulf them rapidly [35]. This natural tendency of the RES provides an excellent way to deliver antiviral and antibody drugs to combat intracellular infections. For example, *Leishmania donovani* infections have been treated by targeting the RES using the amphotericin B liposome (Ambisome) [31].

However, the rapid uptake of drug carriers by such macrophages is a major hurdle in targeting non-macrophage sites. The RES uptake can be avoided through the surface modification of nanoparticles. The hydrophobic or charged surfaces of nanoparticles are more prone to opsonization and are consequently taken up by the RES. In contrast, it has been found that neutral particles have a low opsonization tendency. Therefore, nanoparticles can be modified with groups that can block the hydrophobic and electrostatic interactions, thus, avoiding opsonization. Highly hydrophilic/ampiphilic polymers, such as dextrans and polyethylene glycols (PEGs), can be used for this purpose to shield nanoparticles from interacting with hydrophobic or charged particles in the blood circulation [35]. There has been immense interest in engineering long-circulating nanocarriers that can avoid rapid recognition by the RES after systemic administration. There are two typical approaches to avoid RES uptake: the formulation of nanoparticles with a size less than 200 nm or the PEGylation of nanoparticle surfaces. PEG anchored to the nanocarrier surface avoids macrophage recognition and plasma protein binding, thus, prolonging circulation time.

5.3.3 Active Targeting

Active targeting is the most advanced approach for the targeted delivery of drugs to their designated sites. In this approach, the drug carriers are modified with targeting ligands that can specifically guide the carriers to their target sites (Figure 5.2c). These targeting ligands can be monoclonal antibodies/fragments, peptides, nucleic acids (aptamers), or small molecules (such as sugars and folic acids) that can bind to target receptors or antigens/proteins on target cells (Figure 5.2c). These targets are either uniquely expressed or overexpressed on the diseased cells.

The target receptors may be categorized as internalization (endocytosis) receptors or endothelium receptors (Table 5.2) [33]. The internalization receptors, such as the transferrin receptors, low-density lipoprotein receptors (LDLRs), folate receptors, and epidermal growth factor receptors (EGFRs), help internalize drug carriers rather than enhance their accumulation at the target site. Targeting the internalization receptors on cancer cells is a promising strategy to kill the cancerous cell without affecting normal cells.

On the other hand, cancer cells can be destroyed by inhibiting their growth or nutrient supply via targeting the endothelium receptors, such as vascular endothelium growth factor receptors (VEGFRs) and $\alpha_v\beta_3$ integrin receptors. The essence of this approach is that it does not require the extravasation of nanocarriers into cancer cells but relies on the binding of the nanocarriers to the overexpressed endothelium receptors on tumor tissues. It has been well established that angiogenesis is regulated by vascular endothelium growth factors (VEGFs) and their receptors,

TABLE 5.2 Various Targets and Ligands in Active Targeting [33, 36]

Target Type	Target	Ligand	Mechanism of Internalization
Internalization receptors	Transferrin	Iron	Clathrin-dependent RME
	Folate	Folic acid	Caveolin-assisted
	VLDR	Cholesterol	Caveolin-assisted
	Mannose-6 phosphate receptor (M6PR)	M6P	Clathrin-dependent RME
Endothelium receptors	VEGFR	VEGF	Cell adhesion molecule (CAM) directed
	$\alpha_v\beta_3$ integrin	Arg–Gly–Asp (RGD)	Cell adhesion molecule (CAM) directed

especially VEGFR-1 and VEGFR-2 in tumor tissues. VEGF is largely produced by hypoxic tumors where the expression of VEGFR-2 is also high. Therefore, inhibition of either VEGFR-2 or VEGF can be a straightforward strategy to destruct the endothelium in solid tumors [33]. Similarly, $\alpha_v\beta_3$ integrins are also promising endothelium receptors that are overexpressed in cancer tissues and have been successfully targeted using linear or cyclic RGD (Arg-Gly-Asp) peptides [37].

In another approach, unique antigens/proteins expressed on the cell surface can be used as cellular targets in targeted drug delivery. For example, prostate-specific membrane antigen (PSMA) and erbB2 are overexpressed in prostate and breast cancers, respectively. Any ligands specific to these proteins can be used to achieve direct active targeting. The conjugation of multiple Herceptin (a monoclonal antibody targeting erbB2) molecules to nanoparticles generates multivalent engineered nanoparticles that specifically bind to the erbB2 receptors and subsequently deliver the encapsulated drugs into the cells [38]. Cheng et al. have conjugated an erbB2-specific peptide ligand to TGX-D1, a derivative of TGX221, and have observed a significant enhancement of drug uptake into erbB2-overexpressing cells [39].

Most targeted drug delivery systems enter cells via a process called endocytosis, in which cells engulf or internalize extracellular cargo. Endocytosis is a complex process comprising of three steps: 1) foreign particles are engulfed by cell membrane invaginations followed by the formation of membrane-bound vesicles known as endosomes; 2) the endosome is transported to various intravascular locations that enable the sorting of particles to various intracellular locations in the cells; and 3) endosomes are finally translocated to specific compartments in the cells, recycled to the extracellular space, or transferred across the cells by a process known as transcytosis [40]. In general, endocytosis can be classified into two general types: phagocytosis and pinocytosis. Phagocytosis, also known as "cell eating," is a process by which living cells internalize large solid particles (0.5–20 μm). Phagocytosis is primarily performed by phagocytic cells, such as macrophages, neutrophils, monocytes, and dendritic cells, to exert immunological functions. Phagocytosis also occurs in other mammalian cells but to a lesser extent. Pinocytosis, also known as "cell drinking," is a process by which living cells ingest fluid and solutes from the extracellular environment. Pinocytosis is virtually ubiquitous and exists in all types of cells via different mechanisms. Cell pinocytosis can be divided into clathrin-dependent and clathrin-independent endocytosis [40]. Clathrin-dependent endocytosis, also called receptor-mediated endocytosis (RME), is the most prominent mechanism for the cellular uptake of nanoscale carriers. These pathways are further classified into several subclasses, which are depicted in Figure 5.3. A more detailed discussion of endocytosis can be found in recent reviews [41, 42].

5.4 DELIVERY SYSTEMS FOR DRUG TARGETING

Recent clinical and preclinical studies have demonstrated that targeted drug delivery systems hold tremendous promise for the treatment of various life-threatening diseases. Targeted delivery systems can be classified into nanoscale carriers, prodrugs modified with targeting moieties, and polymer-based delivery systems (Figure 5.1).

5.4.1 Nanoscale Carriers

Recent years have witnessed an unprecedented growth of the research and applications of nanotechnology, especially in the field of cancer therapy. Nanocarrier-based delivery systems are favorable because their dimensions, often ranging from 10 to 1000 nm in diameter, help to improve the therapeutic efficiency of the encapsulated drugs in various types of diseases. As a result of the high surface-to-mass ratio, it is relatively easy to achieve a high density of targeting ligands (e.g., antibodies or antibodies fragments, oligosaccharides, peptides, viral proteins, and aptamers) on the nanocarrier surface. Nanocarriers with a large size or charged surface tend to be captured by phagocytic cells primarily found in the RES (liver, spleen, and lung). This problem can be overcome by surface modification with PEG [43, 44], which minimizes the uptake of nanocarriers by

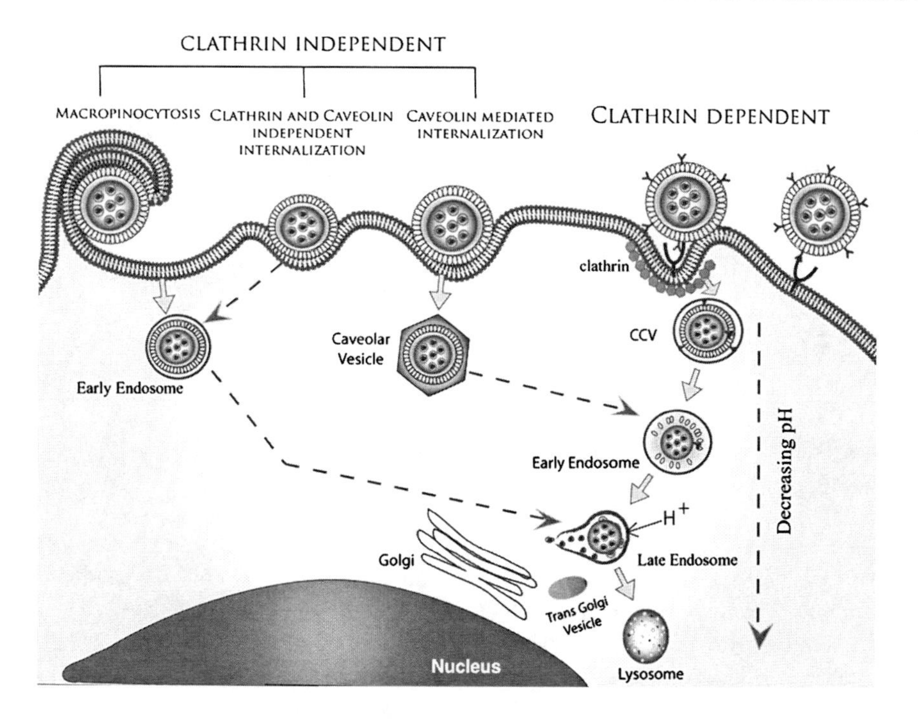

FIGURE 5.3 Schematic illustration of different pathways of endocytosis mechanisms. Pinocytosis is ubiquitously present in all cells and can be further classified in clatherin-dependent and clatherin-independent endocytosis. (See color figure in color plate section.)

macrophages and allows for prolonged systemic circulation. Nanocarriers have been prepared from a variety of materials ranging from natural origin such as albumin and phospholipids to chemically synthesized or modified polymers and metals. In addition, nanocarriers can exert magnetic, optical, or hypothermic properties depending on their ability to accommodate metallic cores and shells [44]. Nanocarriers used as targeted drug delivery systems mainly include liposomes, polymeric nanoparticles, solid lipid nanoparticles, and dendrimers (Figure 5.4) [43, 45].

5.4.1.1 Liposomes Liposomes are by far the most widely studied nanocarriers for targeted drug delivery because they are nontoxic and made of naturally occurring phospholipids. Liposomes are self-assembled circular vesicles composed of one or more bilayers of phospholipids that encapsulate a hydrophilic aqueous environment. The most important feature of liposomes is the ability to carry both hydrophilic and hydrophobic drug molecules. Liposomes are usually made of phospholipids and cholesterol, which are similar to the phospholipid membrane of cells. The phospholipids in liposomes consist of a hydrophobic tail and a hydrophilic head group. The lipid head groups are generally exposed to the aqueous environment, while the hydrophobic tails face each other to form the hydrophobic environment inside the lipid bilayer. The lipids self-assemble in bimolecular lipid layers with extremely low water solubility, and the critical micelle concentration (CMC) decreases four to five orders compared with ordinary lipids. The low water solubility of liposomes is crucial for absorption through the lipid membrane of cells, as it affects the dynamic of lipid exchange between the surrounding media and the lipid bilayer [46, 47].

Commonly used lipids in liposomes are 1) negatively charged lipids such as phosphatidyl glycerol, phosphatidyl ethanolamine, and phosphatidic acid; 2) neutral lipids such as phosphatidyl choline; and 3) positively charged lipids such as stearylamine, *N*-[1-(2,3-dioleoyloxy)propyl]-*N*,*N*,*N*-trimethylammonium Propane methyl-sulfate (DOTAP), and *N*-[1-(2,3-dioleyloxy)propyl]-*N*,*N*,*N*-trimethylammonium chloride (DOTMA). However, the nature of the lipids in liposomes is governed by the hydrophobicity of the lipid chain, particularly the number of double bonds present in the chain [47]. Generally, liposomes are classified depending on their structure and particle size. Morphologically they can be unilamellar or multilamellar as depicted in Figure 5.5. Unilamellar liposomes only contain a single phospholipid bilayer, which encapsulates an aqueous environment, while multilamellar liposomes contain multiple phospholipid bilayers arranged in an onion skin structure that encapsulates water-soluble molecules between the phospholipids bilayers. The unilamellar vesicles are ordinarily preferred for targeted drug delivery because of their facile preparation, easy characterization, and uniformity [46].

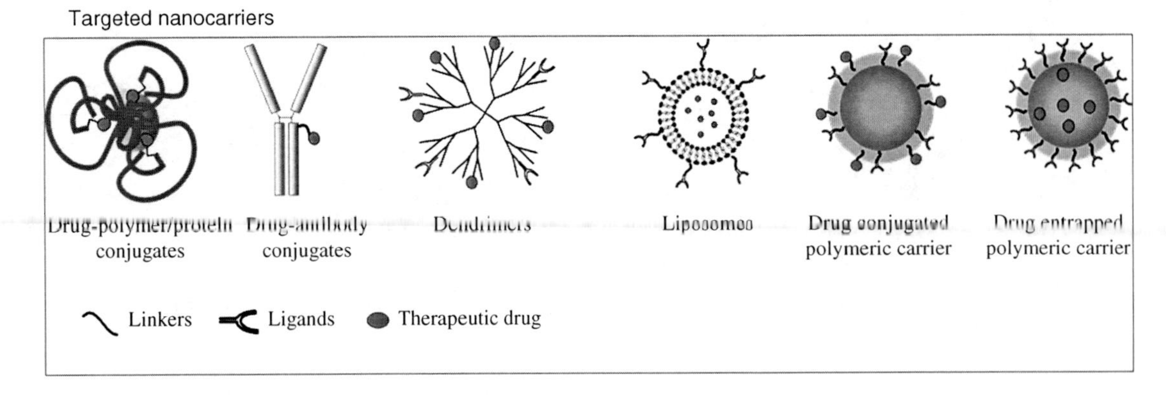

FIGURE 5.4 Schematic representation of numerous nanocarriers used in targeted drug delivery. (See color figure in color plate section.)

5.4.1.2 Polymeric Nanoparticles Polymeric nanoparticles are nanocarriers prepared from biocompatible polymers, which can be used to protect drugs from degradation and control the drug release profile. As a result of their biocompatibility, high drug-loading capability, and protection of drugs from degradation, polymeric nanoparticles have been widely employed for targeted drug delivery. Drugs can be entrapped or linked to the polymeric matrix via covalent bonds. In addition, polymeric nanoparticles allow for easy surface modification, which could improve the pharmacokinetic profile or targetability of the carrier. PEG modification has been extensively adopted for use in polymeric nanoparticles to improve their biodistribution [48]. Polymers used in the preparation of polymeric nanoparticles can be divided into two categories: 1) natural polymers, such as chitosan, albumin, and heparin, and 2) synthetic polymers, such as *N*-(2-hydroxyprpyl)-methacrylamide copolymer (HPMA), poly lactic acid (PLA), poly-L-glutamic acid (PGA), and poly(lactic-co-glycolic acid) (PLGA) [49]. As a result of their biocompatibility and safety, natural polymers are preferred for the delivery of a wide variety of therapeutic agents from macromolecules to small molecules. For example, albumin has been successfully used as the nanocarrier for paclitaxel (Abraxane; Abraxis Bioscience, Los Angeles, CA) to increase its solubility and targetability to tumor cells [50, 51].

Numerous drugs have been encapsulated using biodegradable synthetic polymers (e.g., PGA or PLGA) or non-biodegradable polymers (e.g., HPMA and PEG) for targeted drug delivery. More details can be found in recent

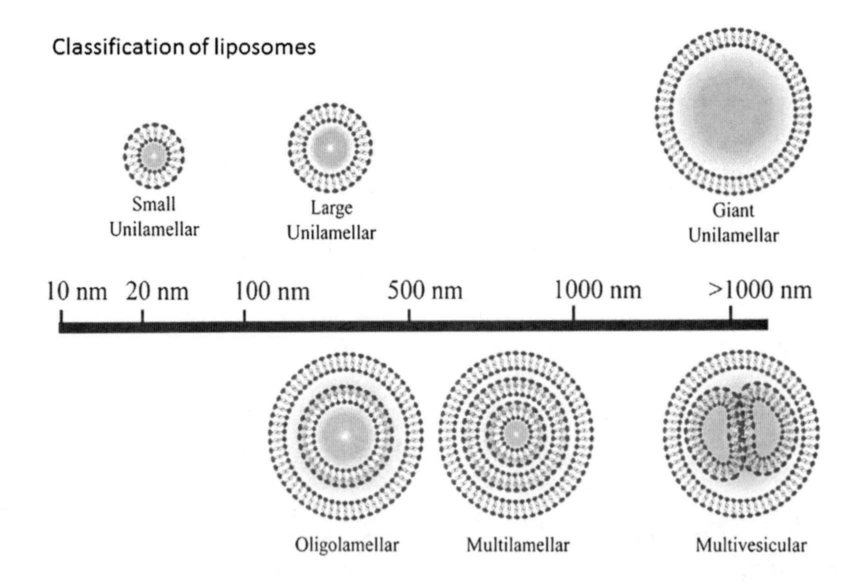

FIGURE 5.5 Schematic illustration depicting types of liposomes used in targeted drug delivery systems along with their nanoscale sizes.

reviews [48, 49]. Both PLA and PLGA are biodegradable polymers that have been approved by the FDA for human use and have been extensively used for nanoparticle formulation. Several methods have been developed to prepare polymeric nanoparticles. For instance, a double emulsion solvent evaporation method using oil and water with poly(vinyl alcohol) is the most widely adopted method for PLGA nanoparticles [48].

5.4.1.3 Solid Lipid Nanoparticles Solid lipid nanoparticles (SLNs) have been used as an efficient and nontoxic alternative to emulsions and liposomes since the 1990s. The formulation of an SLN is generally composed of three basic components: solid lipids (e.g., cholesterol, palmitic acids, and cetylpalmitate), emulsion-stabilizing surfactants (e.g., poloxamer 188, lecithin, and sodium glycolates) and water [45]. In general, SLNs are well tolerated and safer than polymeric nanoparticles because they are prepared from physiologically compatible lipids and exempted from toxic organic solvents during the preparation. Another major advantage of SLNs is the availability of large-scale production, which is the major hurdle for polymeric nanoparticles [52]. SLNs are primarily prepared either through high-pressure homogenization or microemulsion-based methods, which are based on solidified emulsion technology and avoid the use of organic solvents. The high-pressure homogenization technique is the most effective method for the SLN preparation in targeted drug delivery [53, 54].

5.4.1.4 Dendrimers Dendrimers are well-defined, monodisperse, globular, highly branched, tree-shape nanocarriers that are prepared by repetitive coupling reactions. Named as the polymer of the 21st century, dendrimers have been widely used as nanocarriers for various therapeutic entities including small-molecule and macromolecular drugs [55]. A typical dendrimer contains three major architectural components: 1) a central core that is generally a single atom, 2) repeated branch units that emerge from the central core, and 3) terminal functional groups that are present on the exterior surface of dendrimers and can be used for ligand conjugation and other modifications. Dendrimers are synthesized by either a convergent or a divergent method. In the divergent method, the synthesis begins with a central core and extends toward the outer surface. While in the convergent method, synthesis starts from a branched multifunctional structure and builds inward the center. The advantage of the convergent method is that a single dendrimer containing different functional groups on its periphery can be synthesized and used to bind different classes of moieties.

The multivalent targeting ability and uniformly small size (<100 nm) of dendrimers have been extensively explored in drug targeting, especially in tumor targeting [56, 57]. Drug molecules can be either encapsulated inside the dendrimers or directly attached to dendrimer terminal groups via chemical linkers in combination with surface modifications with targeting moieties [58]. A wide variety of compositionally differentiated dendrimers, such as poly (amidoamine) (PAMAM), diaminobutanepoly (propylene imine) (PPI), poly-L-lysine (PLL) dendrimers, melamine-dendrimer, and peptide- or PEG-conjugated dendrimers have been developed for targeted drug delivery. Among them, PAMAM is the most widely used dendrimer as a result of its non-immunogenicity, ability to conjugate with different targeting ligands, and commercial availability [57, 59].

5.4.2 Targeted Prodrugs

Prodrugs are biologically inactive chemical compounds that are converted into their active forms after crossing certain physiological barriers. Traditionally, prodrug approaches have been explored to improve certain pharmaceutical parameters, such as solubility, stability, bioavailability, presystemic metabolism, and toxicity. In recent years, a new class of prodrugs, targeted prodrugs, has attracted great interest. A typical targeted prodrug contains a parent drug or its derivate, an enzymatically or chemically cleavable linker (e.g., amide and ester), a polymer or enzymatically cleavable spacer, and a targeting moiety [60]. The selection of the cleavable linkers and targeting moieties are critical to the success of a targeted prodrug. Commonly used cleavable linkers are amides, esters, disulfide bonds, and phosphate esters. Among them, the amide and ester linkers have been extensively used for the prodrug approach. The ester linkers are relatively unstable and can be cleavable by esterase, which is ubiquitously present in the body. This stability issue can be resolved by replacing carboxyl esters or phosphate esters with carbamate esters [60]. By contrast, the amide linkage is stable and allows for prolonged circulation of targeted prodrugs after systemic administration. With the exception of aromatic amides, amide bonds can be degraded by peptidases and proteases. The amide bonds employed in targeted prodrugs are generally designed to be cleaved by specific enzymes to enhance target efficacy and reduce nonspecific toxicities [60, 61]. For example, the PSA substrate peptide linker SSKYQ is widely used for prostate cancer targeted prodrugs [62].

Other linkers used in targeted prodrugs include oximes/imines and uncleavable thioether bonds. The selection of a linker depends on the application of the prodrug. For example, disulfide linkers are commonly used to target tumor tissues where the overexpressed glutathione can reduce the disulfide linker in tumor cells. Similarly, acid labile hydrazone linkers are used to specifically release parent drugs in the endosome where the pH is low [60].

5.4.3 Cellular Carriers

Recently, various cells including monocytes, macrophages, erythrocytes, neutrophils, dendritic cells, and stem cells have been increasingly exploited as novel carriers for drug delivery. Cell-based targeted drug delivery systems possess several advantages such as biocompatibility, reduced immunogenicity, prolonged drug half-life, and intrinsic targetability to specialized cells including inflamed, injured, and cancer cells. Mononuclear cells such as dendritic cells, monocytes, and macrophages tend to engulf foreign materials and gather at injured, inflamed, and cancerous cells. The cytokines released from these disease sites, especially in hypoxic conditions, attract monocytes and macrophages. Moreover, these cells can migrate through impermeable barriers such as the blood-brain barrier and blood-tumor barrier. Thus, these cells are perfect carriers for targeted drug delivery to enhance and prolong the therapeutic efficacy of a drug without inducing immune responses.

Typically, cells can be used as drug carriers through three different approaches. Therapeutic drugs can be engulfed in cell carriers that are used as "Trojan horses" to deliver carried drugs to the desired disease site. Alternatively, drug molecules can be attached on the surface of cell carriers and released on arrival at the site of disease. The third approach uses genetically modified cells as "biological factories" to produce therapeutically active proteins at the site of action [63]. Despite its promise as a novel targeted drug delivery system, cell-based drug delivery still faces several challenges. First, a sufficient amount of drugs must be engulfed in the host cells without degradation in the intracellular environment. Second, the engulfed drugs cannot cause toxicity to the host cells. Finally, the engulfed drugs must be released at the site of action [63, 64].

The first two challenges can be overcome by encapsulating drug molecules in nanoparticles that are loaded into host cells. The incorporation of drugs into nanocarriers not only protects them from degradation inside the host cells but also increases the loading efficiency in cell carriers. Nanoparticles with optimal morphology, biocompatibility, and controlled release characteristics are preferred for drug encapsulations [64]. Magnetic nanoparticles can be used to encapsulate drugs and guide the cell carriers to target sites with the aid of external magnetic steering [65]. Surface modifications of the nanocarriers may affect their uptake by host cells. It has been observed that charged particles are rapidly taken by phagocytic host cells [63, 66, 67]. Moreover, phagocytic cells contain Fc and mannose receptors that allow for the rapid uptake of opsonized and mannan functionalized nanoparticles, respectively [68]. Drugs encapsulated in nanoparticles have been loaded into host cells for the treatment of several diseases, including Alzheimer's, Parkinson's, and cancer. For example, Batrakova et al. have developed a macrophage-nanozyme delivery system for the efficient delivery of catalase, an enzyme that breaks down microglial hydrogen peroxides, for the treatment of Parkinson's disease. Catalase was encapsulated into a block ionomer complex with a cationic block copolymer prior to loading into bone-marrow–derived macrophages (BMMs). The release of physiologically active catalase was observed for more than 24 h, while naked catalase was rapidly degraded in host cells [69].

By changing the morphology, the drug-containing particles can be attached to the surface of host cells rather than encapsulated inside the cells. This approach provides better control over the release of drugs and avoids interference with the native cellular functions of cell carriers [70].

Cellular carriers can also be genetically engineered to express therapeutic proteins in their native form at disease sites for a prolonged time. These systems have been explored for the treatment of diseases that require long-term treatments such as age-related macular degeneration, diabetes, and some cancers. So far, *in situ* cell-based delivery systems have been used for the delivery of peptides and proteins, thus, circumventing the limitations of other systems that are prone to destabilization during formulation and systemic circulation [71, 72]. In this type of cell-based delivery, donor cells are transfected *ex vivo* with plasmid DNA containing therapeutic genes and then administrated into the host system. Once it reaches the target tissues, the DNA expresses proteins in their natural form. To protect it from host immune responses, cells are encapsulated with different polymers or hydrogels. These encapsulations not only protect the cells from host immune responses but also provide mechanical strength and nutrients. In addition, these encapsulation materials are biodegradable in nature and thus do not exert any toxicity and avoid the need for immunosuppressants [71, 72].

5.5 LIGANDS USED IN DRUG TARGETING

5.5.1 Monoclonal Antibodies/Antibody Fragments

Monoclonal antibodies (MAbs) are immunoglobulin IgG molecules composed of two heavy (H) and two light (L) chains, which are linked by disulfide bonds (Figure 5.6a). The two heavy chains are connected to each other via the interchain disulfide bonds in the hinge region. Generally, the molecular weight of an antibody ranges from 150,000 to 160,000 Da. The heavy chains of all immunoglobulins are attached with polysaccharide chains (mostly at the C_H2 region) and can be exploited for conjugation with other molecules. The structure of an antibody resembles the letter Y, in which the upper part is called the Fab (fragment, antigen binding) of the Y, while the base is known as the Fc (fragment, crystalline). The tip of the Fab region contains the variable region of both heavy and light chains, defined as the F_v (fragment, variable) segments [73].

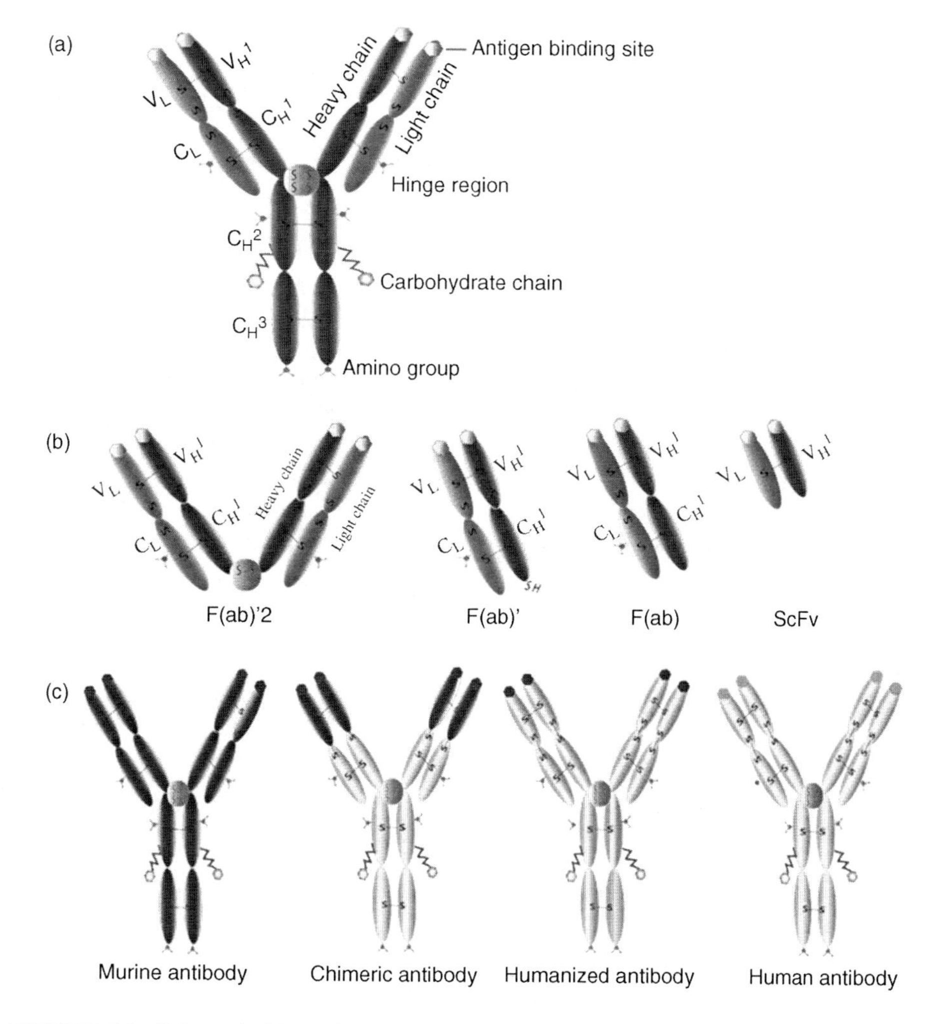

FIGURE 5.6 Schematic illustration of (a) whole IgG antibody, (b) antibody fragments, and (c) antibody body obtained from several sources.

The Fc region of an antibody is responsible for triggering antibody-dependent cellular cytotoxicity in the body. Therefore, the Fc region is preferably removed when antibodies are used as targeting ligands in targeted drug delivery systems. The removal of the Fc region not only avoids immunity but also reduces the molecular weight of the antibody ligands to increase their catabolic rate in the body [74]. Various chemical and enzymatic methods can be used to cleave intact antibodies to generate Fab and Fc for drug targeting purposes.

To develop an effective antibody-mediated delivery system, monoclonal antibodies/fragments can be conjugated directly with drugs or drug-containing carriers via various covalent and noncovalent bonding [75]. The covalent conjugation of antibodies to drugs using cleavable linkers has been used to bring some products to clinical trials [76]. Gemtuzumab ozogamicin (Mylotarg; BDI Pharma, Columbia, SC) was the first FDA-approved antibody-drug conjugate for the treatment of acute myeloid leukemia (AML). It is a conjugate of cytotoxic drug calicheamicin and humanized MAb against CD33 [77]. Although it was withdrawn from the market in 2010, many other antibody-drug conjugates are undergoing late-stage clinical trials, and some of them have shown promising results. On the other hand, antibodies can be anchored to drug carriers. Liposomes are the most extensively studied carrier system used in this regard. Antibodies/fragments can be anchored to lipids via covalent interactions using two strategies: 1) hydrophobic lipids, such as phosphatedyl ethanolamine (PE), are conjugated to antibodies/fragments prior to liposome preparation, or 2) preformulated liposomes are attached *in situ* to antibodies/fragments using hetro-bifunctional reagents, which can form covalent bonds between the amino groups of antibodies and the PE of liposomes [75]. Noncovalent interactions including electrostatic interaction, hydrophobic interaction, or streptavidin–biotin interaction have also been applied to attach targeting antibodies/fragments to therapeutic agents. The streptavidin–biotin interaction is the most commonly used strategy in this approach. For example, biotinylated drugs can form a stable nanocomplex with antibody-conjugated streptavidin [75, 78]. Liposomes containing biotinylated lipids can be easily formulated and subsequently anchored to streptavidin-linked ligands [79, 80].

Antibodies and fragments can be conjugated to drugs or drug carriers at three sites: 1) the ε-amino groups of lysine residues, 2) the disulfides in the hinge region that hold the heavy chains together, and 3) the carbohydrate chains that are attached to the C_H2 domain in the Fc region [73, 74].

5.5.2 Aptamers

The word "aptamer" is derived from the Latin word *aptus*, meaning "fitting," and the Greek word *meros*, meaning "particle" [81, 82]. Aptamers are single-stranded DNA or RNA molecules (6–40 kDa) with numerous three-dimensional arrangements [82, 83]. Such arrangements offer a very high affinity (K_d typically in the nM range) for a wide variety of targets of interest. These nucleic-acid–derived ligands are generated *in vitro* by a process called SELEX (selective expansion of ligands by exponential enrichment). SELEX starts with a random nucleic acid library that contains sequences of 20–100 residues in length along with constant flanking regions on both ends for enzymatic manipulations. The diversity of the library can be calculated by y^N, where N is the number of mutant sequences and y is the alternative monomer (such as A, G, C, and T). For example, the diversity of a library containing 40 random sequences with 4 monomers is $4^{40} = 1.2 \times 10^{24}$ [83].

There are several therapeutic aptamers in clinical trials to treat a number of diseases [84]. Pegaptanib (brand name Macugen) has been approved for the treatment of wet age-related macular degeneration (AMD) [84]. Aptamers have shown promising potential in drug targeting. Both RNA and DNA aptamers can be screened against a molecular target and then conjugated to a drug molecule or a drug carrier. In recent years, aptamers against many important targets such as prostate-specific membrane antigen (PSMA), VEGF, gp120, and EGFR have been successfully used for targeted delivery of various agents [85–89].

5.5.3 Peptides

To circumvent the limitations of high-molecular-weight ligands such as antibodies and their fragments, low-molecular-weight peptides have attracted much attention in recent years. Although their K_d values are not comparable with antibodies or aptamers, their unique structural features, ease of screening, and chemical modifications make them promising alternatives to antibodies in drug targeting. In addition, the absence of tertiary structures in the short-length peptides avoids the chance of physical degradations. Peptides began their journey as a drug delivery in the early 1990s when some transcriptional factor proteins were observed to shuttle into cells or between different cells. Penetratin, the third alpha helix of the Antennapedia homeodomain protein and trans-activating regulator protein (TAT) have been extensively studied as protein transduction domains (PTDs) and cell penetrating peptides (CPPs), respectively [90, 91]. These peptides contain ~30 amino acids comprising mainly basic amino acids, such as arginine and lysine. For example, TAT peptides contain 2-Lys along with 6-Arg residues that facilitate the cellular uptake of their cargo [91]. Positive charges in these peptides are advantageous for the complexation of negatively charged nucleic acids such as siRNA, oligonucleotides, and DNA through charge–charge interactions. Moreover, Arg residues are more important for cellular uptake compared with other positively charged residues, such as Lys or His. Thus, several poly-Arg peptides have been synthesized to exploit this phenomenon. Arg residues are thought to facilitate the uptake by forming hydrogen bonds between the phosphate groups of the membrane with the guanidinium groups of the Arg [92]. The most commonly used peptides are penetratin, TAT, and transportan. Several natural and synthetic peptides (e.g., Pep1, poly-Arg peptides, MPG, and CADY) have also been explored for drug delivery.

Although these cationic peptides have shown very high and promising *in vitro* cellular uptake, none of them has reached to clinical use. There are a number of reasons for this, such as follows: 1) their uptake into several nonspecific tissues when administered via parenteral route and 2) insufficient information regarding the peptide–receptor interaction, cell trafficking, and pharmacokinetic behaviors. Therefore, several researchers have linked cell-surface proteins, such as LHRH, LFA-1, Bombesin, and intracellular adhesion molecules-1 (ICAM-1) to CPPs to deliver therapeutic compounds specifically [93]. Once these CPPs are delivered systemically, receptors overexpressed in the target tissues recognize the peptide sequences and allow the entry of the attached compounds.

In addition, a novel technique called "phage display" has been used to screen peptides of interest. Phage display technology allows for the screening of peptides against any target. Phage display technology is gaining interest in the area of screening peptide ligands for the targeted delivery of potent anticancer drugs and has emerged as an alternative to traditional delivery regimens. Recently, Cheng et al. have used the peptides derived from this strategy to deliver small therapeutic drug and siRNA to prostate cancer cells [94, 95]. For example, Her-2 specific peptide was conjugated to the small-molecule drug TGX-D1 via a PSA cleavable linker [95]. In another example, the same group identified a LnCap cell-specific peptide using phage display and they used it to deliver macromolecules [94].

5.6 INTRACELLULAR TARGETING STRATEGIES

Intracellular targeting refers to the delivery of therapeutic molecules to a specific compartment or an organelle within the cell. Therapeutic agents enter target cells via diffusion or endocytosis. Low-molecular-weight molecules enter cells through the passive diffusion, while macromolecules (e.g., proteins and nucleic acids) and particulate drug carriers (e.g., liposomes and nanoparticles) enter cells via endocytosis. The endocytosis pathway is a complex process that includes several mechanisms, such as clathrin-dependent and clathrin-independent endocytosis, phagocytosis, and macropinocytosis. In general, four intracellular targets have been targeted so far: the cytoplasm, endo-lysosome, nucleus, and mitochondria [96].

5.6.1 Targeting the Cytoplasm

For most therapeutic agents, the primary goal is not only to reach the inside of the cell but also to collect specifically in the cytoplasmic compartments. Cytoplasmic delivery is essential for certain drugs such as glucocorticoids and siRNA therapeutics. Glucocorticoids must reach the cytoplasm to interact with the steroidal receptors, while siRNA induces mRNA degradation in the cytoplasm. Thus, maximum potency for the steroidal drug can be observed only when it reaches the cytoplasm.

Cytoplasmic delivery is not a challenge for small-molecule drugs because they can enter the cytoplasm directly by diffusion. However, for macromolecules and particulate drug carriers, the uptake process is complex. These molecules enter cells via endocytosis and are then entrapped in the endosomes or lysosomes. To achieve cytoplasmic delivery, either macromolecules or particulate drug carriers need to be stable in the endosomes/lysomes and be able to escape from them. Several fusogenic peptides and cationic lipids have been used to deliver macromolecules into the cytoplasm via different mechanisms, such as the proton sponge effect and endosomal disruptions [96].

5.6.2 Targeting the Endo-lysosomes

The second intracellular target is endo-lysosomes, which are beneficial for targeting antibacterial or antiparasitic agents. It has been observed that numerous parasites (e.g., *trypanosome)* and disease-causing bacteria (e.g., *Mycobacterium tuberculosis*) tend to reside in the phagosomal or the endosomal compartments of phagocytic cells [96, 97]. The reduced activity of antibacterials in the acidic pH and their poor absorption into lysosomes and phagosomes illustrate a critical need to develop an effective delivery system that can specifically deliver therapeutic drugs into these acidic compartments. Several nanoscale carriers that simulate the entry of bacteria into phagosomes or lysosomes have been formulated to overcome the low efficacy of antibacterial drugs. For example, polysiohexyl cynoacrylate nanoparticles have been shown to increase the localization of ampicillin in phagosomes [98].

5.6.3 Targeting the Nucleus

Nuclear targeting is another form of intracellular targeting that has been extensively explored for the delivery of macromolecules into the nucleus. In most cases, drug enters the nucleus through the nuclear pore complex (NPC), which are small pores with a diameter of 9 nm. However, the diameter of the NPC may expand up to 26 nm for the active transport of certain molecules [99]. NPCs work as sieves and only allow the entry of molecules with a lower molecular weight (~45 kDa). Large macromolecules such as proteins can only enter the nucleus if they contain a certain nuclear localization signal (NLS) sequence. NLS sequences are the peptide sequences that contain several basic amino acids and are able to form cytosolic complexes with karyopherin α or β. These complexes facilitate the nuclear entry of macromolecules through the NPC channels [100, 101]. It has been suggested that the inclusion of NLS sequences either by mixing with cationic liposomes containing DNA or covalent conjugation to the DNA may enhance the nuclear localization of these macromolecules. A 3.3-kb linear DNA has been capped with a single NLS sequence (PKKKRKVEDPYC) to prove this hypothesis. A 10- to 1000-fold transfection enhancement in the nuclear transport of DNA was observed regardless of cell types and cationic vectors [102].

5.6.4 Targeting Mitochondria

As the "powerhouse" in eukaryotic cells, mitochondria have been established as the primary target of several cyto-protective and cytotoxic agents. The human mitochondrial DNA (16 kbp) encodes for 13 essential proteins that act as the subunits of enzymes participating in oxidative phosphorylation [103]. Any mutations or changes in the mitochondrial DNA sequence directly affect adenosine triiphosphate (ATP) biosynthesis and may cause neural dysfunction and aging [103]. Therefore, gene therapy could be an important tool for overcoming such mutations. Another important aspect of mitochondrial drug delivery is to prevent oxidative damage through the delivery of antioxidant molecules [104]. Mitochondria not only serve as the powerhouse for eukaryotic cells but also regulate the intrinsic pathways of apoptosis. The regulation and activation of apoptotic effector mechanisms are carried out in mitochondria by controlling the translocation of pro-apoptotic proteins between mitochondrial inner membrane spaces and the cytoplasm. Normal mitochondrial function is altered in cancer cells, which exhibit an extensive metabolic reprogramming that makes them more susceptible to mitochondrial perturbation [105].

In normal cells, mitochondria contain a high transmembrane potential in the inner membrane and the low conductance of the permeability transition pore complex (PTPC). The PTPC is structurally complex and composed of three components: adenine nucleotide translocase (ANT) in the inner membrane of mitochondria, voltage-dependent anion channels (VDAC) present in the outer membrane, and cyclophilin D (CYPD) in the mitochondrial matrix. In addition, the PTPC contains some benzodiazepine receptors and hexokinases on the intersurface of the cytosol and the outer mitochondrial surface. Hexokinases play an important role in controlling the permeabilization of mitochondrial membranes in healthy cells [105].

There are two strategies to target mitochondria, especially in cancer cells: 1) the use of lipophilic cations and 2) conjugation with compounds that can interact with PTPC constituents. Cancer cells have a higher membrane potential inside compared with normal cells. This allows for an accumulation of lipophilic cations in the mitochondria, leading to nonspecific disruption of the mitochondrial function. Such lipophilic compounds can be conjugated with anticancer drugs such as cisplatin to kill cancer cells [106, 107].

In recent years, different compounds have been reported that can interact with ANT and induce cell death by mitochondrial apoptosis. 4-(*N*-(*S*-glutathionylacetyl) amino) phenyl arsinoxide (GSAO) has been used as an ANT ligand to interact with the cysteines of ANT (Cys160 and Cys 257). It inhibits the ATP/ADP transporter activity and allows the accumulation of reactive oxygen species (ROS) and mitochondrial apoptosis [108].

5.7 SUMMARY AND FUTURE PERSPECTIVES

The recent progresses in the field of targeted drug delivery have revolutionized pharmaceutical research, and targeted drug delivery has emerged as an efficient tool for the treatment of lethal diseases. Over the last decade, intensive efforts have been made to develop targeted therapies for life-threatening diseases, such as cancer, HIV, diabetes, and central nervous system (CNS) disorders. To reach a distant target organ, a therapeutic agent can be delivered by several routes (e.g., intravenous, oral, intranasal, and inhalation) using polymer, protein, lipid, and peptide-based nanomaterials. Significant developments have been observed using nanoscale systems for the targeted delivery of potent drugs that are susceptible to degradation or toxic to healthy tissues. Recent advances in polymer chemistry have boosted the research by allowing for the bottom-up fabrication of nanocarriers along with their functionalization with targeting ligands. These functionalized nanocarriers for targeted delivery systems are very promising for the delivery of anticancer drugs. Cell-based drug delivery is another revolutionary approach developed in recent years to provide a safe, targeted, and prolonged delivery of therapeutic agents.

Despite recent progress and extensive studies on targeted drug delivery, only a small number of such products is available on the market. The complexity of formulation and the lack of a feasible large-scale production are the two major hurdles that limit the transition of targeted drug delivery systems from the laboratory bench to clinical use. Many pharmaceutical companies are reluctant to invest a huge amount of money in a product line that can only be used for a specific product. Therefore, pharmaceutical scientists should be aware of these challenges during the early stages of the formulation development. In addition, a close collaboration between scientists from the fields of drug delivery, polymer chemistry, and molecular biology is necessary to guarantee the success of product development.

ASSESSMENT QUESTIONS

5.1. What is the most important requirement for a biological active chemical constituent to act as the therapeutic drug?

- **a.** Should have very low IC_{50}
- **b.** Should be very lipophilic
- **c.** Should follow "Lipinski's Rule of Five"
- **d.** None of the above

5.2. Which of the following delivery systems allow active targeting of cancer tissues?

- **a.** Effervesent tablets
- **b.** Capsules
- **c.** Immunoliposomes
- **d.** None of the above

5.3. Describe three important strategies to deliver a therapeutic drug to its site of action.

5.4. Write four ligands for active targeting of a therapeutic drug.

5.5. Match the column for the drug targeting methods and their mechanism used in drug uptake in cells:

Targeting Methods	Mechanism of Drug Entry in Cells
1. Active targeting	A. Folic acid
2. Passive targeting	B. Cell drinking
3. Physical targeting	C. Immunoliposomes
4. Pinocytosis	D. Cell eating
5. Phagocytosis	E. Magnetic liposomes
6. Transferrin receptor	F. EPR effect

REFERENCES

1. Strebhardt, K., Ullrich, A. (2008). Paul Ehrlich's magic bullet concept: 100 years of progress. *Nature Reviews: Cancer, 8(6)*, 473–480.
2. Lipinski, C.A., et al. (2001). Experimental and computational approaches to estimate solubility and permeability in drug discovery and development settings. *Advanced Drug Delivery Reviews, 46(1–3)*, 3–26.
3. Oprea, T.I., et al. (2001). Is there a difference between leads and drugs? A historical perspective. *Journal of Chemical Information and Computer Sciences, 41(5)*, 1308–1315.
4. Paasonen, L., et al. (2010). Gold-embedded photosensitive liposomes for drug delivery: Triggering mechanism and intracellular release. *Journal of Controlled Release, 147(1)*, 136–143.
5. Pradhan, P., et al. (2010). Targeted temperature sensitive magnetic liposomes for thermo-chemotherapy. *Journal of Controlled Release, 142(1)*, 108–121.
6. Liu, Z., et al. (2011). Docetaxel-loaded pluronic p123 polymeric micelles: In vitro and in vivo evaluation. *International Journal of Molecular Sciences, 12(3)*, 1684–1696.
7. Lin, W., Kim, D. (2011). pH-sensitive micelles with cross-linked cores formed from polyaspartamide derivatives for drug delivery. *Langmuir, 27(19)*, 12090–12097.
8. Yu, W., et al. (2010). Mannan-modified solid lipid nanoparticles for targeted gene delivery to alveolar macrophages. *Pharmaceutical Research, 27(8)*, 1584–1596.
9. Liu, C., et al. (2011). Enhanced gene transfection efficiency in CD13-positive vascular endothelial cells with targeted poly (lactic acid)-poly(ethylene glycol) nanoparticles through caveolae-mediated endocytosis. *Journal of Controlled Release, 151(2)*, 162–175.
10. Sethuraman, V.A., Bae, Y.H. (2007). TAT peptide-based micelle system for potential active targeting of anti-cancer agents to acidic solid tumors. *Journal of Controlled Release, 118(2)*, 216–224.
11. Mai, J., et al. (2009). A synthetic peptide mediated active targeting of cisplatin liposomes to Tie2 expressing cells. *Journal of Controlled Release, 139(3)*, 174–181.
12. Bardhan, R., et al. (2010). Tracking of multimodal therapeutic nanocomplexes targeting breast cancer in vivo. *Nano Letters, 114*, 7378–7383.
13. Kumar, A., et al. (2010). Multifunctional magnetic nanoparticles for targeted delivery. *Nanomedicine, 6(1)*, 64–69.
14. Geers, B., et al. (2011). Self-assembled liposome-loaded microbubbles: The missing link for safe and efficient ultrasound triggered drug-delivery. *Journal of Controlled Release, 152(2)*, 249–256.
15. Lin, H.M., et al. (2010). Light-sensitive intelligent drug delivery systems of coumarin-modified mesoporous bioactive glass. *Acta Biomaterialia, 6(8)*, 3256–3263.
16. Oshima, Y., et al. (1999). The comparative benefits of glaucoma filtering surgery with an electric-pulse targeted drug delivery system demonstrated in an animal model. *Ophthalmology, 106(6)*, 1140–1146.
17. Widder, K.J., Senyel, A.E., Scarpelli, G.D. (1978). Magnetic microspheres: A model system of site specific drug delivery in vivo. *Proceedings of the Society for Experimental Biology and Medicine, 158(2)*, 141–146.
18. Pouliquen, D., et al. (1989). Superparamagnetic iron oxide nanoparticles as a liver MRI contrast agent: Contribution of microencapsulation to improved biodistribution. *Magnetic Resonance Imaging, 7(6)*, 619–627.
19. Jung, C.W., Jacobs, P. (1995). Physical and chemical properties of superparamagnetic iron oxide MR contrast agents: Ferumoxides, ferumoxtran, ferumoxsil. *Magnetic Resonance Imaging, 13(5)*, 661–674.
20. Wu, L., et al. (2011). Diagnostic performance of USPIO-enhanced MRI for lymph-node metastases in different body regions: A meta-analysis. *European Journal of Radiology, 80(2)*, 582–589.
21. Yang, F., et al. (2011). Controlled release of Fe3O4 nanoparticles in encapsulated microbubbles to tumor cells via sonoporation and associated cellular bioeffects. *Small, 7(7)*, 902–910.
22. Seip, R., et al. (2010). Targeted ultrasound-mediated delivery of nanoparticles: On the development of a new HIFU-based therapy and imaging device. *IEEE Transactions on Biomedical Engineering, 57(1)*, 61–70.
23. Klibanov, A.L., et al. (2010). Ultrasound-triggered release of materials entrapped in microbubble-liposome constructs: A tool for targeted drug delivery. *Journal of Controlled Release, 148(1)*, 13–17.
24. Deckers, R., Moonen, C.T. (2010). Ultrasound triggered, image guided, local drug delivery. *Journal of Controlled Release, 148(1)*, 25–33.
25. Wang, J.Y., et al. (2010). Photo-sensitive liposomes: Chemistry and application in drug delivery. *Mini Reviews in Medicinal Chemistry, 10(2)*, 172–181.
26. Rai, P., et al. (2010). Development and applications of photo-triggered theranostic agents. *Advanced Drug Delivery Reviews, 62(11)*, 1094–1124.
27. Yavlovich, A., et al. (2011). A novel class of photo-triggerable liposomes containing DPPC:DC(8,9)PC as vehicles for delivery of doxorubcin to cells. *Biochimica et Biophysica Acta, 1808(1)*, 117–126.
28. Caldorera-Moore, M.E., Liechty, W.B., Peppas, N.A. (2011). Responsive theranostic systems: Integration of diagnostic imaging agents and responsive controlled release drug delivery carriers. *Accounts of Chemical Research, 44(10)*, 1061–1070.
29. Putnam, D., Kopeček, J. Polymer conjugates with anticancer activity, in N. Peppas and R. Langer (eds.), *Biopolymers II*, Springer, Berlin/Heidelberg, 1995, pp. 55–123.
30. Yokoyama, M. (2005). Drug targeting with nano-sized carrier systems. *Journal of Artificial Organs, 8(2)*, 77–84.
31. Moghimi, S.M., Hunter, A.C., Murray, J.C. (2001). Long-circulating and target-specific nanoparticles: Theory to practice. *Pharmacological Reviews, 53(2)*, 283–318.

32. Li, S.D., Huang, L. (2008). Pharmacokinetics and biodistribution of nanoparticles. *Molecular Pharmacology*, *5(4)*, 496–504.
33. Danhier, F., Feron, O., Preat, V. (2010). To exploit the tumor microenvironment: Passive and active tumor targeting of nanocarriers for anti-cancer drug delivery. *Journal of Controlled Release*, *148*(2), 135–146.
34. Lamprecht, A., et al. (2001). Biodegradable nanoparticles for targeted drug delivery in treatment of inflammatory bowel disease. *Journal of Pharmacology and Experimental Therapeutics*, *299*(2), 775–781.
35. Nie, S. (2010). Understanding and overcoming major barriers in cancer nanomedicine. *Nanomedicine*, *5(4)*, 523–528.
36. Bareford, L.M., Swaan, P.W. (2007). Endocytic mechanisms for targeted drug delivery. *Advanced Drug Delivery Reviews*, *59(8)*, 748–758.
37. Desgrosellier, J.S., Cheresh, D.A. (2010). Integrins in cancer: Biological implications and therapeutic opportunities. *Nature Reviews: Cancer*, *10(1)*, 9–22.
38. Jiang, W., et al. (2008). Nanoparticle-mediated cellular response is size-dependent. *Nature Nanotechnology*, *3(3)*, 145–150.
39. Tai, W., et al. (2011). Development of a peptide-drug conjugate for prostate cancer therapy. *Molecular Pharmaceutics*, *8* (*3*), 901–912.
40. Sahay, G., Alakhova, D.Y., Kabanov, A.V. (2010). Endocytosis of nanomedicines. *Journal of Controlled Release*, *145*(3), 182–195.
41. Bareford, L.M., Swaan, P.W. (2007). Endocytic mechanisms for targeted drug delivery. *Advanced Drug Delivery Reviews*, *59(8)*, 748–758.
42. Sahay, G., Alakhova, D.Y., Kabanov, A.V. (2010). Endocytosis of nanomedicines. *Journal of Controlled Release*, *145* (*3*), 182–195.
43. De Jong, W.H., Borm, P.J. (2008). Drug delivery and nanoparticles: Applications and hazards. *International Journal of Nanomedicine*, *3*(2), 133–149.
44. van Vlerken, L.E., Amiji, M.M. (2006). Multi-functional polymeric nanoparticles for tumour-targeted drug delivery. *Expert Opinion on Drug Delivery*, *3*(2), 205–216.
45. Zhang, L., et al. (2010). Development of nanoparticles for antimicrobial drug delivery. *Current Medicinal Chemistry*, *17*(*6*), 585–594.
46. Jesorka, A., Orwar, O. (2008). Liposomes: Technologies and analytical applications. *Annual Review of Analytical Chemistry*, *1*, 801–832.
47. Medina, O.P., Zhu, Y., Kairemo, K. (2004). Targeted liposomal drug delivery in cancer. *Current Pharmaceutical Design*, *10*(*24*), 2981–2989.
48. Faraji, A.H., Wipf, P. (2009). Nanoparticles in cellular drug delivery. *Bioorganic & Medicinal Chemistry*, *17*(*8*), 2950–2962.
49. Cho, K., et al. (2008). Therapeutic nanoparticles for drug delivery in cancer. *Clinical Cancer Research*, *14*(*5*), 1310–1316.
50. Schwartzberg, L.S., et al. (2011). Phase II multicenter trial of albumin-bound paclitaxel and capecitabine in first-line treatment of patients with metastatic breast cancer. *Clinical Breast Cancer*.
51. Demeure, M.J., et al. (2012). Preclinical investigation of nanoparticle albumin-bound paclitaxel as a potential treatment for adrenocortical cancer. *Annals of Surgery*, *255*(*1*), 140–146.
52. Shukla, D., et al. (2011). Lipid-based oral multiparticulate formulations—advantages, technological advances and industrial applications. *Expert Opinion on Drug Delivery*, *8*(2), 207–224.
53. Muller, R.H., Mader, K., Gohla, S. (2000). Solid lipid nanoparticles (SLN) for controlled drug delivery—a review of the state of the art. *European Journal of Pharmaceutics and Biopharmaceutics*, *50*(*1*), 161–177.
54. Mehnert, W., Mader, K. (2001). Solid lipid nanoparticles: Production, characterization and applications. *Advanced Drug Delivery Reviews*, *47*(*2–3*), 165–196.
55. Agarwal, A., et al. (2008). Tumour and dendrimers: A review on drug delivery aspects. *Journal of Pharmacy and Pharmacology*, *60*(*6*), 671–688.
56. Paleos, C.M., et al. (2010). Drug delivery using multifunctional dendrimers and hyperbranched polymers. *Expert Opinion on Drug Delivery*, *7*(*12*), 1387–1398.
57. Mullen, D.G., et al. (2011). Design, synthesis, and biological functionality of a dendrimer-based modular drug delivery platform. *Bioconjugate Chemistry*, *22*(*4*), 679–689.
58. Menjoge, A.R., Kannan, R.M., Tomalia, D.A. (2010). Dendrimer-based drug and imaging conjugates: Design considerations for nanomedical applications. *Drug Discovery Today*, *15*(*5–6*), 171–185.
59. Agarwal, A., et al. (2008). Tumour and dendrimers: A review on drug delivery aspects. *Journal of Pharmacy and Pharmacology*, *60*(*6*), 671–688.
60. Mahato, R., Tai, W., Cheng, K. (2011). Prodrugs for improving tumor targetability and efficiency. *Advanced Drug Delivery Reviews*, *63*(*8*), 659–670.
61. D'Souza, A.J., Topp, E.M. (2004). Release from polymeric prodrugs: Linkages and their degradation. *Journal of Pharmaceutical Sciences*, *93*(*8*), 1962–1979.
62. Tai, W., et al. (2011). Development of a peptide-drug conjugate for prostate cancer therapy. *Molecular Pharmaceutics*, *8*(*3*), 901–912.
63. Batrakova, E.V., Gendelman, H.E., Kabanov, A.V. (2011). Cell-mediated drug delivery. *Expert Opinion on Drug Delivery*, *8*(*4*), 415–433.
64. Kelly, C., Jefferies, C., Cryan, S.A. (2011). Targeted liposomal drug delivery to monocytes and macrophages. *Journal of Drug Delivery*, *2011*, 727241.
65. Jain, S., et al. (2003). RGD-anchored magnetic liposomes for monocytes/neutrophils-mediated brain targeting. *International Journal of Pharmaceutics*, *261*(*1–2*), 43–55.
66. Lee, K.D., Hong, K., Papahadjopoulos, D. (1992). Recognition of liposomes by cells: In vitro binding and

endocytosis mediated by specific lipid headgroups and surface charge density. *Biochimica et Biophysica Acta, 1103(2)*, 185–197.

67. Miller, C.R., et al. (1998). Liposome-cell interactions in vitro: Effect of liposome surface charge on the binding and endocytosis of conventional and sterically stabilized liposomes. *Biochemistry, 37(37)*, 12875–12883.
68. Aderem, A., Underhill, D.M. (1999). Mechanisms of phagocytosis in macrophages. *Annual Review of Immunology, 17*, 593–623.
69. Batrakova, E.V., et al. (2007). A macrophage-nanozyme delivery system for Parkinson's disease. *Bioconjugate Chemistry, 18(5)*, 1498–1506.
70. Doshi, N., et al. (2011). Cell-based drug delivery devices using phagocytosis-resistant backpacks. *Advanced Materials, 23(12)*, H105–H109.
71. Balmayor, E.R., Azevedo, H.S., Reis, R.L. (2011). Controlled delivery systems: From pharmaceuticals to cells and genes. *Pharmaceutical Research, 28(6)*, 1241–1258.
72. Murua, A., et al. (2008). Cell microencapsulation technology: Towards clinical application. *Journal of Controlled Release, 132(2)*, 76–83.
73. Manjappa, A.S., et al. (2011). Antibody derivatization and conjugation strategies: Application in preparation of stealth immunoliposome to target chemotherapeutics to tumor. *Journal of Controlled Release, 150(1)*, 2–22.
74. Garnett, M.C. (2001). Targeted drug conjugates: Principles and progress. *Advanced Drug Delivery Review, 53(2)*, 171–216.
75. Vyas, S.P., Singh, A., Sihorkar, V. (2001). Ligand-receptor-mediated drug delivery: An emerging paradigm in cellular drug targeting. *Critical Reviews in Therapeutic Drug Carrier Systems, 18(1)*, 1–76.
76. Webb, S. (2011). Pharma interest surges in antibody drug conjugates. *Nature Biotechnology, 29(4)*, 297–298.
77. Kratz, F., Abu Ajaj, K., Warnecke, A. (2007). Anticancer carrier-linked prodrugs in clinical trials. *Expert Opinion on Investigational Drugs, 16(7)*, 1037–1058.
78. Hauser, P.V., et al. (2010). Novel siRNA delivery system to target podocytes in vivo. *PLoS One, 5(3)*, e9463.
79. Medina, L.A., et al. (2004). Avidin/biotin-liposome system injected in the pleural space for drug delivery to mediastinal lymph nodes. *Journal of Pharmaceutical Sciences, 93(10)*, 2595–2608.
80. Schnyder, A., et al. (2004). Targeting of skeletal muscle in vitro using biotinylated immunoliposomes. *Biochemical Journal, 377(Pt 1)*, 61–67.
81. Ellington, A.D. Szostak, J.W. (1990). In vitro selection of RNA molecules that bind specific ligands. *Nature, 346(6287)*, 818–822.
82. Pan, W., Clawson, G.A. (2009). The shorter the better: Reducing fixed primer regions of oligonucleotide libraries for aptamer selection. *Molecules, 14(4)*, 1353–1369.
83. Keefe, A.D., Pai, S., Ellington, A. (2010). Aptamers as therapeutics. *Nature Reviews Drug Discovery, 9(7)*, 537–550.
84. Esposito, C.L., et al. (2011). New insight into clinical development of nucleic acid aptamers. *Discovery Medicine, 11(61)*, 487–496.
85. Dhar, S., et al. (2008). Targeted delivery of cisplatin to prostate cancer cells by aptamer functionalized Pt(IV) prodrug-PLGA-PEG nanoparticles. *Proceedings of the National Academy of Sciences of the United States of America, 105 (45)*, 17356–17361.
86. Chu, T.C., et al. (2006). Aptamer mediated siRNA delivery. *Nucleic Acids Research, 34(10)*, e73.
87. McNamara, J.O.2nd, et al. (2006). Cell type-specific delivery of siRNAs with aptamer-siRNA chimeras. *Nature Biotechnology, 24(8)*, 1005–1015.
88. Zhou, J., et al. (2008). Novel dual inhibitory function aptamer-siRNA delivery system for HIV-1 therapy. *Molecular Therapy, 16(8)*, 1481–1489.
89. Li, N., et al. (2010). Directed evolution of gold nanoparticle delivery to cells. *Chemical Communications (Cambridge), 46(3)*, 392–394.
90. Crombez, L., et al. (2008). Peptide-based nanoparticle for ex vivo and in vivo drug delivery. *Current Pharmaceutical Design, 14(34)*, 3656–3665.
91. Vives, E., Schmidt, J., Pelegrin, A. (2008). Cell-penetrating and cell-targeting peptides in drug delivery. *Biochimica et Biophysica Acta, 1786(2)*, 126–138.
92. Rothbard, J.B., et al. (2002). Arginine-rich molecular transporters for drug delivery: Role of backbone spacing in cellular uptake. *Journal of Medicinal Chemistry, 45(17)*, 3612–3618.
93. Majumdar, S., Siahaan, T.J. (2010). Peptide-mediated targeted drug delivery. *Medicinal Research Reviews, 32(3)*, 637–658.
94. Qin, B., et al. (2011). Identification of a LNCaP-specific binding peptide using phage display. *Pharmaceutical Research, 28*, 2422–2434.
95. Tai, W., et al. (2011). Development of a peptide-drug conjugate for prostate cancer therapy. *Molecular Pharmacology, 8 (3)*, 901–912.
96. Panyam, J., Labhasetwar, V. (2004). Targeting intracellular targets. *Current Drug Delivery, 1(3)*, 235–247.
97. Scianimanico, S., et al. (1999). Impaired recruitment of the small GTPase rab7 correlates with the inhibition of phagosome maturation by Leishmania donovani promastigotes. *Cellular Microbiology, 1(1)*, 19–32.
98. Pinto-Alphandary, H., et al. (1994). Intracellular visualization of ampicillin-loaded nanoparticles in peritoneal macrophages infected in vitro with Salmonella typhimurium. *Pharmaceutical Research, 11(1)*, 38–46.
99. Dworetzky, S.I., Lanford, R.E., Feldherr, C.M. (1988). The effects of variations in the number and sequence of targeting signals on nuclear uptake. *Journal of Cell Biology, 107(4)*, 1279–1287.
100. Yoneda, Y. (1997). How proteins are transported from cytoplasm to the nucleus. *Journal of Biochemistry, 121(5)*, 811–817.

101. Jans, D.A., Hubner, S. (1996). Regulation of protein transport to the nucleus: Central role of phosphorylation. *Physiological Reviews*, *76*(*3*), 651–685.

102. Zanta, M.A., Belguise-Valladier, P., Behr, J.P. (1999). Gene delivery: A single nuclear localization signal peptide is sufficient to carry DNA to the cell nucleus. *Proceedings of the National Academy of Sciences of the United States of America*, *96*(*1*), 91–96.

103. Wallace, D.C. (1999). Mitochondrial diseases in man and mouse. *Science*, *283*(*5407*), 1482–1488.

104. Halestrap, A.P., et al. (1998). Elucidating the molecular mechanism of the permeability transition pore and its role in reperfusion injury of the heart. *Biochimica et Biophysica Acta*, *1366*(*1–2*), 79–94.

105. Fulda, S., Galluzzi, L., Kroemer, G. (2010). Targeting mitochondria for cancer therapy. *Nature Reviews Drug Discovery*, *9*(*6*), 447–464.

106. Teicher, B.A., Holden, S.A., Cathcart, K.N. (1987). Efficacy of Pt(Rh-123)2 as a radiosensitizer with fractionated X rays. *International Journal of Radiation Oncology*Biology* Physics*, *13*(*8*), 1217–1224.

107. Murphy, M.P. (1997). Selective targeting of bioactive compounds to mitochondria. *Trends in Biotechnology*, *15*(*8*), 326–330.

108. Don, A.S., et al. (2003). A peptide trivalent arsenical inhibits tumor angiogenesis by perturbing mitochondrial function in angiogenic endothelial cells. *Cancer Cell*, *3*(*5*), 497–509.

6

PRODRUG AND BIOCONJUGATION

RAMYA KRISHNA VADLAPATLA, SUJAY SHAH, ASWANI DUTT VADLAPUDI, AND ASHIM K. MITRA

6.1 CHAPTER OBJECTIVES

- To outline the fundamental concepts, rationale, and principles for prodrug design.
- To list the functional groups amenable for prodrug design.
- To explain the major objectives that can be achieved by prodrugs.
- To demonstrate the utility of prodrugs for ocular, dermal, and brain drug delivery as well as the formulation approaches for prodrug delivery.

6.2 INTRODUCTION AND RATIONALE

The term "prodrug" or "promoiety" or "proagent" was first introduced by Adrien Albert in 1958 [1]. Prodrugs are bioreversible derivatives of drug molecules that undergo *in vivo* transformation to release an active parent molecule, which then elicits a desired pharmacological effect. Prodrugs are designed to overcome the physicochemical, biopharmaceutical, or pharmacokinetic barriers of a drug molecule through chemical modifications. In most cases, these prodrugs are simple chemical derivatives and require one or two chemical or enzymatic transformations to release the drug molecule [2]. Sometimes, prodrugs also undergo molecular modifications such as oxidation or reduction to release the active moiety. These are specially referred to as "bioprecursor prodrugs." The prodrug approach in drug discovery is increasing exponentially, representing almost 33% of new small-molecular-weight drugs approved in 2008 [3].

The schematic representation of a prodrug approach is depicted in Figure 6.1. Prodrugs provide a rationale to optimize the "drug-like properties" of a molecule. The fundamental properties associated with drug bioavailability are solubility and permeability. Based on these parameters, drugs are classified into four classes, and this classification scheme is referred to as the biopharmaceutics classification system (BCS) (Figure 6.2). Class I represents high-solubility–high-permeability drugs, class II represents low-solubility–high-permeability drugs, class III represents high-solubility–low-permeability drugs, and class IV represents low-solubility–low-permeability drugs [4]. Prodrugs were successfully being developed to overcome 1) poor aqueous solubility (BCS class II and IV drugs), 2) poor membrane permeation across various biological tissues (BCS class III and IV drugs), 3) rapid presystemic metabolism, and 4) toxicity and local irritation.

6.3 FUNCTIONAL GROUPS FOR PRODRUG DESIGN

The design of a safer and better prodrug depends on the promoiety and functional group of the drug molecule.

Advanced Drug Delivery, First Edition. Edited by Ashim K. Mitra, Chi H. Lee, and Kun Cheng.

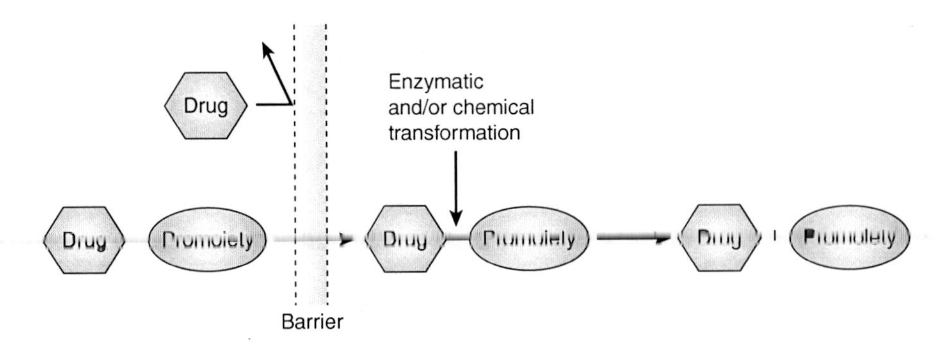

FIGURE 6.1 A simplified illustration of the prodrug concept. Reproduced with permission from Ref. 2.

The promoiety should not have any toxic effects and be eliminated rapidly from the body. The most commonly used functional groups amenable for drug modification include carboxyl, hydroxyl, amine, phosphate, and carbonyl groups. These groups are modified into either simple esters, phosphate esters, carbonates, carbamates, amides, ethers, imines, or oximes (Figure 6.3).

6.3.1 Ester Prodrugs

The presence of a carboxylic or hydroxyl group on a parent moiety often plays an important role in determining the activity by binding to an active site via ionic or hydrogen bonding. However, at physiological pH, these groups are ionizable and pose difficulty in permeating the biological membranes. Hence, ester prodrugs are commonly used to increase the lipophilicity by masking the groups available for hydrogen bonding such as carboxylic acids and phosphates [5]. Esters are the most commonly used prodrugs, accounting for almost 50% of total marketed prodrugs [6]. They are widely preferred as they are easy to synthesize, can be formed from either acids or alcohols, and are hydrolyzed back very easily [7]. The most important enzymes involved in hydrolysis of ester-based prodrugs are carboxylesterase, acetylcholinesterase, butyrylcholinesterase, paraoxonase, and arylesterase [8]. However, the type and amount of esterases present vary from one species to another, making it difficult to predict bioconversion in humans based on animal data [9]. Even within the same species, bioconversion by esterases is affected by age, gender, and diseases, thus, making it more difficult for pharmacokinetic prediction of esterase activity [10–12].

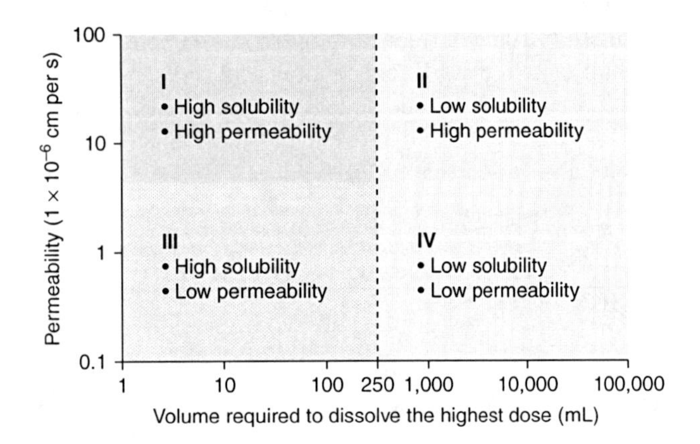

FIGURE 6.2 BCS classification of drug molecules. Reproduced with permission from Ref. 2.

Despite the associated challenges, several ester prodrugs have been developed successfully. Ampicillin is a β-lactam antibiotic used for the treatment of various bacterial infections. The ester prodrugs pivampicillin (pivaloyloxy methyl ester) and bacampicillin (ethoxy carbonyl oxyethyl ester) were superior in terms of bioavailability and absorption rates in both humans and horses [13–15]. The mean plasma-level concentration of ampicillin was higher in both ester forms compared with the drug alone. The bioavailability of these ester prodrugs pivampicillin (92 ± 18%) and bacampicillin (86 ± 11%) was significantly greater than the parent moiety ampicillin (62 ± 17%).

6.3.2 Phosphate Prodrugs

Phosphate prodrugs are used mainly to increase the solubility of a poorly water-soluble drug with hydroxyl and amine functionalities. BCS Class II drugs are considered ideal candidates for phosphate prodrugs [16]. These prodrugs will be biotransformed by alkaline phosphatases abundant at mucosal membrane of the enterocytes and liver [17]. Phosphate prodrugs were shown to be hydrolyzed at the same rates in different species, making it easier to predict pharmacokinetic disposition in humans from animal data [18]. Fosphenytoin, a phosphate ester prodrug of antiepileptic drug phenytoin, is conjugated to the drug via an oxymethylene spacer. This prodrug demonstrated increased solubility (7000 times) compared with the parent drug. Unlike phenytoin, it can be given in more favorable standard IV solution [19, 20]. But increased phosphate concentration at the site of administration may lead to paresthesias and pruritus [21]. Similarly, a phosphate ester prodrug of

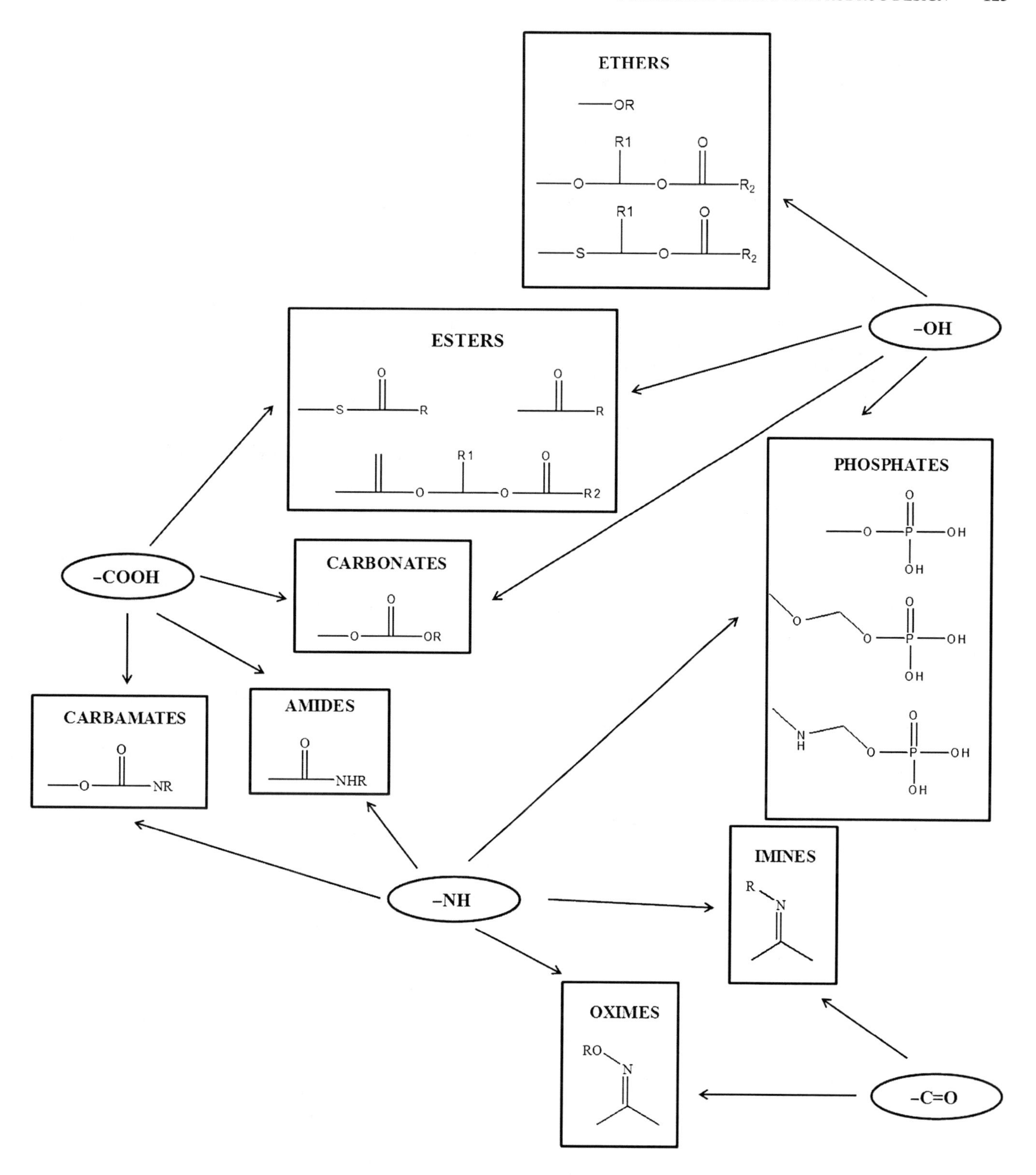

FIGURE 6.3 Common functional groups amenable to prodrug design.

prednisolone has also been developed by conjugating the phosphate moiety directly to the hydroxyl group of the drug. This prodrug enhanced solubility by 30 times, which facilitated the development of an oral liquid formulation [22].

6.3.3 Carbamate and Carbonate Prodrugs

The presence of a nitrogen atom adjacent to the carbonyl group makes the carbamate prodrug unique from esters. These prodrugs are also biotransformed *in vivo* by carboxylesterases and yet are more stable than ester prodrugs [23]. Gabapentin is a structural analog of gamma hydroxyl butyric acid (GABA) indicated in the treatment of epilepsy and neuropathic pain [24–26]. Its corresponding carbamate prodrug (XP13512) showed improved bioavailability and absorption, as well as decreased dose frequency [27, 28]. Since its FDA approval in 1996, irinotecan has been the first-line therapy indicated in the treatment of several cancers such as colorectal, gastrointestinal, small-cell, and non-small-cell lung cancers. This carbamate prodrug exhibited improved solubility with respect to its parent drug, 7-Ethyl-10-hydroxycamptothecin [29, 30]. The carbonate functional group is highly sensitive to hydrolysis, and therefore, it is unstable in biological media. Such poor stability hinders the design of carbonate prodrugs. However, research has been conducted to overcome this instability issue. A series of carbonate prodrugs of zidovudine have been synthesized and evaluated for *in vitro* anti-HIV activity in infected T-cells (MT-4s) and peripheral blood mononuclear cells (PBMCs). A carbonate prodrug bearing a 5′-yl *O*-(4-hydroxybutyl) side chain was found to be 50 and 30 times more potent than the drug itself in both the cells tested. Also, this carbonate prodrug demonstrated an enhanced half-life probably resulting from the formation of a cyclic structure by intramolecular rearrangement [31–33].

6.3.4 Amide Prodrugs

Amide prodrugs are derivatives of carboxylic acids and amines. These prodrugs are more stable than corresponding esters and carbamates. They are hydrolyzed by peptidases or proteases [23, 34]. Their high enzymatic stability *in vivo* accounts for their limited usage. Small peptides constitute an alternative way of derivatizing amide prodrugs. These prodrugs act as substrates of specific transporters and thus enhance absorption [34, 35]. For example, midodrine is an glycyl amide prodrug of 1-(2,5-dimethoxyphenyl)-2-aminoethanol (DMAE), an antihypotensive drug. This prodrug targeting the peptide transporter-1 (PEPT1) increased the bioavailability to almost 97% [36].

6.3.5 Oxime Prodrugs

Besides these commonly used derivatives, prodrugs are also designed for moieties that do not contain hydroxyl, carboxyl, or amine groups. These include derivatization of drugs into oximes such as ketoximes, amidoximes, or gaunidoximes. Oxime prodrugs are highly bioavailable and are metabolized by cytochrome P450 enzymes to release the active drug molecule [37–39]. Ximelagatran is a novel double prodrug developed by AstraZeneca (London, U.K.) [40]. The parent drug, melagatran, is a thrombin inhibitor demonstrating excellent competitive inhibition of human α-thrombin. This molecule contains a strongly basic benzamidine group and an acidic carboxylic group that protonates at intestinal and physiological pH, respectively. The net effect is poor and variable bioavailability of only 3–7%. Ximelagatran protects both functional groups and demonstrates significant improvement in bioavailability (about 20%) [41, 42].

All of the above prodrugs, their functional group modifications, and advantages are summarized in Table 6.1.

6.4 MAJOR OBJECTIVES OF PRODRUG DESIGN

Prodrugs are designed mainly to increase the utility of pharmacologically active molecules by modulating their physicochemical characteristics to optimize ADMET (absorption, distribution, metabolism, excretion, and toxicity) properties. An ideal prodrug should not elicit any pharmacological activity, but it should exhibit high aqueous solubility and chemical stability across a wide pH range. Furthermore, it should also demonstrate good transcellular absorption and rapid enzymatic cleavage to yield the parent moiety. The ultimate rationale for prodrug design is to increase the bioavailability of a drug and site-specific-targeted drug delivery.

6.4.1 Increased Bioavailability

The factors limiting bioavailability include aqueous solubility, passive intestinal absorption, and rapid metabolism.

6.4.1.1 Increased Solubility The aqueous solubility of a molecule depends on two factors: the intramolecular forces in the solid state and the intermolecular forces between the drug molecule and the surrounding fluid. The solubility will be poor if the molecules energetically favor to bind to each other than to the water molecules. Solubility limitations are frequently encountered in the development of new drugs using combinatorial chemistry and high-throughput screening. Almost 40% of new drug molecules designed have a solubility of less than 10 μM. A wide variety of formulation strategies have been developed for successful drug delivery overcoming the solubility limitations. This includes the formation of stable salts and the use of surfactants, co-solvents, solubilizing agents, or complexing agents [43–45]. Despite the availability of many formulation strategies, the design of soluble prodrugs has been widely established in the pharmaceutical industry to improve the aqueous solubility. This design includes derivatization of a drug molecule using either a neutral

TABLE 6.1 Examples of Prodrugs with Specific Functional Group Modification and Their Advantages

Drug	Prodrug and Its Structure	Advantage	References
Ampicillin	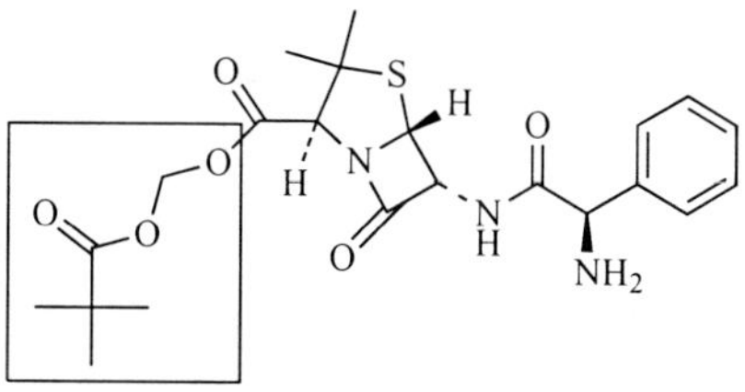 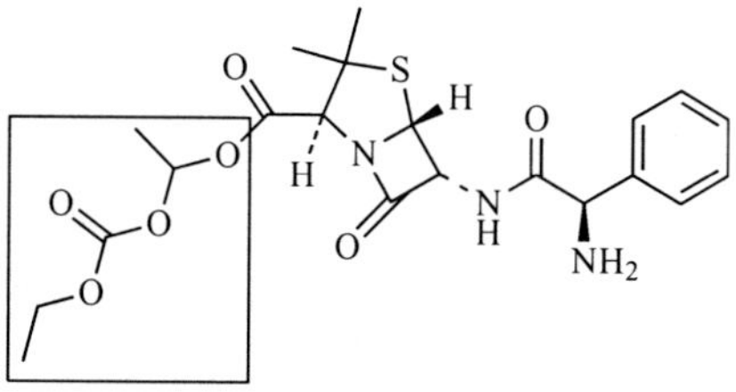 Pivaloyloxymethyl ester prodrug (pivampicillin)	Bioavailability of these prodrugs pivampicillin (92 ± 18%) and bacampicillin (86 ± 11%) was significantly greater than the parent moiety ampicillin (62 ± 17%)	[14]
	Ethoxy carbonyl oxyethyl ester prodrug (bacampicillin)		
Phenytoin	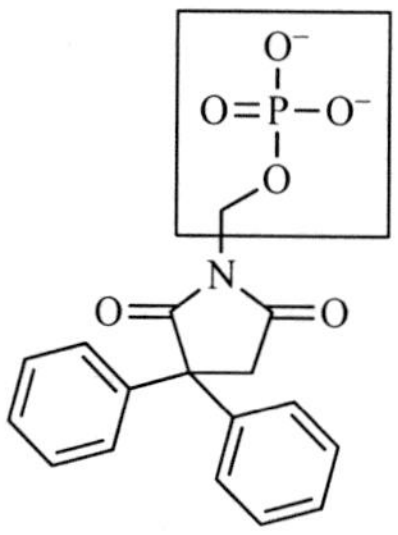 Phosphate prodrug (fosphenytoin)	Solubility increased from 20.5 μg/mL to 75,000 μg/mL	[19, 20]
7-Ethyl-10-hydroxy-camptothecin	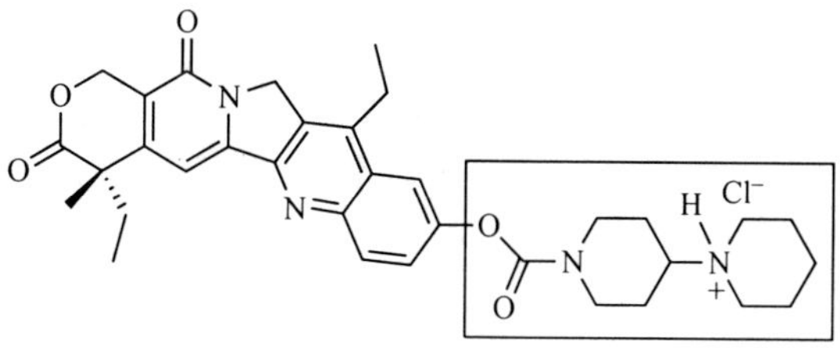 Dipiperidino carbamate prodrug (Irinotecan)	Solubility increased from 2–3 μg/mL to 20 mg/mL	[29, 30]
Zidovudine	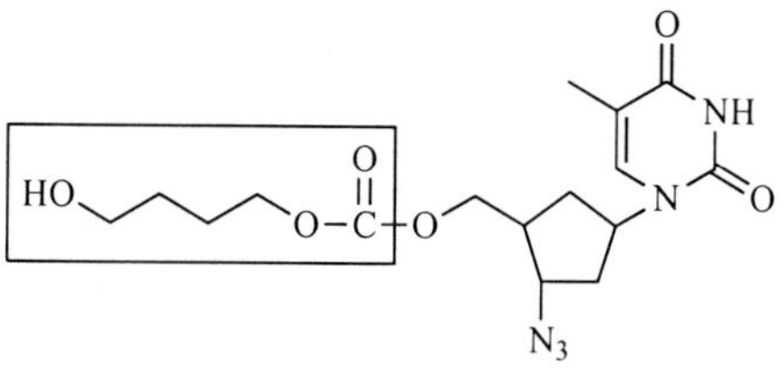 5′-yl *O*-(4-hydroxybutyl) carbonate prodrug	Fifty and thirty times more potent than the drug itself in HIV-infected T-cells (MT-4s) and mononuclear cells (PBMCs), respectively	[31–33]

(*continued*)

TABLE 6.1 (*Continued*)

Drug	Prodrug and Its Structure	Advantage	References
DMAE	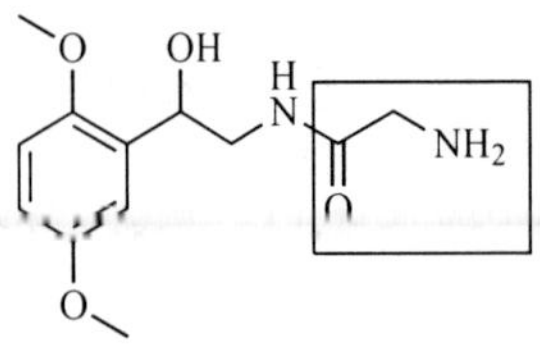 Glycyl amide prodrug (midodrine)	Oral bioavailability improved from 50% (DMAE) to 93% (midodrine)	[36]
Melagatran	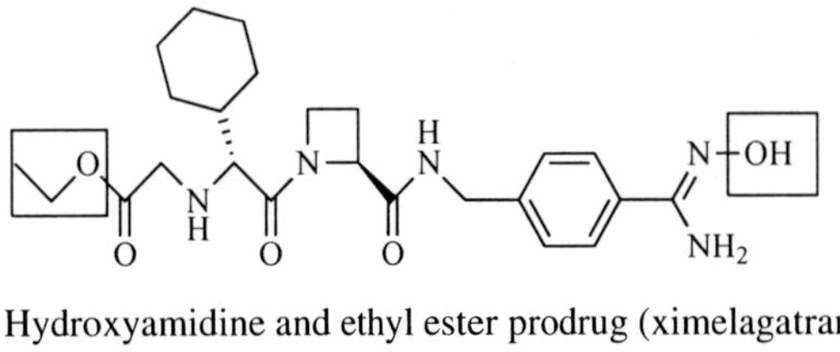 Hydroxyamidine and ethyl ester prodrug (ximelagatran)	Oral bioavailability of melagatran (3–7%) was enhanced by threefold (20%)	[41, 42]

(polyethylene glycol [PEG]) or a charged (phosphate or succinate esters) promoiety.

PEG is a polyether synthesized by anionic polymerization of ethylene oxide. PEG derivatization has been successful for many hydrophobic molecules to impart greater aqueous solubility. PEG is relatively nontoxic, and its hepatic and renal clearance makes it ideal to use in drug delivery applications. Furthermore, it has been approved by FDA for pharmaceutical applications. PEG of higher molecular weight (>2 kDa) should be considered to prevent rapid clearance. Paclitaxel is a potent chemotherapeutic agent used in the treatment of ovarian and breast cancers. Because of its poor aqueous solubility (25 μg/mL), it is administered in a 1:1 concentrate of ethanol and cremophore. A series of 2′-PEG esters with different molecular weights have been designed to increase its solubility. PEG_{40000}-paclitaxel exhibited improved solubility up to 125 mg/mL, rendering it more favorable for intravenous (IV) administration [46]. Similarly, a phosphate ester prodrug has been designed for the HIV protease inhibitor, amprenavir. The poor aqueous solubility (0.04 mg/mL) of the drug rendered it to be administered in the form of soft gelatin capsules, eight times a day. Such a high-dosage regimen often causes patient incompliance. Hence, the drug has been replaced with its highly water-soluble (>0.3 mg/mL) phosphate prodrug, fosamprenavir. This prodrug is delivered as a tablet twice a day, thus, lowering the pill burden and improving patient compliance. In the intestinal epithelium, the charged prodrug is converted rapidly back to the parent drug by the alkaline phosphatases present on the brush border of the enterocytes, which then enters the systemic circulation [47–49].

6.4.1.2 Increased Permeability The most common route of absorption for many drug molecules is an unfacilitated and nonspecific passive transport mechanism. The drug molecule has to permeate through several lipid membranes to elicit its pharmacological action. Hence, the bioavailability of a drug can also be increased by improving the permeability across these biological membranes. The presence of polar functional groups on a molecule accounts for low lipophilicity. Prodrugs can be designed to mask these functional groups, with the aim of increasing membrane permeation. The hydrophilic moieties present on the drug molecule such as hydroxyl, carboxyl, phosphate, and thiol groups can be converted into more lipophilic esters [5]. These esters are then hydrolyzed by esterases to release the active moiety. Similarly, lipidization of a molecule can also increase membrane permeation [50]. In both approaches, increased lipophilicity must be balanced with optimal aqueous solubility to prevent absorption from being dissolution rate limited [6]. A nice example of the prodrug approach to increase permeability is observed in the case of neuraminidase glycoprotein inhibitors. These inhibitors are used in the treatment of influenza type A and type B viruses. The drug Ro 64-0802 is not absorbed because of its high hydrophilicity. The drug is therefore modified into an ethyl ester prodrug, oseltamivir. This prodrug is rapidly absorbed and provides increased plasma drug levels. Bioavailability of this ethyl ester prodrug has increased to 80% as compared with 5% of the free carboxylate form [51]. Likewise, lipidization of a molecule can also enhance the absorption of drug resulting in higher bioavailability [52]. Cidofovir is a potent nucleoside phosphonate antiviral drug. It has poor oral bioavailability. Recently, hexadecyloxypropyl esters of cidofovir have been synthesized. After oral administration, these lipid prodrugs are absorbed readily and converted intracellularly into the corresponding diphosphates. The prodrugs were shown to be more active in animal models of viral infection [53].

TABLE 6.2 Examples of Prodrugs Designed to Enhance the Bioavailability of Therapeutic Molecules

Drug	Prodrug and Its Structure	Advantage	References
	Increased solubility		
Amprenavir	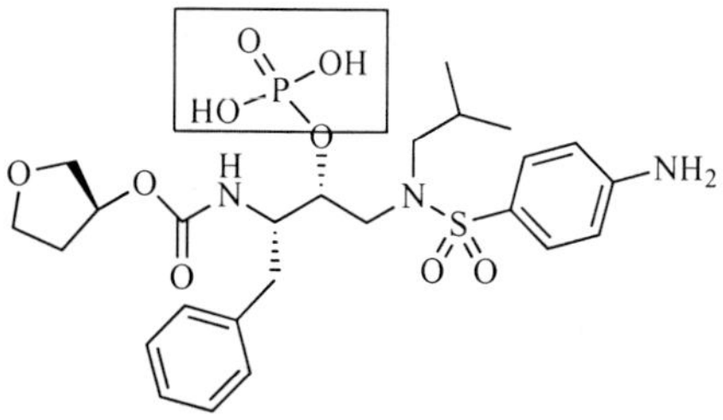 Fosamprenavir	The solubility of the prodrug increased by almost 10-fold from 0.04 mg/mL to >0.3 mg/mL	[47–49]
	Increased permeability		
GS4071/Ro 64-0802	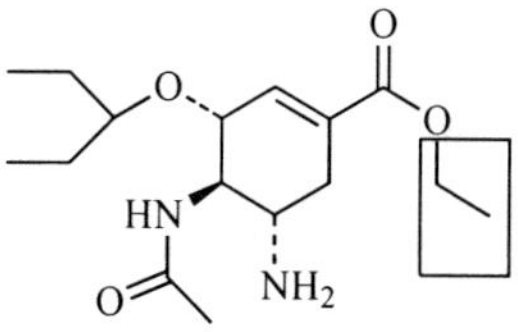 Oseltamivir	The bioavailability of the ester prodrug increased from 5% to 80%	[51]
	Increased half-life		
Terbutaline	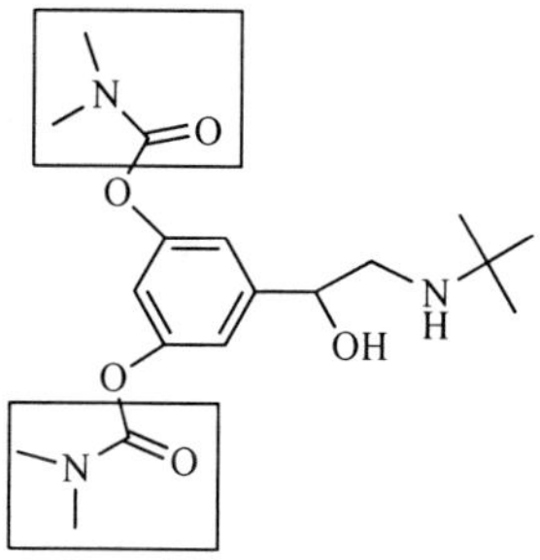 Bambuterol	The increased half-life rendered the dosage regimen to be lowered from thrice a day to once a day	[54, 55]

6.4.1.3 Increased Duration of Action First-pass metabolism greatly reduces the total amount of drug reaching the systemic circulation and thus the bioavailability. Although this problem has been surpassed by the use of sublingual or buccal administration, the use of a prodrug approach has also been prominent. Prodrugs mask the metabolically labile groups to avoid rapid metabolism, hence, prolonging the duration of action of the active moiety. Terbutaline is a bronchodilator and a β_2-agonist. The phenolic groups present on the molecule are susceptible to rapid and extensive presystemic metabolism, rendering it to be administered thrice a day. The respective bisdimethyl carbamate prodrug bambuterol masks the phenolic moieties. This prodrug is biotransformed slowly by butyrylcholinesterases to release the active moiety. As a result of this approach, it is administered once a day with a lower incidence of adverse effects [54, 55]. Another example to increase the duration of therapeutic molecules is by conjugation to macromolecules such as polymers. These macromolecular prodrugs offer increased metabolic stability, prolonged half-life, controlled degradation, and enhanced cellular uptake [56, 57]. Peptide and protein drugs are degraded rapidly by proteolytic enzymes, thus, demonstrating a very short half-life. PEGylation (addition of PEG chains) can overcome the disadvantages associated with peptide and protein therapeutics. The increase in the molecular weight shields them from rapid clearance and degradation, thus, improving their half-life [58]. A 40-kDa branched PEG was conjugated to interferon (IFN)-α2a. This conjugate reduced renal clearance and prolonged half-life from 9 to 77 h. Subsequently, peginterferon-α2a given once a week is more efficient than IFN-α2a given thrice a week in patients with chronic hepatitis C [59].

All the above prodrugs designed to enhance bioavailability are summarized in Table 6.2.

6.4.2 Site-Specific Drug Delivery

The ultimate goal in drug delivery is to deliver the drug at the target site without any adverse reactions. This targeted approach is considered the most exciting accomplishment prodrugs can offer. The selectivity can be accomplished by targeting specific transporters/receptors, antigens, and enzymes. Recent advances in the field of molecular biology allowed researchers to understand more clearly the functional and structural characteristics of various proteins that can be used for drug targeting.

6.4.2.1 Targeting Specific Transporters/Receptors The most important biochemical barrier to the absorption of drugs is the presence of efflux transporters. These efflux transporters secrete drugs back into the lumen, thus, lowering their intracellular concentration. Efflux proteins like P-glycoprotein (P-gp), multidrug resistance protein (MRP), and breast cancer-resistant protein (BCRP) are expressed on the apical surface of intestine and many other tissues. These efflux proteins can act either alone or in a synergistic way to lower the intracellular accumulation of drugs [60–63]. Targeting specific transporters/receptors is the most promising drug delivery strategy. Certain moieties such as amino acids (valine, serine, and leucine), vitamins (biotin, riboflavin, ascorbic acid, and folic acid), monocarboxylic acid-containing moieities (lactic acid and pyruvic acid), and glucose are transported by specific transporters or receptors. The localization of these transporter/receptors in various tissues has been well characterized, studied, and exploited to design prodrugs to treat various diseases. By chemical modification or coupling to a ligand for a known transporter, the parent drug can be transported efficiently. Such transporter-targeted prodrugs also increase the bioavailability, resulting in enhanced therapeutic activity [64–66]. During translocation across cell membranes, the transporter-targeted prodrug is not accessible to bind with efflux transporters. Hence, these site-specific prodrugs offer dual advantage by increasing the absorption and evading efflux proteins simultaneously. The important transporters that are used for drug delivery and examples of some targeted prodrugs are detailed next.

Peptide Transporters Peptide transporters are considered the most versatile transporting systems because of their high capacity and broad substrate specificity. So far, two peptide transporters belonging to the *SLC15A2* class of human genome have been identified: peptide transporter-1 (PEPT1) and peptide transporter-2 (PEPT2). These transporters facilitate the cellular translocation of dipeptides and tripeptides in addition to a wide variety of peptidomimetic molecules such as ACE inhibitors, rennin inhibitors, β-lactam antibiotics, and cephalosporins. The protons generated from the Na^+/H^+ exchanger serve as dynamic force for the absorption of peptides through these transporters. Several prodrugs have been designed to target these transporters, and their numbers are increasing exponentially [65, 67, 68]. Acyclovir (ACV) is a potent antiviral drug indicated in the treatment of the herpes simplex virus (HSV) and herpes zoster (shingles) infections. ACV suffers from limited aqueous solubility and low oral bioavailability (15–30%), resulting in poor accumulation at the target site. A series of amino acid prodrugs of ACV has been synthesized. Among these prodrugs, the L-valyl ester prodrug of ACV demonstrated increased bioavailability by three to fivefold. Such rise in bioavailability is caused by its increased absorption by PEPT1 following rapid hydrolysis back to the parent drug [69–73].

Similarly, prodrugs have been designed for saquinavir (SQV), the first HIV-1 protease inhibitor approved by the U.S. Food and Drug Administration (FDA). It has poor oral bioavailability (4–16%) because of its active efflux by P-gp and MRP2. Dipeptide ester prodrugs of SQV, valine-valine-saquinavir (Val-Val-SQV), and glycine-valine-saquinavir (Gly-Val-SQV) targeting intestinal peptide transporter have been synthesized. These prodrugs demonstrated improved intestinal absorption and bioavailability mediated by peptide transporter. SQV exhibited an efflux ratio of 40 and 7 in MDCK-MDR1 and MDCK-MRP2 cells, respectively. This ratio was decreased significantly to 5 and 2 by Val-Val-SQV and to 6 and 2 by Gly-Val-SQV in both MDCK-MDR1 and MDCK-MRP2 cells, respectively (Figures 6.4a and b). This decrease in efflux ratio has been attributed to increased absorptive flux and decreased secretory flux by the peptide prodrugs [74–76].

Amino Acid Transporters A plethora of amino acid transport systems widely expressed in all living mammalian cells. These systems differ markedly in their substrate specificity and transport mechanism. Because the amino acid requirement differs from cell to cell, the differential expression and activity of these transporters varies between cells. Amino acid transporters have been categorized into subtypes based on their sodium dependence, charge, and substrate specificity. System L and system y+ are sodium-independent systems. System L helps in transporting large neutral amino acids, whereas system y+ helps in translocation of cationic amino acids. Sodium-dependent amino acid transporters include system B, system $B^{0,+}$, IMINO, and β transporters. System B translocates all dipolar amino acids with an amino group in α position and system $B^{0,+}$ accepts all dipolar amino acids (including those with an amino group in α position) and basic amino acids. IMINO systems help in transporting amino acids with imino groups and β systems translocates β-amino acids [77–79]. A series of amino acid ester prodrugs of ACV including L-alanine-ACV (AACV), L-serine-ACV (SACV), L-isoleucine-ACV (IACV),

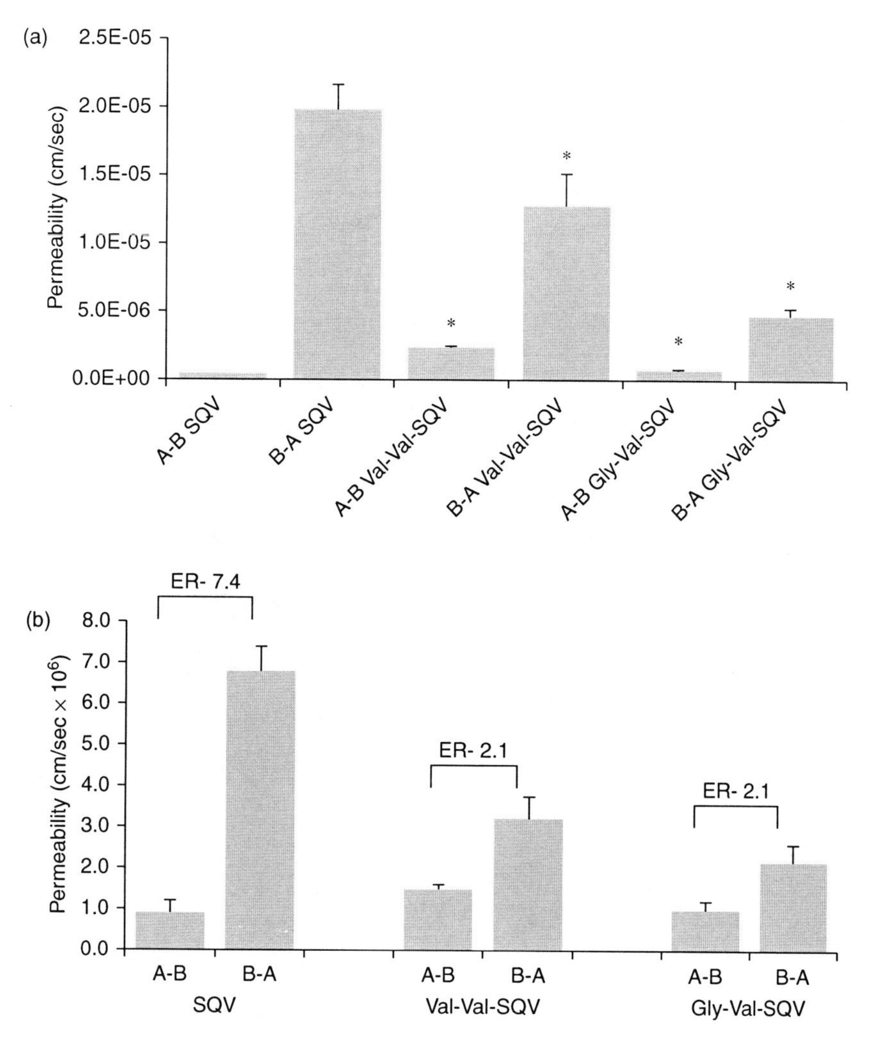

FIGURE 6.4 Apparent permeability of SQV, Val–Val–SQV, and Gly–Val–SQV in apical to basolateral direction (A—B) and basolateral to apical direction (B—A) across MDCK-MDR1 (a) and MDCK-MRP2 (b) cells. Reproduced with permission from Ref. 74 and 76.

γ-glutamate-ACV (EACV) and L-valine-ACV (VACV) have been synthesized. These structures have been depicted in Figure 6.5a. The pharmacokinetic parameters of these prodrugs after oral administration were evaluated in jugular vein cannulated rats. SACV demonstrated an approximately fivefold increase in area under the curve (AUC) values compared with parent moiety, ACV. This increase in the bioavailability of ACV was attributed to the interaction of these prodrugs with intestinal amino acid transporters. The maximum concentration (C_{max}) of ACV in plasma after administering SACV was observed to be 39 ± 2 μM, which is 15 times better than ACV. Furthermore, this C_{max} value was also found to be two times higher than obtained from administering VACV (Figure 6.5b). Results from this study clearly indicated that amino acid ester prodrug SACV seems to be a highly promising candidate for the oral treatment of HSV infections because of its enhanced stability, higher AUC, and better concentration of regenerated ACV than all the other prodrugs tested [80].

Vitamin Transporters The mechanism and regulation of absorption of several water soluble vitamins such as ascorbic acid, biotin, folate, riboflavin, thiamine, and pyridoxine has been significantly explored. These vitamins play a vital role in regulating normal metabolic functions, differentiation and growth of mammalian cells [81–83]. The transporters/receptors specialized in the absorption of these vitamins can be exploited for targeted drug delivery. Luo et al. have synthesized vitamin prodrugs of SQV targeting sodium-dependent vitamin C transporter (SVCT) and sodium-dependent multi vitamin transporter (SMVT) [84, 85]. These prodrugs caused significant evasion of P-gp mediated efflux and CYP3A4 mediated metabolism. Subsequent studies revealed that these nutrient-targeted prodrugs caused

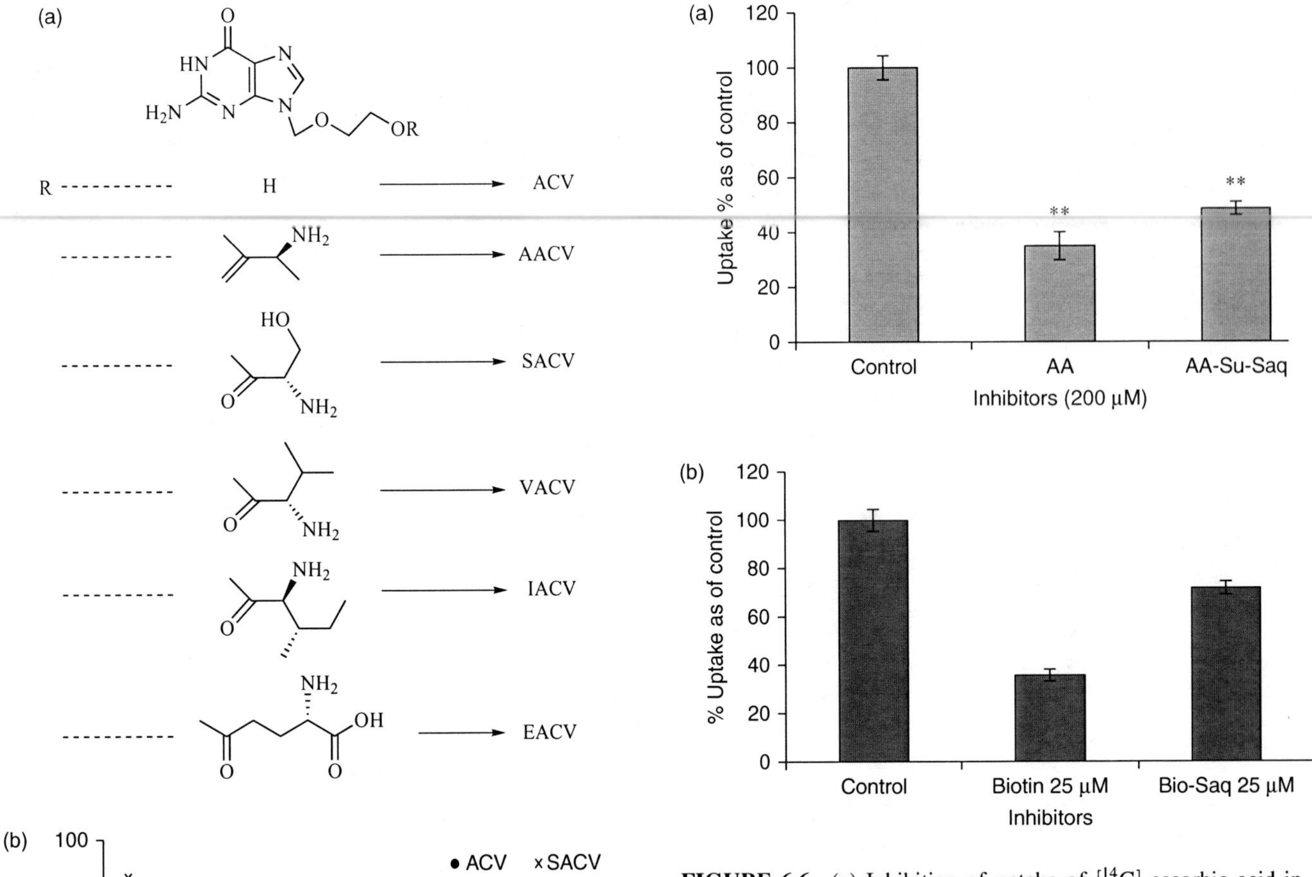

FIGURE 6.5 (a) Structures of amino acid ester prodrugs of acyclovir (ACV). (b) Plasma concentration vs time profile of total concentration of ACV upon oral administration of ACV, SACV, and VACV. Reproduced with permission from Ref. 80.

FIGURE 6.6 (a) Inhibition of uptake of [^{14}C] ascorbic acid in MDCK-MDR1 cells by ascorbic acid (AA) and ascorbate prodrug of SQV (AA-Su-Saq). Reproduced with permission from Ref. 84. (b) Inhibition of uptake of [^{3}H] biotin in MDCK-MDR1 cells by biotin and biotin prodrug of SQV (Bio-Saq). Reproduced with permission from Ref. 85.

significant inhibition in the uptake of ascorbic acid and biotin in MDCK-MDR1 cells suggesting that the prodrugs were translocated by SVCT and SMVT respectively (Figures 6.6a and b). The authors concluded that these prodrugs can be an attractive strategy to enhance the oral absorption and systemic bioavailability of HIV protease inhibitors.

6.4.2.2 Targeting Specific Antigens Targeting surface antigens is recently gaining importance as a highly promising strategy for selective tumor targeting. Because the tumor cells proliferate more rapidly than normal cells, certain enzymes are highly expressed on the surface of these cells, which can be used for targeted drug delivery. The development of monoclonal antibodies (mAbs) against a wide variety of antigens opened a new era for the development of antibody-drug conjugates (ADCs) [86, 87]. The essential components of ADCs are the mAb, a suitable linker, and a drug molecule. A suitable linker must be stable in circulation and cleavable inside the cells. Furthermore, the conjugation of linker must be carried out at mild conditions to avoid denaturation of mAb. The most frequently used linkers are acid labile, proteolytic, disulfide, and hydrolytic linkers. Among these linkers, the disulfide linker is often used in ADCs. This linker is cleaved in the cells by disulfide exchange with glutathione. The concentration of glutathione is 1000-fold higher inside the cells than in the serum and higher especially in the tumor cells when compared with

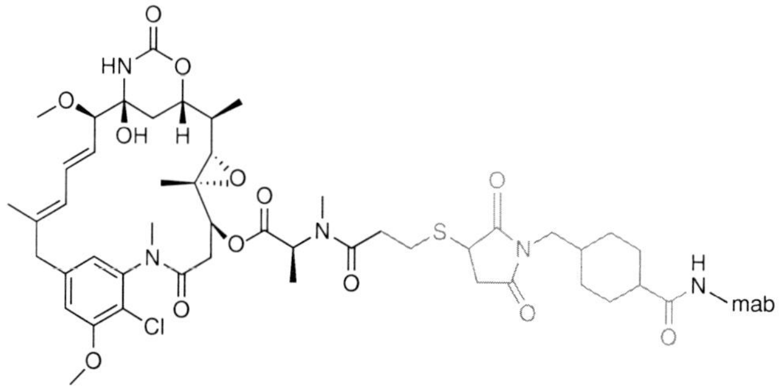

FIGURE 6.7 Structure of antibody-DM1 drug conjugate via SMCC linker. (See color figure in color plate section.)

normal cells [88–91]. Thus, the stability of a disulfide linker at physiological pH coupled with its selective degradation in tumor cells makes it a better choice in the use of ADCs. After administration, these ADCs bind specifically to the antigen and are internalized by receptor-mediated endocytosis. After internalization, an "early endosome" is formed, which then acidifies and gradually becomes "late endosome" and finally fuses to form a "lysosome." Depending on the linker used, various mechanisms occur to release the active moieties inside the cell.

To date, almost 13 ADCs are in clinical trials, with 3 of them in late-stage trials. Maytansine is a macrolide isolated from the plant *Maytenus ovatus* by Kupchan et al. [92, 93]. It inhibits tubulin assembly into microtubules, thus, preventing cell cycle progression. The molecule showed complete or partial response in patients with different types of cancer [94–97]. However, elevated toxic side effects hampered its direct usage in the treatment of cancer [98]. A series of derivatives of maytansine has been developed, out of which $N^{2'}$ -deacetyl-$N^{2'}$ -(3-mercapto-1-oxopropyl)-maytansine (DM1) has been most successful potent candidate [99]. This molecule has been conjugated to an anti-Her2 mAb, namely trastuzumab via a heterobifunctional succinimidyl 4-[*N*-maleimidomethyl] cyclohexane-1-carboxylate (SMCC) linker (Figure 6.7). This ADC (Trastuzumab-SMCC-DM1/ trastuzumab emtansine) is currently in phase III clinical trial for the treatment of metastatic breast cancer. This conjugate dosed at 3.6 mg/kg in a phase II trial, was well tolerated and demonstrated a 41% response rate among 80 patients [100].

6.5 PRODRUGS FOR IMPROVED TOPICAL ADMINISTRATION (OPHTHALMIC AND DERMAL)

Prodrugs have been employed primarily to improve physicochemical, biopharmaceutical, or pharmacokinetic properties of pharmacologically active ophthalmic drugs. Vadlapudi et al. designed a novel prodrug strategy that is more lipophilic and at the same time site specific to increase the cellular absorption of ACV. This study used a lipid raft that is conjugated to the parent drug (ACV) molecule to impart lipophilicity and a targeting moiety (biotin), which can be recognized by a specific transporter/receptor (SMVT) onto the other terminal of lipid raft. Lipophilic prodrugs readily diffuse across the cell membrane by facilitated diffusion whereas transporter/receptor targeted prodrugs translocate compounds across the cell membrane via active transport by transporter recognition. Marginal improvement in cellular uptake was evident from both these approaches. However, this novel approach combines both lipid and transporter/receptor targeted delivery to generate synergistic effect. Compared to ACV, the uptake of targeted lipid prodrugs (B-R-ACV and B-12HS-ACV) increased by ~14 and 13 times, respectively, whereas the uptake of B-ACV, R-ACV, and 12HS-ACV was higher by 4.5, 1.8, and 2 times respectively in human corneal epithelial cells (Figure 6.8). The targeted lipid prodrugs B-R-ACV and B-12HSACV exhibited much higher cellular accumulation than B-ACV, R-ACV, and 12HS-ACV. Both the targeted lipid prodrugs B-R-ACV and B-12HS-ACV demonstrated higher affinity toward SMVT than B-ACV. These exciting results suggested that the lipid raft facilitates enhanced interaction of prodrug with membrane transporters/receptors probably assisting docking of the targeted ligand into the binding domain of transporter/receptor protein. The net effect observed is rapid translocation of the cargo across cell membrane. This novel prodrug design also may allow for enhanced plasma membrane uptake of hydrophilic therapeutic agents such as genes, small interfering RNA, nucleosides, nucleotides, oligonucleotides or antisense oligonucleotides, peptides, and proteins [101].

Dermal administration of drugs holds a high level of interest in pharmaceutical research because it has several advantages over other conventional routes of drug delivery. For example, dermal drug delivery can provide higher concentrations of drug locally than those safely achievable with oral delivery. Unfortunately, most of the skin disorders requiring topical application of such protective/therapeutic medications are localized in the areas of high permeation flux, and in most cases, stratum corneum (SC) barrier resistance is decreased, allowing their easier permeation to attain plasma levels that could sometimes be sufficient to elicit adverse reactions [102]. Also, the dermal drug transport is limited greatly by the unsuitable physicochemical properties of most drugs and the efficient barrier function of the skin, and it is frequently insufficient for medical uses. It is a well-known fact that the barrier properties of skin are mediated by a series of lipid multilayers segregated within SC interstices, and their hydrophobic nature and tortuous, extracellular localization restrict the transport of most compounds across the SC. Therefore, various attempts of improving topical drug absorption

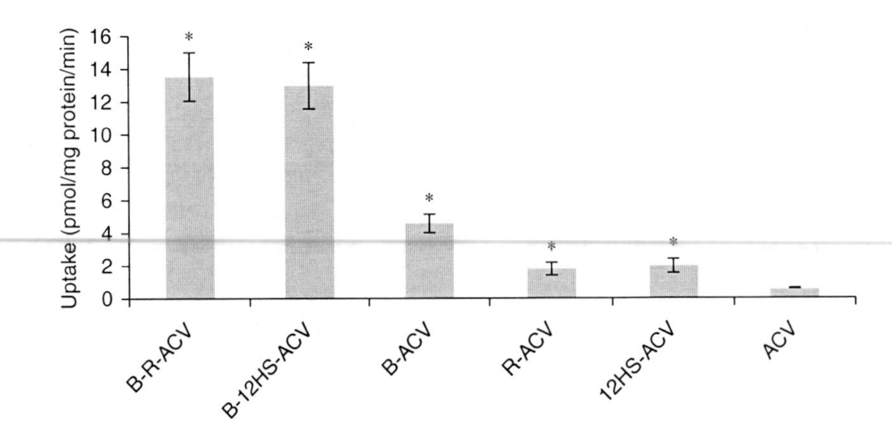

FIGURE 6.8 Cellular accumulation of targeted lipid prodrugs (B-R-ACV and B-12HS-ACV), targeted prodrug (B-ACV), and lipid prodrugs (R-ACV and 12HS-ACV) compared with parent moiety (ACV) on human corneal epithelial cells.

have been investigated, such as the prodrug approach with the aim of altering the pharmaceutical and pharmacokinetic characteristics of the parent drug and enhancing its ability to traverse the skin with high efficiency and also maintain its therapeutic effectiveness.

Naproxen is a nonsteroidal anti-inflammatory drug (NSAID) used widely in the treatment of rheumatoid arthritis and related painful diseases. However, it is poorly absorbed through the percutaneous tissues, and this limits the bioavailability to only 1–2%. Researchers used the prodrug approach to increase the dermal permeation of naproxen and various alkyl esters have been designed. However, the release of naproxen was very slow in both human serum and skin-serum homogenates. Later, Rautio et al. have synthesized acyloxyalkyl esters of naproxen that readily hydrolyzed to the parent drug yet demonstrated poor permeability. This may have been due to low aqueous solubilities of acyloxyalkyl ester prodrugs. This finding led the researchers to investigate aminoacyloxyalkyl ester (amino acids as promoiety) prodrugs of naproxen. The resulting naproxenoxyalkyl diesters of glutamic and aspartic acids showed higher aqueous solubilities and demonstrated a higher flux across the skin compared with naproxen [103].

6.6 PRODRUGS FOR IMPROVED DRUG DELIVERY TO THE BRAIN

Drug delivery to the central nervous system (CNS) has always been a challenging task for scientists. Tight junctions in the blood–brain barrier (BBB) prevent the easy translocation of drug molecules from blood to CNS tissues. Numerous approaches have been attempted to improve bioavailability of drugs for the treatment of diseases affecting the CNS. One of the most popular is the prodrug approach. As mentioned, naproxen is an NSAID, and it finds use as a neuroprotective agent for treatment of several neurodegenerative disorders. However, naproxen has limited brain bioavailability as well. Recently, researchers investigated dihydropyridine and ascorbic acid prodrugs of naproxen to target brain. A twofold increase in naproxen levels occurred with the prodrugs when compared with the drug alone. This increase in drug concentrations can be attributed to a specific carrier system in the brain and also to the reduced plasma protein binding of naproxen [104]. In another study, prodrugs of naproxen were synthesized using either an ester linkage or an amide bond using the dimethylamino moiety as a CNS targeting ligand. It was observed that the dimethyl amino prodrug was highly stable, and the prodrugs with ester bonds were partially hydrolyzed in alkaline media and brain homogenate. IV administration of these prodrugs showed a 15-fold to 30-fold increase in total naproxen concentration. Also, the ester prodrugs had a higher C_{max} than the amide prodrug in the brain [105].

Five ethanolamine-related prodrugs of dexibuprofen were synthesized and administered intravenously, and the brain and plasma concentrations of dexibuprofen were measured. The results showed that the C(brain)/C(plasma) ratios of prodrugs 1, 2, 3, 4, and 5 were 17.0-, 15.7-, 7.88-, 9.31-, and 3.42-fold higher than that of dexibuprofen, respectively. This proves that each of the prodrugs enhanced brain distribution significantly and can be used for efficient transport across the BBB [106].

6.7 FORMULATION APPROACHES FOR SUSTAINED AND CONTROLLED DELIVERY OF PRODRUGS

It is now apparent that prodrug approach is a suitable method for improving drug bioavailability to various tissues. However, in some cases, prodrugs are readily metabolized to their

TABLE 6.3 Some Examples of Prodrugs in Clinical Trials

Prodrug	Drug	Indication	Phase Status	Company
CDX-085	Astaxanthin	Cardiovascular	I	Cardax Pharmaceuticals, Honolulu, Hawaii
SF1126	LY294002	Chronic lymphocytic leukemia (CLL)	I	Semafore Pharmaceuticals, Croydon, U.K.
KP201	Hydrocodone	Pain management	I	KemPharm, Inc., North Liberty, IA
Prodrug of GLPG0187	GLPG0187	Metastasis in solid cancers	I	Galapagos NV, Mechelen, Belgium
TH-302	Bromoisophosphoramide mustard (Br-IPM)	Pancreatic cancer	II	Threshold Pharmaceuticals, South San Francisco, CA
E1224	Ravuconazole	Chagas disease	II	Eisai Co., Ltd., Woodcliff Lake, NJ
BMS-830216	BMS-819881	Obesity	I	Bristol-Myers Squibb, New York, NY
BMS-582664	BMS-540215	Advanced solid tumors	I	Bristol-Myers Squibb
AFP-464	Aminoflavone	Renal cell, breast, and lung cancer	II	Tigris Pharmaceuticals, Inc., Bonita Springs, FL
Tedizolid phosphate (TR-701)	Tedizolid (TR-700)	Gram-positive bacterial infections	I	Trius Therapeutics, Inc., San Diego, CA

parent compound and reduce the time for therapeutic action. Also, there is a need to prolong the duration of action of these prodrugs to administer small doses so as to minimize the side effects. To achieve these objectives formulation of prodrugs is very important. In the past, researchers have studied different formulations with various biocompatible materials to provide a controlled and sustained delivery for prodrugs.

Nalbuphine (NA) is a narcotic analgesic used in the treatment of acute and chronic pain. However, it has very poor oral bioavailability and short elimination half-life. Therefore, patients have to receive several injections, which leads to patient incompliance. It is understood that patient response and therapeutic effectiveness can be improved by maintaining NA blood concentrations. Yen et al. designed a series of NA prodrugs including nalbuphine propionate, nalbuphine pivalate, nalbuphine enanthate, and nalbuphine decanoate. These prodrugs were synthesized via esterification of nalbuphine with various carboxylic acids. Nalbuphine propionate was incorporated into poly(D,L-lactide-co-glycolide) (PLGA)-based microspheres and the *in vitro* and *in vivo* pharmacodynamics were studied. It was observed that PLGA microspheres prolonged the release of drug up to 96 h [107]. L-3,4-dihydroxyphenylalanine (L-DOPA) is used frequently for the treatment of Parkinson's disease. The maleic and fumaric diamide derivatives of (*O,O*-diacetyl)-L-Dopa-methylester [(+)-4, (+)-5] are known to reduce the fluctuations in L-DOPA levels and overcome the problems associated with low bioavailability. These cis dimeric prodrugs of L-DOPA were incorporated into liposomes. All the formulations showed greater stability in buffer solutions at pH 1.3 and 7.4. Also, a relatively slow release of L-DOPA in human plasma was observed. Results demonstrated that the prodrug and prodrug in liposomal formulation improved the release of dopamine [108].

6.8 PRODRUGS IN CLINICAL TRIALS

A successful prodrug design can solve many problems in drug development, including solubility, lipophilicity, permeability, and toxicity. With the discovery of a large number of membrane transporters and receptors, the design of targeted prodrugs seems to have significant therapeutic potential. Numerous ongoing clinical trials are being conducted by biopharmaceutical industries. Table 6.3 lists the drug, its prodrug derivative, therapeutic indication, current clinical status, and company. These data are obtained from Ref. 109.

6.9 CONCLUSIONS AND FUTURE PERSPECTIVES

Prodrug design is a versatile and powerful technique to overcome barriers to a drug's usefulness. Prodrugs are designed mainly to increase the utility of pharmacologically active molecules by modulating their physicochemical characteristics to optimize ADMET (absorption, distribution, metabolism, excretion and toxicity) properties. Clinically, most prodrugs are simple chemical derivates comprising either ester, carbonate, carbamate, amide, ether, imine, or oxime linkages. Prodrug derivatization has been successful in enhancing the chemical and enzymatic stability of various pharmacological active molecules. In the future, an amalgamation of the prodrug approach and nanotechnology-based drug delivery systems may open up a new dimension in providing effective therapy. Accounting for the increased applications of the prodrug approach, this design should be considered in the early phases of drug discovery and not as a post hoc approach.

ASSESSMENT QUESTIONS

6.1. Which of the following represent properties of prodrugs?

a. Bioreversible derivatives
b. Simple chemical linkages
c. Optimizing the "drug-like properties" of a molecule
d. All of the above

6.2. Prodrugs were successfully being developed to overcome poor aqueous solubility for molecules belonging to which class of BCS system?

a. BCS class I
b. BCS class II
c. BCS class I and III
d. BCS class IV
e. BCS class II and IV

6.3. The general order of stability for various functional prodrugs is

a. Ester prodrugs > amide prodrugs > carbonate prodrugs
b. Amide prodrugs > ester prodrugs > carbonate prodrugs
c. Carbonate prodrugs > ester prodrugs > amide prodrugs
d. Amide prodrugs > carbonate prodrugs > ester prodrugs

6.4. Describe briefly the various strategies employed in solubility improvization.

6.5. PEGylation (addition of PEG chains) can offer the following advantages:

a. Shields them from rapid clearance and degradation
b. Improves the half-life
c. Can increase the solubility
d. All of the above

6.6. Explain the various strategies employed for site-specific drug delivery.

6.7. Explain the role of efflux transporters in drug delivery and prodrug evasion of efflux mechanisms.

6.8. A disulfide linker is often used in an antibody-drug conjugate because the

a. Concentration of glutathione is higher inside the cells than the serum
b. Concentration of glutathione is lower inside the cells than the serum
c. Stability of a disulfide linker at physiological pH
d. A and C
e. B and C

6.9. What are the advantages of using nanotechnology-based delivery systems in prodrug delivery?

REFERENCES

1. Albert, A. (1958). Chemical aspects of selective toxicity. *Nature, 182(4633)*, 421–422.
2. Rautio, J., et al. (2008). Prodrugs: Design and clinical applications. *Nature Reviews Drug Discovery, 7(3)*, 255–270.
3. Stella, V.J. (2010). Prodrugs: Some thoughts and current issues. *Journal of Pharmaceutical Sciences, 99(12)*, 4755–4765.
4. Amidon, G.L., et al. (1995). A theoretical basis for a biopharmaceutic drug classification: The correlation of in vitro drug product dissolution and in vivo bioavailability. *Pharmaceutical Research, 12(3)*, 413–420.
5. Beaumont, K., et al. (2003). Design of ester prodrugs to enhance oral absorption of poorly permeable compounds: Challenges to the discovery scientist. *Current Drug Metabolism, 4(6)*, 461–485.
6. Ettmayer, P., et al. (2004). Lessons learned from marketed and investigational prodrugs. *Journal of Medicinal Chemistry, 47(10)*, 2393–2404.
7. Sinkula, A.A., Yalkowsky, S.H. (1975). Rationale for design of biologically reversible drug derivatives: Prodrugs. *Journal of Pharmaceutical Sciences, 64(2)*, 181–210.
8. Liederer, B.M., Borchardt, R.T. (2006). Enzymes involved in the bioconversion of ester-based prodrugs. *Journal of Pharmaceutical Sciences, 95(6)*, 1177–1195.
9. Liederer, B.M., Borchardt, R.T. (2005). Stability of oxymethyl-modified coumarinic acid cyclic prodrugs of diastereomeric opioid peptides in biological media from various animal species including human. *Journal of Pharmaceutical Sciences, 94(10)*, 2198–2206.
10. Draganov, D.I., La Du, B.N. (2004). Pharmacogenetics of paraoxonases: A brief review. *Naunyn-Schmiedeberg's Archives of Pharmacology, 369(1)*, 78–88.

11. Ngawhirunpat, T., et al. (2003). Age dependency of esterase activity in rat and human keratinocytes. *Biological & Pharmaceutical Bulletin*, *26*(*9*), 1311–1314.
12. Moser, V.C., et al. (1998). Age- and gender-related differences in sensitivity to chlorpyrifos in the rat reflect developmental profiles of esterase activities. *Toxicolological Sciences*, *46*(2), 211–222.
13. Sarasola, P., McKellar, Q.A. (1994). Ampicillin and its congener prodrugs in the horse. *British Veterinary Journal*, *150*(2), 173–187.
14. Ehrnebo, M., Nilsson, S.O., Boreus, L.O. (1979). Pharmacokinetics of ampicillin and its prodrugs bacampicillin and pivampicillin in man. *Journal of Pharmacokinetics and Biopharmaceutics*, *7*(*5*), 429–451.
15. von Daehne, W., et al. (1970). Pivampicillin, a new orally active ampicillin ester. *Antimicrobial Agents and Chemotherapy (Bethesda)*, *10*, 431–437.
16. Heimbach, T., et al. (2003). Absorption rate limit considerations for oral phosphate prodrugs. *Pharmaceutical Research*, *20*(*6*), 848–856.
17. Heimbach, T., et al. (2003). Enzyme-mediated precipitation of parent drugs from their phosphate prodrugs. *International Journal of Pharmaceutics*, *261*(*1–2*), 81–92.
18. Herries, D.G. (1981). Alkaline phosphatase: By R.B. McComb, G.N. Bowers, Jr., and S. Posen. *Biochemical Education*, *9*(*2*), 76.
19. Browne, T.R., Kugler, A.R., Eldon, M.A. (1996). Pharmacology and pharmacokinetics of fosphenytoin. *Neurology*, *46*(*6 Suppl 1*), S3–S7.
20. Varia, S.A., et al. (1984). Phenytoin prodrugs III: Water-soluble prodrugs for oral and/or parenteral use. *Journal of Pharmaceutical Sciences*, *73*(*8*), 1068–1073.
21. Luer, M.S. (1998). Fosphenytoin. *Neurological Research*, *20*(2), 178–182.
22. Sousa, F.J. (1991). The bioavailability and therapeutic effectiveness of prednisolone acetate vs. prednisolone sodium phosphate: A 20-year review. *CLAO Journal*, *17*(*4*), 282–284.
23. Potter, P.M., Wadkins, R.M. (2006). Carboxylesterases–detoxifying enzymes and targets for drug therapy. *Current Medicinal Chemistry*, *13*(*9*), 1045–1054.
24. Rice, A.S., Maton, S. (2001). Gabapentin in postherpetic neuralgia: A randomised, double blind, placebo controlled study. *Pain*, *94*(2), 215–224.
25. McLean, M.J. (1999). Gabapentin in the management of convulsive disorders. *Epilepsia*, *40 Suppl 6*, S39–S50, discussion: S73–S74.
26. Rowbotham, M., et al. (1998). Gabapentin for the treatment of postherpetic neuralgia: A randomized controlled trial. *JAMA*, *280*(*21*), 1837–1842.
27. Cundy, K.C., et al. (2004). XP13512 [(+/−)-1-([(alpha-isobutanoyloxyethoxy)carbonyl] aminomethyl)-1-cyclohexane acetic acid], a novel gabapentin prodrug: II. Improved oral bioavailability, dose proportionality, and colonic absorption compared with gabapentin in rats and monkeys. *Journal of Pharmacology and Experimental Therapeutics*, *311*(*1*), 324–333.
28. Cundy, K.C., et al. (2004). XP13512 [(+/−)-1-([(alpha-isobutanoyloxyethoxy)carbonyl] aminomethyl)-1-cyclohexane acetic acid], a novel gabapentin prodrug: I. Design, synthesis, enzymatic conversion to gabapentin, and transport by intestinal solute transporters. *Journal of Pharmacology and Experimental Therapeutics*, *311*(*1*), 315–323.
29. Sanghani, S.P., et al. (2004). Hydrolysis of irinotecan and its oxidative metabolites, 7-ethyl-10-[4-N-(5-aminopentanoic acid)-1-piperidino] carbonyloxycamptothecin and 7-ethyl-10-[4-(1-piperidino)-1-amino]-carbonyloxycamptothecin, by human carboxylesterases CES1A1, CES2, and a newly expressed carboxylesterase isoenzyme, CES3. *Drug Metabolism and Disposition*, *32*(*5*), 505–511.
30. Rothenberg, M.L. (2001). Irinotecan (CPT-11): Recent developments and future directions–colorectal cancer and beyond. *Oncologist*, *6*(*1*), 66–80.
31. Vlieghe, P., et al. (2001). New 3′-azido-3′-deoxythymidin-5′-yl O-(4-hydroxyalkyl or -alkenyl or -alkylepoxide) carbonate prodrugs: Synthesis and anti-HIV evaluation. *Journal of Medicinal Chemistry*, *44*(*18*), 3014–3021.
32. Chamorro, C., et al. (2001). Exploring the role of the 5′-position of TSAO-T. Synthesis and anti-HIV evaluation of novel TSAO-T derivatives. *Antiviral Research*, *50*(*3*), 207–222.
33. Vlieghe, P., et al. (2001). New 3′-azido-3′-deoxythymidin-5′-yl O-(omega-hydroxyalkyl) carbonate prodrugs: Synthesis and anti-HIV evaluation. *Journal of Medicinal Chemistry*, *44*(*5*), 777–786.
34. Yang, C.Y., Dantzig, A.H., Pidgeon, C. 1999. Intestinal peptide transport systems and oral drug availability. *Pharmaceutical Research*, *16*(*9*), 1331–1343.
35. Steffansen, B., et al. (2004). Intestinal solute carriers: An overview of trends and strategies for improving oral drug absorption. *European Journal of Pharmaceutical Sciences*, *21*(*1*), 3–16.
36. Tsuda, M., et al. (2006). Transport characteristics of a novel peptide transporter 1 substrate, antihypotensive drug midodrine, and its amino acid derivatives. *Journal of Pharmacology and Experimental Therapeutics*, *318*(*1*), 455–460.
37. Kumpulainen, H., et al. (2006). Evaluation of hydroxyimine as cytochrome P450-selective prodrug structure. *Journal of Medicinal Chemistry*, *49*(*3*), 1207–1211.
38. Clement, B. (2002). Reduction of N-hydroxylated compounds: Amidoximes (N-hydroxyamidines) as pro-drugs of amidines. *Drug Metabolism Reviews*, *34*(*3*), 565–579.
39. Jousserandot, A., et al. (1998). Microsomal cytochrome P450 dependent oxidation of N-hydroxyguanidines, amidoximes, and ketoximes: Mechanism of the oxidative cleavage of their C=N(OH) bond with formation of nitrogen oxides. *Biochemistry*, *37*(*49*), 17179–17191.
40. Carlsson, S.C., et al. (2005). A review of the effects of the oral direct thrombin inhibitor ximelagatran on coagulation assays. *Thrombosis Research*, *115*(*1–2*), 9–18.

41. Gustafsson, D., Elg, M. (2003). The pharmacodynamics and pharmacokinetics of the oral direct thrombin inhibitor ximelagatran and its active metabolite melagatran: A mini-review. *Thrombosis Research, 109 Suppl 1*, S9–S15.
42. Eriksson, U.G., et al. (2003). Absorption, distribution, metabolism, and excretion of ximelagatran, an oral direct thrombin inhibitor, in rats, dogs, and humans. *Drug Metabolism and Disposition, 31(3)*, 294–305.
43. Strickley, R.G. (2004). Solubilizing excipients in oral and injectable formulations. *Pharmaceutical Research, 21*(2), 201–230.
44. Rao, V.M., Stella, V.J. (2003). When can cyclodextrins be considered for solubilization purposes? *Journal of Pharmaceutical Sciences, 92(5)*, 927–932.
45. Muller, R.H., Jacobs, C., Kayser, O. (2001). Nanosuspensions as particulate drug formulations in therapy. Rationale for development and what we can expect for the future. *Advanced Drug Delivery Reviews, 47(1)*, 3–19.
46. Greenwald, R.B., et al. (1996). Drug delivery systems: Water soluble taxol 2′-poly(ethylene glycol) ester prodrugs-design and in vivo effectiveness. *Journal of Medicinal Chemistry, 39(2)*, 424–431.
47. Wire, M.B., Shelton, M.J., Studenberg, S. (2006). Fosamprenavir: Clinical pharmacokinetics and drug interactions of the amprenavir prodrug. *Clinical Pharmacokinetics, 45*(2), 137–168.
48. Chapman, T.M., Plosker, G.L., Perry, C.M. (2004). Fosamprenavir: A review of its use in the management of antiretroviral therapy-naive patients with HIV infection. *Drugs, 64(18)*, 2101–2124.
49. Furfine, E.S., et al. (2004). Preclinical pharmacology and pharmacokinetics of GW433908, a water-soluble prodrug of the human immunodeficiency virus protease inhibitor amprenavir. *Antimicrobial Agents and Chemotherapy, 48(3)*, 791–798.
50. Lambert, D.M. (2000). Rationale and applications of lipids as prodrug carriers. *European Journal of Pharmaceutical Sciences, 11 Suppl 2*, S15–S27.
51. McClellan, K., Perry, C.M. (2001). Oseltamivir: A review of its use in influenza. *Drugs, 61*(2), 263–283.
52. Trevaskis, N.L., Charman, W.N., Porter, C.J. (2008). Lipid-based delivery systems and intestinal lymphatic drug transport: A mechanistic update. *Advacned Drug Delivery Reviews, 60(6)*, 702–716.
53. Beadle, J.R. (2007). Synthesis of cidofovir and (S)-HPMPA ether lipid prodrugs. *Current Protocols in Nucleic Acid Chemistry*, Chapter 15: Unit 15-2.
54. Tunek, A., Levin, E., Svensson, L.A. (1988). Hydrolysis of 3H-bambuterol, a carbamate prodrug of terbutaline, in blood from humans and laboratory animals in vitro. *Biochemical Pharmacology, 37(20)*, 3867–3876.
55. Svensson, L.A., Tunek, A. (1988). The design and bioactivation of presystemically stable prodrugs. *Drug Metabolism Reviews, 19*(2), 165–194.
56. Murthy, N., et al. (2003). Bioinspired pH-responsive polymers for the intracellular delivery of biomolecular drugs. *Bioconjugate Chemistry, 14*(2), 412–419.
57. Chilkoti, A., et al. (2002). Targeted drug delivery by thermally responsive polymers. *Advanced Drug Delivery Reviews, 54(5)*, 613–630.
58. Harris, J.M., Chess, R.B. (2003). Effect of pegylation on pharmaceuticals. *Nature Reviews Drug Discovery, 2(3)*, 214–221.
59. Zeuzem, S., et al. (2000). Peginterferon alfa-2a in patients with chronic hepatitis C. *New England Journal of Medicine, 343(23)*, 1666–1672.
60. Choudhuri, S., Klaassen, C.D. (2006). Structure, function, expression, genomic organization, and single nucleotide polymorphisms of human ABCB1 (MDR1), ABCC (MRP), and ABCG2 (BCRP) efflux transporters. *International Journal of Toxicology, 25(4)*, 231–259.
61. Cascorbi, I. (2006). Role of pharmacogenetics of ATP-binding cassette transporters in the pharmacokinetics of drugs. *Pharmacology & Therapeutics, 112*(2), 457–473.
62. Katragadda, S., et al. (2005). Role of efflux pumps and metabolising enzymes in drug delivery. *Expert Opinions in Drug Delivery*, *2(4)*, 683–705.
63. Lennernas, H. (2003). Intestinal drug absorption and bioavailability: Beyond involvement of single transport function. *Journal of Pharmacy and Pharmacology, 55(4)*, 429–433.
64. Hosoya, K., Tachikawa, M. (2009). Inner blood-retinal barrier transporters: Role of retinal drug delivery. *Pharmaceutical Research, 26(9)*, 2055–2065.
65. Majumdar, S., Duvvuri, S., Mitra, A.K. (2004). Membrane transporter/receptor-targeted prodrug design: Strategies for human and veterinary drug development. *Advanced Drug Delivery Reviews, 56*(*10*), 1437–1452.
66. Han, H.K. and Amidon, G.L. 2000. Targeted prodrug design to optimize drug delivery. *AAPS PharmSci, 2*(*1*), E6.
67. Janoria, K.G., et al. (2007). Novel approaches to retinal drug delivery. *Expert Opinion on Drug Delivery, 4(4)*, 371–388.
68. Rubio-Aliaga, I., Daniel, H. (2002). Mammalian peptide transporters as targets for drug delivery. *Trends in Pharmacological Sciences, 23(9)*, 434–440.
69. Anand, B.S., Katragadda, S., Mitra, A.K. (2004). Pharmacokinetics of novel dipeptide ester prodrugs of acyclovir after oral administration: Intestinal absorption and liver metabolism. *Journal of Pharmacology and Experimental Therapeutics, 311*(2), 659–667.
70. Guo, A., et al. (1999). Interactions of a nonpeptidic drug, valacyclovir, with the human intestinal peptide transporter (hPEPT1) expressed in a mammalian cell line. *Journal of Pharmacology and Experimental Therapeutics, 289*(*1*), 448–454.
71. Balimane, P.V., et al. (1998). Direct evidence for peptide transporter (PepT1)-mediated uptake of a nonpeptide prodrug, valacyclovir. *Biochemical and Biophysical Research Communications, 250*(2), 246–251.

72. de Vrueh, R.L., Smith, P.L., Lee, C.P. (1998). Transport of L-valine-acyclovir via the oligopeptide transporter in the human intestinal cell line, Caco-2. *Journal of Pharmacology and Experimental Therapeutics*, *286(3)*, 1166–1170.
73. Perry, C.M., Faulds, D. (1996). Valaciclovir. A review of its antiviral activity, pharmacokinetic properties and therapeutic efficacy in herpesvirus infections. *Drugs*, *52(5)*, 754–772.
74. Jain, R., et al. (2008). Interaction of dipeptide prodrugs of saquinavir with multidrug resistance protein-2 (MRP-2): Evasion of MRP-2 mediated efflux. *International Journal of Pharmaceutics*, *362(1–2)*, 44–51.
75. Jain, R., et al. (2007). Intestinal absorption of novel-dipeptide prodrugs of saquinavir in rats. *International Journal of Pharmaceutics*, *336(2)*, 233–240.
76. Jain, R., et al. (2005). Evasion of P-gp mediated cellular efflux and permeability enhancement of HIV-protease inhibitor saquinavir by prodrug modification. *International Journal of Pharmaceutics*, *303(1–2)*, 8–19.
77. Ganapathy, M.E., Ganapathy, V. (2005). Amino acid transporter ATB0,+ as a delivery system for drugs and prodrugs. *Current Drug Targets - Immune, Endocrine & Metabolic Disorders*, *5(4)*, 357–364.
78. Anand, B.S., Dey, S., Mitra, A.K. (2002). Current prodrug strategies via membrane transporters/receptors. *Expert Opinion on Biological Therapy*, *2(6)*, 607–620.
79. Christensen, H.N. (1990). Role of amino acid transport and countertransport in nutrition and metabolism. *Physiological Reviews*, *70(1)*, 43–77.
80. Katragadda, S., et al. (2008). Pharmacokinetics of amino acid ester prodrugs of acyclovir after oral administration: Interaction with the transporters on Caco-2 cells. *International Journal of Pharmaceutics*, *362(1–2)*, 93–101.
81. Vadlapudi, A.D., Vadlapatla, R.K., Mitra, A.K. (2012). Sodium dependent multivitamin transporter (SMVT): A potential target for drug delivery. *Current Drug Targets*, *13(7)*, 994–1003.
82. Rivas, C.I., et al. (2008). Vitamin C transporters. *Journal of Physiology and Biochemistry*, *64(4)*, 357–375.
83. Said, H.M. (2004). Recent advances in carrier-mediated intestinal absorption of water-soluble vitamins. *Annual Review of Physiology*, *66*, 419–446.
84. Luo, S., et al. (2011). Targeting SVCT for enhanced drug absorption: Synthesis and in vitro evaluation of a novel vitamin C conjugated prodrug of saquinavir. *International Journal of Pharmaceutics*, *414(1–2)*, 77–85.
85. Luo, S., et al. (2006). Functional characterization of sodium-dependent multivitamin transporter in MDCK-MDR1 cells and its utilization as a target for drug delivery. *Molecular Pharmacology*, *3(3)*, 329–339.
86. Alley, S.C., Okeley, N.M., Senter, P.D. (2010). Antibody-drug conjugates: Targeted drug delivery for cancer. *Current Opinion in Chemical Biology*, *14(4)*, 5295–5237.
87. Chen, J., et al. (2005). Antibody-cytotoxic agent conjugates for cancer therapy. *Expert Opinion on Drug Delivery*, *2(5)*, 873–890.
88. Saito, G., Swanson, J.A., Lee, K.D. (2003). Drug delivery strategy utilizing conjugation via reversible disulfide linkages: Role and site of cellular reducing activities. *Advanced Drug Delivery Reviews*, *55(2)*, 199–215.
89. Kigawa, J., et al. (1998). Glutathione concentration may be a useful predictor of response to second-line chemotherapy in patients with ovarian cancer. *Cancer*, *82(4)*, 697–702.
90. Vitetta, E.S., Thorpe, P.E., Uhr, J.W. (1993). Immunotoxins: Magic bullets or misguided missiles? *Immunology Today*, *14(6)*, 252–259.
91. Meister, A. (1991). Glutathione deficiency produced by inhibition of its synthesis, and its reversal; applications in research and therapy. *Pharmacology & Therapeutics*, *51(2)*, 155–194.
92. Kupchan, S.M., et al. (1977). The maytansinoids. Isolation, structural elucidation, and chemical interrelation of novel ansa macrolides. *Journal of Organic Chemistry*, *42(14)*, 2349–2357.
93. Kupchan, S.M., et al. (1972). Maytansine, a novel antileukemic ansa macrolide from Maytenus ovatus. *Journal of the American Chemical Society*, *94(4)*, 1354–1356.
94. Issell, B.F., Crooke, S.T. (1978). Maytansine. *Cancer Treatment Reviews*, *5(4)*, 199–207.
95. Eagan, R.T., et al. (1978). Phase II evaluation of maytansine in patients with metastatic lung cancer. *Cancer Treatment Reports*, *62(10)*, 1577–1579.
96. Blum, R.H., Kahlert, T. (1978). Maytansine: A phase I study of an ansa macrolide with antitumor activity. *Cancer Treatment Reports*, *62(3)*, 435–438.
97. Chabner, B.A., et al. (1978). Initial clinical trials of maytansine, an antitumor plant alkaloid. *Cancer Treatment Reports*, *62(3)*, 429–433.
98. Cassady, J.M., et al. (2004). Recent developments in the maytansinoid antitumor agents. *Chemical and Pharmaceutical Bulletin (Tokyo)*, *52(1)*, 1–26.
99. Widdison, W.C., et al. (2006). Semisynthetic maytansine analogues for the targeted treatment of cancer. *Journal of Medicinal Chemistry*, *49(14)*, 4392–4408.
100. Krop, I.E., et al. (In press). A phase II study of trastuzumab emtansine in patients with human epidermal growth factor receptor 2-positive metastatic breast cancer who were previously treated with trastuzumab, lapatinib, an anthracycline, a taxane, and capecitabine. *Journal of Clinical Oncology*.
101. Vadlapudi, A.D., et al. (2012). Targeted lipid based drug conjugates: A novel strategy for drug delivery. *International Journal of Pharmaceutics*, *434(1–2)*, 315–324.
102. Bhandari, K.H., et al. (2007). Evaluation of skin permeation and accumulation profiles of ketorolac fatty esters. *Journal of Pharmacy & Pharmaceutical Sciences*, *10(3)*, 278–287.
103. Rautio, J., et al. (1999). Synthesis and in vitro evaluation of aminoacyloxyalkyl esters of 2-(6-methoxy-2-naphthyl)propionic acid as novel naproxen prodrugs for dermal drug delivery. *Pharmaceutical Research*, *16(8)*, 1172–1178.

104. Sheha, M. (2012). Pharmacokinetic and ulcerogenic studies of naproxen prodrugs designed for specific brain delivery. *Archives of Pharmacal Research*, *35*(*3*), 523–530.

105. Zhang, Q., et al. (2012). Novel brain targeting prodrugs of naproxen based on dimethylamino group with various linkages. *Arzneimittelforschung*, *62*(*6*), 261–266.

106. Zhang, X., et al. (2012). In vitro and in vivo investigation of dexibuprofen derivatives for CNS delivery. *Acta Pharmacologica Sinica*, *33*(2), 279–288.

107. Yen, S.Y., et al. (2001). Controlled release of nalbuphine propionate from biodegradable microspheres: In vitro and in vivo studies. *International Journal of Pharmaceutics*, *220*(*1–2*), 91–99.

108. Di Stefano, A., et al. (2006). Maleic- and fumaric-diamides of (*O*,*O*-diacetyl)-L-Dopa-methylester as anti-Parkinson prodrugs in liposomal formulation. *Journal of Drug Targeting*, *14*(*9*), 652–661.

109. www.clinicaltrials.gov.

Micronized = non-nanoparticulate

7

NANOSCALE DRUG DELIVERY SYSTEMS

MITAN R. GOKULGANDHI, ASHABEN PATEL, KISHORE CHOLKAR, MEGHA BAROT, AND ASHIM K. MITRA

7.1 CHAPTER OBJECTIVES

- To provide an overview of nanoscale delivery systems.
- To elucidate various types and preparation methods of nanoscale carrier systems.
- To illustrate the advantages and limitations of different nanocarriers.
- To summarize the numerous delivery applications of nanocarrier systems.

7.2 INTRODUCTION

The method of drug delivery can have a significant effect on its efficacy and potency for the treatment of various ailments. Different nanoparticulate systems are currently under development to overcome drug delivery challenges such as to minimize drug degradation and loss, to prevent harmful side effects, and to increase drug bioavailability and accumulation at the target site. Nanoparticulate systems such as nanoparticles, liposomes, and nanomicelles have gained a lot of attention in the area of drug delivery. However, designing effective drug delivery system is a challenging task in terms of targeting drug to the specific sites, specifically to the complex tumor microenvironment. Generally, tumor tissue is abnormal with leaky vasculature and nanoparticulate system takes advantage of the enhanced permeation and retention (EPR) effect througty 7h this leaky vasculature to remain in the systemic circulation for long period for high tumor accumulation. This chapter will describe the basic definition and rationale behind developing each carrier system. Moreover, pharmaceutical significance and formulation specification related to each nanocarrier system will be discussed in detail.

7.3 CELLULAR INTERNALIZATION OF NANOPARTICULATE SYSTEMS

Nanoparticulate systems can use multiple uptake pathways for cellular internalization. Various parameters such as physicochemical characteristics of nanoparticulate systems (particle size, shape, surface charge, and ligand density), nature of the target cells, receptor expression levels, and cell properties (phenotype and location) play an important role in the cellular internalization mechanism. Phagocytosis and nonphagocytosis (pinocytosis and endocytosis) are the important cellular internalization pathways of nanoparticulate systems. Phagocytosis plays a vital physiological role in the clearance of dying cells by preventing the efflux of potentially harmful components from the dying cell and thereby limits direct tissue injury by inhibiting secondary immune responses [1]. The shape, size, and presence of various functional groups on the surface of a nanoparticulate system are an important driving force for the phagocytosis process [2]. The phagocytosis process involves recognition of a nanoparticulate system by opsonization followed by adhesion of the opsonized particles to the macrophages and

Advanced Drug Delivery, First Edition. Edited by Ashim K. Mitra, Chi H. Lee, and Kun Cheng.

finally ingestion of the particle. Pinocytosis is a nonphagocytic process that allows internalization of foreign particles via lysosomal degradation. Small-size nanoparticulate systems are more predisposed to get internalized into the cells via pinocytosis [3]. The molecular mechanism of the endocytosis process, which is also known as the nonphagocytic process, is further divided into five subcategories as follows: 1) clathrin-mediated endocytosis (receptor mediated and non–receptor mediated), 2) caveolae-mediated endocytosis, 3) nonclathrin, non–caveolae-mediated endocytosis, 4) macropinocytosis, and 5) nonendocytotic pathway or transduction [3].

7.4 NANOPARTICLES

Nanoparticles are colloidal solid particles with the size range of 1 to 1000 nm. For the purpose of drug delivery, drug can be entrapped within nanoparticles or adsorbed or attached to the nanoparticle surface. Generally, nanoparticles are fabricated from biodegradable or nonbiodegradable materials such as natural or synthetic polymers, lipids, phospholipids, or metals [4–6]. Hence, the different types of nanoparticulate systems that have been studied for the diagnosis and treatment of cancer therapy include quantum dots [7], paramagnetic nanoparticles [8], gold nanoparticles [9], and many others [10, 11]. For example, Nab-paclitaxel (Abraxane; Abraxis Bioscience, Los Angeles, CA), an albumin-bound nanoparticle formulation of paclitaxel, has been developed for the treatment of breast, lung, ovarian, head and neck, and Kaposi's sarcoma [12–14], which shows high patient response (33% vs 19% for cremophore-paclitaxel) and significant disease progression rate (23 weeks vs 16 weeks) [15]. Moreover, Langer et al. have developed the HER2 receptor specific antibody trastuzumab (Herceptin; Genentech, South San Francisco, CA) conjugated gelatin and human serum albumin (HSA) nanoparticles for targeting HER-2 overexpressed cells, which demonstrates that antibody-modified nanoparticles can combine specific tumor targeting with the drug delivery properties for the treatment of cancer. In addition, nanoparticulate systems can also be useful for tissue engineering such as the formation of biocompatible scaffolds [16]. The other applications involve biofabrication of functional epithelial, myocardial, skeletal muscle, skin, liver tissue, and many other tissues [17]. The more advanced applications of nanoparticulate systems involve optical coding for bioassay [18, 19] and protein detections [20].

7.4.1 Nanoparticle Types

Depending on the type of fabricated materials, nanoparticles can be allocated into three major categories: polymeric nanoparticles, solid lipid nanoparticles, and inorganic nanoparticles.

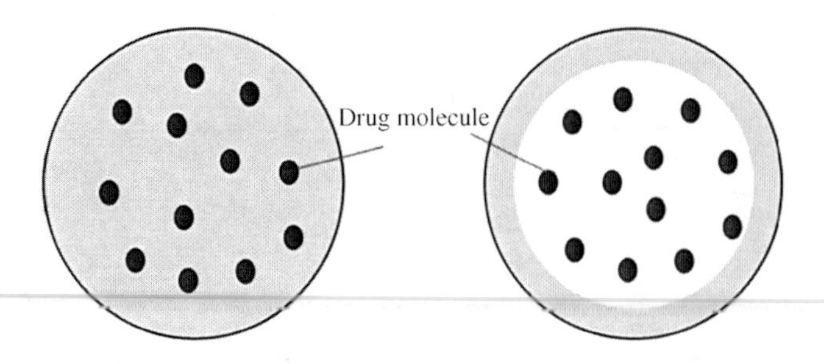

FIGURE 7.1 Nanosphere (left) and nanocapsule (right).

7.4.1.1 ***Polymeric Nanoparticles*** Polymeric nanoparticles are the most common type of nanoparticles employed for drug delivery application. Polymeric nanoparticles are developed from various natural, synthetic biodegradable, as well as nonbiodegradable polymers. Polymers such as chitosan, sodium alginate, poly(lactide-co-glycolide) (PLGA), polycaprolactone (PCL), and polylactic acid (PLA) are prevalent in constructing polymeric nanoparticles. Polymeric nanoparticles can be engineered as nanocapsules or nanospheres (Figure 7.1). With polymeric nanocapsules, drugs are enclosed within the polymeric membrane, whereas with nanospheres, drugs are evenly distributed within the polymeric matrix. These versatile polymeric nanoparticles can be engineered by numerous methods to obtain high drug loading and tunable release kinetics [21].

7.4.1.2 ***Solid Lipid Nanoparticles (SLNs)*** SLNs have been developed as an alternative to other colloidal systems, such as polymeric nanoparticles, liposomes, and emulsions. These colloidal carriers are composed of physiologically compatible solid lipids. The major components of SLNs are solid lipids and surfactants. The most commonly employed solid lipids in SLNs include triglycerides, beeswax, cetyl alcohol, cholesterol, and cholesterol butyrate. Active ingredients can be incorporated into SLNs by various preparation methods including high shear homogenization, hot homogenization, cold homogenization, solvent emulsification/evaporation, and supercritical fluid method. SLNs combine the advantages of both polymeric nanoparticles and liposomes, which include controlled drug release, high entrapment of lipophilic drugs, easy production and scaleup, enhanced drug stability, and bioavailability. Additionally, excellent biocompatibility and biodegradability make SLNs unique over other nanocarriers [4, 22].

7.4.1.3 ***Inorganic Nanoparticles*** The term "inorganic nanoparticle" is generally used for nanoparticles fabricated from metal, metal oxides, or metal sulfides. Inorganic nanoparticles gained immense interest over the past few years because of their unique physicochemical properties, such as small size and inertness. In addition, optical and magnetic properties of some inorganic nanoparticles make them an attractive alternative to organic nanoparticles. Inorganic nanoparticles including magnetic nanoparticles, gold nanoparticles, and quantum dots (QDs) have been successfully developed as contrast agents for bioimaging applications. Recently, inorganic nanoparticles have also been explored for drug delivery, specifically anti-cancer drugs. Furthermore, inorganic nanoparticles can be functionalized to achieve targeted drug delivery [23].

7.4.2 Preparation of Polymeric Nanoparticles

Generally, the methods used for polymeric nanoparticle preparation are categorized depending on whether they are formulated from a preformed polymer or by monomer polymerization. In this section, different polymeric nanoparticle preparation methods are described. Moreover, the advantages and limitations of each method are summarized in Table 7.1.

7.4.2.1 Nanoparticle Preparation from Preformed Polymer Depending on the type of drug and polymer used, nanoparticles from a preformed polymer can be fabricated by different techniques such as single emulsion-solvent evaporation, double emulsion-solvent evaporation, salting out, and nanoprecipitation.

Single Emulsion-Solvent Evaporation It is the most frequently used method for nanoparticle preparation. This method is composed of two steps: 1) emulsion preparation and 2) solvent evaporation. In the first step, drug and polymer are dissolved in a water immiscible organic solvent, such as chloroform and methylene chloride, and then the organic phase is emulsified in an aqueous phase containing stabilizer. High-energy homogenization or sonication is generally employed to induce the formation of nanodroplets during the emulsification process. Subsequently, the organic phase is evaporated under vacuum or continuous overnight stirring, leading to the formation of nanodispersion. Nanoparticles are collected by ultracentrifugation and washed with distilled water to remove free drugs and stabilizer residues [24]. The homogenization speed, types, and amounts of stabilizer, as well as the viscosity of organic and aqueous phases, are the main factors to be considered while preparing the nanoparticle by this method [25].

Double Emulsion-Solvent Evaporation This is the method of choice for encapsulation of hydrophilic drugs into

TABLE 7.1 Advantages and Limitations of Polymeric Nanoparticles Preparation Methods

Nanoparticles Preparation Method	Advantages	Limitations
Single emulsion-solvent evaporation	Higher entrapment of lipophilic drugs. Nanoparticle size can be tuned by adjusting the homogenization speed, amount of stabilizer, and viscosity of organic and aqueous phases	Poor entrapment of hydrophilic drugs and difficult to scale up
Double emulsion-solvent evaporation	Entrapment of hydrophilic drugs	Difficult to scale up. Leakage of the hydrophilic active component into external water phase leads to poor entrapment efficiency
Emulsification or solvent diffusion	Higher entrapment of lipophilic drugs. Use of nontoxic solvents, easy scale-up process, and good batch-to-batch reproducibility	Poor entrapment of hydrophilic drugs, longer time of emulsion agitation, and requirement of a large amount of water for nanoparticles formation
Nanoprecipitation	Simple and fast method uses non–highly toxic solvents and poses high batch-to-batch reproducibility. It can be employed for both hydrophilic and lipophilic small molecules as well as proteins. This process does not require high shear stress	Nanoparticle size mainly depends on polymer concentration
Salting out	It does not require high shear stress and applicable for heat sensitive drugs. High loading efficiency for lipophilic drugs, easy scale-up, and high reproducibility	Extensive nanoparticles washing step and exclusively applicable for only lipophilic drugs
Emulsion polymerization	Fast and scalable	Use of toxic organic solvents and monomers (organic phase methodology) and difficult-to-remove residual monomers, initiators, and surfactants from final product
Interfacial polycondensation	High encapsulation of lipophilic drugs	

nanoparticles. It involves three steps: 1) formation of single (water in oil, w/o) emulsion, 2) formation of double (water in oil in water, w/o/w) emulsion, and 3) solvent evaporation. In the first step, an aqueous solution containing hydrophilic active components is emulsified in an organic continuous phase (e.g., methylene chloride and ethyl acetate) containing a polymer and surfactant (e.g., span 80). The single (w/o) emulsion is formed with the aid of sonication or high-speed homogenization. The single (w/o) emulsion is added into the second aqueous phase containing stabilizer, usually polyvinyl alcohol (PVA), with continuous stirring to form the double (w/o/w) emulsion. The double (w/o/w) emulsion is also subjected to sonication or homogenization for droplet size reduction. Finally, the organic phase is evaporated under vacuum or by overnight continuous stirring. The formed nanoparticles are collected by ultracentrifugation and washed with distilled water to remove free drug and stabilizer residues. The key parameters to be considered are the amounts of drug, polymer concentration, surfactant amount, solvent nature, shear stress, and first/second-phase volume ratios [25–27].

Emulsification/Solvent Diffusion This process is another widely employed method of nanoparticle preparation. Unlike the emulsion-solvent evaporation method, it involves application of partially water miscible organic solvent, such as benzyl alcohol, propylene carbonate, and ethyl acetate. In this method, polymers and drugs are dissolved in a partially water-miscible organic solvent saturated with water, and then this organic phase is emulsified with an aqueous solution containing stabilizer (e.g., PVA and poloxamer 188) under continuous stirring. Nanoparticles are formed by diffusion of the organic solvent and the counterdiffusion of water into the emulsion droplets. Last, the solvent is removed by evaporation or cross-flow filtration. Polymer concentration, amount of stabilizer, miscibility of water with the organic solvent, and stirring rate are the key process parameters that need to be considered while preparing nanoparticles by this method [28–30].

Nanoprecipitation The nanoprecipitation method, also known as the solvent displacement method, is the easiest method for nanoparticle preparation. It employs water-miscible solvent (e.g., acetone, ethanol, dimethyl sulfoxide, and isopropyl alcohol) as a polymer solvent (i.e., solvent for polymer solubilization) and usually water as a nonsolvent. Ethanol, methanol, or propanol can also be employed as nonsolvent depending on the nature of drug and polymer [28]. In this method, drug and polymer are first dissolved in polymer solvent and then the solution is injected or poured into aqueous solution containing surfactants (e.g., poloxamer 407 and povidone k 30) under continuous stirring. The rapid diffusion of polymer solvent in the nonsolvent leads to the instantaneous formation of nanospheres. Finally, the polymer solvent is removed by either evaporation or centrifugation, and nanospheres are washed and lyophilized. Polymer concentration, surfactant type and concentration, solvent nature, viscosity, and nature of active component, are the main factors affecting the physicochemical characteristics of nanoparticles produced by nanoprecipitation method [31, 32].

Salting Out This method is a modified form of the emulsification/solvent diffusion method. It also involves formation of oil/water (o/w) emulsion; however, emulsion is formed from water-miscible polymer solvent and aqueous gel containing the salting out agent and a stabilizer. Acetone and tetrahydrofuran (THF) are generally employed as a polymer solvent and PVA, polyvinyl pyrrolidone, and hydroxyethyl cellulose as a stabilizer. Typically, the concentration of the salting out agent is 60% and the examples of salting out agents include electrolytes such as magnesium chloride, calcium chloride, magnesium acetate, and non-electrolyte such as sucrose. For preparing nanoparticles by this method, drug and polymer are first dissolved in acetone and then solution is emulsified in aqueous gel containing the salting out agent and a stabilizer by vigorous stirring. The formed o/w emulsion is then diluted with an excess of water. The dilution produces a sudden drop in the concentration of salting out agent in the continuous phase of the emulsion, and hence, polymer solvent diffuses out of the emulsion droplets inducing precipitation of the polymer. The nanoparticles dispersion is then purified by eliminating polymer solvent and the salting out agent by cross-flow filtration. The main factors affecting physicochemical characteristics of nanoparticles produced by salting out method are polymer concentration, stirring rate and time, solvent type, and nature of salting out agent [24, 33, 34].

7.4.2.2 Nanoparticle Preparation from Polymerization of Monomer Nanoparticles can be prepared by *in situ* polymerization of monomer. The most commonly employed polymerization methods are emulsion polymerization and interfacial polycondensation. The basic chemical constituents used in nanoparticle preparation by polymerization methods are monomers, polymerization initiators, additives, and solvent.

Emulsion Polymerization Emulsion polymerization can be performed in either aqueous phase or organic phase. In the organic phase methodology, nanoparticles are prepared from polymerization of water-soluble monomers such as acrylamide and *N,N′*-bisacrylaminde, which are polymerized by either chemical initiators or light irradiation. However, the high toxicity of acrylamide monomers and organic solvent made this method less popular. Later on, this method has been used to prepare polyalkylcynoacrylate nanoparticles from cyanoacrylate monomers. Although cyanoacrylate monomers are less toxic, this method is still less popular because of the requirement of a high amount of toxic organic solvent and surfactant.

In aqueous phase methodology, as the name describes, monomers are dissolved in the aqueous phase. The polymerization is initiated on contact of the monomers present in continuous phase with an initiator molecule that can be an ion or a free radical or by high-energy radiation. Polymerization leads to the formation and subsequent precipitation of solid nanoparticles. To prevent excessive rapid polymerization, it is usually carried out at acidic pH. The polymerization time and temperature, as well as surfactant and stabilizer concentration, are the key factors that affect physicochemical properties of nanoparticle prepared by emulsion polymerization [21, 35–37].

Interfacial Polycondensation In this method, nanoparticles with a shell-like wall form at the interface of two nonmiscible phases. To obtain a nanoparticle, the oil phase/organic phase is slowly injected into the aqueous phase with continuous stirring, which leads to the formation of emulsion. Nanocapsules formed spontaneously by hydroxyl-ion–induced polymerization at the oil/water interface. Generally, the oil phase/organic phase contains the lipophilic monomer and a lipophilic drug, while the aqueous phase contains water, the hydrophilic monomer, and a hydrophilic surfactant. The nanocapsule wall thickness and porosity are the key factors affecting drug-loading and release properties. The thickness and porosity of the wall depends on the concentration and molecular weight of the monomers. It is reported that the thickness of the wall is dependent mainly on the lipophilic monomer concentration and not on the hydrophilic monomer. Nanocapsules composed of polyurea and polyamides have been prepared by this method with high encapsulation of alpha-tocopherol [28, 38–40].

7.4.2.3 Advantages of Polymeric Nanoparticles Polymeric nanoparticles can be employed for drug administration via any route (e.g., oral, intravenous, and intraocular). Easy modulation of particle size and surface potential is feasible with polymeric nanoparticles. Moreover, site-specific drug delivery can be achieved by surface decoration with targeting ligand. Polymeric nanoparticles can be employed for delivering small hydrophilic and hydrophobic drugs as well as macromolecules. Furthermore, polymeric nanoparticles can offer controlled and sustained drug delivery and can protect the entrapped drug from enzymatic or acidic degradation. Finally, polymeric nanoparticles can prolong the half-life of a drug in systemic circulation.

7.4.2.4 Limitations of Polymeric Nanoparticles Particle aggregation caused by small size and large surface makes purification and handling difficult for polymeric nanoparticles. Moreover, limited drug loading because of small size and initial burst release are other limitations of polymeric nanoparticles.

7.4.3 Preparation of Solid Lipid Nanoparticles

7.4.3.1 Homogenization The homogenization includes three types of processes: 1) high shear homogenization, 2) hot homogenization, and 3) cold homogenization. The high shear homogenization technique was initially used for the production of solid lipid nanodispersions by melt emulsification [41]. However, the dispersion quality is often compromised by the presence of microparticles. Moreover, different process parameters such as emulsification time, stirring rate, and cooling condition affect the particle size and zeta potential of SLNs.

The hot homogenization, similar to high shear homogenization, is carried out at high temperatures (usually above the melting point of the lipids) to form an emulsion [42]. The hot homogenization process involves formation of the pre-emulsion phase containing drug-loaded lipid melt and the aqueous emulsifier phase, which is obtained by a high-shear mixing device. This is followed by several passes of pre-emulsion through the high-pressure homogenizer [42, 43]. The major limitation of the above process is that it may cause temperature-mediated accelerated degradation of drug payload, partitioning and loss of drug into the aqueous phase during homogenization, and uncertain polymorphic transitions of the lipid, which leads to variation in drug entrapment [44]. Therefore, to avoid the above problems, the cold homogenization process can be used. The cold homogenization process is carried out with the solid lipids at elevated pressure but with an effective temperature controller [45]. This process involves solubilization or dispersion of drug molecules in the lipid melt followed by subsequent cooling (using dry ice or liquid nitrogen) and grounding of microparticles by milling (ball/mortar milling). The large particle size and a broad size distribution of SLNs are the major limitation of the cold homogenization process [45, 46].

7.4.3.2 Solvent Emulsification/Evaporation In this method, the SLNs were prepared by solubilization of lipophilic material in water-immiscible organic solvent (cyclohexane), which is then emulsified in an aqueous phase [47], which is followed by stirring to evaporate the solvent to form nanoparticle dispersion caused by precipitation of the lipid in the aqueous medium. The other methods that are not well known include SLN preparation by using supercritical fluid [48], spray drying [49], and double-emulsion [50] methods.

7.5 MICELLES

Micelles are colloidal structures (5–100 nm) formed from self-assembling of amphiphilic molecules (e.g., surface active agents) (Figure 7.2a) in aqueous solution. These surface-active agents have two distinct groups, a hydrophobic head and a hydrophilic tail. Depending on the concentration (from lower to higher), amphiphiles can exist in three different phases: 1) monomers, 2) an arranged monolayer at interphase, and 3) monomer aggregates or micelles. The formed aggregates at a high amphiphile concentration have two distinct regions, namely, inner hydrophobic core and outer hydrophilic corona. The inner hydrophobic core is formed by van der Waals bonds and can encapsulate lipophilic drugs [51]. The outer hydrophilic corona is in contact with the surrounding water molecules through hydrogen bonds [51, 52]. The hydrophilic corona of micelles has two advantages: 1) It provides steric stability and 2) helps to avoid reticuloendothelial system uptake, which results in prolonged circulation in the body. Micelles are dynamic structures and display high formation and deformation rates with apparent stability ranging from microseconds to seconds [53]. Micelle shape depends on the length of block polymer segments because the larger hydrophilic segment generates spherical micelles, whereas a larger hydrophobic segment forms different micelle structures such as rods, lamellae, etc. [54].

Micelle formulations are mostly employed for delivering anticancer agents by using its high drug encapsulation capacity, small size, and hydrophilic surface that prevents plasma protein binding (Table 7.2) [55–62]. Anticancer drug-loaded micelle formulations have demonstrated improved circulation and therapeutic efficacy over a free drug in tumor-bearing animal models [55, 56]. Moreover, micelles have also demonstrated sufficient drug stability and adequate release kinetics at the targeted site because of the EPR effect [57]. Different pH-sensitive micelles have been also synthesized to protect the anticancer drug from the mononuclear phagocyte system [58]. To improve tumor drug localization, the surface of the micelles can be conjugated with a targeting ligand that can bind to a specific receptor or transporter expressed on the tumor cells. Polymeric micelles conjugated with folate moiety have been developed to study its targeting effect on the tumor cells [59]. Other rapidly emerging alternatives in the micelle formulation are polyionic complex micelles (PICMs). Opposite charges of polymers and macromolecules (peptides and DNA) have been used to develop PICMs because of the charge neutralization process. PICMs have demonstrated improved DNA stability against gastric enzymes such as nucleases [60]. Micelle formulations are also developed to deliver therapeutic agents at the anterior and posterior segments of the eye via noninvasive route [61, 62].

7.5.1 Micelle Types

Two different types of micelles are commonly employed for drug delivery: surfactant micelles and block co-polymer micelles. Different types of surfactant micelles are known depending on the presence or absence of charge on the surfactant head group (Table 7.3) [60, 61]. Block co-polymer micelles are prepared from biocompatible, biodegradable polyester or derivatives of poly amino acid. Different types of block co-polymers used for micelle preparation include diblock (A-B type), triblock (A-B-A type), grafted, or branched co-polymers (Figure 7.2b) [63–65]. Polyethylene glycol (PEG) is commonly employed as a hydrophilic block because of its water solubility, low toxicity, biocompatibility, and ability to provide steric stability [65]. The inner hydrophobic core is generally made of polyesters, polyethers, and polyamino acids (e.g., PCL, PLA, and poloxamers).

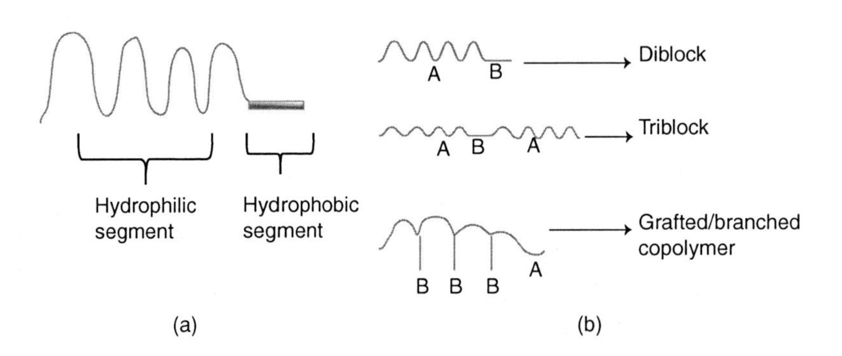

FIGURE 7.2 Structure of amphiphilic monomer (a) and block co-polymers (b).

TABLE 7.2 List of Polymers Used in Micelle Formulation Preparation and Their Applications

Polymer Used in Micelle Preparation	Drug	Application	References
Pluronic (BASF Corporation, NJ, USA)	Doxorubicin	Leukemia P388, Lewis lung carcinoma, breast carcinoma	[55]
Methoxy poly(ethylene oxide)-b-poly (ε-caprolactone)	Cyclosporine	Improved drug solubilization and blood circulation	[56]
PEG-b-PGlu	Cisplatin	Improved blood circulation and drug concentration at target site because of enhanced permeability and retention effect	[57]
Poly (*N*-isopropylacrylamide)	Phtalonine	Antitumor effect against EMT-6-mouse mammary tumor	[58]
Poly(L-histidine)-b-PEG-folic acid and poly(L-lactic acid)-b-PEF-folic acid	Doxorubicin	Targeted micelles into the cytosol polyHis was effective because of its fusogenic activity in delivering drug into cytosol	[59]
poly(ethylene glycol)-poly(L-lysine) (PEG-PLL)	DNA	Improved DNA nuclease resistance and stability with increasing molecular weight of PLL block in the block co-polymer	[60]
Vitamin E TPGS and octoxynol-40	Voclosporine	Improved drug delivery to anterior and posterior segment of the eye	[61, 62]
Vitamin E TPGS and octoxynol-40	Dexamethasone		
Vitamin E TPGS and octoxynol-40	Rapamycin		

7.5.2 Critical Micellar Concentration (CMC)

CMC is a characteristic feature that depends on the surfactant or polymer concentration used during the preparation of micelles. The surfactant or polymer concentration that initiates the formation of micelles in the aqueous phase is referred to as CMC. Generally, a low CMC value indicates micelle formation at low polymer or surfactant concentration, and it offers higher stability to the micelle structure [66–68]. CMC can be determined by evaluating various physicochemical changes during micelle formation. Commonly used techniques include surface tension measurement, conductivity, voltammetry, calorimetry, luminescence probe technique, scattering technique, ultraviolet (UV)/Vis, and fluorescence spectroscopy.

7.5.3 Methods for Micelle Preparation

Drug-loaded micelles can be prepared using different procedures depending on the physicochemical properties of the polymer [69]. Five different methods for micelle preparation are available that can be classified into two different categories: direct dissolution and organic solvent method. The direct dissolution process comprises simple equilibrium, dialysis, o/w emulsion, and solution casting methods, whereas the organic solvent process uses the freeze-drying method for micelle preparation (Figure 7.3) [61]. These methods are described in detail in the next section.

TABLE 7.3 List of Surfactant Used for Micelle Preparation

Surfactant Type	Example
Anionic	Sodium dodecyl sulfate (SDS)
Cationic	Dodecyl trimethyl ammonium bromide (DTAB)
Nonionic	*N*-Dodecyl tetra(ethylene oxide)
Zwitterionic	Dioctanoyl phosphatidyl choline

*7.5.3.1 **Simple Equilibrium*** This method is employed for block co-polymers that are moderately hydrophobic such as poloxamers. In this method, drug and co-polymers both are dissolved in the aqueous solvent. Micelle formation is brought by heating the aqueous solution. The application of heat to the aqueous solution dehydrates the core forming segments and ultimately leads to the development of micelles. This method is also applied to the injectable formulations with slight modifications. Both the polymer and the drug are separately dissolved in the injectable aqueous medium. The two solutions are appropriately mixed considering the polymer–drug charge ratio. A combination of appropriate co-polymer-to-drug charge ratio induces micellization in the aqueous solution [70].

*7.5.3.2 **Dialysis*** Dialysis is a slow process that is employed for the separation of mixtures. This method is applied to the amphiphilic block co-polymers that are not readily soluble in the aqueous medium. Both the co-polymer and the drug are separately dissolved in the water-soluble organic solvent. A typical example of organic solvents includes dimethylsulfoxide (DMSO), *N,N*-dimethylformamide (DMF), acetone, acetonitrile, THF, dimethylacetamide, and ethanol [70–72]. The organic mixture containing co-polymer and drug are loaded into the dialysis membrane bag and dialyzed against water. The process involving slow removal of organic solvent by dialysis against water triggers micelle formation [70–72].

*7.5.3.3 **Oil in Water (o/w) Emulsion*** In this method, the drug is physically entrapped through an o/w emulsification

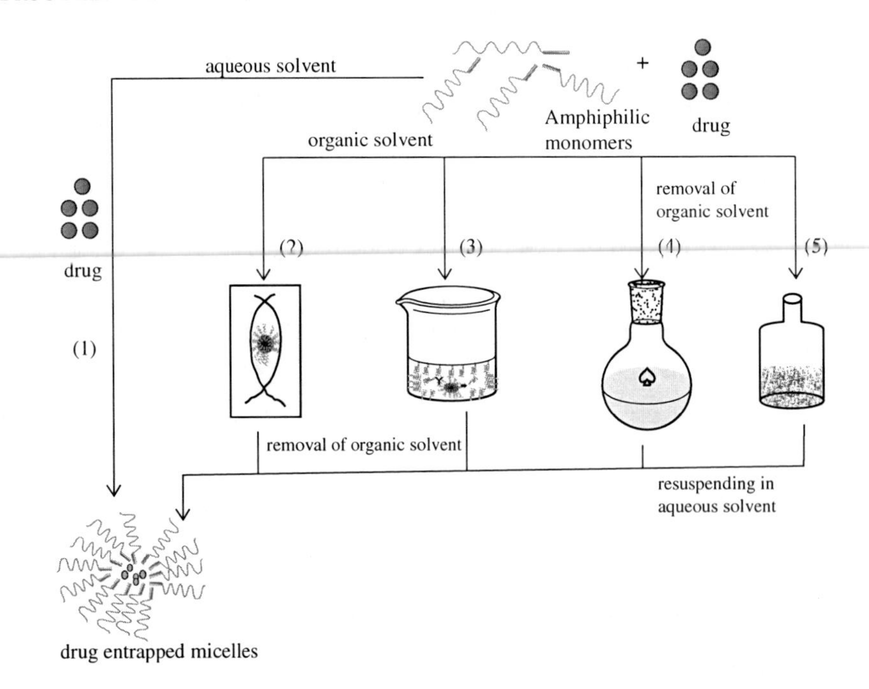

FIGURE 7.3 Pictorial representation of different methods for micelle preparations: (1) simple equilibrium, (2) dialysis, (3) o/w emulsion method, (4) solvent casting, and (5) freeze-drying method.

process. Water-insoluble organic solvents such as dichloromethane and ethyl acetate are used. Both co-polymer and hydrophobic drugs are dissolved in the organic solvent with the addition of some amount of water. Organic solvent is removed by continuous stirring of the mixture. Organic solvent evaporation triggers formation of micelles within aqueous solution. This process assists physical entrapment of hydrophobic drugs in the core of micelles [72].

7.5.3.4 ***Solution Casting*** This method involves the use of organic solvent and heated aqueous solvent. Initially, both polymer and drug are dissolved in the organic solvent to obtain a clear homogenous solution. The organic solvent evaporation causes development of thin polymeric film at the bottom of the container [73]. The evaporation of organic solvent favors polymer–drug interactions. The polymeric thin film is then rehydrated with heated aqueous solvent, which spontaneously develops drug-loaded micelles.

7.5.3.5 ***Freeze Drying*** This is a one-step procedure recently employed for the development of drug-loaded micelles. A mixture of water/tert-butanol (TBA) is used to dissolve the co-polymer and drug. TBA is a water-miscible solvent with high vapor pressure. High vapor pressure accelerates the rate of sublimation, which is helpful in the lyophilization process. The use of excess TBA is found to increase the size of drug-loaded micelles. Therefore, required/low amounts of TBA should be employed in the process. During the freeze drying process, TBA induces the formation of fine ice crystals that rapidly sublime, leaving behind the freeze-dried material. The rehydration of freeze dried cake with an injectable vehicle spontaneously forms drug-loaded polymeric micelles [74].

7.5.4 Advantages

The major advantage of micelles is their simple, easy, and reproducible manufacturing procedure at the small as well as large scale. The monomers can be surface conjugated with a targeting moiety or specific ligand to optimize drug release and achieve specific pharmacological effects because of the targeted delivery [75]. The core forming blocks can accommodate hydrophobic drugs by preventing their exposure to outer aqueous environment. The small size of micelles (5–100 nm) prevents opsonization and subsequent recognition by the macrophages of the reticuloendothelial system. This ultimately causes longer drug circulation and delivery at the desired site [76]. Because of the ability to tailor the hydrophobic and hydrophilic blocks, CMC of the micelle can be reduced up to the millimolar range to improve their stability against dilution. The important advantage of micelles is their ease of sterilization by simple filtration process for safe administration. The inner core or the hydrophobic segment of the micelle can be cross-linked to provide improved stability and delivery [77]. Also, a strong cohesive force of attraction between polymer and drug can confer physical stability to the micelle formulation. Moreover, polymeric micelles with desired release properties can also be prepared to facilitate drug release on biological, environmental, or external stimulation (stimuli-responsive polymeric micelles) [54].

7.5.5 Limitations

Drug-loaded micelle formulations are subjected to extreme dilution on their systemic administration (intravenous injections). Premature drug release, lack of sustained/controlled release, and fragile structure of micelles limits its applications in drug delivery. Another major limitation of micelles is their inability to entrap hydrophilic small as well as macromolecules. Moreover, the application of surfactant micelles in drug delivery is limited by the associated toxicity and tolerability issues. Oral administration of drug-loaded surfactant micelles causes gastric irritation. Intravenous administration of cremophor EL micelle formulation have been found to cause development of biological side effects such as severe anaphylactic hypersensitivity reactions, hyperlipidemia, erythrocyte aggregation, abnormal patterns in lipoprotein structure, and peripheral neuropathy [78–83]. In certain cases, improper hydrophobic drug loading may cause precipitation of drug on administration or dilution with aqueous media. Therefore, careful monitoring of micelle formulation is recommended before administration.

7.6 LIPOSOMES

A liposome is a vesicular structure entirely enclosed by a membraneous lipid bilayer. The basic molecular building block of a typical liposomal membrane is a phospholipid. Phospholipids are built on a glycerol backbone. Phosphorelated molecules are esterified to carbon 3 of the glycerol forming a polar headgroup [e.g., phosphoryl choline (PC), phosphoryl ethanolamine (PE), phosphoryl glycerol (PG), phosphoryl inositol (PI), and phosphoryl serine (PS)]. Fatty acids are esterified to carbon 1 and 2 of the glycerol forming nonpolar tails. Phospholipids are known as polar lipids because the phosphorelated portion is polar or water soluble, whereas fatty acid (saturated or unsaturated) tails of the molecules are nonpolar or fat soluble. In an aqueous environment, phospholipids orient themselves to a thermodynamically stable structure called a bilayer. This flat sheet lipids then curves into a spherical liposomal structure that has no edges. Liposomes can encapsulate both hydrophilic and lipophilic drugs, which are slowly released as liposomes are broken down by enzyme and acids found in tissues and cells especially at the diseased sites [84, 85]. Liposomes can have various molecules attach to their surface. The most common surface modification is pegylation in which PEG can covalently link to the surface of the liposomes. Small pegylated liposomes can circulate in the bloodstream longer than plain liposomes [86, 87]. Antibodies can be attached to the surface of the liposomes for targeting purposes. Many studies have shown that targeting is more effective if the antibody is attached to a spacer arm rather than directly to the liposome surface [88, 89]. Fluorescent liposome can be made by encapsulating fluorescent molecules in the aqueous interior of the liposome or by adding florescent lipid to the bilayer [90, 91]. Liposomes are an important tool for characterizing membrane-associated proteins in the native environment. Liposomes can encapsulate DNA and RNA in their aqueous space for delivery to cells. Another type of liposome containing positive charge lipid such as DOTEP binds negatively charged nucleic acid to its surface through electrostatic interactions. These so-called lipoplexes can be used to deliver nucleic acid to cells. Both liposomes and lipoplexes have been shown to deliver nucleic acid to cells *in vitro* and *in vivo* [92–95].

7.6.1 Liposomes Types

Based on the structural morphology, liposomes can be classified as small unilamellar vesicles (SUVs) or large unilamellar vesicles (LUVs), multilamellar vesicles (MLVs), giant unilamellar vesicles (GUVs) or giant multilamellar vesicles (GMVs), and multivesicular vesicles (MVVs) (Figure 7.4). The bilayers of all MVVs and MLVs have an identical lipid composition, which is their characteristic feature.

7.6.2 Methods for Liposome Preparation

Liposomes are mainly prepared by the passive or active loading method. The passive loading method involves drug loading before or during the liposome formation, whereas drug loading into premade liposomes is known as an active or a remote loading process. The latter process is not widely applicable. Passive drug loading can be performed by mechanical dispersion (thin film hydration or membrane extrusion), solvent dispersion (solvent injection or reversed phase evaporation), or detergent removal method. The selection of the appropriate liposome preparation method can depend on the physicochemical properties of the drug and other constituents. This section summarizes the different liposome preparation methods, their advantages, and their limitations.

7.6.2.1 Mechanical Dispersion Methods

Thin Film Hydration The simplest method for preparing multilamellar liposomes (MLVs) is hydration of dry lipid. The lipid and lipophilic compounds are dissolved in organic solvent, and solvent is removed by rotary evaporation or lyophilization, resulting in a formation of thin lipid film or dried lipid cake, respectively. An aqueous solution containing hydrophilic compounds is then added to the lipid film or cake to hydrate the lipid and must be heated above the phase

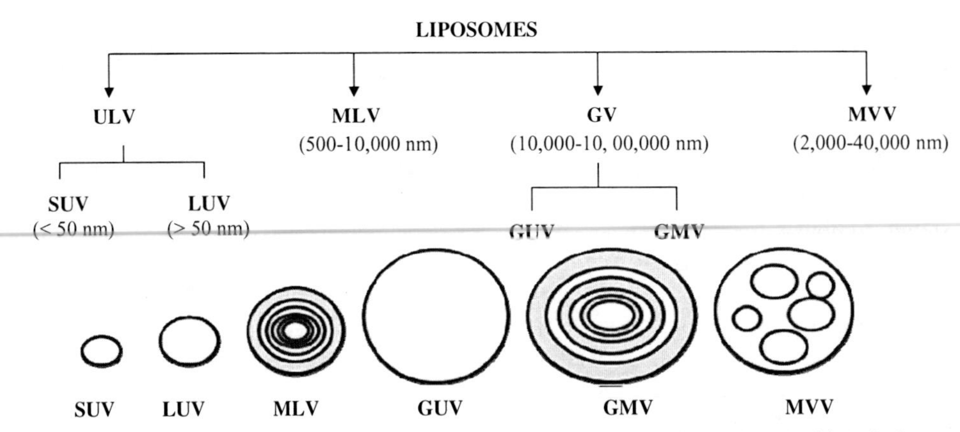

FIGURE 7.4 Classification and pictorial representation of different types of liposomes.

transition of the lipids to form liposomes. The resulting MLVs consist of several concentric lipid bilayers containing lipid-soluble compounds. The entrapment of hydrophilic compound is usually low because of the small captured volume of these MLVs and low aqueous solute penetration across the hydrated bilayer lipid. Repeated freezing and thawing cycles can rupture and reform the MLVs and thereby increase the captured volume of these MLVs because of the increased number of liposomes with fewer lipid layers. These freeze–thaw liposomes can allow higher encapsulation and uniform distribution of aqueous solutes across the hydrated bilayer lipid. Heterogenous size distribution of liposomes is the limitation of the lipid hydration method. Moreover, this process is restricted to only laboratory-scale liposome production [96].

Membrane Extrusion This method can produce liposomes with unimodel size distribution (100-nm range) through membrane-type filters of a fixed pore size. The device used for extrusion must withstand higher internal pressures (up to 1000 psi). Extrusion cannot be performed with standard liquid filtration devices. Larger extruders are pressurized by nitrogen, whereas extruders handling lower volume (<1 mL) can use gas-type syringes to generate pressure manually. Extrusion must be carried out above the phase-transition temperature of the lipids. Liposomes must be passed through the filters multiple times (>10 times) to attain narrow size distribution. The translucent appearance of liposome suspension during the extrusion process indicates the smaller size of the liposomes [97].

7.6.2.2 Solvent Dispersion Methods

Solvent (Ether/Ethanol) Injection In this method, the organic solution (diethyl ether or ethanol) of the lipid is slowly injected into aqueous phase containing water-soluble components and subsequent removal of organic solvent under reduced pressure to form liposomes. The major limitation of this method is the heterogeneous size of the liposomes and the exposure of encapsulated compounds to organic solvents [98, 99].

Reversed Phase Evaporation In this method, lipid and lipophilic components are dissolved in organic solvent and an aqueous component is added to this lipid solution to form water in oil emulsion. This biphasic mixture is then emulsified by high sheer mixing, and organic solvent is evaporated from this emulsion under reduced pressure, forcing the lipid into the aqueous phase where it organizes into liposomes. The temperature of the aqueous phase must be above the phase-transition temperature of the lipid for liposomes to form. Liposome characteristics (size distribution, captured volume, and number of bilayers) can be optimized for particular formulation by systematically varying the process parameters (sovent:water ratio, rate of solvent removal, and size of emulsion particles). Liposomes produced by these methods have a high internal volume/encapsulation efficiency and broad size distribution. Moreover, this process can be used to produce a large volume of liposomes. The major limitation of this process is the heterogeneous size distribution of liposomes, and exposure to organic solvents and sonication may cause denaturation of encapsulated macromolecules or proteins [100].

7.6.2.3 Detergent Removal Method A particular subgroup of surfactants is known as detergents that can solubilize various lipids. Detergents at their CMC can reorganize lipid bilayers to form detergent–lipid aggregates also known as mixed micelles. After removal of detergent, these mixed micelles can spontaneously vesiculate to prepare liposomes.

Various methods to remove detergent in the final processing step include dialysis and gel chromatography. Excellent reproducibility and homogenous size of the liposomes are major advantages of this method. The retention of detergent traces is the main drawback of this process [101].

7.6.3 Advantages

Liposomes can provide selective passive targeting to tumor tissues (liposomal doxorubicin) and can enhance the efficacy and therapeutic index of active drug molecules. Encapsulation of cytotoxic agent inside the liposome offers enhanced drug stability (improved drug circulation) and reduced toxicity. Moreover, liposomes can also offer flexibility to couple site-specific ligands to achieve targeted drug delivery.

7.6.4 Limitations

Although liposomes have great potential, major issues limiting the development of liposomes include stability, batch-to-batch reproducibility, low drug entrapment, and heterogeneous particle size [96].

7.7 CONCLUSION

Nanocarrier systems have gained a lot of popularity in the field of drug delivery systems with great success. These systems have a greater potential for several applications including antitumor therapy, gene therapy, AIDS therapy, radiotherapy, and macromolecule delivery across physiological barriers. The main goals of nanocarriers are to improve drug molecule stability, biodistribution, drug loading, targeting, transport, release, and interaction with biological barriers. Nanocarriers provide distinct advantages regarding drug targeting, delivery, tailor-made release profile, along with diagnosis and therapy. However, there are still major scopes of improvements in the development of efficient nanocarriers and that can be a main concern of future developments. These improvements involve developing nanocarriers that can provide controllable drug release profiles, intelligent drug release devices or bioresponsive triggered systems, and self-regulated delivery systems. Nevertheless, successful nanocarriers will offer new perspectives for the efficient treatment of various diseases.

ASSESSMENT QUESTIONS

7.1. Which of the following is an example of the nanoparticle preparation method by monomer polymerization?

- **a.** Emulsion polymerization
- **b.** Salting out method
- **c.** Nanoprecipitation method
- **d.** None of the above

7.2. List four methods of preparing a nanoparticle from a preformed polymer.

- **a.** Salting out method
- **b.** Single emulsion-solvent evaporation method
- **c.** Double emulsion-solvent evaporation method
- **d.** Emulsification/solvent diffusion

7.3. Define nanoparticles. Mention three main types of nanoparticles.

7.4. Give examples of polymers employed for fabrication of polymeric nanoparticles.

7.5. List five advantages of polymeric nanoparticles.

7.6. List advantages and disadvantages of micelles.

7.7. Define the term "critical micellar concentration."

7.8. What are the different methods of micelle preparations?

7.9. Which one of the following is a Zwitterionic polymer?

- **a.** Dioctanoyl phosphatidyl choline b
- **b.** Dodecyltrimethylammonium bromide (DTAB)
- **c.** Both a and b
- **d.** None of the above

7.10. The process by which the micelles are internalized into cell cytoplasm is__.

- **a.** Passive diffusion
- **b.** Active transport
- **c.** Endocytosis
- **d.** All of the above

7.11. Micelles help to improve the stability of DNA and proteins.

- **a.** True
- **b.** False

7.12. Enlist different types of liposomes.

REFERENCES

1. Ren, Y., Savill, J. (1998). Apoptosis: The importance of being eaten. *Cell Death & Differerentiation*, *5(7)*, 563–568.
2. Devine, D.V., Wong, K., Serrano, K., Chonn, A., Cullis, P.R. (1994). Liposome-complement interactions in rat serum: Implications for liposome survival studies. *Biochimica et Biophysica Acta*, *1191(1)*, 43–51.
3. Perez-Martinez, F.C., Guerra, J., Posadas, I., Cena, V. (2011). Barriers to non-viral vector-mediated gene delivery in the nervous system. *Pharmaceutical Research*, *28(8)*, 1843–1858.

4. Jin, Y. Nanotechnology in pharma-ceutical manufacturing, in S.C. Gad, *Pharma-ceutical Manufacturing Handbook: Production and Processes*, Wiley-Interscience, Hoboken, NJ, 2008, 1264–1265.
5. Sahoo, S.K., Dilnawaz, F., Krishnakumar, S. (2008). Nanotechnology in ocular drug delivery. *Drug Discovery Today, 13 (3–4)*, 144–151.
6. Lockman, P.R., Mumper, R.J., Khan, M.A., Allen, D.D. (2002). Nanoparticle technology for drug delivery across the blood-brain barrier. *Drug Development and Industrial Pharmacy, 28(1)*, 1–13.
7. Cai, W., Chen, K., Li, Z.B., Gambhir, S.S., Chen, X. (2007). Dual-function probe for PET and near-infrared fluorescence imaging of tumor vasculature. *Journal of Nuclear Medicine, 48(11)*, 1862–1870.
8. Thorek, D.L., Chen, A.K., Czupryna, J., Tsourkas, A. (2006). Superparamagnetic iron oxide nanoparticle probes for molecular imaging. *Annals of Biomedical Engineering, 34(1)*, 23–38.
9. Huang, X., Jain, P.K., El-Sayed, I.H., El-Sayed, M.A. (2006). Determination of the minimum temperature required for selective photothermal destruction of cancer cells with the use of immunotargeted gold nanoparticles. *Photochemistry and Photobiology, 82(2)*, 412–417.
10. Grodzinski, P., Silver, M., Molnar, L.K. (2006). Nanotechnology for cancer diagnostics: Promises and challenges. *Expert Review of Molecular Diagnostics, 6(3)*, 307–318.
11. Ferrari, M. (2005). Cancer nanotechnology: Opportunities and challenges. *Nature Reviews Cancer, 5(3)*, 161–171.
12. Luo, C., Wang, Y., Chen, Q., Han, X., Liu, X., Sun, J., He, Z. (2012). Advances of paclitaxel formulations based on nanosystem delivery technology. *Mini Reviews in Medicinal Chemistry, 12(5)*, 434–444.
13. Guarneri, V., Dieci, M.V., Conte, P. (2012). Enhancing intracellular taxane delivery: Current role and perspectives of nanoparticle albumin-bound paclitaxel in the treatment of advanced breast cancer. *Expert Opinion on Pharmacotherapy, 13(3)*, 395–406.
14. Montero, A.J., Adams, B., Diaz-Montero, C.M., Gluck, S. (2011). Nab-paclitaxel in the treatment of metastatic breast cancer: A comprehensive review. *Expert Review of Clinical Pharmacology, 4(3)*, 329–334.
15. Gradishar, W.J., Tjulandin, S., Davidson, N., Shaw, H., Desai, N., Bhar, P., Hawkins, M., O'Shaughnessy, J. (2005). Phase III trial of nanoparticle albumin-bound paclitaxel compared with polyethylated castor oil-based paclitaxel in women with breast cancer. *Journal of Clinical Oncology, 23(31)*, 7794–803.
16. Buyukhatipoglu, K., Chang, R., Sun, W., Clyne, A.M. (2010). Bioprinted nanoparticles for tissue engineering applications. *Tissue Engineering Part C Methods, 16(4)*, 631–642.
17. Thevenot, P., Sohaebuddin, S., Poudyal, N., Liu, J.P., Tang, L. (2008). Magnetic nanoparticles to enhance cell seeding and distribution in tissue engineering scaffolds. *Proceedings IEEE Conference on Nanotechnology, 2008*, 646–649.
18. Wu, T.F., Mei, Z., Pion-Tonachini, L., Zhao, C., Qiao, W., Arianpour, A., Lo, Y.H. (2011). An optical-coding method to measure particle distribution in microfluidic devices. *AIP Advances, 1(2)*, 22155.
19. Han, M., Gao, X., Su, J.Z., Nie, S. (2001). Quantum-dot-tagged microbeads for multiplexed optical coding of biomolecules. *Nature Biotechnology, 19(7)*, 631–635.
20. Cao, Y.C., Jin, R., Nam, J.M., Thaxton, C.S., Mirkin, C.A. (2003). Raman dye-labeled nanoparticle probes for proteins. *Journal of the American Chemical Society, 125(48)*, 14676–14677.
21. Pinto Reis, C., Neufeld, R.J., Ribeiro, A.J., Veiga, F. (2006). Nanoencapsulation I. Methods for preparation of drug-loaded polymeric nanoparticles. *Nanomedicine, 2(1)*, 8–21.
22. Ekambaram, P., Sathali, A.H., Priyanka, K. (2012). Solid lipid nanoparticles: A review. *Scientific Reviews and Chemical Commununications, 2(1)*, 80–102.
23. Cho, E.C., Glaus, C., Chen, J., Welch, M.J., Xia, Y. (2010). Inorganic nanoparticle-based contrast agents for molecular imaging. *Trends in Molecular Medicine, 16(12)*, 561–573.
24. Quintanar-Guerrero, D., Allemann, E., Fessi, H., Doelker, E. (1998). Preparation techniques and mechanisms of formation of biodegradable nanoparticles from preformed polymers. *Drug Development and Industrial Pharmacy, 24(12)*, 1113–1128.
25. Pal S.L., Jana, U., Manna, P.K., Mohanta, G.P. Manavalan, R. (2011). Nanoparticle: An overview of preparation and characterization. *Journal of Applied Pharmaceutical Science, 1 (6)*, 228–234.
26. Bilati, U., Allemann, E., Doelker, E. (2005). Poly(D,L-lactide-co-glycolide) protein-loaded nanoparticles prepared by the double emulsion method–processing and formulation issues for enhanced entrapment efficiency. *Journal of Microencapsulation, 22(2)*, 205–214.
27. Lee, W.K., Park, J.Y., Jung, S., Yang, C.W., Kim, W.U., Kim, H.Y., Park, J.H., Park, J.S. (2005). Preparation and characterization of biodegradable nanoparticles entrapping immunodominant peptide conjugated with PEG for oral tolerance induction. *Journal of Controlled Release, 105(1–2)*, 77–88.
28. Vauthier, C., Bouchemal, K. (2009). Methods for the preparation and manufacture of polymeric nanoparticles. *Pharmaceutical Research, 26(5)*, 1025–1058.
29. Konan, Y.N., Cerny, R., Favet, J., Berton, M., Gurny, R., Allemann, E. (2003). Preparation and characterization of sterile sub-200 nm meso-tetra(4-hydroxylphenyl)porphyrin-loaded nanoparticles for photodynamic therapy. *European Journal of Pharmaceutics and Biopharmaceutics, 55(1)*, 115–124.
30. Quintanar-Guerrero, D., Fessi, H., Allémann, E., Doelker, E. (1996). Influence of stabilizing agents and preparative variables on the formation of poly(-lactic acid) nanoparticles by an emulsification-diffusion technique. *International Journal of Pharmaceutics, 143*, 133–141.
31. Bilati, U., Allemann, E., Doelker, E. (2005). Nanoprecipitation versus emulsion-based techniques for the encapsulation of proteins into biodegradable nanoparticles and process-related stability issues. *AAPS PharmSciTech, 6(4)*, E594–604.

32. Galindo-Rodriguez, S., Allemann, E., Fessi, H., Doelker, E. (2004). Physicochemical parameters associated with nanoparticle formation in the salting-out, emulsification-diffusion, and nanoprecipitation methods. *Pharmaceutical Research, 21(8)*, 1428–1439.

33. Zweers, M.L., Engbers, G.H., Grijpma, D.W., Feijen, J. (2004). *In vitro* degradation of nanoparticles prepared from polymers based on DL-lactide, glycolide and poly (ethylene oxide). *Journal of Controlled Release, 100(3)*, 347–356.

34. Konan, Y.N., Gurny, R., Allemann, E. (2002). Preparation and characterization of sterile and freeze-dried sub-200 nm nanoparticles. *International Journal of Pharmaceutics, 233(1–2)*, 239–252.

35. Reddy, L.H., Murthy, R.R. (2004). Influence of polymerization technique and experimental variables on the particle properties and release kinetics of methotrexate from poly (butylcyanoacrylate) nanoparticles. *Acta Pharmaceutica, 54* (2), 103–118.

36. Puglisi, G., Fresta, M., Giammona, G., Ventura, C.A. (1995). Influence of the preparation conditions on poly(ethylcyanoacrylate) nanocapsule formation. *International Journal of Pharmaceutics, 125*, 283–287.

37. Majuru, S., Oyewumi, M.O. Nanotechnology in drug development and life cycle management, in, Melgardt M.de Villiers, Pornanong Aramwit, and Glen S. Kwon (eds.), *Nanotechnology in Drug Delivery*. Springer, New York, AAPS Press, 2009, pp. 605–606.

38. Fallouh, N.A., Roblot-Treupel, L., Fess, H., Devissaguet, J.P., Puissieux, F. (1986). Development of a new process for the manufacture of polyisobutylcyanoacrylate nanoparticles. *International Journal of Pharmaceutics, 28*, 125.

39. Bouchemal, K., Briancon, S., Perrier, E., Fessi, H., Bonnet, I., Zydowicz, N. (2004). Synthesis and characterization of polyurethane and poly(ether urethane) nanocapsules using a new technique of interfacial polycondensation combined to spontaneous emulsification. *International Journal of Pharmaceutics, 269(1)*, 89–100.

40. Bouchemal, K., Briançon., S., Fessi, H., Chevalier, Y., Bonnet, I., Perrier, E. (2006). Simultaneous emulsification and interfacial polycondensation for the preparation of colloidal suspension of nanocapsules. *Materials Science and Engineering C, 26*, 472–480.

41. Ghosh, I., Vippagunta, R., Li, S., Vippagunta, S. (2012). Key considerations for optimization of formulation and melt-extrusion process parameters for developing thermosensitive compound. *Pharmaceutical Development and Technology, 17(4)*, 502–510.

42. Lander, R., Manger, W., Scouloudis, M., Ku, A., Davis, C., Lee, A. (2000). Gaulin homogenization: A mechanistic study. *Biotechnology Progress, 16(1)*, 80–85.

43. Dingler A, Gohla, S. (2002). Production of solid lipid nanoparticles (SLN): Scaling up feasibilities. *Journal of Microencapsulation, 19(1)*, 11–16.

44. Mukherjee, S., Ray, S., Thakur, R.S. (2009). Solid lipid nanoparticles: A modern formulation approach in drug delivery system. *Indian Journal of Pharmaceutical Sciences, 71(4)*, 349–358.

45. Jahnke, S. The theory of high pressure homogenization, in Rainer H. Muller, Simon Benita, and Bernard H.L. Bohm, *Emulsions and Nanosuspensions for the Formulation of Poorly Soluble Drugs*, Medpharm Scientific Publishers, Stuttgart, Germany, 1998, pp. 177–200.

46. Gohla, S.H., Dingler, A. (2001). Scaling up feasibility of the production of solid lipid nano-particles (SLN). *Pharmazie, 56 (1)*, 61–63.

47. Sjostrom, B., Bergenstahl, B. (1992). Pre-paration of submicron drug particles in lecithin stabilized o/w emulsions. I. Model studies of the precipitation of cholesteryl acetate. *International Journal of Pharmaceutics, 88*, 53–62.

48. Gosselin, P.M., Thibert, R., Preda, M., McMullen, J.N. (2003). Polymorphic properties of micronized carbamazepine produced by RESS. *International Journal of Pharmaceutics, 252(1–2)*, 225–233.

49. Freitas, C., Müllerä, R.H. (1998). Spray-drying of solid lipid nanoparticles (SLN TM). *European Journal of Pharmaceutics and Biopharmaceutics, 46(2)*, 145–151.

50. Cortesi, R., Esposjto, E., Luca, G., Nastruzzi, C. (2002). Production of lipospheres as carriers for bioactive compounds. *Biomaterials, 23(11)*, 2283–2294.

51. Torchilin, V.P. (2007). Micellar nanocarriers: Pharmaceutical perspectives. *Pharmaceutical Research, 24(1)*, 1–16.

52. Jones, M., Leroux, J. (1999). Polymeric micelles - a new generation of colloidal drug carriers. *European Journal of Pharmaceutics and Biopharmaceutics, 48(2)*, 101–111.

53. Aniansson, E.A.G., Wall, S.N., Almgren, M., Hoffmann, H., Kielmann, I., Ulbricht, W., Zana, R., Lang, J., Tondre, C. (1976). Theory of the kinetics of micellar equilibria and quantitative interpretation of chemical relaxation studies of micellar solutions of ionic surfactants. *Journal of Physical Chemistry, 80(9)*, 905–922.

54. Cai, S., Vijayan, K., Cheng, D., Lima, E.M., Discher, D.E. (2007). Micelles of different morphologies--advantages of worm-like filomicelles of PEO-PCL in paclitaxel delivery. *Pharmaceutical Research, 24(11)*, 2099–2109.

55. Alakhov, V.Y., Kabanov, A.V. (1998). Block copolymeric biotransport carriers as versatile vehicles for drug delivery. *Expert Opinion on Investigational Drugs, 7(9)*, 1453–1473.

56. Aliabadi, H.M., Brocks, D.R., Lavasanifar, A. (2005). Polymeric micelles for the solubilization and delivery of cyclosporine A: Pharmacokinetics and biodistribution. *Biomaterials, 26(35)*, 7251–7259.

57. Nishiyama, N., Okazaki, S., Cabral, H., Miyamoto, M., Kato, Y., Sugiyama, Y., Nishio, K., Matsumura, Y., Kataoka, K. (2003). Novel cisplatin-incorporated polymeric micelles can eradicate solid tumors in mice. *Cancer Research, 63(24)*, 8977–8983.

58. Dufresne, M.H., Garrec, D.L., Sant, V., Leroux, J.C., Ranger, M. (2004). Preparation and characterization of water-soluble pH-sensitive nanocarriers for drug delivery. *International Journal of Pharmaceutics, 277(1–2)*, 81–90.

59. Kim, D., Lee, E.S., Park, K., Kwon, I.C., Bae, Y.H. (2008). Doxorubicin loaded pH-sensitive micelle: Antitumoral efficacy against ovarian A2780/DOXR tumor. *Pharmaceutical Research*, *25*(*9*), 2074–2082.
60. Katayose, S., Kataoka, K. (1998). Remarkable increase in nuclease resistance of plasmid DNA through supramolecular assembly with poly(ethylene glycol)-poly(L-lysine) block copolymer. *Journal of Pharmaceutical Sciences*, *87*(2), 160–163.
61. Cholkar, A., Patel, A., Vadlapudi, A.D., Mitra, A.K. (2012). Novel nanomicellar formulation approaches for anterior and posterior segment ocular drug delivery. *Recent Patents on Nanomedicine*, *2*(2), 82–95.
62. Velagaleti, P.R., Anglade, E., Khan, J., Gilger, B.C., Mitra, A. K. (2010). Topical delivery of hydrophobic drugs using a novel mixed nanomicellar technology to treat diseases of the anterior and posterior segments of the eye. *Drug Delivery Technology*, 42–47.
63. Sheng, Y.J., Wang, T.Y., Chen, W.M., Tsao, H.K. (2007). A-B diblock copolymer micelles: Effects of soluble-block length and component compatibility. *Journal of Physical Chemistry B*, *111*(*37*), 10938–10945.
64. Lavasanifar, A., Samuel, J., Kwon, G.S. (2002). Poly(ethylene oxide)-block-poly(L-amino acid) micelles for drug delivery. *Advanced Drug Delivery Reviews*, *54*(2), 169–190.
65. Koo, O.M., Rubinstein, I., Onyuksel, H. (2005). Camptothecin in sterically stabilized phospholipid micelles: A novel nanomedicine. *Nanomedicine*, *1*(*1*), 77–84.
66. Kwon, G.S., Yokoyama, M., Okano, T., Sakurai, Y., Kataoka, K. (1993). Biodistribution of micelle-forming polymer-drug conjugates. *Pharmaceutical Research*, *10*(*7*), 970–974.
67. Slepnev, V.I., Kuznetsova, L.E., Gubin, A.N., Batrakova, E. V., Alakhov, V., Kabanov, A.V. (1992). Micelles of poly (oxyethylene)-poly(oxypropylene) block copolymer (pluronic) as a tool for low-molecular compound delivery into a cell: Phosphorylation of intracellular proteins with micelle incorporated [gamma-32P]ATP. *Biochemistry International*, *26*(*4*), 587–595.
68. Nah, J.W., Cho, C.S. (1998). Norfloxacin release from polymeric micelle of poly(γ benzyl L-glutaate)/poly-(ethyelene oxide)/poly(γ benzyl L-glutamate) block copolymer. *Bulletin of the Korean Chemical Society*, *19*, 962–967.
69. Teagarden, D.L., Baker, D.S. (2002). Practical aspects of lyophilization using non-aqueous co-solvent systems. *European Journal of Pharmaceutical Sciences*, *15*(2), 115–133.
70. Yang, L., Wu, X., Liu, F., Duan, Y., Li, S. (2009). Novel biodegradable polylactide/poly(ethylene glycol) micelles prepared by direct dissolution method for controlled delivery of anticancer drugs. *Pharmaceutical Research*, *26*(*10*), 2332–2342.
71. Cai, L.L., Liu, P., Li, X., Huang, X., Ye, Y.Q., Chen, F.Y., Yuan, H., Hu, F.Q., Du, Y.Z. (2011). RGD peptide-mediated chitosan-based polymeric micelles targeting delivery for integrin-overexpressing tumor cells. *International Journal of Nanomedicine*, *6*, 3499–3508.
72. La, S.B., Okano, T., Kataoka, K. (1996). Preparation and characterization of the micelle-forming polymeric drug indomethacin-incorporated poly(ethylene oxide)-poly(beta-benzyl L-aspartate) block copolymer micelles. *Journal of Pharmaceutical Sciences*, *85*(*1*), 85–90.
73. Mitra, A.K., Velagaleti, P.R., Natesan, S. (2009). Ophthalmic compositions comprising calcineurin inhibitors or mTOR inhibitors. U.S. Patent 2011/0300195 A1.
74. Dufresne, M.H., Fournier, F., Jones, M.C., Ranger, M., Leroux, J.C. (2003). Block copolymer micelles-engineering versatile carriers for drugs and biomacromolecules, in R. Gurny (ed.), *Challenges in Drug Delivery for the New Millennium. Bulletin Technique Gattefosse*, Swiss Federal Institute of Technology Zurich, France, *96*, 87–102.
75. Liu, Y., Sun, J., Cao, W., Yang, J., Lian, H., Li, X., Sun, Y., Wang, Y., Wang, S., He, Z. (2011). Dual targeting folate-conjugated hyaluronic acid polymeric micelles for paclitaxel delivery. *International Journal of Pharmaceutics*, *421*(*1*), 160–169.
76. Lukyanov, A.N., Gao, Z., Mazzola, L., Torchilin, V.P. (2002). Polyethylene glycol-diacyllipid micelles demonstrate increased acculumation in subcutaneous tumors in mice. *Pharmaceutical Research*, *19*(*10*), 1424–1429.
77. Kim, J.O., Kabanov, A.V., Bronich, T.K. (2009). Polymer micelles with cross-linked polyanion core for delivery of a cationic drug doxorubicin. *Journal of Controlled Release*, *138*(*3*), 197–204.
78. Woodburn, K., Kessel, D. (1994). The alteration of plasma lipoproteins by cremophor EL. *Journal of Photochemistry and Photobiology B*, *22*(*3*), 197–201.
79. Windebank, A.J., Blexrud, M.D., de Groen, P.C. (1994). Potential neurotoxicity of the solvent vehicle for cyclosporine. *Journal of Pharmacology and Experimental Therapeutics*, *268*(2), 1051–1056.
80. Adams, J.D., Flora, K.P., Goldspiel, B.R., Wilson, J.W., Arbuck, S.G., Finley, R. (1993). Taxol: A history of pharmaceutical development and current pharmaceutical concerns. *Journal of the National Cancer Institute Monographs*, *15*, 141–147.
81. Kongshaug, M., Cheng, L.S., Moan, J., Rimington, C. (1991). Interaction of cremophor EL with human plasma. *International Journal of Biochemistry*, *23*(*4*), 473–478.
82. Huttel, M.S., Schou Olesen, A., Stoffersen, E. (1980). Complement-mediated reactions to diazepam with Cremophor as solvent (Stesolid MR). *British Journal of Anaesthesia*, *52*(*1*), 77–79.
83. Watkins, J., Milford, W.A., Appleyard, N. (1977). Adverse reactions to intravenous anaesthetic induction agents. *British Medical Journal*, *2*(*6094*), 1084–1085.
84. Alberts, B., Johnson, A., Lewis, J., et al. *Molecular Biology of the Cell*, 4th edition. Garland Science, New York, 2002, Ch. 10. Available from: http://www.ncbi.nlm.nih.gov/books/NBK26871/.
85. Wagner, A., Vorauer-Uhl, K. (2011). Liposome technology for industrial purposes. *Journal of Drug Delivery*, 591325.
86. Huwyler, J., Drewe, J., Krähenbuhl, S. (2008). Tumor targeting using liposomal antineoplastic drugs. *International Journal of Nanomedicine*, *3*(*1*), 21–29.
87. Makwana, K., Tandel, H. (2012). Design and characterization of anionic PEGylated liposomal formulation loaded with

paclitax for ovarian cancer. *Journal of Pharmacy and Bioallied Sciences*, *4* (Suppl 1), S17–S18.

88. Schnyder, A., Huwyler, J. (2005). Drug transport to brain with targeted liposomes. *NeuroRx*, *2(1)*, 99–107.
89. Bendas, G. (2001). Immunoliposomes: A promising approach to targeting cancer therapy. *BioDrugs*, *15(4)*, 2152–24.
90. Mitchell, N., Kalber, T.L., Cooper, M.S., Sunassee, K., Chalker, S.L., Shaw, K.P., Ordidge, K.L., Badar, A., Janes, S.M., Blower, P.J., Lythgoe, M.F., Hailes, H.C., Tabor, A.B. *Biomaterials*, *S0142-9612(12)*, 01093–9.
91. Strieth, S., Dunau, C., Kolbow, K., Knuechel, R., Michaelis, U., Ledderose, H., Eichhorn, M.E., Strelczyk, D., Tschiesner, U., Wollenberg, B., Dellian, M. (2012). Phase I clinical study of vascular targeting fluorescent cationic liposomes in head and neck cancer. *European Archives of Oto-Rhino-Laryngology*, Sep 27.
92. Martino, S., di Girolamo, I., Tiribuzi, R., D'Angelo, F., Datti, A., Orlacchio, A. (2009). *Journal of Biomedicine and Biotechnology*, 410260.
93. Tros de Ilarduya, C., Sun, Y., Düzgüneş, N. (2010). Gene delivery by lipoplexes and polyplexes. *European Journal of Pharmaceutical Sciences*, *40(3)*, 159–170.
94. Smyth Templeton, N. (2002). Liposomal delivery of nucleic acids in vivo. *DNA and Cell Biology*, *21(12)*, 857–867.
95. Immordino, M.L., Dosio, F., Cattel, L. (2006). Stealth liposomes: Review of the basic science, rationale, and clinical applications, existing and potential. *International Journal of Nanomedicine*, *1(3)*, 297–315.
96. Sharma, U.S., Sharma, A. (1997). Liposomes in drug delivery: Progress and limitations. *International Journal of Pharmaceutics*, *154*, 123–140.
97. Olson, F., Hunt, C.A., Szoka, F.C., Vail, W.J., Papahadjopoulos, D. (1979). Preparation of liposomes of defined size distribution by extrusion through polycarbonate membranes. *Biochimica Biophysica Acta*, *557(1)*, 9–23.
98. Batzri, S., Korn, E.D. (1973). Single bilayer liposomes prepared without sonication. *Biochimica Biophysica Acta*, *298(4)*, 1015–1019.
99. Deamer, D.W. (1978). Preparation and properties of ether-injection liposomes. *Annals of the New York Academy of Sciences*, *308*, 250–258.
100. Szoka, F.Jr, Papahadjopoulos, D. (1978). Procedure for preparation of liposomes with large internal aqueous space and high capture by reverse-phase evaporation. *Proceedings of the National Academy of Sciences*, *75(9)*, 4194–4198.
101. Schubert, R. (2003). Liposome preparation by detergent removal. *Methods in Enzymology*, *367*, 46–70.

8

STIMULI-RESPONSIVE TARGET STRATEGIES

CHI H. LEE

8.1 CHAPTER OBJECTIVES

- This chapter reviews the current status and possible future directions in the emerging area of stimuli-responsive advanced carriers with primary attention on the development and evaluation of core shell microparticles as a prototype system.
- Advances in the understanding of the molecular mechanisms of pathological onset along with the novel micro- or nanoparticle technologies should offer various opportunities in development of novel stimuli-responsive delivery systems, which have the potential to enhance the efficacy of existing therapeutic agents at target sites and simultaneously reduce adverse effects in normal tissues.
- Advanced formulations including nano- and microparticles have been exploited as a promising vehicle for stimuli-responsive targeting. Properties like low host response, resistance to degradation, higher expression in target tissue, and rapid elimination after binding significantly contribute to stimuli-responsive targeting efficacy.
- Stimuli-responsive formulations were designed based on both physiological factor and target ligand approaches toward host cells.
  - (i) Physiological-based approaches involve variables, such as pH, temperature, and magnetism, whereas target ligands include monoclonal antibody, peptide, polysaccharide, and transporter.
  - (ii) In target-ligand-based approaches, advanced formulations are linked with stimuli-responsive moieties, such as disease-specific ligands, peptides, or monoclonal antibodies, which offer high affinity and targeting accuracy.
- A combination of advanced formulations and targeting ligands serves as an attractive and challenging therapeutic strategy against tumor or infected diseases.

8.2 INTRODUCTION

One of the major issues of the conventional therapy against tumor or infected diseases is lack of target specificity, which usually lowers drug treatment efficacy. A few organs like the brain, eye, vagina, and fetus have barriers that hinder the accumulation or penetration of the active moiety or therapeutic compounds usually distributed uniformly within the human body [1]. Moreover, the intestinal lining, liver, kidney, and body fluids have enzymes that can inactivate therapeutic agents [2]. As a result, therapeutic agents should be administered at high doses to achieve sufficient concentrations at the target sites. Therefore, one of the important goals of drug therapy lies in enhancement of targeting

Advanced Drug Delivery, First Edition. Edited by Ashim K. Mitra, Chi H. Lee, and Kun Cheng.

efficacy and controlled release of the therapeutic agents to the infected site.

Proteomics and genomics continue to uncover molecular signatures that are unique to infected diseases [3]. Most pathologically defected tissues have affected uptake, detoxification, and efflux of exogenous compounds and their carriers [4]. Overexpression of receptors, antibodies, enzymes, polysaccharides, and vascular system are a few examples of pathologically evolved upnormality [5]. Within a solid defected cell, delivered particles encounter a phenomenon known as the binding site barrier, in which particles tend to bind to cells at the periphery of the infected mass, reducing further diffusion within the cell [6]. Transporter expression [7] and heterogeneity of the infected cell contribute to the low efficacy of the administered drug [8]. High vascular pressure, downregulation of receptors, and absence of lymphatic system further obscure the targeting efficiency [9].

The efficient delivery of the drug to the target tissue depends on the chemical and physical properties of the conjugate as well as on the pathological conditions of the tissue environment [10]. The target delivery may reduce variance or unsuccessful treatment outcome from pharmacogenomic differences of individual patients. Physiological impairment includes a decrease in nutrients and O_2 supply and accumulation of cellular metabolites [11]. Pathological abnormalities like hypoxia, lower pH, and depletion of nutrients are the utilized strategies for enhancement of the pharmacological efficacy through modulating the physical affinity of the carrier systems. Thus, the advanced delivery systems that are responsive to physiological stimulus and simultaneously release the impregnated drug seem to be an ideal approach for enhancement of target specificity [12].

The targeting and controlled release strategies used in chemotherapy were designed based on both physiological factors and target ligand approaches toward pathological organs or tissues. Physiological factors include variables, such as pH, temperature, and magnetism, whereas target ligands include monoclonal antibody, peptide, polysaccharide, and transporter/receptor as their approaches [13]. To date, polymeric formulations intended for target therapy are classified into two strategic pathways: passive and active targeting. Passive targeting involves with localized accumulation of polymeric nanoparticles preferentially in infected tissues by enhanced permeation and retention effects (PREs) of malignant vessels compared with healthy vessels [14, 15]. Passive targeting formulations have stimuli-responsive properties related to mostly physiological variables including pH and temperature, whereas active targeting formulations are involved with numerous biological ligands or chemical ligands that specifically bind to overexpressed receptors in the tumor region [16].

Most studies on active targeting have focused on surface coupling of the novel formulations for enhancement of therapeutic efficacy and/or diagnostic purposes. Nanoparticles with a size of 5 to 250 nm are considered an optimal system for target delivery because of their size, allowing for passive accumulation in target sites because of their ability to carry multiple compounds. Therapies using targeted drug delivery consist of coupling a monoclonal antibody or other high-affinity ligands to deliver conjugated highly potent active pharmaceutical ingredients (HPAPIs) to targeted cells expressing disease-associated biomarkers as in the case of cancer [17]. Various moieties have been examined as targeting ligands including vitamins [18], carbohydrates [19], aptamers [20, 21], peptides (e.g., Arg-Gly-Asp, allatostatin, and **trans**-activating transcriptional activator) [22–25], and proteins (e.g., lectins [26] and transferrin [27, 28]). The active target ability of the nano-carrier systems is dependent on the characteristics of the conjugated ligands [29]. In a conjugated form, a drug exhibits more selective cytotoxicity, thereby sparing nontarget cells from many of the toxic effects [5].

As an example application of this strategy, core shell microparticles consisting of phenethyl isothiocyanate (PEITC) loaded solid-lipid particles and chitosan-based outer shell and folate receptors were developed for chemotherapeutic means, and their target efficacies were demonstrated through the evaluation process.

8.3 PHYSIOLOGICAL-FACTOR-BASED TARGETING FORMULATIONS

Stimuli-sensitive polymers that respond to external variables are of great interest in development of targeting formulations. Physiological factors have affected the targeting efficacy of formulations with stimuli-responsive properties through mechanical changes, such as shape and surface characteristics [30], reversible solubility control [31], and reversible self-assembly into polymeric micelles or vesicles [32].

Formulations made of externally responsive polymers have been developed as drug delivery systems [33–35] as well as for utility in the tissue engineering field [36, 37] based on a variety of types and changes of stimuli, such as pH [38, 39], temperature [40–43], radio frequency [44], or magnetic field [45–49]. Also, modulations in ionic strength, which causes a change in the swelling inside the formulations, and enzyme immobilized radicals have emerged as additional physiological components for stimuli-sensitive advanced carriers [49].

8.3.1 pH-Sensitive Targeting

Most infection sites including tumors seem to have acidic extracellular pH. Angiogenic deficiencies in large tumors cause nutritional insufficiency as a result of inadequate vascularization, which subsequently causes hypoxia and leads to compensative glycolysis [50]. Acidic by-products are produced in cytoplasm as a compensated function of mitochondrial enzymes. To maintain near-normal cytosolic pH, the cell exports protons, causing the surrounding micro-environment to be acidic by at least 0.5 pH units [51]. Considered collectively, this consequence elucidates the crucial importance of pH regulation in the drug targeting process.

(1) *Combinations of polymers:* Polyacrylic acid (PAA) in aqueous solutions are less viscose and acidic in nature and transformed into gels as the pH increases [52]; PAA has demonstrated a long duration of action mainly as a result of the high yield stress that governs the shearing action *in vivo*. pH-sensitive, PAA-based polymers seem to be suited for protein/peptide delivery through intravenous or ophthalmic or mucosal route. An addition of hydroxypropyl methylcellulose (HPMC) affected the rheological properties of aqueous solutions containing PAA in a pH-dependent manner. PAA in the presence of HPMC formed a low-viscosity liquid at pH 4.0 and transformed into stiff gels with a plastic rheological behavior and comparable viscosities at the pH to 7.4 [53], which will be suitable as a liquid delivery system for chemotherapeutic application.

The synthesized polymers conjugated with galactose as a target moiety was introduced to encapsulate paclitaxel for hepatocyte target delivery [54]. The mixture in a combination of pH- and temperature-sensitive co-polymer of *N*-isopropylacrylamide, *N*,*N*-dimethylacrylamide, and 10-undecenoic acid self-assembled in aqueous medium. The hydrophilicity of undecenoic acid rendered the polymer pH-sensitive property. In the target hepatocyte cell line, the stimuli-responsive particles released ~100% of the drug within 24 hours at a pH of 5.0 under 37°C, thus, achieving significantly more toxicity than the non-stimuli-responsive particles as well as the nontargeted particles.

To optimize the polymeric drug delivery system for chemotherapy, a pH-sensitive polymeric carrier, poly(vinylpyrrolidone-co-dimethylmaleic anhydride) (PVD), was prepared through radical synthesis with vinylpyrrolidone and 2,3-dimethylmaleic anhydride under the slightly basic conditions (pH 8.5) [55]. PVD was able to gradually release a native form of drugs, such as Adriamycin with full activity, from the conjugates in response to changes in pH, suggesting that PVD is an effective polymeric carrier for chemotherapy.

Poly(*N*-isopropylacrylamide) (PNIPAM) undergoes a globule transition from a coil when pH is low, allowing for a rapid erosion of the particle, thereby releasing the therapeutic agent [56]. Poly (ethylene oxide)-modified poly(b-amino ester) [57] and diblock co-polymer, poly(methacryloyl sulfadimethoxine) (PSD)-block-PEG (PSD-b-PEG) [58], are a few examples of the pH-sensitive polymers used to encapsulate anticancer drugs.

(2) *Addition of a pH-sensitive functional group: p*-nitrophenyl acrylate (NPA). One of the promising strategies to achieve new synthetic devices with enhanced stimuli-responsive sensitivity and targeting ligands is the chemical fictionalization of nanodevices such as microgels and nanoparticles. *p*-nitrophenyl acrylate (NPA) is an active ester molecule with a group that can be easily cleavaged by the nucleophilic attack of species including amines. This modification consists of an easy chemical reaction that leads to numerous types of functionalized microgels, which are originally made up of NPA as one of their constituent monomers [59].

Microgels made of *p*-nitrophenyl acrylate (NPA)-co-methacrylamide (MeAM) were further modified with two different pyridine derivatives, 2-aminomethylpyridine (2-AMP) and 2-aminopyridine (2-AP), to obtain pH-sensitive microgels with acid pH swelling capacity [60]. The swelling behavior of pH-sensitive microgels was influenced by various physicochemical factors, such as co-polymer composition, accessibility of pendant pyridine groups, and ionic strength. The reaction of these microgels with a linker molecule, monoprotected diamines, makes it easier to attach folic acid molecules, producing folate–microgel conjugates, which subsequently demonstrated its effectiveness for the controlled release in tumors, where the pH is slightly more acid than physiologic pH.

(3) *Sulfonamide:* Several pH-sensitive polymers with the greatest potential of biological applications use weak acid sulfonamide as a trigger for extracellular delivery of exogenous compounds. Sulfonamides derived from *p*-aminobenzenesulfonamide (**1**, Figure 8.1) display pK_a values between 5.0 and 7.4 [61]. Sulfonamide units can be incorporated into the polymer network either by coupling the amine group on the sulfonamide with a polymer functional group such as –COOH or –COCl or by producing polymerizable sulfonamide monomers (**2**, Figure 8.1).

The pH-sensitive polymers were derived from the co-polymerization reaction of sulfonamide-based monomers with water-soluble units, such as acrylamide or acrylic acid monomers. The polymer produced from the radical copolymerization of *N*,*N*-

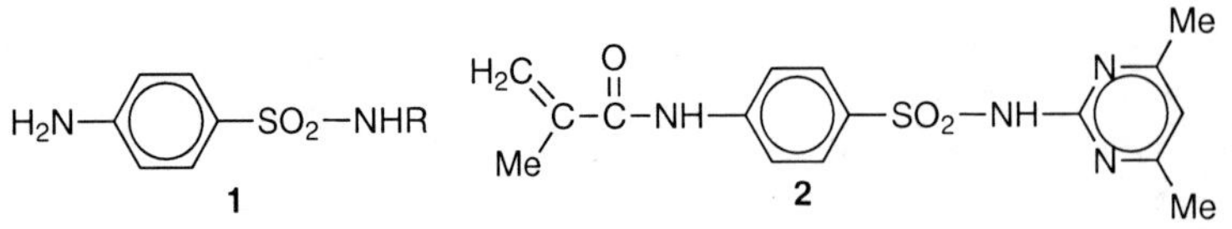

H_2N–C₆H₄–SO_2–NHR (1) H_2C=C(Me)–C(=O)–NH–C₆H₄–SO_2–NH–(dimethylpyrimidinyl) (2)

FIGURE 8.1 *p*-Aminobenzenesulfonamide (**1**) and sulfonamide monomers (**2**).

dimethylacrylamide (DMAA) and a sulfamethazine monomer (SAM, 2) can accommodate a wide ratio of monomer units with SAM/DMAA of 2.5:97.5 to 90:10. The changes in solubility and swelling were found to be dependent on the co-polymer composition and sulfonamide derivative used. When sulfonamide (as a weak acid) was deprotonated upon acidification, the micelle collapsed and was no longer solvated, implying that collapsed nanoparticles with doxorubicin were accumulated in the tumor tissue and subsequently taken up by the cells [62].

(4) *Dimethyl maleic anhydride:* Dimethyl maleic anhydride (Figure 8.2) is a pH-sensitive monomer functional group that has been introduced into the polymer like poly lactic glycolic acid. It is a pH-reversible protective agent popularly used in amino groups in proteins [63, 64]. Dimethyl maleic anhydride at over pH 8 forms an amide bond through its acid anhydride and can reversibly dissociate from the protein at below pH 7. This monomer or polymer modifier when co-polymerized with a polymer of interest can make the polymer pH-sensitive co-block polymer. Conjugates of dimethyl maleic anhydride provide higher accumulation in the tumor cells and extend a drug half-life as compared with unconjugated drugs.

The polyconjugate was constructed for hepatocyte delivery of siRNA by linking the siRNA payload to an amphipathic poly(vinyl ether) through a disulfide linkage [65]. The siRNA–polymer conjugate was reversibly modified with maleic anhydride derivatives synthesized from carboxy dimethylmaleic anhydride containing PEG or *N*-acetylgalactosamine (NAG) groups [66]. PEG enhances solubility and reduces nonspecific interactions, thus, preventing nonaggregating of the resulting siRNA polyconjugate under physiological conditions, whereas the NAG ligand allows for hepatocyte targeting. Dynamic PolyConjugate technology demonstrated effective knockdown of two endogenous genes in mouse liver: apolipoprotein B (*apoB*) and peroxisome proliferator-activated receptor alpha (*ppara*), causing clear phenotypic changes that included a significant reduction in serum cholesterol and increased fat accumulation in the liver.

(5) *PEGylation:* PEGylation is the process of covalent attachment of polyethylene glycol polymer chains to a drug or therapeutic protein. PEGylation is routinely achieved by incubation of a reactive derivative of polyethylene glycol (PEG, as shown in Figure 8.3) with the target macromolecule [67]. The covalent attachment of PEG to a drug or therapeutic protein can protect the agent from the host's immune system and increase the hydrodynamic size of the agent [68].

Poly(L-histidine)-*b*-PEG in combination with PLLA-*b*-PEG was used for an extracellular tumor targeting of adriamycin. This system displayed a very sharp transition from nonionized (nonprotonated) and hydrophobic status at pH 7.4, where the mixed micelles are stable, to ionized and destabilized micelle at about pH 6.6, at which adriamycin is rapidly released from the micelles [69].

Subsequently, a pH-sensitive, mixed-micelle system made of PEG-detachable co-polymers and conjugated with folic acid is prepared to circumvent multidrug resistance (MDR) in cancer cells. The micelles are composed of poly(histidine (His)-co-phenylalanine (Phe))-b-(PEG) and poly(L-lactic

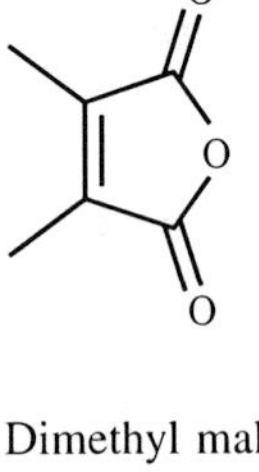

FIGURE 8.2 Dimethyl maleic anhydride.

HO–(CH_2CH_2OCH_2CH_2)$_n$–OH

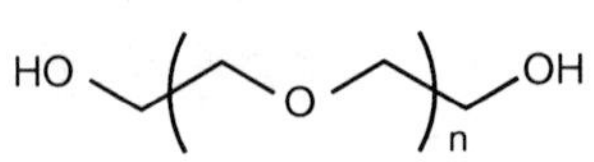

FIGURE 8.3 Polyethylene glycol (PEG).

acid) (PLLA)-b-PEG-folate. The pH sensitivity of the hydrophobic block micelles was controlled by the co-polymer composition and adjusted to early endosomal pH by blending PLLA(3K)-b-PEG(2K)-folate in the presence of a basic anticancer drug, doxorubicin (DOX) [70]. *In vitro* tests showed that a mixed-micelle system composed of poly(His-co-Phe (16 mol%))-b-PEG (80 wt%) and PLLA-b-PEG-folate (20 wt%) targeted early endosomal pH effectively killed both wild-type sensitive (A2780) and DOX-resistant ovarian MDR cancer-cell lines (A2780/DOX(R)) through an instantaneous high dose of DOX in the cytosol. A mixed-micelle system displayed active internalization, accelerated DOX release triggered by endosomal pH, and accomplished an endosomal membranes disruption.

PEG-detachable polyplex micelles based on disulfide-linked block catiomers and PEGylated liposomes modified with a fibronectin-mimetic peptide were effective as bioresponsive nonviral gene vectors [71] or colon-cancer-specific targeting carriers [72], respectively.

8.3.2 Temperature-Sensitive Targeting

Hyperthermia therapy is a type of medical treatment in which body tissue is exposed to high temperatures to damage and kill cancer cells or to make cancer cells more sensitive to the effects of radiation and certain anticancer drugs [73]. Hyperthermia is usually applied with conventional therapies, so it is normally used as an adjuvant therapy. When combined with radiation therapy, it is called thermoradiography. For instance, the thermosensitive nanoparticles show a slow release rate in the body temperature at a normal site, whereas they show large cumulative release at a tumor site by local hyperthermia at about 40–44°C.

As heating or cooling allows a reversible switch between the different forms of aggregation, the co-polymers with both upper critical solution temperature (UCST) and lower critical solution temperature (LCST) are suitable for thermosensitive formulations. Polymers with tunable LCST like pNIPAm are soluble in aqueous solution below their LCST through hydrogen bonding with water molecules, but they become dehydrated and insoluble when heated above the LCST, resulting in abrupt phase separation as shown in Figure 8.4 [74]. Any transition from soluble to emulsion or vice versa (at a given concentration) should be denoted as transition temperature T_{tr}. However, if a phase transition of some polymers like pNIPAm is independent of the concentration or molecular weight, then the T_{tr} at any given concentration is almost identical to the LCST [75]. As the mechanisms and driving forces for the conformational variation in response to external stimuli are unique for each polymer, thermosensitive formulations should be prepared using a proper polymer or a polymer mixture based on targeting priority.

(1) *Combinations of polymers:* Various polymers or their combinations have served as the formulation bases for temperature-responsive targeting of exogenous compounds. Temperature-sensitive formulations including hydrogels are well known for swelling and shrinking reversibly in response to varying environmental temperatures [76, 77]. Further modification of the basic structure by co-polymerization or modulation of hydrophobicity/hydrophilicity has led to the production of suitable thermo-responsive smart materials that have numerous applications.

    Poly(*N*-isopropylacrylamide) (pNIPAAm) synthesized from NIPAM is the most well-known thermosensitive polymer that is also sensitive to pH. It forms a three-dimensional hydrogel when crosslinked with *N,N′*-methylene-bis-acrylamide (MBAm) or *N,N′*-cystamine-bis-acrylamide (CBAm). The polymer exhibits an LCST at 32°C and is soluble below its LCST, but it precipitates above LCST as a result of the reversible formation and cleavage of the hydrogen bonds between –NH and C=O groups of pNIPAAm chains and the surrounding water molecules adjacent to the hydrophobic molecular groups of pNIPAAm [77].

    Prototype polymers with LCST are made up of the combination of poly(*N*-isopropylacrylamide) (pNIPAAm) and *N,N*-diethylacrylamide [78], the combination of methylvinylether and *N*-vinylcaprolactam as monomers [79], or the combination of acrylamide and acrylic acid [80]. Several block co-polymers or polymer conjugates, such as PEO-*b*-PPO-*b*-PEO and PEG-*b*-PLGA-*b*-PEG [81], folate-conjugated thermoresponsive block co-polymers [41], and poly(2-(dimethylamino)ethyl methacrylate-based polymers [82], demonstrated excellent temperature-sensitive properties as well as targeting efficacy.

(2) *pNIPAAm as the strategy of molecular imprinting:* pNIPAAm has been the focus of continuous work and has been applied to the strategy of molecular imprinting, which is a rapidly developing technique for the preparation of the memory template in polymers having a high affinity for a target molecule. A novel temperature-sensitive polymer was developed based on methacrylic acid (MAA), which was chosen to be the functional monomer to recognize the target molecule L-pyroglutamic acid, whereas *N*-isopropylacrylamide (NIPAAm) was chosen to be the temperature-sensitive monomer. A novel

temperature-sensitive imprinted polymer allowed for swelling and shrinking of the gels in response to temperature changes and subsequently released L-pyroglutamic acid [40].

The polymer–biomolecule conjugates made of poly(*N*-isopropylacrylamide) and encapsulated within erythrocyte ghosts made of autologous red blood cells were also used as a temperature-responsive formulation [42]. The manipulation of target proteins inside the cells was demonstrated with polymer–biomolecule conjugates and fusion of differentially labeled erythrocyte ghosts. The properties of such materials to alter the functionality of proteins actively render molecular imprinting and tailoring modes of interference with cellular events.

(3) *Temperature-sensitive liposome:* Liposome has been a popular formulation for various targeting delivery compounds [83, 84]. pNIPAAm incorporated into the membrane of liposome exhibited its thermosensitive responses and enhanced the targeting efficacy of gel formulations [85, 43].

Recently, the Phillips Research Institution [86] successfully developed temperature-sensitive liposomes (TSLs) for delivery of doxorubicin (Adriamycin) to tumor sites (Figure 8.4). The liposomes are stable at a normal body temperature (37°C), stop their drug payload from diffusing into the blood, and therefore exhibit minimal toxicity. The liposomes became leaky and released doxorubicin at the target area as environmental temperatures increased to 42°C by a site-specific heating process using a high-intensity focused ultrasound (HIFU) beam.

8.4 MAGNETIC TARGETING PARTICLES

8.4.1 Sources of Magnetic Response

One approach to overcoming the difficulties in response-based targeting of drugs involves the use of magnetic particles conjugated with various targeting molecules. Magnetic particles offer advantages over conventional drug formulations, localizing targeted agents at the target site and minimizing their systemic circulation [87]. Electromagnets positioned outside the body use electricity to create a temporary on and off magnetic field, which causes magnetic particles to be aggregated, creating areas of non-magnetic holding as the magnetic field is gradually removed as a result of slow degradation. As all alive cells are electrical, that is, the outside of a cell has a negative charge and the inside has a positive charge, this combination of opposite charges allows the cell to function normally and affect the efficacy of magnetic particles. The sustained concentrations at target sites over time supported the importance of magnetic field strength on the tissue distribution of magnetic particles.

Metal ion, Fe_3O_4, is the primary candidate for noncovalent surface modification of nanoparticles, which still has limitations for biological applications because the exposed metal ion on the surface of nanoparticles can produce metal elemental toxicities [88]. Silica (SiO_2) was introduced for surface modification of MNPs because it is a good biocompatible material and is resistant to decomposition *in vivo* [89]. By virtue of magnetic properties, these nanoparticles could serve as a vehicle for the transport of target molecules into cells, while the fluorescent target ligand allows for simultaneous optical detection. The advanced fabrication and surface engineering of the super paramagnetic iron oxide nanoparticles (SPIONs) approach were adapted for

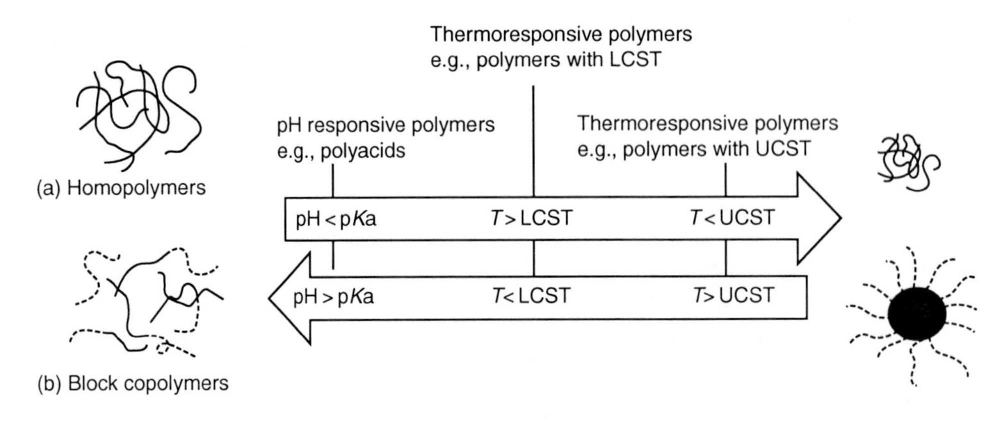

FIGURE 8.4 Conformational changes of polymeric responsive systems with pH and temperature: (a) homopolymers and (b) block co-polymers; solid line, responsive block; dotted line, hydrophilic block [74].

cancer diagnosis and chemotherapy with a main focus on identification and development of nanocarriers by potential malignancy-targeting ligands [90].

Along with the magnetic systems using uncharged particles, those with bioadhesive cationic microspheres achieved an enhanced particle retention time at the target site [91]. Cationic magnetic microspheres have been hypothesized to bind electrostatically with anionic glycosaminoglycans (GAGs) on the luminal surface of the capillary endothelial cells as well as of the tumor cells. A novel cationic bioadhesive magnetic microsphere, magnetic aminodextran microsphere (MADM), was introduced and shown to be endocytized *in vitro* to a greater extent by rat glioma-2 (RG-2) cells than neutral magnetic dextran particles (MDM). These cationic particles were intended to target a brain tumor selectively *in vivo*, delivering the drug at a brain tumor with a significantly greater amount than neutral MDM particles [92].

8.4.2 Application of Magnetic Targeting Particles

Magnetic particles were introduced to deliver cytotoxic drugs (i.e., doxorubicin), achieving a distinctive remission at the sarcomas as compared with no remission in the control group of rats without magnetic targeting, even though the control was administered with the ten times greater dose. It was also demonstrated that transfection efficacy of astrocytes loaded in magnetic nanoparticles (MNPs) was enhanced by static and oscillating magnetic fields [93]. The magnetic-mediated technique has demonstrated its targeting efficacy through numerous animal models including swine [94], rabbits [95], and rats [96, 97].

Preclinical models using magnetic drug delivery systems showed enhanced target selectivity and efficacy in varying tumors including a brain tumor [98]. Magnetic particles were employed to target cytotoxic drugs to brain tumors that have been a challenging task as a result of the presence of the blood–brain barrier. It was demonstrated that a significantly higher amount of magnetic particles was captured at the tumor site using a locally applied magnetic field and concentrated at the site of intra-cerebral rat glioma-2 (RG-2) tumors than nonmagnetic particles [97], supporting the usefulness of magnetic particles in drug delivery to various sites including a brain tumor.

8.4.3 Theranostic Approach of Magnetic Response

Magnetic nanaoparticles were used as cellular tracking or identification of receptors or protein separation. The development of novel nanosystems that synergistically incorporate multiple functionalities including targeting and imaging properties is considered an ideal means to deliver simultaneously traditional therapeutic drugs as well as imaging agents [99]. This new approach is emerging as "theranostic," which entails the efficient integration of therapeutic and diagnostic moieties into a single nanosystem to obtain improved detection, site-specific treatment, and longitudinal monitoring [100].

The immobilization of polyinosinic-polycytidylic acid [poly(IC)] on γ-Fe_2O_3 magnemite nanoparticles made of a multifunctional polymer via the phosphor-amidate route and coupled with dsRNA was used to visualize the Toll-like (TLR3) receptors in the Caki-1 cell line [101]. A flow-through quartz crystal microbalance (QCM) immunoassay method developed using aflatoxin B_1 antibody (anti-AFB_1)-functionalized magnetic core-shell Fe_3O_4/SiO_2 composite nanoparticles (bionanoparticles) has added to the evidence that the QCM immunoassay system was simple and rapid without multiple labeling and separation steps [102].

Monodisperse magnetic nanoparticles conjugated with virus-surface-specific antibodies self-assemble in the presence of specific viral particles and create supramolecular structures with enhanced magnetic properties, which enables them to detect adenovirus-5 and herpes simplex virus-1 at concentrations of 5 viral particles/10 μL [103]. A novel gold nanoshell–based complex (nanocomplex) intended for multipurpose applications, such as targeting, dual modal imaging, and photothermal therapy, was developed [104]. The results of immunofluorescence staining and magnetic resonance imaging studies demonstrated that nanocomplex–anti-HER2 conjugates not only bind to ovarian cancer OVCAR3 cells as compared with the control but also selectively destructed cancer cells through photothermal ablation.

The self-assembled manganese(III)-labeled nanobialys is a toroidal-shaped magnetic resonance (MR) theranostic nanoparticle, which was used as an MR molecular imaging agent for targeted detection of fibrin, a major biochemical feature of thrombus [105]. The nanobialys offered the potential of site-specific molecular imaging with manganese (as opposed to gadolinium) as well as local delivery of potent chemotherapy agents. A secondary ability of nanobialys to incorporate chemotherapeutic compounds with greater than 98% efficiency and to retain more than 80% of these drugs after infinite sink dissolution successfully proved the theranostic potential of this platform technology.

8.4.4 QD-Based Formulations for Magnetic Resonance Responsive Theranostic Modalities

It was reported that quantum dots (QDs), luminescent semiconductor nanocrystals, served not only as an imaging agent but also as a nanoscaffold catering to magnetic resonance responsive therapeutic modalities [46]. Much of the initial progress for QD-based formulations in biology and medicine has focused on developing new biosensing formats with enhanced sensitivity, involving magnetic semiconductors based on interactions between magnetic dopants and charge carriers [106]. The nanoparticles may contain dual-mode agents, permitting the combination of positive features associated with optical magnetic resonance imaging. The high surface-to-volume ratio of QDs enables the construction of a smart multifunctional nano-platform, where the QDs can be more than passive bioprobes or labels for biological imaging and cellular studies [107].

8.5 LIGAND-BASED TARGETING FORMULATIONS

When linked with tumor-targeting moieties, such as tumor-specific ligands or monoclonal antibodies, nanometer-sized particles can be used to target cancer-specific receptors, tumor antigens, and tumor vasculatures with high affinity and precision [15]. As previously reported receptor-targeted particles are uptaken by the tumor cell through endocytosis [108]. Various ligands used for target strategies are highlighted in this chapter.

8.5.1 Monoclonal Antibodies Coupled Targeting

At present, monoclonal antibodies are the most widely used ligand in a targeting application. Rapid progress in molecular biology has revealed that various antigens can be used to enhance the target efficacy of chemotherapeutic drugs on target cells [109, 110]. The rationale behind the use of antibodies for the treatment of infected diseases including cancer is based on antigenic moieties that are overexpressed on tumor cells but not expressed or minimally present on normal cells.

Only a few of the antigens in the market are truly tumor specific, and they bind to transferrin receptor, folic acid receptor, and CD19, CD20, and CD33 (Cluster of Differentiation 19, 20, and 33 are proteins that in humans are encoded by the CDI9, CD20, or CD33 gene, respectively) [111, 112]. Antigens like ganglioside GM3 on melanoma, mucin antigen 1 (MUC1), MUC2, and MUC3 on the surfaces of breast, lung, and prostate cancer, and Lewis X on the surface of digestive cancer were found to be tumor-type specific [113]. The immunoglobulin was also shown to be specific on the surface of malignant B cells and on the T-cell antigen receptor protein [114].

Liposomes conjugated to monoclonal antibody (MAb) have been a popular choice in antibody coupled targeting as a result of their ease of conjugation and preparation. Immuno-liposomes can be easily constructed using a modular strategy in which components are optimized for internalization and intracellular drug delivery. Liposomes [115] or nanoparticles [116], conjugated to anti-HER2 monoclonal antibody (MAb) fragments, served as a drug targeting carrier to HER2-overexpressing cells. The HER2 immunliposomes increased target specificity by 700-fold as compared with untargeted liposomes [115]. Liposomal doxorubicin (Doxil; ALZA Corporation, Mountain View, CA) incorporated with an antibody that targets breast tumors (ErbB2) overexpressed with a growth factor exerted a faster and greater regression at target sites as compared with unmodified Doxil [117]. Another attempt was made to enhance the tumor accumulation and therapeutic effect of doxorubicin-loaded, long-circulating liposomes (Doxil) by coupling to their surface the anticancer monoclonal antibody 2C5 (mAb 2C5) with nucleosome (NS)-restricted activity, which can recognize the surface of various tumors but not normal cells [118]. Antibody-targeted liposomes demonstrated significantly enhanced accumulation in primary Lewis lung carcinoma (LLC) tumors in mice and were more effective in inhibiting tumor growth and metastatic processes.

Biodegradable microspheres conjugated to MAb for E- and P-selectin were developed based on polycaprolactone as a drug targeting carrier considering that endothelial E- and P-selectin expressions were enhanced in various disease conditions including tumor growth [119]. These Mab conjugated microspheres were found to adhere to the cell surface even in high shear conditions, at which fluid-flow type systems were used to simulate blood flow in tumors [119, 120].

Immunonanoparticles synthesized by conjugation of an anti-transferrin receptor MAb to maleimide-grafted pegylated nanoparticles prepared from poly(lactic acid) (PLA) and a bi-functional polyethyleneglycol (PEG) successfully displayed tumor specificity [121]. Subsequently, nanoparticles or microparticles made of PLGA [122] or poly(lactide-co-glycolide) [123] and conjugated with antibodies through peripheral attachment have been used for target-specific drug delivery of various chemotherapeutic agents including camptothecin.

Recently, novel surface-functionalized crosslinked nanogels, made of diblock co-polymers via condensation of PEG-b-PMA with Ca^{2+} ions into micelle-like aggregates, were developed using a simple one-step approach as a platform to allow conjugation of monoclonal MAb for targeted drug delivery [124]. The mAb retained the binding affinity to bovine submaxillary mucin after conjugation as demonstrated by surface plasmon resonance (SPR), supporting the finding that aldehyde functionalized nanogels could have a potential for targeted delivery of diagnostic and therapeutic agents to tumors.

8.5.2 Pretargeting Approach

Even though directly labeled antibodies, fragments, and subfragments (minibodies and other constructs) have shown their potential in both imaging and therapy applications, their clinical usage has not been successful as a result of either poor image resolution in scanning or insufficient concentrations delivered to target sites. An alternative method to antibody mediated delivery is to provide targeted Mab to tumors known as pretargeting. Pretargeting involves two subsequent processes: the tumor localization with an anticancer antibody and the delivery of the imaging or therapeutic radionuclide [125]. In the first step, a Mab conjugate that binds to tumor-associated antigens is administered. When the tumor-to-nontumor conjugate ratio becomes relatively high, an antigen conjugated delivery system is administered [126]. This approach effectively prevents the slow distribution of the Mab moiety from rapid binding and elimination of the extra ligand at the tumor site, leading to a very high ratio of particle uptake in the tumor as compared with normal tissue.

Advanced technologies offer greatly improved feasibility in the clinical usage of pretargeting properties. For instance, the antiTAG-72 antibody B72.3 was conjugated with an 18 mer MORF, while the cMORF was radio-labeled with ^{99m}Tc, specifically targeting the CWR22 tumor, which was known to be TAG-72-positive [127]. The maximum percentage tumor accumulation (MPTA) of the labeled cMORF in the CWR22 tumor was 2.22%ID/g as compared with only 0.12%ID/g in control mice without the pretargeting moiety. Both the planar and tomographic images confirmed the success of the CWR22 pretargeting efficacy. The use of bispecific trimeric (3 Fabs) recombinant constructs made by a modular method of antibody and protein engineering of fusion molecules called Dock and Lock (DNL) [125] also significantly improved molecular imaging of cancer and further validated the approach with a bi-specific monoclonal antibody (bsMAb). Pretargeting therapy combined with new molecular imaging techniques may pave the way to an individual patient-specific treatment for chemotherapy.

8.5.3 Avidin- and Biotin-Mediated Pretargeting

Avidin (Figure 8.5: a highly glycosylated, positively charged protein found in egg white) is a structurally and functionally analogous protein that contains terminal N-acetylglucosamine and mannose residues. Avidin and streptavidin are stable against heat, denaturants, pH, and the activity of proteolytic enzymes, rendering (strept)avidins an outstanding tool for the various disciplines of bioscience and biomedicine [128]. The applications of avidin include labeling, separation, and targeting, constructing self-assembling nanostructures for the target of various manipulations [129].

Avidin showed a high affinity toward biotin (a B vitamin, Figure 8.5) and some lectins (proteins that bind specific sugar molecules on glycoproteins and glycolipids) that are expressed at various levels on the surface of tumor cells [130]. Avidin injected 1–24 hours before the injection of radioactive biotin (avidin pretargeting; avidin-biotin conjugates formed *in vivo*) displayed localized highly and rapidly in the tumors [131]. More than 50% of the administered dose of avidin–biotin conjugate accumulated per gram of tumor tissue 2 hours after injection, demonstrating the ability of avidin, labeled through conjugation to radioactive biotin, to target intraperitoneal tumors.

An interesting targeting approach of the streptavidin–biotin interaction is site-specific conjugation of stimuli-responsive polymers to streptavidin through mutation of the desired linking residues into cysteines or lysines [132]. These stimuli-responsive polymers respond to environmental stimuli, such as changes in temperature, pH, and light, by altering their conformation, concomitantly affecting the biotin-binding activity of the polymer-conjugated streptavidin [132]. Applications for these (strept)avidin polymers are found in biomedical applications, ranging from targeted drug delivery, controlled enzyme function and gene delivery, or expression to cell-adhesion mediators [133]. For example, the release of an internalized antibody from the endosomal system into the cytoplasm using the acidic environment in lysosomes was displayed using a pH-sensitive streptavidin–polymer conjugate [132]. Streptavidin coupled nanoparticles using natural and synthetic polymers with pretargeting biotinylated targeting

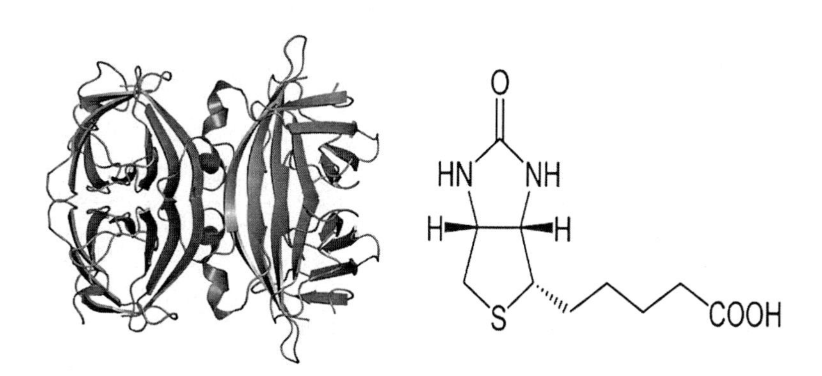

FIGURE 8.5 Structures of avidin and biotin (vitamin B6).

ligands were made available as a tumor-selective drug delivery system [134].

Applications for avidin targeting ability also include gene transduction to specific targeting tissues through local or intravenous injection that has been the ultimate preferred method of gene delivery [135]. A dual-imaging strategy based on the avidin–biotin system was developed by incorporating avidin and streptavidin fused to the transmembrane anchor of vesicular stomatitis virus G protein on gp64-pseudotyped envelopes, which consequently showed binding to biotin in ELISA [136]. These vectors conjugated to biotinylated radionuclides and engineered to express a ferritin transgene allowed for easy exchange of the surface ligand on an HIV-derived lentivirus envelope. It was demonstrated *in vitro* that this vector was retargeting to cancer cells overexpressing CD46, the epidermal growth factor, and transferrin receptors using biotinylated ligands and antibodies, enabling dual imaging of virus biodistribution and transduction pattern.

8.5.4 Peptide and Protease Coupled Targeting

The use of peptides, proteases, and protein domains with amphipathic sequences has attracted increasing attention in the area of drug and gene delivery across cellular membranes [137, 138]. Some peptide pharmaceuticals use peptides to deliver a chemotherapeutic agent or a tracer to the tumor and allow sensitive imaging or targeted therapy. [139]. The internalization of peptides by cells is independent of energy and free from the endocytic pathway [140]. The disadvantages in peptide design, such as short half-life, fast proteolytic cleavage and low oral bioavailability, have been overcame by advanced technologies including peptide PEGylation, lipidization or multimerization (i.e., the introduction of peptidomimetic elements into the sequences) and innovative uptake strategies through formulation approaches, such as liposomal, capsule or subcutaneous injectables [141].

Proteases, which are known to be involved in various physiological processes, such as tissue remodeling, wound healing, and tumor invasion, have been identified as potential candidates to control the drug release *in vivo*. As the binary β-sheet peptides are able to form a self-assembled matrix via β-sheet stacking, the protease-sensitive matrix is developed by building blocks, which contain a protease-sensitive motif and two weak β-sheet forming peptide sequences [142]. The cleavage of the protease-sensitive sequence dissembles the building blocks, that in turn weakens the β-sheet interactions and leads to matrix degradation and controlled drug release.

By combining the enhanced permeation and duration effect with cancer-associated protease (CAP) sensitivity, a cholesterol-anchored graft co-polymer composed of a short peptide sequence for urokinase plasminogen activator (uPA) and poly(acrylic acid) was synthesized and incorporated into liposomes prepared at high osmolarities [143]. The protease-triggered caged liposomes, upon crosslinking of the polymers, showed resistance to osmotic swelling and achieved substantial enhancement of protease-sensitive delivery in the presence of uPA as compared with a bare liposome.

8.5.5 Peptide Coupled to Cell-Penetrating Peptides (CPPs) for Target Delivery

Cell-penetrating peptides (CPPs) have been used to transport a variety of molecules, such as proteins, plasmids, peptide nucleic acids, short interfering RNA (siRNA), liposomes, and nanoparticles, across the cell membranes [144–146]. Penetratins, one of the most studied CPPs, enhanced the translocation efficiency of liposomes, which was proportional to the number of peptides attached to liposome surface [147].

Although CPPs provide a means through which cell-impermeable compounds can reach intracellular targets, conventional CPPs, like trans-activator of transcription (TAT), MAPs, transportans, and penetratins were unable to deliver chemotherapeutic agents with desirable cell specificity, displaying a lack of sensitivity [148]. As they are a powerful nonimmunogenic tool for delivery of cell-impermeable drugs to cancer cells, nonspecific CPPs have been widely investigated and their target efficiency has been continuously improved [149–151].

TAT peptides, the synthetic peptides containing an arginine-glycine-aspartate (RGD) sequence motif, emerged as a versatile CPP. The HIV Tat-derived peptide has successfully delivered a large variety of cargoes from small particles to proteins, peptides, and nucleic acids. The transduction domain or region conveying the cell penetrating properties seems to be confined to a small (nine amino acids) stretch of basic amino acids. The HIV-Tat transduction domain and polyamines are essential for tumor cell growth, and their pathway represents an attractive target for cancer treatment. The HIV-Tat transduction domain and polyamines can enter cells through a common pathway, which can be used to target polyamine-dependent tumor growth [138].

The N-terminal region (2–147 amino acids) of *Esherichia* coif-derived mucin antigen 1 (MUC1)-N fused to the protein transduction domain of HIV was tested for dendritic cell (DC)-based cancer immunotherapy [115]. Tat-MUC1-N-loaded DCs efficiently induced type 1 T-cell responses as well as cytotoxic T lymphocytes. Compared with DCs pulsed with unconjugated MUCI-N, DCs loaded with Tat-conjugated MUC1-N could delay tumor growth more effectively in the transgenic tumor model as well as in the tumor injection model, suggesting that the recombinant Tat-conjugated N-terminal part of MUC1 could be used as an effective tumor antigen for DC-based cancer immunotherapy.

TAT conjugated liposomes enhanced the delivery of metabolic inhibitors in human breast cancer cells [152–154]. Although a TAT peptide linked to a suicide protein, herpes simplex virus type I thymidine kinase (HSV-TK), could be a useful booster, any enhancement by TAT was shown in only a few tumor cells *in vitro* [155]. It was also found that the triple fusion protein HIV-1 transactivator protein transduction domain–thymidine kinase suicide gene–green fluorescent protein marker gene (TAT-TK-GFP) increased GCV cytotoxicity only in 3/12 of different human tumor cell lines [156]. Therefore, it is integral to go through broad and extensive examination of the clinical adaptation of the TAT-mediated targeting approach in the treatment of infected diseases and cancers.

8.5.6 Cyclic RGD Peptides and Integrin

Integrins are a large family of heterodimeric transmembrane glycoproteins that readily interact with extracellular ligands and play a vital role in angiogenesis, leukocytes function, and tumor development, positioning integrin as an excellent target for chemotherapy treatment [157]. Integrins contain large (α) and small (β) subunits of sizes 120–170 kDa and 90–100 kDa, respectively, and form several subfamilies sharing common β subunits that associate with different α subunits. Integrins contain binding sites for divalent cations Mg^{2+} and Ca^{2+}, which are necessary for their adhesive function.

Synthetic or natural peptides with the Arg-Gly-Asp (RGD) sequence motif are active modulators of cell adhesion for drug carriers [158] or viruses [159]. As RGD peptides found in proteins of the extracellular matrix interact with the integrin receptor sites, they can initiate cell-signaling processes and influence various different diseases [160]. Therefore, the inhibition of the alpha beta subunits of integrin by RGD peptide-mediated cell-matrix interaction could lead to apoptosis of activated endothelial cells and disrupt blood vessel formation in tumor cells [161–163].

Interleukin 24 (IL-24), which is a novel cancer growth-suppressing and apoptosis-inducing cytokine, was coupled with RGD-4C (ACDCRGDCFCG peptide) at the N-terminus of IL-24. Cell proliferation and adhesion experiments revealed that RGD-IL-24 specifically binds to MCF-7 cancer cells [158], supporting the effectiveness of the RGD-IL-24 protein in tumor-targeting therapy.

8.5.7 Formulations Based on Integrin and Cyclic RGD Peptides

Integrins and RGD-based ligands for integrins are intensively used in the area of imaging and target drug delivery. RGD-targeted drugs have been developed either by direct conjugation of the homing peptide to the drug or by conjugation of the RGD-peptide to a carrier device containing drug molecules [164]. Cyclic RGD peptide anchored sterically stabilized liposomes (RGD-SLs) were investigated for targetability and controlled delivery of carrier contents at angiogenic endothelial cells overexpressing integrins on and around tumor tissue. In tumor models, inhibition of blood vessel formation using alpha beta integrin antagonists (cyclic RGDs) not only blocked tumor-associated angiogenesis but in some cases caused tumor regression. A 5 fluorouracil in A cyclic RGD peptide was more active against the tumor than that in a plain liposome or free drug [165, 166].

A cyclic RGD peptide-conjugated block co-polymer, cyclo[RGDfK(CX-)]−poly(ethylene glycol)−polylysine (c(RGDfK)−PEG−PLys), was synthesized from acetal-PEG−PLys under mild acidic conditions and spontaneously associated with plasmid DNA (pDNA) to form a polyplex micelle in aqueous solution [167]. The cyclic RGD peptide recognizes $\alpha_v\beta_3$ and $\alpha_v\beta_5$ integrin receptors, which play a pivotal role in the proliferation of malignant tumors. The c (RGDfK)−PEG−PLys/pDNA polyplex micelle showed higher transfection efficiency (TE) compared with the PEG−PLys/pDNA polyplex micelle for the cultured HeLa cells possessing $\alpha_v\beta_3$ and $\alpha_v\beta_5$ integrins. These results indicate that the increase in the TE induced by the introduction of the c(RGDfK) peptide ligand was a result of an increase in cellular uptake as well as facilitated intracellular trafficking of micelles toward the perinuclear region via $\alpha_v\beta_3$ and $\alpha_v\beta_5$ integrin receptor-mediated endocytosis.

Five conjugates of poly(ethylene glycol) modified polyethylenimine (PEG-PEIs) coupled in two different synthesis routes to a nonpeptidic pentacyclic RDG-mimetic were developed and characterized for integrin receptor-targeted gene delivery [168]. The binding, uptake, and transfection efficiency in receptor-positive cells were dependent on the degree of peptide substitution and significantly increased upon enhanced conjugation of the RGD-mimetic to AB-block-co-polymers of PEG-PEI. It can be concluded that the conjugates of PEG-PEI AB-block-co-polymers with low ligand density of the RGD-mimetic could be a promising candidate for *in vivo* cancer gene therapy.

8.5.8 Peptide Ligand Targeting for Tumor Angiogenesis and Vascular

(1) *NGR sequence for chemotoxic drug targeting:* Angiogenesis is the development of new blood vessels from existing ones and plays a critical role in controlling tumor growth and metastasis. Tumor growth requires the elaboration of a vascular network to supply nutrients and oxygen avoiding hypoxia and tumor cell apoptosis [169].

Similar to the RGD-sequence, the asparagine–glycine–argininen (NGR) sequence was used to target drugs, proapoptotic peptides, or cytokines like tumor necrosis factor (TNF), to tumor vasculature

[170]. Cyclic as well as linear peptides containing the NGR sequence have high selectivity to tumor vessels; yet the specificity of the cyclic sequence is much higher [171]. Human endostatin, which was modified genetically to introduce an NGR motif (NGR-endostatin), showed increased binding to endothelial cells compared with the native protein, demonstrating improved tumor localization and, as a consequence, effectively inhibited ovarian carcinoma growth in athymic nude mice [172].

Although the changes typically have negative effects on protein function, recent studies have suggested that isoAsp formation at certain Asn-Gly-Arg (NGR) sites in ECM proteins have a gain-of-function effect because the resulting isoAsp-Gly-Arg (isoDGR) sequence can mimic Arg-Gly-Asp (RGD), a well-known integrin-binding motif [173]. Substantial experimental evidence suggests that the NGR-to-isoDGR transition can occur *in vitro* in natural proteins and drugs containing this motif, thereby promoting integrin recognition and cell adhesion.

It was shown that very low concentrations of TNF targeted with the NGR homing motif altered the vessel barrier function and improved the chemotoxicity of anticancer drugs [174]. By stabilizing the homing peptide through a disulfide bond (sequence CNGRC), the conformational changes increased the tumor targeting efficiency and lowered systemic toxicity. Significant preclinical synergy chemotherapeutic activity was observed with low doses of NGR-TNF in the presence of doxorubicin [175]. Moreover, the NGR sequence is useful for delivering nanoparticles like liposomes loaded with chemotoxic drugs to the tumor vasculature [176].

Aminopeptidase N (APN, also termed CD13) was expressed exclusively on newly formed vessels, but not on normal vasculature, and was identified to play an important role in angiogenesis [177]. Subsequently, enhanced expression of APN in tumor vascular endothelium offered an opportunity to target NGR peptide-linked therapeutic reagents to tumors. Peptides that contain an NGR motif, such as CNGRC and GNGRG, facilitated delivery of APN to tumor vasculature, suggesting that peptide-phage libraries could be used for generating ligands for the tumor vasculature targeting peptides with low immunogenicity [178].

(2) *CBO-P11, a cyclo-peptide:* Angiogenesis is regulated by a balance of positive and negative mediators, such as a vascular endothelial growth factor (VEGF), which regulates endothelial cell proliferation, permeability and survival. CBO-P11, a 17-amino-acid molecule designated a cyclo-peptidic vascular endothelial growth inhibitor (cyclo-VEGI or CBO-P11), has proven to bind specifically to VEGF receptors and has showed potential to be used as a targeting ligand for tumor angiogenesis.

Novel poly(vinylidene fluoride) (PVDF) nanoparticles conjugated to CBO-P11 were developed to target the tumor site specifically (Figure 8.6) [179]. Fluorescence highlighted the specific interaction of these functionalized nanoparticles with VEGF receptors, suggesting that the targeting peptide bioactivity was retained. Therefore, they could be potentially used as a multifunctional platform for the treatment of tumor angiogenesis, if coupled with therapeutic agents.

(3) *Platelet-targeted formulations:* Platelet integrin alpha(IIb)beta(3) (GP IIb/IIIa) serves as a receptor for various proteins, such as fibrinogen, fibronectin,

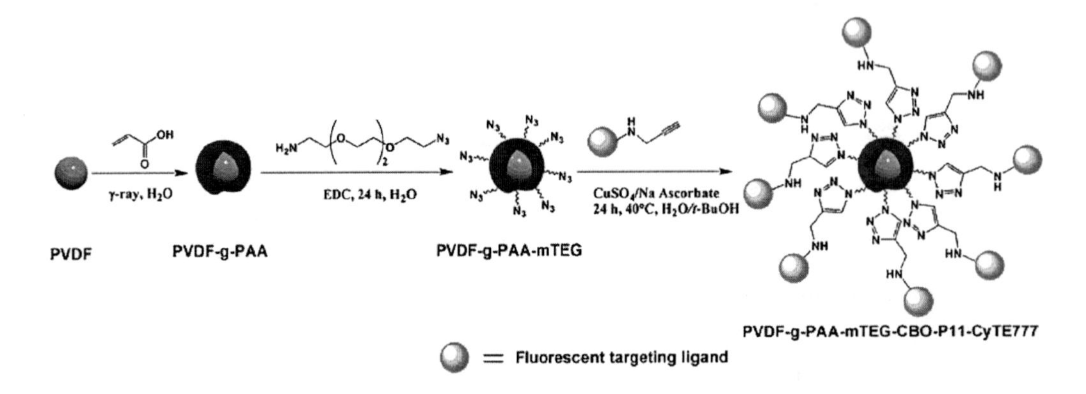

FIGURE 8.6 Functionalization of novel poly(vinylidene fluoride) (PVDF) nanoparticles conjugated to CBO-P11. Radio-grafting of PAA, coupling with azido spacer arm (mTEG), and "click" conjugation of fluorescent targeting ligand (CBO-P11-CyTE777) [179]. (See color figure in color plate section.)

and vitronectin, as well as contributes to the adhesion and aggregation of platelets in pathological status [180]. This integrin is upregulated and stimulated into a ligand-binding conformation on the surface-activated platelets. Activated-platelet adhesion and aggregation are primary events in atherosclerosois, thrombosis, and restenosis. Hence, platelet-targeted formulations have enormous potential to be used as vascular site-selective delivery of drugs and imaging probes.

Examples of potential fields of application include liposome nanoparticles whose surfaces were modified by RGD peptide ligands having targeting specificity to integrin GPIIb-IIIa present in vascular [181]. The *in vitro* SEM results allowed for visualization of nanoscopic liposomes attached to activated platelets, and *in vivo* studies demonstrated successful platelet targeting by the peptide-modified liposomes.

8.5.9 Folate Conjugated Particle

Folic acid (Figure 8.7) is a nutrient for dividing cells in the synthesis of various amino acids and nucleic acids. The cellular uptake of folic acid is mediated by both reduced folate carriers and folate receptors [182]. As a result of a small molecular size and high binding affinity for cell-surface folate receptors (FRs), folate conjugates have the ability to deliver a variety of molecular complexes to pathologic cells without causing any damages to normal tissues [183].

FRs are expressed in very low amounts in normal cells except for dividing tissues like reticular endothelial cells, kidney, spleen, and bone marrow [184]. FRs are highly expressed in lung, brain, ovarian, colon, and renal cancers [185]. FRs are on the apical side of the epithelial cells where they are not supplied with folate via vascular tissue. The internal proton gradient facilitates the removal of folate from the receptor and allows for the nutrient to permeate across the membrane. FRs are expressed at 10^7/cell in tumor tissue [186] and have a relatively high binding affinity in tumor cells ($K_D = 110\,pM$) [187, 188]. Folate receptors internalize their substrates by phagocytosis [189], and internalized folate conjugates are stable in the cytoplasm.

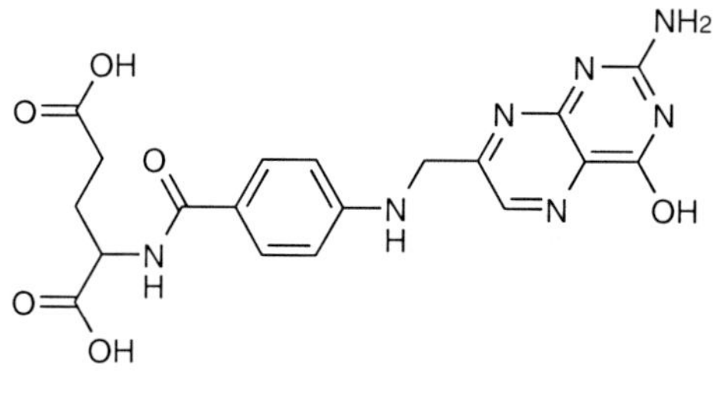

OH O O N H OH N H N N N NH2 N OH

FIGURE 8.7 Folic acid.

FRs generally require highly potent drugs for direct coupling with folate (IC_{50} value greater than 10 nM). The problem related to relatively lower potent drugs can be overcome by encapsulation and coupling with folate. Folate-linked formulations, such as liposome and solid-lipid particle and nanoparticle [190–192], have demonstrated excellent tumor selectivity and have enhanced the drug residence time in tumors. Although the folate receptor shows great potential to be clinically used, the expression of folate on the epithelial cells of the tumor hinders the drug penetration into the inner layers of a solid tumor [193].

As a result of the cationic nature of the amine groups, chitosan was widely tested for folate conjugated drug carriers. Chitosan can absorb to oppositely charged molecules, metal ions, and peptides [194, 195]. Folate bears two carboxylate functional groups leading to a negative charge, which can easily adsorb onto the cationic chitosan surface as a result of the amine groups. Folate conjugated N-trimethyl chitosan (folate-TMC) was synthesized and characterized using Fourier transform infrared (FTIR) and spectroscopy [196]. The enhancement of cellular uptake of TMC-nanoparticles (NP) by SKOV3 cells was observed and attributed to the folate-receptor-mediated endocytosis. The results of this study revealed that TMC-NP could be a promising carrier for tumor-specific target delivery of various proteins. Later, the same group synthesized folate-poly(ethylene glycol)-grafted-trimethyl chitosan for gene delivery [197].

The polyelectrolyte nanogels made of diblock co-polymer poly(ethylene oxide)-b-poly(methacrylic acid) (PEO-b-PMA) with the proper degree of crosslinking are conjugated to folic acid (FA) and loaded with different types of drugs (cisplatin and doxorubicin) [198]. This nanogel exhibited a tumor-specific targeted delivery and superior antitumor effects of an anticancer drug *in vivo*, guaranteeing the use of nanogels conjugated to FA for the therapy of ovarian and other cancers, where the folate receptor is overexpressed.

8.5.10 siRNA Approach for Targeting

In addition to antibody-based treatments, targeted cancer therapy by RNA interference (RNAi)-based treatments is one of frontier approaches that can be used to silence reversibly targeting genes *in vivo* [199–201]. RNAi is a system within living cells that takes part in controlling which genes are active and how much active they are [202]. Small interfering RNA (siRNA) that acts as a genetic on/off switch could serve as anticancer material by blocking the cancer cells from producing proteins, thus, killing them [203]. It was demonstrated that when EphA2-targeting siRNA was combined with paclitaxel (Taxol; Bristol-Myers Squibb, New York, NY), tumor growth was dramatically reduced as compared with treatment with paclitaxel only [204], demonstrating the feasibility of siRNA as a clinically applicable therapeutic modality.

The efficacy of the siRNA approach was tested in mice with an ovarian cancer cell line known to be resistant to taxane-based drugs including docetaxel. Interleukin-8 (IL-8) is a pro-angiogenic cytokine that is overexpressed in various human cancers. Mice that received both IL-8 siRNA plus the taxane-based drug docetaxel (Taxotere; Aventis, Bridgewater, NJ) had a median tumor weight reduction of 90% and 98% in the two cell lines [205]. Mice with control siRNA plus docetaxel saw reductions of 67% and 84%, suggesting that the tested combination resensitizes a resistant tumor to taxanes. The impact of IL-8 siRNA on tumor blood supply was assessed by measuring the density of the tumor, in which the IL-8 siRNA alone reduced blood vessel density by 34% and 39% in two cancer lines.

siRNA approaches were also tested against cervical and ovarian cancer. Dendrosome-based delivery of siRNA was effective against E6 and E7 oncogenes in cervical cancer [206]. siRNA loaded in liposome was administered to mice to target an ovarian cancer protein known as focal-adhesion kinase (FAK) [207]. The siRNA in a liposome travels into cells through the blood supply and dispense its activities through the so-called "Trojan Horse" effect. Adding chemotherapy to the siRNA treatment boosted tumor weight reduction in the range of 94% to 98%.

Core/shell hydrogel nanoparticles (nanogels) functionalized with peptides that specially target the EphA2 receptor were developed to deliver small interfering RNAs (siRNAs) targeting the epidermal growth factor receptor (EGFR) [208, 209]. Treatment of EphA2-positive Hey cells with siRNA-loaded, peptide-targeted nanogels decreased EGFR expression levels and significantly increased the sensitivity of this cell line to docetaxel ($P < 0.05$). However, SK-OV-3 cells, which are negative for EphA2 expression, neither reduced EGFR levels upon nanogel treatment nor increased docetaxel sensitivity ($P > 0.05$), revealing the target specificity of siRNA.

As previously shown with dimethyl maleic anhydride, a pH-sensitive monomer functional group involved in target delivery, the poly-conjugate developed for siRNA by linking the siRNA payload to an amphipathic poly(vinyl ether) also displayed its effectiveness in hepatocyte target delivery [66]. Based on the successful outcomes of *in vivo* siRNA delivery with dendritic poly(L-lysine) for the treatment of hypercholesterolemia [210], environment-responsive block copolymer micelles with a disulfide crosslinked core prepared through the assembly of iminothiolane-modified poly(ethylene glycol)-block-poly(L-lysine) [PEG-b-(PLL-IM)] and siRNA at a characteristic optimum mixing ratio were developed. The micelles achieved enhanced transfection efficacy at the intracellular reductive environment [211].

8.5.11 Polysaccharide-Anchored Targeting

Among the polymeric micelles, hydrophobicized polysaccharides have currently become one of the hottest areas of research in the field of nanosystems for drug delivery. It is attributable to such appealing properties as small particle size and narrow size distribution, distinctive core-shell structure, high solubilization capacity and structural stability, tumor passive localization by enhanced permeability and retention (EPR) effect, active targeting ability via tailored targeting promoiety, long-circulation property, and facile preparation [212]. These polysaccharides include pectin, guar gum, amylose, inulin, dextran, chitosan, and chondroitin sulphate.

Saccharides have been used as ligands for surface-modified nanocarriers, possesing the receptor-mediated targeting properties and showing the potential for cell-specific delivery of drugs and genes. Target efficacy was dependent on ligand types, targeting properties, therapeutic effects, and methods for administering the nanocarriers [213]. As polysaccharidases are bacterial enzymes that are available in a sufficient quantity to be exploited in colon targeting of drugs, various polysaccharides have been investigated for colon-specific drug release [214].

Polysaccharide-anchored liposomes have been exploited as a carrier equipped with a targeting ligand, where the polysaccharide coating stabilizes the system both *in vitro* and *in vivo* while the anchored recognition ligand confers target selectivity [215]. The polysaccharide-anchored liposomes have been studied extensively as targetable and stable drug carriers in chemotherapy especially for introducing chemotherapeutics into tumor cell lines. Studies conducted using tumor recognition ligand 1-amino-lactose, anchored to liposomes containing adriamycin on A66 hepatoma in nude mice, revealed that anticancer drug carriers can be tailored for the active targeting to tumor cells. As carbohydrate ligands can confer anchoring cell recognition elements to liposomes, making the drug delivery more precise and target specific [214], approaches like ligand-anchored to liposomes could be potentially used for delivering antitumor drugs to breast cancer cells.

Along with encapsulation of water-insoluble drugs, hydrophobicized polysaccharide polymeric micelles can complex with charged proteins or peptide drugs through electrostatic force or hydrogen bond and can serve as an effective nonviral vector for gene delivery. A natural polysaccharide called schizophyllan (SPG) was used as an effective CpG (i.e., the phosphodiester bond between the cytosine and the guanine) DNA carrier because SPG can complex with CpG DNA and the resultant complex showed the nuclease resistance of the bound DNA [217]. The complexes made of the chemically modified SPG and CpG DNA having a phosphorothioate (PS) or phosphodiester (PO) backbone caused an increase in cytokine secretion of about 4- to 15-fold compared with the uncomplexed dose [218], suggesting that unmodified SPG could effectively deliver PO *in vivo* as a result of the electrically neutral nature of unmodified SPG. The modified polysaccharide condenses DNA and is capable of transforming it into cells, not only markedly protecting these macromolecules from degradation by protease or ribozymes, but also increasing the gene transfection efficiency [219]. The cationized polysaccharide also demonstrated its potential as a nonviral carrier of plasmid DNA for mesenchymal stem cells (MSCs) [220].

8.6 FORMULATIONS APPROACH BASED ON HOST RECEPTOR TARGETING

8.6.1 Peptides Targeting the Epidermal Growth Factor Receptor (EGFR)

One of the major target receptors by protease inhibitors is the epidermal growth factor receptor (EGFR), which plays a key role in numerous cellular processes and in sustaining neutrophil inflammation [221]. EGFR is a transmembrane protein consisting of an extracellular ligand-binding domain to which EGFR ligands such as transforming growth factor α (TGFα) and epidermal growth factor (EGF) bind for activation [222]. Immunological targeting of protease inhibitors for EGFR were achieved with various formulations, such as nanoparticles [223, 224, 225], dendrimers [226], and liposomes [143], from whom, upon enzymatic treatment, protease-mediated drug release of a model therapeutic peptide was feasible.

8.6.2 Peptides Targeting G-Protein–Coupled Receptors (GPCRs)

G-protein–coupled receptors (GPCRs) constitute the largest family of intercellular signaling molecules and are estimated to be the target of more than 50% of all modern drugs [227]. As a result of the high density of GPCRs on immune cells that are activated by small peptides or chemokines, peptides targeting GPCRs are a promising tool for target delivery of drug candidates or that have recently entered the pharmaceutical market. It was shown that HIV required CC chemokine receptor (CCR)5 or CXC chemokine receptor (CXCR)4 co-receptors to enter the cell [228]. Both receptors are class-A GPCRs and recognize chemokines as endogenous ligands. Accordingly, more than 20 clinical studies on chemokine antagonists have been reported [229] since the proof of inhibiting virus entry with peptides was demonstrated with a drug called enfuvirtide (Fuzeon; Hoffman-La Roche, Basel, Switzerland).

The overexpression of peptide GPCRs in tumor cells compared with the original tissue they are derived from is exploited in direct or indirect therapeutic concepts. In indirect approaches, the peptide hormone is used as a carrier to direct chemotherapeutics, radiodiagnostics, or radiotherapeutics to the tumor [230]. The tumor takes up the peptide–drug complex by endocytosis, which leads to intracellular enrichment of the toxic compounds. Only Octreoscan (Mallinckrodt, Inc., Hazelwood, MO), an octreotide analog coupled to diethylenetriaminepentaacetic acid that chelates radioactive indium-111, has reached the market and is a standard diagnostic in the imaging of neuroendocrine tumors [231] and radio-guided surgery [232].

8.6.3 Targeting Calcium-Sensing Receptor (CaR)

The discovery of a G-protein–coupled, calcium-sensing receptor (CaR) and of diseases caused by CaR mutations has provided formidable evidence of the CaR's role in the maintenance of systemic calcium homeostasis [233]. As a change in the concentration of Ca^{+2} ions through the extracellular CaR causes the cell to differentiate uncontrollably, the regulation of the CaR could potentially serve as an efficient targeting means in cancer or other disease treatment [234, 235].

8.7 DESIGN OF A CORE SHELL MICROPARTICLE: AN EXAMPLE OF FORMULATION DEVELOPMENT

Nanotechnology, whose size range (5–250 nm) is smaller than the diameter of human cells spans (10–20 μm), could offer a less invasive approach, readily interacting with biomolecules on the cell surface and localizing in the cells in a noninvasive manner, leaving the biochemical properties of those molecules intact [236].

8.7.1 Specific Aim

The objective of this study was to develop a core shell microparticle (CSM: Figure 8.8) as a tumor targeted drug delivery system consisting of solid-lipid particles (SLNs) inside loaded with phenethyl isothiocyanate (PEITC) and chitosan outer shell conjugated with folic acid (cyclic RGD (PC1-3986-PI). This formulation is designed to transport

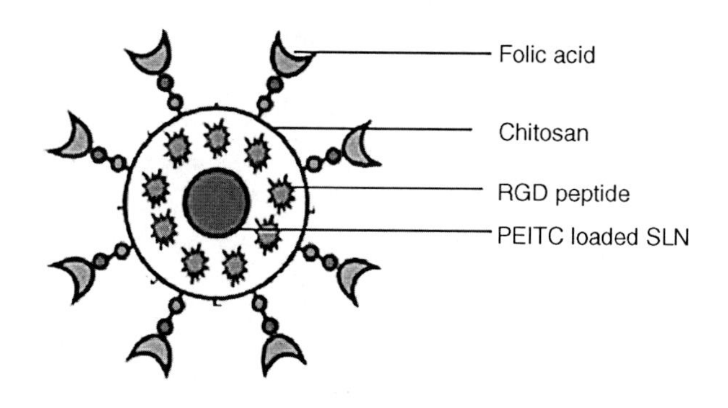

FIGURE 8.8 Design of a core shell microparticle (CSM).

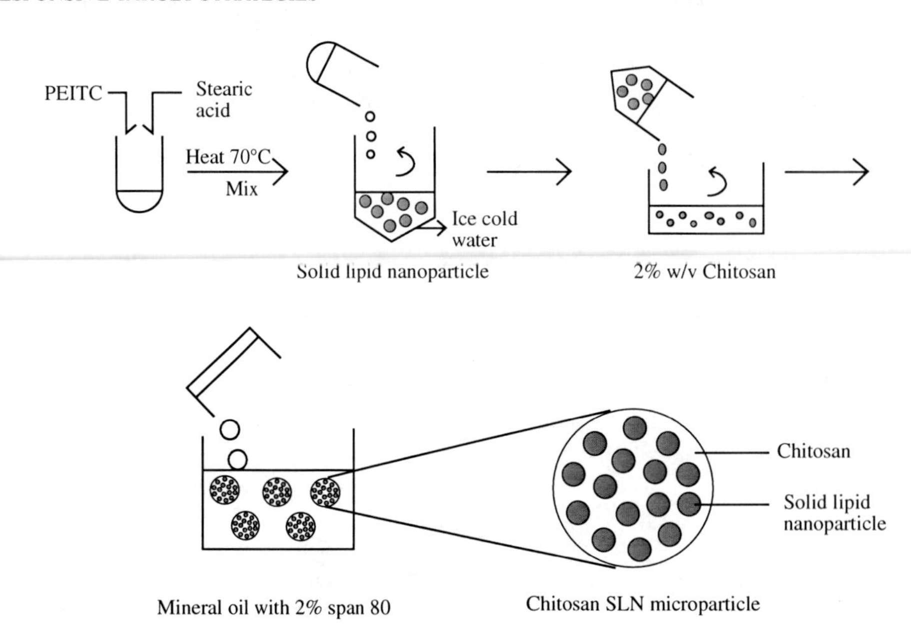

FIGURE 8.9 Schematic representation of preparation of chitosan-SLN microparticles.

SLNs actively through the cell and achieve enhanced pharmacological activity of PEITC. Active cell targeting was expected to be enhanced by using folate adsorbed CSM after intravenous administration of CSM.

The main objects of this study have been as follows:

(1) To determine the adsorption of the folate on the CSM (i.e., binding property, association constant, and stability) and bio-reversion profiles of the folate-receptor.
(2) To study the *in vitro* release characteristics of PEITC from folate-coupled CSM, the *in vitro* cell uptake, and anti-angiogenetic biomarkers.
(3) To investigate the optimal combination of folic acid (cyclic RGD peptide) and PEITC in the CSM formulation.

In a core shell microparticle, RGD peptides are hypothesized to act on the tumor in two mechanisms:

(1) RGD peptides facilitate the entry of therapeutic agent PEITC [237].
(2) RGD peptides act as an anti-angiogenetic agent on chronic or large dose administration (10 mg/kg of body weight) [238].

8.7.2 Formulation Development

The formulation was prepared in two stages (Figure 8.9). In the first stage, SLN was prepared using stearic acid and Tween 80 (Sigma-Aldrich, St. Louis, MO). In the second stage, the SLN solution was dispersed in chitosan solution to produce core shell microparticles (Figure 8.10).

8.7.3 Preparation of SLN

PEITC was completely solubilized in stearic acid at 70°C, followed by the addition of Tween 80 and sodium taurocholate, whose mixture was melted at 70°C. To the melt, 1 mL of triple distilled water was added at 70°C. An

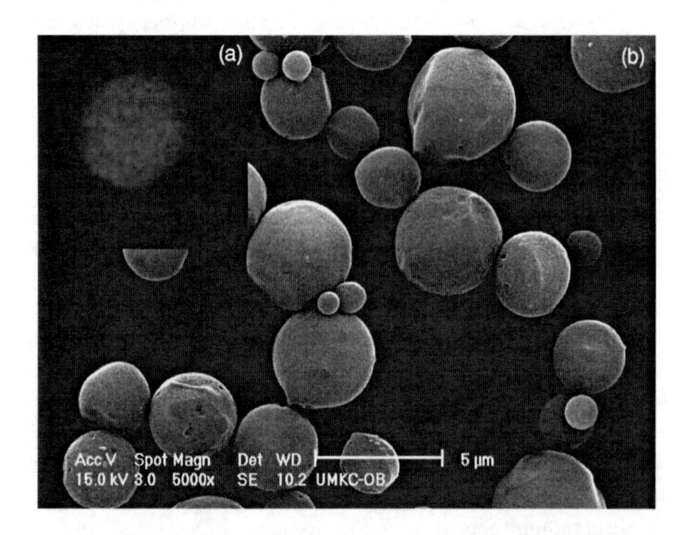

FIGURE 8.10 SEM results of chitosan mean particle sizes (b) and CSM (a).

optically transparent micro-emulsion was obtained from a mixture by stirring at 3000–4000 rpm. The obtained micro-emulsion was dispersed in 10 mL of water at 2–3°C and stirred for 15 min. SLNs were formed and freeze dried until further usage.

8.7.4 Preparation of Core Shell Microparticles (CSMs)

Low-molecular-weight chitosan was dispersed in 1% acetic acid with cyclic RGD peptide. To this solution, 50 mg of SLN were added and a mixture was stirred until a uniform solution was obtained. The chitosan–SLN dispersion was dropped into span 80 (2% in light mineral oil) and stirred at 3000 rpm for 10 min. The CSMs were crosslinked by the addition of 0.1% glutaraldehyde followed by stirring at 1000 rpm. The crosslinked CSMs will be incubated with an excess amount of folate (1 M) overnight and freeze dried until further use. The loading dose was optimized for RGD to deliver 1 : 4 ratios (10 mg per 40 mg) of RGD peptide to PEITC dose/kg body weight. RGD peptides and PEITC have a threshold or an optimized dosage for pharmacological activity at 10-mg and 40-mg/kg body weight, respectively [239]. Further dose adjustments were followed to decrease toxicity as a result of potential synergistic effects.

8.7.5 Radioactive Ligand Assay

The binding of radioactive folate to chitosan was estimated using a radioactive ligand assay [240]. The chitosan microparticles were washed with organic solvent (Hexane) and subsequently with distilled water to remove unbound radioactive folic acid. The filtered and weighed chitosan microparticles were suspended in Scintisafe (Fisher Scientific Company, Pittsburgh, PA) fluid and estimated for the radioactivity. The bound folic acid was targeted at least 0.03% of the total polymer weight to be effective for targeted delivery [241].

8.7.6 Cellular Uptake

Folate receptor expressing cells CD163+ were selected for the cellular uptake studies. Briefly, cells were grown to confluence on cover slips and were placed on a sterile culture plate. At 70% confluence, the cover slips were washed with folate-free buffer and incubated with CSM in the presence of folate or the absence of folate. The cells were then treated with 4,6 diamidino 2 phenyl indole dilactate (DAPI). DAPI, which emits fluorescence, was attached to the minor grove of the DNA. The cells were mounted on a microscope and assessed for the intensity of fluorescence, which reflected the amount of the intact DNA, as fragmented DNA did not emit any fluorescence. The emitted fluorescence was quantified for estimation of the amounts of cellular uptake.

8.7.7 Competitive Inhibition Studies

To estimate the folate linkage, the CSM were co-incubated with free radioactive folate. The uptake amount of radiolabeled folate was assessed for the binding coefficient of folate adsorbed into CSM and compared with those from CSM without free radioactive folate.

8.7.8 The Model for Receptor Binding

The modeling approach was used to evaluate the effects of basic parameters including tumor ligand binding affinity, injected dose, particle size, and normal tumor tissue receptor quantity on host factor values. Those factors affecting a targeted system were evaluated individually, as each factor is independently and complicatedly involved with the targeting processes in practice.

The modeling process was also capable of predicting the effects of the novel strategies, such as two-step targeting, and theoretical approaches including tumor ligand binding with a target carrier and modes of tumor uptake like reversible receptor binding. The kinetics of the binding reaction to a receptor was closely correlated with tumor-reducing capabilities. A linear binding model also elucidated the effects of a computable free and bound ligand receptor system on chemotherapeutic activities. When the injected dose of ligand is smaller than those of tissue receptor expression, the equilibrium did not take place, even though binding to the target was maximally achieved.

Although higher affinity is not directly correlated with greater efficiency, it is integral that receptor expression in the tumor should be greater than those in normal tissues. As the folate receptor is a saturable system, the loading doses of a ligand have to be within the regeneration levels of the receptor. In some occasions, low affinity allows for more *in vivo* tissue penetration and for avoiding trapping of a tightly bound ligand at the tumor surface. Therefore, the optimal binding affinity of various ligands for tumor targeting has yet to be identified. If the particle is assumed to have a single binding site, then a reversible ligand receptor complex can be represented by the following equation [242]:

$$K_a[\mathrm{L}][\mathrm{R}] = K_d[\mathrm{L} - \mathrm{R}]$$

where

K_a = association rate constant
K_d = dissociation rate constant
[L] = concentration of dosing ligand
[R] = receptor expression in tumor cells
[L-R] = ligand-to-receptor association or binding affinity

8.7.9 Results and Conclusions

Therapeutic inefficiency and building resistance to chemotherapy by cancer cells have been attributed to the lack of ability for an individual chemotherapeutic agent to penetrate solid tumors. The efficacy of chitosan-SLN microparticles (CSMs) for delivery of PEITC was evaluated by assessing the release profiles of loaded PEITC and its cytotoxicity in the presence of efflux-transporter inhibitors—tamoxifen, verapamil, or nifedipine. An initial burst release of inhibitors, followed by gradual, sustained release of PEITC and subsequent increase in cytotoxicity, indicated that the PEITC uptake rate by the Calu 3 cell line was significantly influenced the efflux inhibitors.

The receptors in tumor cells, when they are bound to substrate, tend to be saturated and regenerated by releasing the ligand into the cycled cytoplasm [243]. The RGD peptide has cell membrane penetrating capabilities, which can aid in PEITC accumulation in cancer cells to a greater extent. The RGD peptide in conjunction with PEITC displayed its potential to penetrate solid tumors and synergistically exerted the tumor suppression. Nanoparticles impregnated with target moieties seem to be an innovative and effective method in target delivery of chemotherapeutic agents to tumor cells.

ASSESMENT QUESTIONS

8.1. What are the major factors determining the efficacy of drug delivery to the target tissue?

8.2. What are the physiological/pathological impairments in individual patients that may contribute to an unsuccessful treatment outcome of target delivery?

8.3. Stimuli-responsive formulations were designed on both physiological-factor-based and target-ligand-based approaches toward host cells. What are physiological-based approaches and target-ligand-based approaches?

REFERENCES

1. Touitou, E., Barry, B.W. eds. *Enhancement in Drug Delivery*, Culinary and Hospitality Industry Publications, Weimar, TX, 2006.
2. Deshpande, N., et al. (1991). Tumor enzymes and prognosis in transitional cell carcinoma of the bladder: prediction of risk of progression in patients with superficial disease. *The Journal of Urology.*, *146*(*5*), 1247–1251.
3. Soman, C., Giorgio, T. (2009). Sensitive and multiplexed detection of proteomic antigens via quantum dot aggregation. *Nanomedicine*, *5*, 402–409.
4. Alexis, F., et al. (2008). Factors affecting the clearance and biodistribution of polymeric nanoparticles. *Molecular Pharmacology*, *5*, 505–515.
5. Jain, K.K. (2005). Targeted drug delivery for cancer. *Technology in Cancer Research & Treatment*, *4*(*4*).
6. Weinstein, J.N., Van Osdol, W. (1992). Early intervention in cancer using monoclonal antibodies and other biological ligands: Micropharmacology and the "binding site barrier." *Cancer Research*, *52*, 2747s–2751s.
7. Ghaghada, K.B., et al. (2005). Folate targeting of drug carriers: A mathematical model. *Journal of Controlled Release*, *104*, 113–128.
8. Saul, J.M., et al. (2003). Controlled targeting of liposomal doxorubicin via the folate receptor in vitro. *Journal of Controlled Release*, *92*, 49–67.
9. Witte, M.H. (2011). Lymphangiogenesis and hemangiogenesis: Potential targets for therapy. *Journal of Surgical Oncology*, *103*(*6*), 489–500.
10. Roth, J.M., et al. (2005). Recombinant alpha2(IV)NC1 domain inhibits tumor cell-extracellular matrix interactions, induces cellular senescence, and inhibits tumor growth in vivo. *American Journal of Pathology*, *166*, 901–911.
11. Siemann, D.W. *Vascular-Targeted Therapies in Oncology*, Wiley, New York, NY, 2006.
12. Lim, J., et al. (2009). Design, synthesis, characterization, and biological evaluation of triazinedendrimers bearing paclitaxel using ester and ester/disulfide linkages. *Bioconjugate Chemistry*, *20*, 2154–2161.
13. Jain, S., et al. (2003). RGD-anchored magnetic liposomes for monocytes/neutrophils-mediated brain targeting. *International Journal of Pharmacy*, *261*, 43–55.
14. Matsumura, Y., Maeda, H. (1986). A new concept for macromolecular therapeutics in cancer chemotherapy: Mechanism of tumoritropic accumulation of proteins and the antitumor agent Smancs. *Cancer Research*, *46*(*12*), 6387–6392.
15. Kim, G.J., Nie, S. (2005). Targeted cancer nanotherapy. *Materials Today*, *8*(*8*), 28–33.
16. Ruoslahti, E. (2000). Targeting tumor vasculature with homing peptides from phage display. *Semin Cancer Biology*, *10* (*6*), 435–442.
17. Sudimack, J., Lee, R.J. (2000). Targeted drug delivery via the folate receptor. *Advanced Drug Delivery Reviews*, *41*, 147–162.
18. Zhang, Z, Huey, L.S., Feng, S.S. (2007). Folate-decorated poly(lactide-co-glycolide)-vitamin E TPGS nanoparticles for targeted drug delivery. *Biomaterials*, *28*, 1889–1899.
19. Eliaz, R.E., Szoka, F.C.Jr., (2001). Liposome-encapsulated doxorubicin targeted to CD44: A strategy to kill CD44-overexpressing tumor cells. *Cancer Research*, *61*, 2592–2601.
20. Farokhzad, O.C., et al. (2006). Targeted nanoparticle-aptamerbioconjugates for cancer chemotherapy *in vivo*. *Proceedings of the National Academy of the USA*, *103*, 6315–6320.

21. Dhar, S., et al. (2008). Targeted delivery of cisplatin to prostate cancer cells by aptamer functionalized Pt(IV) prodrug–PLGA–PEG nanoparticles. *Proceedings of the National Academy of the USA, 105*, 17356–17361.

22. Lu, J., Shi, M., Shoichet, M.S. (2009). Click chemistry functionalized polymeric nanoparticles target corneal epithelial cells through RGD-cell surface receptors. *Bioconjugate Chemistry, 20*, 87–94.

23. Singh, S.R., et al. (2009). Intravenous transferrin, RGD peptide and dual-targeted nanoparticles enhance anti-VEGF intraceptor gene delivery to laser-induced CNV. *Gene Therapy, 16*, 645–659.

24. Hu, Z., et al. (2008). Arg-Gly-Asp (RGD) peptide conjugated poly(lactic acid)–poly(ethylene oxide) micelle for targeted drug delivery. *Journal of Biomedical Materials Research Part A., 85*, 797–807.

25. Gao, X., et al. (2007). UEA I-bearing nanoparticles for brain delivery following intranasal administration. *International Journal of Pharmacy, 340(1–2)*, 207–215.

26. Gupta, P.N., et al. (2006). Lectin anchored stabilized biodegradable nanoparticles for oral immunization 1. Development and *in vitro* evaluation. *International Journal of Pharmacy, 318*, 163–173.

27. Ulbrich, K., et al. (2009). Transferrin- and transferrin-receptor-antibody-modified nanoparticles enable drug delivery across the blood–brain barrier (BBB). *European Journal of Pharmaceutics and Biopharmaceutics, 71*, 251–256.

28. Wang, J., et al. (2010). The complex role of multivalency in nanoparticles targeting the transferrin receptor for cancer therapies. *Journal of the American Chemical Society, 132*, 11306–11313.

29. Aillon, K.L., et al. (2009). Effects of nanomaterial physicochemical properties on *in vivo* toxicity. *Advanced Drug Delivery Reviews, 61*, 457–466.

30. Borgman, M.P., et al. (2008). Tumor-targeted HPMA copolymer-(RGDfK)-(CHX-A″-DTPA) conjugates show increased kidney accumulation. *Journal of Controlled Release, 132(3), 18*, 193–199.

31. Ito, Y., et al. (1999). Enzyme modification by polymers with solubilities that change in response to photoirradiation in organic media. *Nature Biotechnology, 17*, 73–75.

32. Oya, T., et al. (1999). Reversible molecular adsorption based on multiple-point interaction by shrinkable gels. *Science, 286 (5444)*, 1543–1545.

33. Dincer, S., Tuerk, M., Piskin, E., (2005). Intelligent polymers as nonviral vectors. *Gene Therapy, 12*, S139–S145.

34. Bajpai, A.K., et al. (2008). Responsive polymers in controlled drug delivery. *Progress in Polymer Science, 33*, 1088–1118.

35. Gavini, E., et al. (2009). Frontal polymerization as a new method for developing drug controlled release systems (DCRS) based on polyacrylamide. *European Polymer Journal, 45*, 690–699.

36. Langer, R., Tirrell, D.A. (2004). Designing materials for biology and medicine. *Nature, 428*, 487–492.

37. Chan, G., Mooney, D.J. (2008). New materials for tissue engineering: Towards greater control over the biological response, *Trends in Biotechnology, 26*, 382–392.

38. Dai, S., Ravi, P., Tam, K.C. (2008). pH-Responsive polymers: Synthesis, properties and applications. *Soft Matter, 4*, 435–449.

39. Kim, B.S., et al. (2009). All-star polymer multilayers as pH-responsive nanofilms. *Macromolecules, 42*, 368–375.

40. Liu, X.Y., et al. (2004). Design of temperature sensitive imprinted polymer hydrogels based on multiple-point hydrogen bonding. *Macromolecular Bioscience, 4(7)*, 680–684.

41. De, P., Gondi, S.R., Sumerlin, B.S. (2008). Folate-conjugated thermoresponsive block copolymers: Highly efficient conjugation and solution self-assembly. *Biomacromolecules, 9*, 1064–1070.

42. Pelah, A., Bharde, A., Jovin, T.M. (2009). Protein manipulation by stimuli-responsive polymers encapsulated in erythrocyte ghosts. *Soft Matter, 5*, 1006–1010.

43. Antunes, F., et al. (2009). Rheological characterization of the thermal gelation of poly(N-isopropylacrylamide) and poly (N-isopropylacrylamide)co-acrylic acid. *Applied Rheology, 19(4)*, 42064–42069.

44. Glazer, E.S., et al. (2010). Pancreatic carcinoma cells are susceptible to noninvasive radio frequency fields after treatment with targeted gold nanoparticles. *Surgery, 148*, 319–324.

45. Gonda, K., et al. (2010). *In vivo* nano-imaging of membrane dynamics in metastatic tumor cells using quantum dots. *Journal of Biological Chemistry, 285*, 2750–2757.

46. Dubertret, B., et al. (2002). *In vivo* imaging of quantum dots encapsulated in phospholipid micelles. *Science, 298*, 1759–1762.

47. Chang, E., et al. (2006). Evaluation of quantum dot cytotoxicity based on intracellular uptake. *Small, 2*, 1412–1417.

48. Benkoski, J.J., et al. (2008). Self-assembly of polymer-coated ferromagnetic nanoparticles into mesoscopic polymer chains. *Journal of Polymer Science Part B: Polymer Physics, 46*, 2267–2277.

49. Torchilin V. (2009). Multifunctional and stimuli-sensitive pharmaceutical nanocarriers. *European Journal of Pharmaceutics and Biopharmaceutics, 71(3)*, 431–444.

50. Rajashekhar, G., et al. (2005). Hypoxia up-regulated angiogenin and down-regulated vascular cell adhesion molecule-1 expression and secretion in human placental trophoblasts. *Journal of the Society for Gynecologic Investigation, 12*, 310–319.

51. Gerweck, L.E., Vijayappa, S., Kozin, S. (2006). Tumor pH controls the in vivo efficacy of weak acid and base chemotherapeutics. *Molecular Cancer Therapeutics, 5*, 1275–1279.

52. Hartmann, V., Keipert, S. (2000). Physico-chemical, in vitro and in vivo characterization of polymers for ocular use. *Pharmazie 55(6)*, 440–443.

53. Kumar, S., Himmelstein, K.J. (1995). Modification of in situ gelling behavior of carbopol solutions by hydroxypropyl methyl cellulose. *Journal of Pharmacy & Pharmaceutical Sciences, 84(3)*, 344–348.

54. Zaman, N.T., Yang, Y.Y., Ying, J.Y. (2010). Stimuli-responsive polymers for the targeted delivery of paclitaxel to hepatocytes. *Nanotoday*, *5*, 9–14.
55. Kamada, H., et al. (2004). Design of a pH-sensitive polymeric carrier for drug release and its application in cancer therapy. *Clinical Cancer Research*, *i10*, 2545–2550.
56. Dufresne, M.H., et al. (2004). Preparation and characterization of water-soluble pH-sensitive nanocarriers for drug delivery. *International Journal of Pharmacy*, *277*, 81–90.
57. Shenoy, D., et al. (2005). Poly(ethylene oxide)-modified poly (beta-amino ester) nanoparticles as a pH-sensitive system for tumor-targeted delivery of hydrophobic drugs: Part 2. In vivo distribution and tumor localization studies. *Research in Pharmacy*, *22*, 2107–2114.
58. Sethuraman, V.A., Na, K., Bae, Y.H. (2006). pH-responsive sulfonamide/PEI system for tumor specific gene delivery: An in vitro study. *Biomacromolecules*, *7*, 64–70.
59. Grainger, S.J., El-Sayed, M.E.H. Stimuli-sensitive particles for drug delivery, In: Stephanie J. Grainger and Mohamed E. H. El-Sayed (eds.), *Biologically-Responsive Hybrid Biomaterials*, 2010.
60. Sáez-Martínez, V., et al. (2008). Macromolecular nanotechnology: pH-sensitive microgels functionalized with folic acid. *European Polymer Journal*, *44(5)* 1309–1322.
61. Park, S.Y., Bae, Y.H., (1999). pH-sensitive polymers containing sulfonamide groups. *Macromolecular Rapid Communication*, *20*, 269–273.
62. Na K., Bae, Y.H. pH-sensitive polymers for drug delivery, in G.S. Kwon (ed.), *Polymeric Drug Delivery Systems*, Taylor & Francis, Boca Raton, FL, 2005, pp. 129–194.
63. Butler, P.J., et al. (1969). The use of maleic anhydride for the reversible blocking of amino groups in polypeptide chains. *Biochemical Journal*, *112*, 679–689.
64. Butler, P.J., et al. (1967). Reversible blocking of peptide amino groups by maleic anhydride. *Biochemical Journal*, *103*, 78P–79P.
65. Wakefield, D.H., et al. (2005). Membrane activity and transfection ability of amphipathic polycations as a function of alkyl group size. *Bioconjugate Chemistry*, *16*, 1204–1208.
66. Rozema, D.B., et al. (2007). Dynamic polyconjugates for targeted in vivo delivery of siRNA to hepatocytes. *Proceedings of the National Academy of the USA*, *104(32)*, 12982–12987.
67. Hatakeyama, H., et al. (2007). Tumor targeting of doxorubicin by anti-MT1-MMP antibody-modified PEG liposomes. *International Journal of Pharmacy*, *342*, 194–200.
68. Andreopoulou, E., et al. (2007). Pegylated liposomal doxorubicin HCL (PLD; Caelyx/Doxil): Experience with long-term maintenance in responding patients with recurrent epithelial ovarian cancer. *Annals of Oncology*, *18*, 716–721.
69. Lee, E.S., Na, K., Bae, Y.H. (2003). Polymeric micelle for tumor pH and folate-mediated targeting. *Journal of Controlled Release*, *91*, 103–113.
70. Kim, D., et al. (2008). Doxorubicin-loaded polymeric micelle overcomes multidrug resistance of cancer by double-targeting folate receptor and early endosomal pH. *Small*, *4(11)*, 2043–2050.
71. Takae, S., et al. (2008). PEG-detachable polyplex micelles based on disulfide-linked block catiomers as bioresponsive nonviral gene vectors. *Journal of the American Chemical Society*, *130*, 6001–6009.
72. Garg, A., et al. (2009). Targeting colon cancer cells using PEGylated liposomes modified with a fibronectin-mimetic peptide. *International Journal of Pharmacy*, *366*, 201–210.
73. Bicher, H.I., Al-Bussam, N. (2006). Thermoradiotherapy with curative intent–Breast, head, neck and prostate tumors. *Deutsche Zeitschrift für Onkologie*, *38(3)*, 116–122.
74. Lee, H.I., et al. (2010). Stimuli-responsive molecular brushes. Special Issue on Stimuli-Responsive Materials. *Progress in Polymer Science*, *35(1–2)*, 24–44.
75. Schmaljohann, D. (2006). Thermo- and pH-responsive polymers in drug delivery. *Advanced Drug Delivery Reviews*, *58(15)*, 1655–1670.
76. Alvarez-Lorenzo, C., et al. (2000). Polymer gels that memorize elements of molecular conformation. *Macromolecules*, *33*, 8693.
77. Ono, Y., Shikata, T. (2007). Contrary hydration behavior of N-Isopropylacrylamide to its polymer, P(NIPAm), with a lower critical solution temperature. *Journal of Physics Chemistry B Condensed Matter Materials Surface Interfaces Biophysics*, *111(7)*, 1511–1513.
78. Schild, H.G., (1992). Poly (N-isopropylacrylamide): Experiment, theory and application. *Progress in Polymer Science*, *17*, 163–249.
79. Van Durme, K., et al. (2004). *Macromolecules*, *37*, 1054.
80. Aoki, T., et al. (1994). *Macromolecules 27*, 947.
81. Kwon, Y.M., Kim, S.W. Thermosensitive biodegradable hydrogels for the delivery of therapeutic agents, in G.S. Kwon (ed.), *Polymeric Drug Delivery Systems*, Taylor & Francis, Boca Raton, FL, 2005, pp. 251–274.
82. Huang, J., et al. (2007). Synthesis and in situ atomic force microscopy characterization of temperature-responsive hydrogels based on poly(2-(dimethylamino)ethyl methacrylate) prepared by atom transfer radical polymerization. *Langmuir*, *8*, 241–249.
83. Kontermann, R.E. (2006). Immunoliposomes for cancer therapy. *Current Opinion in Molecular Therapeutics*, *8*, 39–45.
84. Bertrand, N., et al. (2010). Transmembrane pH-gradient liposomes to treat cardiovascular drug intoxication. *ACS Nano*, *4*, 7552–7558.
85. Ichikawa, H., Fukumori, Y. (2000). A novel positively thermosensitive controlled-release microcapsule with membrane of nano-sized poly(N-isopropylacrylamide) gel dispersed in ethylcellulose matrix. *Journal of Controlled Release*, *63*, 107–119.
86. Phillips Research Institution. (2011). New method combines MRI, HIFU. temperature-senaitive liposomes for chemo delivery directly to tumor report on Feb 9.
87. Veiseh, O., et al. (2005). Optical and MRI multifunctional nanoprobe for targeting gliomas. *Nano Letters*, *5*, 1003–1008.

88. Kirchner, C., et al. (2005). Cytotoxicity of colloidal CdSe and CdSe/ZnS nanoparticles. *Nano Letters*, *5*, 331–338.
89. Rossi, L.M., et al. (2005). Synthesis of monodispersed luminescent silica nanoparticles for bioanalytical assays. *Langmuir*, *21*, 4277–4280.
90. Lin, M.M., et al. (2010). Surface activation and targeting strategies of superparamagnetic iron oxide nanoparticles in cancer-oriented diagnosis and therapy. *Nanomedicine*, *5(1)*, 109–133.
91. Hassan, E.E., Gallo, J.M. (1993). Targeting anticancer drugs to the brain. I: Enhanced brain delivery of oxantrazole following administration in magnetic cationic microspheres. *Journal of Drug Targeting*, *1*, 7–14.
92. Walsh, D., et al. (2003). Dextran templating for the synthesis of metallic and metal oxide sponges. *Nature Materials*, *2*, 386–90.
93. Pickard, M., Chari, D. (2010). Enhancement of magnetic nanoparticle-mediated gene transfer to astrocytes by "magnetofection": Effects of static and oscillating fields. *Nanomedicine*, *5*(*2*), 217–232.
94. Avilés, M.O., et al. (2008). Isolated swine heart ventricle perfusion model for implant assisted-magnetic drug targeting. *International Journal of Pharmaceutics*, *361*(*1–2*), 202–208.
95. Alexiou, C., et al. (2000). Locoregional cancer treatment with magnetic drug targeting. *Cancer Research*, *60*, 6641–6648.
96. Widder, K.J., et al. (1983). Selective targeting of magnetic albumin microspheres containing low-dose doxorubicin–total remission in Yoshida sarcoma-bearing rats. *European Journal of Cancer & Clinical Oncology*, *19*, 135–139.
97. Pulfer, S.K., Gallo, J.M., (1999). Enhanced brain tumor selectivity of cationic magnetic polysaccharide microspheres. *Journal of Drug Targeting*, *6*, 215–228.
98. Devineni, D., Klein-Szanto, A., Gallo, J.M. (1995). Tissue distribution of methotrexate following administration as a solution and as a magnetic microsphere conjugate in rats bearing brain tumors. *Journal of Neuro-Oncology*, *24*, 143–152.
99. Lucignani, G. (2009). Nanoparticles for concurrent multimodality imaging and therapy: The dawn of new theragnostic synergies. *European Journal of Nuclear Medicine and Molecular Imaging*, *36*(*5*), 1619–7070.
100. McCarthy, J.R. (2009). The future of theranostic nanoagents. *Nanomed*, *4*, 693–5.
101. Shukoor, M.I., et al. , (2007). *Chem Commun (Camb), Superparamagnetic—Fe2O3 Nanoparticles with Tailored Functionality for Protein Separation*, *44*, 4677.
102. Wang, L., Gan, X.X. (2009). Biomolecule-functionalized magnetic nanoparticles for flow-through quartz crystal microbalance immunoassay of aflatoxin B_1. *Bioprocess and Biosystems Engineering*, *32(1)*, 1615–7591.
103. Perez, J.M., et al. (2003). Viral-induced self-assembly of magnetic nanoparticles allows the detection of viral particles in biological media. *Journal of the American Chemical Society*, *125(34)*, 10192–10193.
104. Chen, W., et al. (2010). A molecularly targeted theranostic probe for ovarian cancer. *Molecular Cancer Therapeutics*, *9*, 1028.
105. Pan, D., et al. (2008). Ligand-directed nanobialys as theranostic agent for drug delivery and manganese-based magnetic resonance imaging of vascular targets. *Journal of the American Chemical Society*. *130*, 9186–9187.
106. Wood, J. (2006). Charging up magnetic quantum dots for spintronics. *Nanotechnology Materials Today*, *9*(*5*), 13.
107. Ho, Y.P., Leong, K.W. (2010). Quantum dot-based theranostics. *Nanoscale*, *2*, 60–68.
108. Pastan, I., Willingham, M.C. *Endocytosis*, Plenum Press, Plattsburg, NY, 1985.
109. Elbayoumi, T.A., Torchilin, V.P. (2008). Tumor-specific antibody-mediated targeted delivery of Doxil reduces the manifestation of auricular erythema side effect in mice. *International Journal of Pharmacy*, *357*, 272–279.
110. Cruz, L.J., et al. (2010). Targeted PLGA nano- but not microparticles specifically deliver antigen to human dendritic cells via DC-SIGN in vitro. *Journal of Controlled Release*, *144*, 118–126.
111. Sorokin, P. (2000). Mylotarg approved for patients with $CD33^+$ acute myeloid leukemia. *Clinical Journal of Oncology Nursing*, *4*, 279–280.
112. Sapra, P., Allen, T.M., (2004). Improved outcome when B-cell lymphoma is treated with combinations of immunoliposomal anticancer drugs targeted to both the CD19 and CD20 epitopes. *Clinical Cancer Research*, *10*, 2530–2627.
113. Yang, H., Cho, N.H., Seong, S.Y. (2009). The Tat-conjugated N-terminal region of mucin antigen 1 (MUC1) induces protective immunity against MUC1-expressing tumours. *Clinical and Experimental Immunology*, *158*(*2*), 174–185.
114. Miller, J., Bothwell, A., Storb. U. (1981). Physical linkage of the constant region genes for immunoglobulins λ_I and λ^{III}. *Proceedings of the National Academy of Science of the USA*, *78*, 3829–3933.
115. Park, J.W., et al. (2001). Tumor targeting using anti-her2 immunoliposomes. *Journal of Controlled Release*, *74*, 95–113.
116. Cirstoiu-Hapca, A., et al. (2010). Benefit of anti-HER2-coated paclitaxel-loaded immuno-nanoparticles in the treatment of disseminated ovarian cancer: Therapeutic efficacy and biodistribution in mice. *Journal of Controlled Release*, *144*, 324–331.
117. Nielsen, U.B., et al. (2002). Therapeutic efficacy of anti-ErbB2 immunoliposomes targeted by a phage antibody selected for cellular endocytosis. *Biochimica et Biophysica Acta*, *1591*, 109–118.
118. Elbayoumi, T.A., Torchilin, V.P. (2009). Tumor-specific anti-nucleosome antibody improves therapeutic efficacy of doxorubicin-loaded long-circulating liposomes against primary and metastatic tumor in mice. *Molecular Pharmaceutics*, *6*(*1*), 246–254.
119. Blackwell, J.E., et al. (2001). Ligand coated nanosphere adhesion to E- and P-selectin under static and flow conditions. *Annals of Biomedical Engineering*, *29*, 523–533.
120. Dickerson, J.B., et al. (2001). Limited adhesion of biodegradable microspheres to E- and P-selectin under flow. *Biotechnology and Bioengineering*, *73*, 500–509.

121. Olivier, J.C., et al. (2002). Synthesis of pegylated immunonanoparticles. *Research in Pharmacy, 19,* 1137–1143.
122. McCarron, P.A., et al. (2008). Antibody targeting of camptothecin-loaded PLGA nanoparticles to tumor cells. *Bioconjugate Chemistry, 19,* 1561–1569.
123. Scott, C.J., et al. (2008). Immunocolloidal targeting of the endocytotic siglec-7 receptor using peripheral attachment of siglec-7 antibodies to poly(lactide-co-glycolide) nanoparticles. *Research in Pharmacy, 25,* 135–146.
124. Nukolova, N.V., et al. (2011). Polyelectrolyte nanogels decorated with monoclonal antibody for targeted drug delivery. *Reactive and Functional Polymers, 71(3),* 315–323.
125. Goldenberg, D.M., et al. (2007). Cancer imaging and therapy with bispecific antibody pretargeting. *Cancer Therapy, 2(1),* 19–31.
126. Goodwin, D.A., et al. (1992). Pretargeted immunoscintigraphy: Effect of hapten valency on murine tumor uptake. *Journal of Nuclear Medicine, 33,* 2006–2013.
127. Liu, G., et al. (2008). Pretargeting CWR22 prostate tumor in mice with MORF-B72.3 antibody and radiolabeled cMORF. *European Journal of Nuclear Medicine and Molecular Imaging, 35(2),* 272–280.
128. Howarth, M. et al., (2005). Targeting quantum dots to surface proteins in living cells with biotin ligase. *Proceedings of the National Academy of Science of the USA, 102,* 7583–7588.
129. Laitinen, O.H., et al. (2007). Brave new (strept)avidins in biotechnology. *Trends in Biotechnology, 25(6),* 269–277.
130. Wilchek, M., et al. (2006). Essentials of biorecognition: The (strept)avidin–biotin system as a model for protein–protein and protein–ligand interaction. *Immunology Letters, 103,* 27–32.
131. Yao, Z., et al. (1998). Avidin targeting of intraperitoneal tumor. *Xenografts, 90(1),* 25–29.
132. Stayton, P.S., et al. (2004). Smart polymer–streptavidin conjugates. *Methods in Molecular Biology, 283,* 37–43.
133. De Las Heras Alarcon, C., et al. (2005). Stimuli responsive polymers for biomedical applications. *Chemical Society Reviews, 34,* 276–285.
134. Dinauer, N., et al. (2005). Selective targeting of antibody-conjugated nanoparticles to leukemic cells and primary T-lymphocytes. *Biomaterials, 26,* 5898–5906.
135. Waehler, R., Russell, S.J., Curiel, D.T. (2007). Engineering targeted viral vectors for gene therapy. *Nature Reviews Genetics, 8,* 573–587.
136. Kaikkonen, M.U., et al. (2009). (Strept)avidin-displaying lentiviruses as versatile tools for targeting and dual imaging of gene delivery. *Gene Therapy, 16,* 894–904.
137. Schwartz, J.J., Zhang, S. (2000). Peptide-mediated cellular delivery. *Current Opinion in Molecular Therapeutics, 2,* 162–167.
138. Mani, K., et al. (2007). HIV-Tat protein transduction domain specifically attenuates growth of polyamine deprived tumor cells. *Molecular Cancer Therapeutics, 6(2),* 782–8.
139. Fawell, S., et al. (1994). Tat-mediated delivery of heterologous proteins into cells. *Proceedings of the National Academy of Science of the USA, 91,* 664–668.
140. Vives, E., Brodin, P., Lebleu, B. (1997). A truncated HIV-1 Tat protein basic domain rapidly translocates through the plasma membrane and accumulates in the cell nucleus. *Journal of Biological Chemistry, 272,* 16010–16017.
141. Bellmann-Sickert, K., Beck-Sickinger, A.G. (2010). Peptide drugs to target G protein-coupled receptors. *Trends in Pharmacological Sciences 31(9),* 434–441.
142. Law, B., Weissleder, R., Tung, C.H. (2006). Peptide-based biomaterials for protease-enhanced drug delivery. *Biomacromolecules, 7(4),* 1261–1265.
143. Basel, M.T., et al. (2011). Protease-sensitive, polymer-caged liposomes: A method for making highly targeted liposomes using triggered release. *ACS Nano, 5(3),* 2162–2175.
144. Järver, P., Langel, Ü. (2006). Cell-penetrating peptides-A brief introduction. *Biochimica et Biophysica Acta, 1758,* 260–263.
145. Torchilin, V.P. (2007). Tatp-mediated intracellular delivery of pharmaceutical nanocarriers. *Biochemical Society Transactions, 35,* 816–820.
146. Endoh, T., Ohtsuki, T. (2009). Cellular siRNA delivery using cell-penetrating peptides modified for endosomal escape. *Advanced Drug Delivery Reviews, 61,* 704–709.
147. Tseng, Y.L., Liu, J.J., Hong, R.L. (2002). Translocation of liposomes into cancer cells by cell-penetrating peptides penetratin and tat: A kinetic and efficacy study. *Molecular Pharmacology, 62,* 864–872.
148. Sebbage, V. (2009). Cell-penetrating peptides and their therapeutic applications. *Bioscience Horizons, 2,* 64–72.
149. Hassane, F.S. et al. (2009). Cell-penetrating-peptides: Overview and applications to the delivery of oligonucleotides. *Cellular and Molecular Life Sciences,* 715–726.
150. Andaloussi, S.E., Guterstam, P., Langel, U. (2007). Assessing the delivery efficacy and internalization route of cell-penetrating peptides. *Nature Protocols, 2(8),* 2043–2047.
151. Martin, I. Teixidó, M., Giralt, E. (2010). Review building cell selectivity into CPP-mediated strategies. *Pharmaceuticals, 3(5),* 1456–1490.
152. Torchilin, V.P. (2002). TAT peptide-modified liposomes for intracellular delivery of drugs and DNA. *Cellular and Molecular Biology Letters, 7,* 265–267.
153. Torchilin, V.P., Levchenko, T.S. (2003). TAT-liposomes: A novel intracellular drug carrier. *Current Protein & Peptide Science, 4,* 133–140.
154. Torchilin, V.P., et al. (2001). TAT peptide on the surface of liposomes affords their efficient intracellular delivery even at low temperature and in the presence of metabolic inhibitors. *Proceedings of the National Academy of Science of the USA, 98,* 8786–8791.
155. Rautsi, O., et al. (2008). Characterization of HIV-1 TAT peptide as an enhancer of HSV-TK/GCV cancer gene therapyUtility of TAT-TK-GFP in HSV-TK/GCV therapy. *Cancer Gene Therapy, 15,* 303–314.
156. Sorriento, D., et al. (2009). A new synthetic protein, TAT-RH, inhibits tumor growth through the regulation of NFκB activity. *Molecular Cancer, 8,* 97.

157. Chen, K., Chen, X. (2011). Review: Integrin targeted delivery of chemotherapeutics. *Theranostics*, *1*, 189–200.

158. Xiao, B., et al. (2009). RGD-IL-24, A novel tumor-targeted fusion cytokine: Expression, purification and functional evaluation. *Molecular Biotechnology*, *41*(2), 138–144.

159. Rothwangl, K.B., Rong, L. (2009). Analysis of a conserved RGE/RGD motif in HCV E2 in mediating entry. *Virology Journal*, *6*, 12.

160. Kantlehner, M., et al. (2000). Surface coating with cyclic RGD peptides stimulates osteoblast adhesion and proliferation as well as bone formation. *Chembiochem*, *1*, 107–114.

161. Haubner, R., et al. (1999). Radiolabeled alpha(v)beta3 integrin antagonists: A new class of tracers for tumor targeting. *Journal of Nuclear Medicine*, *40*, 1061–1071.

162. Haubner, R., et al. (2001). Glycosylated RGS-containing peptides: Tracer for tumor targeting and angiogenesis imaging with improved biokinetics. *Journal of Nuclear Medicine*, *42*, 326–336.

163. Kumar, C.C., et al. (2000). Targeting integrins alpha v beta 3 and alpha v beta 5 for blocking tumor-induced angiogenesis. *Advances in Experimental Medicine & Biology*, *476*, 169–180.

164. Vyas, S.P., Vaidya, B. (2009). Targeted delivery of thrombolytic agents: Role of integrin receptors. *Expert Opinion on Drug Delivery*, *6*(*5*), 499–508.

165. Dubey, P.K., et al. (2004). Liposomes modified with cyclic RGD peptide for tumor targeting. *Journal of Drug Targeting*, *12*, 257–264.

166. Jain, S., et al. (2003). RGD-anchored magnetic liposomes for monocytes/neutrophils-mediated brain targeting. *International Journal of Pharmacy*, *261*, 43–55.

167. Oba, M., et al. (2007). Cyclic RGD peptide-conjugated polyplex micelles as a targetable gene delivery system directed to cells possessing $\alpha_v\beta_3$ and $\alpha_v\beta_5$ integrins. *Bioconjugate Chemistry*, *18*(*5*), 1415–1423.

168. Merkel, O.M., et al. (2009). Integrin $\alpha_v\beta_3$ targeted gene delivery using RGD peptidomimetic conjugates with copolymers of PEGylated poly(ethylene imine). *Bioconjugate Chemistry*, *20*(*6*), 1270–1280.

169. Folkman, J. (1971). Tumor angiogenesis: therapeutic implications. *New England Journal of Medicine*, *285*, 1182–1186.

170. Moffatt, S., Cristiano, R.J. (2006). Uptake characteristics of NGR-coupled stealth PEI/pDNA nanoparticles loaded with PLGA–PEG–PLGA tri-block copolymer for targeted delivery to human monocyte-derived dendritic cells. *International Journal of Pharmacy*, *321*, 143–154.

171. Colombo, G., et al. (2002). Structure-activity relationships of linear and cyclic peptides containing the NGR tumor-homing motif. *Journal of Biological Chemistry*, *277*, 47891–47897.

172. Yokoyama, Y., Ramakrishnan S., (2005). Addition of an aminopeptidase N-binding sequence to human endostatin improves inhibition of ovarian carcinoma growth. *Cancer*, *104*(2), 321–331.

173. Corti, A., Curnis, F., (2011). Isoaspartate-dependent molecular switches for integrin–ligand recognition. *Journal of Cell Science*, *124*, 515–522.

174. Curnis, F., et al. (2005). Targeted delivery of IFNgamma to tumor vessels uncouples antitumor from counter-regulatory mechanisms. *Cancer Research*, *65*, 2906–2913.

175. Gregorc, V., et al. (2009). Phase Ib study of NGR–hTNF, a selective vascular targeting agent, administered at low doses in combination with doxorubicin to patients with advanced solid tumours. *British Journal of Cancer*, *101*, 219–224.

176. Grifman, M., et al. (2001). Incorporation of tumor-targeting peptides into recombinant adeno-associated virus capsids. *Molecular Therapeutics*, *3*, 964–975.

177. Pasqualini, R., et al. (2000). Aminopeptidase N is a receptor for tumor-homing peptides and a target for inhibiting angiogenesis. *Cancer Research*, *60*, 722–727.

178. Matteo, P.D., et al. (2006). Immunogenic and structural properties of the Asn-Gly-Arg (NGR) tumor neovasculature-homing motif. *Molecular Immunology*, *43*(*10*), 1509–1518.

179. Deshayes, S., et al. (2011). "Click" conjugation of peptide on the surface of polymeric nanoparticles for targeting tumor angiogenesis. *Pharmaceutical Research*, *28*, 1631–1642.

180. Bennett, J.S. (2005). Structure and function of the platelet integrin alphaIIbbeta3. *Journal of Clinical Investigation*, *115* (*12*), 3363–3369.

181. Srinivasan, R., Marchant, R.E., Gupta, A.S. (2010). In vitro and in vivo platelet targeting by cyclic RGD-modified liposomes. *Journal of Biomedical Materials Research Part A*, *93*(*3*), 1004–1015.

182. Stevens, P.J., Sekido, M., Lee, R.J. (2004a). A folate receptor-targeted lipid nanoparticle formulation for a lipophilic paclitaxel prodrug. *Research in Pharmacy*, *21*, 2153–2157.

183. Hilgenbrink, A.R., Low, P. (2005). Folate receptor-mediated drug targeting: From therapeutics to diagnostics. *Journal of Pharmaceutical Sciences*, *94*(*10*), 2135–2146.

184. Ross, J.F., Chaudhuri, P.K., Ratnam, M. (1994). Differential regulation of folate receptor isoforms in normal and malignant tissues in vivo and in established cell lines. Physiologic and clinical implications. *Cancer*, *73*, 2432–2443.

185. Franzen, S.A. (2011). Comparison of peptide and folate receptor targeting of cancer cells: From single agent to nanoparticle. *Expert Opinion on Drug Delivery*, *8*(*3*), 281–298.

186. Parker, N., et al. (2005). Folate receptor expression in carcinomas and normal tissues determined by a quantitative radioligand binding assay. *Analytical Biochemistry*, *338*, 284–293.

187. Kamen, B.A., Capdevila, A. (1986). Receptor-mediated folate accumulation is regulated by the cellular folate content. *Proceedings of the National Academy of Science of the USA*, *83*, 5983–5987.

188. Antony, A.C. (1996). Folate receptors. *Annual Review of Nutrition*, *16*, 501–521.

189. Rothberg, K.G., et al. (1990). The glycophospholipid-linked folate receptor internalizes folate without entering the clathrin-coated pit endocytic pathway. *The Journal of Cell Biology*, *110*, 637–649.

190. Lee, R.J., Huang, L. (1996). Folate-targeted, anionic liposome-entrapped polylysine-condensed DNA for tumor cell-

specific gene transfer. *Journal of Biological Chemistry*, *271*, 8481–8487.

191. Kim, S.H., et al. (2005). Target-specific cellular uptake of PLGA nanoparticles coated with poly(L-lysine)-poly(ethylene glycol)-folate conjugate. *Langmuir*, *21*, 8852–8857.
192. Stevens, P.J., Sekido, M., Lee, R.J. (2004b). Synthesis and evaluation of a hematoporphyrin derivative in a folate receptor-targeted solid-lipid nanoparticle formulation. *Anticancer Research*, *24*, 161–165.
193. Rogers, L.M., et al. (1997). A dual-label stable-isotopic protocol is suitable for determination of folate bioavailability in humans: Evaluation of urinary excretion and plasma folate kinetics of intravenous and oral doses of [13C5] and [2H2] folic acid. *Journal of Nutrition*, *127*, 2321–2327.
194. Schatz, C., et al. (2003). Typical physicochemical behaviors of chitosan in aqueous solution. *Biomacromolecules*, *4*, 641–648.
195. Schatz, C., et al. (2005). Formation of polyelectrolyte complex particles from self-complexation of N-sulfated chitosan. *Biomacromolecules*, *6*, 1642–1647.
196. Zheng, Y., et al. (2009). Preparation and characterization of folate conjugated N-trimethyl chitosan nanoparticles as protein carrier targeting folate receptor: In vitro studies. *Journal of Drug Targeting*, *17(4)*, 294–303.
197. Zheng, Y., et al. (2010). Receptor-mediated gene delivery by folate-poly(ethylene glycol)-grafted-trimethyl chitosan in vitro. *Journal of Drug Targeting*, *19(8)*, 647–656.
198. Nukolova, N.V., et al. (2011). Folate-decorated nanogels for targeted therapy of ovarian cancer. *Biomaterials*, *32(23)*, 5417–5426.
199. Pardridge, W.M. (2007). shRNA and siRNA delivery to the brain. *Advanced Drug Delivery Reviews*, *59*, 141–152.
200. Feng, C., et al. (2010). Silencing of the MYCN gene by siRNA delivered by folate receptor-targeted liposomes in LA-N-5 cells. *Pediatric Surgery International*, *26*, 1185–1191.
201. Davis, M.E., et al. (2010). Evidence of RNAi in humans from systemically administered siRNA via targeted nanoparticles. *Nature*, *464*, 1067–1070.
202. Chen, Y., et al. (2010). Multifunctional nanoparticles delivering small interfering RNA and doxorubicin overcome drug resistance in cancer. *Journal of Biological Chemistry*, *285*, 22639–22650.
203. Geusens, B., et al. (2009). Ultradeformable cationic liposomes for delivery of small interfering RNA (siRNA) into human primary melanocytes. *Journal of Controlled Release*, *133(3)*, 214–220.
204. Landen, C.N., et al. (2005). The therapeutic EphA2 gene targeting in vivo using neutral liposomal small interfering RNA delivery. *Cancer Research*, *65*, 6910–6918.
205. Merritt, W.M., et al. (2008). Effect of interleukin-8 gene silencing with liposome-encapsulated small interfering RNA on ovarian cancer cell growth. *Journal of the National Cancer Institute*, *100(5)*, 359–372.
206. Dutta, T., et al. (2010). Dendrosome-based delivery of siRNA against E6 and E7 oncogenes in cervical cancer. *Nanomedicine*, *6(3)*, 463–470.
207. Tilghman, R.W., et al. (2005). Focal adhesion kinase is required for the spatial organization of the leading edge in migrating cells. *Journal of Cell Science*, *118*, 2613–2623.
208. Blackburn, W.H., et al. (2009). Peptide functionalized nanogels for targeted siRNA delivery. *Bioconjugate Chemistry*, *20(5)*, 960–968.
209. Dickerson, E.B., et al. (2010). Chemosensitization of cancer cells by siRNA using targeted nanogel delivery. *BMC Cancer*, *10*, 10.
210. Watanabe, K., et al. (2009). In vivo siRNA delivery with dendritic poly(L-lysine) for the treatment of hypercholesterolemia. *Molecular Biosystems*, *5(11)*, 1306–1310.
211. Matsumoto, S., et al. (2009). Environment-responsive block copolymer micelles with a disulfide cross-linked core for enhanced siRNA delivery. *Biomacromolecules*, *10*, 119–127.
212. Liu, Y., et al. (2011). Amphiphilic polysaccharide-hydrophobicized graft polymeric micelles for drug delivery nanosystems. *Current Medicinal Chemisty*, *18(17)*, 2638–2648.
213. Zhang, Y.W., Changjun, N.L. (2009). Saccharide modified pharmaceutical nanocarriers for targeted drug and gene delivery. *Current Pharmaceutical Design*, *15(32)*, 3826–3836.
214. Chourasia, M.K., Jain, S.K. (2004). Polysaccharides for colon targeted drug delivery. *Drug Delivery*, *11(2)*, 129–148.
215. Sihorkar, V., Vyas, S.P. (2001). Potential of polysaccharide anchored liposomes in drug delivery, targeting and immunization. *Journal of Pharmacy & Pharmaceutical Sciences*, *4*, 138–158.
216. Jones, M.N., et al. (1994). The targeting of phospholipid liposomes to bacteria. *Biochimica et Biophysica Acta*, *1196*, 57–64.
217. Mizu, M., et al. (2004). A polysaccharide carrier for immunostimulatory CpG DNAs to enhance cytokine secretion. *Journal of the American Chemical Society*, *126(27)*, 8372–8373.
218. Shimada, N., et al. (2007). A polysaccharide carrier to effectively deliver native phosphodiester CpG DNA to antigen-presenting cells. *Bioconjugate Chemistry*, *18(4)*, 1280–1286.
219. Yudovin-Farber, I., Dombm A.J. (2007). Cationic polysaccharides for gene delivery. *Materials Science and Engineering C*, *27(3)*, 595–598.
220. Jo, J., et al. (2010). Preparation of cationized polysaccharides as gene transfection carrier for bone marrow-derived mesenchymal stem cells. *Journal of Biomaterials Science, Polymer Edition*, *21*(2), 185–204.
221. Gleysteen, J.P., et al. (2008). Fluorescent labeled anti-EGFR antibody for identification of regional and distant metastasis in a preclinical xenograft model. *Head Neck*, *30(6)*, 782–789.
222. Talavera, A., et al. (2009). Nimotuzumab, an antitumor antibody that targets the epidermal growth factor receptor, blocks ligand binding while permitting the active receptor conformation. *Cancer Research*, *69*, 5851–5859.
223. Mamot, C., et al. (2006). EGFR-targeted immunoliposomes derived from the monoclonal antibody EMD72000 mediate specific and efficient drug delivery to a variety of colorectal cancer cells. *Journal of Drug Targeting*, *14*, 215–223.

224. El-Sayed, I.H., Huang, X., El-Sayed, M.A. (2006). Selective laser photo-thermal therapy of epithelial carcinoma using anti-EGFR antibody conjugated gold nanoparticles. *Cancer Letters*, *239*, 129–135.

225. Acharya, S., Dilnawaz, F., Sahoo, S.K. (2009). Targeted epidermal growth factor receptor nanoparticle bioconjugates for breast cancer therapy. *Biomaterials*, *30*, 5737–5750.

226. Wu, G., et al. (2007). Molecular targeting and treatment of an epidermal growth factor receptor-positive glioma using boronatedcetuximab. *Clinical Cancer Research*, *13*, 1260–1268.

227. Klammt, C., et al. (2011). Polymer-based cell-free expression of ligand-binding family B G-protein coupled receptors without detergents. *Protein Science*, *20(6)*, 1030–1041.

228. Suresh, P., Wanchu, A. (2006). Chemokines and chemokine receptors in HIV infection: Role in pathogenesis and therapeutics. *Journal of Postgraduate Medicine*, *52*, 210–217.

229. Pease, J.E., Horuk, R. (2009). Chemokine receptor antagonists: Part 1. *Expert Opinion on Therapeutic Patents*, *19*, 39–58.

230. Zwanziger, D., Beck-Sickinger, A.D. (2008). Radiometal targeted tumor diagnosis and therapy with peptide hormones. *Current Pharmaceutical Design*, *14*, 2385–2400.

231. Delpassand, E.S., et al. (2008). Safety and efficacy of radionuclide therapy with high-activity In-111 pentetreotide in patients with progressive neuroendocrine tumors. *Cancer Biotherapy and Radiopharmaceuticals*, *23*, 292–300.

232. Dammers, R., et al. (2009). Radioguided improved resection of a cranial base meningioma. *Neurosurgery*, *64*, 84–85.

233. Rodland, K. (2004). The role of the calcium-sensing receptor in cancer. *Cell Calcium*, *35*, 291–295.

234. Gavalas, N.G., et al. (2007). The calcium-sensing receptor is a target of autoantibodies in patients with autoimmune polyendocrine syndrome type 1. *The Journal of Clinical Endocrinology and Metablism*, *92(6)*, 2107–2114.

235. Marie, P.J. (2010). The calcium-sensing receptor in bone cells: A potential therapeutic target in osteoporosis. *Bone*, *46(3)*, 571–576.

236. Dharmala, K, Yoo, J.W., Lee, C.H. (2008). Development of Chitosan-SLN microparticles for chemotherapy: In vitro approach through efflux transporter modulation. *Journal of Controlled Release*, *131*, 190–197.

237. Bayless, K.J., Salazar, R., Davis, G.E. (2000). RGD-dependent vacuolation and lumen formation observed during endothelial cell morphogenesis in three-dimensional fibrin matrices involves the alpha(v)beta(3) and alpha(5)beta(1) integrins. *American Journal of Pathology*, *156*, 1673–1683.

238. Chen, X., et al. (2004). Pegylated Arg-Gly-Asp peptide: 64Cu labeling and PET imaging of brain tumor alphavbeta3-integrin expression. *Journal of Nuclear Medicine*, *45*, 1776–1783.

239. Kelloff, G.J., et al. (1996). Clinical development plan: Phenethyl isothiocyanate. *Journal of Cellular Biochemistry – Supplement*, *26*, 149–157.

240. Kehle, T., Herzog, V. (1987). Interactions between protein-gold complexes and cell surfaces: a method for precise quantitation. *European Journal of Cell Biology*, *45*, 80–87.

241. Reddy, J.A., et al. (2002). Folate-targeted, cationic liposome-mediated gene transfer into disseminated peritoneal tumors. *Gene Therapy*, *9*, 1542–1550.

242. Weiland, G.A., Molinoff, P.B. (1981). Quantitative analysis of drug-receptor interactions: I. Determination of kinetic and equilibrium properties. *Life Sciences*, *29(4)*, 313–330.

243. Colombo, R., et al. (2004) Overall clinical outcomes after nerve and seminal sparing radical cystectomy for the treatment of organ confined bladder cancer. *Journal of Urology*, *171*, 1819–1822.

9

IMPLANTS

Aswani Dutt Vadlapudi, Ashaben Patel, Ramya Krishna Vadlapatla, Durga Paturi, and Ashim K. Mitra

9.1 CHAPTER OBJECTIVES

- To outline fundamental concepts, rationale, and principles associated with the design of implantable controlled-release drug delivery systems.
- To facilitate sound knowledge of various polymers and polymeric membranes for achieving controlled drug release in biological systems.
- To provide a comprehensive overview of the mechanical pumps that provide external control of drug release through a pump-type mechanism.
- To illustrate the clinical and therapeutic applications of polymeric and mechanical pump systems.
- To discuss the importance of biocompatibility issues related to implantable drug delivery systems.

9.2 INTRODUCTION

Rapid enhancements in the development of drug delivery systems drastically changed the field of pharmacotherapy. Maintaining therapeutic drug concentration levels *in vivo* has always been a major problem. Intravenous or oral administration of drugs may either generate high plasma concentrations causing toxicity or low drug levels leading to subtherapeutic blood levels (Figure 9.1) [1, 2]. Repeated administrations may also cause drug resistance. In the past, drugs are administered via intravenous infusion at a constant rate to achieve therapeutic concentration; i.e., the drug concentration lies in between the minimum effective concentration and the maximum toxic concentration. However, this type of therapy requires continuous monitoring of the drug concentration by clinicians, which cannot be performed at home and turns out be very expensive. In a biological system, several mechanisms exist to prevent exposure to xenobiotics and protect the cell from toxins. Physiological, biochemical, and chemical barriers hinder absorption of drug molecule before reaching the site of action. Physiological barriers such as intestinal membrane and blood–brain barrier protect the body from various toxins by preventing their entry. Biochemical barriers constitute metabolizing enzymes that can convert the drug into its inactive form via degradation. Nevertheless, the drug should also possess optimal physicochemical properties for efficient permeation across biological membranes. Successful drug therapy involves overcoming these biological barriers to achieve desired concentration at the site of action and sufficiently sustain drug release besides lowering the side effects. This could be achieved by delivering drug to its specific site

Advanced Drug Delivery, First Edition. Edited by Ashim K. Mitra, Chi H. Lee, and Kun Cheng.

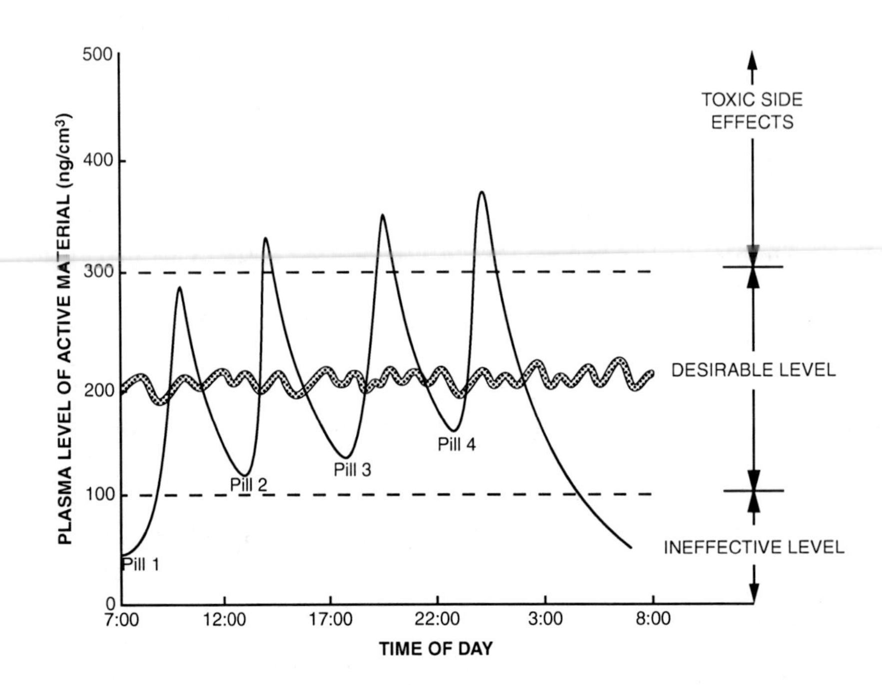

FIGURE 9.1 Plasma drug concentration versus time profile of a drug upon oral administration when compared with a sustained release drug delivery system. Reproduced with permission from Ref. 2.

of action via drug delivery systems such as suppositories, eye drops, creams, ointments, inhalation aerosols, injections, and so on. But drug administration with these delivery systems frequently leads to fluctuations in drug blood levels, side effects, and noncompliance.

To lessen these problems, a system with greater site specificity, less dosing frequency, and providing sustained release for longer periods was essential. This can be accomplished through the design of implantable controlled-release drug delivery systems. The systematic and scientific concepts of implantable drug delivery systems were instigated in 1937 by R. Deansby and A.S. Parkes, who presented a paper at the Royal Society of Medicine in London. They described the effects of various hormone preparations on the growth of livestock [3]. Within a year, similar technology was used by P.M.F. Bishop at Guy's Hospital in London for implantation of compressed estrogen pellets subcutaneously to treat a young woman afflicted with premature menopausal conditions. The results from this study showed that the estrogen replacement was for about 5 weeks after implantation. The rapid spread of this technique instigated the researchers to implant solid-compressed pellets of pure drug, particularly steroid hormones. After subcutaneous implantation, these pellets release active constituents by slow erosion and diffusion process. The surface area of the implant, particle size, and drug solubility in the physiological fluids determine the release rate. Subsequent investigations by J. Folkman and D.M. Long scrutinized the use of silicone rubber as a potential carrier for prolonged drug therapy [4]. Silicone rubber capsules implanted in the cardiac muscle of dogs controlled the release of various drugs and showed fewer signs of inflammation. Later on, tremendous improvements in the development of implantable drug delivery systems have been observed. Implants are single-unit drug delivery systems designed to deliver drug molecules at a therapeutically desired rate over a prolonged period of time and offer sustained drug release [1, 5]. The advantages and disadvantages associated with implants and its drug delivery related aspects are described in the next sections.

9.2.1 Advantages

(1) Targeted drug delivery can be achieved with the use of implants. This reduces the dosage requirements, and thus, systemic toxicities associated with undesirable side effects can be minimized.
(2) The use of implants facilitates greater therapeutic efficacy compared with conventional routes of administration. Peaks and troughs observed from uneven and frequent dosing intervals also can be eliminated by these systems.
(3) Macromolecules such as proteins and peptides with poor permeability characteristics, shorter *in vivo* half-life, and/or susceptible to enzymatic degradation can also be delivered successfully.
(4) Drug release from implantable delivery systems usually follows zero-order kinetics facilitating controlled drug levels at the target site.

(5) Therapeutic compounds that cannot be administered by other routes can preferably be delivered by implantable systems.
(6) Drugs that require frequent dosing can be administered through implants to provide sustained drug release ranging from 1 week to 1 year.
(7) A wide range of flexibility can be feasible with these systems in the selection of supplies, materials, methods of manufacturing, formulating, extent of drug loading, modulation of drug release, etc.

9.2.2 Disadvantages

The disadvantages of these systems are as follows:

(1) Implantation is often associated with a major or a minor surgery to place at the respective target site.
(2) Surgical procedure generally requires expert personnel and physicians. It may be traumatic and cause some surgery-associated complications. Moreover, scars could be developed at the site of implantation in most patients.
(3) The use of nonbiodegradable polymeric systems requires surgical removal of the implant immediately after the therapy is terminated.
(4) Although biodegradable polymeric systems do not have to be removed, the byproducts generated from them may be harmful sometimes.
(5) Implants are usually designed to be small and patient compliant with reduced discomfort. But this reduced size may limit the drug loading capacity of the delivery system.
(6) Implantable drug delivery systems, if not properly placed, may move, and fail to operate, alter drug release profile, eventually leading to adverse reactions.
(7) These drug delivery systems are generally sophisticated and require careful attention during its design. Also, the design of implants is time consuming and very expensive.

9.3 POLYMERIC IMPLANTABLE SYSTEMS

This class of implants exploits the application of polymer and polymeric membranes for achieving controlled drug release in biological systems. Depending on the property of polymer used, polymeric implantable drug delivery systems are subclassified in two categories: 1) nonbiodegradable implant systems and 2) biodegradable implant systems [1, 6].

9.3.1 Nonbiodegradable Implant Systems

Nonbiodegradable polymeric implants are usually composed of ethylene vinyl acetate (EVA), silicon, polyvinyl alcohol (PVA), and polysulfone polymers. Different kinds of nonbiodegradable implant systems are available for the treatment of chronic conditions requiring long-term therapy. The major disadvantage of the nonbiodegradable implant is the requirement of surgery for implantation and removal. Although the surgical procedures are a major disadvantage of these systems, implants can be removed easily if early termination is required because of side effects. Such systems have been employed for the administration of various anticancer agents, ophthalmic drugs, and contraceptives [7, 8]. Nonbiodegradable implant systems available in the market can be categorized into two main classes: reservoir systems and matrix systems.

9.3.1.1 Reservoir Systems In the reservoir systems, the drug core is surrounded by permeable polymeric membrane that functions as a rate-controlling membrane (Figure 9.2). The rate of drug release depends on the thickness and permeability properties of the membrane, and hence, the desired rate can be obtained by tailoring properties of polymeric membrane. The major advantages of this system are simplicity, longevity, and steady-state pharmacokinetics. However, it is difficult to design a reservoir-type system that can provide continuous release of macromolecules because of their poor diffusion through the polymeric membrane. Disadvantages of these systems include high manufacturing cost and requirement of surgery to remove implant because of its nonbiodegradable nature. Moreover, there is also a

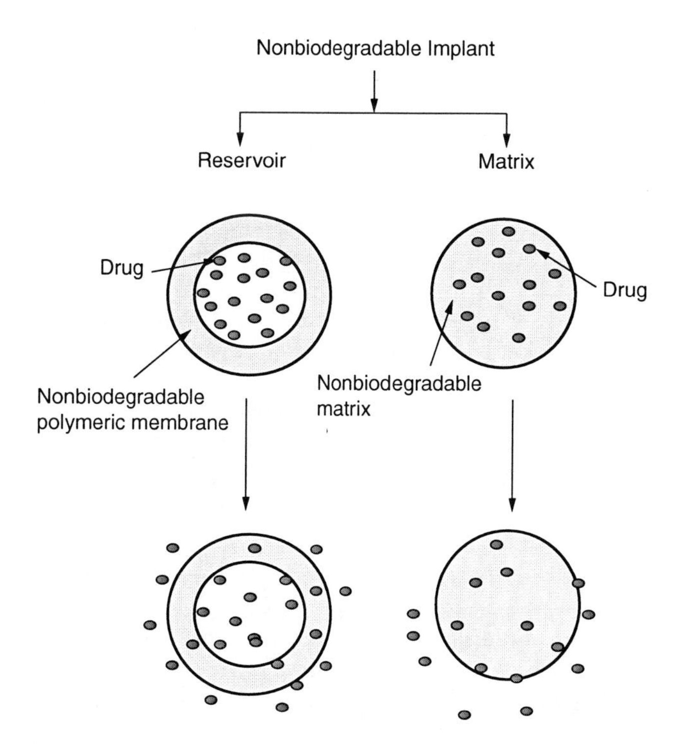

FIGURE 9.2 Schematic diagram of reservoir and matrix nonbiodegradable implant systems.

potential risk of "drug dumping" with reservoir systems resulting from rupture of polymeric membrane, which makes them less popular as drug delivery systems [1, 6].

9.3.1.2 Matrix Systems Matrix systems, also known as monolithic systems, consist of uniform dispersion of drug inside the nonbiodegradable polymer matrix (Figure 9.2). The drug release form matrix system is driven by slow diffusion of drug through the nonbiodegradable fibrous network of the polymer. If the drug is less soluble in polymeric matrix, then drug release is governed by a solution diffusion mechanism, and in the case of insoluble drug, leaching through intergranular openings in the matrix is considered to be the main mechanism of drug release. Advantages of matrix systems include the low cost of manufacturing and offers relative safety in case of leakage. Moreover, tortuous interconnecting pores in polymeric matrix allow continuous release of macromolecules such as insulin, enzymes and antibodies for prolonged period. However, the drug release from matrix system is driven by Fickian diffusion, and hence, release is not constant. The drug release rate declines continuously with time because of the increase in the diffusion path and decrease in drug concentration. Similar to reservoir systems, matrix systems also need minor surgery for implantation and removal, causing poor patient compliance [1, 6].

9.3.2 Biodegradable Implant Systems

Biodegradable implants are gaining more popularity over nonbiodegradable systems. These implants employ inert polymer, which can be degraded within biological system into nontoxic metabolites that are excreted by the body. The most frequently used biodegradable polymers for fabricating these systems include polyglycolic acid (PGA), polylactic acid (PLA), poly(lactic-co-glycolic acid) (PLGA), polyaspartic acid (PAA), polyanhydride, hydroxypropyl methyl cellulose (HPMC), and poly (ε-caprolactone) (PCL). Two different types of biodegradable implant systems are common: reservoir and matrix. Unlike nonbiodegradable reservoir systems, this reservoir system consists of a drug solution surrounded by a biodegradable polymeric membrane that degrades at a slower rate than the rate of drug release. While in matrix systems, the drug is dispersed uniformly into biodegradable polymeric matrix *in vivo*, which degrades at a controlled rate. The main mechanism for drug release from biodegradable polymer matrix includes erosion, diffusion, and cleavage of covalent linkage in the polymer (Figure 9.4). The main advantage of biodegradable system is that it alleviates the need for surgical removal at the end of therapy, leading to increased patient compliance. However, it is more complicated to develop biodegradable implant systems as many critical variables such as pH and temperature can affect the degradation kinetics of polymer, which could affect the drug release rate. Furthermore, bioerosion of polymer leads to changes in the shape and surface area of implant thus affecting drug release kinetics. Therefore, to attain more uniform and constant drug release, it is required to consider all these factors while fabricating a biodegradable implant system [1, 7–9]. Examples of nonbiodegradable and biodegradable polymers are shown in Figure 9.3.

9.4 CLINICAL AND THERAPEUTIC APPLICATIONS OF POLYMERIC IMPLANT SYSTEMS

Several biodegradable and nonbiodegradable implants using different types of release mechanisms have been developed to provide long-term sustained release of diverse therapeutic agents for treating chronic diseases. Major clinical applications of polymeric implant systems involve delivery of contraceptive steroids, anticancer agents, narcotic analgesics, and ocular therapeutics.

9.4.1 Contraceptive Steroids

A hormonal contraceptive implant is a birth control device and it provides an effective and safe way of preventing pregnancy. Usually, it is inserted beneath the skin and offers sustained release of hormone into the bloodstream for more than 1 year. Both biodegradable and nonbiodegradable systems have been developed as contraceptive implants. Examples of contraceptive implants include Norplant (Wyeth Pharmaceuticals, Madison, NJ), Jadelle (Schering Oy, Turku, Finland), Implanon (Organon International, Oss, the Netherlands), and Nexplanon (Merck, Whitehouse Station, NJ) [10].

9.4.1.1 Norplant Norplant, a first contraceptive implant, is a reservoir system made up of nonbiodegradable silicone elastomer (Silastic; Dow Corning, Midland, MI). It involves the insertion of six capsules each 3.4 cm in length and each having 36 mg of crystalline levonorgestrel mixed with polymer under the skin of the upper arm. After insertion, levonorgestrel releases into the blood stream by slow diffusion through the capsule wall over a period of 5 years. At the initial time point, the release rate of levonorgestrel from Norplant® system is 85 μg per 24 h, which gradually declines at the end to 25–50 μg per 24 h [10, 11, 12]. The released levonorgestrel prevents pregnancy by inhibiting ovulation and thickening of the cervical mucus.

9.4.1.2 Implanon Implanon is the single-rod subdermal implant developed by Organon International. It was first marketed in Indonesia in 1998 and is currently available in more than 30 countries. Implanon was approved by the U.S. Food and Drug Administration (FDA) in July 2006.

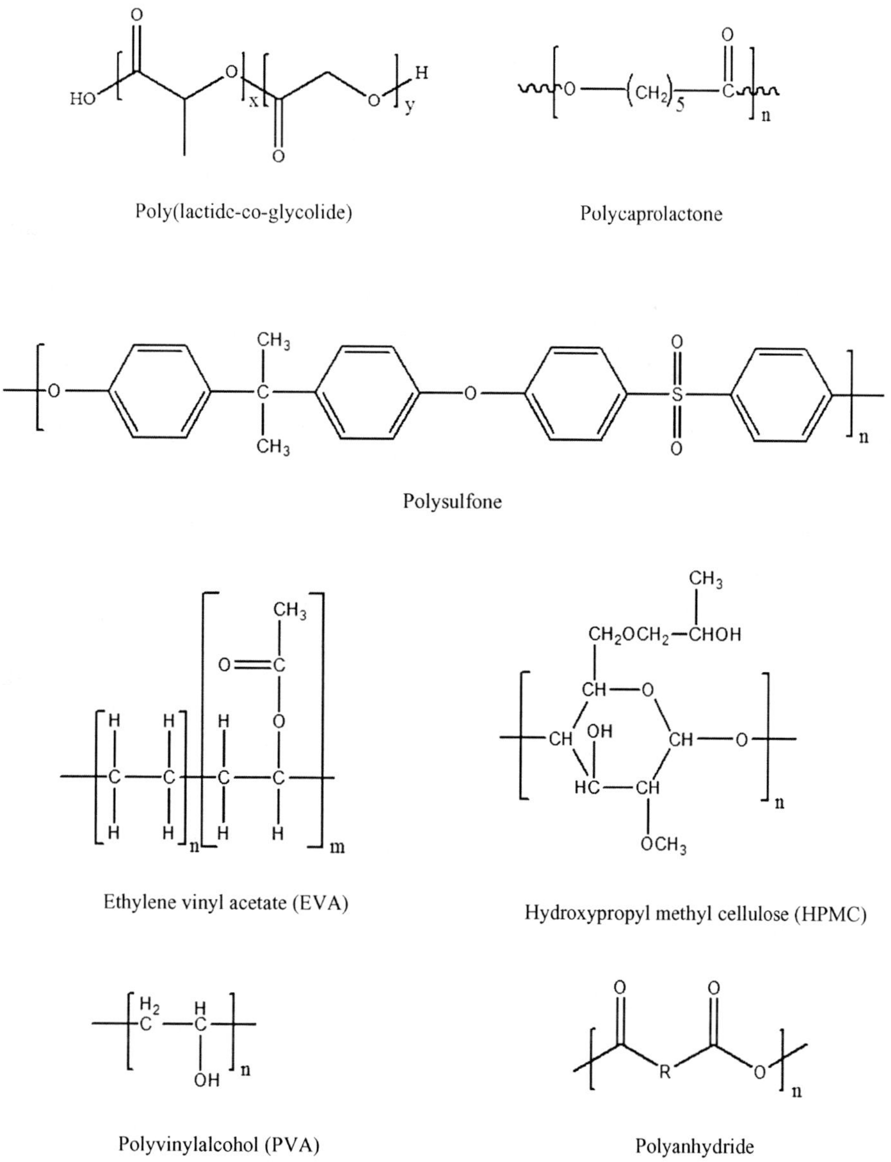

Poly(lactide-co-glycolide)
Polycaprolactone
Polysulfone
Ethylene vinyl acetate (EVA)
Hydroxypropyl methyl cellulose (HPMC)
Polyvinylalcohol (PVA)
Polyanhydride

FIGURE 9.3 Chemical structures of the most commonly used polymers.

Matrix
Drug dispersed in biodegradable matrix

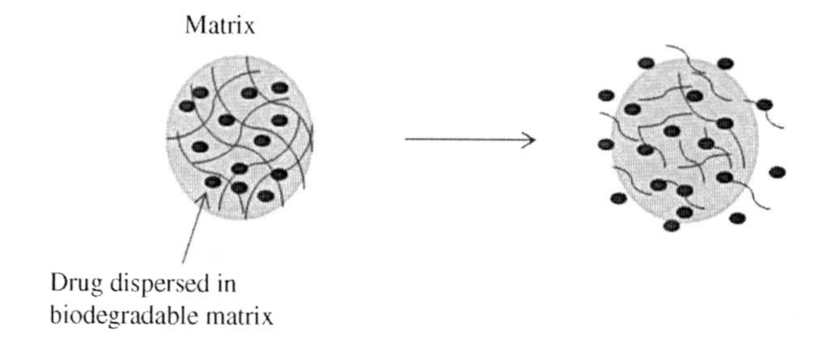

FIGURE 9.4 Schematic diagram of a matrix biodegradable implant system.

Implanon has 68 mg of etonogestrel (active metabolite of desogestrel) enclosed in 4 cm by 2 mm implantable rod made up of nonbiodegradable polymer EVA. The implant is preloaded in a trocar to facilitate subdermal insertion. Once implanted, it can sustain the release of etonogestrel over a 3-year period. The reported serum levels of etonogestrel are 813 pg/mL at early stage of implantation and 156 pg/mL at 3 years. The released etonogestrel provides contraceptive protection by inhibiting ovulation, increasing the viscosity of cervical mucus, and inhibiting endometrial proliferation [10, 13–15].

9.4.2 Ocular Therapeutics

The eye represents an ideal organ for localized sustained drug delivery using implantable devices because of the chronic nature of various ocular diseases such as glaucoma, cytomegalovirus retinitis, macular degeneration, uveitis, etc., and the ease of implantation and removal. Currently, several ocular implants are available on the market, which include Ocusert Pilo (ALZA Corporation, Mountain View, CA), Vitrasert (Bausch & Lomb, Inc., Rochester, NY), Retisert (Bausch & Lomb), Surodex (Allergan, Inc., Irvine, CA), Ozurdex (Allergan Inc.), and Lacrisert (Valeant Pharmaceuticals North America LLC, Aliso Viego, CA) [7, 8]. Some of them are briefly discussed in the next sections.

9.4.2.1 Ocusert Pilo Ocusert was the first ocular implant developed by ALZA Corporation and commercially available since 1974. It is a reservoir-type system that consists of antiglaucoma drug, pilocarpine, in the core surrounded by nonbiodegradable EVA copolymer membrane. It is placed beneath the tarsus of lower eyelid and provides pilocarpine release for 1 week. The advantages of Ocusert Pilo include patient compliance, easy insertion, easy removal, and fewer side effects. However, the high cost over topical eye drops impeded its use in the treatment of glaucoma [1, 8, 16].

9.4.2.2 Vitrasert Vitrasert is an intravitreal implant developed for the treatment of AIDS-associated cytomegalovirus retinitis (CMV). It was approved by the U.S. FDA in 1996. It contains 4.5 mg of ganciclovir (GCV) in its core covered with polymeric membrane composed of PVA and EVA. The combination of EVA and PVA helps in achieving well-controlled zero-order release without a burst effect. It is positioned transsclerally by making an incision (5.5 mm) at pars plana. It releases GCV at a rate of approximately 1 μg/h over a 6–8-month period. After the depletion of GCV, the implant is removed by surgery. The device provides long-term sustained release without systemic toxicity at a reduced cost. However, it is associated with potential disadvantages such as the risk of endophthalmitis and retinal detachment [7, 8].

9.4.2.3 Retisert The U.S. FDA approved Retisert in 2005 for the treatment of chronic, noninfectious uveitis affecting the posterior segment of the eye. It is a nonbiodegradable reservoir device containing 0.59 mg of fluocinolone acetonide surrounded with PVA and silicone laminates. It is implanted at pars plana through an incision. The implanted device delivers 0.6 μg of drug per day up to first month, followed by 0.3–0.4 μg/day for approximately 30 months. The implant had effectively controlled inflammation, reduced uveitis recurrences and improved vision acuity. The associated side effects are cataract formation and elevated intraocular pressure (IOP) [7, 17–19].

9.4.2.4 Surodex Surodex is a biodegradable matrix implant developed for treating postoperative inflammation after cataract surgery. It is a rod-shaped device containing 60 μg of dexamethasone (DEX) dispersed in polymeric matrix composed of PLGA and HPMC. The implant is inserted in anterior chamber and delivers DEX over a period of 7 days. It has demonstrated equal effectiveness as of 0.1% DEX topical eye drops in reducing intraocular inflammation after cataract surgery [7, 20, 21].

9.4.2.5 Ozurdex Ozurdex is a biodegradable intravitreal injectable implant consisting of 0.7 mg DEX. It was approved by U.S. FDA in June 2009 for the treatment of macular edema (ME) associated with retinal vein occlusion. It contains a PLGA polymer matrix that degrades slowly to lactic acid and glycolic acid allowing prolonged release of DEX up to 6 months. The rod-shaped implant (6 mm) is inserted by 22-gauge pars plana injection. Randomized clinical trials have demonstrated its potency in reducing vision loss and improving vision acuity in eyes with ME associated with branch retinal vein occlusion (BRVO) or central retinal vein occlusion (CRVO). Also, several clinical studies indicate that Ozurdex is a promising treatment option for patients with other ocular conditions such as diabetic retinopathy, uveitis, and Irvine-Gass Syndrome [7, 22–25].

9.4.3 Cancer Chemotherapy

Polymeric implants represent an ideal approach for minimally invasive and localized cancer chemotherapy. The implants can be placed directly into tumor, inserted subcutaneously or intramuscularly (palliative). The intratumoral implant provides localized drug delivery without systemic toxicity, whereas palliative implant provides sustained delivery obviating the need of repeated injections. The currently available anticancer drugs eluting polymeric implants are Zoladex (AstraZeneca Pharmaceuticals, London, U.K.), Lupron Depot (Abbott Laboratories, Abbott Park, IL), Gliadel (Eisai Inc., Woodcliff Lake, NJ), Eligard (Sanofi-Synthelabo Inc., Bridgewater, NJ), and OncoGel (Protherics, a BTG PLC Company, UT) [26]. Some of them are briefly discussed in the next sections.

9.4.3.1 Zoladex Zoladex is a biodegradable implant consisting of goserelin acetate (a gonadotropin releasing hormone agonist) dispersed in PLGA matrix. It is intended for treating hormone-responsive prostate cancer. The cylinder-shaped (1.5 mm diameter) device consisting of 10.8 mg of drug is inserted subcutaneously into the anterior abdominal wall at every 12 weeks using aseptic techniques. Another device with 3.6 mg of goserelin acetate is administered subcutaneously every 28 days. After implantation, the drug releases via diffusion through aqueous pores produced by the degradation of polymer matrix.

9.4.3.2 Eligard Eligard, an injectable leuprolide acetate depot formulation, is marketed as a palliative treatment for prostate cancer. It is an *in situ* forming implant in which biodegradable PLGA polymer is dissolved in a biocompatible solvent, *N*-methyl-2-pyrrolidone. Leuprolide acetate is admixed with polymer solution prior to administration, and this mixture is injected subcutaneously via a 20-gauge needle. Inside body, the solvent diffuses away and water penetrates into the system, leading to the precipitation of polymer resulting in formation of an implant depot. Multiple Eligard depot systems are available on the market providing 1 (7.5 mg), 3 (22.5 mg), 4 (30 mg), and 6 (45 mg) months sustained release of leuprolide acetate. A sustained suppression of testosterone is achieved with all Eligard depot systems [27, 28].

9.4.3.3 Gliadel Gliadel wafer (MGI Pharma, Inc., Woodcliff Lake, NJ) is approved by U.S. FDA in 1996 for the treatment of malignant glioma. It is a solid, biodegradable implant containing 7.7 mg of carmustine in 192.3 mg of biodegradable polyanhydride co-polymer (Polifeprosan 20). The round wafer of approximately 14 mm in diameter and 1 mm thickness is placed in surgical cavities created after brain tumor removal. As the wafer erodes, it releases carmustine slowly in the tumor area for a period of approximately 3 weeks [29, 30].

9.5 IMPLANTABLE PUMP (MECHANICAL) SYSTEMS

The second most important type of implantable systems include mechanical pumps that provide external control of drug release through a pump-type mechanism. Implantable pump systems are particularly useful for those drugs where biodegradable or nonbiodegradable delivery systems cannot offer controlled drug delivery. Advancements in microtechnology have produced miniature pump systems that can be implanted subcutaneously for drug delivery. These systems can regulate drug release devoid of an external pump system. Unlike other implantable systems such as polymeric controlled drug delivery systems, drug release from the implantable pumps is different. Drug release is mainly caused by a pressure difference that results in the bulk flow of a drug at convenient and controllable rates. Differences in pressure can be produced by pressurizing a drug reservoir, by osmotic action, or by direct mechanical actuation [31].

The superlative characteristics of an ideal implantable pump include the following [32, 33]:

(1) The pump should be capable of delivering the drug at a controlled and sustained rate for prolonged periods of time.
(2) The pump should provide a wide range of drug delivery rates. Accuracy and precision of drug delivery should be preferably less than $\pm 5\%$ based on *in vitro* measurements.
(3) It should offer protection against physical, chemical, and biological degradation of drug within the pump.
(4) It should be safe, noninflammatory, nontoxic, nonallergic, nonmutagenic, noncarcinogenic, and nonthrombogenic.
(5) It should be leak free, offer overdose protection and convenient to use.
(6) It should possess a sufficient drug reservoir, whose life is evaluated by drug requirement and the maximum drug concentration.
(7) It should also possess a long battery life, be easily monitored, be easy to program, and be capable of adjusting the parameters as and when required.
(8) It should be preferably implanted under local anesthesia rather than general anesthesia because of frequent and regular complications by the latter.
(9) It should be sterilized easily to reduce the exposure of microorganisms after implantation.

The next sections discuss different types of implantable pumps.

9.5.1 Infusion Pumps

Infusion pumps are implantable controlled-release systems which employ a fluorocarbon propellant to administer the drug. Infusaid (Infusaid Corp., Norwood, MA) infusion pumps were one of the first to be developed commercially for this purpose. These pumps were used initially to administer insulin to diabetic patients. These pumps were intended to reduce the requirement of multiple insulin injections and control the peaks and troughs in blood glucose levels. Diabetic complications were often associated with abnormal changes in blood glucose levels [34]. These pumps were designed to abolish such types of risk factors. The pump encompasses a disk-shaped canister made with lightweight biocompatible titanium consisting of a collapsible welded bellows [35]. The bellow partitions the interior canister into two separate chambers. The first chamber consists of fluorocarbon propellant and the second consists of either the drug or its formulation (Figure 9.5). The fluorocarbon propellant exerts a vapor pressure above atmospheric pressure at body

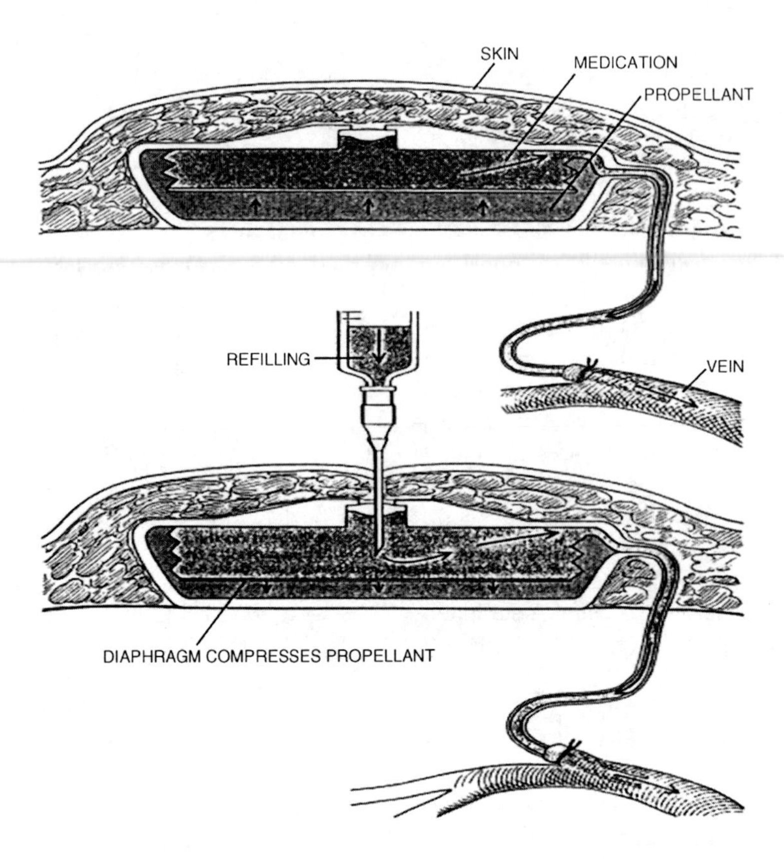

FIGURE 9.5 An implantable propellant-driven infusion pump system while in operation (top) and during refilling (bottom). Reproduced with permission from Ref. 1.

temperature. The drug-containing chamber is filled by administering an injection through a membrane consisting of a self-sealing silicone rubber and Teflon septum. This injection pressure causes expansion of drug-containing chamber and compression of fluorocarbon propellant to condense the vapor to initiate drug delivery. The gas formed by vaporization of fluorocarbon drives the drug through a filter and fine-bore capillary tubing, which acts as a flow regulator, thus providing a steady rate of drug administration at a given temperature. Drug concentration in the pump reservoir can be altered to achieve the desired delivery rate [31]. No external energy input is required for this system to drive the pump action. Later on, to refill the pump reservoir, drug/medication is injected through the membrane again. The force generated during injection process recompresses the fluorocarbon propellant and recharges the system.

In more advanced and newer systems, the valve is lodged in a small module attached to the side of a pump collectively with an infusion regulator, to balance the effects of changes in ambient pressure and temperature. In some designs, an auxiliary injection port and companion check valve are also provided for allowing direct access to the feed cannula. A transducer and transmitter can also be integrated to make pressure data accessible for determining flow rate and reservoir volume levels. Besides insulin therapy, pumps of this type have also been successfully implanted subcutaneously under the infraclavicluar fossa and sutured to the underlying fascia for an anticoagulant heparin therapy. Also, this pump system has been employed to deliver chemotherapeutic agents by placing them in the abdominal wall [36, 37].

9.5.2 Osmotic Pumps

Osmotic pumps are energy-modulated devices that are the most popular type of implantable drug delivery systems studied so far [38]. These pumps were first portrayed by Theeuwes and Yum, and unconfined for use by Alza Corporation [31, 39, 40]. Constant rate delivery and preprogrammed delivery of therapeutic agents was achieved by the use of Alza osmotic pumps (ALZET osmotic pump). Because pressure difference is the major driving force for drug release from the drug reservoir, a controlled rate is achieved via modulation of the osmotic pressure gradient. The pump consists of a drug or drug solution surrounded by a semipermeable membrane, which permits a steady invasion of water molecules into the reservoir via osmosis. An increase in hydrostatic pressure generated by this influx of

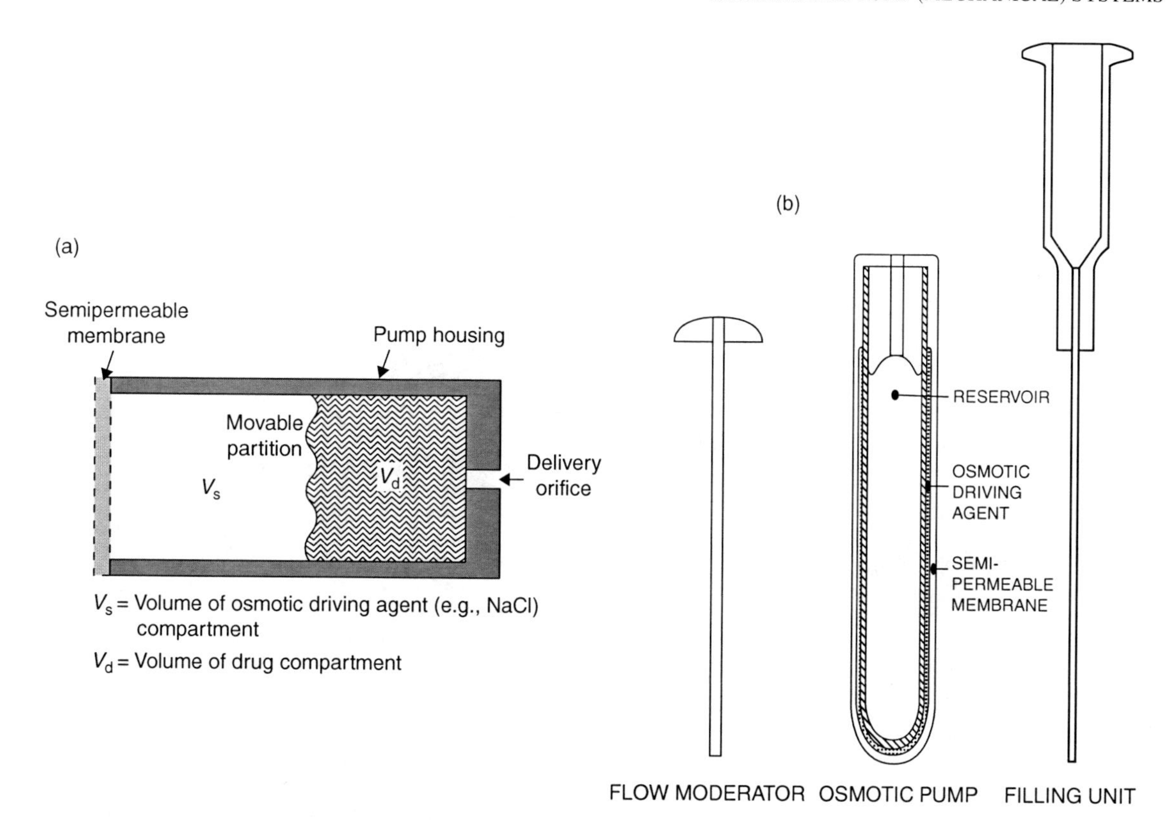

FIGURE 9.6 (a) Schematic representation of an osmotic pump. Reproduced with permission of John Wiley & Sons, Inc. from Ref. 41. (b) Osmotic pump and components. Reproduced with permission from Ref. 39.

water produces a constant drug release through an orifice known as the drug portal (Figure 9.6) [39, 41]. Constant zero-order drug release can be attained until the drug reservoir is exhausted completely [6, 31, 34]. The rate of drug administration can be altered only by changing the semipermeable membrane [42]. Some of the semi-permeable membranes used in implantable osmotic pumps include cellulose acetate, plasticized cellulose triacetate, cellulose acetate methyl carbamate, cellulose acetate ethylcarbamate, cellulose acetate phthalate, and cellulose acetate succinate. Polymers such as poly(ethylene-vinyl acetate), polyvinyl chloride, acrylic acid and methacrylic acid polyesters, polyvinylalkyl ethers, polymeric epoxide, and polystyrenes can also be used as semipermeable membranes. Several organic and inorganic carbohydrates and swelling hydrogels can be employed as osmotic agents. Some of them include sodium chloride, sodium carbonate, sodium sulfate, calcium sulfate, monobasic and dibasic potassium phosphate, magnesium chloride, magnesium sulfate, lithium chloride, calcium lactate, magnesium succinate, tartaric acid, choline chloride, glucose, lactose, mannitol, sorbitol, sucrose, and sodium carbopol.

The mechanistic action of these pumps is based on the principle of osmosis. The flow rate (dV/dT) generated from the water influx into the osmotic agent containing solution is determined by both osmotic pressure ($\Delta\pi$) as well as the back pressure (ΔP) created during this process. The volume influx of water can be calculated by:

$$dV/dT = A\,L_p(\sigma\,\Delta\pi - \Delta P)/h$$

where A is the effective surface area of the membrane, h is the thickness of the membrane, L_p is the permeability coefficient of the membrane, and σ is the osmotic reflection coefficient, which illustrates the selectivity of the membrane towards water and an osmotic agent. A σ value of 1 is generally a characteristic of an ideal semipermeable membrane.

Other osmotic pumps have also been designed with a freely movable piston that can maintain constant pressure in a low-osmotic-pressure solution reservoir divided from high osmotic fluid by a semipermeable membrane. Movement of either solvent or biological fluid through the membrane builds pressure on that side of the membrane, pumping drug from the drug reservoir out of a chamber alienated from a high-osmotic-pressure solution by another freely moving piston. The freely moving piston on the low-osmotic-pressure compartment moves to decrease the

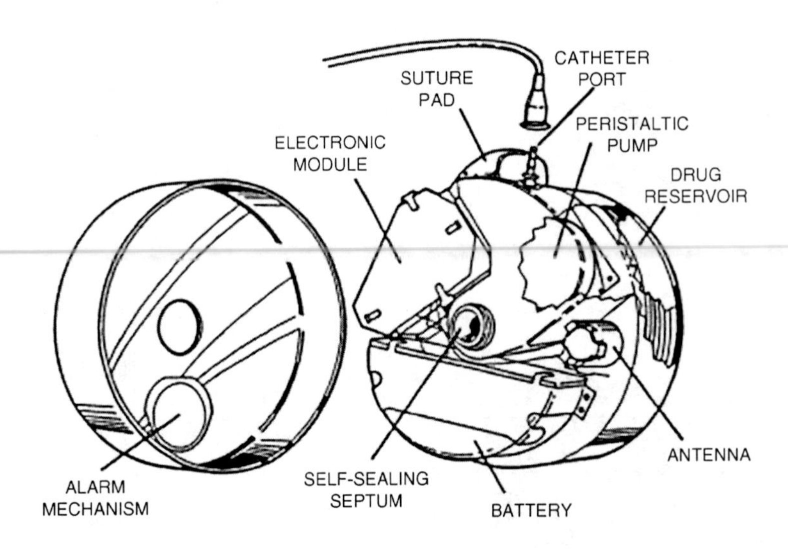

FIGURE 9.7 Cross-sectional view of a peristaltic pump. Reproduced with permission from Ref. 1.

volume of that reservoir as the solvent passes through the membrane. These pumps assume that the piston is exposed to a source of atmospheric pressure on the other side.

9.5.3 Peristaltic Pumps

Peristaltic pumps are a type of rotary, solenoid-driven systems based on the principle of a portable pump [43]. These pumps were designed initially to be implanted in diabetic patients by Sandia Laboratories (Albuquerque, NM). Unlike the stainless steel casing that was used originally, laser-welded titanium chamber is currently being employed to house the entire pump (including electronics and battery). These pumps run by means of an external power source, usually a battery [6]. The chambers of the pump are usually coated with silicone polymers and silicone rubber pouches are used as drug reservoirs. The pumps are refilled by means of silicone rubber septum and can be used for many years depending on the battery life span. The cross-sectional view of a model implantable peristaltic pump systems is provided in Figure 9.7. Backflow of physiological/biological fluids is prevented by a low-pressure valve that is present in the catheter. These pumps can offer accurate delivery, and the pump rate, flow rate, and drug administration rate can be controlled by an electronic external remote control system. They are also considered safe because the drug delivery can be halted in case of any electrical malfunction [44]. But these systems are found to be expensive and their practical usage seems to be very limited or rare [43].

9.5.4 Positive Displacement Pumps

Positive displacement pumps were fabricated to offer continuous delivery of insulin in diabetic populations. Most systems employ piezoelectric disk benders [45] and delicate disks of these benders are connected to brass and subsequently fastened to a flexible tubing, which then forms a bellow type of structure [6, 31, 34]. Piezoelectric disks bend to form spherical surfaces when a particular voltage is applied. Connecting this bellow type structure to the drug reservoir through a three-way solenoid driven valve and application of certain voltage subsequently causes opening or closing of the pump valve. This modulation is based on the direction of the pulse generated. This type of action releases the active medicament in a controlled manner depending on the electrical pulse rate. Other types of positive displacement pump systems use a solenoid type of diaphragm. After activation of the solenoid, drug localized in the reservoir gets pressurized, causing the outlet valve to open into a delivery catheter. An inlet valve prevents backflow into the reservoir. Also, other pumps using similar technology and design are under investigation for delivery of insulin and other drugs.

9.5.5 Controlled-Release Micropumps

Controlled-release micropumps work on a diffusion phenomenon across a rate-controlling membrane, whereas a rapidly oscillating piston acts on a compressible disk of foam augments the drug delivery rate [6, 31]. A major advantage of this type of system is that it does not require any kind of external power source. The difference in concentration gradient between the drug reservoir and the site of action is adequate to cause diffusion of the drug (also termed as basal delivery) to the target site. A current is applied across the solenoid coil, which actually compresses the foam disk via a steel piston and generates a pressure gradient sufficient enough to improve drug delivery. Previous studies revealed that such pumps can administer average daily flow rates essential for adequate insulin therapy with commercially available insulin solutions of 100 U/mL [46]. These pumps could possibly be used up to 1 year depending on the endurance of the foam disk [31].

9.6 CLINICAL AND THERAPEUTIC APPLICATIONS OF IMPLANTABLE PUMP SYSTEMS

The accuracy and predictability of drug release from the implantable pumps is evident from the fact that these have been used for determining the pharmacokinetic and pharmacodynamic properties of current and emerging drug molecules during the preliminary developmental stages. Several pumps for experimental research in human and veterinary use, including ALZET osmotic pump (DURECT Corporation, Cupertino, CA), OSMET, L-OROS SOFTCAP, L-OROS HARDCAP (Alza Corporation, Vacaville, CA), SCOT (Andrx Pharmaceuticals, Fort Lauderdale, FL), EnSoTrol (Supernus Pharmaceuticals, Inc., Rockville, MD), Osmodex (Osmotica Pharmaceutical, Wilmington, NC), controlled porosity osmotic pump, DUROS (DURECT Corporation, Cupertino, CA), Veterinary Implantable Therapeutic System (VITS), and Ruminal Therapeutic System (RUTS) (Alza Corporation, Vacaville, CA), are available. However, this chapter discusses only the clinically important and widely used pumps.

9.6.1 ALZET Osmotic Pumps

ALZET osmotic pumps are miniature implantable pumps used for research purposes (Figure 9.8). These pumps are capable of delivering drugs, hormones, and other therapeutic agents at controlled rates ranging from 1 day to 6 weeks exclusive of any external connections or frequent handling. Their unattended operation and controlled release eliminates the need for repeated dosing [47]. These pumps function on an osmotic pressure gradient between compartments within the pump, called the salt sleeve, and the tissue environment in which the pump is implanted. Osmolarity differences will cause influx of water into the pump through a semipermeable membrane. The entry of water compresses the flexible reservoir and displaces the drug solution from the pump at a controlled and predetermined rate [39, 48]. Because the compressed reservoir cannot be refilled, the pumps are designed for single-use only. The delivery rate is controlled by the water permeability of the pump's external membrane and therefore do not depend on the drug formulation dispensed. The operating mechanism of these pumps enables delivery of compounds with any molecular weight predictably at controlled rates, independent of their physical and chemical properties. ALZET osmotic pumps could

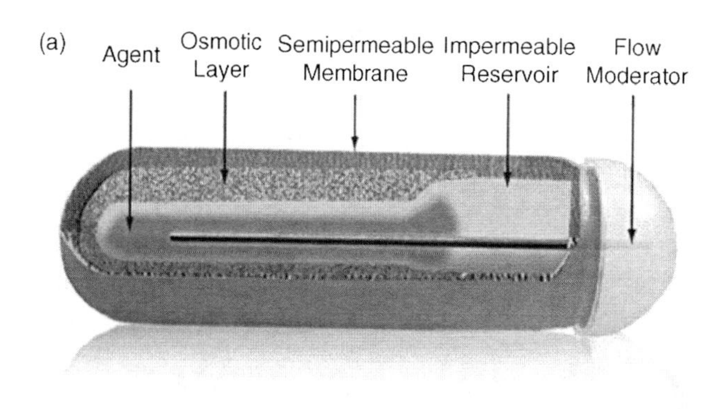

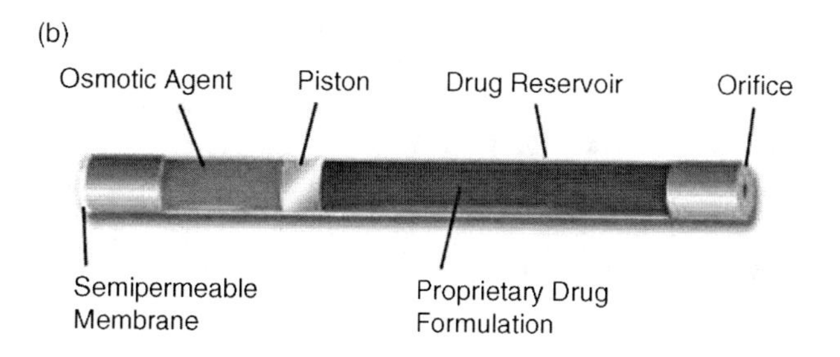

FIGURE 9.8 Cross-sectional view of (a) ALZET and (b) DUROS pumps. Reproduced with permission from ALZET Osmotic Pumps and DURECT Corporation. (See color figure in color plate section.)

deliver drugs at a rate of 0.11–10 μL/h, which can deliver between 1 day and 6 weeks [49].

9.6.2 DUROS Pumps

The DUROS osmotic pumps are shaped in the form of a small rod with titanium housing, which can be as small as a matchstick, designed to enable sustained drug release. These pumps bear resemblance to a small syringe in which drug is pressurized out in highly controlled, minute dosages. Water from the body is slowly drawn into the pump through the semipermeable membrane by an osmotic agent located in the engine compartment. Drug formulation from the drug reservoir is dispensed slowly and continuously through the orifice because of the displacement of the piston by the water drawn from the engine compartment [49, 50]. One major advantage associated with these pumps is that they do not require batteries, switches, or other electromechanical parts to operate. The pumps are designed to deliver up to 1 g concentrated drug from months to a year. The titanium shell in this system prevents the drug formulation from contact with any body fluids, thus protecting the formulation from enzymatic, hydrolytic degradation and other metabolic clearance processes within the body. This technology was approved by the U.S. FDA in 2000 in the form of Viadur (leuprolide acetate implant; Bayer Healthcare, Leverkusen, Germany) for the palliative treatment of prostate cancer [51, 52].

9.7 CLINICAL APPLICATION OF IMPLANTS FOR DELIVERY OF NARCOTIC ANALGESICS

Pain is often the hallmark of progressive malignant diseases, as 60–90% of the patients with terminal cancer experience pain [53, 54]. Narcotic analgesics are usually administered orally or intravenously to alleviate pain; however, side effects such as sedation, nausea, vomiting, and constipation are commonly observed. Additional studies have shown that epidural administration of opioid at lower doses can produce potent analgesia compared with oral or parenteral administrations. Moreover, the epidural route is associated with less central side effects [55–57]. Advantages associated with implantable systems have led to the development of PORT-A-CATH (Smiths Medical, Dublin, OH) implantable epidural access system. This system is generally used to relieve intractable cancer pain by delivering preservative-free morphine sulfate into the epidural space. The PORT-A-CATH epidural system is composed of a portal with a 60-micron filter, a catheter, a catheter connector, and a guide wire. Implantable-grade stainless steel is used to make the portal housing and screen filter. Below the portal's chamber is the screen filter, which filters the infused drug and prevents the entry of large particulate matter into the catheter and the epidural space. Drugs enter the catheter through the portal outlet tube. The catheter is made of polyurethane and includes four markings, 5 cm apart from the catheter tip, to aid in positioning of the catheter during implantation. The catheter contains a preassembled guide wire, which offers stiffness to facilitate the introduction of catheter into the epidural space. Clinical studies have shown that the PORT-A-CATH implantable epidural access system is safe and effective for the delivery of morphine sulfate, a narcotic analgesic indicated for the palliative management of chronic pain in cancer patients. The major advantages of a PORT-A-CATH system include quick reliable venous access, low maintenance, fewer restrictions on lifestyle, and low frequency of infection and malfunction when compared with externalized systems [58, 59].

Similarly, a controlled-release, implantable rod-type drug delivery system composed of two co-polymers of a biodegradable polymer PLGA was developed and investigated for the delivery of either an analgesic or anesthetic type of pain reliever. Zero-order release kinetics were observed for codeine, hydromorphone, and bupivacaine from PLGA (85:15) rods [60]. This polymeric system has shown interesting results in animal models where a significant alleviation of chronic and severe neuropathic pain was observed for about 3–4 days when rods for two drugs, "dual drug" (analgesic-anesthetic), were used. Moreover, these implantable rods sustained the release of hydromorphone from PLGA (85:15) rods, thereby minimizing systemic analgesia than the more rapidly eroding PLGA (50:50) rods of hydromorphone [61].

9.8 BIOCOMPATIBILITY ISSUES OF IMPLANTABLE DRUG DELIVERY SYSTEMS

During the past two decades, much research in drug delivery has been focused on achieving pharmacologically active drug at the target site and maintaining therapeutic drug levels for prolonged periods of time. Controlled-release technology has progressed to such an extent that the zero-order delivery can be achieved easily for up to several years. Subsequently, many controlled-release implantable systems have been commercially successful. Because the controlled-release implantable devices have to be implanted in the target site, it is very important to consider the biocompatibility issues of these systems. Various materials ranging from biodegradable collagen to nonbiodegradable titanium metal have been investigated. Biomaterials are generally considered as nonviable materials that constitute a part of the body either temporarily or permanently to restore, replace, and/or augment the natural functions of the living/target tissues in the body [62]. When these biomaterials are suitably placed in the target site or body, they are expected to produce desirable host responses and be compatible with the body without causing any side effects. Biocompatibility is a two-way dynamic process that involves the time-dependent effects of the host on material and the material on the host. It is considered as a measure of either local or systemic biological performance of a given implant in a specific application [63–66].

The International Organization for Standardization (ISO) has developed some guidelines for the biological evaluation of biomaterials that are employed for implantable devices. Some of the important and desirable criteria for such biomaterials include the following:

(1) The biomaterial should be compatible with various drugs and should not alter the pharmacological activity of the respective drug.
(2) The biomaterial should be easily sterilizable without altering its physical, chemical, and mechanical properties.
(3) The biomaterial should be molded into different shapes depending on the need. After implantation, it should not lose it shape and be stable enough because these delivery systems are placed for a long period of time.
(4) Biodegradable biomaterials should be capable of degrading in a controlled fashion when exposed to the tissue environment.
(5) The biomaterial should be chemically inert and not be altered by any physical or chemical stresses caused by local tissues. Post implantation, the biomaterial should not interact with surrounding tissues.

(6) The biomaterial should be devoid of any toxicity and must not elicit allergic or hypersensitivity reactions or inflammatory and immunogenic responses. The biomaterial itself or the breakdown products should not be carcinogenic and not cause any thrombogenicity.

(7) Most importantly, the biomaterial should be easily removed from the implanted site after its use or easily replaced in case of nonbioerodible materials.

9.8.1 Biological Response to an Implant Device

The implantation of a device results in a series of events which include tissue injury, blood–material interactions, matrix formation, acute inflammation and chronic inflammation, formation of granulomatous tissue, foreign body reaction, and fibrous capsule development. After implantation, blood and material interactions occur leading to protein adsorption and provisional matrix formation. A highly vascularized granulation tissue composed of fibroblasts and vascular endothelial cells is formed at the end of chronic inflammatory phase, which is replaced by the extracellular matrix. Finally, a 50–200 μm thick fibrous and collagenous capsule is formed around the implant, which prevents further interactions with the surrounding environment. Understanding the mechanism of this response may have a significant impact on the safety, biocompatibility, and function of an implant [65, 67, 68].

9.8.2 *In Vitro* Tests

In vitro tests provide sensitive, rapid, reliable, and inexpensive data of the biological environment and minimize the number of animals used for research. Also, *in vitro* tests generate data that can predict whether the implant need to be further evaluated *in vivo*. Cell culture tests are generally employed to determine the biocompatibility of an implant *in vitro*. These tests stimulate the biological response of the body environment on which the biomaterial is placed and predict its functional performance. Primary cell lines are also commonly used to screen the biocompatibility of an implant. L-929 mouse fibroblast cell line and rat primary culture of osteoblasts are commonly used for evaluating the biocompatibility *in vitro*. ISO guidelines include the criteria for *in vitro* testing as well as the positive and negative control materials, extraction methods, choice of cell lines, and media used [69]. Direct contact, agar diffusion, and elution are the three primary cell culture assays that are used for determining the biocompatibility of the implant.

9.8.3 *In Vivo* Tests

When compared with *in vitro* cellular biocompatibility tests, *in vivo* animal models (sheep, pig, and rat) can better reflect the impact of implants on the surrounding environment.

TABLE 9.1 Different Tests Used for Determining *In Vitro* and *In Vivo* Biocompatibility

In Vitro Tests	*In Vivo* Tests
Cytotoxicity	Sensitization
Mutagenesis/carcinogenesis	Irritation
Biofunctionality	Systemic acute toxicity
Hemocompatibility	Genotoxicity
	Implantation
	Hemocompatibility
	Subchronic toxicity
	Carcinogenicity
	Reproductive and developmental toxicity
	Chronic toxicity
	Biodegradation
	Immune response
	Microvascularization
	Pathohistological examination of tissues

Animal models mimic the biological environment while predicting the clinical behavior, safety, and biocompatibility of the implant. Table 9.1 shows the different tests used for determining *in vitro* and *in vivo* compatibility. Initial tests such as cytotoxicity, carcinogenicity, sensitization, and irritation determine the effects of the implant and its products on surrounding tissue. Biodegradation and implantation test study the effect of biological environment on the implant [70, 71]. Various natural, synthetic, and semisynthetic biodegradable and biocompatible polymers are currently used in the formulation of coatings for the implants. However, tests should be performed to determine the compatibility of the leachable products released from the implants.

The development of novel biomaterials is a very long and complex process, and the biocompatibility characteristics form a major aspect of their utilization. Reliable methods must be devised to evaluate their biocompatibility, possibly during the initial stages of development. This would reduce the expenditure and minimize wastage to time. Some tests that have been widely employed to evaluate the biocompatibility of biomaterials for implants are detailed in the next sections.

9.8.4 Blood Compatibility Testing

The most common method used to test blood compatibility of bioerodible materials is the kinetic clotting test (KCT). This test involves the entry of venous blood from an animal model (for example, dog) into the chamber that contains the biomaterial to be tested via a short segment of silicone rubber tubing. The amount of free hemoglobin and bold clot is measured at a wavelength of 254 nm at periodic intervals by spectrophotometer. Though this test is reliable and useful, it does not take into account the factors determining blood compatibility. As a result, this test does not ensure that the tested biomaterial is entirely blood compatible even when there is no blood coagulation. Moreover, silicone itself possesses the capability of activating coagulation factors when the venous blood comes into contact with the silicone tubing before the test biomaterial [72].

Another test that is widely employed to evaluate the *ex vivo* measurement of thrombus formation and platelet and fibrin content is the radiotracer technique. Carotid arterial blood to the jugular vein of a dog is connected *ex vivo* to two stainless steel chambers (i.e., one coated with test biomaterial and the other will serve as a control). The chambers are connected by 20-cm long silicone rubber tubing. The silicone rubber tubing, the centrifugal force of the rotating stainless steel shafts, and the complexity of coating could generate problems in interpreting the results and ultimately the suitability of the biomaterial [6]. Many biomaterials including polymers, ceramics, and metals are known to cause surface-induced thrombosis because of the activation of adherent platelets. Thrombus formation on the surface of drug delivery device would affect the drug release profile and may lead to undesirable and detrimental effects. To prevent thrombus formation, the biomaterials are surfaces modified with polyethylene oxide, polyurethane, heparin, albumin, or other hydrophilic polymer chains. This surface modification would prevent or minimize protein adsorption and/or platelet adhesion, possibly by the steric repulsive mechanism that arises from the increased osmotic pressure and elastic forces of the compressed molecules [73–76].

Other tests to evaluate the blood compatibility of biomaterials include 1) critical surface tension test, 2) hemolysis and shear stress test, and 3) caval ring implant test.

9.8.5 Tissue Compatibility Testing

It is very important that the degree of biodegradation needs to be critically evaluated when developing either a biostable or a biodegradable implantable drug delivery system. Inflammation is a serious result of tissue damage caused during implantation. The degree of tissue toxicity of the biomaterials, the implant itself, and the metabolic products should be estimated accurately before implantation into patients. Hegyeli [77] developed a chick embryo organ culture test to evaluate biodegradation and biocompatibility of polymer implant materials. Under aseptic conditions, the organs of 8–14-day-old Leghorn chick embryos are immediately decapitated, removed, cleaned, and minced into fragments of 0.5 cm × 0.5 cm each. Subsequently, the fragments are washed with basic salt in roller tubes containing Trowell TS medium, supplemented with 10% chick serum, 5% chick embryo extract, 125 IU/mL of penicillin/streptomycin mixture, and 2 mM of L-glutamine. The radiolabeled biomaterials (preferably in amorphous form) are added to the culture, incubated in carbon monoxide at 37°C, and rotated at a rate of 1 rpm for different periods of time. Biomaterial degradation is then estimated by centrifugation of biomaterial and filtration through a filter paper. Also, histological and electron microscopic examination could be performed to assess the nuclear changes, chromatin patterns, cytoplasmic vacuolization, epithelial encapsulation, and presence of acellular fluids [77].

An *in vivo* method to screen the biomaterials for biocompatibility evaluation was also developed [78]. This test evaluates acute and subacute tissue reactions at 1 week and 4 weeks, respectively, after implantation in rats. This method is reproducible and reliable, and it was found to be an excellent screen for many polymers during early investigations. The tissue responses and a series of defensive reactions such as 1) extent of muscle damage; 2) total thickness of tissue; 3) overall cell density; 4) number of polymorphonuclear leucocytes (neutrophils) and erythrocytes; 5) number of eosinophils, macrophages, lymphocytes, and foreign body giant cells; and 6) number of fibrocytes and mononuclear phagocytes can be determined.

Langer et al. studied *in vivo* host responses to specific implants on rabbit cornea to evaluate the tissue compatibilities of polymeric drug delivery systems [79]. They reported that cornea as an implantation site is advantageous than other organs because of its clarity, avascularity, sensitivity, and ease of access. This test served as a first basis for assessing the inflammatory response of biomaterials and lead to the development of several intraocular implants.

Another method to perform biological tests directly on biomaterials and material extracts was developed, which measures the response and scores arithmetically. Thus, a cumulative toxicity index can be obtained to enable grading of materials. Acute toxicological screening tests include 1) cell/tissue culture of biomaterial and extracts, 2) hemolytic induction and erythrocyte osmotic fragility, 3) systemic toxicity and *in vitro* mutagenicity, 4) isolated heart test, and 5) subacute and chronic intramuscular implantation.

Many materials have been claimed to be biocompatible without suitable evaluation. For example, silicone rubber that was initially thought to be entirely biocompatible turned out to be causing some detrimental effects. Although the tests discussed previously can be extremely useful, no single test can provide conclusive evidence of biocompatibility. Because the major issue associated with implantable delivery systems is the biocompatibility, it could be solved only by conducting several tests involved with multidisciplinary efforts. However, the current tests are very useful in the short term to screen various potential biomaterials during preliminary or early stages of development. Eventually, conclusive knowledge about the biocompatibility of candidate biomaterials can be derived only from long-term human clinical trials.

9.9 CONCLUSION

Advances in drug delivery systems progressed to achieve controlled drug delivery, particularly using implantable drug delivery systems. Although pharmacologically effective, many drugs are considered to be potentially toxic because of the lack of adequate formulation development and the variability of blood levels over the period of prophylaxis. Hopefully, such drugs could be delivered within the therapeutic window, achieving adequate therapeutic concentrations by means of reformulating them into implantable drug delivery systems. Also, most of the emerging molecules including macromolecular drugs, proteins and peptides are highly susceptible to enzymatic degradation, thus rendering them unstable. It is anticipated that these sustained/controlled-release drug delivery systems will deliver such molecules at constant rates over a prolonged period of time. This would reduce the need for multiple dosing, decrease the cost of drug therapy, increase drug efficacy, and most importantly enhance patient compliance. This advancement should be accompanied with advances in biocompatibility of the materials employed in designing implants. Despite significant advances, much work still needs to be performed to evaluate novel biodegradable and biocompatible polymers, examine drug release kinetics, and expand future development. Biocompatible tests that require shorter duration and wider application need to be developed, which would result in speedy approval for the devices from the U.S. FDA. Hopefully, many new implantable drug delivery systems would rush into the pharmaceutical market that could sustain and provide ideal zero-order release kinetics profiles over prolonged periods of time and at controlled rates.

ASSESSMENT QUESTIONS

9.1. Define implantable drug delivery systems.

9.2. What characteristics can be achieved with implantable drug delivery systems?

a. Greater site specificity
b. Less dosing frequency
c. Sustained release for longer periods
d. All of the above

9.3. What are polymeric implantable systems? How are they classified?

9.4. Which of the following is an example of reservoir-type nonbiodegradable implant?

a. Surodex™
b. Zoladex®
c. Eligard®
d. Retisert®
e. None of the above

9.5. Give examples of polymers employed for fabrication of biodegradable implant systems.

9.6. Give examples of polymers employed for fabrication of nonbiodegradable polymeric implant systems.

9.7. What is the main difference between reservoir and matrix-type implantable systems?

9.8. What are the ideal characteristics of an implantable pump?

9.9. What are the most widely employed tests to evaluate the biocompatibility of biomaterials for implants?

a. Blood compatibility testing
b. Tissue compatibility testing
c. Both of them

9.10. Describe the desirable criteria that the International Organization for Standardization (ISO) has developed for biological evaluation of biomaterials employed for implantable devices.

REFERENCES

1. Dash, A.K., Cudworth, 2nd, G. C. (1998). Therapeutic applications of implantable drug delivery systems. *Journal of Pharmacological and Toxicological Methods*, *40(1)*, 1–12.
2. Graham, N.B. (1978). Polymeric inserts and implants for the controlled release of drugs. *British Polymer Journal*, *10(4)*, 260–266.
3. Blackshear, P.J. (1979). Implantable drug-delivery systems. *Scientific American*, *241(6)*, 66–73.
4. Folkman, J., Long, D.M. (1964). The use of silicone rubber as a carrier for prolonged drug therapy. *The Journal of Surgical Research*, *4*, 139–142.
5. Holzapfel, B.M., et al. (2012). How smart do biomaterials need to be? A translational science and clinical point of view. *Advanced Drug Delivery Reviews*.
6. Danckwerts, M., Fassihi, A. (1991). Implantable controlled release drug delivery systems: A review. *Drug Development and Industrial Pharmacy*, *17(11)*, 1465–1502.
7. Christoforidis, J.B., et al. (2012). Intravitreal devices for the treatment of vitreous inflammation. *Mediators of Inflammation*, *2012*, 126463.
8. Bourges, J.L., et al. (2006). Intraocular implants for extended drug delivery: Therapeutic applications. *Advanced Drug Delivery Reviews*, *58(11)*, 1182–1202.
9. Rodrigues da Silva, G., et al. (2010). Implants as drug delivery devices for the treatment of eye diseases. *Brazilian Journal of Pharmaceutical Sciences*, *46(3)*.

10. Meckstroth, K.R., Darney, P.D. *Implantable Contraception in Gynecology & Obstetrics*. Lippincott Williams & Wilkins, Philadelphia, PA, 2004.
11. Shastri, P.V. (2002). Toxicology of polymers for implant contraceptives for women. *Contraception, 65(1)*, 9–13.
12. Lahteenmaki, P., Jukarainen, H. (2000). Novel delivery systems in contraception. *British Medical Bulletin, 56(3)*, 739–748.
13. Funk, S., et al. (2005). Safety and efficacy of Implanon, a single-rod implantable contraceptive containing etonogestrel. *Contraception, 71(5)*, 319–326.
14. Darney, P.D. (2000). Implantable contraception. *The European Journal of Contraception & Reproductive Health Care, 5 Suppl 2*, 2–11.
15. Darney, P.D. (1995). The androgenicity of progestins. *The American Journal of Medicine, 98(1A)*, 104S–110S.
16. Yasukawa, T., et al. (2006). Drug delivery from ocular implants. *Expert Opinion on Drug Delivery, 3(2)*, 261–273.
17. Mohammad, D.A., Sweet, B.V., Elner, S.G. (2007). Retisert: Is the new advance in treatment of uveitis a good one? *The Annals of Pharmacotherapy, 41(3)*, 449–454.
18. Jaffe, G.J., et al. (2006). Fluocinolone acetonide implant (Retisert) for noninfectious posterior uveitis: Thirty-four-week results of a multicenter randomized clinical study. *Ophthalmology, 113(6)*, 1020–1027.
19. Jaffe, G.J., et al. (2005). Long-term follow-up results of a pilot trial of a fluocinolone acetonide implant to treat posterior uveitis. *Ophthalmology, 112(7)*, 1192–1198.
20. No author. (2002). Dexamethasone ophthalmic-oculex. Surodex. *Drugs in R&D, 3(3)*, 152–153.
21. Tan, D.T., et al. (1999). Randomized clinical trial of a new dexamethasone delivery system (Surodex) for treatment of post-cataract surgery inflammation. *Ophthalmology, 106(2)*, 223–231.
22. London, N.J., Chiang, A., Haller, J.A. (2011). The dexamethasone drug delivery system: Indications and evidence. *Advances in Therapy, 28(5)*, 351–366.
23. Herrero-Vanrell, R., Cardillo, J.A., Kuppermann, B.D. (2011). Clinical applications of the sustained-release dexamethasone implant for treatment of macular edema. *Clinical Ophthalmology, 5*, 139–146.
24. Lee, S.S., et al. (2010). Biodegradable implants for sustained drug release in the eye. *Pharmaceutical Research, 27(10)*, 2043–2053.
25. Haller, J.A., et al. (2010). Randomized, sham-controlled trial of dexamethasone intravitreal implant in patients with macular edema due to retinal vein occlusion. *Ophthalmology, 117(6)*, 1134–1146e3.
26. Exner, A.A., Saidel, G.M. (2008). Drug-eluting polymer implants in cancer therapy. *Expert Opinion on Drug Delivery, 5(7)*, 775–788.
27. Sethi, R., Sanfilippo, N. (2009). Six-month depot formulation of leuprorelin acetate in the treatment of prostate cancer. *Clinical Interventions in Aging, 4*, 259–267.
28. Sartor, O. (2003). Eligard: Leuprolide acetate in a novel sustained-release delivery system. *Urology, 61 (2 Suppl 1)*, 25–31.
29. Attenello, F.J., et al. (2008). Use of Gliadel (BCNU) wafer in the surgical treatment of malignant glioma: A 10-year institutional experience. *Annals of Surgical Oncology, 15 (10)*, 2887–2893.
30. Panigrahi, M., Das, P.K., Parikh, P.M. (2011). Brain tumor and Gliadel wafer treatment. Indian Journal of Cancer. *48(1)*, 11–16.
31. Ranade, V.V. (1990). Drug delivery systems. 4. Implants in drug delivery. *Journal of Clinical Pharmacology, 30(10)*, 871–889.
32. Sefton, M.V. (1987). Implantable pumps. *Critical Reviews in Biomedical Engineering, 14(3)*, 201–240.
33. Sefton, M., Implantable pumps, in R.S. Langer and D.L. Wise (eds.), *Medical Applications of Controlled Release*. CRC Press, Boca Raton, FL, 1984, pp. 129–158.
34. Langer R, Implantable controlled release systems, in G. Ihler (ed.), *Methods of Drug Delivery*. Pergamon Press, New York, 1986, pp. 121–137.
35. Blackshear, P.J., Rhode, T.H. Artificial devices for insulin infusion in the treatment of patients with diabetes mellitus, in S. Burk (ed.), *Controlled Drug Delivery, Vol. 2 Clinical Applications*. CRC Press, Boca Raton, FL, 1983, p. 11.
36. Buchwald, H., et al. (1980). Long-term, continuous intravenous heparin administration by an implantable infusion pump in ambulatory patients with recurrent venous thrombosis. *Surgery, 88(4)*, 507–516.
37. Buchwald, H., et al. (1980). Intraarterial infusion chemotherapy for hepatic carcinoma using a totally implantable infusion pump. *Cancer, 45(5)*, 866–869.
38. Ranade, V.V., M.A. Hollinger. Implants in drug delivery, in V.V. Ranade and M.A. Hollinger (eds.), *Drug Delivery Systems, Second Edition*. CRC Press, Boca Raton, FL, 2003.
39. Theeuwes, F., Yum, S.I. (1976). Principles of the design and operation of generic osmotic pumps for the delivery of semisolid or liquid drug formulations. *Annals of Biomedical Engineering, 4(4)*, 343–353.
40. Martin, A., Bustamante, P., Chun, A. in G. H. Mundorff and P. Malvern (eds.), *Physical Pharmacy*. Lea & Febiger Press, Philadelphia, PA, 1993, pp. 534–536.
41. Wright, J.C., Stevenson, C.L. Pumps/osmotic: Introduction, in E. Mathiowitz (ed.), *Encyclopedia of Controlled Drug Delivery*. John Wiley & Sons, New York, 1999, p. 898.
42. Fara, J.W., R.N, Osmotic pumps, in P. Tyle (ed.), *Drug Delivery Devices: Fundamentals and Applications*. Marcel Dekker, New York, 1988, p. 1–41.
43. Schade, D.S., et al. (1982). A remotely programmable insulin delivery system. Successful short-term implantation in man. *The Journal of the American Medical Association, 247(13)*, 1848–1853.
44. G. A. Clarson, et al. (1979). A new low-power, high-reliability infusion pump. *7th Annu. New England (Northeast) Bioengineering Conf., Troy, NY.*

45. Thomas, L.J., Jr., Bessman, S.P. 1975. Prototype for an implantable micropump powdered by piezoelectric disk benders. *Transactions - American Society for Artificial Internal Organs*, *21*, 516–522.
46. Uhlig, E.L., Graydon, W.F., Zingg, W. (1983). The electro-osmotic actuation of implantable insulin micropumps. *Journal of Biomedical Materials Research*, *17*(*6*), 931–943.
47. Fara, J.W. Osmotic delivery systems for research, in R.G. Kenneth and J. Widder (eds.), *Methods in Enzymology*. Academic Press, New York, 1985, pp. 470–484.
48. Keraliya, R.A., et al. (2012). Osmotic drug delivery system as a part of modified release dosage form. *ISRN Pharmaceutics*, *2012*, 528079.
49. Herrlich, S., et al. (2012). Osmotic micropumps for drug delivery. *Advanced Drug Delivery Reviews*, *64*(*14*), 1617–1627.
50. Wright, J.C., Culwell, J. Long-term controlled delivery of therapeutic agents by the osmotically driven DUROS® implant, in M.J. Rathbone, J. Hadgraft, and M.S. Roberts (eds.), *Modified-Release Drug Delivery Technology, Volume 2*. CRC Press, Boca Raton, FL, pp. 143–149.
51. Fowler, J.E., Jr., (2001). Patient-reported experience with the Viadur 12-month leuprolide implant for prostate cancer. *Urology*, *58*(*3*), 430–434.
52. Fowler, J.E., et al. (2000). Evaluation of an implant that delivers leuprolide for 1 year for the palliative treatment of prostate cancer. *Urology*, *55*(*5*), 639–642.
53. Ballantyne, J.C. (2012). "Safe and effective when used as directed": The case of chronic use of opioid analgesics. *Journal of Medical Toxicology*, *8*(*4*), 417–423.
54. Manchikanti, L., et al. (2012). Opioid epidemic in the United States. *Pain Physician*, *15* (*3 Suppl*), ES9–38.
55. Rauck, R.L., et al. (2003). Long-term intrathecal opioid therapy with a patient-activated, implanted delivery system for the treatment of refractory cancer pain. *The Journal of Pain*, *4*(*8*), 441–447.
56. Pybus, D.A., Torda, T.A. (1982). Dose-effect relationships of extradural morphine. *British Journal of Anaesthesia*, *54*(*12*), 1259–1262.
57. Gustafsson, L.L., et al. (1982). Extradural and parenteral morphine: Kinetics and effects in postoperative pain. A controlled clinical study. *British Journal of Anaesthesia*, *54*(*11*), 1167–1174.
58. Bothwell, J.E., et al. (2001). Port-A-Cath use in refractory seizure disorders. *Archives of Disease in Childhood*, *85*(*6*), 510.
59. Bow, E.J., Kilpatrick, M.G., Clinch, J.J. (1999). Totally implantable venous access ports systems for patients receiving chemotherapy for solid tissue malignancies: A randomized controlled clinical trial examining the safety, efficacy, costs, and impact on quality of life. *Journal of Clinical Oncology*, *17*(*4*), 1267.
60. Sendil, D., Wise, D.L., Hasirci, V. (2002). Assessment of biodegradable controlled release rod systems for pain relief applications. *Journal of Biomaterials Science*, *13* (*1*), 1–15.
61. Sendil-Keskin, D., et al. (2003). In vivo pain relief effectiveness of an analgesic-anesthetic carrying biodegradable controlled release rod systems. *Journal of Biomaterials Science*, *14*(*6*), 497–514.
62. Duncan, E. (1990). Biomaterials. What is a biomaterial? *Medical Device & Diagnostic Industry*, *12*, 138–142.
63. Shard, A.G., Tomlins, P.E. (2006). Biocompatibility and the efficacy of medical implants. *Regenerative Medicine*, *1*(*6*), 789–800.
64. Marchant, R.E. (1989). The cage implant system for determining in vivo biocompatibility of medical device materials. *Fundamental and Applied Toxicology*, *13*(*2*), 217–227.
65. Anderson, J.M. (1988). Inflammatory response to implants. *ASAIO Transactions/American Society for Artificial Internal Organs*, *34*(*2*), 101–107.
66. Coleman, D.L., King, R.N., Andrade, J.D. (1974). The foreign body reaction: A chronic inflammatory response. *Journal of Biomedical Materials Research*, *8*(*5*), 199–211.
67. Onuki, Y., et al. (2008). A review of the biocompatibility of implantable devices: Current challenges to overcome foreign body response. *Journal of Diabetes Science and Technology*, *2* (*6*), 1003–1015.
68. Nuss, K.M., von Rechenberg, B. (2008). Biocompatibility issues with modern implants in bone - a review for clinical orthopedics. *The Open Orthopaedics Journal*, *2*, 66–78.
69. Helmus, M.N., D.F. Gibbons, and D. Cebon, (2008). Biocompatibility: Meeting a key functional requirement of next-generation medical devices. *Toxicologic Pathology*, *36* (*1*), 70–80.
70. Morais, J.M., Papadimitrakopoulos, F., Burgess, D.J. (2010). Biomaterials/tissue interactions: Possible solutions to overcome foreign body response. *AAPS Journal*, *12*(*2*), 188–196.
71. Anderson, J.M., *4.402* - Biocompatibility and the relationship to standards: Meaning and scope of biomaterials testing, in D. Paul (ed.), *Comprehensive Biomaterials*. Elsevier, Oxford, U. K., 2011, pp. 7–26.
72. Kambic, H.E., Kiraly, R.J., Nose, Y. (1976). A simple in vitro screening test for blood compatibility of materials. *Journal of Biomedical Materials Research*, *10*(*4*), 561–570.
73. Peng, T., et al. (1996). Role of polymers in improving the results of stenting in coronary arteries. *Biomaterials*, *17*(*7*), 685–694.
74. Lambert, T.L., et al. (1994). Localized arterial wall drug delivery from a polymer-coated removable metallic stent. Kinetics, distribution, and bioactivity of forskolin. *Circulation*, *90*(*2*), 1003–1011.
75. Amiji, M., Park, K. 1993. Surface modification of polymeric biomaterials with poly(ethylene oxide), albumin, and heparin for reduced thrombogenicity. *Journal of Biomaterials Science*, *4*(*3*), 217–234.

76. Park, K., Cooper, S.L. (1985). Importance of composition of the initial protein layer and platelet spreading in acute surface-induced thrombosis. *Transactions–American Society for Artificial Internal Organs*, *31*, 483–488.
77. Hegyeli, A.F. (1973). Use of organ cultures to evaluate biodegradation of polymer implant materials. *Journal of Biomedical Materials Research*, *7*(2), 205–214.
78. Gourlay, S.J., et al. (1978). Biocompatibility testing of polymers: In vivo implantation studies. *Journal of Biomedical Materials Research*, *12*(2), 219–232.
79. Langer, R., Brem, H., Tapper, D. (1981). Biocompatibility of polymeric delivery systems for macromolecules. *Journal of Biomedical Materials Research*, *15*(2), 267–277.

10

APTAMERS IN ADVANCED DRUG DELIVERY

WEIWEI GAO, OMID C. FAROKHZAD, AND NAZILA KAMALY

10.1 CHAPTER OBJECTIVES

- To review aptamers in the context of advanced drug delivery, with a primary focus on their applications as targeting ligands in nanoparticle-based drug delivery systems.
- To introduce the principles of the SELEX technique of which the binding targets have advanced from biochemically purified molecules to whole living cells and animals.
- To summarize key concepts of aptamers as targeting ligands, including their molecular characteristics, engineering strategies to improve their stability, and mechanisms of nanoparticle targeting.
- To select representative aptamers and review their recent developments as targeting ligands, particularly for nanoparticle drug delivery systems.
- To highlight novel applications of aptamers in building complex biomaterials and devices for both drug delivery and disease diagnosis.

10.2 INTRODUCTION

Nucleic acids, in addition to their well-known ability for storing genetic information, can also fold into complex structures that bind to specific targets, including small molecules and proteins [1, 2]. In nature, this vital ability allows nucleic acids to transmit genetic information and direct protein synthesis [3–5]. The study of interactions between biological nucleic acids and their binding targets also intrigued the search for synthetic nucleic acids that possess similar properties. Given a specific protein target, if such binding nucleic acids can be found easily, then they can become valuable tools for researchers to unlock some of the deepest biological mysteries [6, 7], develop useful probes to aid molecular biology studies [8], and discover novel drugs to treat devastating diseases [9]. However, most protein targets are too complex to allow determination of their binding sites. Even if such knowledge is available, the number of individual nucleic acid molecules necessary to do a thorough screen to identify all possible binding sequences is prohibitively large. In addition, the structural changes that might occur to nucleic acids on ligand binding remain largely unpredictable. As a result, a rational approach to designing nucleic acids with tertiary structures complementary to a given protein target was once an unattainable task.

In the last few decades, nucleic acid research has achieved tremendous technological breakthroughs. In particular, large quantities of degenerate oligonucleotides can now be synthesized at a relatively low cost. Through polymerase chain reaction (PCR), a small quantity of nucleic acid can be rapidly amplified into an amount that can be manipulated easily. Meanwhile, novel separation techniques have continued to emerge and have allowed oligonucleotides to be partitioned according to their binding or catalytic activities. These technological advances intertwined and

Advanced Drug Delivery, First Edition. Edited by Ashim K. Mitra, Chi H. Lee, and Kun Cheng.

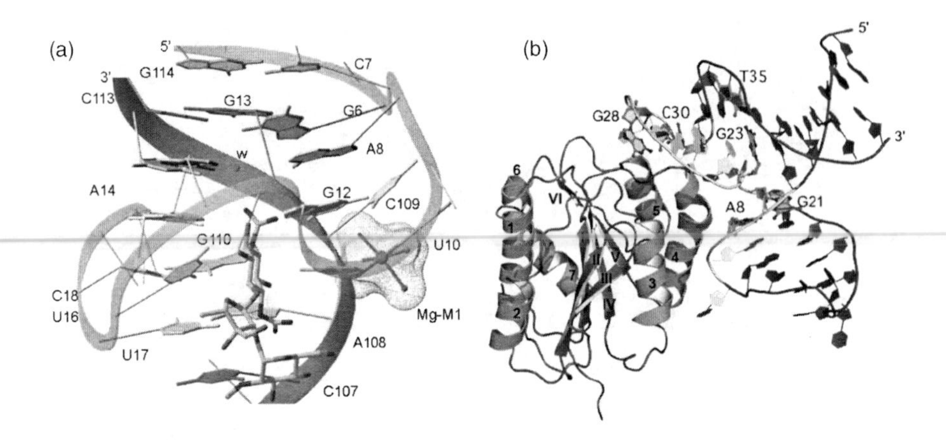

FIGURE 10.1 By using X-ray diffraction combined with theoretical analysis, researchers now can look deep into the binding structure of a protein-aptamer complex: (a) the binding pocket of a 40-mer RNA that binds to streptomycin; and (b) crystal structure of Arc1172 bound to the A1 domain of von Willebrand factor. Figures adapted from Refs. 14, 15, respectively.

eventually led to the invention of systemic evolution of target-specific ligands by exponential enrichment (SELEX) in the early 1990s, a technique that could fast produce oligonucleotides of single-stranded RNA or DNA from a large combinatorial oligonucleotide library with high binding specificity and affinity to the target [10–13]. Oligonucleotides produced from the SELEX process have been termed "aptamers," a term derived from the Latin *aptus* meaning "to fit." Since the invention of SELEX, researchers have discovered numerous aptamers that can bind to a broad range of targets, including small organic molecules, proteins, protein domains, whole living cells, and animals. Aptamers that distinguish between closely related but non-identical members of a protein family or between the different functional and conformational states of the same protein can now be routinely selected, and the fundamental understanding of aptamer-target binding interactions continues to grow (Figure 10.1) [14, 15]. As a result, aptamers have become a family of materials applied in numerous molecular biology studies. Meanwhile, various aptamers bind with target proteins of therapeutic interest, acting as antagonists to inhibit protein–protein interactions. Interestingly, several aptamers are also found to function as agonists that promote bioactivities such as the editing responses of RNA synthetase [16] and hetero-dimerization between human epidermal growth factor receptor-2 and -3 [17]. Although the first aptamer-based drug was approved by the U.S. Food and Drug Administration (FDA) in 2006 as a treatment for age-related macular degeneration [18], many have been identified as drug candidates and have entered different stages of development.

Together with these advances comes the increasing use of aptamers in numerous nanotechnology-enabled drug delivery platforms that take advantage of the superior binding affinity and specificity of aptamers to protein targets. In particular, modification of nanoparticles by using aptamers or other families of ligands that bind to the surface receptors of target cells can improve on the therapeutic outcomes by altering drug pharmacokinetics and biodistribution profiles [19–21]. Consequently, the aptamer-targeted nanoparticles useful to a broad range of therapeutic applications have entered different stages of development.

In this chapter, we review aptamers in the context of advanced drug delivery, including their selection techniques, chemical and biological characteristics, engineering strategies, and current development, with a primary focus on their applications as targeting ligands in nanoparticle-based drug delivery systems. Articles with an excellent review of aptamers used as molecular biology probes and therapeutic drugs [8, 22, 23] can be found elsewhere. This chapter is organized as follows: First, the principles of the SELEX technique are introduced and recent progress made using SELEX to isolate highly functional aptamers is assessed; second, key chemical and biological characteristics of aptamers related to their applications in drug delivery are discussed; third, the discovery and applications of aptamers frequently used as targeting ligands are reviewed and the underlying strategies in formulating aptamer-targeted drug delivery systems are highlighted; and fourth, additional roles besides that of targeting ligand played by aptamers that are beneficial for developing advanced drug delivery systems are also reviewed.

10.3 APTAMER DISCOVERY USING SELEX

Although several aptamers were discovered serendipitously, most aptamers are selected strategically based on similar principles developed in the original SELEX process. According to the physicochemical characteristics of binding targets, aptamer selections can be categorized into three distinct groups: conventional SELEX, cell SELEX, and *in vivo* SELEX. Conventional SELEX uses purified small molecules and proteins as targets under cell-free conditions. In contrast, cell SELEX uses whole living cells as target under *in vitro* conditions, in most cases, bypassing the molecular information of cell surface markers. Taking aptamer selection one step further by using tumor-bearing mice as a target, *in vivo* SELEX was performed to generate aptamers that could recognize their targets in an *in vivo* context.

10.3.1 Conventional SELEX

SELEX was initially developed as an iterative process to identify, isolate, and enrich aptamers from a large pool of nucleic acids binding to a chosen molecular target of specific biochemical activity (Figure 10.2). This process starts with a combinatorial library of nucleotide sequences generated from standard automated oligonuleotide synthesis. The typical length of the random sequences is 20–40 bases, resulting in a library that contains approximately 10^{12}–10^{15} oligonucleotides, each with a unique sequence that can, in principle, adopt a unique three-dimensional structure. Subsequently, the nucleotide library is incubated with the target molecule. The sequences in the library with weak or no affinity for the target tend to remain free in solution, allowing for the separation of the sequences strongly bound to the target molecule. The sequences bound to the target are then eluted and amplified using the PCR for DNA and reverse transcriptase (RT)-PCR for RNA sequences; thus, a new library of sequences is created and a new selection cycle can start. After 5–15 cycles of a complete SELEX process, the library contains several nucleotide sequences capable of strong binding to the target with a dissociation constant (Kd) in the range of picomolar to nanomolar. At this stage, the nucleotide sequences of individual members from the library can be determined, and the binding affinity and specificity of selected sequences can be carefully measured and compared.

Since the invention of the SELEX process, high-affinity aptamers that can bind to numerous protein families including cytokines, proteases, kinases, cell-surface receptors, and cell-adhesion molecules have been identified. Traditional SELEX relies on soluble and purified targets; however, if the proper folding of target proteins requires the presence of the cell membrane (e.g., G-protein–coupled receptors and ion channels) or a co-receptor, it is difficult to perform SELEX with purified, soluble protein targets. With novel separation techniques available allowing for facile partitioning of nucleotides from nonbinders, aptamers can now be isolated from complex mixtures such as human plasma [24] and cell-surface proteins [25]. In addition, when full proteins are either unstable or unavailable, structurally constrained peptides and protein domains or fragments can also been used to generate aptamers [26, 27].

10.3.2 Cell-SELEX

Following the invention of SELEX, researchers have also developed "cell-SELEX" processes, where whole living cells rather than biochemically purified molecules are used as targets (Figure 10.3). Compared with conventional SELEX, cell-SELEX can identify aptamers that recognize target cells without requiring prior surface marker information. This unique advantage has enabled efficient discovery

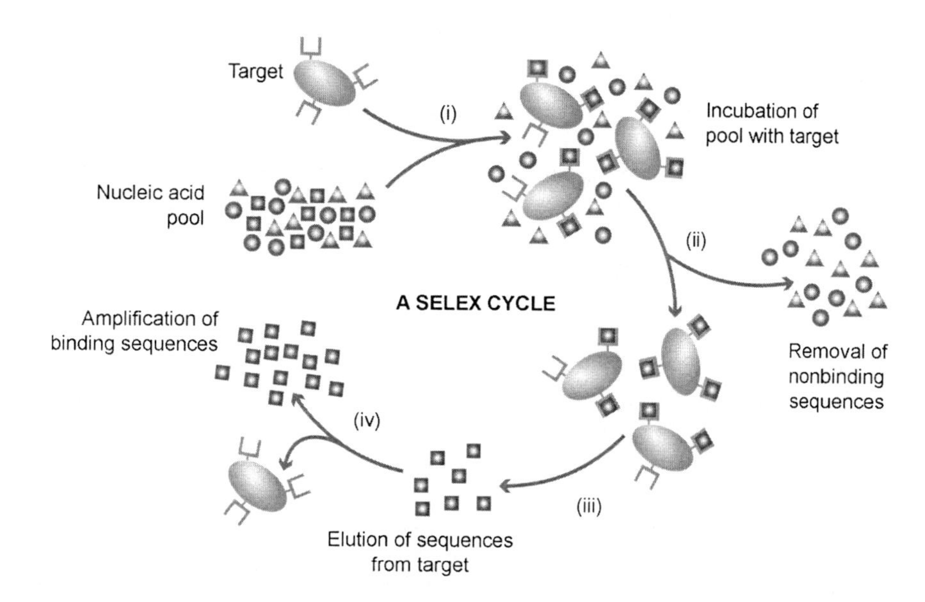

FIGURE 10.2 Scheme of a conventional SELEX cycle: (i) sequence binding, (ii, iii) partitioning, and (iv) amplifying isolated nucleotides. (See color figure in color plate section.)

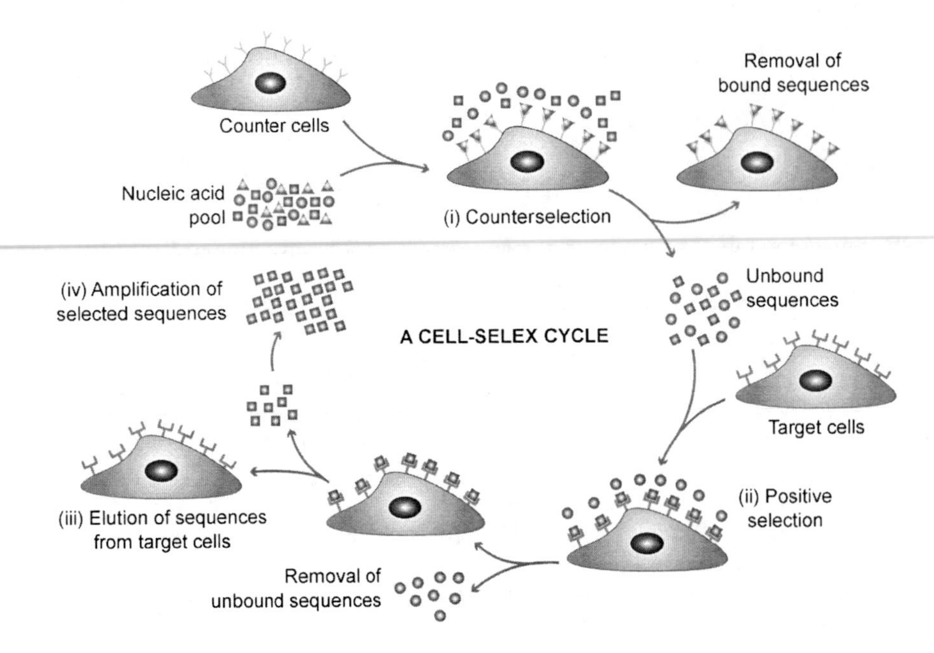

FIGURE 10.3 Scheme of a cell-SELEX cycle: (i) counterselection, (ii) positive selection, and (iii) elution of sequences from targeted cells, and (iv) amplification of selected sequences. (See color figure in color plate section.)

of a wide range of aptamers recognizing and binding with cell surface proteins that would otherwise prove impractical by using conventional SELEX [28–32]. Even when the surface target is known, the purified membrane protein might not have the native conformation as that presented on the cell membrane; therefore, using living cells as targets reflects a more physiological condition where the protein is displayed on the cell surface rather than isolated in its purified form. The implementation of complex targets in SELEX also represents a shift in the paradigm of ligand discovery in which new probes and techniques can be developed regardless of the level of understanding of the disease markers. Particularly in cancer, heterogeneous complexes of diseases develop in a sequential manner through a multistep carcinogenic process, and therefore, distinguishing tumors with similar molecular background can be challenging. Bypassing the knowledge of cancer cell-specific surface markers allows cell-SELEX to identify aptamers that discriminate between two closely related targets, for example, a cancerous cell and an untransformed cell of the same tissue type, making aptamers suitable for a wide range of sophisticated applications in targeting leukemia [33], liver cancer [34], small-cell lung cancer [35], ovarian cancer [36], colorectal cancer [37], and breast cancer [38].

As the cell-SELEX process involves steps where target cells are labeled by progressively enriched aptamers, the results of cell-SELEX can in turn facilitate the extraction and identification of cell-surface markers unknown prior to the selection process. For example, by using cell-SELEX, one selected aptamer, sgc8, preferentially binds to most of the T-cell acute lymphoblastic leukemia (T-ALL) cells, acute myeloid leukemia (AML) cells, and some B-cell acute lymphoblastic leukemia (B-ALL) cells; yet it shows no detectable level of binding to either lymphoma cells or normal human bone marrow cells. The elevated expression of the target of the sgc8 aptamer on leukemia cells implies the existence of a leukemia-specific membrane biomarker potentially useful for disease detection and drug delivery. Once the sgc8 aptamers were isolated, they were conjugated with magnetic beads and then used to capture and purify their binding targets on the leukemia cell surface. Using this strategy, protein tyrosine kinase 7 (PTK7) was identified as a membrane marker for the aforementioned leukemia cells [33]. This two-step strategy, that is, first selecting cancer cell-specific aptamers and then identifying their binding target proteins, is promising where it can improve the overall effectiveness of biomarker discovery substantially.

Using the whole living cell as a target, the cell-SELEX process allows aptamer isolation and enrichment in each cycle to be accomplished by implementing specific cell functions, thus, generating cell-specific aptamers that can also distinguish certain cell functions. In an example of using the cell-SELEX process to identify neutralizing aptamers that inhibit the RET receptor tyrosine kinase, two counterselection steps were coupled to avoid selecting for aptamers that nonspecifically recognize the cell surface that involved a first step against parental PC12 cells to eliminate nonspecific binders, followed by a second step against PC12/MEN2B cells that expressed an allele of RET (RETM918T) mutated in the intracellular tyrosine kinase domain. Aptamers that specifically recognize the dimeric form of the extracellular domain on PC12/MEN2A cells are enriched. As a result, this process generates aptamers that not only recognize the extracellular domain of RET but also block RET downstream signaling and subsequent molecular and cellular events. Another interesting example is the selection of aptamers that can be internalized inside living cells for aptamer functional studies and for targeted intracellular delivery [39]. In this strategy, only aptamers internalized by the target cells are enriched for each subsequent cell-SELEX cycle. As a result, aptamers selected through this process not only can bind preferentially to the target cells but also are taken up by the target cells. These examples suggest that cell-SELEX is a useful tool to select aptamers that indicate or modulate certain cell functions in the absence of a specific selective pressure [40].

The principle of cell-SELEX has also been applied to infectious diseases to exploit intrinsic differences between uninfected and infected cell surfaces [41, 42] or closely related pathogenic viruses or bacteria [43, 44], allowing for the selection of highly antigenic aptamers and then the elucidation of potential biomarkers for a particular pathogen. In these living organisms, membrane proteins play crucial roles in a variety of cellular processes that controls the exchange of membrane impermeable molecules and communication between cells through signal transduction. In this respect, the cell-SELEX process is particularly powerful in identifying and targeting upregulated membrane proteins that play essential roles in disease progression and in transforming healthy cells into diseased cells. Hence, aptamers generated here can become promising drugs or targeting ligands against a broad range of infectious diseases.

10.3.3 *In Vivo* SELEX

Both conventional SELEX and cell-SELEX isolate aptamers under *in vitro* conditions by using either biologically purified proteins or whole living cells as targets. However, aptamer binding depends on the conformation of its target, which in turn is largely influenced by the target's physiological environment. Therefore, conventional SELEX and cell-SELEX may not generate the most relevant aptamers capable of localizing to specific tissues *in vivo*.

In an effort to target the *in vivo* context of disease-specific moieties, an *in vivo* selection process was developed by using an animal model as target [45]. In this process, mice bearing hepatic tumors were injected intravenously with a random library of 2′-fluropyrimidine-modified RNA sequences. Subsequently, tumors were harvested and the injected RNA molecules were extracted and amplified using primers specific for the starting library. The resulting pool of RNA was then reinjected and the process was repeated. After 14 rounds of selections, a 39-bp aptamer capable of *in vivo* homing and targeting an intracellular protein (p68, an RNA helicase) within the tumor compartment was identified. Compared with conventional SELEX and cell-SELEX, the *in vivo* selection recognizes the *in situ* context of potential targets and leads to aptamers that may be less likely to bind with nontarget proteins *in vivo*.

Using conventional SELEX, cell SELEX, and *in vivo* SELEX, researchers now can search aptamers with their binding targets under a wide range of environments. Despite the differences in practice, the SELEX technique allows for aptamer discovery unrestrained by the complexity of nucleic acid–target interactions and thus can generate aptamers with unpredictable and unimaginable molecular configurations and targeted functions.

10.4 CHARACTERISTICS OF APTAMERS AS TARGETING LIGANDS IN DRUG DELIVERY SYSTEMS

Aptamers comprising wild-type DNA and RNA are susceptible to nuclease-mediated degradation. One strategy to enhance aptamer stability is through proprietary post-SELEX modifications [46, 47]; however, these modifications may cause structural changes and in turn compromise the binding affinity between aptamers and their targets. An alternative strategy is to use chemically modified nucleic acids inherently stable to chemical and enzymatic degradations to perform SELEX [23]. These chemical modifications include 1) replacing the 2′ position with either a fluoro- (-F), amino- (-NH_2), or *O*-methyl (-OCH_3) group to enhance nuclease resistance; 2) substituting phosphodiester linkage with boranophosphate or phosphorothioate internucleotide linkages; 3) conjugating stealth polymers such as polyethylene glycol (PEG) to the 5′-ends; and 4) using end caps that involve reversing the polarity of the chain (Figure 10.4). From the perspective of drug development, selective protection of nuclease-sensitive sites in oligonucleotides could induce toxicity and require careful assessment [48]. In addition, applying these nucleic acids to SELEX requires that the chemically modified oligonucleotide libraries be amenable to enzymatic manipulations. Therefore, efforts have been made to develop more permissive polymerases to accept modified nucleotides [49].

As nucleases are highly stereoselective, another strategy to generate highly stable aptamers is to replace D-ribose of the sugar moiety in the wild-type nucleic acid with L-ribose. Such aptamers are named Spiegelmers (in German Spiegel means mirror) and show nuclease-resistance several orders of magnitude higher than the corresponding wild-type RNA sequences (Figure 10.5) [50, 51]. However, because wild-type RNA polymerases do not recognize L-ribonucleotide triphosphates as substrates and enantiomeric RNA polymerases (D-amino acids) are yet available, Spiegelmers to date have been generated using the wild-type RNA on the

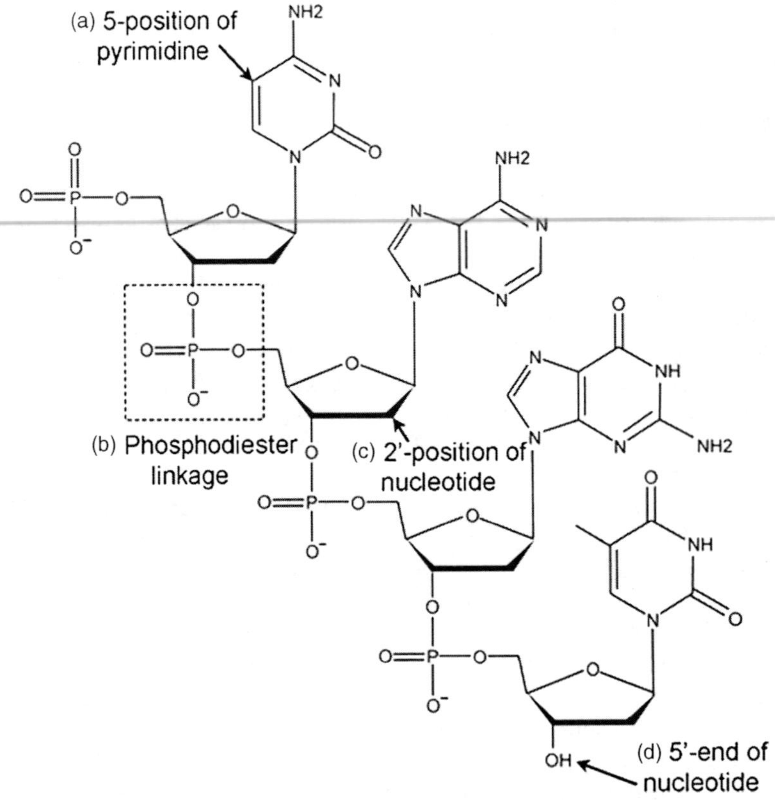

FIGURE 10.4 Nucleotide structure and positions often modified to enhance stability, including (a) 5-position of pyrimidine, (b) phosphodiester linkage, (c) 2′-position of nucleotide, and (d) 5′-end of nucleotide. Figure adapted from Ref. 28.

enantiomer of the desired target. When synthesized with L-ribose, the wild-type RNA transcripts that bind to the enantiomer of the target will bind to the desired target in the same manner. Such an approach has limited the production of Spiegelmers to a relatively small number of protein domains or peptides of which their enantimoeric targets can be prepared synthetically by using D-amino acids instead of the naturally occurring L-amino acids [52–55].

In developing specific nanoparticle formulations, the choice of targeting ligands in a specific nanoparticle drug delivery platform depends on multiple factors including the basis of diseases and indications, the physicochemical properties of drugs, the administration routes, and the engineering principles of delivery vehicles [56]. Nevertheless, aptamers possess a variety of desirable characteristics, which has resulted in their increasing applications as targeting ligands in nanoparticle drug delivery.

For example, aptamers are versatile and can target a wide range of molecules including proteins, nucleotides, organic dyes, amino acids, and metal ions, demonstrating their large potential as targeting ligands. In addition, aptamers can consistently achieve binding affinities comparable with therapeutic antibodies with less immunogenicity and are of smaller sizes (~1–2 nm and ~10 kDa vs ~10 nm and ~155 kDa). Meanwhile, by advancing from using biochemically purified molecules to whole living cells and animal models as targets, SELEX protocols now discover aptamers with significantly improved biological relevance and binding specificity. Additional strategies have also been applied to enhance aptamers' binding specificity. For example, counterselection against closely related targets together with selection against the desired target can effectively reduce cross binding that could compromise binding specificity [57]. By "toggling" the targets between human-derived and animal-derived proteins during alternating rounds of selection, SELEX can yield aptamers that bind to the target in both animal models as well as in humans, which may facilitate the preclinical evaluation of potential therapeutic effects of aptamers in animal models [58]. Alternatively, iteratively toggling between full-length protein target and isolated protein domains can drive aptamer binding to a particular epitope [59].

Once an aptamer is selected, it can be manufactured on a large scale through standard and cost-effective chemical synthesis with minimal batch-to-batch bioactivity difference. In contrast to the *in vivo* production of other targeting

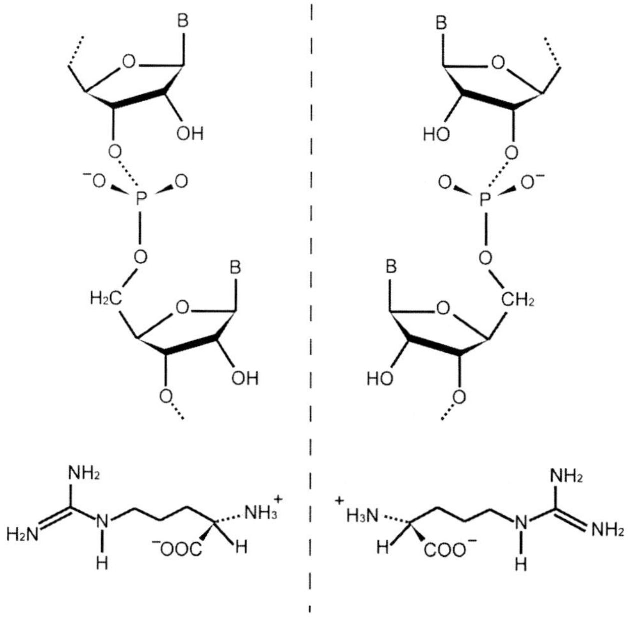

FIGURE 10.5 Mirror-design of L-RNA ligands that bind to Dadenosine. High-affinity D-RNA ligands binding to the enantiomeric form of D-adenosine were identified by *in vitro* selection. Truncated aptamers containing the binding motif were prepared by solid-phase synthesis in the D- and Lforms. While the selected D-RNA is able to recognize the unnatural adenosine enantiomer, the mirror-image RNA binds to naturally occurring D-adenosine. Figure adapted from Ref. 50.

molecules such as antibodies, the chemical production process of aptamers is not prone to viral or bacterial contamination. In addition, the stability of nucleic acid backbones allow aptamers to adapt to diverse chemical environments and engineering processes; show tolerance to heat, pH, and organic solvents; and can be denatured and renatured multiples times without significant loss of activity. In addition, aptamers can be easily conjugated to various delivery platforms. The ability to attach fluorescent dyes or chemical groups allows aptamers to bring rich functionalities and integrate with advanced drug delivery systems.

Taken together, these distinct characteristics have made aptamers useful additions to the arsenal of targeting ligands for drug delivery applications.

10.5 APPLICATIONS OF APTAMERS AS TARGETING LIGANDS IN DRUG DELIVERY

Cell-specific drug delivery can be achieved by directly conjugating aptamers to drug molecules. In addition to conventional drugs, a myriad of organic/inorganic nanomaterials and devices has been used as delivery vehicles to develop effective therapeutic modalities with clinical applications ranging from oncologic to cardiovascular disease [19, 60] (Figure 10.6). These nanomedicines, partly because of their unique ability to selectively accumulate at disease sites, improve existing treatments through their altered

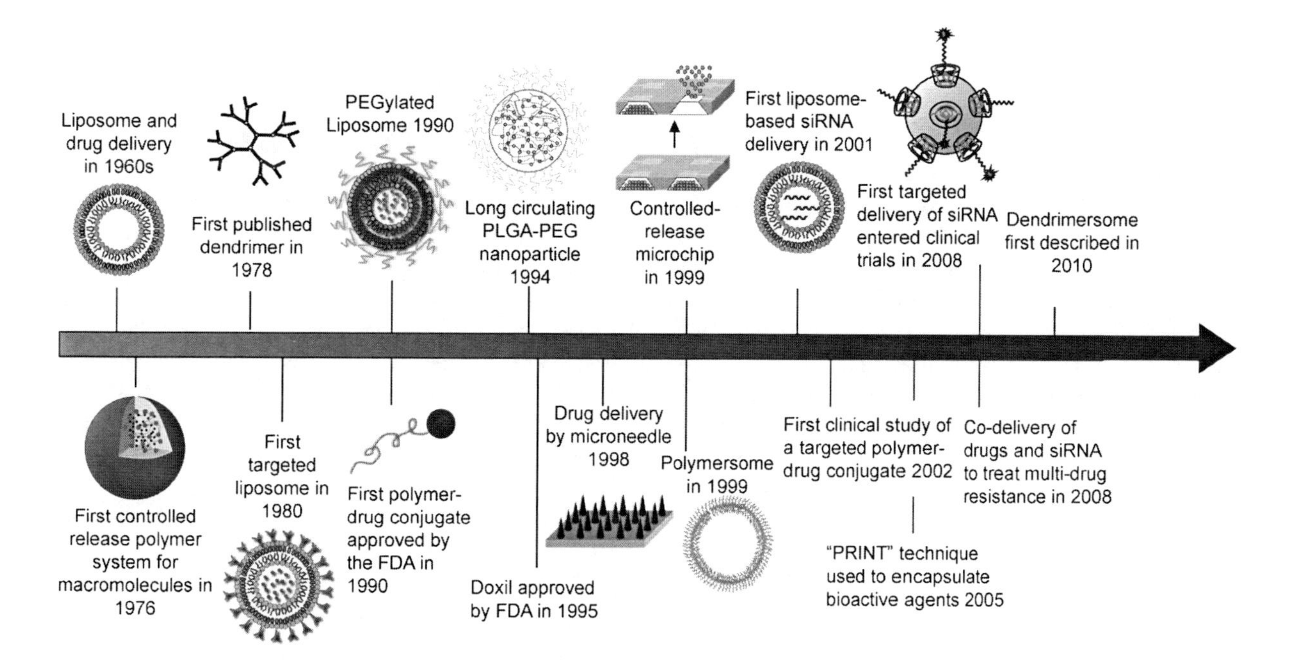

FIGURE 10.6 Timeline of nanotechnology-based drug delivery. Here, we highlight some delivery systems that serve as important milestones throughout the history of drug delivery. Figure adapted from Ref. 60.

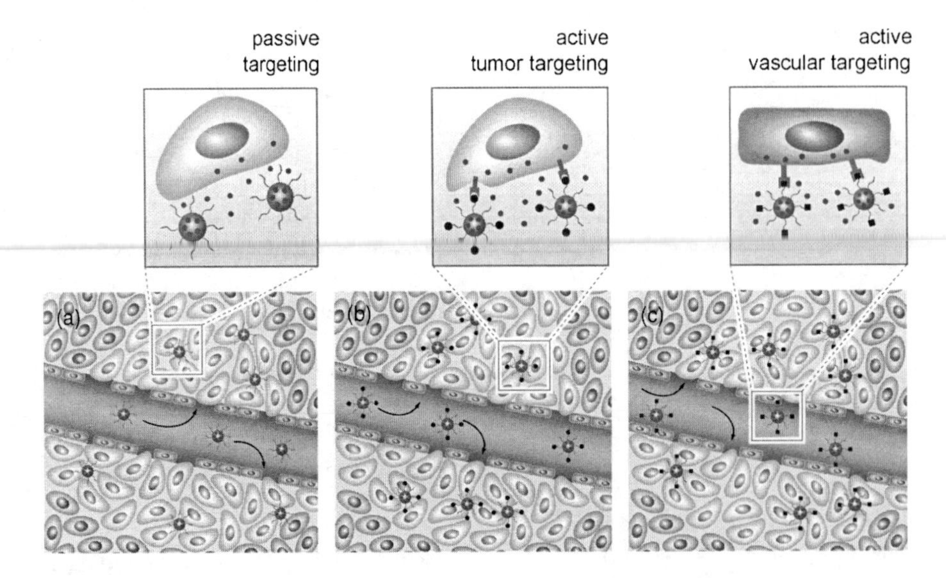

FIGURE 10.7 Passive versus active targeting. Figure adapted from Ref. 61. (See color figure in color plate section.)

pharmacokinetics and biodistribution profiles [56, 61]. Using aptamers as targeting ligands can further increase the benefit of these nanomedicines.

Nanoparticles tend to extravasate passively through the leaky vasculature, which is characteristic of solid tumors and inflamed tissue, and they accumulate preferentially through the enhanced permeability and retention effect (Figure 10.7a). In this case, the drug may be released in the extracellular matrix and diffuse throughout the tissue for bioactivity. Once particles have extravasated in the target tissue, the presence of ligands on the particle surface can result in active targeting of particles to receptors that are present on target cell or tissue resulting in enhanced accumulation and cell uptake through receptor-mediated endocytosis (Figure 10.7b). This process, referred to as "active targeting," can enhance the therapeutic efficacy of drugs, especially those that do not readily permeate the cell membrane and require an intracellular site of action for bioactivity. Alternatively, nanoparticles can be engineered for vascular targeting by incorporating ligands that bind to endothelial cell-surface receptors (Figure 10.7c). Whereas the presence of leaky vasculature is not required for vascular targeting, when present as is the case in tumors and inflamed tissue, this strategy may potentially work synergistically for drug delivery to target both the vascular tissue and target cells within the diseased tissue for enhanced therapy.

With the rapid development of nanotechnologies for drug delivery, aptamers together with other molecules that can target diseases with high specificity and affinity have been used increasingly as targeting ligands in numerous delivery platforms. In this section, we review several aptamers frequently used as targeting ligands with a primary emphasis on the engineering principles of implementing these molecules in a wide range of multifunctional delivery platforms.

10.5.1 Aptamers Targeting the Prostate-Specific Membrane Antigen (PSMA)

PSMA is a well-characterized cell-surface marker of prostate cancer, which is highly upregulated in prostate carcinomas [62, 63]. Its expression increases with disease progression, becoming highest in metastatic hormone-refractory disease. Different from other secretory prostate-specific proteins such as prostate specific antigen and prostatic acid phosphatase, PSMA is an integral membrane glycoprotein whose expression is largely restricted to the prostate epithelial cells. In addition, PSMA is abundantly expressed on the neovasculature of multiple nonprostate solid tumors, including breast, lung, gastric, and colorectal cancers, but not on normal vasculature [64–67]. Thus, the highly restricted presence of PSMA on prostate cancer and nonprostate solid tumor neovasculature makes it an attractive target for anticancer drug delivery applications [68–70].

PSMA-binding aptamers were selected from an initial 40mer library of $\sim 6 \times 10^{14}$ random-sequence RNA molecules according to their ability to bind to a recombinant protein representing the extracellular 706 amino acids of PSMA, termed xPSM [71]. By monitoring aptamer inhibition of xPSM *N*-acetyl-α-linked acid dipeptidase (NAALADase) enzymatic activity, six rounds of *in vitro* selection resulted in an aptamer pool consisting of two sequences, termed A9 and A10 aptamers, which share no consensus sequences and bind to distinct extracellular epitopes of xPSM. The A10 aptamer was further truncated into a shorter version, termed A10-3 aptamer, which retained PSMA binding ability. These three aptamers showed binding affinity to LNCaP human prostate cancer cells expressing PSMA but not PSMA-devoid PC-3 human prostate cancer cells. As PSMA is an internalizing receptor for its ligand [72], PSMA-binding aptamers have attracted attention in a broad range of drug delivery applications.

PSMA-binding aptamers have been used to formulate aptamer-small interfering RNA (siRNA) chimeras and are studied for targeted siRNA delivery. This strategy appears attractive because the formulation of aptamer-siRNA chimeras only requires simple hybridization or co-synthesis. Aptamer-siRNA chimeras inhibited PMSA-expressing LNCaP cells *in vitro* by regulating gene expression [73] and in a LNCaP xenograft mouse model using intratumoral injection [74], respectively. The chimeras in the latter study were further modified by adding 2-nucleotide 3′-overhangs to promote cellular processing and conjugating with PEG moieties to improve circulating half-life, which together led to pronounced inhibition of LNCaP tumor in an xenograft athymic mouse model after systemic administration [75]. In another study, A10-3 aptamer-siRNA chimeras were used to inhibit nonsense-mediated messenger RNA decay (NMD) in subcutaneous and metastatic prostate tumor models and successfully led to immune-mediated tumor rejection and growth inhibition [76], thus providing an alternative approach to the conventional cancer vaccination normally aimed at stimulating a systemic immune response. In these studies, the underlying mechanisms by which siRNA molecules escape from endosomes into the cytoplasm for bioactivity is not clear, as most of the internalized siRNA-aptamer chimeras are presumably trapped inside the endosomes and face degradation [72, 77].

Using aptamers as targeting ligands to deliver nanoparticles in a cell-specific manner was first attempted by conjugating A10-3 aptamers to the surface of nanoparticles formulated by using an amphiphilic diblock co-polymer poly lactic acid-block-PEG (PLA-PEG), where PLA allows for the controlled drug release and PEG provides "stealth" properties to decrease immune evasion [77]. Compared with nontargeted nanoparticles, with the presence of aptamers on the nanoparticle surfaces, the number of nanoparticles taken up by the PMSA (+) LNCaP cells significantly increased. When the same experiments were performed on PSMA(−) PC3 cells, the presence of A10-3 aptamers did not improve nanoparticle uptake, indicating a positive role played by aptamers to enhance nanoparticle cell uptake. When administered via intratumoral injection, the nanoparticles targeted by A10-3 aptamer showed a largely improved antitumor effect and reduced toxicity in LNCaP xenograft nude mice [78]. Together, these studies demonstrate that using aptamers as targeting ligands can be beneficial for the efficient delivery of nanoparticles in a cell-, tissue-, or disease-specific manner.

By using PLGA-PEG nanoparticles targeted by A10-3 aptamer as a model system, several engineering strategies have been explored, which can be generally applied to improve nanoparticle drug delivery. For example, in addition to aptamer targeting, nanoparticle size optimization through systematically altering formulation parameters, including polymer concentration, drug loading, water miscibility of solvent, and the water-to-solvent ratio, is a general strategy to achieve drug biodistribution profiles that favor clinically relevant targeted therapies [79]. In a attempt to engineer nanoparticle surface properties precisely and to minimize batch-to-batch variations in nanoparticles' biophysicochemical properties, tri-block co-polymers composed of end-to-end linkages of PLGA, PEG, and A10 aptamer were synthesized, followed by self-assembly to form targeted nanoparticles [80]. In contrast to the conventional method where nanoparticles were first formulated followed by the aptamer conjugation, this new approach controls nanoparticle composition and aptamer surface density through premixing of co-polymers with and without aptamers, thus allowing for the fine tuning of formulation parameters. By using this strategy, a narrow range of aptamer density was determined, resulting in most efficient cell uptake both *in vitro* and *in vivo*. Furthermore, to improve on drug delivery efficiency and safety, a "prodrug" strategy was developed to deliver cisplatin with A10-3 aptamer-targeted PLGA-PEG nanoparticles [81]. This approach used cisplatin molecules in an inactive form and obtained higher drug loading yield because of the better solubility of prodrug in organic solvents. After release from the nanoparticles, the prodrug underwent hydrolysis and was activated at the disease site. *In vivo* studies using LNCaP xenograft mouse models showed enhanced drug tolerability and efficacy when compared with cisplatin administered in its conventional form. Moreover, by using the same delivery platform, combination delivery with precisely controlled drug ratios was achieved by first conjugating drug molecules or imaging agents to PLA backbones, followed by blending different drug-attached polymers to formulate nanoparticles. In addition, encapsulation of drug-attached polymers, as opposed to directly encapsulating free drug molecules, can minimize undesired drug leakage from the polymer matrices during circulation and improve on delivery efficiency [82]. Co-delivery of docetaxel (Dtxl) and cisplatin using A10-3 aptamer targeted nanoparticles resulted in drug synergy *in vivo*. Collectively, these studies using A10 aptamer-targeted PLGA-PEG nanoparticles imply that an integrated approach, by combining aptamer targeting with other engineering strategies, can achieve safer and more effective drug delivery.

Whereas A10 aptamer folds into its tertiary conformation through intramolecular base pairing, a short double stranded region forms near the stem, which in turn can serve as a binding site to non-covalently intercalate drug molecules containing flat aromatic rings such as doxorubicin (Dox) and donarubicin. This physical intercalation does not require additional modifications of drug or aptamer molecules nor interferes with the subsequent chemical conjugations of the aptamers to nanoparticle carriers [83]. Therefore, as a convenient method to achieve co-delivery of multiple drugs, A10-3 aptamers intercalated with Dox have been conjugated to a wide range of nanoparticle delivery systems including polymeric nanoparticles [84], superparamagnetic iron oxide nanoparticles [85], gold nanoparticles [86], quantum dots [87, 88], radioactive nanoparticles [89], and polyplexes [90].

10.5.2 Aptamers Targeting PTK7 on Leukemia Cells

Knowledge regarding molecular characteristics of leukemia cells is limited, especially at the proteomic level. As mentioned, the discovery of PTK7 as a molecular signature on leukemia cells was accomplished by a two-step process: cell-SELEX to enrich aptamers that could distinguish leukemia cells followed by target identification. In cell-SELEX processes, CCRF-CEM, a cultured precursor T-ALL cell line, was used as the target cell line, whereas Ramos cells, a B cell line from human Burkitt's lymphoma, were used as counter cell line to reduce the collection of DNA sequences that could bind to common surface molecules present on both types of cells [91]. Cell-SELEX generated a panel of 10 aptamers that could recognize specifically leukemia cells with Kd in the nanomolar-to-picomolar range. One selected aptamer, Sgc8, shows the highest binding affinity in the panel, which was further truncated into a shorter sequence, namely sgc8c, with a comparable binding affinity with that of the full-length Sgc8 and a single loop–stem structure [92]. In a series test using cultured cell lines and clinical patient samples, Sgc8 aptamer was found to bind preferentially with most T-ALL cells, AML cells, and some B-ALL cells but not lymphoma cells or normal human bone marrow cells [30]. Following cell-SELEX, the selected aptamers were conjugated with magnetic streptavidin beads to capture and purify their binding targets on the leukemia cell surface [33]. Assisted by mass spectrometry, PTK7 was ultimately identified as the target of Sgc aptamers on T-ALL cells. This two-step approach to identify cell surface markers is generally applicable to distinguish the differences between any two types of cells at the molecular level. In addition, the two-step approach by first selecting cell-specific aptamers and then identifying their binding target is promising to substantially improve the overall effectiveness of biomarker discovery.

As an sgc8 aptamer can be internalized through receptor-mediated endocytosis, conjugation of sgc8 to small-molecule drugs allows for cell-specific drug delivery [39]. For example, conjugation of sgc8c aptamer to daunorubicin showed significantly improved drug potency on PTK7-positive Molt-4 cells, a human acute lymphoblastic leukemia cell line [93]. Drug potency can be further enhanced by conjugating aptamers to drug molecules through environment-responsive chemical linkers that are cleaved in endosomes [94]. In one study, sgc8c aptamer conjugated to Dox via a malamide-hydrazone bond, a pH-labile cross-linker, resulted in preferential delivery of drug molecules to CCRF-CEM cells and responsive drug release after internalization [95], which together led to improved drug potency.

Although the targeting ability of an aptamer is preserved, it can be further engineered to integrate additional functionalities that favor drug release at the target site. For example, sgc8 aptamer was modified by adding a short DNA probe, which was complementary to a 14-mer oligonucleic acid attached with a quenched fluorescence resonance energy transfer (FRET) reporter and a dithiothreitol (DTT) molecule [96]. This 14-mer oligonucleic acid can recognize cell surface-bound sgc8 aptamer, and the hybridization of two DNA templates releases the quencher from the incoming complementary DNA (cDNA) probe and restores the fluorescence. This study suggests a useful strategy to activate photosensitizers or fluorochromes at the tumor site, which may aid the development of novel delivery strategies for a variety of cancer tumor therapies.

Sgc8 and sgc8c aptamers have also been conjugated to several nanoparticle platforms for targeted delivery. For example, a sgc8c aptamer modified with a carboxyl group was conjugated to the surface of ultrasmall ($\sim$26 nm) chitosan nanoparticles through water-soluble carbodiimide chemistry [97]. As chitosan is biocompatible and biodegradable, nanoparticles developed in this study with ultrasmall sizes can find many applications in drug delivery. As another example, a liposome system was formulated by hydrogenated soy phosphatidyl choline, cholesterol, and methoxypoly(ethylene glycol)-distearoyl-phosphatidylethanolamine (mPEG-DSPE). By adding maleimide-terminated PEG-DSPE, a thiol-modified sgc8 aptamer was conjugated to the liposome surface, allowing for preferential targeting to CCRF-CEM leukemia cells [98]. Similarly, a thiol-modified sgc8 aptamer was also conjugated to the surface of mesoporous silica nanoparticles (MSNs) coated with thiolated poly(methacrylic acid) (PMASH) [99]. MSNs are attractive drug containers because of the inherent large surface area and high loading capacity. Sequential deposition of polyelectrolyte multilayers on the particle surface can prevent the premature drug leakage and achieve controlled drug release under reducing conditions. Thiol-modification of sgc8c aptamer also allows for its conjugation to Au-Ag nanorods used for photothermal therapy, which led to enhanced hyperthermia efficiency to targeted CEM cells in cell mixtures [100]. Using the same principle, sgc8c aptamer was modified by an amine group at the 5-prime end during the aptamer synthesis and conjugated to carboxyl-terminated poly(amidoamine) (PAMAM) of the fifth generation [101]. This model targeted dendrimer platform showed enhanced uptake in CCRF-CEM cells compared with PTK7-negative Ramos cells.

Sgc8c aptamer was also applied to develop viral capsid-aptamer conjugates as multivalent cell-targeting vehicles [102]. By using the protein shell of bacteriophage MS2, aniline groups were first installed on the outer surface of the capsid a short synthetic amino acid (*p*-aminophenylalanine) into position 19 of the MS2 coat protein. The short amino acids presented on the capsid surface were used to attach up to 60 sgc8c molecules in mild conditions without apparent loss of recognition capabilities. Subsequently, the interior surface of the vehicle could attach up to 180 porphyrins and generate cytotoxic singlet oxygen on illumination [103]. The doubly modified capsids killed Jurkat cells selectively even when mixed with erythrocytes, therefore suggesting the possible applications to target blood-borne cancers or other pathogens in the blood.

10.5.3 Aptamers Targeting Ramos Cells

Burkitt's lymphoma is an acute blood cell cancer among the most progressive of all human cancers [104]. As Burkitt's lymphoma is immunophenotypically indistinguishable from many other large B-cell lymphomas, the lack of molecular probes that can recognize cell surface molecular signatures has hindered the development of its early diagnosis and targeted therapy. Motivated by the significance to discover biomarkers that can recognize Burkitt's lymphoma, a group of aptamers was selected to recognize Ramos cells, a Burkitt's lymphoma cell line, and CCRF-CEM and Toledo cells (CRL-2631, B lymphocyte, and human diffuse large cell lymphoma) were used as counter cells. Three aptamers, namely TD05, TD02, and TE03, showed specific binding to Ramos cells but not CCRF-CEM or Toledo cells. These aptamers have been subsequently applied in different drug delivery applications.

The TD05 aptamer was modified by an amine group and subsequently conjugated with chlorin e6, a porphyrin-based photosensitizer, which could generate reactive oxygen species after irradiation with light of an appropriate wavelength [105]. The toxicity of a photosensitizer mainly results from the reactive oxygen species produced through the interaction of excited photosensitizer with neighboring oxygen. Therefore, cell-photosensitizer co-localization achieved by conjugating the aptamer directly to photosensitizer can significantly improve the efficiency of photodynamic therapy. Conjugation of the aptamer to the photosensitizer also overcomes the hydrophobic nature of most photosensitizers, further broadening their applications in biological fluids.

Studies also suggest that TD05 aptamer is an efficient targeting ligand for potential *in vivo* applications. For example, TD05 aptamer was directly conjugated with Cy-5 and injected through tail vein to Ramos xenograft nude mice. Cy5-TD05 conjugate produced localized florescent signal in the tumor region with high signal-to-background ratio [106]. A TD05 aptamer was also conjugated to a simple lipid tail phosphomidite with diacyl chains. The amphiphilic conjugates can self-assemble into spherical micelles with an average diameter in the sub-100 nm range [107]. The micelles could permeate cells through both membrane fusion and aptamer-mediated internalization. To prove the potential ability in detection and delivery of this aptamer–micelle in biological living systems, a tumor site in the bloodstream was mimicked by immobilizing tumor cells onto the surface of a flow channel device. Flushing the aptamer–micelles through the channel demonstrated their selective recognition ability under flow circulation comparable with physiological conditions.

10.5.4 AS1411, a Guanosine-Rich Aptamer Targeting the Nucleolin

Early studies found that a group of guanosine-rich oligonucleotides (GROs) bound to a specific cellular protein and exhibited anti-proliferative properties against certain cancer cells [18, 108]. Later, among these oligonucleotides, a 26-mer DNA aptamer named AS1411 was isolated and nucleolin was identified as its binding target [109, 110]. AS1411 aptamer showed promising anti-tumor activity without serious systemic toxicity and became the first aptamer entering human clinical trials for cancer treatment [111]. Studies also found that nucleolin, one of the major proteins of the nucleolus, was abundantly expressed on tumor cell surfaces where it serves as a binding protein and mediates calcium-dependent internalization for various ligands implicated in tumorigenesis and angiogenesis [112, 113]. Therefore, in parallel to its development as an anticancer drug, applications of AS1141 in drug delivery have also been explored.

Amine-modified AS1411 aptamer was conjugated to carboxyl-terminated quantum dots (QDs), and the QD-AS1141 conjugates showed enhanced uptakes in several cancer cell lines including HeLa (human cervical cancer cells), MDA-MB-231 (human breast cancer cells), and C6 cells (a rat glioma cell line) [114, 115]. The mixture of QD-AS1411 and quantum dots conjugated with different targeting moieties can simultaneously monitor different cancer biomarkers, a useful strategy for assessing cancer bioactivities. AS1411 aptamer folds into a dimeric G-quadruplex structure and can intercalate with six molecules of a porphyrin-derived photosensitizer for targeted photodynamic therapy [116]. The combination of loading and targeting of photosensitizers provides a convenient strategy to enhance therapeutic efficiency.

Using AS1411 as a targeting ligand, a liposome formulation composed of hydrogenated soybean phosphatidylcholine

(HSPC), cholesterol, and mPEG2000–DSPE was developed to deliver cisplatin to breast cancer cells [117]. AS1411 aptamer allows for an enhanced and specific targeting on MCF-7 cells (nucleolin positive) compared with LNCaP cells (nucleolin negative). In addition, in this study, a complementary 20-base sequence composed of all 2′-O-methyl-modified RNA bases was employed as antidotes to disrupt selectively the G-quadruplex structure of AS1411 and delete its binding ability to the nucleolins. This "reversible cell-specific delivery strategy" demonstrates the ability of modulating molecular targeting for desired drug delivery applications.

10.5.5 Other Aptamers Used as Targeting Ligands for Drug Delivery

To date, using aptamers that target PSMA, PTK7, Ramos cells, and nucleolin has resulted in a plethora of drug delivery platforms with numerous designs and applications. Aptamers have been established as robust targeting ligands to improve on drug delivery specificity and efficiency. Meanwhile, additional aptamers targeting a diverse range of biomarkers are developed and applied for drug delivery applications. Some examples include aptamers that target the transferrin receptor [118], adenosine triphosphate (ATP) [119–121], human α-thrombin [122], surface glycoprotein 120 (gp120) on type-1 HIV-infected cells [123, 124], epidermal growth factor receptor (EGFR) [125], Tenascin-C receptor on glioma cells [126], platelet-derived growth factor-BB [127, 128], and mouse liver hepatoma cell line BNL 1 ME A.7R.1 (MEAR) cells [129, 130] (Table 10.1).

TABLE 10.1 Selected Examples of Aptamers Used as Targeting Ligand in Nanoparticle-Based Drug Delivery

Target	Reference
Prostate specific membrane antigen (PSMA)	[71–90]
Protein tyrosine kinase 7 (PTK7) on leukemia cells	[30, 33, 39, 91–93, 95–103]
Ramos cells	[104–107]
Nucleoline	[18, 108–117]
Transferrin receptor	[118]
Adenosine triphosphate (ATP)	[119–121]
Human α-thrombin	[122]
Surface glycoprotein 120 (gp120) on type-1 HIV-infected cells	[123, 124]
Epidermal growth factor receptor (EGFR)	[125]
Tenascin-C receptor on glioma cells	[126]
Platelet-derived growth factor-BB	[127, 128]
Mouse liver hepatoma cell line BNL 1 ME A.7R.1 (MEAR) cells	[129, 130]

10.6 NOVEL APPLICATIONS OF APTAMERS IN ADVANCED DRUG DELIVERY

Over the past two decades, three-dimensional DNA and RNA nanoscaffolds with various architectures have been constructed and extensively explored for drug delivery applications [131, 132]. The ability of nucleic acid molecules including DNA and RNA to recognize and hybridize with their complement sequences in a highly accurate manner allows these nanoscaffolds to achieve sophisticated design with precise positioning of therapeutic agents and fine tuning of their releases to specific areas of the body [133]. In this respect, aptamers are attractive building blocks. Because of their relatively short sequences, aptamers are particularly suitable to construct nanoscaffolds of small sizes, simple geometries, and large numbers of participating modules [134]. In addition, aptamers convey intrinsic advantages of nucleic acids with an additional ability of providing direct binding interactions with protein molecules, thus, offering unique functionalities in a variety of nucleic acid-based nanoscaffolds. For example, aptamers can be grafted to the surface of streptavidin-coated polystyrene particles and then embedded into an injectable poloxamer hydrogel [127]. Through aptamer-mediated protein binding interactions, the hydrogel could prolong protein release and the release rates could be tailored by choosing individual aptamer sequences from an aptamer library selected to bind to the same protein target but with different binding affinities. Furthermore, the addition of complementary oligonucleotides to the system could trigger the release of the bound proteins in a pulsatile manner at predetermined time points, therefore providing a useful strategy to develop pulsatile protein delivery systems [128].

The high selectivity and affinity of aptamers has also attracted broad interests in using these molecules to develop sensors and devices for effective disease diagnosis and detection. For example, by changing the doping ratio of different fluorescent dyes, FRET nanoparticles exhibited multiple colors after excitation with a single wavelength [135]. When the FRET nanoparticles were conjugated with aptamers specific for different cancer cell lines, the resulting aptamer-conjugated FRET nanoparticles achieved simultaneous and sensitive detection of multiple cancer cells from complex living samples.

Aptamers have also been exploited to develop rapid, specific, sensitive, and low-cost detection of circulating tumor cells (CTCs). CTCs contain key information on how tumor genotypes evolve during cancer progression. Therefore, technologies that can yield purer CTC populations from blood samples are powerful tools to provide early and noninvasive detection of cancer, along with the prediction of treatment responses and tumor progression [136]. Despite these significances, in reality, CTCs are extremely rare. A few CTCs shed from metastatic tumors mingle with approximately 10 million leukocytes and 5 billion erythrocytes in 1 mL of blood, making their detection and isolation a formidable technological challenge [137]. In a two-step approach to achieve economic and fast CTC detection, circulating Ramos cells as model cells were first labeled by using TD05 aptamer-functionalized gold nanoparticles [138], followed by flowing the sample over a two-dimensional stripe functionalized by TE02 aptamer, another aptamer that binds with Ramos cells, thus, allowing for the isolation and capture of Ramos cells from the sample. Several Au-NPs attached to the captured cells then accumulate on the test zone and produce a characteristic red band, which can be used for both qualitative and quantitative analysis. A similar strategy was also applied to developing square capillary channels for CTC isolation [139]. To explore the possibilities of using aptamers to manipulate rare circulating cells, a poly(dimethylsiloxane)-based microfluidic device was developed and contained separate regions functionalized by using aptamers that could bind each cell line of interest [140]. By combining cell-affinity chromatography, the microfluidic device allowed for capturing and sorting mixed cells in the sample and yielded an enrichment of rare cells more than two orders of magnitude in a single run. These aptamer-based strategies have resulted in prototype devices and are under further development. Continuing discovery of aptamers that target specific subtypes of disease cells and development of automated devices that incorporate intelligent operation mechanisms will advance our ability in early disease diagnosis and detection.

10.7 SUMMARY

Aptamers have been established as a useful class of molecules with distinct molecular characteristics and superior binding properties. Since the birth of SELEX, aptamers have been selected to bind targets ranging from pure small organic molecules to the entire organisms or animals. An aptamer database (http://aptamer.icmb.utexas.edu/) has been established to contain comprehensive sequence information on aptamers and unnatural ribozymes generated by *in vitro* selection methods [141]. The database is not only useful for categorizing what aptamers and unnatural ribozymes already exist but also for garnering aptamer information as a whole to understand more completely the distribution of functional nucleic acids in sequence space and the topographies of fitness landscapes.

Aptamers have been increasingly used as biomolecular probes, therapeutic drugs, and targeting ligands. Rapid technology advances continue to lower the cost of aptamer manufacturing and provide a better understanding of their pharmacokinetic properties [23]. Novel concepts in aptamer development are also emerging. For example, bivalent aptamers engaging more than one target are attractive for applications where both recruitment and targeting are needed [142]. Meanwhile, the progress of nanotechnology has also resulted in complex and advanced drug delivery strategies that call for further exploration of functional molecules including aptamers [94, 143]. With collaborative and sustained efforts, aptamers will play a significant role in next-generation nanomedicines that have extensive medical applications.

ASSESSMENT QUESTIONS

10.1. By using SELEX, aptamers can be selected against a variety of targets including biochemically purified molecules, the whole living cells, and animals. What are the advantages and disadvantages of these targets for selecting aptamers?

10.2. Compared with other targeting ligands such as small molecules, antibodies, antibody fragments, and short peptides, what are the advantages and disadvantages of aptamers when used as a targeting ligand for drug delivery applications?

10.3. What are the major criteria in choosing a targeting ligand for a specific drug delivery system?

ACKNOWLEDGMENTS

This work was supported by National Institutes of Health Grants CA119349 and EB003647 and David Koch–Prostate Cancer Foundation Award in Nanotherapeutics.

REFERENCES

1. Hermann, T., Patel, D.J. (2000). Adaptive recognition by nucleic acid aptamers. *Science*, *287*, 820–825.
2. Schlünzen, F., Zarivach, R., Harms, J., Bashan, A., Tocilj, A., Albrech, R., Yonath, A., Franceschi, F. (2001). Structural basis for the interaction of antibiotics with the peptidyl transferase centre in eubacteria. *Nature*, *413*, 814–821.
3. Cech, T.R., Bass, B.L. (1986). Biological Catalysis by RNA. *Annual Review of Biochemistry*, *55*, 599–629.
4. Werstuck, G., Green, M.R. (1998). Controlling gene expression in living cells through small molecule-RNA interactions. *Science*, *282*, 296–298.
5. Pan, T., Sosnick, T. (2006). RNA folding during transcription. *Annual Review of Biophysics and Biomolecular Structure*, *35*, 161–175.
6. Strobel, S.A. (2001). Repopulating the RNA world. *Nature*, *411*, 1003–1006.

7. Michalak, P. (2006). RNA world – the dark matter of evolutionary genomics. *Journal of Evolutionary Biology, 19*, 1768–1774.
8. Rimmele, M. (2003). Nucleic acid aptamers as tools and drugs: Recent developments. *ChemBioChem, 4*, 963–971.
9. Yang, Y., Yang, D., Schluesener, H.J., Zhang, Z. (2007). Advances in SELEX and application of aptamers in the central nervous system. *Biomolecular Engineering, 24*, 583–592.
10. Ellington, A.D., Szostak, J.W. (1990). In vitro selection of RNA molecules that bind specific ligands. *Nature, 346*, 818–822.
11. Ellington, A.D., Szostak, J.W. (1990). Selection in vitro of single-stranded DNA molecules that fold into specific ligand-binding structures. *Nature, 355*, 850–852.
12. Famulok, M., Szostak, J.W. (1992). In vitro selection of specific ligand-binding nucleic acids. *Angewandte Chemie International Edition in English, 31*, 979–988.
13. Bock, L.C., Griffin, L.C., Latham, J.A., Vermaas, E.H., Toole, J.J. (1992). Selection of single-stranded DNA molecules that bind and inhibit human thrombin. *Nature, 355*, 564–566.
14. Tereshko, V., Skripkin, E., Patel, D.J. (2003). Encapsulating streptomycin within a small 40-mer RNA. *Chemistry & Biology, 10*, 175–187.
15. Huang, R., Fremont, D.H., Diener, J.L., Schaub, R.G., Sadler, J.E. (2009). A structural explanation for the antithrombotic activity of ARC1172, a DNA aptamer that binds von Willebrand factor domain A1. *Structure, 17*, 1476–1484.
16. Hale, S.P., Schimmel, P. (1996). Protein synthesis editing by a DNA aptamer. *Proceedings of the National Academy of Sciences, 93*, 2755–2758.
17. Chen, C.B., Chernis, G.A., Hoang, V.Q., Landgraf, R. (2003). Inhibition of heregulin signaling by an aptamer that preferentially binds to the oligomeric form of human epidermal growth factor receptor-3. *Proceedings of the National Academy of Sciences, 100*, 9226–9231.
18. Ireson, C.R., Kelland, L.R. (2006). Discovery and development of anticancer aptamers. *Molecular Cancer Therapeutics, 5*, 2957–2962.
19. Peer, D., Karp, J.M., Hong, S., Farokhzad, O.C., Margalit, R., Langer, R. (2007). Nanocarriers as an emerging platform for cancer therapy. *Nature Nanotechnology, 2*, 751–760.
20. Davis, M.E., Chen, Z., Shin, D.M. (2008). Nanoparticle therapeutics: An emerging treatment modality for cancer. *Nature Review Drug Discovery, 7*, 771–782.
21. Petros, R.A., DeSimone, J.M. (2010). Strategies in the design of nanoparticles for therapeutic applications. *Nature Reviews Drug Discovery, 9*, 615–627.
22. Lee, J.-O., So, H.-M., Jeon, E.-K., Chang, H., Won, K., Kim, Y.H. (2008). Aptamers as molecular recognition elements for electrical nanobiosensors. *Analytical and Bioanalytical Chemistry, 390*, 1023–1032.
23. Keefe, A.D., Pai, S., Ellington, A. (2010). Aptamers as therapeutics. *Nature Reviews Drug Discovery, 9*, 537–550.
24. Fitter, S., James, R. (2005). Deconvolution of a complex target using DNA aptamers. *The Journal of Biological Chemistry, 280*, 34193–34201.
25. Shamah, S.M., Healy, J.M., Cload, S.T. (2008). Complex target SELEX. *Accounts of Chemical Research, 41*, 130–138.
26. Biroccio, A., Hamm, J., Incitti, I., Francesco, R.D., Tomei, L. (2002). Selection of RNA aptamers that are specific and high-affinity ligands of the hepatitis C virus RNA-dependent RNA polymerase. *Journal of Virology, 76*, 3688–3696.
27. Vo, N., Tuler, J.R., Lai, M.M.C. (2004). Enzymatic characterization of the full-length and C-terminally truncated hepatitis C virus RNA polymerases: Function of the last 21 amino acids of the C terminus in template binding and RNA synthesis. *Biochemistry, 43*, 10579–10591.
28. Daniels, D.A., Chen, H., Hicke, B.J., Swiderek, K.M., Gold, L. (2003). A tenascin-C aptamer identified by tumor cell SELEX: Systematic evolution of ligands by exponential enrichment. *Proceedings of the National Academy of Sciences, 100*, 15416–15421.
29. Tang, Z., Shangguan, D., Wang, K., Shi, H., Sefah, K., Mallikratchy, P., Chen, H.W., Li, Y., Tan, W. (2007). Selection of aptamers for molecular recognition and characterization of cancer cells. *Analytic Chemistry, 79*, 4900–4907.
30. Shangguan, D., Cao, Z., Li, Y., Tan, W. (2007). Aptamers evolved from cultured cancer cells reveal molecular differences of cancer cells in patient samples. *Clinical Chemistry, 53*, 1153–1158.
31. Cerchia, L., Esposito, C.L., Jacobs, A.H., Tavitian, B., Franciscis, V.d. (2009). Differential SELEX in human Glioma cell lines. *PLoS One, 4*, e7917.
32. Shi, H., Tang, Z., Kim, Y., Nie, H., Huang, Y., He, X., Deng, K., Wang, K., Tan, W. (2010). In vivo fluorescence imaging of tumors using molecular aptamers generated by cell-SELEX. *Chemistry – An Asian Journal, 5*, 2209–2213.
33. Shangguan, D., Cao, Z., Meng, L., Mallikaratchy, P., Sefah, K., Wang, H., Li, Y., Tan, W. (2008). Cell-specific aptamer probes for membrane protein elucidation in cancer cells. *Journal of Proteome Research, 7*, 2133–2139.
34. Shangguan, D., Meng, L., Cao, Z., Xiao, Z., Fang, X., Li, Y., Cardona, D., Witek, R.P., Liu, C., Tan, W. (2008). Identification of liver cancer-specific aptamers using whole live cells. *Analytical Chemistry, 80*, 721–728.
35. Chen, H.W., Medley, C.D., Sefah, K., Shangguan, D., Tang, Z., Meng, L., Smith, J.E., Tan, W. (2008). Molecular recognition of small-cell lung cancer cells using aptamers. *ChemMedChem, 3*, 991–1001.
36. Simaeys, D.V., López-Colón, D., Sefah, K., Sutphen, R., Jimenez, E., Tan, W. (2010). Study of the molecular recognition of aptamers selected through ovarian cancer cell-SELEX. *PLoS One, 5*, e13770.
37. Sefah, K., Meng, L., Lopez-Colon, D., Jimenez, E., Liu, C., Tan, W. (2010). DNA aptamers as molecular probes for colorectal cancer study. *PLoS One, 5*, e14269.
38. Kang, H.S., Huh, Y.M., Kim, S., Lee, D. (2009). Isolation of RNA aptamers targeting HER-2-overexpressing breast cancer cells using cell-SELEX. *The Bulletin of the Korean Chemical Society, 30*, 1827–1831.

39. Xiao, Z., Shangguan, D., Cao, Z., Fang, X., Tan, W. (2008). Cell-specific internalization study of an aptamer from whole cell selection. *Chemistry – A European Journal*, *14*, 1769–1775.
40. Cerchia, L., Ducongé, F., Pestourie, C., Boulay, J., Aissouni, Y., Gombert, K., Tavitian, B., Franciscis, V.d., Libri, D. (2005). Neutralizing aptamers from whole-cell SELEX inhibit the RET receptor tyrosine kinase. *PLoS*, *3*, e123.
41. Mallikaratchy, P., Tang, Z., Kwame, S., Meng, L., Shangguan, D., Tan, W. (2007). Aptamer directly evolved from live cells recognizes membrane bound immunoglobin heavy Mu chain in Burkitt's lymphoma cells. *Molecular & Cellular Proteomics*, *6*, 2230–2238.
42. Parekh, P., Tang, Z., Turner, P.C., Moyer, R.W., Tan, W. (2010). Aptamers recognizing glycosylated hemagglutinin expressed on the surface of vaccinia virus-infected cells. *Analytical Chemistry*, *82*, 8642–8649.
43. Nitsche, A., Kurth, A., Dunkhorst, A., Pänke, O., Sielaff, H., Junge, W., Muth, D., Scheller, F., Stöcklein, W., Dahmen, C., Pauli, G., Kage, A. (2007). One-step selection of Vaccinia virus-binding DNA aptamers by MonoLEX. *BMC Biotechnology*, *7*, article number 48.
44. Dwivedi, H.P., Smiley, R.D., Jaykus, L. (2010). Selection and characterization of DNA aptamers with binding selectivity to Campylobacter jejuni using whole-cell SELEX. *Applied Microbiology and Biotechnology*, *87*, 2323–2334.
45. Mi, J., Liu, Y., Rabbani, Z.N., Yang, Z., Urban, J.H., Sullenger, B.A., Clary, B.M. (2010). In vivo selection of tumor-targeting RNA motifs. *Nature Chemical Biology*, *6*, 22–24.
46. Floege, J., Ostendorf, T., Janssen, U., Burg, M., Radeke, H.H., Vargeese, C., Gill, S.C., Green, L.S., Janjic, N. (1999). Novel approach to specific growth factor inhibition in vivo - Antagonism of platelet-derived growth factor in glomerulonephritis by aptamers. *American Journal of Pathology*, *154*, 169–179.
47. Adler, A., Forster, N., Homann, M., Goringer, H.U. (2008). Post-SELEX chemical optimization of a trypanosome-specific RNA aptamer. *Combinatorial Chemistry & High Throughput Screening*, *11*, 16–23.
48. Volkov, A.A., Kruglova, N.S., Meschaninova, M.I., Venyaminova, A.G., Zenkova, M.A., Vlassov, V.V., Chernolovskaya, E.L. (2009). Selective protection of nuclease-sensitive sites in siRNA prolongs silencing effect. *Oligonucleotides*, *19*, 191–202.
49. Keefe, A.D., Cload, S.T. (2008). SELEX with modified nucleotides. *Current Opinion in Chemical Biology*, *12*, 448–456.
50. Klußmann, S., Nolte, A., Bald, R., Erdmann, V.A., Fürste, J.P. (1996). Mirror-image RNA that binds D-adenosine. *Nature Biotechnology*, *14*, 1112–1115.
51. Nolte, A., Klußmann, S., Bald, R., Erdmann, V.A., Fürste, J.P. (1996). Mirror-design of L-oligonucleotide ligands binding to L-arginine. *Nature Biotechnology*, *14*, 1116–1119.
52. Helmling, S., Maasch, C., Eulberg, D., Buchner, K., Schröder, W., Lange, C., Vonhoff, S., Wlotzka, B., Tschöp, M.H., Rosewicz, S., Klussmann, S. (2004). Inhibition of ghrelin action in vitro and in vivo by an RNA-Spiegelmer. *Proceedings of the National Academy of Sciences*, *101*, 13174–13179.
53. Becskei, C., Bilik, K.U., Klussmann, S., Jarosch, F., Lutz, T. A., Riediger, T. (2007). The anti-Ghrelin Spiegelmer NOX-B11-3 blocks ghrelin- but not fasting-induced neuronal activation in the hypothalamic arcuate nucleus. *Journal of Neuroendocrinology*, *20*, 85–92.
54. Ninichuk, V., Clauss, S., Kulkarni, O., Schmid, H., Segerer, S., Radomska, E., Eulberg, D., Buchner, K., Selve, N., Klussmann, S., Anders, H. (2008). Late onset of Ccl2 blockade with the spiegelmer mNOX-E36-3PEG prevents glomerulosclerosis and improves glomerular filtration rate in db/db mice. *The American Journal of Pathology*, *172*, 628–637.
55. Maasch, C., Vater, A., Buchner, K., Purschke, W.G., Eulberg, D., Vonhoff, S., Klussmann, S. (2010). Polyetheylenimine-polyplexes of Spiegelmer NOX-A50 directed against intracellular high mobility group protein A1 (HMGA1) reduce tumor growth in vivo. *Journal of Biological Chemistry*, *285*, 40012–40018.
56. Farokhzad, O.C., Langer, R. (2009). Impact of nanotechnology on drug delivery. *ACS Nano*, *3*, 16–20.
57. White, R.R., Shan, S., Rusconi, C.P., Shetty, G., Dewhirs, M. W., Kontos, C.D., Sullenger, B.A. (2003). Inhibition of rat corneal angiogenesis by a nuclease-resistant RNA aptamer specific for angiopoietin-2. *Proceedings of the National Academy of Sciences*, *100*, 5028–5033.
58. White, R., Rusconi, C., Scardino, E., Wolberg, A., Lawson, J., Hoffman, M., Sullenger, B. (2001). Generation of species cross-reactive aptamers using "Toggle" SELEX. *The American Society of Gene Therapy*, *4*, 567–573.
59. Diener, J.L., Lagassé, H.A.D., Duerschmied, D., Merhi, Y., Tanguay, J.-F., Hutabarat, R., Gilbert, J., Wagner, D.D., Schaub, R. (2009). Inhibition of von Willebrand factor-mediated platelet activation and thrombosis by the anti-von Willebrand factor A1-domain aptamer ARC1779. *Journal of Thrombosis and Haemostasis*, *7*, 1155–1162.
60. Shi, J., Votruba, A.R., Farokhzad, O.C., Langer, R. (2010). Nanotechnology in drug delivery and tissue engineering: from discovery to applications. *Nano Letters*, *10*, 3223–3230.
61. Timko, B.P., Whitehead, K., Gao, W., Kohane, D.S., Farokhzad, O.C., Anderson, D., Langer, R. (2011). Advanced in drug delivery. *Annual Review of Materials Research*, *41*, 3.1–3.20.
62. Rajasekaran, A.K., Anilkumar, G., Christiansen, J.J. (2005). Is prostate-specific membrane antigen a multifunctional protein. *American Journal of Physiology*, *288*, C975–C981.
63. Bühler, P., Wolf P., Elsässer-Beile, U. (2009). Targeting the prostate-specific membrane antigen for prostate cancer therapy. *Immunotherapy*, *1*, 471–481.
64. Milowsky, M.I., Nanus, D.M., Kostakoglu, L., Sheehan, C.E., Vallabhajosula, S., Goldsmith, S.J., Ross, J.S., Bander, N.H. (2007). Vascular targeted therapy with anti–prostate-specific membrane antigen monoclonal antibody J591 in advanced solid tumors. *Journal of Clinical Oncology*, *25*, 540–547.
65. Morris, M.J., Pandit-Taskar, N., Divgi, C.R., Bender, S., O'Donoghue, J.A., Nacca, A., Smith-Jones, P., Schwartz, L., Slovin, S., Finn, R., Larson, S., Scher, H.I. (2007). Phase I evaluation of J591as a vascular targeting agent in progressive solid tumors. *Clinical Cancer Research*, *13*, 2707–2713.

66. Haffner, M.C., Kronberger, I.E., Ross, J.S., Sheehan, C.E., Zitt, M., Mühlmann, G., Öfner, D., Zelger, B., Ensinger, C., Yang, X.J., Geley, S., Margreiter, R., Bander, N.H. (2009). Prostate-specific membrane antigen expression in the neovasculature of gastric and colorectal cancers. *Human Pathology*, *40*, 1754–1761.
67. Liu, T.C., Jabbes, M., Nedrow-Byers, J.R., Wu, L.Y., Bryan, J. N., Berkman, C.E. (2011). Detection of prostate-specific membrane antigen on HUVECs in response to breast tumor conditioned medium. *International Journal of Oncology*, *38*, 1349–1355.
68. Sonpavde, G., Spencer, D.M., Slawin, K.M. (2007). Vaccine therapy for prostate cancer. *Urologic Oncology: Seminars and Original Investigations*, *25*, 451–459.
69. Elsässer-Beile, U., Bühler, P., Wolf, P. (2009). Targeted therapies for prostate cancer against the prostate specific membrane antigen. *Current Drug Targets*, *10*, 118–125.
70. Tagawa, S.T., Beltran, H., Vallabhajosula, S., Goldsmith, S.J., Osborne, J., Matulich, D., Petrillo, K., Parmar, S., Nanus, D. M., Bander, N.H. (2010). Anti–prostate-specific membrane antigen-based radioimmunotherapy for prostate cancer. *Cancer*, *116*, 1075–1083.
71. Lupold, S.E., Hicke, B.J., Lin, Y., Coffey, D.S. (2002). Identification and characterization of nuclease-stabilized RNA molecules that bind human prostate cancer cells via the prostate-specific membrane antigen. *Cancer Research*, *62*, 4029–4033.
72. Liu, H., Rajasekaran, A.K., Moy, P., Xia, Y., Kim, S., Navarro, V., Rahmati, R., Bander, N.H. (1998). Constitutive and antibody-induced internalization of prostate-specific membrane antigen. *Cancer Research*, *58*, 4055–4060.
73. Chu, T.C., Twu, K.Y., Ellington, A.D., Levy, M. (2006). Aptamer mediated siRNA delivery. *Nucleic Acids Research*, *34*, e73.
74. McNamara, J.O., Andrechek, E.R., Wang, Y., Viles, K.D., Rempel, R.E., Gilboa, E., Sullenger, B.A., Giangrande, P.H. (2006). Cell type–specific delivery of siRNAs with aptamer-siRNA chimeras. *Nature Biotechnology*, *24*, 1005–1015.
75. Dassie, J.P., Liu, X., Thomas, G.S., Whitaker, R.M., Thiel, K. W., Stockdale, K.R., Meyerholz, D.K., McCaffrey, A.P., McNamara, J.O., Giangrande, P.H. (2009). Systemic administration of optimized aptamer-siRNA chimeras promotes regression of PSMA expressing tumors. *Nature Biotechnology*, *27*, 839–849.
76. Pastor, F., Kolonias, D., Giangrande, P.H., Gilboa, E. (2010). Induction of tumour immunity by targeted inhibition of nonsense-mediated mRNA decay. *Nature*, *465*, 227–231.
77. Farokhzad, O.C., Jon, S., Khademhosseini, A., Tran, T.T., LaVan, D.A., Langer, R. (2004). Nanoparticle-aptamer bioconjugates: a new approach for targeting prostate cancer cells. *Cancer Research*, *64*, 7668–7672.
78. Farokhzad, O.C., Cheng, J., Teply, B.A., Sherifi, I., Jon, S., Kantoff, P.W., Richie, J.P., Langer, R. (2006). Targeted nanoparticle-aptamer bioconjugates for cancer chemotherapy in vivo. *Proceedings of the National Academy of Sciences*, *103*, 6315–6320.
79. Cheng, J., Teply, B.A., Sherifi, I., Sung, J., Luther, G., Gu, F. X., Levy-Nissenbaum, E., Radovic-Moreno, A.F., Langer, R., Farokhzad, O.C. (2007). Formulation of functionalized PLGA–PEG nanoparticles for in vivo targeted drug delivery. *Biomaterials*, *28*, 869–876.
80. Gu, F., Zhang, L., Teply, B.A., Mann, N., Wang, A., Radovic-Moreno, A.F., Langer, R., Farokhzad, O.C. (2008). Precise engineering of targeted nanoparticles by using self-assembled biointegrated block copolymers. *Proceedings of the National Academy of Sciences*, *105*, 2586–2591.
81. Dhara, S., Gu, F.X., Langer, R., Farokhzad, O.C., Lippard, S. J. (2008). Targeted delivery of cisplatin to prostate cancer cells by aptamer functionalized Pt(IV) prodrug-PLGA–PEG nanoparticles. *Proceedings of the National Academy of Sciences*, *105*, 17356–17361.
82. Kolishetti, N., Dhar, S., Valencia, P.M., Lin, L.Q., Karnik, R., Lippard, S.J., Langer, R., Farokhzad, O.C. (2010). Engineering of self-assembled nanoparticle platform for precisely controlled combination drug therapy. *Proceedings of the National Academy of Sciences*, *107*, 17939–17944.
83. Bagalkot, V., Farokhzad, O.C., Langer, R., Jon, S. (2006). An aptamer–doxorubicin physical conjugate as a novel targeted drug-delivery platform. *Angewandte Chemie International Edition*, *45*, 8149–8152.
84. Zhang, L., Radovic-Moreno, A.F., Alexis, F., Gu, F.X., Basto, P.A., Bagalkot, V., Jon, S., Langer, R., Farokhzad, O.C. (2007). Co-delivery of hydrophobic and hydrophilic drugs from nanoparticle–aptamer bioconjugates. *ChemMedChem*, *2*, 1268–1271.
85. Wang, A.Z., Bagalkot, V., Vasilliou, C.C., Gu, F., Alexis, F., Zhang, L., Shaikh, M., Yuet, K., Cima, M.J., Langer, R., Kantoff, P.W., Bander, N.H., Jon, S., Farokhzad, O.C. (2008). Superparamagnetic iron oxide nanoparticle–aptamer bioconjugates for combined prostate cancer imaging and therapy. *ChemMedChem*, *3*, 1311–1315.
86. Kim, D., Jeong, Y.Y., Jon, S. (2010). A drug-loaded aptamer-gold nanoparticle bioconjugate for combined CT imaging and therapy of prostate cancer. *ACS Nano*, *4*, 3689–3696.
87. Chua, T.C., Shieh, F., Lavery, L.A., Levy, M., Richards-Kortum, R., Korgel, B.A., Ellington, A.D. (2006). Labeling tumor cells with fluorescent nanocrystal–aptamer bioconjugates. *Biosensors and Bioelectronics*, *21*, 1859–1866.
88. Bagalkot, V., Zhang, L., Levy-Nissenbaum, E., Jon, S., Kantoff, P.W., Langer, R., Farokhzad, O.C. (2007). Quantum dot-aptamer conjugates for synchronous cancer imaging, therapy, and sensing of drug delivery based on bi-fluorescence resonance energy transfer. *Nano Letters*, *7*, 3065–3070.
89. Wang, A.Z., Yuet, K., Zhang, L., Gu, F.X., Huynh-Le, M., Radovic-Moreno, A.F., Kantoff, P.W., Bander, N.H., Langer, R., Farokhzad, O.C. (2010). ChemoRad nanoparticles: A novel multifunctional nanoparticle platform for targeted delivery of concurrent chemoradiation. *Nanomedicine*, *5*, 361–368.
90. Kim, E., Jung, Y., Choi, H., Yang, J., Suh, J., Huh, Y., Kim, K., Haam, S. (2010). Prostate cancer cell death produced by the co-delivery of Bcl-xL shRNA and doxorubicin using an aptamer-conjugated polyplex. *Biomaterials*, *31*, 4529–4599.

91. Shangguan, D., Li, Y., Tang, Z., Cao, Z., Chen, H., Mallikaratchy, P., Sefah, K., Yang, C., Tan, W. (2006). Aptamers evolved from live cells as effective molecular probes for cancer study. *Proceedings of the National Academy of Sciences*, *103*, 11838–11843.
92. Shangguan, D., Tang, Z., Mallikaratchy, P., Xiao, Z., Tan, W. (2007). Optimization and modifications of aptamers selected from live cancer cell lines. *ChemBioChem*, *8*, 603–606.
93. Taghdisi, S.M., Abnous, K., Mosaffa, F., Behravan, J. (2010). Targeted delivery of daunorubicin to T-cell acute lymphoblastic leukemia by aptamer. *Journal of Drug Targeting*, *18*, 277–281.
94. Gao, W., Chan, J.M., Farokhzad, O.C. (2010). pH-Responsive nanoparticles for drug delivery. *Molecular Pharmaceutics*, *7*, 1913–1920.
95. Huang, Y., Shangguan, D., Liu, H., Phillips, J.A., Zhang, X., Chen, Y., Tan, W. (2009). Molecular assembly of an aptamer–drug conjugate for targeted drug delivery to tumor cells. *ChemBioChem*, *10*, 862–868.
96. Mallikaratchy, P., Liu, H., Huang, Y., Wang, H., Lopez-Colon, D., Tan, W. (2009). Using aptamers evolved from cell-SELEX to engineer a molecular delivery platform. *Chemical Communications*, *21*, 3056–3058.
97. Tallury, P., Kar, S., Bamrungsap, S., Huang, Y., Tand, W., Santra, S. (2009). Ultra-small water-dispersible fluorescent chitosan nanoparticles: synthesis, characterization and specific targeting. *Chemical Communications*, *17*, 2347–2349.
98. Kang, H., O'Donoghue, M.B., Liu, H., Tan, W. (2010). A liposome-based nanostructure for aptamer directed delivery. *Chemical Communications*, *46*, 249–251.
99. Zhu, C., Song, X., Zhou, W., Yang, H., Wen, Y., Wang, X. (2009). An efficient cell-targeting and intracellular controlled-release drug delivery system based on MSN-PEM-aptamer conjugates. *Journal of Materials Chemistry*, *19*, 7765–7770.
100. Huang, Y.-F., Sefah, K., Bamrungsap, S., Chang, H.-T., Tan, W. (2008). Selective photothermal therapy for mixed cancer cells using aptamer-conjugated nanorods. *Langmuir*, *24*, 11860–11865.
101. Zhou, J., Soontornworajit, B., Martin, J., Sullenger, B.A., Gilboa, E., Wang, Y. (2009). A hybrid DNA aptamer–dendrimer nanomaterial for targeted cell labeling. *Macromolecular Bioscience*, *9*, 831–835.
102. Tong, G.J., Hsiao, S.C., Carrico, Z.M., Francis, M.B. (2009). Viral capsid DNA aptamer conjugates as multivalent cell-targeting vehicles. *Journal of the American Chemical Society*, *131*, 11174–11178.
103. Stephanopoulos, N., Tong, G.J., Hsiao, S.C., Francis, M.B. (2010). Dual-surface modified virus capsids for targeted delivery of photodynamic agents to cancer cells. *ACS Nano*, *4*, 6014–6020.
104. Rochford, R., Cannon, M.J., Moormann, A.M. (2005). Endemic Burkitt's lymphoma: A polymicrobial disease? *Nature Review Microbiology*, *3*, 182–187.
105. Mallikaratchy, P., Tang, Z., Tan, W. (2008). Cell specific aptamer–photosensitizer conjugates as a molecular tool in photodynamic therapy. *ChemMedChem*, *3*, 425–428.
106. Shi, H., Tang, Z., Kim, Y., Nie, H., Huang, Y.F., He, X., Deng, K., Wang, K., Tan, W. (2010). In vivo fluorescence imaging of tumors using molecular aptamers generated by cell-SELEX. *Chemistry An Asian Journal*, *5*, 2209–2213.
107. Wu, Y., Sefah, K., Liu, H., Wang, R., Tan, W. (2010). DNA aptamer–micelle as an efficient detection/delivery vehicle toward cancer cells. *Proceedings of the National Academy of Sciences*, *107*, 5–10.
108. Bates, P.J., Kahlon, J.B., Thomas, S.D., Trent, J.O., Miller, D. M. (1999). Antiproliferative-activity of G-rich oligonucleotides correlates with protein binding. *The Journal of Biological Chemistry*, *274*, 26369–26377.
109. Dapic, V., Bates, P.J., Trent, J.O., Rodger, A., Thomas, S.D., Miller, D.M. (2002). Antiproliferative activity of G-quartet-forming oligonucleotides with backbone and sugar modifications. *Biochemistry*, *41*, 3676–3685.
110. Soundararajan, S., Wang, L., Sridharan, V., Chen, W., Courtenay-Luck, N., Jones, D., Spicer, E.K., Fernandes, D.J. (2009). Plasma membrane nucleolin is a receptor for the anticancer aptamer AS1411 in MV4-11 leukemia cells. *Molecular Pharmacology*, *76*, 984–991.
111. Soundararajan, S., Chen, W., Spicer, E.K., Courtenay-Luck, N., Fernandes, D.J. (2008). The nucleolin targeting aptamer AS1411 destabilizes Bcl-2 messenger RNA in human breast cancer cells. *Cancer Research*, *68*, 2358–2365.
112. Hovanessian, A.G., Soundaramourty, C., Khoury, D.E., Nondier, I., Svab, J., Krust, B. (2010). Surface expressed nucleolin is constantly induced in tumor cells to mediate calcium dependent ligand internalization. *PLoS ONE*, *5*, e15787.
113. Reyes-Reyes, E.M., Teng, Y., Bates, P.J. (2010). A new paradigm for aptamer therapeutic AS1411 action: uptake by macropinocytosis and its stimulation by a nucleolin-dependent mechanism. *Cancer Research*, *70*, 8617–8629.
114. Ko, M.H., Kim, S., Kang, W.J., Lee, J.H., Kang, H., Moon, S. H., Hwang, D.W., Ko, H.Y., Lee, D.S. (2009). In vitro derby imaging of cancer biomarkers using quantum dots. *Small*, *5*, 1207–1212.
115. Ko, H.Y., Choi, K.J., Lee, C.H., Kim, S. (2011). A multimodal nanoparticle-based cancer imaging probe simultaneously targeting nucleolin, integrin avb3 and tenascin-C proteins. *Biomaterials*, *32*, 1130–1138.
116. Shieh, Y., Yang, S., Wei, M., Shieh, M. (2010). Aptamer-based tumor-targeted drug delivery for photodynamic therapy. *ACS Nano*, *4*, 1433–1442.
117. Cao, Z., Tong, R., Mishra, A., Xu, W., Wong, G., Cheng, J., Lu, Y. (2009). Reversible cell-specific drug delivery with aptamer-functionalized liposomes. *Angewandte Chemie International Edition*, *48*, 6494–6498.
118. Chen, C.B., Dellamaggiore, K.R., Ouellette, C.P., Sedano, C. D., Lizadjohry, M., Chernis, G.A., Gonzales, M., Baltasar, F. E., Fan, A.L., Myerowitz, R., Neufeld, E.F. (2008). Aptamer-based endocytosis of a lysosomal enzyme. *Proceedings of the National Academy of Sciences*, *105*, 15908–15913.
119. Nutiu, R., Li, Y. (2003). Structure-switching signaling aptamers. *Journal of the American Chemical Society*, *125*, 4771–4778.

120. Tang, Z., Zhu, Z., Mallikaratchy, P., Yang, R., Sefah, K., Tan, W. (2010). Aptamer–target binding triggered molecular mediation of singlet oxygen generation. *Chemistry An Asian Journal*, *5*, 783–786.

121. Wang, Y., Li, Z., Hu, D., Lin, C.-T., Li, J., Lin, Y. (2010). Aptamer/graphene oxide nanocomplex for in situ molecular probing in living cells. *Journal of the American Chemical Society*, *132*, 9274–9276.

122. Levy, M., Cater, S.F., Ellington, A.D. (2005). Quantum-dot aptamer beacons for the detection of proteins. *ChemBioChem*, *6*, 2163–2166.

123. Kim, D., Behlke, M.A., Rose, S.D., Chang, M., Choi, S., Rossi, J.J. (2005). Synthetic dsRNA Dicer substrates enhance RNAi potency and efficacy. *Nature Biotechnology*, *23*, 222–226.

124. Zhou, J., Li, H., Li, S., Zaia, J., Rossi, J. J. (2008). Novel dual inhibitory function aptamer–siRNA delivery system for HIV-1 therapy. *Molecular Therapy*, *16*, 1481–1489.

125. Li, N., Larson, T., Nguyen, H.H., Sokolov, K.V., Ellington, A. D. (2010). Directed evolution of gold nanoparticle delivery to cells. *Chemical Communications*, *46*, 392–394.

126. Nair, B.G., Nagaoka, Y., Morimoto, H., Yoshida, Y., Maekawa, T., Kumar, D.S. (2010). Aptamer conjugated magnetic nanoparticles as nanosurgeons. *Nanotechnology*, *21*, 455102.

127. Soontornworajit, B., Zhou, J., Zhang, Z., Wang, Y. (2010). Aptamer-functionalized in situ injectable hydrogel for controlled protein release. *Biomacromolecules*, *11*, 2724–2730.

128. Soontornworajit, B., Zhou, J., Wang, Y. (2010). A hybrid particle–hydrogel composite for oligonucleotide-mediated pulsatile protein release. *Soft Matter*, *6*, 4255–4261.

129. Shangguan, D., Meng, L., Cao, Z.C., Xiao, Z., Fang, X., Li, Y., Cardona, D., Witek, R.P., Liu, C., Tan, W. (2008). Identification of liver cancer-specific aptamers using whole live cells. *Analytical Chemistry*, *80*, 721–728.

130. Zhang, J., Jia, X., Lv, X., Deng, Y., Xie, H. (2010). Fluorescent quantum dot-labeled aptamer bioprobes specifically targeting mouse liver cancer cells. *Talanta*, *81*, 505–509.

131. Aldaye, F.A., Palmer, A.L., Sleiman, H.F. (2008). Assembling materials with DNA as the guide. *Science*, *321*, 1795–1799.

132. Guo, P. (2010). The emerging field of RNA nanotechnology. *Nature Nanotechnology*, *5*, 833–842.

133. Seeman, N.C. (2010). Nanomaterials based on DNA. *The Annual Review of Biochemistry*, *79*, 65–87.

134. Afonin, K.A., Bindewald, E., Yaghoubian, A.J., Voss, N., Jacovetty, E., Shapiro, B.A., Jaeger, L. (2010). In vitro assembly of cubic RNA-based scaffolds designed in silico. *Nature Nanotechnology*, *5*, 676–682.

135. Chen, X., Estévez, M., Zhu, Z., Huang, Y., Chen, Y., Wang, L., Tan, W. (2009). Using aptamer-conjugated fluorescence resonance energy transfer nanoparticles for multiplexed cancer cell monitoring. *Analytic Chemistry*, *81*, 7009–7014.

136. Yu, M., Stott, S., Toner, M., Maheswaran, S., Haber, D.A. (2011). Circulating tumor cells: approaches to isolation and characterization. *Journal of Cell Biology*, *192*, 373–382.

137. Yap, T.A., Sandhu, S.K., Workman, P., deBono, J.S. (2010). Envisioning the future of early anticancer drug development. *Nature Reviews Cancer*, *10*, 514–523.

138. Liu, G., Mao, X., Phillips, J.A., Xu, H., Tan, W., Zeng, L. (2009). Aptamer-nanoparticle strip biosensor for sensitive detection of cancer cells. *Analytic Chemistry*, *81*, 10013–10018.

139. Martin, J.A., Phillips, J.A., Parekh, P., Sefah, K., Tan, W. (2011). Capturing cancer cells using aptamer-immobilized square capillary channels. *Molecular BioSystems*, *7*, 1720–1727.

140. Xu, Y., Phillips, J.A., Yan, J., Li, Q., Fan, Z.H., Tan, W. (2009). Aptamer-based microfluidic device for enrichment, sorting, and detection of multiple cancer cells. *Analytical Chemistry*, *81*, 7436–7443.

141. Lee, J.F., Hesselberth, J.R., Meyers, L.A., Ellington, A.D. (2004). Aptamer database. *Nucleic Acids Research*, *32*, D95.

142. Zhou, J., Rossi, J.J. (2008). Bivalent aptamers deliver the punch. *Chemistry & Biology*, *15*, 644–645.

143. Dvir, T., Timko, B.P., Kohane, D.S., Langer, R. (2011). Nanotechnological strategies for engineering complex tissues. *Nature Nanotechnology*, *6*, 13–22.

11

NANOFIBER

MEGHA BAROT, MITAN R. GOKULGANDHI, ANIMIKH RAY, AND ASHIM K. MITRA

11.1 CHAPTER OBJECTIVES

- To provide introduction and benefits of nanofibers.
- To elucidate various polymer classes used for nanofiber preparation.
- To illustrate different methods for nanofiber fabrication.
- To summarize numerous biomedical applications of nanofibers.

11.2 INTRODUCTION

Nanofibers provide a connection between the nanoscale and the macroscale world, as the diameters are in the range of 1–100 nanometers and the lengths are in the range of several meters [1, 2]. Polymeric nanofiber, an important class of nanostructured materials, has gained growing attention in the last decade. Nanofibers are biocompatible and biodegradable polymeric fibers having diameters of less than 100 nanometers. Moreover, fibers produced by an ultrafine fiber manufacturing process with diameters of less than 1000 nanometers are also referred to as nanofibers. The large surface-area-to-mass ratio (10–1000 m^2/g) combined with the porous structure of nanofibers make them appropriate for a wide range of applications in the field of biomedicine and biotechnology [2, 3].

The development of nanosized fibers offers unique benefits [2–5]:

(1) The higher catalytic efficiency results from high surface-to-mass ratios.
(2) The controlled pore size of polymeric nanofibers provides higher porosity and permeability, which facilitates efficient exchange of nutrient and metabolic waste between a scaffold and the environment.
(3) The porous structure of nanofibers in conjugation with its higher surface area favors desired features useful for tissue engineering:
    (i) Cell adhesion
    (ii) Proliferation
    (iii) Migration
    (iv) Differentiation
(4) The fibrous structure offers enhanced cellular interactions, including selective endocytosis, adhesion, and orientation.
(5) The small physical dimension of nanofibers enhances the scope to mimic a biological microenvironment at the nanoscale.
(6) The unique physical, optical, electrical, chemical, and biochemical properties of nanofibers offer a wide range of application in regenerative medicine (tissue engineering), as well as controlled and local delivery of biological agents (e.g., proteins and nucleic acids).
(7) The ability to incorporate a wide range of drugs within the fibers with the ease of fabricating the delivery vehicle in the required form.

Advanced Drug Delivery, First Edition. Edited by Ashim K. Mitra, Chi H. Lee, and Kun Cheng.

(8) The surface modification of nanofiber offers modulation of several properties such as aqueous solubility, biocompatibility, and biorecognition.

11.3 POLYMERS FOR NANOFIBER PREPARATION

Several biodegradable, synthetic, and natural polymers have been used for the development of nanofibers (Table 11.1). Synthetic polymers are biocompatible and cheap, and because of the diversity of their physicochemical properties, these polymers have been extensively used in soft tissue regeneration and, as carriers, for controlled drug delivery [4, 6]. However, synthetic polymers cannot mimic a biological environment, and hence, the use of naturally derived polymers is more appealing to process biomimetic nanofibers that can retain cell-binding sites and emulate natural cell and tissue responses [7]. Natural polymers propose the benefit of being very similar to the macromolecular substances present in the human body. Therefore, the biological environment is ready to identify and interact with natural polymers favorably. The harvesting and processing of natural polymers are complicated relative to synthetic polymers. The origin and forms of animal-based natural polymers can significantly affect the physical and biological properties of nanofiber [8]. In addition, animal-originated polymeric nanofibers also hold the risk of batch variability, antigenicity, and disease transmission. Nanofibers that originated from non-animal-based natural polymers such as chitosan and alginate offer considerable advantage in overcoming the preceding challenges and, hence, are considered a promising alternative for the preparation of nanofibers [4]. Various combinations of polymeric blends have also been used for the preparation of nanofibers (Table 11.2 [9–20]) such as 1) synthetic polymer blends, 2) natural polymer blends, 3) natural–synthetic polymer blends, and 4) hydrophilic and hydrophobic polymer blends.

TABLE 11.1 Commonly Used Polymers for the Development of Nanofibers

Natural	Synthetic
Collagen (hydrophilic)	PLA (hydrophobic)
Gelatin (hydrophilic)	PGA (hydrophilic)
Elastin (hydrophilic)	PLGA (variable)
Chitosan (hydrophilic)	PVA (hydrophilic)
Silk fibroin (hydrophilic)	PEO (hydrophilic)
Alginate (hydrophilic)	PCL (hydrophobic)

Polymers: PLA, polylactic acid; PGA, poly(glycolic acid); PLGA, poly (lactic-co-glycolic acid); PVA, polyvinyl alcohol; PEO, polyethylene oxide; PCL, polycaprolactone.

11.3.1 Synthetic Polymer Blends

The primary aim of synthetic polymeric blends is to modulate the nanofiber degradation rate. Most synthetic polymers are biodegradable in nature and hence allows for designing a fiber system that disintegrates once their drug payloads are released. The biodegradation of synthetic labile groups (e.g., esters, amides, anhydrides, and carbonates) are site specific (hydrolytic or enzymatic) in nature, which favors generation of nontoxic metabolites. The rate of biodegradation can alter by changing the different polymeric ratios; for instance, hydrophilic PGA degrades faster relative to slowly degrading hydrophobic PLA. The fast degrading synthetic polymers (PGA, PLA) are well suitable for tissue engineering, whereas the slow degrading polymers (PCL) are more appealing for long-term implants. Combinations of various synthetic co-polymers, e.g., PLLA–CL (PLA and PCL) and PLGA (PLA and PGA), or polyblends of similar polymers are other useful alternatives to modulating degradation rates of polymeric nanofibers [4].

11.3.2 Natural Polymer Blends

Nanofibers prepared from natural polymeric blends have the ability to mimic an extracellular matrix as a result of similar biochemical composition. Besides such advantage, rigid chemical processing during isolation and purification can disrupt native structures of nanofibers prepared from natural polymers. In addition, natural polymers are normally soluble in water and utilization of crosslinking agents can not only prevent such dissolution but also stabilize and strengthen nanofibrous structures. *N*-Hydroxysuccinimide or 1-ethyl-3-(3-dimethyl aminopropyl) carbodiimide are more safer crosslinking agents relative to glutaraldehyde as the latter can increase the risk of material cytotoxicity and calcification [4].

11.3.3 Natural–Synthetic Polymer Blends

Hybrid polyblends containing both natural and synthetic polymers are more widely investigated than natural–natural and synthetic–synthetic polyblends for nanofiber preparations. This is primarily because nanofibers can be engineered to retain the mechanical strength and durability of a synthetic component and the biological functionality of a natural polymer. Moreover, these combinations do not require additional processing such as chemical crosslinking to retain sufficient mechanical strength [4].

11.3.4 Hydrophilic and Hydrophobic Polymer Blends

Polymeric blends of hydrophilic and hydrophobic material are mostly used for the preparation of biodegradable nanofibers. In this system, a hydrophobic polymer serves as a

TABLE 11.2 Polymeric Blends Used for the Preparation of Nanofibers

Polymeric Blend		Application	Reference
Synthetic–synthetic polyblends	PLGA and PLGA	Articular cartilage reconstruction	[9]
	PCL and PLGA	Peripheral nerve regeneration	[10]
	PLGA and PLA–polyethylene glycol (PEG)	Gene delivery for tissue engineering	[11]
Natural–natural polyblends	Collagen and chitosan	Vascular and nerve tissue engineering	[12]
	Collagen and collagen	Tissue engineering	[13]
	Collagen and elastin	Cardiovascular tissue engineering	[14]
Natural–synthetic polyblends	Chitosan and PEO	Wound dressings, drug delivery	[15]
	Chitosan and PCL	Peripheral nerve regeneration	[16]
	Collagen and PCL	Vascular tissue engineering	[17]
	Gelatin, elastin, and PLGA	Vascular, cardiac, and pulmonary tissue engineering	[18]
	Gelatin and PLLA–CL	Human skin tissue engineering	[19]
	Dextran and PLGA	Tissue engineering	[20]

backbone that degrades over a long period of time, whereas a hydrophilic polymer relatively degrades at a faster rate. The choice of such polymeric blends plays an important role in designing a controlled delivery system [21].

11.4 METHODS FOR NANOFIBER FABRICATION

Polymeric nanofibers can be processed using several techniques such as electrospinning, self-assembly, phase separation, and template synthesis.

11.4.1 Electrospinning

Electrospinning is the most widely investigated, highly flexible, polymeric fiber-processing technology. This process allows for fiber production with diameters ranging from 3 nm to 5 μm using an electrostatically charged jet of polymer melt or solution [22, 23]. The basic principle of electrospinning involves creation of an electric field between the collector and the syringe filled with a polymeric solution. High direct current voltage (10–20 kV) provides a surface charge to the polymer solution. At a critical voltage, repulsive surface charges overcome the surface tension of the polymer solution, which will lead to the elongation of solution at the tip of a syringe to form a Taylor cone. The charged jet of a polymer solution ejects from the tip of the Taylor cone and progressively thins in air as a result of elongation and solvent evaporation. Eventually, solidification of the polymer jet will lead to the formation of nanodimension fibers that can be collected at the surface of a metallic collector (stationary or rotating) [24–26]. Several system and process parameters controlling nanofiber preparation by electrospinning processes are listed in Table 11.3. Several biodegradable, nonbiodegradable, and custom-made polymers have been electrospun into nanofibers for various biomedical applications [23].

Advantages: Electrospinning is the simplest, most cost-effective, most efficient, and most preferred process for nanofiber fabrication. It is the only technique appropriate for large-scale nanofiber production for industrial applications. A wide range of polymers can be successfully electrospun into long and continuous nanofibers with variety of cross-sectional shapes and alignments.

Limitations: Drug release from conventional electrospun nanofibers cannot be controlled independently. Because of poor drug entrapment, most of the drug rapidly diffuses out of the nanofibers (burst release), especially when a linear drug release pattern is required. However, recent advancements have explored the modification in basic electrospun technique to overcome this limitation [27, 28].

11.4.2 Self-Assembly

Self-assembly is the autonomous organization of natural or synthetic, atoms, or molecules via weak and noncovalent forces (hydrogen bonding, electrostatic, and hydrophobic interactions) into well-defined, stable nanoscale functionalities [25, 29]. This method has been used to develop structural variations (films, membranes, nanoparticles, fibers, micelles, and unilamellar and multilamellar vesicles) with the major intent to use as an *in vivo* scaffold for mimicking the extracellular matrix using biomaterials [24, 23, 30]. Several polymeric configurations including diblock co-polymers [31], triblock from peptide amphiphile [32], and dendrimers [33] have been self-assembled into nanofibers.

Advantages: Self-assembly can generate thinner nanofibers (with a few nanometers in diameter) relative to the electrospinning process. It is an attractive technique in terms of fabricating versatile materials into a variety of structures

TABLE 11.3 Factor Affecting Electrospinning Process During Nanofiber Preparation [22, 29]

	Parameters	Controlling Effect
System parameters	Polymer molecular weight, distribution and architecture (branched, linear, etc.)	– Rate of nanofibers degradation
	Polymer solution properties (surface tension, conductivity, elasticity, and viscosity)	– Nanofiber diameter and possibility for bead formation – Higher solution viscosity associates with formation of larger diameter fibers
Process parameters	Orifice diameter, flow rate of polymer, and electric potential	– Fiber diameter
	Distance between capillary and metal collector	– Extent of evaporation of solvent from the nanofibers and deposition on the collector – Increasing the distance or decreasing the electrical field decreases the bead density, regardless of the polymer solution concentration
	Motion of collector	– Pattern formation during fiber deposition
Ambient parameters	Solution temperature, humidity, air velocity, and static electricity	– Increasing the temperature associates with decrease fiber diameter due to reduced polymer solution viscosity – Increasing the humidity results in the appearance of small circular pores on the surface of the fibers

including layered and lamellar structures with great flexibility and low polydispersity that cannot be achieved by conventional techniques [24].

Limitations: Self-assembly involves more complex and elaborated methodology with relatively less productivity [26].

11.4.3 Phase Separation

The principle behind the phase separation process involves thermodynamic demixing of homogeneous polymer–solvent solution into a polymer-rich phase and solvent-rich phase, usually either by exposure of solution to another immiscible solvent or by cooling of solution below a binodal solubility curve. Phase separation can be induced either using thermal energy (thermally induced phase separation) or by introducing nonsolvent to the polymer solution (nonsolvent-induced phase separation) [25, 26, 29, 34]. Several porous structures with microscale spherical pores can be fabricated by this process by regulating thermodynamic and kinetic parameters for three-dimensional tissue-engineering scaffolds. Solvent, polymer concentration, gelation temperature, and gelation time are the important parameters for regulating the phase separation process [35, 36], Nanofibers with a size (50–500 nm) similar to the natural collagen of the extracellular matrix can be developed using the phase separation process. In general, this process involves five basic steps, including 1) polymer dissolution, 2) liquid–liquid phase separation, 3) polymer gelation, 4) solvent extraction from the gel with water, and 5) freezing and freeze drying [24]. Various nanofibrous scaffolds have been developed using this process for tissue engineering application with enhanced cell adhesion, migration, proliferation, and differentiation function than traditional scaffolds [37].

Advantages: It is a simple technique and requires minimum processing equipment compared with other techniques. This process allows for direct fabrication of a scaffold for a preferred anatomical shape of a body part. It will generate nanoarchitecture and macroarchitecture simultaneously that can have a dual advantage in terms of cell response at the nanofiber level, as well as cell distribution and tissue architecture at the macroporosity level [24, 38].

Limitations: It is a laboratory-scale process that is restricted to the transformation of a particular polymer directly into the nanofiber scaffold [25].

11.4.4 Template Synthesis

This method has been used for the preparation of polymeric nanofibers using polypyrrole, poly(3-methylthiophene), polyaniline, poly(*p*-phenylene), and poly(3,4-ethylenedioxythiophene) [25, 39, 40]. This process involves electrochemical or chemical template synthesis of nanofibers using oxidative polymerization. Electrochemical template synthesis involves metal film coating on one part of the template membrane, which serves as an anode for electrochemical synthesis of polymeric nanofibers within the pores of the template membrane. Chemical template synthesis involves simple membrane soaking into the solution of an anticipated monomer and oxidizing agent [25].

Advantages: It is a simple process and requires standard laboratory equipment. Different templates can be used for the synthesis of nanofiber with desired diameter.

Limitations: It is a laboratory-scale process that is restricted to the conversion of a particular polymer directly into nanofiber [25].

11.5 BIOMEDICAL APPLICATIONS

Nanofibers are a distinct class among numerous nanomaterials available today as it can be arranged into porous fiber architectures similar to natural biological tissues. This property allows nanofibers to be useful for numerous applications. They have biomedical applications for the following reasons [41]:

(1) High surface area and surface energy compared with bulk materials. This is useful for enhanced adhesion with cells, proteins, and drugs.
(2) It is possible to customize to a large extent the properties of nanofiber assemblies, like flexibility. A large number of polymers can be electrospun for numerous applications.

In this chapter, the following biomedical applications of nanofiber will be discussed in detail:

(1) Tissue engineering
(2) Drug delivery
(3) Nanofiber-enzyme biocatalyst conjugates

11.5.1 Tissue Engineering

Tissue engineering is an emerging discipline that involves an interdisciplinary approach encompassing biological, chemical, and engineering sciences. It usually involves isolation of healthy cells from patients, following which they are cultured *in vitro*. These cultured cells are then seeded onto a three-dimensional biodegradable scaffold that will act as a structural support and function as a reservoir for bioactive molecules like growth factors. The scaffold slowly degrades and is replaced by newly grown tissues from the cultured cells (Figure 11.1) [24].

Nanofibers can mimic the architecture of natural human tissue at the nanometer scale. The large surface-area-to-volume ratio of the nanofibers along with their microporous structure is ideal for cell adhesion, proliferation, migration, and differentiation necessary properties for tissue engineering applications. They provide an excellent micro/nano environment, which allows the cells to grow and perform their functions.

11.5.1.1 Bone Tissue Engineering The physical properties of bone tissues like physical strength, pore size, porosity, hardness, and overall three-dimensional configurations are the considerations that need to be taken into account while designing scaffolds for bone tissue engineering.

Nonwoven PCL scaffolds can be used to engineer bone tissue (Figure 11.2) [42]. Mesenchymal stem cells (MSCs, which can differentiate into bone cells and cartilage cells among other cells types) derived from neonatal rat bone marrow when seeded into the scaffolds the cells migrate inside the matrix and produce an extracellular matrix in abundance inside the scaffolds. In an *in vivo* study performed in a rat model with PCL nanofibers along with MSCs, extracellular matrix formation was observed throughout the scaffold with mineralization and type I collagen formation [43].

11.5.1.2 Skeletal Muscle Generation Voluntary movements are caused by skeletal muscles and are difficult to

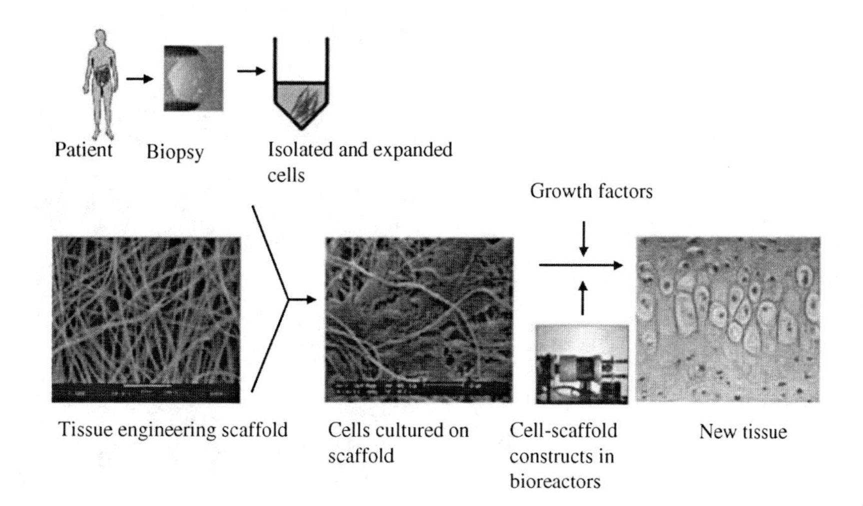

FIGURE 11.1 Main aspects of tissue regeneration scaffold system. Reproduced with permission from Ref. 41.

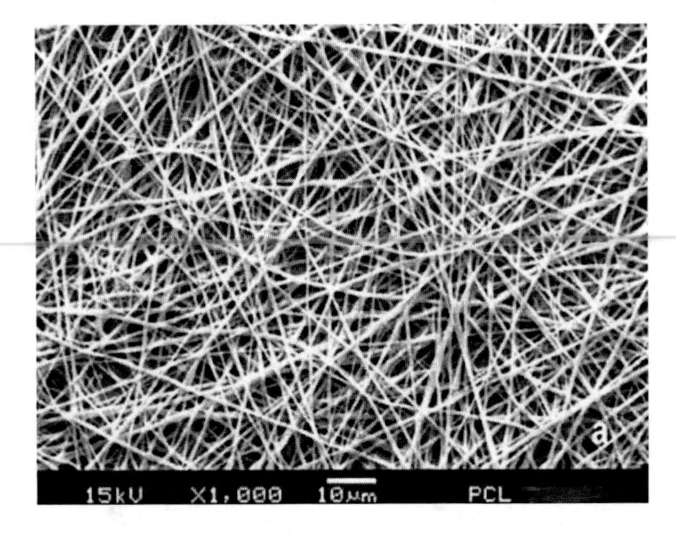

FIGURE 11.2 Scanning electron micrograph (SEM) of random PCL nanofibers. Reproduced with permission from Ref. 44.

regenerate if damaged. This is the reason tissue engineering of skeletal muscle is significant. Electrospun nanofibers obtained from degradable polyester urethane (PEU) have been investigated as scaffolds for skeletal muscle [45]. Primary human satellite cells, murin, and rat myoblast cells have been seeded in PEU nanofibrous scaffolds. It was observed that satisfactory mechanical properties and required cellular responses like adhesion and differentiation were obtained with electrospun PEU nanofibers.

11.5.1.3 Neural Tissue Engineering When tissues of the nerve are destroyed or the extracellular matrix of the neural tissues is degenerated, it leads to a wide variety of clinical disorders. Irreversible functional loss occurs from injuries of the neural tissues. Engineering of neural tissue is a challenge to scientists, which they aim to address by employing normal or genetically engineered cells and extracellular matrix equivalents along with the design of scaffolds.

Poly(L-lactic acid) (PLLA)-based electrospun nanofibrous scaffolds may be used for neural tissue engineering (Figure 11.3) [46]. It has been observed that randomly oriented nanofibers (150–300 nm) have the capacity of supporting neural stem cell adhesion and can promote neural stem cell differentiation. Therefore, PLLA-based nanofibrous scaffolds can potentially be used for neural tissue engineering.

11.5.1.4 Blood Vessel Tissue Engineering Aligned biodegradable poly(L-lactide-co-ε-caprolactone) (PLLA-CL) (75:25) nanofibrous scaffolds have been used to create a tubular scaffold that can then be used to engineer blood vessels (Figure 11.4) [48, 49]. It has been observed that nanosized fibers have dimensions similar to the natural extracellular matrix, which can simulate the mechanical

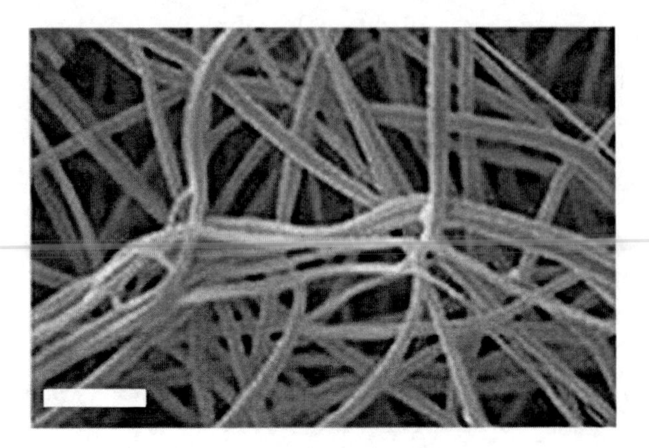

FIGURE 11.3 Scanning electron micrograph (SEM) of electrospun PLLA nanofibers. Reproduced with permission from Ref. 47.

properties of the human coronary artery and can form a defined architecture that allows smooth muscle cells to proliferate and differentiate. Aligned nanofibers also provide necessary mechanical strength, which would allow withstanding the high pressure generated by the human circulatory system.

11.5.2 Drug Delivery

An electrospun nanofiber is a promising platform for the development of different kinds of drug delivery systems for three important reasons. First, an enhanced surface-area-to-volume ratio of polymeric nanofibers allows the delivery of hydrophobic drugs. Recent advances in high-throughput screening of potential therapeutic agents have led to an enormous increase in the number of poorly water-soluble drug candidates. The formulation of these poorly soluble compounds for oral delivery is a major challenge. Second, it

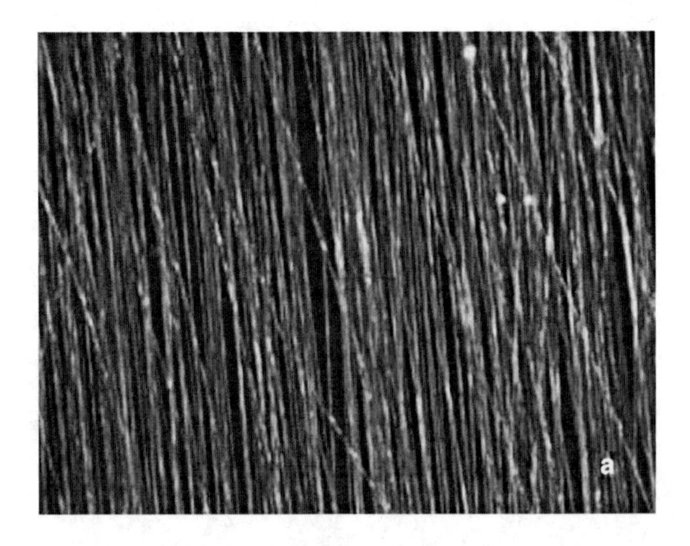

FIGURE 11.4 Scanning electron micrograph (SEM) of aligned PLLA-CL nanofibers. Reproduced with permission from Ref. 49.

is easy to fine-tune the drug release profile by modulating the composition as well as morphology of the nanofibers. Third, there is a definite advantage of flexibility in using nanofibers while designing various dosage forms to achieve maximum drug bioavailability for different delivery routes.

11.5.2.1 Small-Molecule Delivery Nanofibers have been used for the delivery of drugs that have unfavorable pharmacokinetics. Hussain and Ramkumar investigated the delivery of phenytoin using nanofibers [50]. Phenytoin is an antiepileptic drug that has slow-absorption and low-dissolution properties when it is administered orally. To overcome these unfavorable characteristics, phenytoin was incorporated into PEG and PCL nanofibers. The results show that phenytoin-loaded PEG and PCL nanofiber has the potential to overcome the barriers mentioned previously.

A study by Zeng et al. [51] investigated the encapsulation and release kinetics of hydrophobic (paclitaxel) and hydrophilic (doxorubicin hydrochloride) drugs with electrospun PLLA fiber mats. It was observed that paclitaxel was encapsulated better than doxorubicin. This may be because of its better compatibility with PLLA and solubility in chloroform/acetone solvent. On the other hand, doxorubicin was observed on or almost near the surface of the PLLA. This is the reason for differential release kinetics of the two drugs from PLLA nanofibers. The release of paclitaxel follows nearly zero-order kinetics because of the degradation of the fibers. However, in the case of doxorubicin, a burst release observed was caused by the diffusion of a drug from the surface [51]. Therefore, it was concluded that solubility as well as compatibility of drugs in drug/polymer/solvent system play an important role in the preparation of the electrospun fiber formulation. To achieve encapsulation of drugs inside the polymer fibers and to acquire a constant and stable drug release profile, a lipophilic polymer should be chosen as the fiber material for a lipophilic drug. Similarly, a hydrophilic polymer should be employed for a hydrophilic drug and the solvents used should be suitable for both the drug and the polymer.

Electrospun nanofibers have also been used extensively to load insoluble drugs to improve its dissolution. This has been made possible because of the high surface area per unit mass of the nanofibers. Tungprapa et al. [52] have prepared ultrafine fiber mats of cellulose acetate (CA) for four different types of model drugs, namely, naproxen (NAP), indomethacin (IND), ibuprofen (IBU), and sulindac (SUL). The observed maximum release of the drugs from loaded fiber mats when arranged in a decreasing order was as follows: NAP > IBU > IND > SUL. The interesting aspect of this profile was that it did not correspond to their solubility properties. Taepaiboon et al. [53] have further explained this behavior with the explanation that the molecular weight of the drugs plays a critical role on both the rate and the total amount of drugs released from the prepared drug-loaded electrospun nanofibers. Tungprapa et al. and Taepaiboon et al. have also confirmed by ^{1}H-nuclear magnetic resonance that the electrospinning process does not affect the chemical integrity of drugs. Taepaiboon et al. [53] demonstrated that drug-loaded electrospun mats exhibited superior release characteristics of model drugs when compared with drug-loaded cast films. Tungprapa et al. [52] showed that the release of drugs from CA drug-loaded films was mainly caused by the slow dissolution of drug aggregates from the film surfaces. The diffusion of drugs incorporated within the films occurred to a lesser extent. However, in the case of drug-loaded CA fibers, a complete absence of drug aggregates was observed on the surface of the fibers. As a result, the release of drugs from drug-loaded fiber mats was mainly caused by the diffusion of the drug from the fibers. The probable reason was that fiber mats swell in the testing medium.

Paclitaxel-loaded biodegradable implants in the form of microfiber disks and sheets were developed using electrospinning to treat malignant glioma *in vitro* and *in vivo*. The fibrous matrices have offered a greater surface-area-to-volume ratio for effective drug release and necessary implantability into the tumor-resected cavity of a postsurgical glioma [54].

11.5.2.2 Macromolecule Delivery **Small-Interfering RNA (siRNA) Delivery:** Nanofibers have also been used for gene delivery (Figure 11.5). In recent years, RNA interference is being investigated as an important therapeutic agent against genetic diseases. The delivery of siRNA has been very challenging because of its short *in vivo* half-life. Nanofibers have the potential to function as a delivery vehicle for these macromolecules. siRNA can be encapsulated within nanofibers made of PCL with a diameter in the range of 300–400 nm [55]. It was observed that under physiological conditions, the controlled release of intact siRNA was obtained for 28 days. HEK 293 cells were successfully transfected with GAPDH siRNA released from nanofibrous scaffolds at days 5, 10, 15, and 30. The results have explained that siRNA molecules encapsulated within the nanofibers remained bioactive throughout its period of release. Silencing efficiency was observed to be between 61% and 81%, which is comparable with regular siRNA transfection. The cells seeded directly onto the scaffolds have shown enhanced uptake and transfection efficiency. This work showed the applicability of nanofibers as potential delivery vehicles for gene delivery [56].

DNA Delivery PLGA and PLA-PEG block co-polymer-based nanofibrous scaffolds have been investigated to deliver plasmid DNA [56]. It was observed that electrospun nanofiber scaffolds can deliver the gene in a sustained manner at the target site, which leads to efficient transfection and required bioactivity. This mode of delivery can achieve higher transfection efficiency when compared with naked

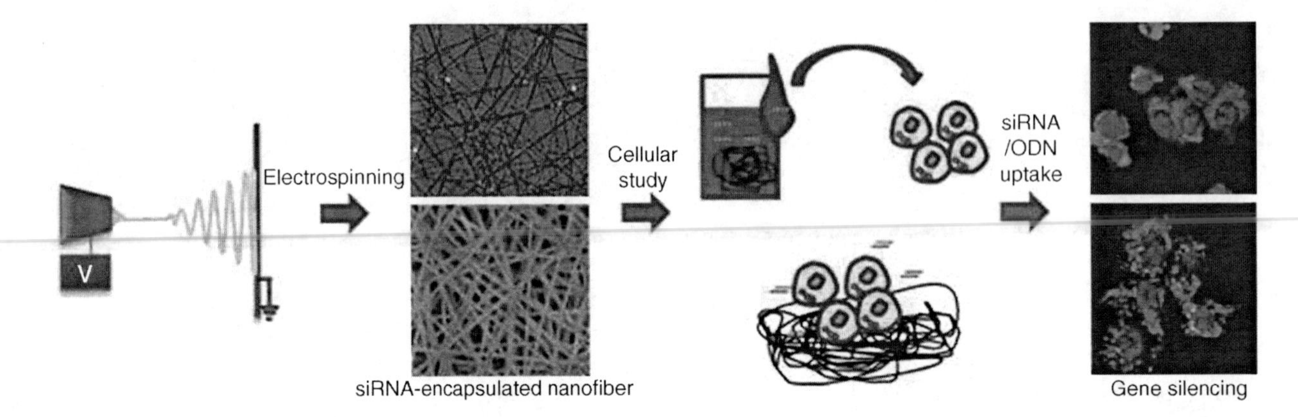

FIGURE 11.5 Diagrammatic representation of siRNA delivery by nanofibrous scaffold. Reproduced with permission from Ref. 55. (See color figure in color plate section.)

DNA. The properties of the scaffold and its architecture control the rate of DNA release. Therefore, the release profile of the DNA can be manipulated by controlling the parameters of the scaffold-like diameter, pore size, and degradation profile of the polymer [56]. By manipulating these parameters, it is possible to achieve release of the DNA for a longer duration. This system seems to be ideal for the sustained release of DNA.

Protein Delivery Electrospun nanofibers have been used also for protein delivery. Bovine serum albumin or luciferase enzyme-loaded nanofibrous scaffolds made of PVA have been studied. It has been observed that an intact protein/enzyme was constantly released from the nanofibrous scaffolds without affecting its bioactivity (Figure 11.6) [57].

11.5.3 Nanofiber-Enzyme Biocatalyst Conjugates

Nanofibers as a support for enzyme immobilization function well because of 1) high surface-area-to-volume ratio, 2) reduced mass transfer resistance, 3) effective loading, and 4) easier recycling [58]. Compared with other nanomaterials, as a support for enzyme immobilization, nanofibers can provide a better platform and can balance above parameters influencing the catalytic performance of immobilized enzymes [59]. It is easy to control and manipulate properties of nanofibers. Parameters such as size and surface morphology, which are necessary for enzyme immobilization supports, can be modulated during the nanofiber preparation by the electrospinning process.

Enzyme immobilization has been investigated by researchers in different disciplines including chemistry, biomedicine, and pharmaceutics. The activity of immobilized enzyme is mainly dependent on the structure of support. It is believed that nanostructured supports can retain the catalytic activity and ensure that the immobilization efficiency of an enzyme is retained to a large extent. Electrospinning is a simple and versatile method to fabricate nanofibrous supports. Compared with other nanostructured supports (e.g., mesoporous silica nanoparticles), nanofibrous supports offer several advantages for their high porosity and interconnectivity.

Enzymes can be coated onto nanofibers to generate biocatalyst conjugates; for example, electrospun polystyrene–poly(styrene-co-maleic anhydride) (PS–PSMA) nanofibers coated with trypsin appeared as stable nanobiocatalytic systems [60].

Silk fibroin (SF) nanofibers have also been prepared by electrospinning, and an attempt has been made to use them as a support for enzyme immobilization [61]. The activity of immobilized α-chymotrypsin (CT) on an SF nanofiber has been observed to be almost eight times higher compared with silk fiber. This efficiency has been found to be enhanced as the diameter of the nanofiber has been decreased.

Marx et al. developed a type of biosensor made of gold nanofibers. Fructose dehydrogenase was immobilized on these nanofibers. The sensor has been found to be accurate and precise in the detection of both serum and popular beverages sweetened with high-fructose corn syrup [62].

Regeneration of nerves after injury to the spinal cord remains suboptimal despite recent advances. One important roadblock that remains to be overcome is the clearance of drugs from the injury site. This process prevents effective therapeutic outcomes. Nanofiber scaffolds might be ideal for enhancing nerve regeneration because of its architecture. In a promising study, the feasibility of incorporating neurotrophin-3 (NT-3) and chondroitinase ABC (ChABC) onto electrospun collagen nanofibers for the treatment of spinal cord injury has been investigated. Biofunctional nanofiber constructs like these can be promising in spinal injury treatment by providing topographical signals and multiple biochemical cues. These will, in turn, aid in the promotion of nerve regeneration while antagonizing axonal growth inhibition for central nervous system regeneration [63].

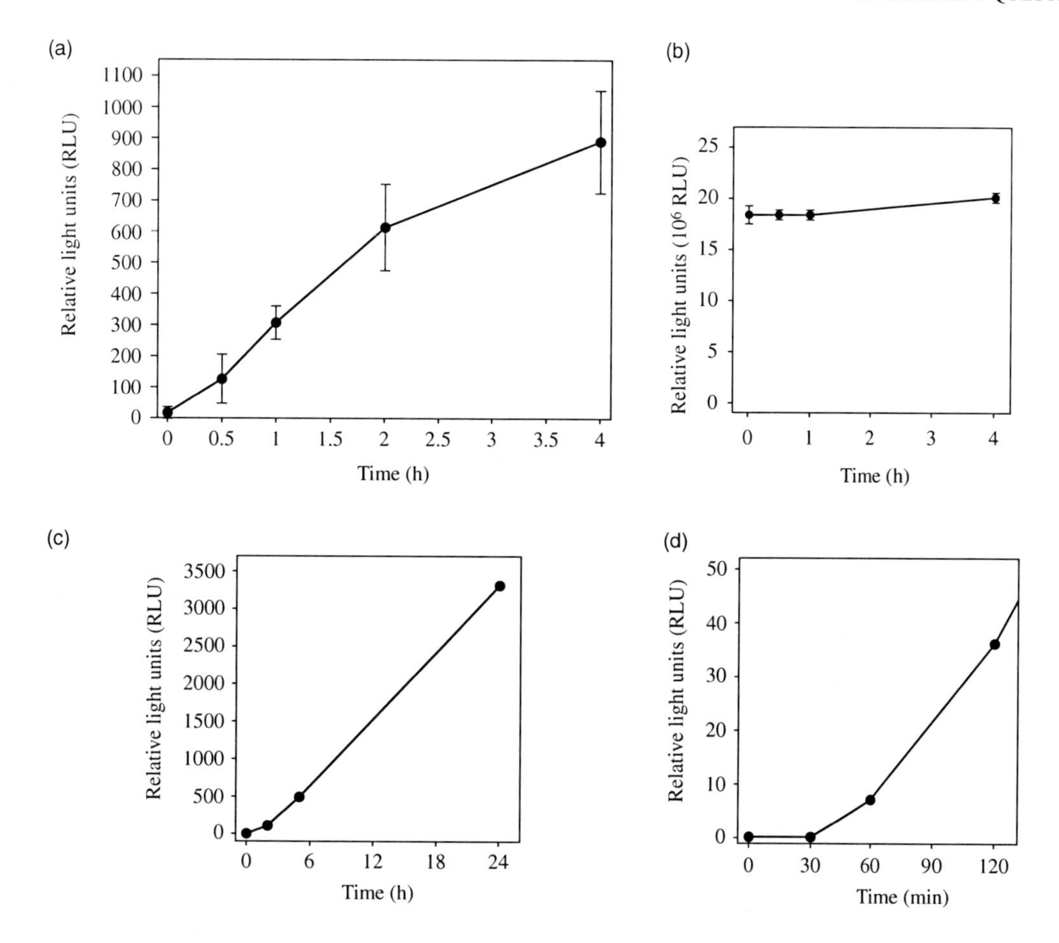

FIGURE 11.6 (a) Time-dependent release of luciferase from luciferase-loaded PVA nanofibers at 4 °C as determined by enzyme activity. (b) The parallel determination of luciferase activity in solution confirms that luciferase activity remained stable under these experimental conditions for at least 4 h. (c) The linearity of the luciferase release is observed also at an extended time scale. (d) Time-dependent release of luciferase from luciferase-loaded PPX-coated PVALuc composite fibers. The figures show the combination of multiple experiments (bars = SD) or the results of one representative experiment. Reproduced with permission from Ref. 57.

ASSESSMENT QUESTIONS

11.1. Define nanofibers and describe a few unique benefits offered by nanofibers.

11.2. What are the various combinations of polymeric blends used for the preparation of nanofibers?

11.3. What are the different techniques used to prepare polymeric nanofibers?

11.4. Discuss various factors affecting the electrospinning process during nanofiber preparation.

11.5. What are the different applications of nanofibers?

a. Tissue engineering

b. Drug delivery

c. Biocatalyst conjugate

d. All of the above

11.6. What is the main reason for the use of nanofiber in drug delivery?

11.7. Which kind of polymer has been used for blood vessel tissue regeneration?

a. Poly(L-lactide-co-ε-caprolactone)

b. Polylactide-co-glycolide

c. Polyethylene glycol

d. All of the above

11.8. Which physical property of bone tissue is considered while designing a scaffold for bone tissue engineering?

a. Elasticity

b. Plasticity

c. Porosity

d. Two of the above

11.9. Which pharmacokinetic parameter of siRNA is the reason for its delivery being a challenge?

- **a.** Maximum or peak concentration (C_{max})
- **b.** Half-life
- **c.** Area under curve (AUC)
- **d.** None of the above

REFERENCES

1. Venugopal, J., Ramakrishna, S. (2005). Applications of polymer nanofibers in biomedicine and biotechnology. *Applied Biochemistry and Biotechnology, 125(3)*, 147–158.
2. Venugopal, J., Zhang, Y.Z., Ramakrishna, S. (2005). Electrospun nanofibres: Biomedical applications. *IMechE, 218*, 35–44.
3. Venugopal, J., Low, S., Choon, A.T., Ramakrishna, S. (2008). Interaction of cells and nanofiber scaffolds in tissue engineering. *Journal of Biomedical Materials Research Part B: Applied Biomaterials, 84(1)*, 34–48.
4. Gunn, J., Zhang, M. (2010). Polyblend nanofibers for biomedical applications: Perspectives and challenges. *Trends in Biotechnology, 28(4)*, 189–197.
5. Kumbar, S.G., Nair, L.S., Bhattacharyya, S., Laurencin, C.T. (2006). Polymeric nanofibers as novel carriers for the delivery of therapeutic molecules. *Journal of Nanoscience and Nanotechnology, 6(9–10)*, 2591–2607.
6. Li, W.J., Laurencin, C.T., Caterson, E.J., Tuan, R.S., Ko, F.K. (2002). Electrospun nanofibrous structure: A novel scaffold for tissue engineering. *Journal of Biomedical Materials Research, 60(4)*, 613–621.
7. Dang, J.M., Leong, K.W. (2006). Natural polymers for gene delivery and tissue engineering. *Advanced Drug Delivery Reviews, 58*, 487–499.
8. Matthews, J.A., Wnek, G.E., Simpson, D.G., Bowlin, G.L. (2002). Electrospinning of collagen nanofibers. *Biomacromolecules, 3*, 232–238.
9. Shin, H.J., Lee, C.H., Cho, I.H., Kim, Y.J., Lee, Y.J., Kim, I.A., Park, K.D., Yui, N., Shin J.W. (2006). Electrospun PLGA nanofiber scaffolds for articular cartilage reconstruction: Mechanical stability, degradation and cellular responses under mechanical stimulation *in vitro*. *Journal of Biomaterials Science, Polymer Edition, 17(1–2)*, 103–119.
10. Panseri, S., Cunha, C., Lowery, J., Del Carro, U., Taraballi, F., Amadio, S., Vescovi, A., Gelain, F. (2008). Electrospun micro- and nanofiber tubes for functional nervous regeneration in sciatic nerve transections. *BMC Biotechnology, 8*, 39.
11. Luu, Y.K., Kim, K., Hsiao, B.S., Chu, B., Hadjiargyrou, M. (2003). Development of a nanostructured DNA delivery scaffold via electrospinning of PLGA and PLA-PEG block copolymers. *Journal of Controlled Release, 89(2)*, 341–353.
12. Chen, Z.G., Wang, P.W., Wei, B., Mo, X.M., Cui, F.Z. (2010). Electrospun collagen-chitosan nanofiber: a biomimetic extracellular matrix for endothelial cell and smooth muscle cell. *Acta Biomaterialia, 6(2)*, 372–382.
13. Matthews, J.A., Wnek, G.E., Simpson, D.G., Bowlin, G.L. (2002). Electrospinning of collagen nanofibers. *Biomacromolecules, 3(2)*, 232–238.
14. Heydarkhan-Hagvall, S., Schenke-Layland, K., Dhanasopon, A.P., Rofail, F., Smith, H., Wu, B.M., Shemin, R., Beygui, R. E., MacLellan, W.R. (2008). Three-dimensional electrospun ECM-based hybrid scaffolds for cardiovascular tissue engineering. *Biomaterials, 29(19)*, 2907–2914.
15. Bhattarai, N., Edmondson, D., Veiseh, O., Matsen, F.A., Zhang, M. (2005). Electrospun chitosan-based nanofibers and their cellular compatibility. *Biomaterials, 26(31)*, 6176–6184.
16. Bhattarai, N., Li, Z., Gunn, J., Leung, M., Cooper, A., Edmondson, D., Veiseh, O., Chen, M., Zhang, Y., Ellenbogen, R.G., Zhang, M. (2009). Natural-synthetic polyblend nanofibers for biomedical applications. *Advanced Materials, 21*, 2792–2797.
17. Lee, S.J., Liu, J., Oh, S.H., Soker, S., Atala, A., Yoo, J.J. (2008). Development of a composite vascular scaffolding system that withstands physiological vascular conditions. *Biomaterials, 29(19)*, 2891–2898.
18. Li, M., Mondrinos, M.J., Chen, X., Gandhi, M.R., Ko, F.K., Lelkes, P.I. (2006). Co-electrospun poly(lactide-co-glycolide), gelatin, and elastin blends for tissue engineering scaffolds. *Journal of Biomedical Materials Research, A 79*, 963–973.
19. Jeong, S.I., Lee, A.Y., Lee, Y.M., Shin, H. (2008). Electrospun gelatin/poly(L-lactide-co-epsilon-caprolactone) nanofibers for mechanically functional tissue-engineering scaffolds. *Journal of Biomaterials Science, Polymer Edition, 19(3)*, 339–357.
20. Pan, H., Jiang, H., Chen, W. (2006). Interaction of dermal fibroblasts with electrospun composite polymer scaffolds prepared from dextran and poly lactide-co-glycolide. *Biomaterials, 27(17)*, 3209–3220.
21. Heunis, T.D., Dicks, L.M. (2010). Nanofibers offer alternative ways to the treatment of skin infections. *Journal of Biomedicine and Biotechnology*, article ID 510682.
22. Pham, Q.P., Sharma, U., Mikos, A.G. (2006). Electrospinning of polymeric nanofibers for tissue engineering applications: a review. *Tissue Engineering, 12(5)*, 1197–1211.
23. Venugopal, J., Low, S., Choon, A.T., Ramakrishna, S. (2008). Interaction of cells and nanofiber scaffolds in tissue engineering. *Journal of Biomedical Materials Research Part B: Applied Biomaterials, 84(1)*, 34–48.
24. Vasita, R., Katti, D.S. (2006). Nanofibers and their applications in tissue engineering. *International Journal of Nanomedicine, 1(1)*, 15–30.
25. Jayaraman, K., Kotaki, M., Zhang, Y., Mo, X., Ramakrishna, S. (2004). Recent advances in polymer nanofibers. *Journal of Nanoscience and Nanotechnology, 4(1–2)*, 52–65.
26. Ma, Z., Kotaki, M., Inai, R., Ramakrishna, S. (2005). Potential of nanofiber matrix as tissue-engineering scaffolds. *Tissue Engineering, 11(1–2)*, 101–109.
27. Greiner, A., Wendorff, J.H., Yarin, A.L., Zussman, E. (2006). Biohybrid nanosystems with polymer nanofibers and

nanotubes. *Applied Microbiology and Biotechnology*, *71(4)*, 387–393.

28. Zeng, J., Aigner, A., Czubayko, F., Kissel, T., Wendorff, J.H., Greiner, A. (2005). Poly(vinyl alcohol) nanofibers by electrospinning as a protein delivery system and the retardation of enzyme release by additional polymer coatings. *Biomacromolecules*, *6(3)*, 1484–1488.
29. Venugopal, J., Low, S., Choon, A.T., Ramakrishna, S. (2008). Interaction of cells and nanofiber scaffolds in tissue engineering. *Journal of Biomedical Materials Research Part B: Applied Biomaterials*, *84(1)*, 34–48.
30. Hartgerink, J.D. (2004). Covalent capture: A natural complement to self-assembly. *Current Opinion in Chemical Biology*, *8 (6)*, 604–609.
31. Liu, G.J., Qiao, L.J., Guo, A. (1996). Diblock copolymer nanofibers. *Macromolecules*, *29*, 5508.
32. Hartgerink, J.D., Beniash, E., Stupp, S.I. (2001). Self-assembly and mineralization of peptide-amphiphile nanofibers. *Science*, *294(5547)*, 1684–1688.
33. Liu, D.J., Feyter, S.D., Cotlet, M., Wiesler, U.M., Weil, T., Herrmann, A., Müllen, K., Schryver, F.CD. (2003). Fluorescent self-assembled polyphenylene dendrimer nanofibers. *Macromolecules*, *36*, 8489.
34. Nam, Y.S., Park, T.G. Porous biodegradable polymeric scaffolds prepared by thermally induced phase separation. (1999). *J Biomed Mater Res.*, *47(1)*, 8–17.
35. Hua, F.J., Kim, G.E., Lee, J.D., Son, Y.K., Lee, D.S. (2002). Macroporous poly(L-lactide) scaffold 1. Preparation of a macroporous scaffold by liquid--liquid phase separation of a PLLA-dioxane-water system. *Journal of Biomedical Materials Research*, *63(2)*, 161–167.
36. Nam, Y.S., Park, T.G. (1999). Biodegradable polymeric microcellular foams by modified thermally induced phase separation method. *Biomaterials*, *20(19)*, 1783–1790.
37. Smith, L.A., Ma, P.X. (2004). Nano-fibrous scaffolds for tissue engineering. *Colloids and Surfaces B Biointerfaces*, *39(3)*, 125–131.
38. Ma, P.X., Choi, J.W. (2001). Biodegradable polymer scaffolds with well-defined interconnected spherical pore network. *Tissue Engineering*, *7(1)*, 23–33.
39. Martin, C.R. (1994). Nanomaterials: A membrane-based synthetic approach. *Science*, *266(5193)*, 1961–1966.
40. Wu, C.G., Bein, T. (1994). Conducting polyaniline filaments in a mesoporous channel host. *Science*, *264(5166)*, 1757–1759.
41. Leung, V., Ko, F. (2011). Biomedical applications of nanofibers. *Polymers for Advanced Technologies*, *22(3)*, 350–365.
42. Yoshimoto, H., Shin, Y.M., Terai, H., Vacanti, J.P. (2003). A biodegradable nanofiber scaffold by electrospinning and its potential for bone tissue engineering. *Biomaterials*, *24(12)*, 2077–2082.
43. Shin, M., Yoshimoto, H., Vacanti, J.P. (2004). *In vivo* bone tissue engineering using mesenchymal stem cells on a novel electrospun nanofibrous scaffold. *Tissue Engineering*, *10(1–2)*, 33–41.
44. Venugopal, J., Zhang, Y.Z., Ramakrishna, S. (2004). Electrospun nanofibres: Biomedical applications. *Journal of Nanoengineering and Nanosystems*, *218(1)*, 35–45.
45. Riboldi, S.A., Sampaolesi, M., Neuenschwander, P., Cossu, G., Mantero, S. (2005). Electrospun degradable polyesterurethane membranes: Potential scaffolds for skeletal muscle tissue engineering. *Biomaterials*, *26(22)*, 4606–4615.
46. Yang, F., Xu, C.Y., Kotaki, M., Wang, S., Ramakrishna, S. (2004), Characterization of neural stem cells on electrospun poly(L-lactic acid) nanofibrous scaffold. *Journal of Biomaterials Science, Polymer Edition*, *15(12)*, 1483–1497.
47. Li, W.J., Tuan, R.S. (2009). Fabrication and application of nanofibrous scaffolds in tissue engineering. *Current Protocols in Cell Biology*, *42*, 25.2.1–25.2.12.
48. Mo, X., Weber, H. (2004). Electrospinning P(LLA-CL) nanofiber: A tubular scaffold fabrication with circumferential alignment. *Macromolecular Symposia, Special Issue: Contributions from 6th Austrian Polymer Meeting*, *217(1)*, 413–416.
49. Xu, C.Y., Inai, R., Kotaki, M., Ramakrishna, S. (2004). Aligned biodegradable nanofibrous structure: A potential scaffold for blood vessel engineering. *Biomaterials*, *25(5)*, 877–886.
50. Hussain, M.M., Ramkumar, S.S. (2006). Physicochemical characteristics of drug-laden nanofibers for controlled drug delivery. *The 2006 Annual Meeting*, 323b.
51. Zeng, J., Yang, L., Liang, Q., Zhang, X., Guan, H., Xu, X., Chen, X., Jing, X. (2005). Influence of the drug compatibility with polymer solution on the release kinetics of electrospun fiber formulation. *Journal of Controlled Release*, *105(1–2)*, 43–51.
52. Tungprapa, S., Jangchud, I., Supaphol, P. (2007). Release characteristics of four model drugs from drug-loaded electrospun cellulose acetate fiber mats. *Polymer*, *48*, 5030–5041.
53. Taepaiboon, P., Rungsardthong, U., Supaphol, P. (2006). Drug-loaded electrospun mats of poly(vinyl alcohol) fibers and their release characteristics of four model drugs. *Nanotechnology*, *17*, 2317–2329.
54. Ranganath, S.H., Wang, C.H. (2008). Biodegradable microfiber implants delivering paclitaxel for post-surgical chemotherapy against malignant glioma. *Biomaterials*, *29(20)*, 2996–3003.
55. Cao, H., Jiang, X., Chai, C., Chew, S.Y. (2010). RNA interference by nanofiber-based siRNA delivery system. *Journal of Controlled Release*, *144(2)*, 203–212.
56. Luu, Y.K., Kim, K., Hsiao, B.S., Chu, B., Hadjiargyrou, M. (2003). Development of a nanostructured DNA delivery scaffold via electrospinning of PLGA and PLA-PEG block copolymers. *Journal of Controlled Release*, *89(2)*, 341–353.
57. Zeng, J., Aigner, A., Czubayko, F., Kissel, T., Wendorff, J.H., Greiner, A. (2005). Poly(vinyl alcohol) nanofibers by electrospinning as a protein delivery system and the retardation of enzyme release by additional polymer coatings. *Biomacromolecules*, *6(3)*, 1484–1488.
58. Wang, Z.G., Wan, L.S., Liu, Z.M., Huang, X.J., Xu, Z.K. (2009). Enzyme immobilization on electrospun polymer nanofibres: An overview. *Journal of Molecular Catalysis: Enzymatic B*, *56*, 189–195.
59. Jia, H. (2011). Enzyme-carrying electrospun nanofibers. *Methods in Molecular Biology*, *743*, 205–212.

60. Lee, S.M., Nair, S., Ahn, H., Kim, B.S., Jun, S.H., An, H.J., Hsiao, E., Kim, S.H., Koo, Y.M., Kim, J. (2010). Property control of enzyme coatings on polymer nanofibers by varying the conjugation site concentration. *Enzyme and Microbial Technology*, *47*(*5*), 216–221.

61. Lee, K.H., Ki, C.S., Baek, D.H., Kang, G.D., Ihm, D., Park, Y.H. (2005). Application of electrospun silk fibroin nanofibers as an immobilization support of enzyme. *Fibers and Polymers*, *6*(*3*), 181–185.

62. Marx, S., Jose, M.V., Andersen, J.D., Russell, A.J. (2011). Electrospun gold nanofiber electrodes for biosensors. *Biosensors and Bioelectronics*, *26*(*6*), 2981–2986.

63. Liu, T., Xu, J., Chan, B.P., Chew, S.Y. (2012). Sustained release of neurotrophin-3 and chondroitinase ABC from electrospun collagen nanofiber scaffold for spinal cord injury repair. *Journal of Biomedical Materials Research Part A*, *100*(*1*), 236–242.

12

BIOMIMETIC SELF-ASSEMBLING NANOPARTICLES

Maxim G. Ryadnov

12.1 CHAPTER OBJECTIVES

- To stimulate the understanding of biomimetic nanoparticles as nanostructured protein and peptide self-assembling systems that are structurally reminiscent of native proteinaceous cages.
- To outline examples of biomimetic designs with a main emphasis given to their design rationale rather than to their biological properties. Certainly, such designs can be presented from a technological perspective and assessed against their utility and performances in different applications, with gene delivery being an obvious example.
- However, because self-assembled nanoparticles remain in infancy, it is important to provide and systematize generic principles for their construction that will serve a long-standing goal of advancing contemporary biomedical approaches including gene therapy, regenerative medicine, and molecular diagnostics.
- To highlight existing links between the structure of native and biomimetic nanoparticles, which may not be precise or evident.
- Therefore, it is essential to seek an insight into how known strategies for engineering self-assembling nanoparticles are selected and why they are preferred over somewhat more straightforward approaches of complexing nucleic acids with synthetic macromolecules.
- To develop a sound grasp on key factors guiding native assemblies necessary for an independent assessment of biomimetic designs, both known and probable.

For these reasons, this chapter gives a basic introduction to virus architecture as an example of a native symmetry-driven self-assembly and makes an attempt to generalize biomimetic designs into one category of self-assembling spherical shells.

12.2 INTRODUCTION

Engineered nanoscale particles have attracted growing attention as novel biological materials. The trend is not surprising because nanoparticles exhibit unique physicochemical properties making them advantageous over other materials. An exemplar characteristic is the high surface-area-to-volume ratio of nanoparticles, which affords reaction rates significantly faster than those of polymeric or colloidal monolithic materials, multiplies the surface exposure of an antigen supporting robust immune responses, and enhances adsorption selectivity through chemical tailoring [1–3]. Collectively, such properties can give rise to promising technology platforms allowing for the encapsulation and conversion of specific analytes at desired concentrations. These properties can be used as efficient macromolecular delivery vehicles into cells and tissues [4].

However, it is becoming increasingly clear that all these properties are strongly dependent on other specific requirements inherent for nanoparticles. These are dominated by monodispersity, agglomeration, stability, and structural

Advanced Drug Delivery, First Edition. Edited by Ashim K. Mitra, Chi H. Lee, and Kun Cheng.

reproducibility, which are particularly important for the validation of nanoparticle materials in dynamic and mechanically aggressive environments [5].

One route to address these and other potential issues is to use nanostructured particles as opposed to merely nanosized particles. In other words, to afford reproducible, robust, and stimuli-responsive materials, it is necessary to develop particles whose very ultrastructure and morphology are maintained at the nanoscale. Native biomolecular systems provide excellent examples. Many are well characterized with their structures resolved to the atomistic level of detail, and all the systems are conserved and highly reproducible assemblies, which taken together may underpin efficient design rationales.

Various approaches for different nanoparticle formulations aimed at a variety of applications have been proposed and covered in many specialist reviews [6–8]. This chapter highlights those strategies that deliberately focus on the development of self-assembled mimetics of native nanostructured systems.

12.3 BODY

12.3.1 Native Nanoparticles

Native nanoparticles can be of different origins and can have different functions. However, they all are replicable protein-based supramolecular architectures. Indeed, all nanoparticles belonging to one virus type are uniform in size, whereas molecular storage and transport cages such as clathrin or ferritin complexes are readily reconstituted protein assemblies, so are primitive bacterial organelles that arrange from geometrically defined macromolecular structures [9–12].

These examples provide design fundamentals for biomimetic nanoparticles. In the context of gene and drug delivery, nanoparticles are defined by their abilities to target specific cells and tissues, also known as host tropism, which occurs at a single-cell level and requires biocompatible architectures that can traverse across biological barriers and function at biomolecular interfaces. Given that nanoparticles are essentially vehicles whose main purpose is to deliver macromolecular cargo and deliver safely, an additional requirement for biomimetic nanoparticles as gene delivery systems is to protect cargo material during transport through encapsulation or complexation. This in turn determines the choice of potential vector formulations that can maintain robust architectures, encapsulate delivered material, and target host cells; one particular characteristic is a prerequisite for the structural and functional uniformity of all native nanoparticles. This is self-assembly. It is therefore logical to assume that the most efficient strategy to mimic biological nanoparticles is to mimic the way they are constructed.

Native nanoparticles are little more than protein capsules loaded with a genetic or inorganic material. The cargo often sets size limits for a particular capsule that can vary from a few nanometers, for example, ferritin cages or satelliviruses [9, 10], to several hundreds of nanometers, for example, megavirus [13]. Despite such an apparent diversity in sizes and functions, all self-assembled capsules are discrete symmetry-driven architectures [9–14]. Thus, a desired nanocapsule can be engineered to encapsulate, assemble, or wrap around a size-defined material. Native encapsulating nanoparticles and principles of their assembly are sufficiently described in the literature to aid in the design of biomimetic nanoparticles. However, the current pace with which artificial self-assemblies are being introduced remains to be improved dramatically. Perhaps the main reasons for this are 1) the lack of robust structure prediction methods, which would otherwise afford a set of generic rules for de novo construction, and 2) the traditional notion of the entry efficiency of nanoparticles into host cells and tissues, which is being taken as an overriding design criterion. The structural and physicochemical properties representative of native architectures have been of a much lesser concern, which has created a clear gap for the predictable design of biomimetic nanoparticles. Nevertheless, evidence exists for technologically promising biomimetic systems designed as geometric or symmetry-driven proteinaceous cages.

This is what distinguishes such designs from all other synthetic systems: whether these are based on other molecular classes such as polymers, carbohydrates or lipids, or are of different formulation types such as poly-, peptide-, or lipoplexes.

Admittedly, nanoparticle formulations are most sought for gene and drug delivery to enable molecular therapy. Among other issues pertaining to efficient macromolecular delivery including drug administration and side effects, the structural heterogeneity of delivery vehicles continues to be a major obstacle for delivery technologies on the path to clinic. Viruses remain dominant technological platforms for gene delivery. Certainly, the transfection efficiency of viruses is difficult to match. However, viruses are intrinsically associated with properties that are undesirable for gene delivery which include insertional mutagenesis that can lead to cancers, the lack of cell-specificity, and most of all viral hosts (i.e., human tissues) exhibit conserved immune mechanisms against viral infections, which severely compromises the systemic use of viral vectors. However, viruses represent unchallenged examples of robust structural uniformity in the dynamic nanoscale assembly. In marked contrast, most, if not all, artificial systems suffer from the same set of drawbacks including polydispersity, aggregation, poor surface chemistry, and poorly controlled drug release in response to external stimuli.

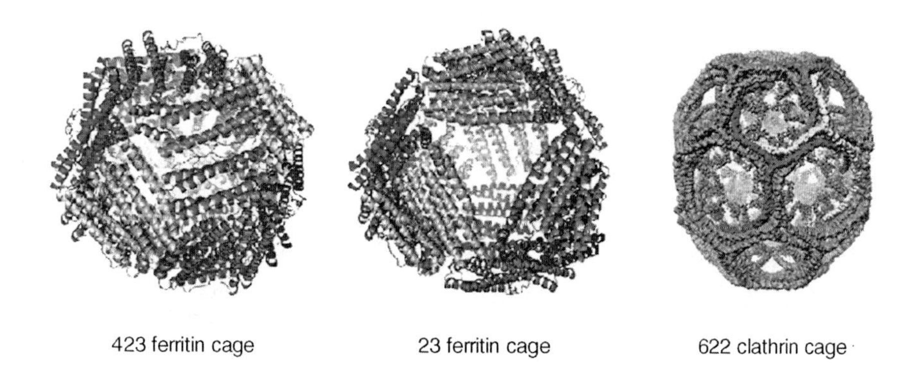

FIGURE 12.1 Native nanoparticles: ribbon diagrams of 423 and 23 ferritin cages (reproduced with permission from Ref. 10) and a cryoelectron image reconstruction of a clathrin cage with three overlapping triskelions shown in different colors (reproduced with permission from Ref. 11). (See color figure in color plate section.)

Taken together, this stimulates the search for designs that first of all are structurally as reproducible as native systems, i.e., biomimetic designs.

12.3.2 Native Nanoparticle Assembly

Native nanoparticles are noncovalent assemblies or ordered copious collections of identical building blocks. The blocks are conserved polypeptide chains that follow precise folding and assembly pathways to form spherical encapsulants [15]. The concept of quasi-equivalent positions introduced by Caspar and Klug for the virus architecture can give a generic description of this type of nanoparticle self-assembly [16]. The concept builds on the main criteria developed by Crick and Watson in the theory of identical subunits [17], which can describe the blocks as follows:

- Closed up into a sphere with a cubic symmetry (minimum energy structure)
- Positioned in similar, quasi-equivalent environments with respect for each other

This implies that the blocks themselves are asymmetric three-dimensional structures that assemble in a hierarchical manner into closed supramolecular networks and that the structure of resulting nanoparticle assemblies can be thought of in terms of solid geometry. This is true for all biological assemblies. Notwithstanding structural differences between various building blocks of different systems, native self-assembling nanoparticles exhibit point-group symmetries [18].

This can be illustrated in a few examples. For instance, ferritin, an iron-storage protein cage, can be described as a 432 cube. One, fourfold symmetry axis of the cube is in the middle of one square flat face, with other, threefold and twofold, symmetry axes being formed by three and two square faces, respectively. Ferritin is a nanoscale cage assembled from 24 building blocks, each folded as a four-helix bundle (Figure 12.1) [10]. One block can be viewed as placed on squares or corners. Because the cube has six faces and eight corners, there would be four blocks in each square and three blocks at each corner. Some ferritins adopt a 23 symmetry allowing them to form outsized pores (Figure 12.1).

A similar example is clathrin. This cross-shaped protein is involved in the intracellular transport of molecular cargo, and in structural terms it is usually referred to as triskelion. The protein assembles into polyhedral cages and lattices (Figure 12.1). Clathrin cages can be described as 622 barrels. The design basis of a clathrin cage is a hexagonal lattice that to be fully closed needs at least 12 pentagon and 8 hexagon faces arranged by 36 triskelion building blocks [11].

Spherical viruses that represent perhaps the most abundant class of self-assembled nanoparticles can be viewed as 532 icosahedra. An icosahedron has 20 faces of equilateral triangles or 20 threefold axes that are arranged around a sphere with 12 fivefold axes and 30 twofold axes. Each face can have smaller triangular facets. The number of these facets describes a given virus and its size and is defined by a triangulation number T [19–21].

T can be found graphically from an equilateral triangular net (Figure 12.2a) and using the following equation:

$$\mathrm{T} = f^2 P$$

where f is any integer and $P = (k^2 + h^2 + k \times h)$. P relates to a particular icosahedron class and can take a limited number of values: 1, 3, 4, 7, 9, 12, etc., with k and h being zero or any positive integer with no common factor [9, 14, 20–22].

Triangulation number 1, $T = 1$, describes an icosahedron consisting of 20 triangular facets hosting 60 identical building blocks, three blocks per facet. $T = 3$ and $T = 4$ viruses will have each of their facets split into three and four smaller triangles, which in total gives 180 and 240 building blocks, respectively (Figure 12.2a). Thus, any icosahedron can be described as having $20T$ facets.

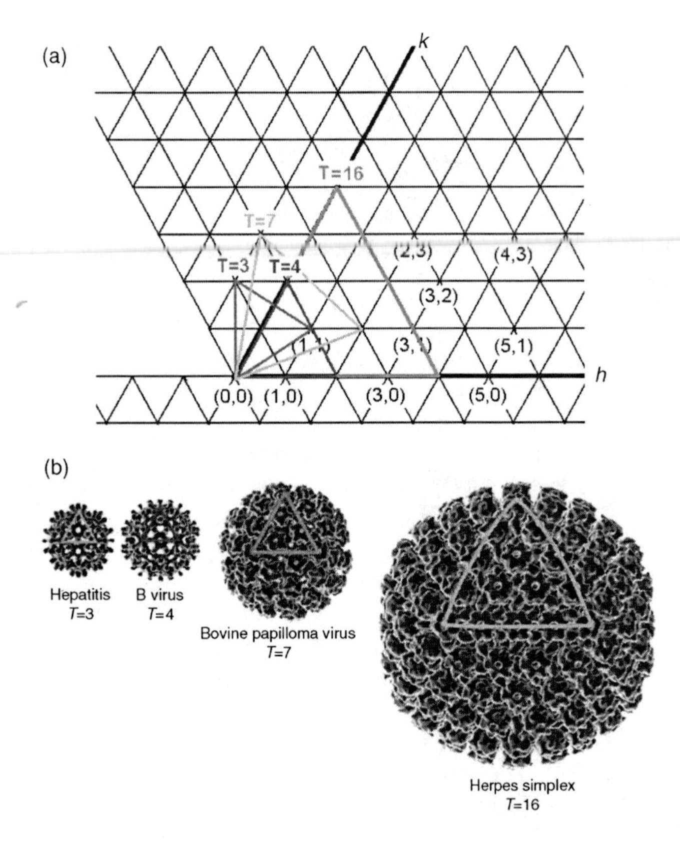

FIGURE 12.2 Virus architecture. (a) Triangulation numbers on a hexagonal p6 net. (0,0) indicates the origin of a fivefold vertex and the placement of a pentamer. T number is calculated from (h,k) and denotes the number of smaller triangles, arranged around local quasi-sixfolds, in one triangular icosahedron facet. (b) cryoelectron image reconstructions of different viruses showing corresponding T numbers with highlighted icosahedral facets. Reproduced with permission from Ref. 21.

However, not all facets are the same.

An icosahedron can be folded from a uniform hexagonal lattice, where each hexagon comprises six equilateral triangles, hence the triangular net. When folded, the icosahedron has vertices that are convex structures with a five-fold symmetry. Hexagons in contrast are flat. To generate a convex vertex one triangle has to be removed to give two free edges that can be fused together only in three dimensions (Figure 12.2). Pentamers are constructed in such a way and placed at the vertices.

The number of vertices is 12 and is constant. Therefore, only a few building blocks assemble into 12 pentameric units, whereas the others arrange into hexamers. In this notation, $20T$ faces are split between 12 pentamers and $10(T-1)$ hexamers. For $T=4$ viruses, for example, this means that 60 blocks arrange into 12 pentamers and 180 blocks assemble into 30 hexamers, $10(4-1)=30$.

In general, for all $T>1$ viruses, individual blocks will have different numbers of neighbors and none in any given pair will be in a strictly equivalent environment (Figure 12.2b).

These principles can provide generic guidance for the construction of self-assembled nanoparticles. More importantly, they imply that building blocks in every architectural unit of a nanoparticle have to be the same. This concerns the primary and secondary levels of polypeptide structure. An alternative approach of using nonidentical blocks would require an efficient means for predicting their mutual stoichiometric bonding, which although possible in principle is questionable in practical terms [18, 22]. The quasi-equivalence concept can also be extended to include pseudo-equivalence relations by adjusting triangulation numbers of non–quasi-equivalent viruses with their structural resemblances in quasi-equivalent viruses. This however requires further assumptions to exclude complications associated with mixed or defective structures, or assembly "mutants" of distorted icosahedra, and it is hardly useful for biomimetic designs [21–25].

Nonetheless, the progress in designing self-assembling nanoparticles so far has been limited to systems that seem to be virus-like but primarily demonstrate their spheroidal morphologies. Most of the reported designed structures are micellar aggregates or capsule-type materials rather than delineated convex deltahedra. All these designs can be grouped into a category of supramolecular encapsulation or caging with a certain preference given to symmetry-driven approaches.

12.3.3 Biomimetic Nanoparticles

One of the first attempts to combine symmetry with self-assembly into one design rationale for self-assembling nanoparticles was made in a nanohedra concept [26]. Two different oligomerization domains, bromoperoxidase (dimerizing domain) and the M1 matrix protein of influenza virus (trimerizing domain), were coupled into one asymmetric block (Figure 12.3a). Each block was expected to oligomerize with other blocks through the domains that assemble asymmetrically. Virtual symmetry axes, one per domain, provide a symmetric arrangement. This is further enforced with the help of a rigid α-helical linker introduced to form a continuous secondary structure stretch with the domains (Figure 12.3a). The resulting chimera assembled into spherical particles with the predicted edge lengths of 15 nm. The sizes of the nanoparticles varied, suggesting polymorphism of the assembly, which can also be observed in native cages (clathrins). The design offers a promising approach for the fabrication of small nanoparticles that are of particular interest for those applications where overcoming blood-brain barrier is a prerequisite. A limitation here remains in sequence-based designs of such cages and the validation of their encapsulation and delivery properties.

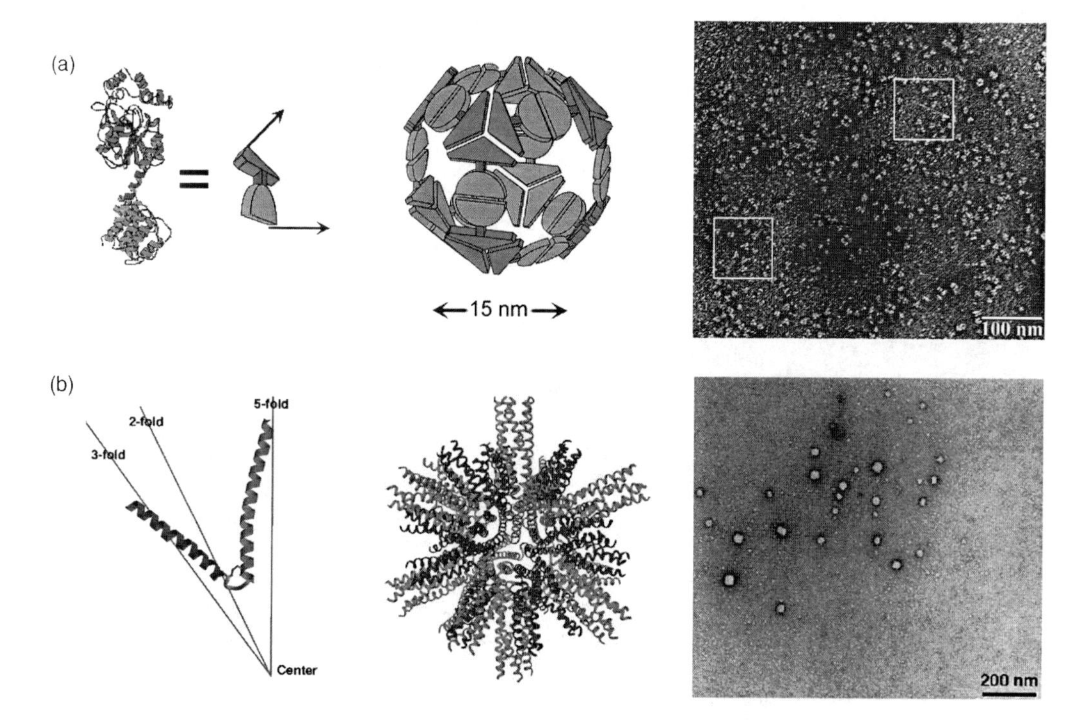

FIGURE 12.3 Polyhedra designs. Schematics of asymmetric building blocks composed of two protein domains (a) and two coiled-coil domains (b) that self-oligomerize into regular nanoparticles, shown both schematically and in electron micrographs. Reproduced with permission from Refs. 26 and 27. (See color figure in color plate section.)

One strategy to overcome this, at least partially, can be provided by the design of regular polyhedral nanoparticles [27]. In this design, nanoparticles were assembled from multiple copies of one asymmetric block, which also comprises two different oligomerization domains. The number of the copies is defined by the least common multiple of the domains that when superimposed onto the edges of a tripyramidal arrangement and linked together should assemble into a sphere (Figure 12.3b). The domains were designed as α-helical coiled-coil motifs that arranged into pentamers and trimers along fivefold and threefold symmetry axes of a polyhedron. This way, 15 block copies formed an "even unit" with several units affording nanoparticle structures. Similar to the nanohedra design, structural polymorphism for these assemblies was also apparent. Irregularities in the geometry of the units and in their packing led to various sizes ranging from 15 to 45 nm. It was also possible to obtain more uniform assemblies after making structural adjustments of the domains. This suggests that responsive sequence- and unit-based reconstruction of nanoparticles can be rationally designed and may be achieved by relating polypeptide sequence with the topology of a self-assembling unit.

This conjecture can be illustrated using two strategies.

One represents a C_3-symetric conjugation of a β-sheet-forming peptide [28]. Individually, the peptide assembles into antiparallel β-sheets. In contrast, when configured into a triskelion it is forced to interact with other triskelions leading to the formation of intermolecular networks closing up into spheres of 20 nm in diameter. This is consistent with a ball structure (26 nm) or a dodecahedron (16 nm) with a 6-nm side of a polyhedron formed by a two-arm sheet of two triskelions (Figure 12.4a).

Another approach is a dendrimer-like peptide assembly. In this concept peptides were designed to self-arrange in a dendrimer fashion with the formation of multiple cavities (Figure 12.4b) [29]. Having two opposite polar faces the sequences formed a complex branching network thereby making assembled structures porous. Pores or cavities of approximately 5 nm in diameter were formed in the juxtapositions of interacting units such that branching cores of otherwise a covalent dendrimer architecture were converted into hollow cavities (Figure 12.4b). Thus, unlike most nanocapsule assemblies, which carry only one cavity, this design can exhibit multivalent encapsulation. To demonstrate this, ionic silver ($AgNO_3$) was converted into colloidal silver within the multiple cavities. Each cavity thus should host one silver nanoparticle, and given that one nanocapsule assembly comprises many cavities, a formation of many silver nanoparticles should be expected. Indeed, an enzymatic degradation of the assembly to remove nanocapsule completely following the reaction revealed microscopic

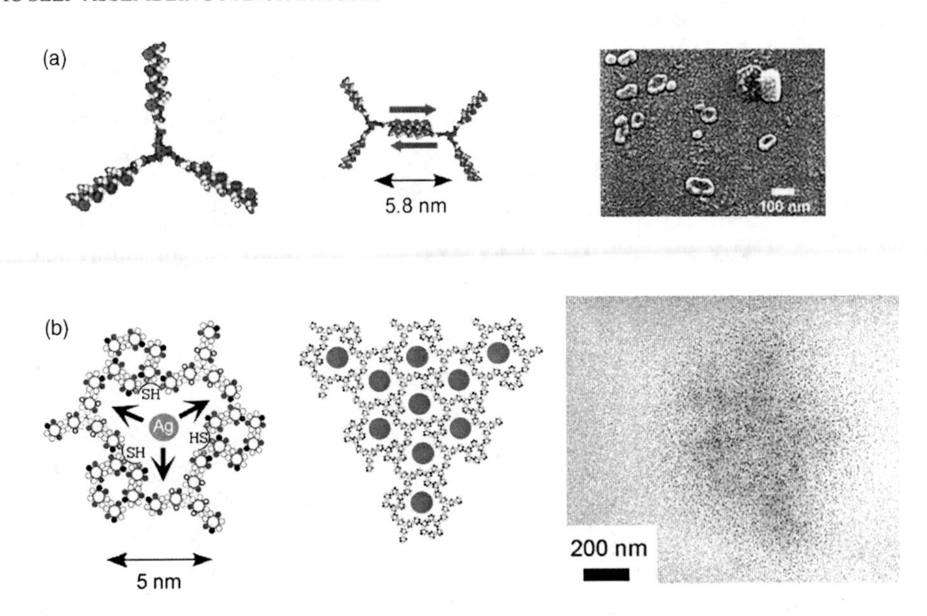

FIGURE 12.4 Biomimetic cages. (a) Schematic and electron micrograph of a C_3-symetric conjugation of a β-sheet peptide into nanoscale cages. Reproduced with permission from Ref. 28. (b) A helical-wheel representation of a dendrimer-like assembly of a helical block into polynanocages. Electron micrograph of silver nanoparticles formed in one polynanocage after its enzymatic degradation. The mean diameters of individual cavities and nanoparticles are ~5 nm. Reproduced with permission from Ref. 29.

spreads of uniform 5-nm silver particles. The sizes of both silver nanoparticles and their spreads were consistent with the diameters of cavities and self-assembled nanocapsules, respectively.

An interesting feature of this design is the formation of regular ring-like cavities that may be viewed as intermediate assembly units analogous to viral capsomeres or proteinaceous pores of primitive bacterial organelles. Thus, the polymerization of monomeric nanoscale rings, if designed rationally, can provide a controllable route for polyhedra construction. Monomeric nanorings are abundant in biology and may include ring-shaped tryptophan RNA-binding attenuation proteins, phage recombinases, or DNA helicases. However, designing discrete nanorings as building blocks requires fairly stable components that to date have been demonstrated only as fully folded proteins. For instance, dimerized dihydrofolate reductase can spontaneously self-assemble into discrete rings of <40 nm in diameter [30]. The assembly did not lead to larger associations, suggesting that the formed rings were stable autonomous structures. The strategy was as efficient for the construction of nanorings from antibodies and enzymes [31, 32], which implies that it can offer a generic strategy for the controlled assembly of monodisperse nanoparticles. However, nanoring structures assembled from artificial sequences or, in other words, deliberately defined at the sequence level have yet to emerge. This is observed in the moderate progress of designing nanoparticles assembled from de novo sequences for which symmetry-driven approaches will continue to be a sought and ultimately answered. As our understanding of such designs improves, more robust concepts can be anticipated. It is also reasonable to expect that this will advance nonviral gene delivery despite scarce information on delivery efficiencies of biomimetic nanoparticles. Alternative and more general routes exist that are not as dependent on precise sequence-folding relationships.

Typical examples include the design of diblock and facile amphiphiles (Figure 12.5). These peptides contain two explicit parts or faces: polar and hydrophobic. Unlike in secondary structures, in which polar and hydrophobic clusters form after folding along the peptide backbone, the clusters in these amphiphiles are two sequence segments or two sides of a constrained framework or a covalent plane, for example, a cyclopeptide. The main goal is the generation of vesicular assemblies with a much lesser stress made on the structural cooperativity and uniformity of resulting nanoparticles. For instance, a diblock co-polypeptide amphiphile can be made of a cationic poly-arginine block and a hydrophobic poly-leucine block (Figure 12.5a) [33]. Leucine residues have high propensity for helix formation, whereas polyarginines and oligoarginines are active promoters of intracellular uptake. In water, the hydrophobic helical segments clustered together in an antiparallel manner to drive the formation of outer and inner arginine layers of vesicular particles. Similar vesicles can be assembled from

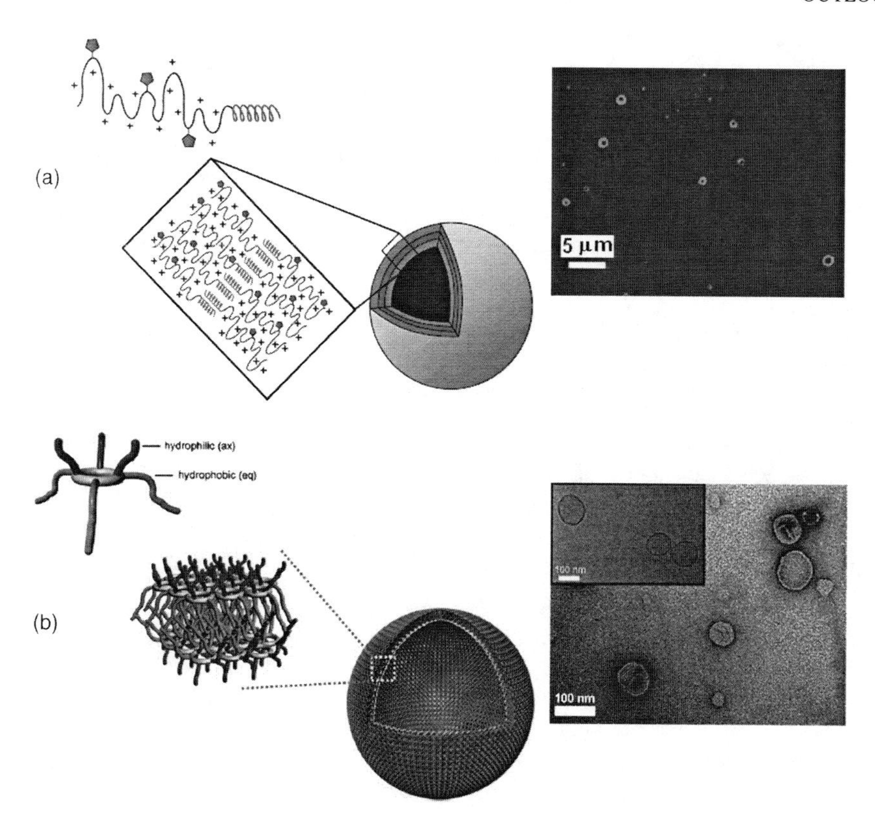

FIGURE 12.5 Facile amphiphiles. Schematics and micrographs of vesicular assemblies from a diblock co-polypeptide amphiphile (a) and a cyclic peptide facial amphiphile (b). Reproduced with permission from Refs. 33 and 34.

small cyclic peptides with alternating hydrophobic and cationic residues that also cluster into one hydrophobic interface separating two polar wall surfaces of the vesicles (Figure 12.5b) [34]. These and similar designs were shown to traverse efficiently across cell membranes, which can be attributed to cationic surfaces mimicking self-promoted delivery of oligoarginines. However, size distributions of the particles tend to be fairly broad, and although they can be controlled by extrusion after the assembly, the need for size separation attests to the main drawback of these vesicular types—polydispersity in the assembly—which can lead to aggregation or fibrillation [34]. These shortcomings reemphasize the promise and technological potential of symmetry designs. Yet again, more compelling evidence is needed before any substantial progress can be witnessed as a truly biomimetic attempt to self-assembled nanoparticles.

12.4 OUTLOOK SUMMARY

The outlined designs represent the main trends in engineering biomimetic nanoparticles and certainly do not cover all reported developments to date. It is apparent, however, that spherical shells will continue to inspire new designs and will dominate the thinking in the field. Structurally reproducible and stable assemblies will not cease as principle requirements for future biomimetic designs. These are primary requirements for efficient synthetic systems with the potential to challenge native nanoparticles. Specific impacts of symmetry itself on the functional behavior of assembled nanoparticles are secondary in this regard as the focus on symmetry designs offers a highly amenable construction approach. Because symmetry-based designs are bottom-up assemblies of identical building blocks, different modular strategies can be developed to give nanoparticles of virtually any size, morphology, and surface chemistry. Modular strategies open up new avenues for 1) control over nanoparticle loading efficiencies and over more efficient delivery into important tissues that impose size restrictions (e.g., <20-nm particles), 2) surface charge redistributions to circumvent electrostatic barriers such as the blood-brain barrier, 3) molecular surface decoration to enhance intracellular uptake or render cell specificity (e.g., receptor mediated or receptor independent), and 4) promoting drug encapsulation as opposed to surface adsorption and the like. Ultimately, geometric parameters that are universal for all native proteinaceous

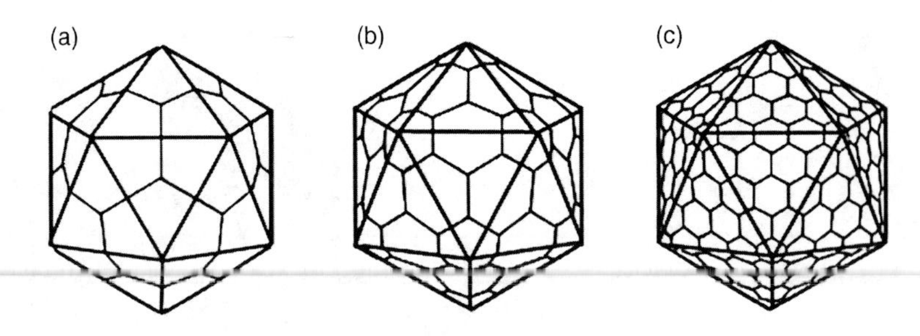

FIGURE 12.6 Folded hexagonal nets of hypothetical viruses.

nanoparticles serve the goal of providing a rationale for dynamic encapsulating systems capable of tailored responses to environmental stimuli. Admittedly, the current progress in this particular direction is extremely limited. To some extent, this can be attributed to the uncertainties of ensuring directed assembly of designed building blocks, which could otherwise lead to misassembly or aggregation. Although protein aggregation is a universal problem applicable to protein folding and self-assembly as a whole, remedies for more predictable self-assembly are set in polypeptide sequences themselves and are linked directly to our yet limited ability to relate protein structure to function. Alternatively, the use of native folding motifs and folded proteins as building blocks can provide at least a partial answer to this by enabling monodisperse assemblies. Therefore, it should be expected that the emergence of more efficient and creative strategies leading to more technically robust systems is likely to be based on better and applied understanding of native self-assembling designs.

ASSESSMENT QUESTIONS

12.1. Hypothetical viruses depicted in Figure 12.6 were assembled using the equilateral triangular net shown in Figure 12.2a. Deduce the triangulation numbers corresponding to each nanoparticle and the number of protein blocks in each icosahedral facet.

12.2. Deduce the triangulation numbers for each of the unfolded icosahedra given in Figure 12.7.

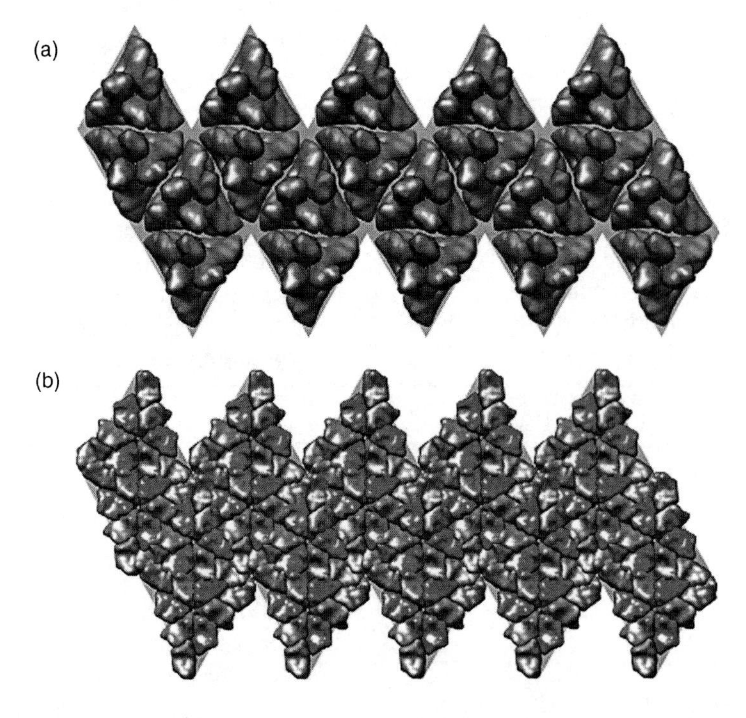

FIGURE 12.7 Hexagonal nets for *Avibirnavirus* (a) and *Sobemovirus* (b). Reproduced with permission from Ref. 35. (See color figure in color plate section.)

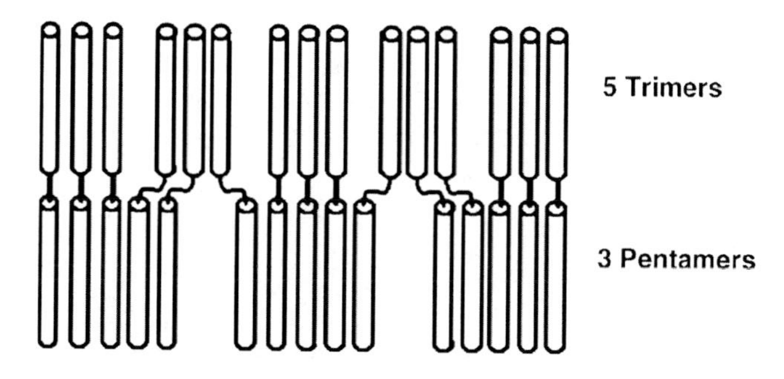

FIGURE 12.8 An even unit comprising 15 monomeric blocks of trimers and pentamers. Reproduced with permission from Ref. 27.

12.3. The building block shown in Figure 12.3b first assembles into even units (see Figure 12.8). Based on the least-common multiple of the oligomerization states of the domains of the block, deduce the number of the blocks in one even unit and show an arrangement of the domains schematically.

12.4. All native nanoparticles have conserved precise dimensions and can be described using generic principles of solid geometry. What is the underlying parameter that makes it possible to construct and design proteinaceous assemblies at the nanoscale?

REFERENCES

1. Vriezema, D.M., Comellas Aragonès, M., Elemans, J.A., Cornelissen, J.J., Rowan, A.E., Nolte, R.J. (2005). Self-assembled nanoreactors. *Chemical Reviews*, *105*, 1445–1489.
2. Boato, F., Thomas, R.M., Ghasparian, A., Freund-Renard, A., Moehle, K., Robinson, J.A. (2007). Synthetic virus-like particles from self-assembling coiled-coil lipopeptides and their use in antigen display to the immune system. *Angewandte Chemie International Edition*, *46*, 9015–9018.
3. Rosi, N.L., Mirkin, C.A. (2005). Nanostructures in biodiagnostics. *Chemical Reviews*, *105*, 1547–1562.
4. Lin, B.F., Marullo, R.S., Robb, M.J., Krogstad, D.V., Antoni, P., Hawker, C.J., Campos, L.M., Tirrell, M.V. (2011). De novo design of bioactive protein-resembling nanospheres via dendrimer-templated peptide amphiphile assembly. *Nano Letters*, *11*, 3946–3350.
5. Cavalli, S., Albericio, F., Kros, A. (2010). Amphiphilic peptides and their cross-disciplinary role as building blocks for nanoscience. *Chemical Society Reviews*, *39*, 241–263.
6. Grzelczak, M., Vermant, J., Furst, E.M., Liz-Marzán, L.M. (2010). Directed self-assembly of nanoparticles. *ACS Nano*, *4*, 3591–3605.
7. Mastrobattista, E., van der Aa, M.A., Hennink, W.E., Crommelin, D. J. (2006). Artificial viruses: A nanotechnological approach to gene delivery. *Nature Reviews Drug Discovery*, *5*, 115–121.
8. Kostarelos, K., Miller, A.D. (2005). Synthetic, self-assembly ABCD nanoparticles; a structural paradigm for viable synthetic non-viral vectors. *Chemical Society Reviews*, *34*, 970–994.
9. Fauquet, C.M., Mayo, M.A., Maniloff, J., Desselberger, U., Ball, L.A. (eds.). *Virus Taxonomy: VIIIth Report of the International Committee on the Taxonomy of Viruses*. Elsevier Academic Press, New York, 2005.
10. Tatur, J., Hagen, W.R., Matias, P.M. (2007). Crystal structure of the ferritin from the hyperthermophilic archaeal anaerobe *Pyrococcus furiosus*. *Journal of Biological Inorganic Chemistry*, *12*, 615–630.
11. Fotin, A., Cheng, Y., Sliz, P., Grigorieff, N., Harrison, S.C., Kirchhausen, T., Walz, T. (2004). Molecular model for a complete clathrin lattice from electron cryomicroscopy. *Nature*, *432*, 573–539.
12. Tanaka, S., Sawaya, M.R., Yeates, T.O. (2010). Structure and mechanisms of a protein-based organelle in Escherichia coli. *Science*, *327*, 81–84.
13. Arslan, D., Legendre, M., Seltzer, V., Abergel, C., Claverie, J.M. (2011). Distant Mimivirus relative with a larger genome highlights the fundamental features of Megaviridae. *Proceedings of the National Academy of Sciences U S A*, *108*, 17486–17491.
14. Raoult, D., Forterre, P. (2008). Redefining viruses: Lessons from Mimivirus. *Nature Reviews Microbiology*, *6*, 315–319.
15. Horne, R.W., Wildy, P. (1961). Symmetry in virus architecture. *Virology*, *15*, 348–373.
16. Caspar, D.L., Klug, A. (1962). Physical principles in the construction of regular viruses. *Cold Spring Harbor Symposia on Quantitative Biology*, *27*, 1–24.
17. Crick, F.H.C., Watson, J. D. (1956). Structure of small viruses. *Nature*, *177*, 473–475.
18. Caspar, D.L., Fontano, E. (1996). Five-fold symmetry in crystalline quasicrystal lattices. *Proceedings of the National Academy of Sciences U S A*, *93*, 14271–14278.
19. Baker, T.S., Olson, N.H., Fuller, S.D. (1999). Adding the third dimension to virus life cycles: three-dimensional reconstruction of icosahedral viruses from cryo-electron micrographs. *Microbiology and Molecular Biology Reviews*, *63*, 862–922.
20. Natarajan, P., Lander, G.C., Shepherd, C.M., Reddy, V.S., Brooks, C.L. 3rd, Johnson, J. E. (2005). Exploring icosahedral virus structures with VIPER. *Nature Reviews Microbiology*, *3*, 809–817.
21. Zlotnick, A. (2004). Viruses and the physics of soft condensed matter. *Proceedings of the National Academy of Sciences U S A*, *101*, 15549–15550.
22. Klug, A. (1983). Architectural design of spherical viruses. *Nature*, *303*, 378–379.
23. Twarock, R. (2006). Mathematical virology: A novel approach to the structure and assembly of viruses. *Philosophical Transactions. Series A, Mathematical, Physical, and Engineering Sciences*, *364*, 3357–3373.
24. Bruinsma, R.F. Gelbart, W.M., Reguera, D., Rudnick, J., Zandi, R. (2003). Viral self-assembly as a thermodynamic process. *Physical Review Letters*, *90*, 248101.

25. Zandi, R., Reguera, D., Bruinsma, R.F., Gelbart, W.M., Rudnick, J. (2004). Origin of icosahedral symmetry in viruses. *Proc. Nat. Acad. Sci. USA*, *101*, 15556–15560.
26. Padilla, J.E., Colovos, C., Yeates, T.O. (2001). Nanohedra: Using symmetry to design self -assembling protein cages, layers, crystals, and filaments. *Proceedings of the National Academy of Sciences U S A*, *98*, 2217–2221.
27. Raman, S., Machaidze, G., Lustig, A., Aebi, A., Burkhard, P. (2006). Structure-based design of peptides that self-assemble into regular polyhedral nanoparticles. *Nanomedicine*, *2*, 95–102.
28. Matsuura, K., Murasato, K., Kimizuka, N. (2005). Artificial peptide-nanospheres self-assembled from three-way junctions of beta-sheet-forming peptides. *Journal of the American Chemical Society*, *127*, 10148–10149.
29. Ryadnov, M.G. (2007). A self-assembling peptide polynanoreactor. *Angewandte Chemie International Edition*, *46*, 969–972.
30. Carlson, J.C.T., Jena, S.S., Flenniken, M., Chou, T., Siegel, R. A., Wagner, C.R. (2006). Chemically controlled self-assembly of protein nanorings. *Journal of the American Chemical Society*, *128*, 7630–7638.
31. Li, Q., So, C.R., Fegan, A., Cody, V., Sarikaya, M., Vallera, D. A., Wagner, C.R. (2010). Chemically self-assembled antibody nanorings (CSANs): Design and characterization of an anti-CD3 IgM biomimetic. *Journal of the American Chemical Society*, *132*, 17247–17257.
32. White, B.R., Li, Q., Wagner, C.R. (2011). Chemically induced self-assembly of enzyme nanorings. *Methods in Molecular Biology*, *743*, 17–26.
33. Holowka, E.P., Sun, V.Z., Kamei, D.T., Deming, T.J. (2007). Polyarginine segments in block copolypeptides drive both vesicular assembly and intracellular delivery. *Nature Materials*, *6*, 52–57.
34. Chung, E. K., Lee, E., Lim, Y. B., Lee, M. (2010). Cyclic peptide facial amphiphile preprogrammed to self-assemble into bioactive peptide capsules. *Chemistry—A European Journal*, *16*, 5305–5309.
35. Carrillo-Tripp, M., Shepherd, C.M., Borelli, I.A., Venkataraman, S., Lander, G., Natarajan, P., Johnson, J.E., Brooks, C.L. 3rd, Reddy, V. S. (2009). VIPERdb2: An enhanced and web API enabled relational database for structural virology. *Nucleic Acids Research*, *37*, D436–D442.

13

PROTEIN AND PEPTIDE DRUG DELIVERY

MITESH PATEL, MEGHA BAROT, JWALA RENUKUNTLA, AND ASHIM K. MITRA

13.1 CHAPTER OBJECTIVES

- To provide an overview on challenges in protein and peptide drug delivery.
- To outline various mechanisms for protein transport across absorptive membrane.
- To highlight various strategies used for enhancing peptide and protein absorption.
- To present various novel drug delivery systems developed for improving peptide and protein drug delivery.

13.2 INTRODUCTION

Proteins and peptides have gained considerable attention in the treatment of several diseases because of their high potency, specificity, and selectivity. Despite their potent activities, the delivery of peptides and proteins faces several challenges such as large size, poor absorption, rapid degradation, and high cost of manufacturing. In recent years, extensive research work has been conducted for improving the delivery of proteins to their target site of action. Poor oral bioavailability and patient incompliance because of the injections led to exploration of noninvasive routes such as buccal, pulmonary, nasal, and transdermal. Recent advances in biotechnology and development of inhalation devices and novel drug delivery systems have further raised research interest in the field of protein and peptide drug delivery. In this chapter, various mechanisms and strategies that have attempted to improve protein drug absorption will be discussed. This chapter will also focus on various particulate and nonparticulate systems designed for improving protein and peptide drug bioavailability.

13.3 CHALLENGES FOR PROTEIN AND PEPTIDE DRUG DELIVERY

The development of macromolecules such as proteins is a more tedious and challenging task than traditional small-molecule drug development. The organic and synthetic chemistry of proteins needs to be considered while developing protein-based therapeutics. These macromolecules with secondary and tertiary structures are highly susceptible to physical and chemical degradation [1]. Proteins can be easily denatured when exposed to higher temperature and humidity. Moreover, frequent exposure to organic solvents may cause structural changes in proteins. Development of immune response, poor cell entry, and rapid systemic clearance are other major challenges associated with protein delivery [2].

Oral delivery is highly preferred for protein therapeutics; however, tight intracellular junctions of intestinal epithelium and high enzymatic degradation pose a formidable barrier for intestinal absorption [3]. After oral administration, proteins are required to permeate through intestinal epithelial cells to generate high systemic concentrations. Unfortunately, the phospholipid bilayer of intestinal membrane acts as a primary barrier for the transport of proteins because of their large size

Advanced Drug Delivery, First Edition. Edited by Ashim K. Mitra, Chi H. Lee, and Kun Cheng.

and high hydrophilicity. Tight junctions in the intestinal cell membrane also hinder protein transport through intercellular spaces [4, 5]. Moreover, the pH of gastrointestinal fluids varies significantly, which may result in pH-dependent hydrolysis of proteins [6].

Poor systemic bioavailability of proteins after oral administration led to the exploration of several noninvasive routes such as buccal, transdermal, nasal, and pulmonary. Several absorption enhancers including protease inhibitors, cell-penetrating peptides, surfactants, and tight junction modulators have been investigated to improve absorption and stability of proteins. Drug delivery systems such as liposomes, microparticles, and nanoparticles have also been used to enhance protein absorption. Furthermore, protein and nucleic acid combinatorial libraries have facilitated the development of novel lead molecules that enhanced site-specific delivery of proteins.

13.4 MECHANISM OF ABSORPTION

Poor protein permeation across intestinal membrane is one of the major reasons for lower oral bioavailability. Depending on physicochemical properties, proteins can permeate the absorptive membrane paracellularly, transcellularly, or by transcytosis (Figure 13.1) [7]. Proteins can either diffuse paracellularly or can transport actively or passively by a transcellular route. In the paracellular pathway, proteins permeate through the intercellular spaces or through the epithelial tight junctions. However, low surface area and the presence of tight epithelial junctions significantly restricts the paracellular diffusion of proteins [8]. Hence, transient opening of tight junctions can considerably enhance protein absorption. Chitosan has been proposed to enhance drug transport by loosening epithelial tight junctions [9]. Proteins can also transport transcellularly by passive diffusion or can be translocated by specific transporters present on the cell membrane. In transcytosis, protein molecules are internalized in vesicles and are transported to the cytoplasm [7]. In receptor-mediated endocytosis, protein molecules interact with specific receptors expressed on the cell membrane. In adsorptive-mediated endocytosis, positively charged groups in proteins undergo electrostatic interactions with negatively charged groups in the phospholipid bilayer of cell membrane. Lang et al. [10] had mathematically derived the effective permeability coefficient under steady-state conditions using thymocartin across excised bovine nasal mucosa [Equation (13.1)]:

$$P_{\mathrm{eff}} = (dc/dt)_{\mathrm{ss}} V/ (A \times C_{\mathrm{D}}) \qquad (13.1)$$

where $(dc/dt)_{ss}$ represents change in concentration with time at steady state, A is permeation area, V is volume of receiver compartment, and C_D is the initial concentration in the donor compartment [10].

13.5 STRATEGIES TO ENHANCE PROTEIN AND PEPTIDE ABSORPTION

Two strategies are commonly used to enhance protein and peptide permeation across absorptive membrane. The first strategy involves alteration of physicochemical properties such as solubility and partition coefficient by chemically modifying the structure of these molecules. The second strategy involves the use of permeation enhancers to improve protein absorption by altering the properties of physiological barriers such as loosening of tight junctions

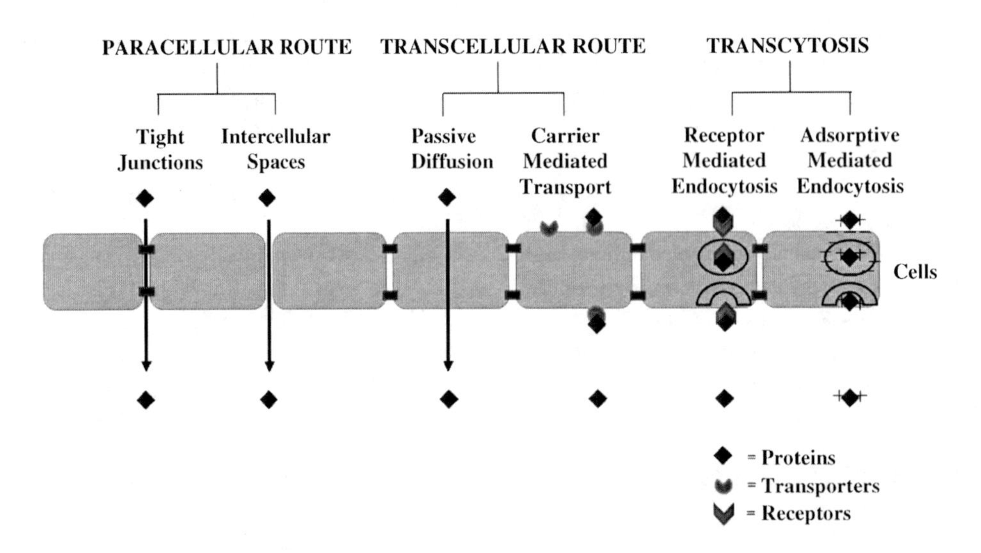

FIGURE 13.1 Various protein transport mechanisms. (See color figure in color plate section.)

or inhibition of proteolytic enzymes. These include the use of absorption enhancers such as protease inhibitors, surfactants, bile salts, and fusidic acid derivatives. In addition to absorption enhancers, several particulate systems such as nanoparticles and microparticles, emulsions, and suspensions have been used recently for improving protein and peptide drug delivery.

13.5.1 Absorption Promoters

Absorption enhancers such as surfactants, chelating agents, bile salts, and lipids have been investigated previously for improving protein absorption. The mechanism by which these promoters increase protein absorption is not understood clearly; however, these agents are known to increase either paracellular or transcellular transport of proteins.

13.5.1.1 Surfactants Surfactants interact with the hydrophobic domain of the membrane or tight junctions, thereby increasing the formation of pores and channels. This effect increases the transepithelial transport of protein across the absorptive membrane along the concentration gradient. A natural pulmonary surfactant and an artificial derivative, phospholipid hexadecanol tyloxapol, generated significant improvement in the absorption of human recombinant insulin in diabetic rats [11]. These surfactants generated a 2-fold to 3-fold higher area under concentration time (AUC) profile of insulin. Furthermore, alkaline phosphatase, lactate dehydrogenase, and *N*-acetyl-β-D-glucoaminidase activities in bronchial fluid remained unaltered, indicating the suitability of these surfactants in enhancing pulmonary delivery of peptides and proteins. Hence, the use of surfactants in protein formulation can be a viable strategy to enhance absorption in poorly permeable tissues.

13.5.1.2 Bile Salts The enhancement of protein absorption by bile salts and their derivatives has been proposed in several mechanisms. These enhancers may improve protein absorption by increasing the formation of hydrophilic pores or channels by undergoing reverse micellar formation with the cell membrane or tight junctions [12]. In another proposed mechanism, bile salts and their derivatives may improve paracellular protein permeability by binding with the luminal calcium ions [13]. Selected bile acid derivatives may also enhance protein absorption by inhibiting proteolytic enzymes [14]. Yamamoto et al. investigated the effects of sodium glycocholate, sodium caprate, linoleic acid-surfactant mixed micelles, *N*-lauryl-β-D-maltopyranoside, and ethylenediaminetetraacetic acid (EDTA), as well as protease inhibitors such as aprotinin, bacitracin, and soybean trypsin inhibitors on the pulmonary absorption of insulin [15]. Insulin powder containing sodium taurocholate or sodium deoxycholate generated significant plasma glucose level reductions in rats [16]. A similar improvement in the absorption of insulin was generated in the presence of sodium glycocholate, bestatin, and aprotinin across a rabbit trachea [17]. Sodium glycocholate has also been reported to enhance the absorption of thyrotropin-releasing hormone by 3-fold across a rabbit trachea [17]. These studies clearly demonstrate the potential of bile salts, protease inhibitors, and surfactants in improving protein absorption.

13.5.1.3 Fusidic Acid Derivatives The potential of the fusidic acid derivative sodium tauro-24,25-dihydrofusidate in improving the rectal absorption of desglycinamide arginine vasopressin was investigated in rats [18]. The mean bioavailability of desglycinamide arginine generated after infusion with 4% of sodium tauro-24,25-dihydrofusidate was $47 \pm 12\%$. Rectal bolus delivery of desglycinamide arginine with 4% of sodium tauro-24,25-dihydrofusidate produced a mean bioavailability of $27 \pm 6\%$. These results signify the potential of fusidic acid derivatives in improving the absorption of peptides and proteins.

13.5.1.4 Cyclodextrins In addition to bile salts, fusidic acid derivatives, and surfactants, cyclodextrins have also been widely used to enhance protein absorption. Several cyclodextrins including alpha-, beta-, and gamma-cyclodextrin, dimethyl-beta-cyclodextrin, and hydroxypropyl-beta-cyclodextrin have been investigated for their efficacy in improving nasal absorption of insulin [19]. Co-administration of insulin with 5% w/v alpha-cyclodextrin generated bioavailability of $27.7 \pm 11.5\%$. Bioavailability was significantly elevated to $108.9 \pm 36.4\%$ with intranasal administration of insulin solution containing 5% dimethyl-beta-cyclodextrin. These results clearly demonstrate the efficacy of cyclodextrins in improving protein bioavailability.

13.5.1.5 Chelating Agents Chelating agents enhance protein absorption by binding to the luminal calcium ions of epithelial cells thereby opening tight intercellular junctions. This effect increases the paracellular transport of proteins [20]. Co-administration of insulin with sodium salicylate or 5-methoxysalicylate significantly improved rectal absorption of insulin [21]. Chitosan has also been investigated previously for improving protein absorption. Insulin-chitosan conjugates generated high pharmacodynamic bioavailability relative to subcutaneously injected insulin [22]. EDTA disodium salt is another chelating agent that has been used for enhancing absorption of insulin. However, promising results with EDTA were not successfully generated when co-administered with insulin [14, 16, 23].

13.5.1.6 Cell-Penetrating Peptides Cell-penetrating peptides such as penetratin, Tat, and octaarginine have been previously examined for determining their potential in enhancing protein absorption. A recent study showed that

L-penetratin produced significantly higher nasal absorption of insulin relative to D-penetratin and octaarginine [24]. Nasal administration of this formulation produced significantly higher bioavailability and pharmacological availability of insulin (50.7% and 76.7%) compared wiith subcutaneous administration in rats. A similar enhancement in the intestinal absorption of insulin was obtained when co administered with L-penetratin [25]. Other cell-penetrating peptides including R8, pVEC, and RRL helices can also generate significant intestinal absorption of insulin relative to insulin solution alone. However, the effect was more pronounced when insulin was co-administered with L-penetratin relative to other cell-penetrating peptides. The absorption of insulin across intestinal mucosa was significantly elevated in the presence of octaarginine relative to insulin solution alone [26]. Furthermore, the exposure of octaarginine had no toxic effect on the intestinal mucosa, as observed in lactate dehydrogenase activity assay. This observation clearly indicates that cell-penetrating peptides such as oligoarginines can be a powerful tool for enhancing the oral delivery of proteins such as insulin. Similarly, Tat and pip2b cell-penetrating peptides have demonstrated high efficiency in delivering BH4 anti-apoptotic peptide in mouse with myocardial IR injury [27].

13.5.2 Chemical/Structural Modification Approach

Several attempts have been made to improve the chemical and enzymatic stability of proteins by chemically modifying few amino acids in the peptide chain. Such modifications may not only improve pharmacokinetic profile but also generate excellent pharmacodynamic effects. These modifications include derivatization of proteins for specific transporter and receptor recognition, conjugation with synthetic or natural polymers for efficient delivery, and structural manipulations on amino acid chains to reduce enzyme affinity and immunogenicity.

13.5.2.1 Simple Modifications Major objectives of synthesizing prodrugs are to enhance protein lipophilicity, permeability, *in vivo* stability, and half-life [28]. The chemical modification of C-terminal peptide bond with N-hydroxymethylation provided significant resistance to degradation by carboxypeptidase A [29]. Similarly, enzymatic degradation had been overcome with prodrug modification on pyroglutamyl group, α-aminoamide moiety, the peptide bond itself, C-terminal amide group in peptide amides, the tyrosine phenol group in tyrosyl peptides, and the N-terminal amino group [30]. Acetyl, propionyl, and pivaloyl ester prodrugs of Leu-enkephalin generated a 2-fold, 7-fold, and 18-fold increase in permeability relative to Leu-enkephalin in intestinal cells [31]. This improvement in the transport of ester prodrugs can be attributed to increase in lipophilicity of parent drug Leu-enkephalin. Lipophilic prodrugs can improve transdermal delivery of the thyrotropin-releasing hormone significantly [30, 32].

13.5.2.2 Cyclic Prodrugs In addition to chemical modification on single functional groups of small linear peptides, cyclic prodrugs have also been investigated previously. These prodrugs provide better enzymatic stability because of conjugation of the C-terminal carboxylic group to the N-terminal amino group. Moreover, these prodrugs are bioreversible and reduce hydrogen bonding with aqueous solvents, thereby enhancing cell permeation [6]. The cyclic prodrug of hexapeptide (H-Trp-Ala-Gly-Gly-Asp-Ala-OH) generated a 76-fold increase in permeability relative to linear peptide in intestinal cells. The apparent permeability values for cyclic and linear hexapeptide were reported to be $1.30 \pm 0.15 \times 10^{-7}$ cm/s and 0.17×10^{-8} cm/s, respectively [33]. Similarly, a 5 to 6-fold rise in permeability was generated by coumarin-based cyclic prodrugs of RGD (Arg-Gly-Asp) peptidomimetics relative to parent RGD peptidomimetics [34]. Recently, N-methylation of cyclic hexapeptides has been proposed as an alternative strategy to enhance intestinal permeability [35].

13.5.2.3 Lipidation Approach This approach involves linking of fatty acids or lipids to peptides and proteins in order to enhance lipophilicity. This type of conjugation will facilitate the interaction of peptides and proteins with the cell membrane resulting in increased absorption. Lipid prodrugs of several peptide drugs with reversible aqueous lipidization (REAL) technology have been investigated. It has been reported that peptide-REAL prodrugs increases transcellular permeability, enzymatic stability, and half-life of peptides [36]. Conjugation of *N*-palmitoyl cysteinyl 2-pyridyl disulfide to salmon calcitonin (REAL-salmon calcitonin) generated a 4-fold increase in AUC relative to salmon calcitonin solution on subcutaneous administration [36]. After oral administration, the conjugation generated a 19-fold increase in AUC relative to salmon calcitonin solution with plasma levels detectable for 12 h. A similar conjugation to desmopressin produced a 250-fold increase in antidiuretic property relative to desmopression solution [37]. Conjugation of fatty acids such as lauric acid has been proposed as a potential strategy to enhance transmembrane permeation of peptides such as thyrotropin-releasing hormone (TRH), tetragastrin (TG), calcitonin, and insulin [38, 39].

13.5.2.4 PEGylation The structural properties of proteins or peptides are primarily responsible for unfavorable physicochemical properties that ultimately limit their intestinal absorption. Structural modifications have been potentially employed to improve physicochemical properties of macromolecules such as proteins and peptides [6]. PEGylation is the covalent attachment of PEG (polyethylene glycol) moieties to therapeutic drug molecules. These moieties are repeating units of ethylene glycol that are both inert and amphiphilic in nature [40]. PEGylation technique has been previously attempted to improve delivery by enhancing stability, pharmacokinetics, and therapeutic utility of proteins and peptides [41, 42]. It improves the efficacy of protein and peptides by altering various physicochemical properties such as size, molecular weight, conformation, steric hindrance, and hydrophilicity [41]. Prolonged circulation time of PEGylated proteins is achieved because of reduced rate of clearance and protection from proteolytic enzymes are other benefits of this modification. In addition, PEGylation masks hydrophobic sites on protein molecules that would otherwise lead to aggregation, loss of activity, or increased immunogenicity [43].

Notwithstanding potential benefits, PEGylation can sometimes compromise the therapeutic activity of proteins. For instance, steric hindrance caused by higher PEGylation can significantly reduce the binding affinity of larger proteins [44]. Polydispersity is another major complication associated with PEGylation [45]. Overall, in the past two decades, PEGylation has been emerged as a viable strategy to improve the absorption and bioavailability of proteins as well as its formulation (hydrogels, nanoparticles, and microparticles) [46]. An example of PEGylated proteins is summarized in Table 13.1.

13.5.2.5 Hyperglycosylation Hyperglycosylation is a technique in which protein molecules are chemically conjugated to carbohydrate moieties. This modification has demonstrated significant potential in improving the structural, functional, immunogenic, and pharmacokinetic properties of therapeutic proteins [47]. It closely resembles PEGylation and, hence, shares similar principle and advantages in the field of protein and peptide drug delivery. Similar to PEGylation, hyperglycosylation can improve protein circulation time and stability, and minimize immunogenicity. Importantly, as a result of the biodegradable nature of oligosaccharides, this approach is more beneficial over PEGylated molecules. Therefore, chronic administration of PEGylated molecules may accumulate in tissues, whereas in hyperglycosylated forms, endogenous carbohydrates are digested readily [48]. Moreover, stealth properties of oligosaccharides such as polysialic acid, hyperglycosylation is clinically considered as a non-immunogenic process [49]. Unfortunately, compromised activity or unwanted conformational changes generated by covalent protein modification is a major limitation of this approach [48]. An example of hyperglycosylation is summarized in Table 13.1 [50–52].

13.5.2.6 Transporter-Mediated Targeted Delivery In addition to passive diffusion, peptides can also permeate through specific transporters expressed on the plasma membrane. Two peptide specific transporters, PEPT1 and PEPT2, with a high capacity and broad substrate specificity, are expressed in human small intestine [53, 54]. Several dipeptides, tripeptides, and amino β-lactam antibiotics have been demonstrated to be transported through peptide transporters [55]. KPV, an anti-inflammatory tripeptide (Lys-Pro-Val), is transported by PEPT1 transporter in intestinal cells [56]. Recently, two different broad-specificity oligopeptide transporters, capable of transporting oligopeptides containing five or more amino acids, have been reported to be expressed in intestinal cells [57]. Such transporter systems can be used for enhancing oral absorption of small peptide drugs.

13.5.2.7 Receptor-Mediated Peptide Delivery Peptides and proteins can also permeate the phospholipid bilayer of the cell membrane through a process known as receptor-mediated endocytosis (RME). RME is highly specific and one of the major transport mechanisms for macromolecules such as proteins. The interaction of ligand (proteins) with receptors expressed on cell membranes causes the folding of the cell membrane to form intracellular vesicles known as endosomes. The encapsulated proteins are eventually released into the cell cytoplasm after endosomal escape.

Epidermal growth factors have been reported to be internalized by specific receptors in liver cells [58, 59]. Murine monoclonal antibodies of IgG2 (Immunoglobulin G) type having a high affinity toward epidermal growth factor receptors have been previously targeted for gene delivery [60]. Keratinocyte growth factor receptors demonstrated clathrin-dependent RME of fibroblast growth factors in epithelial tumor cells [61]. Similarly, the RME of several proteins such as insulin [62, 63], insulin-like growth factors [64], low-density lipoproteins [65], immunoglobulins [66], and transferrin [67, 68] has been reported previously. The use of these receptors to improve protein delivery can be beneficial; however, *in vivo* stability might be a major concern. For enhanced stability and efficient delivery,

TABLE 13.1 PEGylated and Hyperglycosylated Proteins in the Market

Drug (Brand Name and Manufacturer)	Indication	Parent Protein (Structural Modification)	References
Darbepoetin alfa (Aranesp; Amgen, Thousand Oaks, CA)	Increases red blood cell levels in anemia	Synthetic form of erythropoietin (hyperglycosylation)	[50, 51]
PEG-Certolizumab pegol (Cimzia; UCB Inc., Smyrna, GA)	Rheumatoid arthritis and Crohn's disease	Humanized tumor necrosis factor antibody Fab fragment (PEGylation)	[52]

proteins can be encapsulated and administered in carrier systems such as nanoparticles, microparticles, liposomes, and micelles. Furthermore, the efficiency can be maximized by modifying the surface of these carrier systems with targeting moieties such as antibodies or aptamers to ensure site-specific delivery. Recently, bioadhesive or mucoadhesive systems such as hydrogels, patches, and tablets have also been explored widely for enhancing protein absorption.

13.5.3 Formulation Technologies

13.5.3.1 Bioadhesive Systems Drug delivery systems that can adhere to the biological surfaces such as gastrointestinal mucosa are referred to as bioadhesive systems. The term "mucoadhesion" is alternatively used when the adhesive bond forms between mucus layer and delivery system. However, interactions between the adhesive system and cell surface are referred as cytoadhesion [6, 69]. Bioadhesive systems are mainly designed for the following reasons:

(1) To increase the residence time and interaction of drug delivery systems at the absorptive surface
(2) To increase the concentration gradient and instant absorption of therapeutic agents
(3) To prevent active drug dilution or biodegradation in luminal fluids
(4) To enhance drug/delivery system localization at the target site
(5) To promote membrane permeation or inhibit proteolytic enzymes [6, 70, 71]

Several modified as well as unmodified hydrophilic polymers such as chitosan, polyacrylates and cellulose derivatives have been used for preparing bioadhesive systems. The hydrophilic groups of bioadhesive systems (e.g., carboxyl, amide, hydroxyl, and sulfate) bind to the mucus or cell surface by different types of interactions such as hydrogen bond formation, hydrophobic, or ionic interactions. Ideally, bioadhesive polymers should meet the following criteria:

(1) Should be biodegradable, nontoxic, and nonirritant
(2) The ability to bind tightly to the mucus or cell surface
(3) Should offer higher encapsulation of therapeutic agents
(4) Should not restrict drug release from final dosage from
(5) Should be economic and stable during shelf life of the final dosage form

The properties of polymers that can affect bioadhesion include hydrophilicity, molecular weight, concentration, spatial conformation, crosslinking, and swelling ability [72]. Typical examples of the bioadhesive systems used for protein drug delivery includes hydrogels and mucoadhesive tablets and patches.

Hydrogels A hydrogel is a three-dimensional network composed of hydrophilic polymers capable of imbibing large amounts of water or biological fluids while maintaining its shape [73]. This network is fairly insoluble because of the presence of chemical and/or physical crosslinks [73, 74]. Hydrogels were introduced as soft contact lenses in 1960s. However, their use has grown significantly in pharmaceutical and biomedical applications [69, 75, 76]. Hydrogels can be classified as neutral and ionic based on the nature of side groups. Depending on the origin of polymers used to generate hydrogels, these compounds can be classified into two groups: natural or synthetic. Natural polymers have gained considerable attention over the past few decades because of their biocompatibility and presence of biologically recognizable groups to support cellular activities. The major disadvantages of using natural polymers include weak mechanical properties and batch-to-batch variability [77]. Natural polymers frequently used for the preparation of hydrogels include chitosan [74, 78], hyaluronic acid [79, 80], alginate [81, 82], gelatin [83], and dextran [77, 84].

Synthetic polymers generate hydrogels with high mechanical strength and offer considerable opportunities to tailor network properties (release behavior) in a reproducible way. The most common synthetic polymers used for generating hydrogels are PEG [85, 86] and poly(hydroxyethyl methacrylate) (pHEMA) [87, 88]. A summary of monomers/polymers commonly used in the preparation of polymeric hydrogels for oral protein delivery is given in Table 13.2. Considerable attention has been paid to hydrogels for delivering therapeutic agents in the form of controlled release delivery systems [89–91], bioadhesive devices [92–94], or targetable devices [95, 96]. Apart from rectal, ocular, epidermal, and subcutaneous applications, hydrogels have been selected for oral delivery of proteins. Hydrogel responsive properties such as changes in network structure or swelling

TABLE 13.2 Hydrogels Used for Oral Protein Delivery

Monomer/Polymer	Protein	References
Hydroxyethyl methacrylate (HEMA)	Bovine serum albumin	[87]
Ethylene glycol	Insulin	[99]
Acrylic acid (AA)	Bovine serum albumin	[100, 101]
Methacrylic acid	Growth hormone, insulin	[102, 103]
Chitosan	Bovine serum albumin, insulin	[104, 105]
Alginate	Bovine serum albumin	[105]
Gelatin	Bone morphogenetic proteins	[106]
Dextran	Recombinant human bone morphogenetic protein-2	[107]

behavior in response to body temperature, gastrointestinal variation in pH, electric field, or ionic strength may allow targeted delivery of proteins to their site of absorption [97, 98].

Mucoadhesive Tablets and Patches Mucoadhesive polymers in the form of tablets have been established as efficient carriers for poorly absorbed proteins (Table 13.3) [108]. Thiolated polymers have generated strong mucoadhesive properties. These polymers contain thiol groups that produce disulfide bonds with cysteine-rich subdomains of mucus glycoproteins [109]. Among these polymers, chitosan-4-thiobutylamidine conjugate (chitosan-TBA) have exhibited the strongest mucoadhesion properties determined with a rotating cylinder method [110, 111]. Theses polymers generate intimate contact with intestinal mucosa and provide sustained protein release [108]. Mucoadhesive polyacrylates such as carbopol and polycarbophil have been reported to improve intestinal absorption of peptides by reducing the metabolic activity of proteolytic enzymes and opening tight intracellular junctions [112].

Multilayered patch system is a well-established oral delivery system that not only generates higher levels of protein absorption but also provides stability at the intestinal epithelium. These protective, rate-controlling, and adhesiveness properties are considered to be ideal features for the oral delivery of protein and peptides [113, 114]. Previously, intestinal patches consisting of carbopol have been developed for the oral delivery of insulin. These systems not only localized insulin near intestinal mucosa but also protected it from proteolytic degradation [115].

Table 13.3 represents various proteins that have been delivered in tablet dosage forms.

13.5.3.2 Particulate Carrier Systems The use of drug delivery systems for protein and peptide drugs is a promising approach as they can overcome various disadvantages such as premature degradation, poor absorption, and uncontrolled drug release. Important particulate systems used so for include submicron emulsions and suspensions, liposomes, polymeric nanoparticles and microparticles, and polymeric micelles [6].

Polymeric Particles (Nanoparticles and Microparticles) Nanoparticles and microparticles are solid colloidal polymeric particles ranging in size from 10 to 1000 nm and 1 to 250 μm, respectively. These particles consist of macromolecular material in which the active ingredient is either dissolved, dispersed, encapsulated, adsorbed, or chemically attached to the surface [120–122]. Polymeric particles have emerged as potential carriers for proteins because of their facile transformation and modulation of properties such as subcellular size, biodegradability, and biocompatibility [123, 124]. Such delivery systems not only can improve the biological properties of proteins (e.g., targeting, bioadhesion, improved cellular uptake) but also can provide additional stability against enzymatic degradation [125, 126]. Submicron size and large surface area significantly improve the absorption of proteins relative to larger carrier systems. Moreover, surface modification of these particles with chemical grafting of certain molecules such as PEG, poloxamers, and lectins may further improve uptake at their site of absorption [127, 128].

Proteins can be encapsulated into the nanoparticles and microparticles using double emulsion, spray drying, or phase separation methods [129]. Protein release from polymeric particles is attributed to diffusion through the polymer matrix followed by degradation and dissolution of particle itself. Usually, there is an initial "burst" release of the protein adsorbed on the surface of the particle. The degradation profile and crosslink density of polymer chains determine protein diffusion, which in turn is dependent on individual polymer molecular weights, co-polymer ratios, and their resulting glass transition temperature, crystallinity, and hydrophilicity [130, 131]. Hence, protein-release profiles can be controlled significantly through alteration of these properties. Polymeric particles have been designed to deliver a wide array of soluble proteins for different applications in various systems, both *in vitro* and *in vivo*. Some of these important applications include the delivery of encapsulated antigens for vaccination, enzymes, hormones, growth factors, and mitogens in tissue-engineering constructs. Representative oral polymeric particles employed for oral protein delivery are shown in Table 13.4.

Micelles Although polymeric particles have demonstrated significant potential for protein and peptide drug delivery, they poses few inherent disadvantages such as protein

TABLE 13.3 Therapeutic Proteins Delivery as Tablet Dosage Form

Protein	Polymer/Excipient	Observation	Reference
Insulin	Thiolated chitosan	Controlled release of insulin over 8 h with significant reduction in blood glucose level	[116]
Insulin	Hydroxypropyl methylcellulose (HPMC)	System was thus proven suitable for yielding two-pulse release profiles	[117]
Soy proteins	Succinylation	Succinylated soy protein tablets were found gastro-resistant	[118]
Insulin	Chitosan-aprotinin conjugate	Mean blood glucose level decreased to 84 ± 6%	[119]

TABLE 13.4 Oral Administration of Therapeutic Proteins Encapsulated in Polymeric Particles

Polymer	Protein	Size (nm)	Observation	Reference
Poly(lactic-co-glycolic acid) (PLGA)	Insulin	150	Significant reduction in plasma glucose level	[132]
Poly(methyl methacrylate)	Insulin	200–300	Pharmacological bioavailability ~9.7%	[133]
Poly(isobutylcyanoacrylate)	Insulin	220–300	Strong hypoglycemic response	[134]
Chitosan	Insulin	270–340	Effective reduction of glycemia	[135]
Alginate, albumin, chitosan	Insulin	396	Sustained hypoglycemic effect over 24 h	[136]
Chitosan/alginate	Bovine serum albumin	200	pH-dependent release	[137]
Dextran/gelatin	Bone morphogenetic protein	20–100	Fulfilled the basic prerequisites for growth factor delivery	[138]

denaturation caused by exposure to organic solvents and small-scale processing of expensive recombinant proteins [139, 140]. However, the delivery of these macromolecules in micelles can be a viable strategy because of its ability 1) to encapsulate therapeutic protein or peptide in miceller core, 2) to ensure chemical and physical stability of protein during and after processing of final formulation, 3) to encapsulate small amount of proteins over a wide batch sizes in reproducible manner, and 4) to offer a narrow size distribution of final formulation. Typical micelle structure includes a hydrophobic core (to solubilize hydrophobic drugs) and a hydrophilic outer shell (to stabilize micelles) [139, 141]. A wide range of polymeric, surfactant, and phospholipid micelles has been explored for the protein and peptide delivery (Table 13.5).

Liposomes Liposomes are spherical, self-closed vesicles formed by one or more concentric lipid (natural or synthetic) bilayers with an encapsulated aqueous phase in the center and between the bilayers. Liposomes vary in size from 100 nm small unilamellar to 200–800 nm large unilamellar to 500–5000 nm multilamellar vesicles [146]. Generally, proteins and peptides can be either encapsulated within the liposome or chemically conjugated to the surface groups. Passive loading can be achieved by incubating protein or peptide with liposomes at or slightly below the transition temperature of lipids. On the other hand, liposomes are subjected to elevated temperatures for active encapsulation of proteins [48]. Protein conjugation on the surface of liposomes can generate advanced liposomal systems with special properties such as 1) immunoliposomes (conjugated to antibodies or antibody fragments) [147], 2) stealth liposomes (conjugated with protective layer of PEG to prevent opsonins recognition and rapid clearance) [148], 3) long circulating immune-liposomes (conjugated with both a protective polymer and antibody) [149], and 4) surface-modified liposomes (surface modification using stimuli-responsive lipids, cell-penetrating peptides, and diagnostic agents) [48]. Liposomal size, surface charges, and hydrophobicity are predominant factors that control release kinetics and biodistribution of proteins [150]. Liposomal formulations can improve pharmacokinetics as well as the therapeutic efficacy of protein and peptides. The biocompatible and amphiphilic nature of phospholipids incorporated in liposomal formulation can improve protein stability throughout its storage and handling without generating any adverse effects. Moreover, unlike PEGylation or hyperglycosylation, liposomal formulation eliminates the requirement of covalent modifications and may therefore prevent any loss in protein activity [48]. The representative liposomal formulations employed for protein delivery are shown in Table 13.6.

TABLE 13.5 Micelle Delivery of Protein and Peptides

Peptide/Protein	Micelle	Reference
Glucagon-like peptide-1	PEGylated phospholipid micelles	[142]
Glucose-dependent insulinotropic peptide (GIP)	Sterically stabilized phospholipid nanomicelles	[143]
Neuropeptide Y (NPY)	Sterically stabilized phospholipid micelles	[144]
Salmon calcitonin	Polyion complex micelles	[145]
Ovalbumin	Disulfide-crosslinked polyion micelles	[139]

TABLE 13.6 Liposomal Delivery of Protein

Protein	Species	Observation	References
Superoxide dismutase	Rat	Increase activity, prolong circulation, and decrease membrane peroxidation	[151]
Asparginase	Mice	Improved survival and reduced neutralizing antibodies generation	[152, 153]
Plasminogen activating factor	Rabbit	Higher degree of lysis	[154]
Recombinant interleukin-2	Mice	Eightfold higher plasma circulation time	[155]
Muramyl dipeptide	Mice	Significant inhibition of liver metastasis	[156]
Insulin	Rat	Sustained suppression of glucose levels	[157]

13.6 CONCLUSION

Macromolecules such as proteins and peptides have gained significant attention in the treatment of various diseases because of their high potency and specificity. However, oral delivery of proteins and peptides has been a challenging task because of high proteolytic degradation in the gastrointestinal tract prior to absorption. The development of novel formulation approaches to enhance the oral bioavailability of proteins and peptides remains an active field of research. With recent advances in drug delivery devices and biotechnology, potential opportunity exists in the development of novel protein and peptide delivery systems to promote absorption across poorly permeable membranes. Several of these approaches have shown significant potential in clinical studies. Chemical modification approaches and the application of bioadhesive polymers have demonstrated promising outcomes in improved oral delivery of protein and peptides. Several noninvasive routes, such as pulmonary and nasal delivery, have been explored thoroughly to enhance the systemic bioavailability of proteins and peptides. These routes have demonstrated a potential for improving systemic absorption of proteins and peptides. Particulate systems have been employed widely for modulating physicochemical properties, sustaining protein release, and thereby prolonging the desired pharmacological responses. Targeted delivery of proteins and peptides by chemically modifying the surface of drug delivery systems with aptamers, antibodies, and cell-penetrating peptides can further improve the efficiency of such formulation. Despite significant success in protein and peptide drug delivery, continuous research efforts are still required to develop improved strategies in order to deliver these macromolecules in a noninvasive, patient-compliant manner.

ASSESSMENT QUESTIONS

13.1. List the various routes used for peptide and protein drug delivery.

13.2. What are the major factors that can affect oral absorption of peptides and proteins?

13.3. Proteins can permeate absorptive membrane by which of the following mechanisms?

- **a.** Paracellular transport
- **b.** Transcellular transport
- **c.** Transcytosis
- **d.** All of the above

13.4. Name a few enzymes that can degrade peptides and proteins.

13.5. Which of the following absorption enhancers can enhance protein bioavailability?

- **a.** Fusidic acid derivatives
- **b.** Cyclodextrins
- **c.** Bile salts
- **d.** Surfactants
- **e.** All of the above

13.6. What are prodrugs?

13.7. List a few prodrug approaches that have been used to increase protein absorption.

13.8. How does lipidation help in increasing protein absorption?

13.9. Name two endogenous transporters that can transport di- and tripeptides.

13.10. Which of the following have been used to enhance protein absorption?

- **a.** Nanoparticles
- **b.** Liposomes
- **c.** Emulsions
- **d.** Mucoadhesive systems
- **e.** All of the above

13.11. What is a bioadhesive system? What are the important functions of bioadhesive systems?

13.12. List five monomers/polymers most commonly used in the preparation of polymeric hydrogels for oral protein delivery.

13.13. What are the advantages of micelles over other particulate systems for protein and peptide drug delivery?

13.14. What are the different advanced liposomal forms used for protein delivery?

REFERENCES

1. Brown, L.R. (2005). Commercial challenges of protein drug delivery. *Expert Opinion on Drug Delivery*, *2(1)*, 29–42.
2. Torchilin, V.P., Lukyanov, A.N. (2003). Peptide and protein drug delivery to and into tumors: Challenges and solutions. *Drug Discovery Today*, *8(6)*, 259–66.
3. Shah, R.B., Ahsan, F., Khan, M.A. (2002). Oral delivery of proteins: Progress and prognostication. *Critical Reviews in Therapeutic Drug Carrier Systems*, *19(2)*, 135–169.
4. Fasano, A. (1998). Innovative strategies for the oral delivery of drugs and peptides. *Trends in Biotechnology*, *16(4)*, 152–157.
5. Hochmana, J., Artursson, P. (1994). Mechanisms of absorption enhancement and tight junction regulation. *Journal of Controlled Release*, *29(3)*, 253–267.

6. Hamman, J.H., Enslin, G.M., Kotze, A.F. (2005). Oral delivery of peptide drugs: Barriers and developments. *BioDrugs*, *19(3)*, 165–177.
7. Ozsoy, Y., Gungor, S., Cevher, E. (2009). Nasal delivery of high molecular weight drugs. *Molecules*, *14(9)*, 3754–3779.
8. Salamat-Miller, N., Johnston, T.P. (2005). Current strategies used to enhance the paracellular transport of therapeutic polypeptides across the intestinal epithelium. *International Journal of Pharmaceutics*, *294(1–2)*, 201–216.
9. Dodane, V., Amin Khan, M., Merwin, J.R. (1999). Effect of chitosan on epithelial permeability and structure. *International Journal of Pharmaceutics*, *182(1)*, 21–32.
10. Lang, S., Langguth, P., Oschmann, R., Traving, B., Merkle, H. P. (1996). Transport and metabolic pathway of thymocartin (TP4) in excised bovine nasal mucosa. *Journal of Pharmacy and Pharmacology*, *48(11)*, 1190–1196.
11. Zheng, J., Zhang, G., Lu, Y., Fang, F., He, J., Li, N., Talbi, A., Zhang, Y., Tang, Y., Zhu, J., Chen, X. (2010). Effect of pulmonary surfactant and phospholipid hexadecanol tyloxapol on recombinant human-insulin absorption from intratracheally administered dry powders in diabetic rats. *Chemical and Pharmaceutical Bulletin (Tokyo)*, *58(12)*, 1612–1616.
12. Gordon, G.S., Moses, A.C., Silver, R.D., Flier, J.S., Carey, M. C. (1985). Nasal absorption of insulin: Enhancement by hydrophobic bile salts. *Proceedings of the National Academy of Sciences U S A*, *82(21)*, 7419–7423.
13. McMartin, C., Hutchinson, L.E., Hyde, R., Peters, G.E. (1987). Analysis of structural requirements for the absorption of drugs and macromolecules from the nasal cavity. *Journal of Pharmaceutical Sciences*, *76(7)*, 535–540.
14. Yamamoto, A., Hayakawa, E., Kato, Y., Nishiura, A., Lee, V. H. (1992). A mechanistic study on enhancement of rectal permeability to insulin in the albino rabbit. *Journal of Pharmacology and Experimental Therapeutics*, *263(1)*, 25–31.
15. Yamamoto, A., Umemori, S., Muranishi, S. (1994). Absorption enhancement of intrapulmonary administered insulin by various absorption enhancers and protease inhibitors in rats. *Journal of Pharmacy and Pharmacology*, *46(1)*, 14–18.
16. Yang, D.B., Zhu, J.B., Zhu, H., Zhang, X.S. (2005). Deposition of insulin powders for inhalation in vitro and pharmacodynamic evaluation of absorption promoters in rats. *Yao Xue Xue Bao*, *40(12)*, 1069–1074.
17. Morimoto, K., Uehara, Y., Iwanaga, K., Kakemi, M. (2000). Effects of sodium glycocholate and protease inhibitors on permeability of TRH and insulin across rabbit trachea. *Pharmaceutica Acta Helvetiae*, *74(4)*, 411–415.
18. van Hoogdalem, E.J., Heijligers-Feijen, C.D., Mathot, R.A., Wackwitz, A.T., van Bree, J.B., Verhoef, J.C., de Boer, A. G., Breimer, D.D. (1989). Rectal absorption enhancement of cefoxitin and desglycinamide arginine vasopressin by sodium tauro-24, 25-dihydrofusidate in conscious rats. *Journal of Pharmacology and Experimental Therapeutics*, *251(2)*, 741–744.
19. Merkus, F.W., Verhoef, J.C., Romeijn, S.G., Schipper, N.G. (1991). Absorption enhancing effect of cyclodextrins on intranasally administered insulin in rats. *Pharmaceutical Research*, *8(5)*, 588–592.
20. Noacha, A.B.J., Kurosakia, Y., Blom-Roosemalena, M.C.M., de Boera, A.G., Breimera, D.D. (1993). Cell-polarity dependent effect of chelation on the paracellular permeability of confluent caco-2 cell monolayers. *International Journal of Pharmaceutics*, *90(3)*, 229–237.
21. Nishihata, T., Rytting, J.H., Kamada, A., Higuchi, T., Routh, M., Caldwell, L. (1983). Enhancement of rectal absorption of insulin using salicylates in dogs. *Journal of Pharmacy and Pharmacology*, *35(3)*, 148–151.
22. Lee, E., Lee, J., Jon, S. A novel approach to oral delivery of insulin by conjugating with low molecular weight chitosan. *Bioconjugate Chemistry*, *21(10)*, 1720–1723.
23. Yamamoto, A., Tanaka, H., Okumura, S., Shinsako, K., Ito, M., Yamashita, M., Okada, N., Fujita, T., Muranishi, S. (2001). Evaluation of insulin permeability and effects of absorption enhancers on its permeability by an in vitro pulmonary epithelial system using Xenopus pulmonary membrane. *Biological & Pharmaceutical Bulletin*, *24(4)*, 385–389.
24. Khafagy el, S., Morishita, M., Isowa, K., Imai, J., Takayama, K. (2009). Effect of cell-penetrating peptides on the nasal absorption of insulin. *Journal of Controlled Release*, *133(2)*, 103–108.
25. Kamei, N., Morishita, M., Eda, Y., Ida, N., Nishio, R., Takayama, K. (2008). Usefulness of cell-penetrating peptides to improve intestinal insulin absorption. *Journal of Controlled Release*, *132(1)*, 21–25.
26. Morishita, M., Kamei, N., Ehara, J., Isowa, K., Takayama, K. (2007). A novel approach using functional peptides for efficient intestinal absorption of insulin. *Journal of Controlled Release*, *118(2)*, 177–184.
27. Boisguerin, P., Redt-Clouet, C., Franck-Miclo, A., Licheheb, S., Nargeot, J., Barrere-Lemaire, S., Lebleu, B. (2011). Systemic delivery of BH4 anti-apoptotic peptide using CPPs prevents cardiac ischemia-reperfusion injuries in vivo. *Journal of Controlled Release*, *156(2)*, 146–153.
28. Gangwar, S., Pauletti, G.M., Wang, B., Siahaan, T.J., Stella, V.J., Borchardt, R.T. (1997). Prodrug strategies to enhance the intestinal absorption of peptides. *Drug Discovery Today*, *2(4)*, 148–155.
29. Friis, G.J., Bak, A., Larsen, B.D., Frokjaer, S. (1996). Prodrugs of peptides obtained by derivatization of the C-terminal peptide bond in order to effect protection against degradation by carboxypeptidases. *International Journal of Pharmaceutics*, *136(1–2)*, 61–69.
30. Bundgaard, H. (1992). (C) Means to enhance penetration: (1) Prodrugs as a means to improve the delivery of peptide drugs. *Advanced Drug Delivery Reviews*, *8(1)*, 1–38.
31. Fredholt, K., Adrian, C., Just, L., Larsen, D.H., Weng, S., Moss, B., Friis. G.J. (2000). Chemical and enzymatic stability as well as transport properties of a Leu-enkephalin analogue and ester prodrugs thereof. *Journal of Controlled Release*, *63(3)*, 261–273.

32. Bundgaard, H. (1992). The utility of the prodrug approach to improve peptide absorption. *Journal of Controlled Release, 21(1–3)*, 63–72.
33. Pauletti, G.M., Gangwar, S., Okumu, F.W., Siahaan, T.J., Stella, V.J., Borchardt, R.T. (1996). Esterase-sensitive cyclic prodrugs of peptides: Evaluation of an acyloxyalkoxy promoiety in a model hexapeptide. *Pharmaceutical Research, 13(11)*, 1615–1623.
34. Camenisch, G.P., Wang, W., Wang, B., Borchardt, R.T. (1998). A comparison of the bioconversion rates and the Caco-2 cell permeation characteristics of coumarin-based cyclic prodrugs and methylester-based linear prodrugs of RGD peptidomimetics. *Pharmaceutical Research, 15(8)*, 1174–1181.
35. Ovadia, O., Greenberg, S., Chatterjee, J., Laufer, B., Opperer, F., Kessler, H., Gilon, C., Hoffman, A. (2011). The effect of multiple N-methylation on intestinal permeability of cyclic hexapeptides. *Molecular Pharmacology, 8(2)*, 479–487.
36. Wang, J., Chow, D., Heiati, H., Shen, W.C. (2003). Reversible lipidization for the oral delivery of salmon calcitonin. *Journal of Controlled Release, 88(3)*, 369–380.
37. Wang, J., Shen, D., Shen, W.C. (1999). Preparation, purification, and characterization of a reversibly lipidized desmopressin with potentiated anti-diuretic activity. *Pharmaceutical Research, 16(11)*, 1674–1679.
38. Yamamoto, A. (1998). [Improvement of intestinal absorption of peptide and protein drugs by chemical modification with fatty acids]. *Nihon Rinsho, 56(3)*, 601–607.
39. Muranishi, S., Sakai, A., Yamada, K., Murakami, M., Takada, K., Kiso, Y. (1991). Lipophilic peptides: Synthesis of lauroyl thyrotropin-releasing hormone and its biological activity. *Pharmaceutical Research, 8(5)*, 649–652.
40. Veronese, F.M., Harris, J.M. (2002). Introduction and overview of peptide and protein pegylation. *Advanced Drug Delivery Reviews, 54(4)*, 453–456.
41. Harris, J.M., Chess, R.B. (2003). Effect of pegylation on pharmaceuticals. *Nature Reviews Drug Discovery, 2(3)*, 214–221.
42. Harris, J.M., Martin, N.E., Modi, M. (2001). Pegylation: A novel process for modifying pharmacokinetics. *Clinical Pharmacokinetics, 40(7)*, 539–551.
43. Rajan, R.S., Li, T., Aras, M., Sloey, C., Sutherland, W., Arai, H., Briddell, R., Kinstler, O., Lueras, A.M., Zhang, Y., Yeghnazar, H., Treuheit, M., Brems, D.N. (2006). Modulation of protein aggregation by polyethylene glycol conjugation: GCSF as a case study. *Protein Science, 15 (5)*, 1063–1075.
44. Muller, A.F., Kopchick, J.J., Flyvbjerg, A., van der Lely, A.J. (2004). Clinical review 166: Growth hormone receptor antagonists. *The Journal of Clinical Endocrinology & Metabolism, 89(4)*, 1503–1511.
45. Veronese, F.M. (2001). Peptide and protein PEGylation: A review of problems and solutions. *Biomaterials, 22(5)*, 405–417.
46. Veronese, F.M., Pasut, G. (2005). PEGylation, successful approach to drug delivery. *Drug Discovery Today, 10(21)*, 1451–1458.
47. Sinclair, A.M., Elliott, S. (2005). Glycoengineering: The effect of glycosylation on the properties of therapeutic proteins. *Journal of Pharmaceutical Sciences, 94(8)*, 1626–1635.
48. Pisal, D.S., Kosloski, M.P., Balu-Iyer, S.V. (2010). Delivery of therapeutic proteins. *Journal of Pharmaceutical Sciences, 99(6)*, 2557–2575.
49. Gregoriadis, G., Jain, S., Papaioannou, I., Laing, P. (2005). Improving the therapeutic efficacy of peptides and proteins: A role for polysialic acids. *International Journal of Pharmaceutics, 300(1–2)*, 125–130.
50. McKoy, J.M., Stonecash, R.E., Cournoyer, D., Rossert, J., Nissenson, A.R., Raisch, D.W., Casadevall, N., Bennett, C.L. (2008). Epoetin-associated pure red cell aplasia: Past, present, and future considerations. *Transfusion, 48(8)*, 1754–1762.
51. Egrie, J.C., Browne, J. K. (2002). Development and characterization of darbepoetin alfa. *Oncology (Williston Park), 16* (10 Suppl 11), 13–22.
52. Wakefield, I., Stephens, S., Foulkes, R., Nesbitt, A., Bourne, T. (2011). The use of surrogate antibodies to evaluate the developmental and reproductive toxicity potential of an anti-TNFalpha PEGylated Fab' monoclonal antibody. *Toxicological Sciences, 122(1)*, 170–176.
53. Adibi, S.A. (1997). The oligopeptide transporter (Pept-1) in human intestine: Biology and function. *Gastroenterology, 113(1)*, 332–340.
54. Leibach, F.H., Ganapathy, V. (1996). Peptide transporters in the intestine and the kidney. *Annual Review of Nutrition, 16*, 99–119.
55. Liang, R., Fei, Y.J., Prasad, P.D., Ramamoorthy, S., Han, H., Yang-Feng, T.L., Hediger, M.A., Ganapathy, V., Leibach, F. H. (1995). Human intestinal H+/peptide cotransporter. Cloning, functional expression, and chromosomal localization. *The Journal of Biological Chemistry, 270(12)*, 6456–6463.
56. Dalmasso, G., Charrier-Hisamuddin, L., Nguyen, H.T., Yan, Y., Sitaraman, S., Merlin, D. (2008). PepT1-mediated tripeptide KPV uptake reduces intestinal inflammation. *Gastroenterology, 134(1)*, 166–178.
57. Chothe, P., Singh, N., Ganapathy, V. (2011). Evidence for two different broad-specificity oligopeptide transporters in intestinal cell line Caco-2 and colonic cell line CCD841. *American Journal of Physiology Cell Physiology, 300(6)*, C1260–C1269.
58. Dunn, W.A., Connolly, T.P., Hubbard, A.L. (1986). Receptor-mediated endocytosis of epidermal growth factor by rat hepatocytes: Receptor pathway. *The Journal of Cell Biology, 102(1)*, 24–36.
59. Burwen, S.J., Barker, M.E., Goldman, I.S., Hradek, G.T., Raper, S.E., Jones, A.L. (1984). Transport of epidermal growth factor by rat liver: Evidence for a nonlysosomal pathway. *The Journal of Cell Biology, 99(4 Pt 1)* 1259–1265.
60. Chen, J., Gamou, S., Takayanagi, A., Shimizu, N. (1994). A novel gene delivery system using EGF receptor-mediated endocytosis. *FEBS Letters, 338(2)*, 167–169.
61. Marchese, C., Mancini, P., Belleudi, F., Felici, A., Gradini, R., Sansolini, T., Frati, L., Torrisi, M.R. (1998). Receptor-

mediated endocytosis of keratinocyte growth factor. *Journal of Cell Science, 111(Pt 23)*, 3517–3527.

62. Roberts, R.L., Sandra, A. (1992). Receptor-mediated endocytosis of insulin by cultured endothelial cells. *Tissue and Cell, 24(5)*, 603–611.
63. Fan, J.Y., Carpentier, J.L., Gorden, P., Van Obberghen, E., Blackett, N.M., Grunfeld, C., Orci, L. (1982). Receptor mediated endocytosis of insulin: Eole of microvilli, coated pits, and coated vesicles. *Proceedings of the National Academy of Sciences U S A, 79(24)*, 7788–7791.
64. Auletta, M., Nielsen, F. C., Gammeltoft, S. (1992). Receptor-mediated endocytosis and degradation of insulin-like growth factor I and II in neonatal rat astrocytes. *Journal of Neuroscience Research, 31(1)*, 14–20.
65. Stitt, A.W., Anderson, H.R., Gardiner, T.A., Bailie, J.R., Archer, D.B. (1994). Receptor-mediated endocytosis and intracellular trafficking of insulin and low-density lipoprotein by retinal vascular endothelial cells. *Investigative Ophthalmology & Visual Science, 35(9)*, 3384–3392.
66. Lovdal, T., Andersen, E., Brech, A., Berg, T. (2000). Fc receptor mediated endocytosis of small soluble immunoglobulin G immune complexes in Kupffer and endothelial cells from rat liver. *Journal of Cell Science, 113(Pt 18)*, 3255–3266.
67. Roberts, R.L., Fine, R.E., Sandra, A. (1993). Receptor-mediated endocytosis of transferrin at the blood-brain barrier. *Journal of Cell Science, 104(Pt 2)*, 521–532.
68. Harding, C., Heuser, J., Stahl, P. (1983). Receptor-mediated endocytosis of transferrin and recycling of the transferrin receptor in rat reticulocytes. *Journal of Cell Biology, 97(2)*, 329–339.
69. Chickering, D.E., Mathiowitz, E. (1999). Definitions, mechanisms and theories of bioadhesion, in E. Mathiowitz, D.E. Chickering, and C.-M. Lehr (eds.), *Bioadhesive Drug Delivery Systems Fundamentals, Novel Approaches and Development.* Marcel Dekker Inc., New York, pp. 1–10.
70. Hejazi, R., Amiji, M. (2003). Chitosan-based gastrointestinal delivery systems. *Journal of Controlled Release, 89(2)*, 151–165.
71. Lehr, C.M. (2000). Lectin-mediated drug delivery: The second generation of bioadhesives. *Journal of Controlled Release, 65(1–2)*, 19–29.
72. Shaikh, R., Raj Singh, T.R., Garland, M.J., Woolfson, A.D., Donnelly, R.F. (2011). Mucoadhesive drug delivery systems. *Journal of Pharmacy and Bioallied Sciences, 3(1)*, 89–100.
73. Peppas, N.A., Bures, P., Leobandung, W., Ichikawa, H. (2000). Hydrogels in pharmaceutical formulations. *European Journal of Pharmaceutics and Biopharmaceutics, 50 (1)*, 27–46.
74. Berger, J., Reist, M., Mayer, J. M., Felt, O., Peppas, N.A., Gurny, R. (2004). Structure and interactions in covalently and ionically crosslinked chitosan hydrogels for biomedical applications. *European Journal of Pharmaceutics and Biopharmaceutics, 57(1)*, 19–34.
75. Kashyap, N., Kumar, N., Kumar, M.N. (2005). Hydrogels for pharmaceutical and biomedical applications. *Critical Reviews in Therapeutic Drug Carrier Systems, 22(2)*, 107–149.
76. Hoffman, A.S. (2002). Hydrogels for biomedical applications. *Advanced Drug Delivery Reviews, 54(1)*, 3–12.
77. Van Tomme, S.R., Hennink, W.E. (2007). Biodegradable dextran hydrogels for protein delivery applications. *Expert Review of Medical Devices, 4(2)*, 147–164.
78. Obara, K., Ishihara, M., Ishizuka, T., Fujita, M., Ozeki, Y., Maehara, T., Saito, Y., Yura, H., Matsui, T., Hattori, H., Kikuchi, M., Kurita, A. (2003). Photocrosslinkable chitosan hydrogel containing fibroblast growth factor-2 stimulates wound healing in healing-impaired db/db mice. *Biomaterials, 24(20)*, 3437–3444.
79. Peattie, R.A., Nayate, A.P., Firpo, M.A., Shelby, J., Fisher, R. J., Prestwich, G.D. (2004). Stimulation of in vivo angiogenesis by cytokine-loaded hyaluronic acid hydrogel implants. *Biomaterials, 25(14)*, 2789–2798.
80. Zheng Shu, X., Liu, Y., Palumbo, F.S., Luo, Y., Prestwich, G. D. (2004). In situ crosslinkable hyaluronan hydrogels for tissue engineering. *Biomaterials, 25(7–8)*, 1339–1348.
81. Leonard, M., De Boisseson, M.R., Hubert, P., Dalencon, F., Dellacherie, E. (2004). Hydrophobically modified alginate hydrogels as protein carriers with specific controlled release properties. *Journal of Controlled Release, 98(3)*, 395–405.
82. Wee, S., Gombotz, W.R. (1998). Protein release from alginate matrices. *Advanced Drug Delivery Reviews, 31(3)*, 267–285.
83. Sutter, M., Siepmann, J., Hennink, W.E., Jiskoot, W. (2007). Recombinant gelatin hydrogels for the sustained release of proteins. *Journal of Controlled Release, 119(3)*, 301–312.
84. Ferreira, L., Gil, M.H., Cabrita, A.M., Dordick, J.S. (2005). Biocatalytic synthesis of highly ordered degradable dextran-based hydrogels. *Biomaterials, 26(23)*, 4707–4716.
85. van de Wetering, P., Metters, A.T., Schoenmakers, R.G., Hubbell, J.A. (2005). Poly(ethylene glycol) hydrogels formed by conjugate addition with controllable swelling, degradation, and release of pharmaceutically active proteins. *Journal of Controlled Release, 102(3)*, 619–627.
86. Quick, D.J., Anseth, K.S. (2004). DNA delivery from photocrosslinked PEG hydrogels: Encapsulation efficiency, release profiles, and DNA quality. *Journal of Controlled Release, 96(2)*, 341–351.
87. He, H., Guan, J., Lee, J.L. (2006). An oral delivery device based on self-folding hydrogels. *Journal of Controlled Release, 110(2)*, 339–346.
88. Lu, S., Anseth, K.S. (1999). Photopolymerization of multilaminated poly(HEMA) hydrogels for controlled release. *Journal of Controlled Release, 57(3)*, 291–300.
89. Singh, V., Bushetti, S.S., Raju, S.A., Ahmad, R., Singh, M., Ajmal, M. (2011). Polymeric ocular hydrogels and ophthalmic inserts for controlled release of timolol maleate. *Journal of Pharmacy and Bioallied Sciences, 3(2)*, 280–285.
90. Soontornworajit, B., Zhou, J., Snipes, M.P., Battig, M.R., Wang, Y. (2011). Affinity hydrogels for controlled protein release using nucleic acid aptamers and complementary oligonucleotides. *Biomaterials, 32(28)*, 6839–6849.

91. Bhattarai, N., Gunn, J., Zhang, M. (2010). Chitosan-based hydrogels for controlled, localized drug delivery. *Advanced Drug Delivery Reviews*, *62(1)*, 83–99.
92. Romero, V.L., Manzo, R.H., Alovero, F.L. (2010). Enhanced bacterial uptake and bactericidal properties of ofloxacin loaded on bioadhesive hydrogels against Pseudomonas aeruginosa. *Journal of Chemotherapy*, *22(5)*, 328–334.
93. Collaud, S., Warloe, T., Jordan, O., Gurny, R., Lange, N. (2007). Clinical evaluation of bioadhesive hydrogels for topical delivery of hexylaminolevulinate to Barrett's esophagus. *Journal of Controlled Release*, *123(3)*, 203–210.
94. Peppas, N.A., Sahlin, J.J. (1996). Hydrogels as mucoadhesive and bioadhesive materials: A review. *Biomaterials*, *17(16)*, 1553–1561.
95. Kim, S.H., Kiick, K.L. (2010). Cell-mediated delivery and targeted erosion of vascular endothelial growth factor-cross-linked hydrogels. *Macromolecular Rapid Communications*, *31(14)*, 1231–1240.
96. Wang, Y.C., Wu, J., Li, Y., Du, J.Z., Yuan, Y.Y., Wang, J. (2010). Engineering nanoscopic hydrogels via photo-cross-linking salt-induced polymer assembly for targeted drug delivery. *Chemical Communications (Cambridge)*, *46(20)*, 3520–3522.
97. Soppimath, K.S., Aminabhavi, T.M., Dave, A.M., Kumbar, S. G., Rudzinski, W.E. (2002). Stimulus-responsive "smart" hydrogels as novel drug delivery systems. *Drug Development and Industrial Pharmacy*, *28(8)*, 957–974.
98. Qiu, Y., Park, K. (2001). Environment-sensitive hydrogels for drug delivery. *Advanced Drug Delivery Reviews*, *53(3)*, 321–339.
99. Perakslis, E., Tuesca, A., Lowman, A. (2007). Complexation hydrogels for oral protein delivery: An in vitro assessment of the insulin transport-enhancing effects following dissolution in simulated digestive fluids. *Journal of Biomaterials Science, Polymer Edition*, *18(12)*, 1475–1490.
100. El-Sherbiny, I.M., Salama, A., Sarhan, A.A. (2011). Ionotropically cross-linked pH-sensitive IPN hydrogel matrices as potential carriers for intestine-specific oral delivery of protein drugs. *Drug Development and Industrial Pharmacy*, *37(2)*, 121–130.
101. Yin, L., Zhao, X., Cui, L., Ding, J., He, M., Tang, C., Yin, C. (2009). Cytotoxicity and genotoxicity of superporous hydrogel containing interpenetrating polymer networks. *Food and Chemical Toxicology*, *47(6)*, 1139–1145.
102. Carr, D.A., Gomez-Burgaz, M., Boudes, M.C., Peppas, N.A. (2010). Complexation hydrogels for the oral delivery of growth hormone and salmon calcitonin. *Industrial & Engineering Chemistry Research*, *49(23)*, 11991–11995.
103. Wood, K.M., Stone, G.M., Peppas, N.A. (2008). Wheat germ agglutinin functionalized complexation hydrogels for oral insulin delivery. *Biomacromolecules*, *9(4)*, 1293–1298.
104. Cui, F., He, C., He, M., Tang, C., Yin, L., Qian, F., Yin, C. (2009). Preparation and evaluation of chitosan-ethylenediaminetetraacetic acid hydrogel films for the mucoadhesive transbuccal delivery of insulin. *Journal of Biomedical Materials Research Part A*, *89(4)*, 1063–1071.
105. Lin, Y.H., Liang, H.F., Chung, C.K., Chen, M.C., Sung, H.W. (2005). Physically crosslinked alginate/N, O-carboxymethyl chitosan hydrogels with calcium for oral delivery of protein drugs. *Biomaterials*, *26(14)*, 2105–2113.
106. Chen, F.M., Zhao, Y.M., Sun, H.H., Jin, T., Wang, Q.T., Zhou, W., Wu, Z.F., Jin, Y. (2007). Novel glycidyl methacrylated dextran (Dex-GMA)/gelatin hydrogel scaffolds containing microspheres loaded with bone morphogenetic proteins: Formulation and characteristics. *Journal of Controlled Release*, *118(1)*, 65–77.
107. Chen, F., Wu, Z., Wang, Q., Wu, H., Zhang, Y., Nie, X., Jin, Y. (2005). Preparation and biological characteristics of recombinant human bone morphogenetic protein-2-loaded dextran-co-gelatin hydrogel microspheres, in vitro and in vivo studies. *Pharmacology*, *75(3)*, 133–144.
108. Bernkop-Schnurch, A., Schwarz, V., Steininger, S. (1999). Polymers with thiol groups: A new generation of mucoadhesive polymers? *Pharmaceutical Research*, *16(6)*, 876–881.
109. Leitner, V.M., Walker, G.F., Bernkop-Schnurch, A. (2003). Thiolated polymers: Evidence for the formation of disulphide bonds with mucus glycoproteins. *European Journal of Pharmaceutics and Biopharmaceutics*, *56*(2), 207–214.
110. Bernkop-Schnurch, A., Hornof, M., Zoidl, T. (2003). Thiolated polymers--thiomers: Synthesis and in vitro evaluation of chitosan-2-iminothiolane conjugates. *International Journal of Pharmaceutics*, *260*(2), 229–237.
111. Bernkop-Schnurch, A., Guggi, D., Pinter, Y. (2004). Thiolated chitosans: Development and in vitro evaluation of a mucoadhesive, permeation enhancing oral drug delivery system. *Journal of Controlled Release*, *94(1)*, 177–186.
112. Luessen, H.L., de Leeuw, B.J., Langemeyer, M.W., de Boer, A.B., Verhoef, J.C., Junginger, H.E. (1996). Mucoadhesive polymers in peroral peptide drug delivery. VI. Carbomer and chitosan improve the intestinal absorption of the peptide drug buserelin in vivo. *Pharmaceutical Research*, *13(11)*, 1668–1672.
113. Grabovac, V., Foger, F., Bernkop-Schnurch, A. (2008). Design and in vivo evaluation of a patch delivery system for insulin based on thiolated polymers. *International Journal of Pharmaceutics*, *348(1–2)*, 169–174.
114. Tao, S.L., Desai, T.A. (2005). Gastrointestinal patch systems for oral drug delivery. *Drug Discovery Today*, *10 (13)*, 909–915.
115. Schmitz, T., Leitner, V.M., Bernkop-Schnurch, A. (2005). Oral heparin delivery: Design and in vivo evaluation of a stomach-targeted mucoadhesive delivery system. *Journal of Pharmaceutical Sciences*, *94(5)*, 966–973.
116. Krauland, A.H., Guggi, D., Bernkop-Schnurch, A. (2004). Oral insulin delivery: The potential of thiolated chitosan-insulin tablets on non-diabetic rats. *Journal of Controlled Release*, *95(3)*, 547–555.
117. Del Curto, M.D., Maroni, A., Palugan, L., Zema, L., Gazzaniga, A., Sangalli, M.E. (2011). Oral delivery system for two-pulse colonic release of protein drugs and protease inhibitor/absorption enhancer compounds. *Journal of Pharmaceutical Sciences*, *100(8)*, 3251–3259.

118. Caillard, R., Petit, A., Subirade, M. (2009). Design and evaluation of succinylated soy protein tablets as delayed drug delivery systems. *International Journal of Biological Macromolecules*, *45(4)*, 414–420.
119. Werle, M., Loretz, B., Entstrasser, D., Foger, F. (2007). Design and evaluation of a chitosan-aprotinin conjugate for the peroral delivery of therapeutic peptides and proteins susceptible to enzymatic degradation. *Journal of Drug Targeting*, *15(5)*, 327–333.
120. Malik, D.K., Baboota, S., Ahuja, A., Hasan, S., Ali, J. (2007). Recent advances in protein and peptide drug delivery systems. *Current Drug Delivery*, *4(2)*, 141–151.
121. Kreuter, J., Alyautdin, R.N., Kharkevich, D.A., Ivanov, A.A. (1995). Passage of peptides through the blood-brain barrier with colloidal polymer particles (nanoparticles). *Brain Research*, *674(1)*, 171–174.
122. Kreuter, J. Nanoparticles, in J. Swarbrick and J. C. Boylan (eds.), *Encyclopedia of Pharmaceutical Technology*, vol. *10*, Marcel Dekker, New York, 1994, pp. 165–190.
123. Chavanpatil, M.D., Khdair, A., Panyam, J. (2006). Nanoparticles for cellular drug delivery: Mechanisms and factors influencing delivery. *Journal of Nanoscience and Nanotechnology*, *6(9–10)*, 2651–2663.
124. Gref, R., Minamitake, Y., Peracchia, M.T., Trubetskoy, V., Torchilin, V., Langer, R. (1994). Biodegradable long-circulating polymeric nanospheres. *Science*, *263(5153)*, 1600–1603.
125. Galindo-Rodriguez, S.A., Allemann, E., Fessi, H., Doelker, E. (2005). Polymeric nanoparticles for oral delivery of drugs and vaccines: A critical evaluation of in vivo studies. *Critical Reviews in Therapeutic Drug Carrier Systems*, *22(5)*, 419–464.
126. Lowe, P.J., Temple, C.S. (1994). Calcitonin and insulin in isobutylcyanoacrylate nanocapsules: Protection against proteases and effect on intestinal absorption in rats. *Journal of Pharmacy and Pharmacology*, *46(7)*, 547–552.
127. Bhattarai, N., Ramay, H.R., Chou, S.H., Zhang, M. (2006). Chitosan and lactic acid-grafted chitosan nanoparticles as carriers for prolonged drug delivery. *International Journal of Nanomedicine*, *1*(2), 181–187.
128. Rodrigues, J.S., Santos-Magalhaes, N.S., Coelho, L.C., Couvreur, P., Ponchel, G., Gref, R. (2003). Novel core(polyester)-shell(polysaccharide) nanoparticles: Protein loading and surface modification with lectins. *Journal of Controlled Release*, *92(1–2)*, 103–112.
129. Kobsa, S., Saltzman, W.M. (2008). Bioengineering approaches to controlled protein delivery. *Pediatric Research*, *63(5)*, 513–519.
130. Freiberg, S., Zhu, X.X. (2004). Polymer microspheres for controlled drug release. *International Journal of Pharmaceutics*, *282(1–2)*, 1–18.
131. Sinha, V.R., Trehan, A. (2003). Biodegradable microspheres for protein delivery. *Journal of Controlled Release*, *90(3)*, 261–280.
132. Pan, Y., Xu, H., Zhao, H.Y., Wei, G., Zheng, J.M. (2002). [Study on preparation and oral efficacy of insulin-loaded poly (lactic-co-glycolic acid) nanoparticles]. *Yao Xue Xue Bao*, *37(5)*, 374–377.
133. Cui, F., Qian, F., Zhao, Z., Yin, L., Tang, C., Yin, C. (2009). Preparation, characterization, and oral delivery of insulin loaded carboxylated chitosan grafted poly(methyl methacrylate) nanoparticles. *Biomacromolecules*, *10(5)*, 1253–1258.
134. Damge, C., Michel, C., Aprahamian, M., Couvreur, P. (1988). New approach for oral administration of insulin with polyalkylcyanoacrylate nanocapsules as drug carrier. *Diabetes*, *37* (2), 246–251.
135. Ma, Z., Lim, T.M., Lim, L.Y. (2005). Pharmacological activity of peroral chitosan-insulin nanoparticles in diabetic rats. *International Journal of Pharmaceutics*, *293(1–2)*, 271–280.
136. Woitiski, C.B., Neufeld, R.J., Veiga, F., Carvalho, R.A., Figueiredo, I.V. (2010). Pharmacological effect of orally delivered insulin facilitated by multilayered stable nanoparticles. *European Journal of Pharmaceutical Sciences*, *41(3–4)*, 556–563.
137. Li, T., Shi, X.W., Du, Y.M., Tang, Y.F. (2007). Quaternized chitosan/alginate nanoparticles for protein delivery. *Journal of Biomedical Materials Research Part A*, *83*(2), 383–390.
138. Chen, F.M., Ma, Z.W., Dong, G.Y., Wu, Z.F. (2009). Composite glycidyl methacrylated dextran (Dex-GMA)/gelatin nanoparticles for localized protein delivery. *Acta Pharmacologica Sinica*, *30(4)*, 485–493.
139. Heffernan, M.J., Murthy, N. (2009). Disulfide-crosslinked polyion micelles for delivery of protein therapeutics. *Annals of Biomedical Engineering*, *37(10)*, 1993–2002.
140. Tamber, H., Johansen, P., Merkle, H.P., Gander, B. (2005). Formulation aspects of biodegradable polymeric microspheres for antigen delivery. *Advanced Drug Delivery Reviews*, *57(3)*, 357–376.
141. Francis, M.F., Cristea, M., Winnik, F.M. (2004). Polymeric micelles for oral drug delivery: Why and how. *Pure and Applied Chemistry*, *76(7–8)*, 1321–1335.
142. Lim, S.B., Rubinstein, I., Sadikot, R.T., Artwohl, J.E., Onyuksel, H. (2011). A novel peptide nanomedicine against acute lung injury: GLP-1 in phospholipid micelles. *Pharmaceutical Research*, *28(3)*, 662–672.
143. Lim, S.B., Rubinstein, I., Onyuksel, H. (2008). Freeze drying of peptide drugs self-associated with long-circulating, biocompatible and biodegradable sterically stabilized phospholipid nanomicelles. *International Journal of Pharmaceutics*, *356(1–2)*, 345–350.
144. Kuzmis, A., Lim, S.B., Desai, E., Jeon, E., Lee, B.S., Rubinstein, I., Onyuksel, H. (2011). Micellar nanomedicine of human neuropeptide Y. *Nanomedicine*, *7(4)*, 464–471.
145. Li, N., Li, X.R., Zhou, Y.X., Li, W.J., Zhao, Y., Ma, S.J., Li, J. W., Gao, Y.J., Liu, Y., Wang, X.L., Yin, D.D. (2012). The use of polyion complex micelles to enhance the oral delivery of salmon calcitonin and transport mechanism across the intestinal epithelial barrier. *Biomaterials*, *33(34)*, 8881–8892.
146. Torchilin, V.P. (2005). Recent advances with liposomes as pharmaceutical carriers. *Nature Reviews Drug Discovery*, *4*(2), 145–160.

147. Mastrobattista, E., Koning, G.A., van Bloois, L., Filipe, A.C., Jiskoot, W., Storm, G. (2002). Functional characterization of an endosome-disruptive peptide and its application in cytosolic delivery of immunoliposome-entrapped proteins. *The Journal of Biological Chemistry, 277(30)*, 27135–27143.

148. Moghimi, S.M., Szebeni, J. (2003). Stealth liposomes and long circulating nanoparticles: Critical issues in pharmacokinetics, opsonization and protein-binding properties. *Progress in Lipid Research, 42(6)*, 463–478.

149. Zhang, Y.F., Xie, S.S., Hou, X.P., Gao, X., Zhang, S., Chen, Z. S. (2000). [Study on preparation and biodistribution of PEG-immunoliposomes with active carboxylic terminals]. *Yao Xue Xue Bao, 35(11)*, 854–859.

150. Drummond, D.C., Meyer, O., Hong, K., Kirpotin, D.B., Papahadjopoulos, D. (1999). Optimizing liposomes for delivery of chemotherapeutic agents to solid tumors. *Pharmacological Reviews, 51(4)*, 691–743.

151. Stanimirovic, D.B., Markovic, M., Micic, D.V., Spatz, M., Mrsulja, B.B. (1994). Liposome-entrapped superoxide dismutase reduces ischemia/reperfusion "oxidative stress" in gerbil brain. *Neurochemical Research, 19(12)*, 1473–1478.

152. Gaspar, M.M., Perez-Soler, R., Cruz, M.E. (1996). Biological characterization of L-asparaginase liposomal formulations. *Cancer Chemotherapy and Pharmacology, 38(4)*, 373–377.

153. Jorge, J.C., Perez-Soler, R., Morais, J.G., Cruz, M.E. (1994). Liposomal palmitoyl-L-asparaginase: Characterization and biological activity. *Cancer Chemotherapy and Pharmacology, 34(3)*, 230–234.

154. Heeremans, J.L., Prevost, R., Bekkers, M.E., Los, P., Emeis, J.J., Kluft, C., Crommelin, D.J. (1995). Thrombolytic treatment with tissue-type plasminogen activator (t-PA) containing liposomes in rabbits: A comparison with free t-PA. *Journal of Thrombosis and Haemostasis, 73(3)*, 488–494.

155. Kanaoka, E., Takahashi, K., Yoshikawa, T., Jizomoto, H., Nishihara, Y., Hirano, K. (2001). A novel and simple type of liposome carrier for recombinant interleukin-2. *Journal of Pharmacy and Pharmacology, 53(3)*, 295–302.

156. Opanasopit, P., Sakai, M., Nishikawa, M., Kawakami, S., Yamashita, F., Hashida, M. (2002). Inhibition of liver metastasis by targeting of immunomodulators using mannosylated liposome carriers. *Journal of Controlled Release, 80(1–3)*, 283–294.

157. Kisel, M.A., Kulik, L.N., Tsybovsky, I.S., Vlasov, A.P., Vorob'yov, M.S., Kholodova, E.A., Zabarovskaya, Z.V. (2001). Liposomes with phosphatidylethanol as a carrier for oral delivery of insulin: Studies in the rat. *International Journal of Pharmaceutics, 216(1–2)*, 105–114.

14

DELIVERY OF NUCLEIC ACIDS

SHAOYING WANG, BIN QIN, AND KUN CHENG

14.1 CHAPTER OBJECTIVES

- To describe and compare the mechanisms, advantages, and drawbacks of different types of nucleic acids.
- To illustrate the major challenges and biological barriers faced by nucleic acid delivery.
- To illustrate the rationale of designing nucleic acid delivery systems.
- To review nonviral and viral delivery systems adopted in nucleic acid delivery.

14.2 INTRODUCTION

Nucleic acids, including DNA and RNA, are the genetic material of all known organisms. Nucleic acids are composed of chemically linked sequences of nucleotides. Each nucleotide consists of a sugar, a phosphate group, and a nitrogenous base. Since the discovery of DNA in the 1950s, nucleic acids have revolutionized not only our ability to understand the fundamental basis of life but also our capability to develop novel therapeutics. The sequencing of the human genome and the elucidation of a wide variety of disease-associated molecular pathways provide extraordinary opportunities for the advancement of nucleic-acid-based therapies. Compared with small-molecule drugs, nucleic acids have a high therapeutic potential because a large number of human diseases is caused by aberrant gene expression. Therapeutic nucleic acids include plasmids, oligonucleotides, ribozymes, aptamers, and small interfering RNAs (siRNAs) (Table 14.1). Through introducing therapeutic nucleic acids into diseased cells, the defective genes can be corrected, replaced, or silenced [1]. Most nucleic acids exhibit their biological activity at either the transcriptional or the posttranscriptional level within the cell; however, the aptamer acts extracellularly by blocking cell signal transduction by binding to membrane proteins [2] (Figure 14.1). Although tremendous efforts have been devoted to the development of therapeutic nucleic acids, only two nucleic acid drugs are available in the market: Vitravene (ISIS Pharmaceuticals, Inc., Carlsbad, CA), an antisense oligonucleotide targeting a viral gene, and Macugen (Pfizer, New York, NY), a chemically modified DNA aptamer that binds to the vascular endothelial growth factor (VEGF). Both of these nucleic acid drugs are applied to ocular diseases by intravitreal injection rather than by systematic administration, which is the preferred route for most nucleic acid therapies [3, 4].

The major hurdle that limits the clinical application of nucleic acids is the lack of a safe and efficient delivery system to transport the nucleic acids to the target cells. To be effective, nucleic acids must overcome a series of biological barriers before reaching their site of action within the body.

Advanced Drug Delivery, First Edition. Edited by Ashim K. Mitra, Chi H. Lee, and Kun Cheng.

TABLE 14.1 Characteristics of Different Types of Nucleic Acids

Nucleic Acid	Length	Type	Site of Action
siRNA	21–23 bp	Double-stranded RNA	Cytoplasm
Oligonucleotide	13–35 nt	Single-stranded DNA	Cytoplasm/nucleus
Aptamer	12–30 nt	Single-stranded DNA or RNA	Cell surface
Plasmid	1–1000 kbp	Double-stranded circle DNA	Nucleus
Ribozyme	400–600 nt	Single-stranded RNA	Cytoplasm

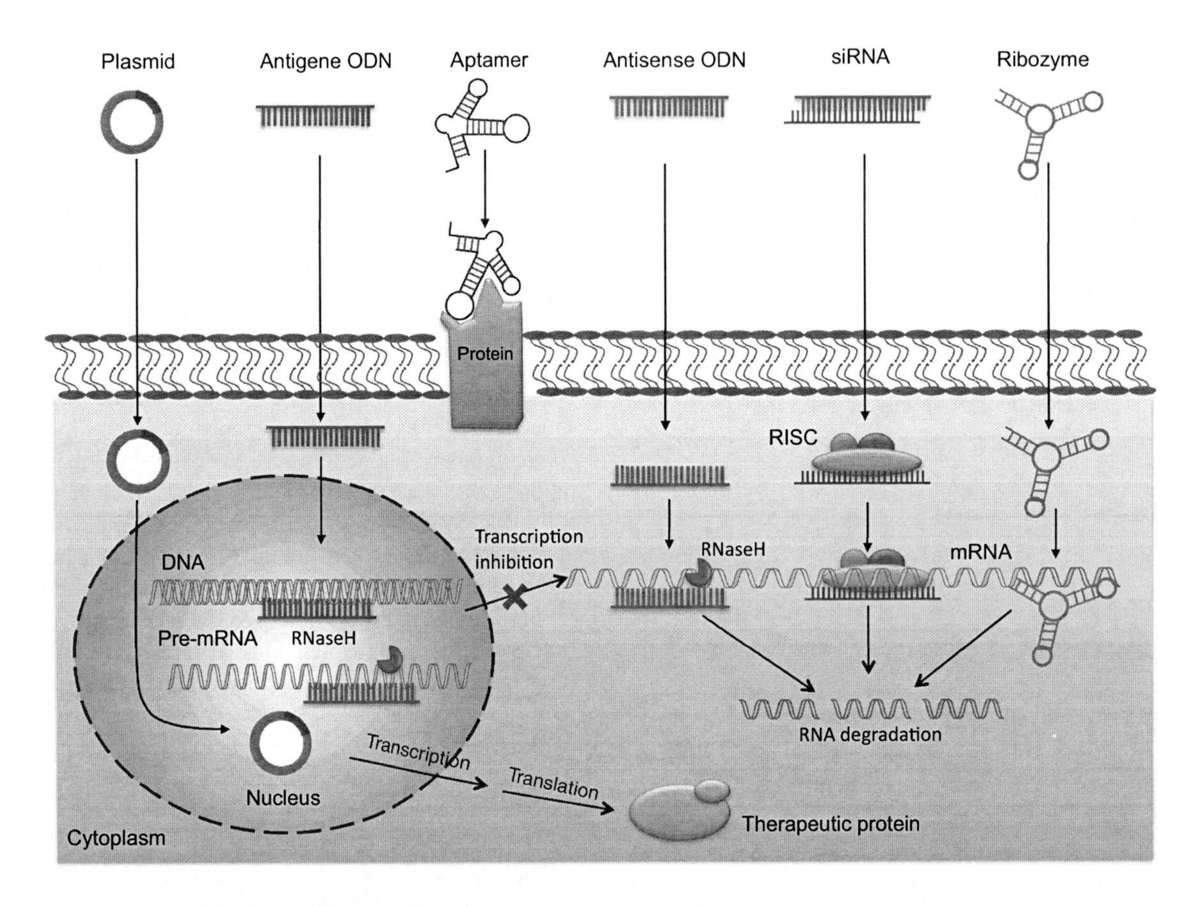

FIGURE 14.1 Different types of nucleic acids and their mechanisms. (i) Plasmids must be delivered into the cell nucleus to express encoded transgenes. (ii) Antigene ODNs exhibit activities at the transcriptional level by forming a triplex with genomic DNA in a sequence-specific manner on the polypurine-polypyrimidine tracts. (iii) Aptamers act extracellularly by binding to membrane proteins. (iv) siRNAs induce the breakdown of target mRNAs in the cytoplasm. (v) Antisense ODNs inhibit gene expressions at the posttranscriptional level. (vi) Ribozymes bind to substrate RNAs in the cytoplasm via Watson-Crick base pairing and cleave the target RNA in a nonhydrolytic reaction. (See color figure in color plate section.)

However, nucleic acids are very unstable in the physiological environment because of the widely distributed nucleases. In addition, their high molecular weight and negative charge make it difficult for nucleic acids to pass through cell membranes. This chapter provides an overview of therapeutic nucleic acids, the biological barriers faced by nucleic acid delivery, and various strategies that have been employed to deliver nucleic acids.

14.3 TYPES OF NUCLEIC ACIDS AND THEIR MECHANISMS

14.3.1 Plasmids

Plasmids are circular double-stranded DNA molecules that have been widely used to introduce recombinant DNA into cells [5]. The plasmids used in genetic engineering are also

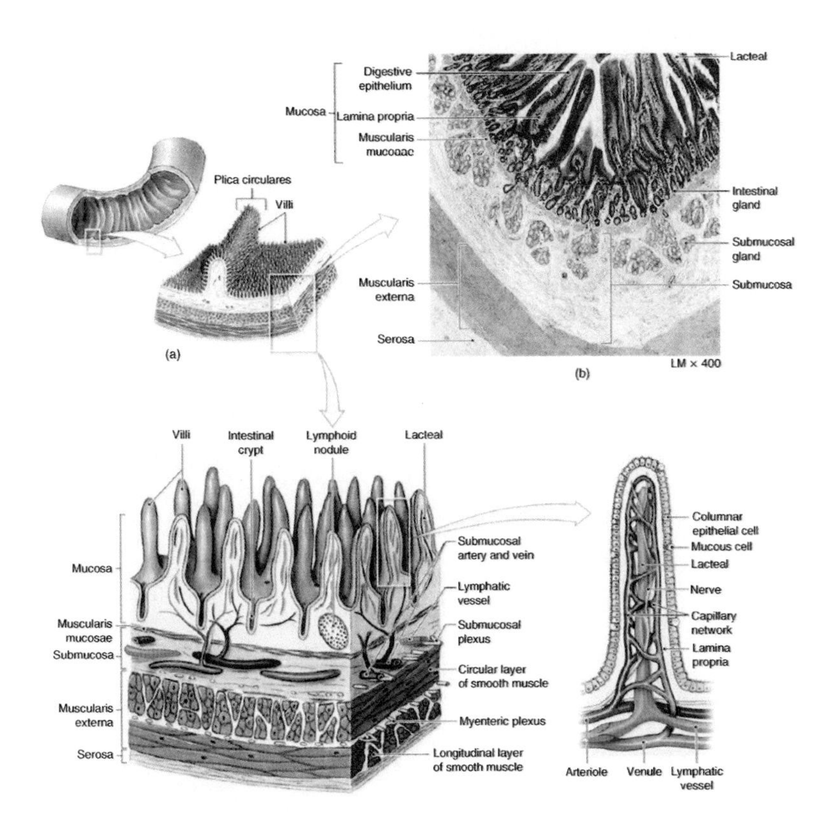

FIGURE 1.2 Gastrointestinal anatomy [8].

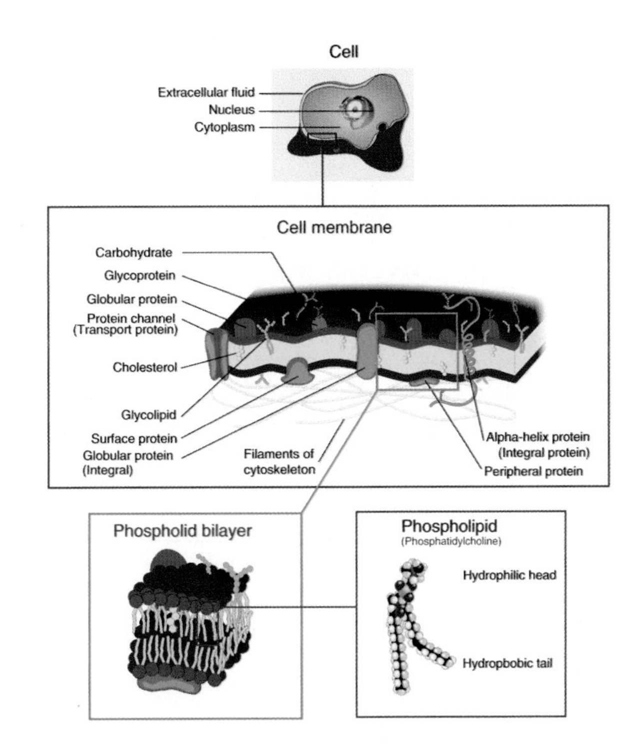

FIGURE 1.5 Illustration of a eukaryotic cell membrane. The cell membrane is a biological membrane that separates the interior of all cells from the outside environment [46].

Advanced Drug Delivery, First Edition. Edited by Ashim K. Mitra, Chi H. Lee, and Kun Cheng.

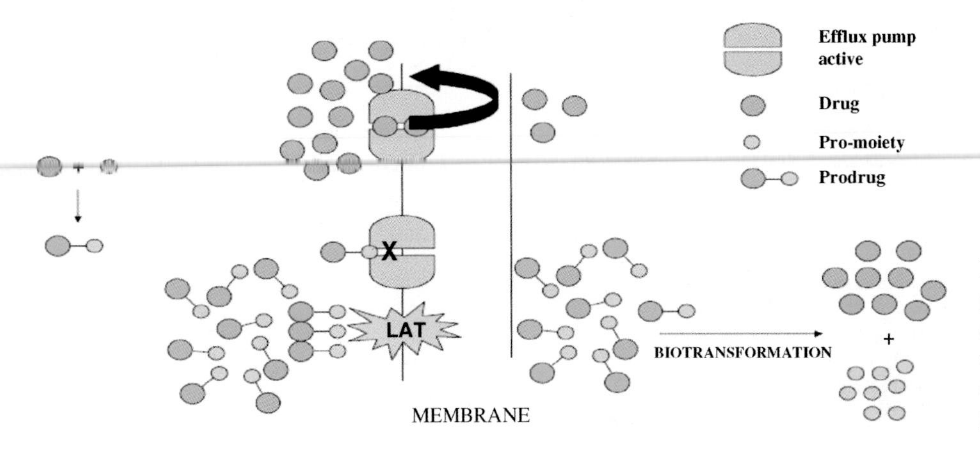

FIGURE 3.5 Transporter-targeted prodrug strategy: Improved permeability could be achieved by overcoming MDR efflux transporters during chemical modification of the parent drug molecule.

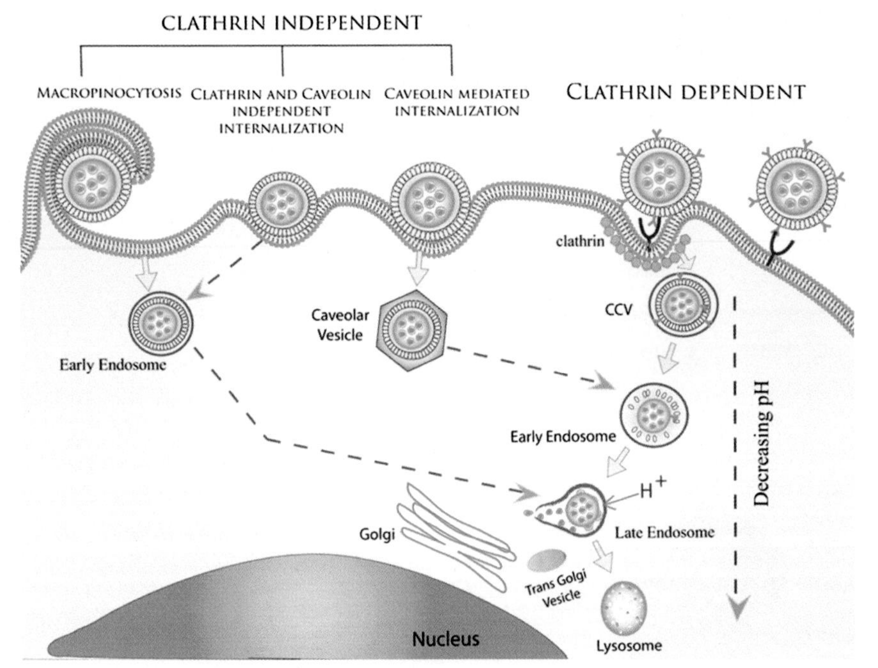

FIGURE 5.3 Schematic illustration of different pathways of endocytosis mechanisms. Phagocytosis and pinocytosis are the two main classes of endocytosis. Pinocytosis can be further classified in clatherin-dependent and clatherin-independent endocytosis.

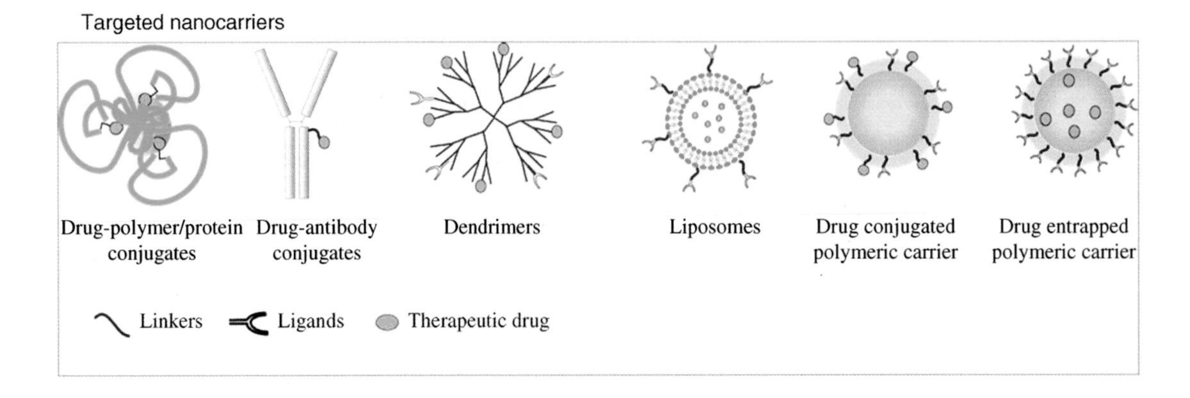

FIGURE 5.4 Schematic representation of numerous nanocarriers used in targeted drug delivery.

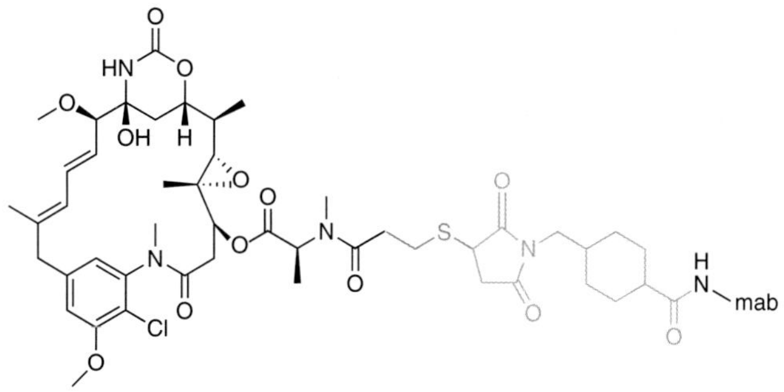

FIGURE 6.7 Structure of antibody-DM1 drug conjugate via SMCC linker.

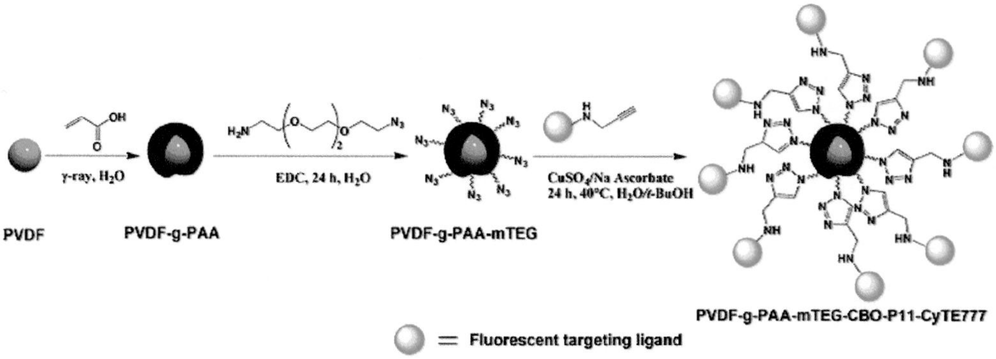

FIGURE 8.6 Functionalization of novel poly(vinylidene fluoride) (PVDF) nanoparticles conjugated to CBO-P11. Radio-grafting of PAA, coupling with azido spacer arm (mTEG), and "click" conjugation of fluorescent targeting ligand (CBO-P11-CyTE777) [179].

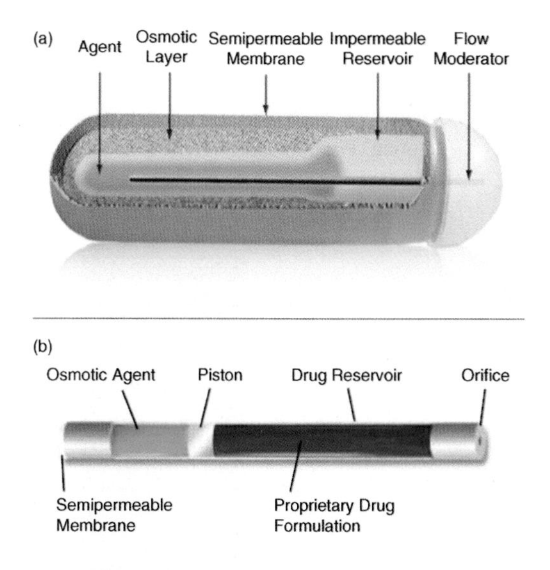

FIGURE 9.8 Cross-sectional view of (a) ALZET and (b) DUROS pumps. Reproduced with permission from ALZET Osmotic Pumps and DURECT Corporation.

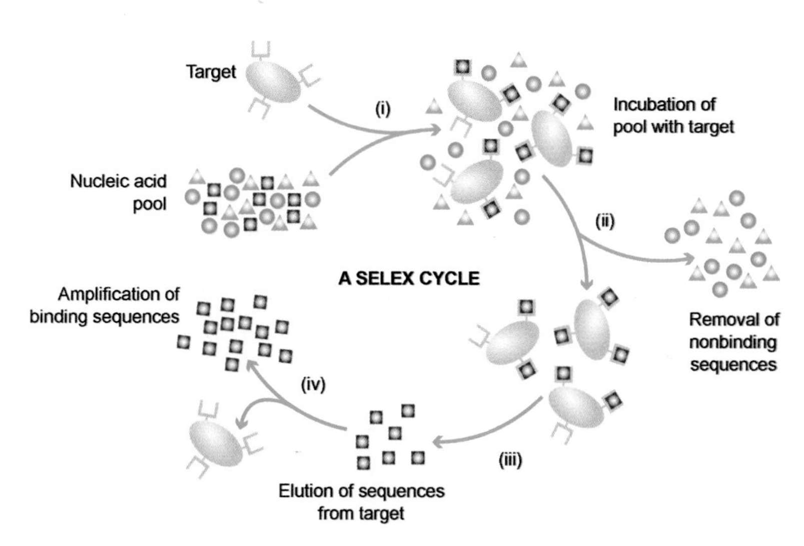

FIGURE 10.2 Scheme of a conventional SELEX cycle: (i) sequence binding, (ii, iii) partitioning, and (iv) amplifying isolated nucleotides.

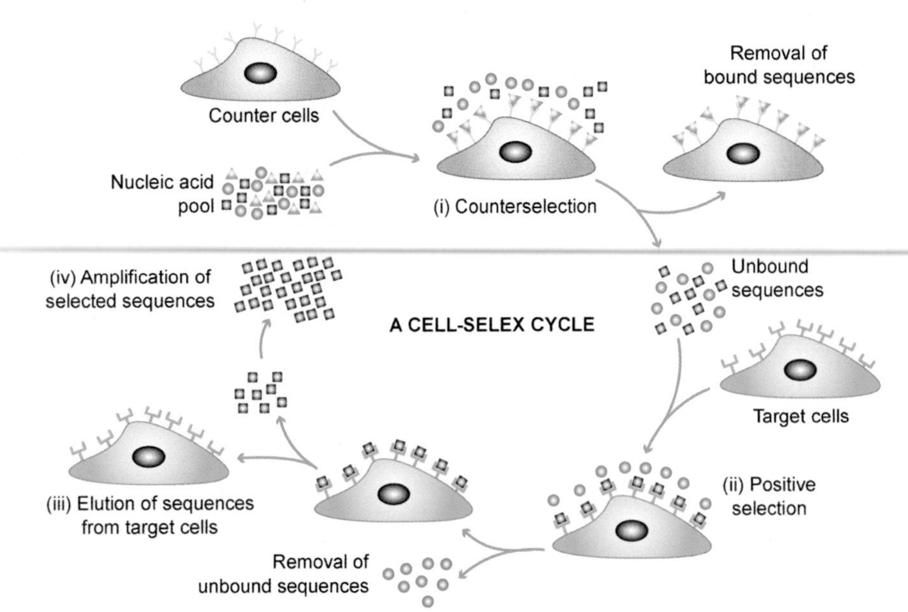

FIGURE 10.3 Scheme of a cell-SELEX cycle: (i) counterselection, (ii) positive selection, and (iii) elution of sequences from targeted cells, and (iv) amplification of selected sequences.

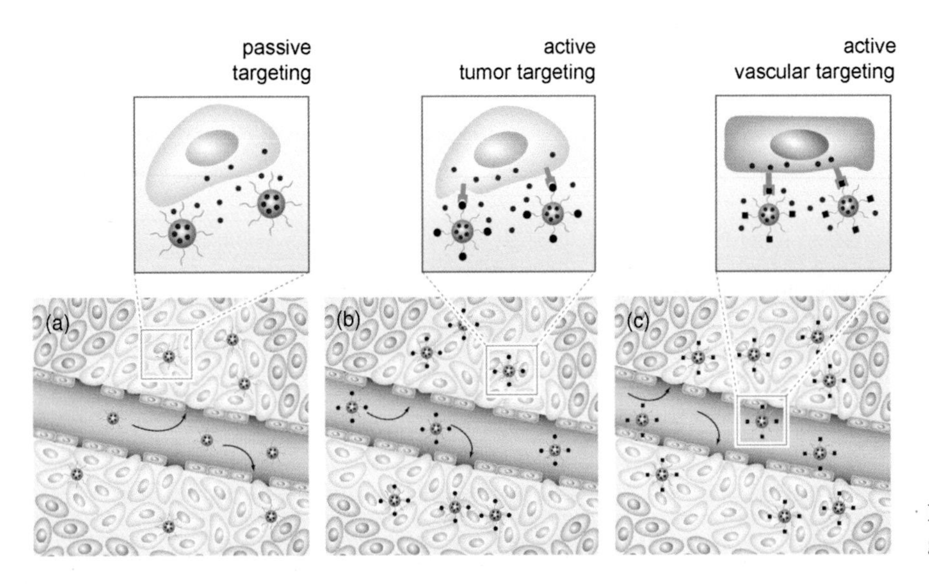

FIGURE 10.7 Passive versus active targeting. Figure adapted from Ref. 61.

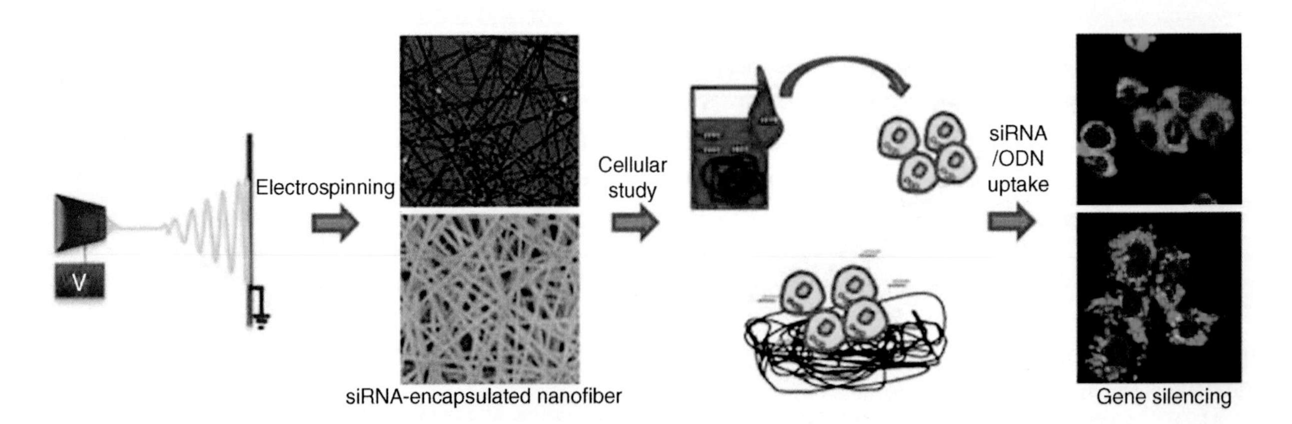

FIGURE 11.5 Diagrammatic representation of siRNA delivery by nanofibrous scaffold [55].

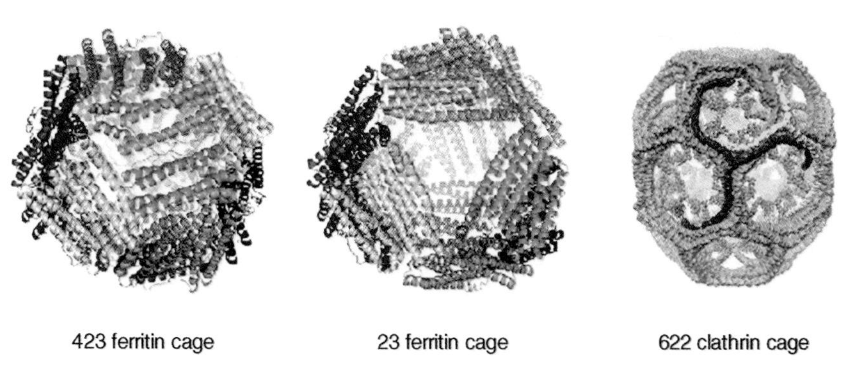

FIGURE 12.1 Native nanoparticles: ribbon diagrams of 423 and 23 ferritin cages (reproduced with permission from Ref. 10) and a cryoelectron image reconstruction of a clathrin cage with three overlapping triskelions shown in different colors (reproduced with permission from Ref. 11).

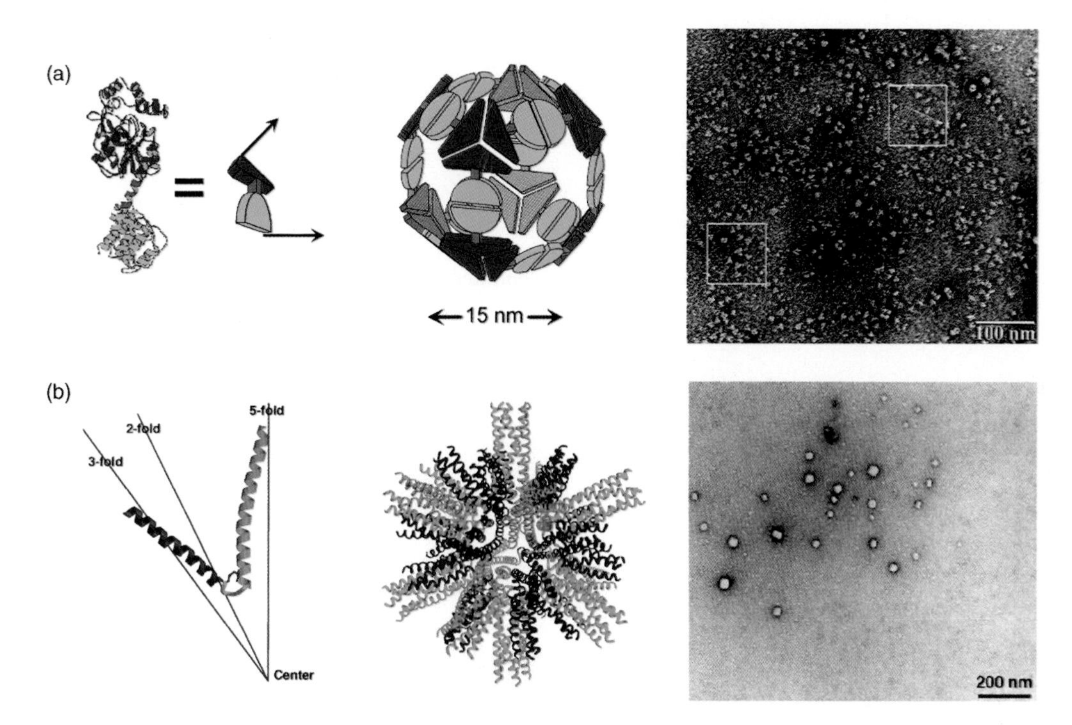

FIGURE 12.3 Polyhedra designs. Schematics of asymmetric building blocks composed of two protein domains (a) and two coiled-coil domains (b) that self-oligomerize into regular nanoparticles, shown both schematically and in electron micrographs. Reproduced with permission from Refs. 26 and 27.

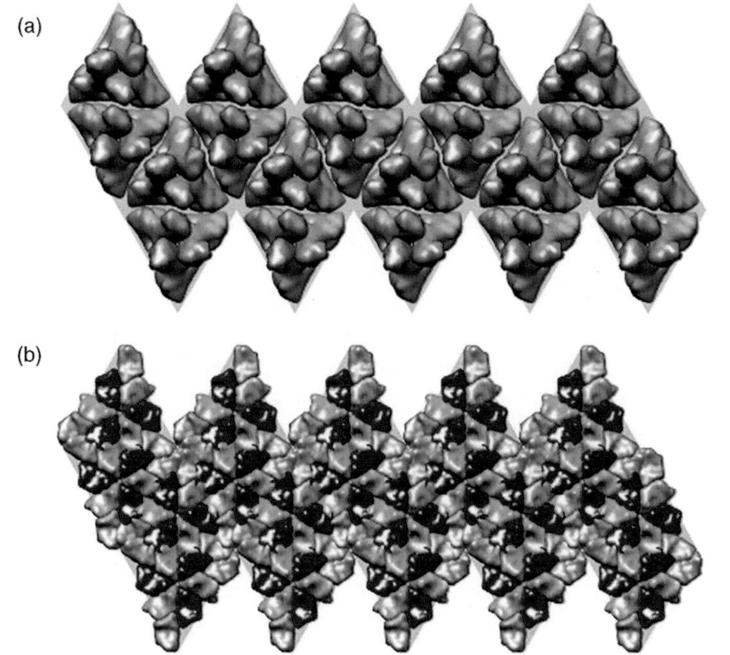

FIGURE 12.7 Hexagonal nets for *Avibirnavirus* (a) and *Sobemovirus* (b). Reproduced with permission from Ref. 35.

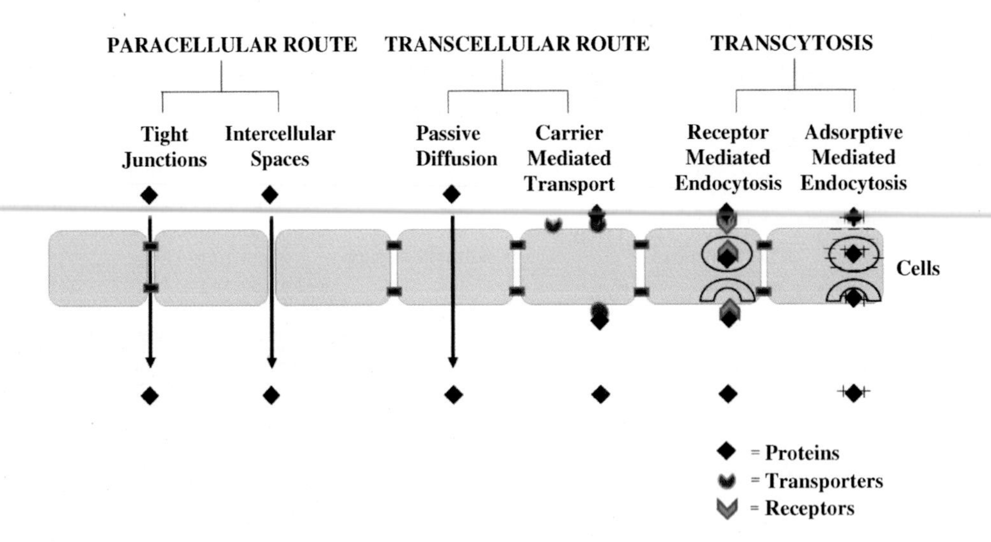

FIGURE 13.1 Various protein transport mechanisms.

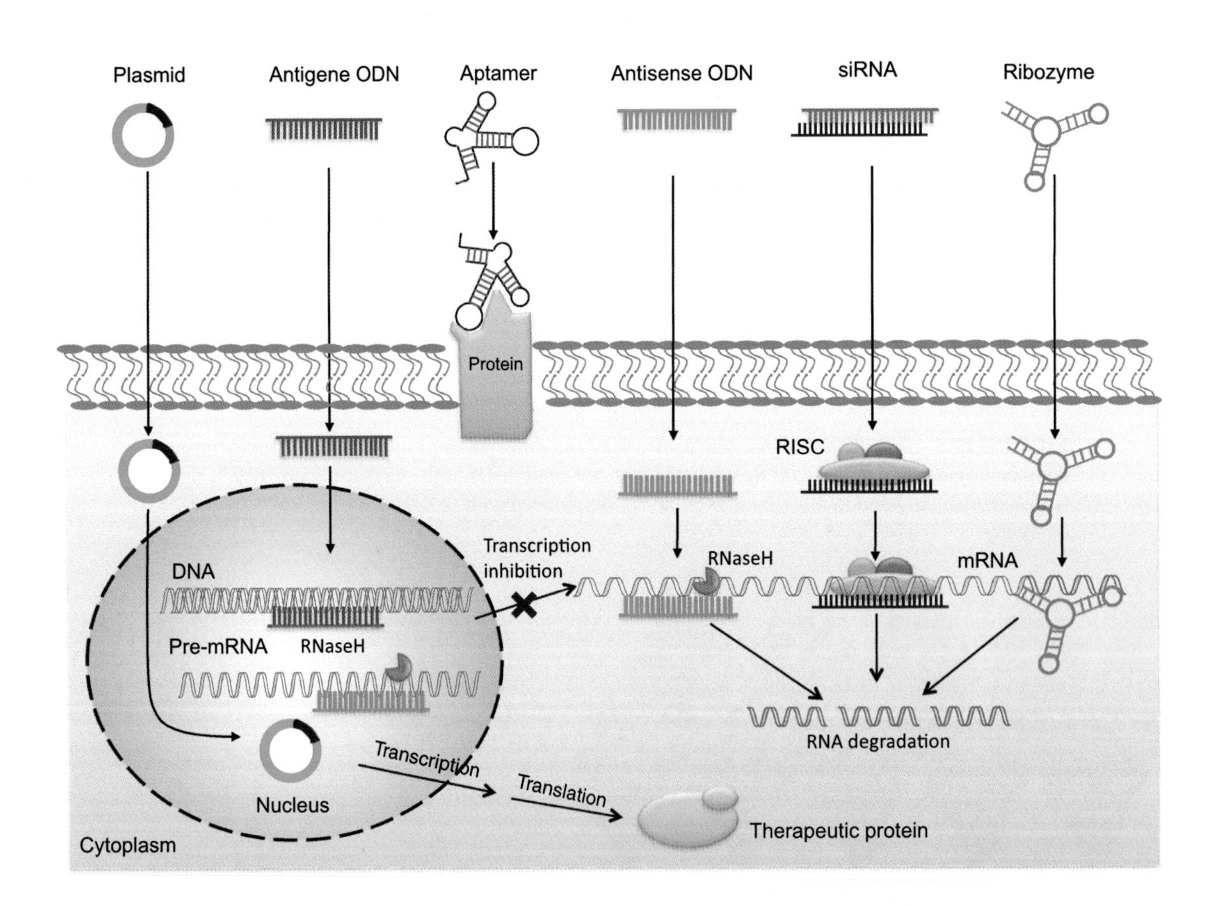

FIGURE 14.1 Different types of nucleic acids and their mechanisms. (i) Plasmids must be delivered into the cell nucleus to express encoded transgenes. (ii) Antigene ODNs exhibit activities at the transcriptional level by forming a triplex with genomic DNA in a sequence-specific manner on the polypurine-polypyrimidine tracts. (iii) Aptamers act extracellularly by binding to membrane proteins. (iv) siRNAs induce the breakdown of target mRNAs in the cytoplasm. (v) Antisense ODNs inhibit gene expressions at the posttranscriptional level. (vi) Ribozymes bind to substrate RNAs in the cytoplasm via Watson-Crick base pairing and cleave the target RNA in a nonhydrolytic reaction.

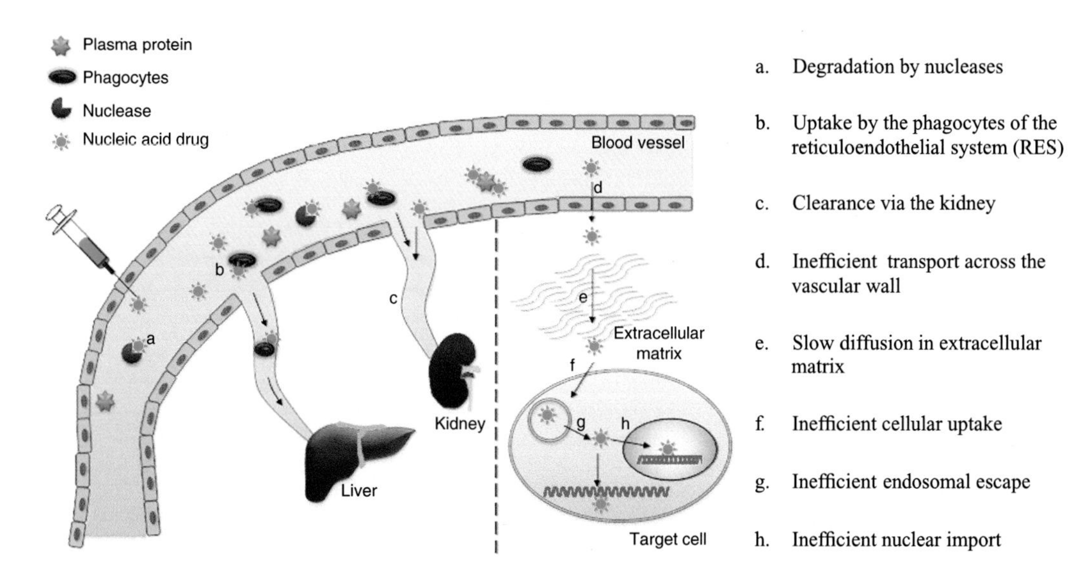

FIGURE 14.2 Various biological barriers faced by nucleic acids *in vivo*. (a) Naked nucleic acids are readily degraded by ubiquitous nucleases in the blood stream and tissues. (b) Nucleic acids are taken up by phagocytes of the RES in the liver and spleen. (c) Nucleic acids are rapidly cleared via the kidney. (d) Inefficient transport across the vascular wall. (e) Extracellular matrix hinders the movement of nucleic acids. (f) Inefficient cellular uptake. (g) Inefficient endosomal escape. (h) Inefficient nuclear import.

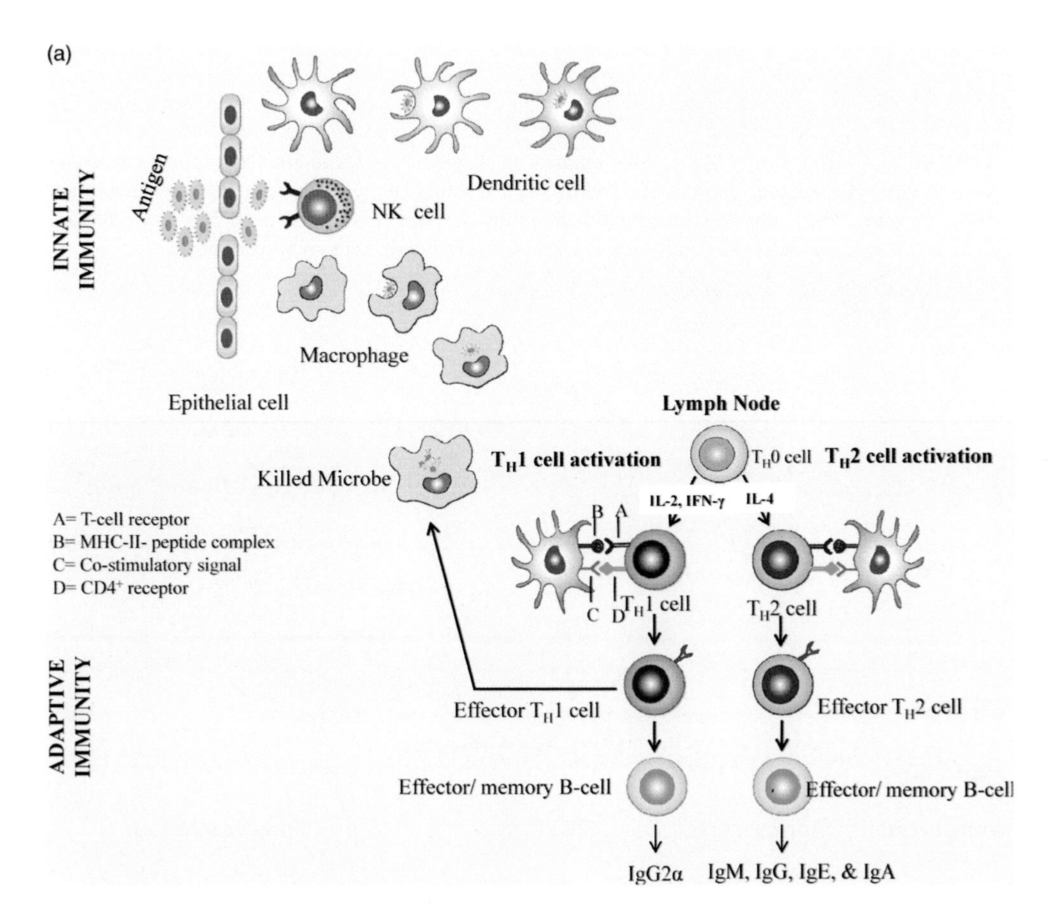

FIGURE 15.1 (a) During a bacterial infection, immature dendritic cells capture vaccine antigens and migrate from infection sites to afferent lymph nodes to become mature dendritic cells. During dendritic cell maturation, ingested antigen undergoes degradation in acidic endosomes to produce small peptides. As a result of an exchange mechanism in the endoplasmic reticulum, antigenic-peptide fragments bound to MHC molecules are translocated to the dendritic cell surface. These mature dendritic cells differentiate naïve T cells into T_H1 and T_H2 cells, which further differentiate naïve B cells to plasma and memory B cells. Distinct classes of cytokines trigger antibody production as well as class switching of antibodies in plasma B cells.

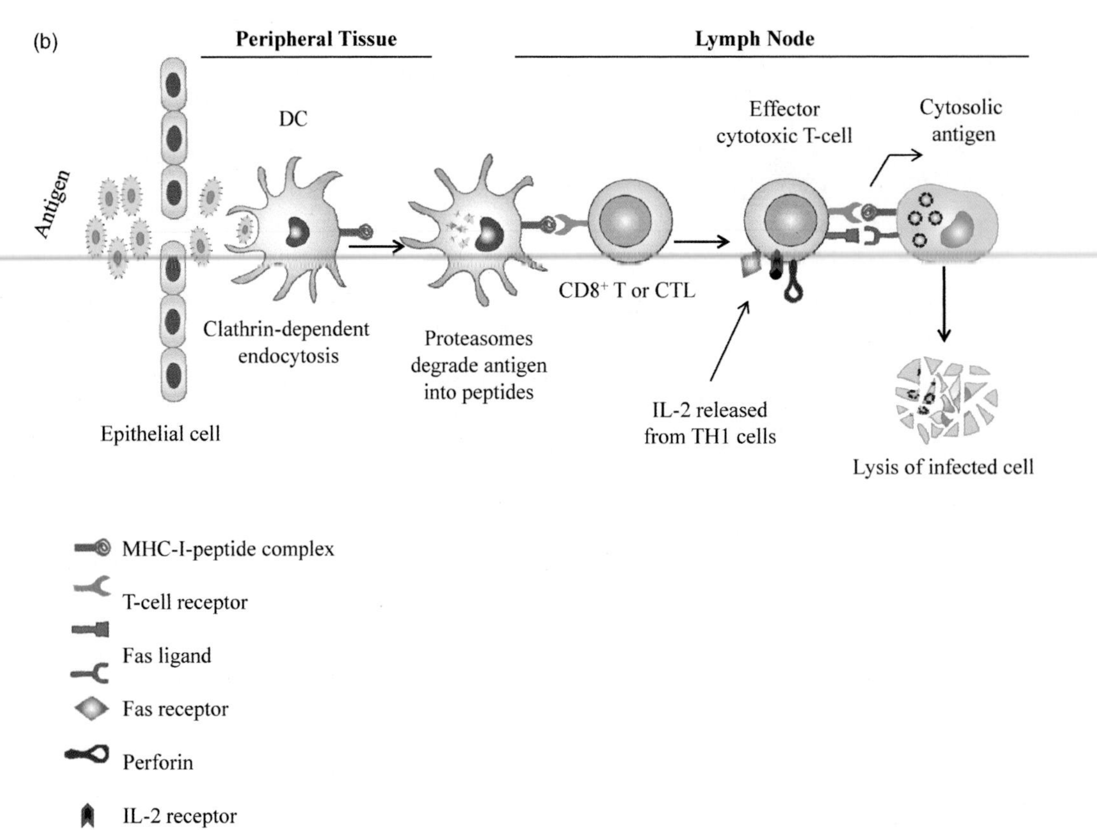

FIGURE 15.1 (b) Demonstrates cellular immune mechanism. Specific internalized antigens, such as viruses, virus-like antigens, intracellular pathogens, and soluble proteins are retained inside dendritic cell endosomes. The internalized antigens escape endosomes and cross into cytosol. Now, the effector cytotoxic T cells cause lysis of pathogen loaded cells through distinct cell-death mechanisms.

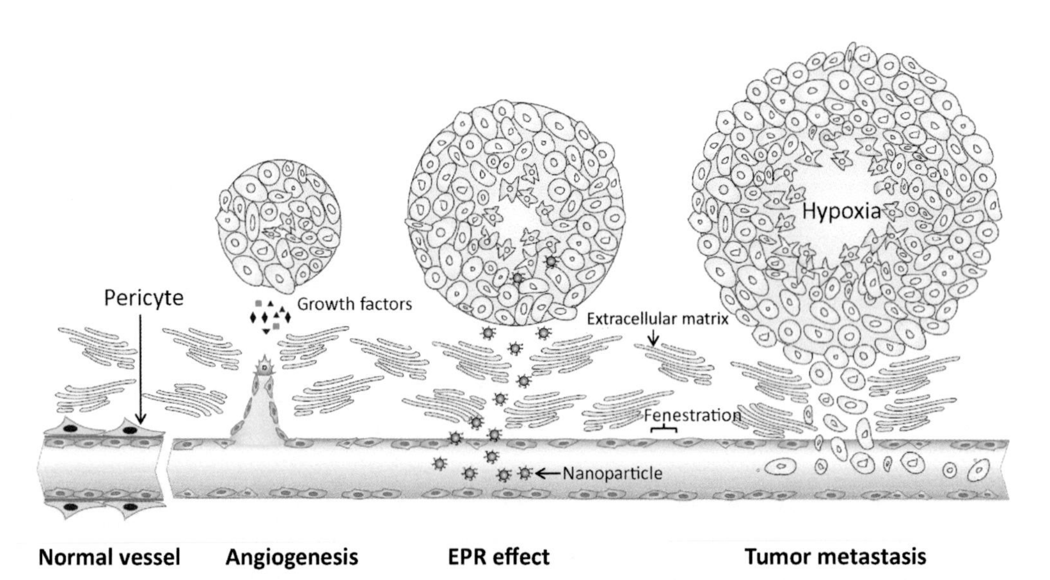

FIGURE 17.1 Tumor microenvironment. The tumor vasculature is structurally different from normal vessels in healthy tissues. In normal vessels, endothelial cells are well aligned along the vessel wall, which is surrounded by pericytes. The walls of tumor vessels have fenestrations and they are not protected by pericytes. The abnormal structure of tumor vasculature leads to the accumulation of macromolecules or particles in tumor tissue, which is called the EPR effect. Tumor cells secrete endothelial growth factors and induce the angiogenesis. Tumor cells also metastasize to other organs through tumor vessels.

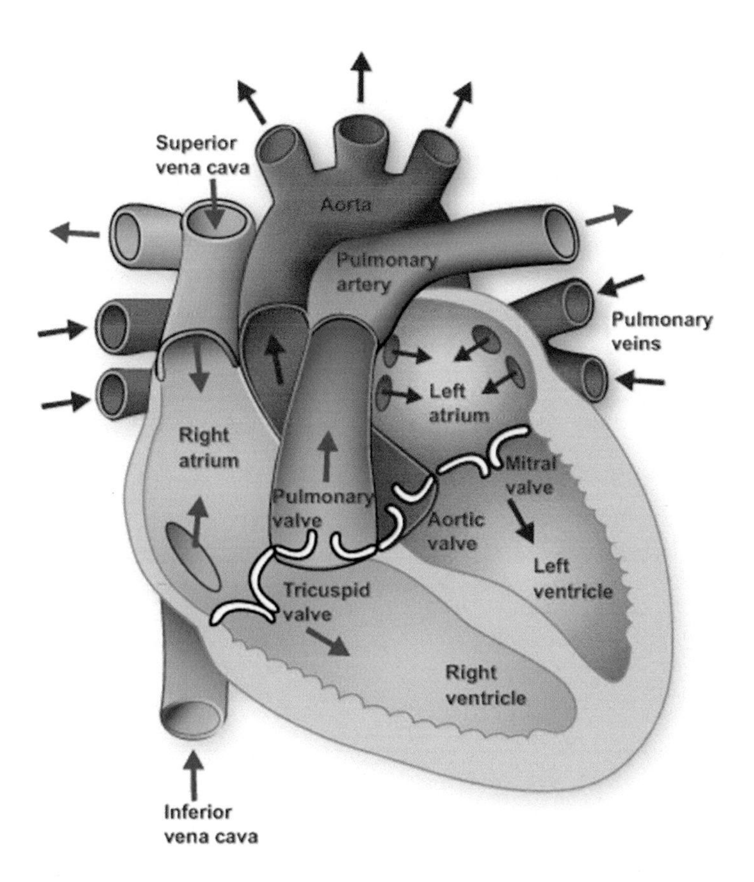

FIGURE 18.1 A cross-section of human heart showing internal chambers and valves. The right chambers, in blue, contain deoxygenated blood. The left heart chambers, in blue, contain oxygenated blood. Reproduced with permission from the Texas Heart Institute.

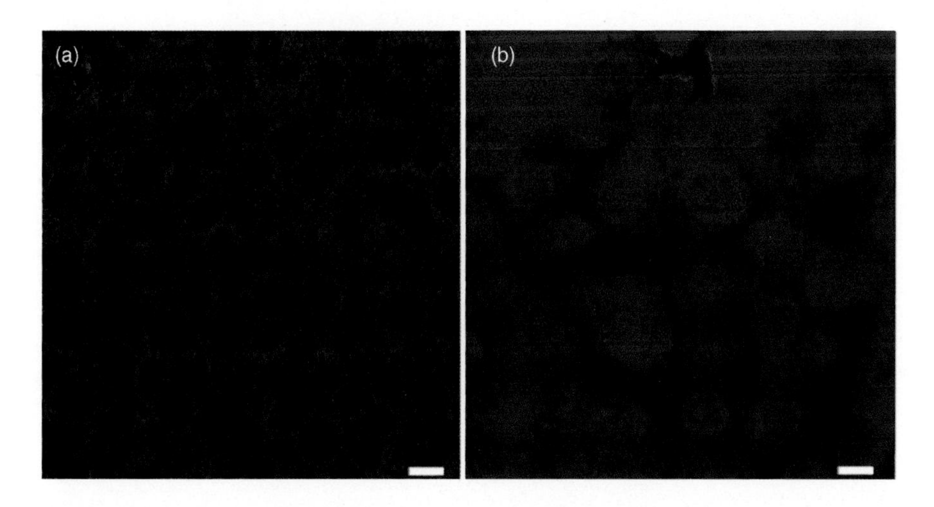

FIGURE 20.8 Cellular uptake profiles of ES nanoparticles in vaginal cells. (a) Nile red solution. Nile red bound on the cell membrane but not crossing the membrane. (b) Nile red-loaded ES nanoparticles. Vaginal cells internalized ES nanoparticles containing nile red and nile red distributed in entire cells, implying that nile red was released from ES nanoparticles in cytosol. Scale bar = 10 μm [173].

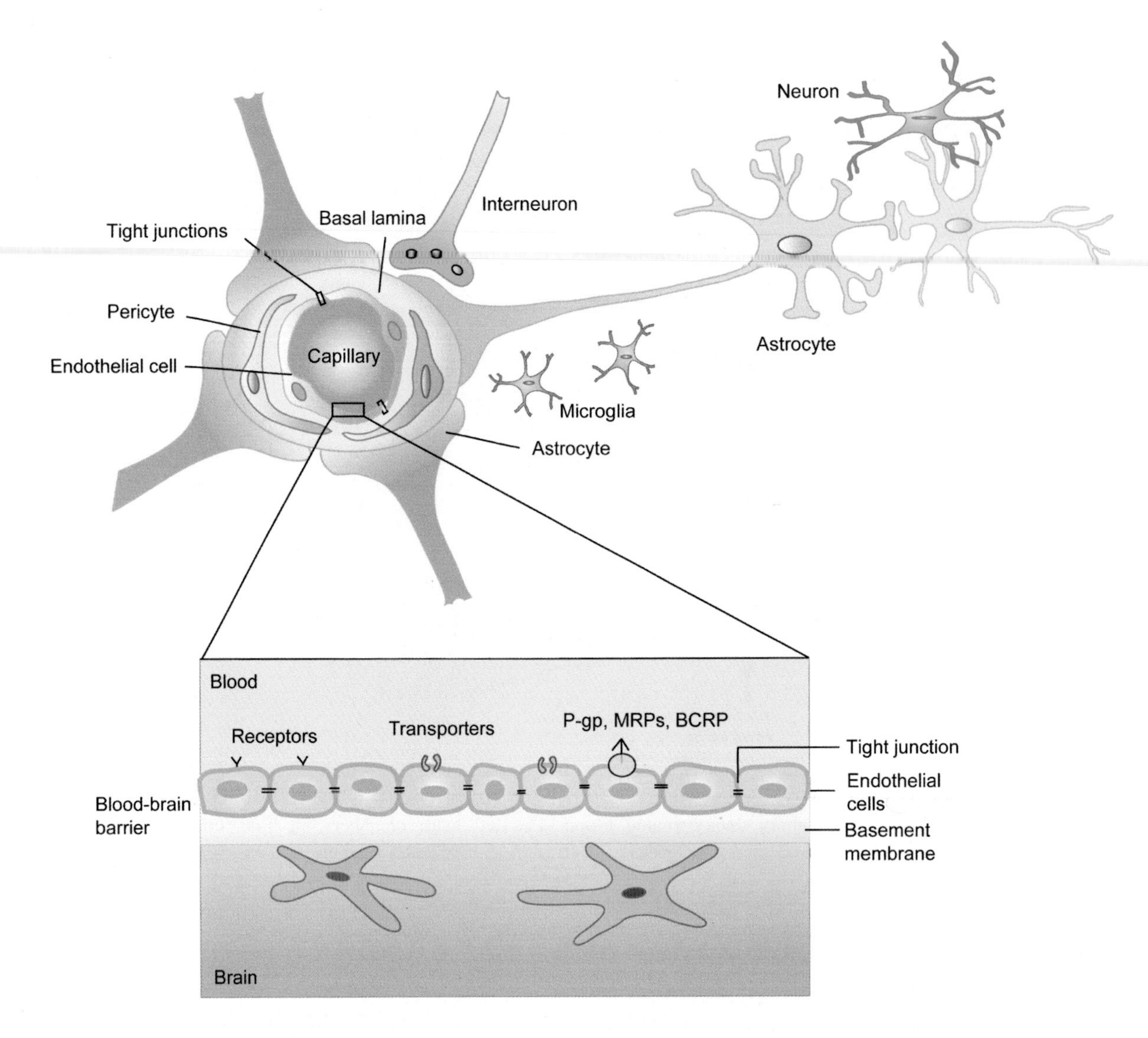

FIGURE 21.1 Schematic representation of the blood–brain barrier.

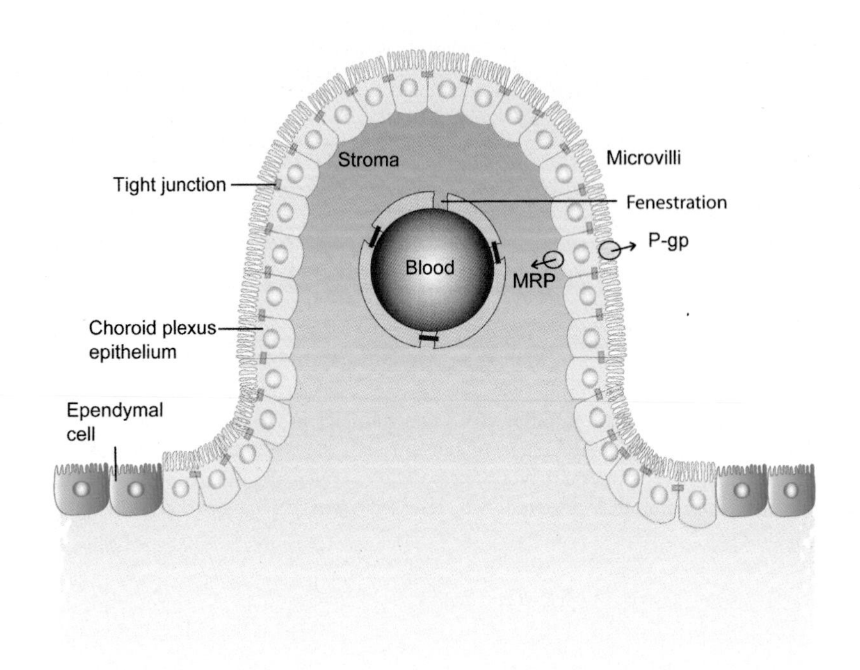

FIGURE 21.2 Schematic representation of the blood–CSF barrier.

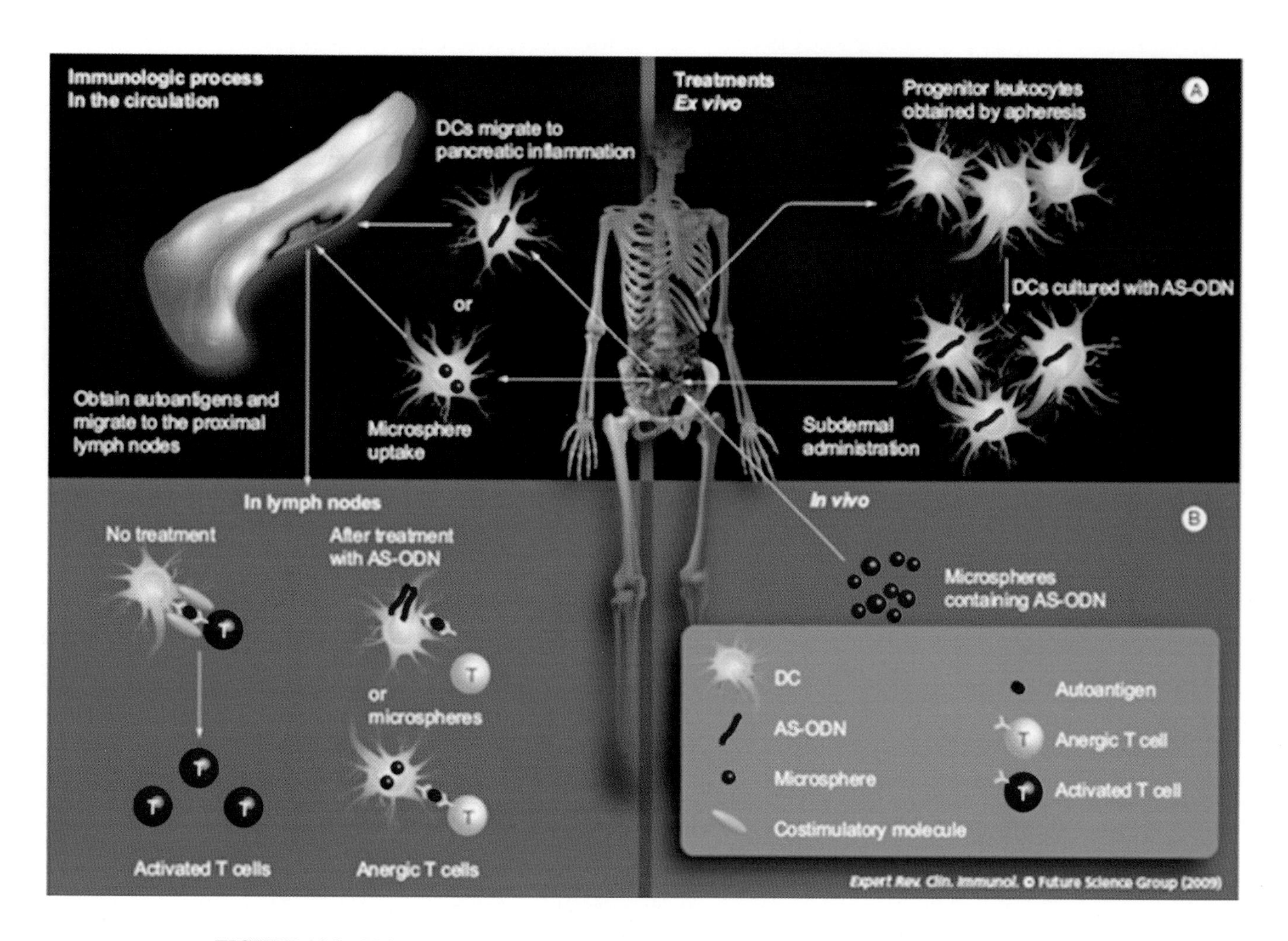

FIGURE 22.2 Using dendritic cells to treat type I diabetes. Reproduced with permission from Ref. 21.

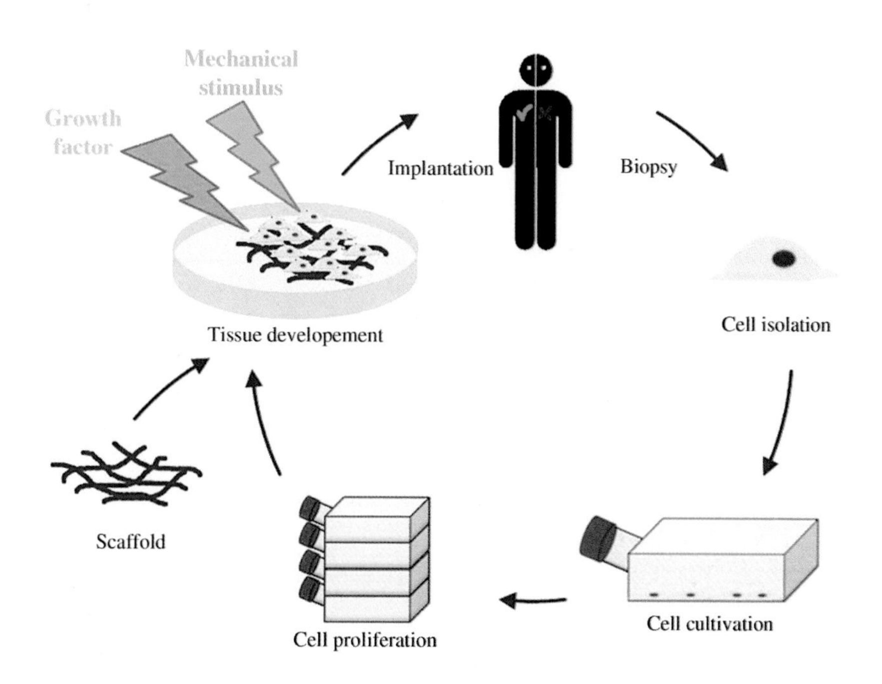

FIGURE 23.2 Tissue engineering in biomedical applications (cited from Wikipedia).

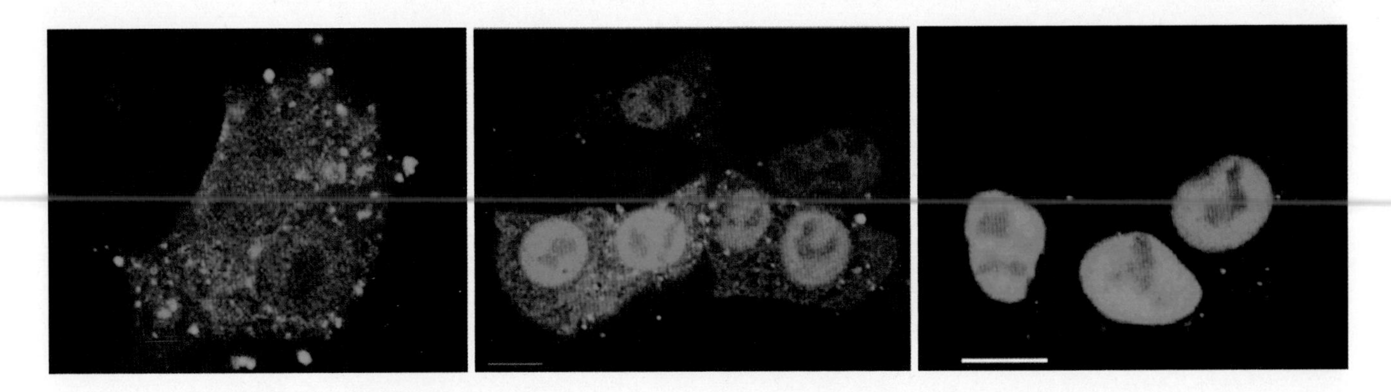

FIGURE 24.2 Confocal images of Hep G2 cells at 15 min (left), 60 (middle) min, and 24 h (right) after cytoplasmic injection of fluorescein-labeled HPMA co-polymers. Adapted from Ref. 76.

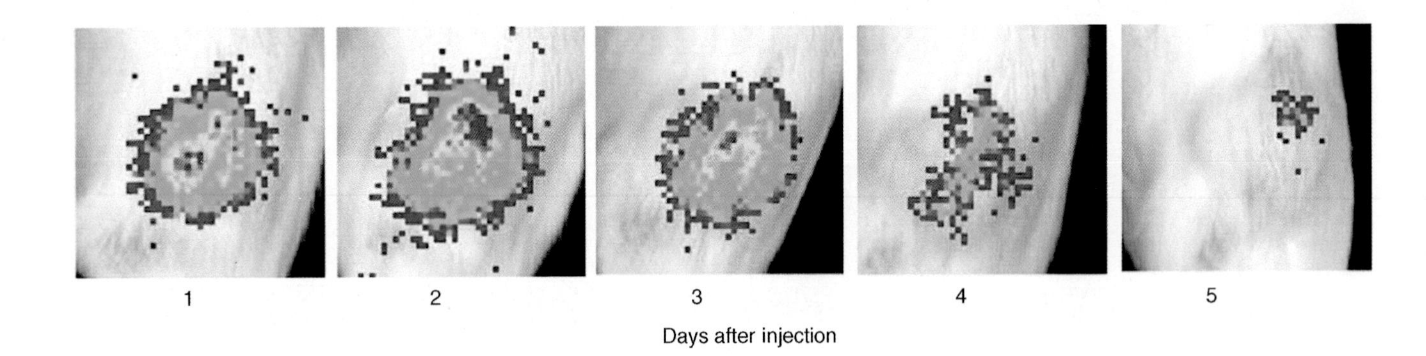

FIGURE 24.7 Color-coded dynamic bioluminescence images of an A/J mouse bearing Neuro2a tumor xenograft at different days after intravenous injection of pCpG-hCMV-Luc/PAMAM G5 polyplexes. Blue color represents the lowest intensity and red for the highest intensity. Adapted from Ref. 115.

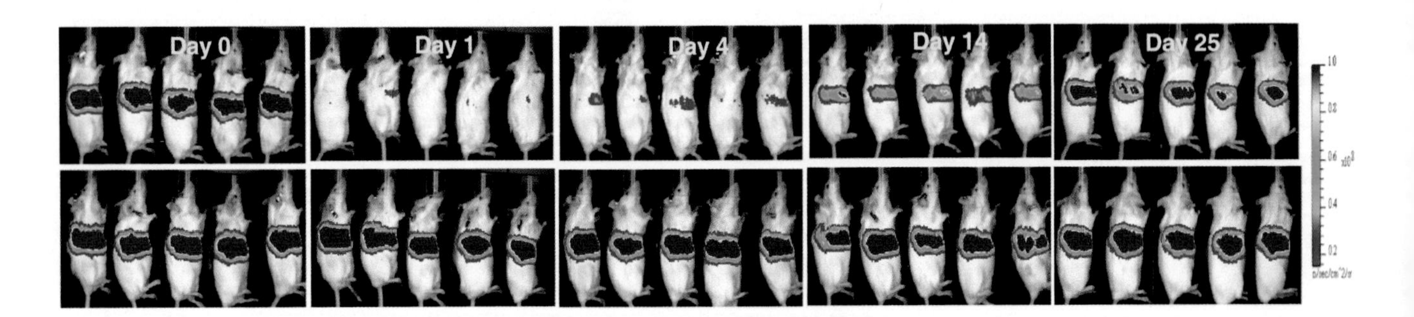

FIGURE 24.8 Color-coded bioluminescence images of a group of mice with constitutive expression of luciferase in the liver before and after the treatment with a lipid nanoparticle of antiluciferase siRNA at 3 mg/kg. Blue color represents the lowest intensity and red for the highest intensity. Adapted from Ref. 123.

called vectors. A plasmid sequence contains several basic components: a promoter, an enhancer, an origin of replication, a transgene, a polyadenylation (polyA) signal, and an antibiotic resistance gene [6]. The promoter is located upstream of a transgene and facilitates the transcription of this transgene. The enhancer is a region that can be bound by enhancer-binding proteins to enhance the transcription of the transgene. The origin of replication is a particular sequence at which replication is initiated. The transgene is a complementary DNA (cDNA) sequence that encodes a protein of interest. The cDNA fragment can be inserted into the plasmid at the multiple cloning site (MCS), a short region containing numerous restriction enzyme sites. The polyA signal is a sequence located at the 3′ end of the eukaryotic messenger RNA (mRNA). The function of the polyA signal is to terminate transcription and stabilize the mRNA. The antibiotic resistance gene encodes a protein that protects bacteria from a specific antibiotic, thus, allowing the selection of plasmid transformed bacteria in a selective growth medium. In general, a proper combination of these components is essential for maximizing the gene-transfer efficiency. The subcellular localization of plasmids is another critical factor for their gene-transfer efficiency. To express encoded proteins efficiently, plasmids must be delivered into the cell nucleus.

14.3.2 Antisense and Antigene Oligodeoxynucleotides (ODNs)

ODNs are short, synthetic, single-stranded DNA or RNA molecules that can inhibit gene expression [7]. Based on the site of action, ODNs can be classified into antisense ODNs and antigene ODNs. Antisense ODNs are single-stranded DNA molecules that inhibit gene expression at the post-transcriptional level. Antisense ODNs can be designed to be complimentary to either mRNA or pre-mRNA to block the translation machinery sterically or to inhibit pre-mRNA splicing at the ODN-RNA complex site. Another widely accepted mechanism of antisense ODNs is the triggering of mRNA degradation at the ODN binding site by RNase H, an endonuclease that binds specifically to the RNA-DNA hybrid and catalyzes the hydrolysis of the RNA strand. In contrast, antigene ODNs exhibit activities at the transcriptional level. Antigene ODNs block gene transcription by forming a triplex with genomic DNA in a sequence-specific manner on the polypurine-polypyrimidine tracts. Antigene ODNs hybridize with the target genome sequences via reverse Hoogsteen hydrogen bonds. Therefore, antigene ODNs might not be available for many genes because a highly specific polypurine-polypyrimidine sequence is required for the triplex formation [8]. Theoretically, antigene ODNs are more effective than antisense ODNs because each cell has only two copies of each gene but thousands of copies of each mRNA, which are the targets of antisense ODNs.

14.3.3 Small Interfering RNA

Synthetic siRNA is a double-stranded RNA oligonucleotide of 21–23 nucleotides that can silence its target mRNA specifically in eukaryotic cells. Long double-stranded RNA (dsRNA) or short-hairpin RNA (shRNA) can be cleaved into siRNAs of 21–23 nucleotides by the dicer enzyme in cells [9]. Once inside the cells, the siRNA is unwound by an adenosine triphosphate (ATP)-dependent helicase, and its antisense strand is incorporated into the RNA-induced silencing complex (RISC) [10]. Subsequently, the antisense strand guides the RISC to its complementary mRNA, and the Argonaute protein (AGO), a catalytic component of the RISC, triggers the degradation of the mRNA [11]. Because of its potent knockdown efficiency, siRNA has been applied extensively to the investigation of gene functions or used to identify new drug targets. Most importantly, its ability to down-regulate a variety of undruggable targets makes the use of siRNA an attractive therapeutic strategy. As of December 2011, there were more than 12 ongoing siRNA clinical trials targeting various conditions, including ocular diseases, acute renal failure, solid tumor, and pachyonychia congenital (www.clinicaltrial.gov).

14.3.4 Aptamers

Aptamers are short, artificial, single-stranded DNA or RNA oligonucleotides that can bind to a specific macromolecule or a small-molecule target with a high affinity (K_d in the nM to pM range) [12]. Aptamers are identified using an *in vitro* process called systematic evolution of target-specific ligands by exponential enrichment (SELEX), which uses repeated cycles of affinity capture, washing, elution, and amplification, to enrich sequences specifically with high binding affinity to the target molecule from a random single-stranded DNA or RNA oligonucleotide library [13–15]. The binding capability of aptamers is a result of their secondary or tertiary structures that allow the specific interactions with target molecules to occur in a complementary manner [16]. Compared with antibodes, aptamers represent a very promising targeting moiety because of their small molecular weight, good physical-chemical stability, lack of immunogenicity, ease of production, high synthetic accessibility, and flexibility in chemical conjugation. Therefore, aptamers are not only used as therapeutic agents, but also they are commonly used as alternatives to antibodies for the targeted delivery of various molecules including nucleic acids.

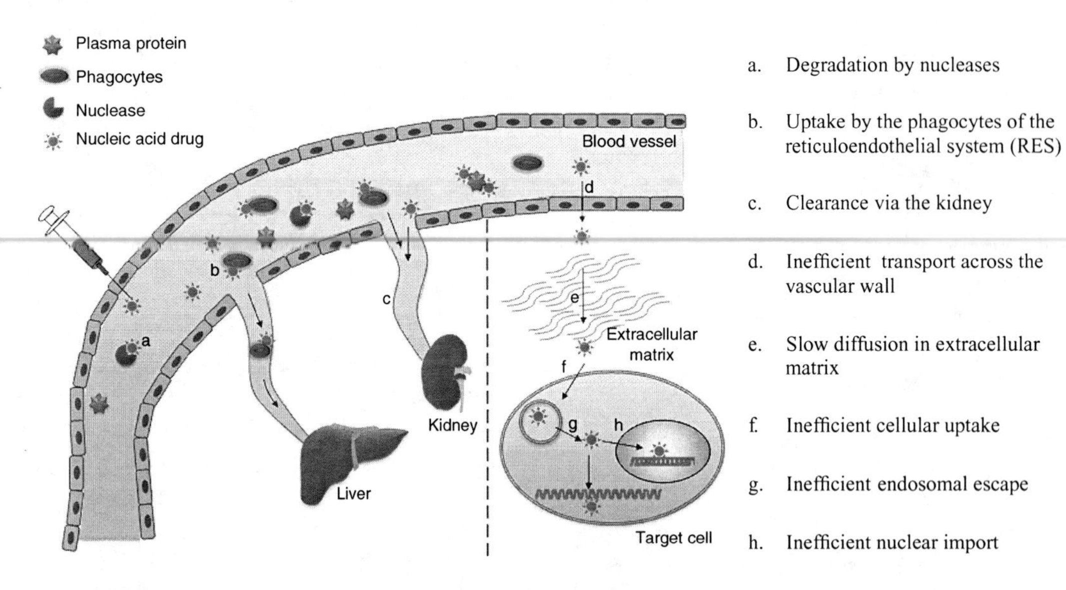

FIGURE 14.2 Various biological barriers faced by nucleic acids *in vivo*. (a) Naked nucleic acids are readily degraded by ubiquitous nucleases in the blood stream and tissues. (b) Nucleic acids are taken up by phagocytes of the RES in the liver and spleen. (c) Nucleic acids are rapidly cleared via the kidney. (d) Inefficient transport across the vascular wall. (e) Extracellular matrix hinders the movement of nucleic acids. (f) Inefficient cellular uptake. (g) Inefficient endosomal escape. (h) Inefficient nuclear import. (See color figure in color plate section.)

14.3.5 Ribozymes

Ribozymes (also called RNA enzymes) are catalytically active RNA molecules that can catalyze a chemical reaction of their substrates, most of which are RNA molecules [17]. The most extensively studied ribozyme is the hammerhead ribozyme, which is composed of two regions: a catalytic core and two flanking sequences for RNA binding [18]. Ribozymes bind to their substrate RNAs via Watson-Crick base pairing, and they cleave the target RNAs via a nonhydrolytic reaction [19]. Because ribozymes can rebind and degrade the mRNAs of the same gene multiple times, ribozyme-induced mRNA cleavage occurs in a concentration- and time-independent manner [20]. Ribozymes can also be used to splice mutant RNA targets in normal sequences, which provides a potential approach to correct the genetic information in the mRNA transcribed from a mutant gene [21].

14.4 BARRIERS FOR NUCLEIC ACIDS DELIVERY

Nucleic acids are characterized by their large molecular weight, negative charge, and hydrophilicity, which make them unfavorable for therapeutic applications. The molecular weight of nucleic acids, ranging from 5 kDa (ODNs) to more than 2 MDa (plasmid DNA), is one of the primary unfavorable features preventing their passage across the vascular endothelial barrier and cell membrane. Another major adverse property of nucleic acids is the negatively charged phosphate backbone, which prevents the interaction of the nucleic acids with the negatively charged biological membrane. Apart from these unwanted physicochemical characteristics, the susceptibility of nucleic acids to nucleases also limits the potential applications of nucleic acids as therapeutics. All of these unfavorable features of nucleic acids in nature combined with a series of biological barriers in the human body prevent the successful translation of nucleic acids from bench to bedside. In this section, we will briefly introduce various biological barriers faced by either naked or formulated nucleic acids after systematic administration (Figure 14.2). For the local delivery of nucleic acids, several of the major barriers in the systematic delivery, including the reticuloendothelial system (RES) clearance and renal clearance, are bypassed. However, the cellular and subcellular barriers are unavoidable for all nucleic acid therapeutics.

14.4.1 Barriers to Systemic Delivery *In Vivo*

Systemic administration is the preferred route for clinically applied nucleic acids because this route provides the most effective distribution of the therapeutic agents. However, it is also the most challenging route for nucleic acids because the efficacy of the nucleic acids is greatly limited by a series of biological barriers, which function as a defense mechanism to protect the body from external toxins and invaders. After systemic administration, the first biological barrier is the presence of a large amount of endonucleases and exonucleases in the plasma and tissues that can readily degrade naked nucleic acids. Another major hurdle is the ready clearance of naked nucleic acids by the RES. The RES is mainly composed of phagocytic cells, including tissue macrophages and circulation monocytes. The normal physiological role of the RES is to remove foreign pathogens and cellular debris [22]. Unfortunately, macromolecules such as nucleic acids and nanoscale drug carriers can be detected and removed by the phagocytic cells of the RES, such as splenic macrophages and Kupffer cells in the liver [23]. The liver and spleen are the organs that contain the highest number of macrophages. Both organs are characterized by a fenestrated vasculature and high blood flow. Therefore, nucleic acids are generally accumulated in the liver and spleen after systemic administration. For naked nucleic acids and their small conjugates, rapid excretion by the kidney is another major barrier after systemic administration. Molecules with mass less than 5 kDa are rapidly ultrafiltered and accumulated in the urine unless there is a reuptake mechanism [24]. However, the interaction between nucleic acids and plasma proteins may retard the renal filtration because of the increased apparent molecular weight of the complex [24, 25].

The vascular endothelial wall constitutes another major barrier that prevents the escape of nucleic acids from the bloodstream into the interstitial space of their target cells. Endothelial cells lining the lumen of the vasculature adhere to the underlying extracellular matrix tightly via integrins and form interendothelial junctions with each other using a variety of cell–cell adhesion molecules. The endothelial permeability is regulated by the extracellular matrix (ECM) and various mediators involved in some signaling pathways [26]. It is postulated that molecules with a diameter greater than 45 Å cannot readily traverse the capillary endothelium and will be degraded in the blood circulation and ultimately cleared from the body [27]. Large molecules cross the endothelial barrier primarily through the transcellular vesicular pathway. However, certain tissues, such as the liver and spleen, allow for the paracellular egress of macromolecules and nanoscale carriers up to 200 nm in diameter because of their relatively large fenestrations [28]. This unique physiological structure makes the liver one of the major organs that takes up both free nucleic acids and nanoscale carriers. In addition, tumor tissues share this physiological feature, allowing for the paracellular permeation and selective accumulation of macromolecules and nanoscale carriers in a certain size range. This feature is a result of the large fenestrations between the endothelial cells caused by the abnormal tumor angiogenesis. Another major characteristic that distinguishes tumor tissues from normal tissues is the poor lymphatic system that allows the extravasated molecules to remain in the interstitial tumor space longer than they remain in normal tissues [29]. The relative leaky nature of the tumor endothelium and the poor lymphatic drainage allows for the selective passage of macromolecules into tumor tissues. This phenomenon is called the enhanced permeability and retention (EPR) effect and has been widely employed in cancer therapy to deliver drugs to tumors specifically [30]. After exiting the vasculature, naked nucleic acids or their carrier still must pass though the ECM in the interstitial tumor space to reach the target cells. The ECM consists of a dense meshwork of proteoglycans and proteins, which can retard the diffusion of nucleic acids and may even to bind them tightly in some cases [31].

14.4.2 Cellular and Subcellular Barriers

After crossing the endothelial barrier and reaching the target cells, nucleic acids face another major barrier that is caused by their negative charge. Both naked nucleic acids (without a delivery agent) and the nanoscale nucleic acid carriers are taken up by cells via endocytosis. Endocytosis is a broad term that consists of macropinocytosis, clathrin-mediated endocytosis, non–clathrin-mediated endocytosis, the caveolar pathway, and phagocytosis [32]. In general, the uptake process is termed receptor-mediated endocytosis if the molecule is bound to a membrane receptor. The uptake process is referred to as pinocytosis when the molecule being taken up is dissolved in the surrounding liquid. After endocytosis, nucleic acids must escape from the endosomes to reach their subcellular sites of action, which is either the cytoplasm or the nucleus. Failure to be released from the endosomal compartments ultimately will lead to the degradation of the nucleic acids by the nucleases in the lysosome in a low-pH environment. Endosomal trapping represents one of the major rate-limiting steps in nucleic acid delivery, and attention must be paid to the enhancement of the endosomal release when designing a delivery system for nucleic acids. After they are released from the endosome, nucleic acids that function in the cytoplasm will reach their target sites to trigger appropriate effects. However, after the endosomal release, plasmid DNA faces an additional intracellular barrier, namely the nuclear envelope, before it can exhibit its activity in the nucleus.

14.5 STRATEGIES TO OVERCOME THE BIOLOGICAL BARRIERS

To overcome the biological barriers described and to fully achieve the potential therapeutic effect of nucleic acids *in vivo*, a wide variety of strategies has been developed over the last two decades. Some of these strategies have already been employed in clinical trials and have exhibited promising results. Generally, these strategies can be classified into three groups: 1) the selection of administration routes, 2) chemical modification, and 3) the use of viral or nonviral delivery systems. The nonviral delivery systems can be further divided into lipid-, polymer-, peptide-, and protein-based delivery systems.

14.5.1 Mode of Administration

The local delivery of nucleic acids is regarded as the simplest and most effective strategy to bypass the biological barriers associated with systemic administration. The advantages of local administration include the reduced dose of nucleic acids, the reduced degradation of nucleic acids, the reduced risk of an immune response, fewer side effects because of the lack of nonspecific delivery, and an improved therapeutic effect. Not surprisingly, then, the only two approved nucleic acid drugs use local administration to the eyes, and many of the promising candidates in clinical trials also employ local administration. However, despite its success in the clinical settings, local delivery is only feasible for a very limited number of diseases, such as ocular and pulmonary disorders. Systemic administration is the desired route for most therapeutic nucleic acids.

14.5.2 Chemical Modification

Chemical modifications of nucleic acids have been studied thoroughly since the therapeutic potential of nucleic acids was realized in the 1980s. Usually, this method is regarded as an effective way to increase the stability and reduce the toxicity of nucleic acids. The two U.S. Food and Drug Administration (FDA)-approved nucleic acid-based drugs in the market and most of the therapeutic nucleic acids in clinical trials employ various chemical modification strategies. As a result of the similar structures shared by all types of nucleic acids, any effective chemical modification strategy can be applied to all other types of nucleic acids. The three basic structural units of nucleic acids, including the sugar group, the phosphate group, and the nucleobase, have been explored extensively for a great variety of modifications (Figure 14.3). The phosphodiester linkage of nucleic acids is the first site that was chemically modified because of its susceptibility to nucleases. The substitution of the oxygen in the phosphodiester linkage with a sulfur results in a phosphorothioate (PS), which is one of the most widely adopted modifications in therapeutic nucleic acids. The PS modification improves the resistance of nucleic acids dramatically against serum nucleases and subsequently increases the half-life of the nucleic acids *in vivo*. The PS modification of antisense oligonucleotides not only increases their nuclease resistance but also improves the activity of RNase H to cleave target RNA molecules and prevents the rapid renal excretion via binding to plasma proteins [33, 34]. Because of these advantages, the only FDA-approved antisense oligonucleotide and many of the ongoing antisense therapeutics in clinical trials employ this modification strategy [35, 36]. Recently, efforts have also been made to exploit the PS modification in siRNA therapeutics, indicating that the modification does not interfere with the silencing effect and that the stability of the siRNA

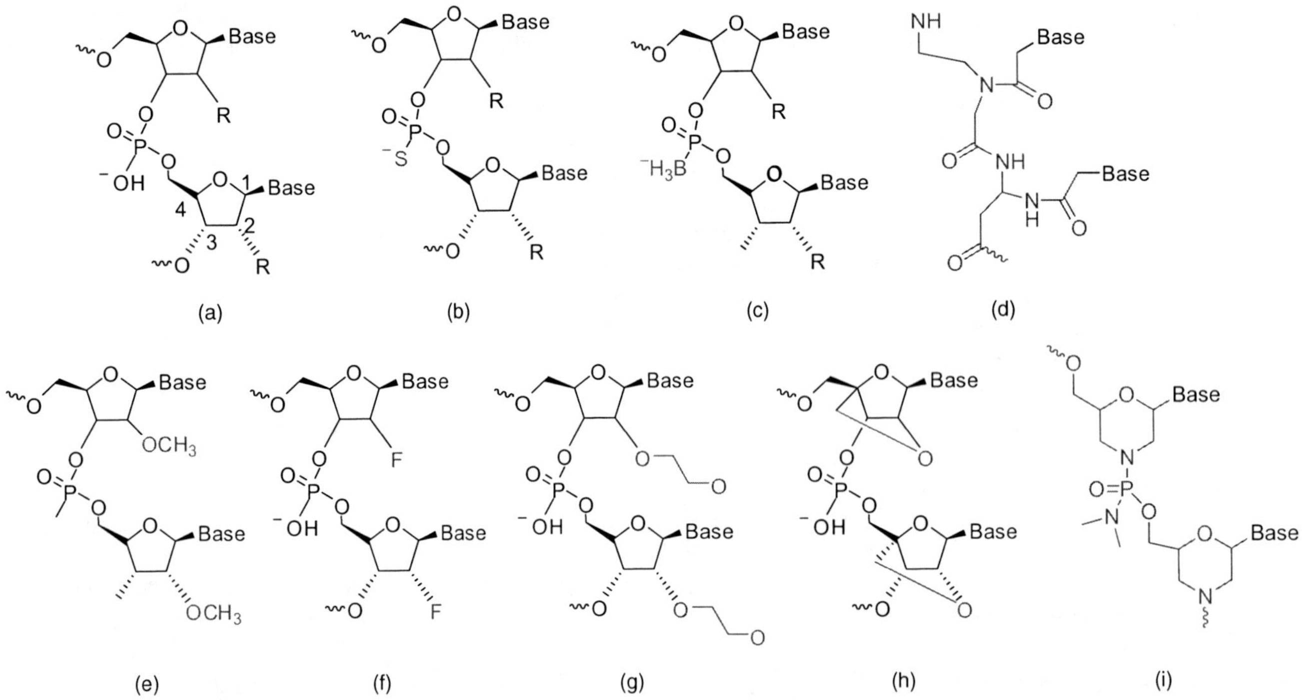

FIGURE 14.3 Chemical modifications of nucleic acids. (a) Unmodified DNA or RNA (R = H, OH), (b) phosphorothioate, (c) boranophosphate, (d) peptide nucleic acid, (e) 2′-*O*-methyl, (f) 2′-*O*-fluoro, (g) 2′-*O*-methoxyethyl (MOE), (h) locked nucleic acid, and (i) morpholino.

can be enhanced [37–39]. The nonbridging oxygen atom of the phosphate backbone can also be replaced with a boron atom. The preliminary studies of this modification in an siRNA demonstrate improved resistance to nuclease degradation and an enhanced silencing effect at lower concentrations compared with either the native siRNA or the PS-modified siRNA [40].

Another commonly modified site is the 2′-position of the sugar moiety, including substitutions of the hydroxyl groups with 2′-*O*-methyl, 2′-*O*-methoxyethyl, and 2′-fluoro groups [41–44]. These modifications have demonstrated an improved resistance to nucleases and an enhanced affinity to complementary DNA or RNA sequences. The siRNAs containing the 2′-modifications (2′-fluoro and 2′-*O*-methyl) maintain the same or an increased silencing effect compared with that of the native siRNAs [45]. The 2′-*O*-methyl modification of the nucleotides near the termini of the RNA guided strand can reportedly reduce the off-target effect of nucleic acids, which is a major concern of siRNA and antisense ODN in the clinic [46, 47].

An locked nucleic acid (LNA) is a type of conformationally restricted oligonucleotide analogue that consists of an oxymethylene bridge between the 2′ and 4' carbons of the ribose ring. An LNA is also regarded as a constrained analog of the 2′-*O*-methyl RNA [48, 49]. The oxy-methylene bridge creates a bicyclic structure that "locks" the ribose in the 3'-*endo* (North) formation, providing an ideal conformation for an A-type duplex. The locked ribose conformation strengthens the backbone preorganization and base stacking, which greatly enhances the affinity of the LNA for its complementary nucleotide sequences [50]. Compared with the classic 20-mer ODNs, the high affinity of the LNA allows for the use of short sequences, also to referred as tiny LNAs [51]. This modification also exhibits improved nuclease resistance and enhanced stability in different tissues *in vivo*. However, it is reported that this modification might induce liver toxicity in mouse models [52]. An understanding of the origins of this toxicity and the discovery of solutions to minimize this toxicity are critical for transforming the LNAs from bench to clinic in the future. Since they were first synthesized in 1998 [53], several LNA-based ODNs have entered phase I and phase II clinical trials, showing promising results [54].

Peptide nucleic acids (PNAs) are single-stranded nucleic acid analogs in which the phosphodiester backbone is substituted with polyamide groups. As a result of their uncharged nature and unique structure, PNAs exhibit higher binding affinity with DNA/RNA and higher resistance to nucleases and proteases than do DNA and RNA. The limitation of PNAs is their poor ability to penetrate cell membranes. Therefore, the conjugation of PNAs with a short cationic peptide or the introduction of charged amino acids into the PNA sequence are common methods used to overcome this problem [55, 56]. Other promising nucleic acid analogs include morpholino oligonucleotides [57], phosphoramidate DNA [58], and hexitol nucleic acid (HNA) [59].

14.6 NUCLEIC ACID DELIVERY SYSTEMS

Generally, nucleic acid delivery systems can be classified into two groups: viral and nonviral systems. Viral vectors are the most efficient methods to deliver nucleic acids to different types of cells. However, the risk of insertional mutagenesis and complications associated with the immune response are the two major concerns for viral vectors in clinical trials. In contrast, nonviral vehicles, including cationic lipids, cationic polymers, proteins, and peptides, have attracted much attention because of their low immunogenicity, low toxicity, ease of manipulation to meet various requirements in manufacturing and clinical use. There are also other delivery strategies using physical forces, such as electricity or pressure, to deliver nucleic acids into target cells. Commonly used physical methods in nucleic acids delivery include needle injection [60], hydrodynamic gene transfer [61], gene gun [62], electroporation [63], and sonoporation [64]. However, we will focus primarily on the viral and nonviral delivery systems in this chapter.

Cationic lipids or polymers can condense polyanionic nucleic acids to form nanoscale lipoplexes or polyplexes. The formation of the nanoscale particles not only facilitates nucleic acid uptake via their interaction with negatively charged cellular membranes but also protects nucleic acids from degradation. Particle size and zeta potential are considered the two most important parameters of the nanoscale complexes that determine the biodistribution of the complexes and their interaction with biological membranes and plasma proteins [65, 66]. To enhance the cellular uptake of nucleic acids or to achieve selective cell targeting, the complexes can be decorated with various targeting ligands that can specifically bind to cell surface receptors. A wide variety of targeting ligands including polypeptides [67], antibodies [68], aptamers [69], and small molecules have been used. To evade uptake by the RES, the surfaces of the lipoplexes or polyplexes are commonly coated with hydrophilic molecules, such as polyethylene glycol (PEG). PEGylation creates a "brush" layer on the surface of the complexes, which sterically stabilizes the complexes and decreases their aggregation and nonspecific interaction with the components of the bloodstream, thus allowing a prolonged circulation time [70, 71]. However, the aqueous "brush" may inhibit the interaction of the complex with a target cell surface and endosome membrane, resulting in lower a cellular uptake and endosomal escape compared with the complexes without the PEG modification [72, 73]. This phenomenon is also known as the "PEG dilemma."

14.6.1 Lipid-Based Delivery System

Lipid-based delivery systems generally include liposomes, solid lipid nanoparticles, microemulsions, and micelles [74]. Cationic lipids are the major components in all lipid-based systems. Commonly used cationic lipids include 1,2-dioleoyl-3-trimethylammonium-propane (DOTAP), *N*-[1-(2,3-dioleyloxy)propyl]-*N*,*N*,*N*-trimethylammonium (DPTMA), 2,3-dioleyloxy-*N*-[2-spermine carboxamide] ethyl-*N*,*N*-dimethyl-1-propanammonium trifluoroacetate (DOSPA), 3-β-[*N*-(*N*,*N*'-dimethylaminoethane) carbamoyl] cholesterol (DC-Chol), and dioctadecyl amidoglyceryl spermine (DOGS) (Figure 14.4). These lipids are amphiphiles with positive charges, and they consist of a cationic head group, a hydrophobic lipid group, and a linker. The transfection efficiency and toxicity of cationic lipids largely depend on the type of the cationic head group, the length

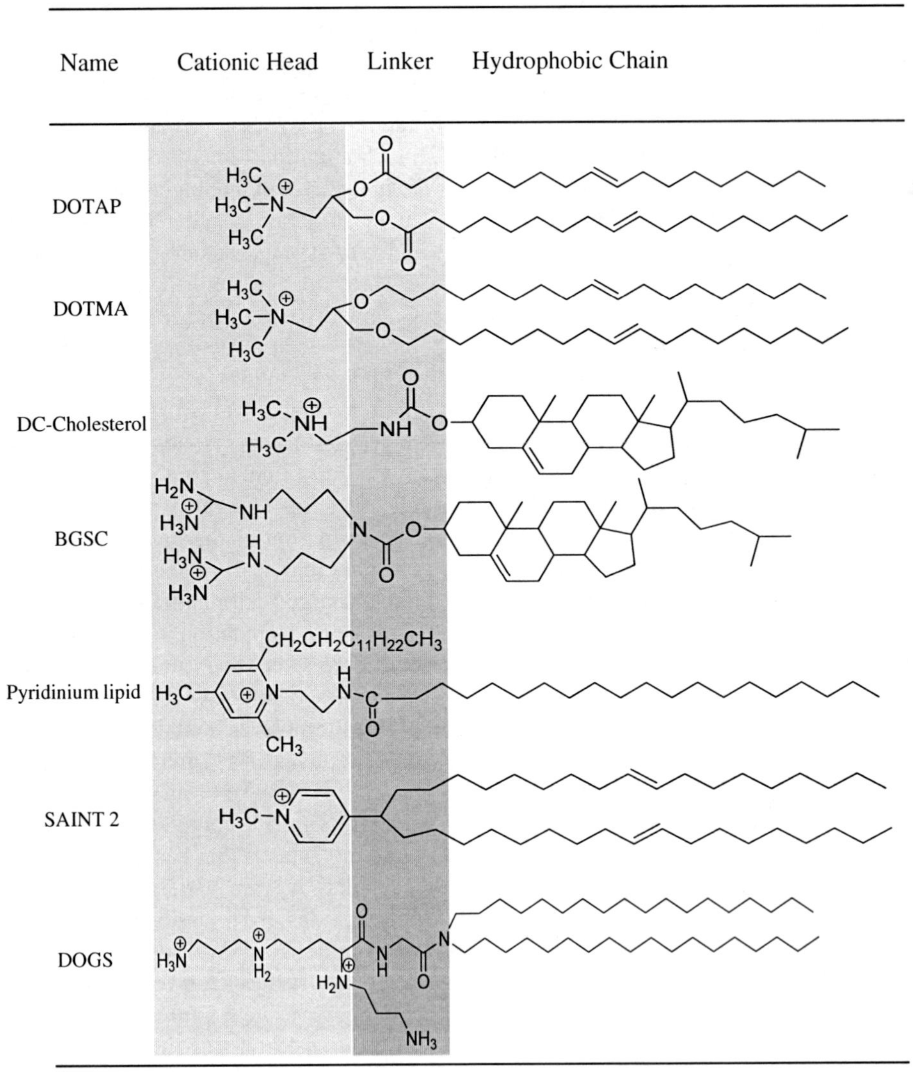

FIGURE 14.4 The structures of commonly used cationic lipids. (i) DOTAP, composed of monoamine, ether linker, two unsaturated fatty acid chains; (ii) DOTMA, composed of monoamine, ester linker, two unsaturated fatty acid chains; (iii) DC-Chol, composed of monoamine, carbamate linker, and cholesterol; (iv) bis-guanidiniumspermidinecholesterol (BGSC), composed of polyamine, carbamate linker, and cholesterol; (v) pyridinium lipid, composed of pyridinium ring, amide linker, and saturated fatty acid chains; (vi) *N*-methyl-4(dioleyl) methylpyridiniumchloride (SAINT-2), composed of pyridinium ring, aliphatic linker, and two unsaturated fatty acid chains; and (vii) DOGS, composed of polyamine, amide linker, and two saturated fatty acid chains.

of the carbon chain in the tail group, and the nature of the linker [75]. Cationic lipids interact easily with the negatively charged phosphate backbone of nucleic acids to form nanoscale lipoplexes. By adjusting the ratio of cationic lipids to nucleic acids, the zeta potential and particle size can be optimized to enhance the interaction between the lipoplex and cell membranes to facilitate cellular internalization. The formation of lipoplexes protects the nucleic acids from degradation by nucleases and prevents their excretion by the kidney. Lipoplexes containing cationic lipids can interact with negatively charged endosome membranes and exert the endosome destabilizing effect to release the nucleic acids into the cytoplasm [76].

Cationic liposomes are currently the most common carriers employed in the delivery of nucleic acids. Liposomes are globular vesicles with a phospholipid bilayer and an aqueous core. They are formed by mixing cationic lipids, cholesterol, and neutral helper lipids in different ratios. As a result of their amphipathic nature, a wide variety of hydrophobic and hydrophilic agents can be loaded into liposomes. Several commercial cationic liposomes, such as lipofectamine-2000 and oligofectamine, are available for the *in vitro* transfection of nucleic acids. One problem associated with the lipid-based system is the short circulation time in the blood because of the excessive surface charge, which can lead to an interaction with plasma proteins and then elimination by the RES [77]. Lipoplexes administrated via systemic administration tend to accumulate first in the capillary bed of the lung [78], and this is followed by redistribution from the lung to the phagocytic Kupffer cells in the liver [79]. To circumvent the RES clearance and increase the circulation time of lipoplexes, PEG has been employed successfully to shield the positive charge of the system and prolong the circulation half-life of lipoplexes [80]. In addition, a variety of neutral or zwitterionic lipids have been introduced into liposomes to reduce the positive zeta potential, therefore prolonging the circulation time and reducing toxicities. However, the introduction of neutral or zwitterionic lipids may lead to a reduced condensing capacity and result in a lower transfection efficiency [81]. Despite the unique advantages of lipid-based systems in nucleic acids delivery, numerous drawbacks, including the transfection efficiency *in vivo*, the high toxicity, and the nonspecific immune response, limit the application of these systems in the clinic.

14.6.2 Polymer-Based Delivery System

Cationic polymers comprise another class of carriers that has been widely exploited for the delivery of nucleic acids. Among these polymers, poly-ethyleneimine (PEI), cationic dendrimers, and chitosan are the three most commonly used carriers (Figure 14.5). Similar to cationic lipids, these cationic polymers can condense nucleic acids to form nanoscale polyplexes. The molar ratio of nitrogen in the cationic polymers to phosphate in the nucleic acid (often called the N/P ratio) is an important indicator of the complex formation. Some cationic carriers such as PEI and polyamidoamine dendrimers can help nucleic acids escape from the endosome via a so-called "proton sponge effect." As the polyplexes enter the endosome compartment, the large buffering capacity of nonprotonated amino groups, such as the secondary amino groups, causes a large influx of protons, which is followed by the influx of chloride anions to maintain the electro-neutrality. To maintain the osmotic pressure inside the endosome, water also diffuses into the endosome, leading to the swelling and burst of the endosome and, consequently, the release of the endosomal content into the cytoplasm [82].

14.6.2.1 Poly-ethyleneimine PEI is one of the most commonly used synthetic polymers in nucleic acid delivery. It has a high positive charge and exists in either a linear or a branched form with a wide range of molecular weights from 1 kDa to more than 1000 kDa [83] (see Figure 14.5c and d). Linear PEIs mainly contain secondary amines, whereas branched PEIs contain primary, secondary, and tertiary amine groups in nearly equal amounts [84]. Because the amine groups with different p*K*a values can be protonated in different quantities at a given pH, PEIs have a strong buffering capacity over a wide range of pH values. The buffering capacity of a PEI can protect its content from degradation in the endosomes/lysosomes and result in an early endosomal escape via the "proton sponge effect." The transfection efficiency and toxicity of PEIs are primarily determined by their molecular weight. In general, both the transfection efficiency and the cytotoxicity increase with the molecular weight of the PEI [85]. It has been reported that the most appropriate molecular weight of a PEI for DNA delivery is approximately 5–25 kDa [86]. In addition to the effect of molecular mass, branched and linear PEIs also have different influences on the characteristics of polyplexes and transfection efficiency. Broadly speaking, branched PEIs have a higher DNA condensing efficiency, a higher zeta potential, and a smaller particle size than linear PEIs because of their strong electrostatic interaction with DNA [87]. Similar to lipoplexes, PEI polyplexes are inclined to aggregate to form large complexes. In addition, the problems associated with the clearance by the RES after systemic administration also restrict the application of PEIs in the clinic. To reduce the nonspecific interactions and prolong the circulation time, the modification of PEIs with inert polymers such as PEG, dextran, or pluronic triblock polymers is widely employed [88]. In addition, many researchers have tried to encapsulate the PEI polyplexes inside neutral or anionic liposomes, polymer-based hydrogel, or other biodegradable nanoparticles, obtaining promising results including a reduced cytotoxicity and an improved transfection efficiency.

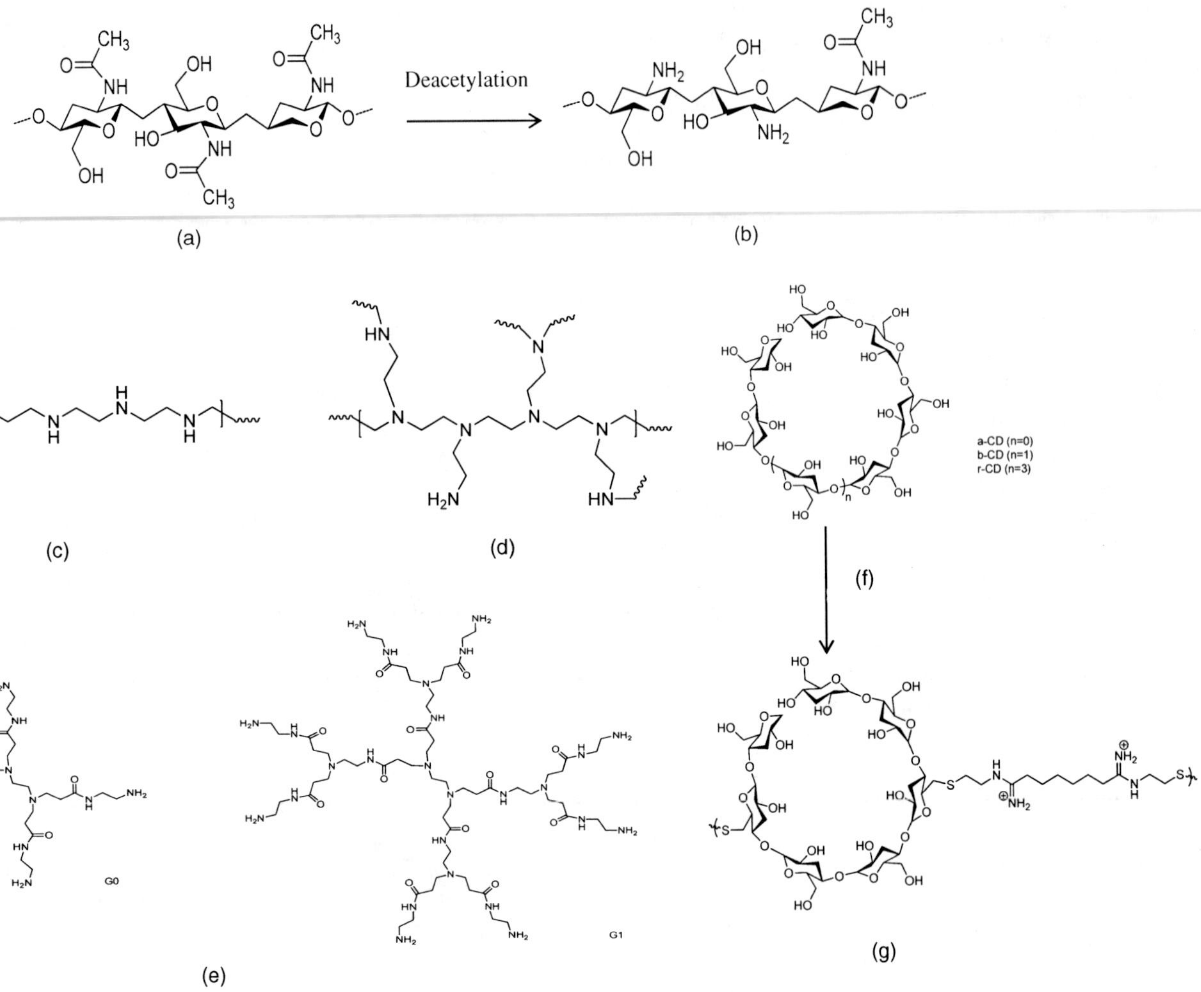

FIGURE 14.5 The structure of commonly used cationic polymers: (a) structure of the naturally occurring chitin, (b) chitosan, (c) linear PEI, (d) branched PEI, (e) different generation PAMAM dendrimer, (f) cyclodextrin, and (g) cationic cyclodextrin.

14.6.2.2 Chitosan Chitosan is derived from the partial deacetylation of chitin, which is abundant in nature and comes primarily from the exoskeletons of crustaceans, such as crab and shrimp shell wastes. Chitosan is a linear amino polysaccharide composed of randomly distributed *N*-acetyl-D-glucosamine and D-glucosamine (Figure 10.5b. It has been widely applied in the delivery of various nucleic acids because of its biocompatibility, biodegradability, low toxicity, and low immunogenicity [89, 90]. The primary amine groups in chitosan can form positively charged helicoidal stiff chains in acidic aqueous medium that can interact with negatively charged nucleic acids. Because the positive charge of chitosan is a result of deacetylation, the degree of deacetylation is an important factor that determines the condensing capacity of a chitosan. Generally, the chitosans that are commonly used in nucleic acid delivery are highly deacetylated, approximately 80% or greater [91, 92]. In comparison with PEI, chitosan exhibits a lower transfection efficiency because of its low buffering capacities, which results in a relatively weak "proton sponge effect." The physical-chemical properties of the chitosan/nucleic acid complex, including size, zeta potential, morphology, stability, and transfectability, are largely determined by the molecular mass, N/P ratio, preparation method, and the degree of deacetylation of the chitosan [93].

14.6.2.3 Dendrimers A dendrimer is a repeatedly branched polymer with a tree-like structure. The unique architecture of a dendrimer is usually composed of three parts: the center core, the interior branches consisting of tertiary amine groups, and the periphery [94]. The tertiary amine groups in the interior branches play an important role in the endosome escape. The periphery of a dendrimer can be modified with various functional groups. Based on the number of repeated branching cycles in the synthesis, dendrimers can be classified by generation. The molecular

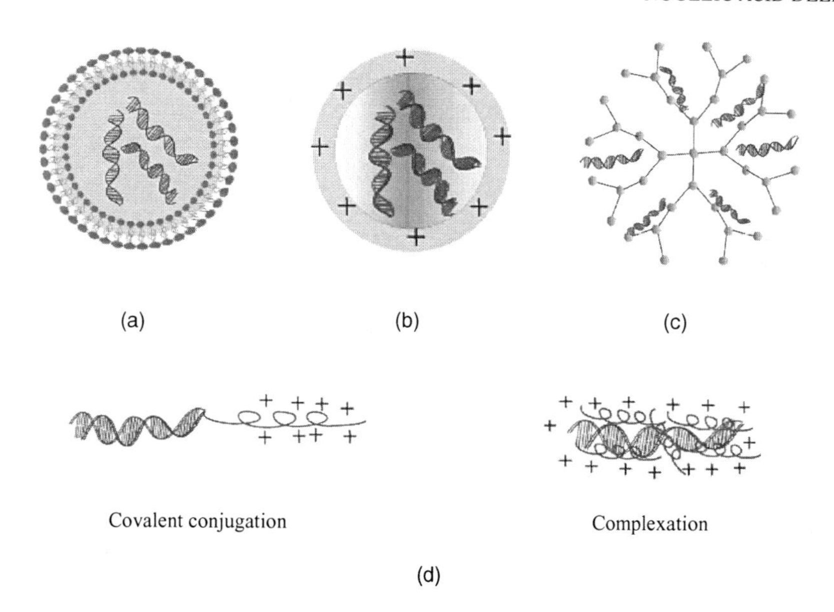

FIGURE 14.6 Carrier systems for nucleic acids: (a) liposome-based carrier, (b) cationic polyplex-based carrier, (c) dendrimer-based carrier, and (d) peptide-based carrier.

weight can be doubled from the previous generation after each successful generation. High-generation dendrimers expose more functional groups on the surface, which can be customized for a specific application. Because the molecular weight, shape, and size can be precisely controlled, dendrimers have been investigated widely for drug and nucleic acid delivery as well as for bioengineering and diagnostics applications. The space inside a dendrimer is suitable for the encapsulation of small molecule drugs. However, this space is not appropriate for nucleic acids because of their large molecular weight. Cationic dendrimers are commonly employed for nucleic acid delivery. Nucleic acids can be condensed and compacted into nanosize particles by the primary amine at the surface of the dendrimer. Endosome escape can be achieved by the internal tertiary amino groups via the proton sponge effect. A high transfection efficiency can be achieved using a high charge density or a high generation. However, this type of dendrimer is always associated with high cytotoxicity compared with low-generation dendrimers [94, 95]. Polyamidoamine (PAMAM) and polypropylenimine (PPI) are the two most commonly used dendrimers. Because of their high transfection efficiency, several dendrimer-based transfection reagents are commercially available, such as Priostar dendrimers (Dendritic Nanotechnologies, Mount Pleasant, MI), PolyFect and SuperFect (QIAGEN, Valencia, CA), Astramol (DSM, Netherlands), and Starburst PAMAM dendrimers (Aldrich Chemical Co, Milwaukee, WI).

14.6.2.4 Cyclodextrin-Containing Cationic Polymers

Cyclodextrins (CDs) are natural cyclic oligosaccharides composed of six, seven, or eight glucose units (referred as α-, β-, and γ-cyclodextrin, respectively). These molecules have a cage-like structure that consists of a hydrophilic exterior and a hydrophobic inner cavity and impacts the water solubility of the CDs. This unique structure has been explored extensively by the pharmaceutical industry to enhance the solubility of hydrophobic molecules by incorporating them into the inner cavity of CDs. To deliver nucleic acids, CDs need to be grafted or modified with cationic moieties including PEI, chitosan, and dendrimers [96] because negatively charged nucleic acids cannot be incorporated into the CD cavities as hydrophobic small molecules. One of the promising CD-containing cationic carriers for nucleic acid delivery was developed by Davis's group and is currently undergoing clinical trials [97]. This is a linear β-CD-containing polycation synthesized by the polymerization of a bifunctional β-CD monomer with a second bifunctionalized monomer via a cationic dimethyl suberimidate linage [98].

An important feature of CD-containing polymers is their low toxicities *in vitro* and *in vivo* compared with other non–CD-containing polymers [99]. Another important feature of CD-based polymers is their ability to form inclusion complexes that can be further modified with various functional moieties. A simple and innovative method to modify the complex surface and impart new functions is to introduce an adamantine (AD) conjugate, which can self-assemble with cyclodextrins (Figure 14.5f and g). This approach has several advantages. First, the AD conjugate and the cyclodextrins can be synthesized and purified separately, which simplifies the manufacturing process and the quality control. Second, the formation of the cyclodextrin/AD complex is self-assembled using a simple and reproducible procedure.

Third, multiple functionalities can be endowed by simply formulating the complex with different AD conjugates, such as AD-PEG for particle stabilization and Tf-PEG-AD for tumor targeting [100].

14.6.2.5 ***Peptide-Based Delivery Systems*** Since the phenomenon that the HIV-1-transactivting protein Tat can be taken up by mammalian cells was first observed approximately two decades ago [34, 101], tremendous work has been performed to explore the application of similar peptides in the delivery of macromolecules, such as proteins and nucleic acids. Cell-penetrating peptides (CPPs), also known as protein transduction domains (PTDs), are a class of peptides composed of basic amino acids that carry a net positive charge at a physiological pH. According to the traditional definition [102], a peptide can be classified as a CPP if: 1) it contains fewer than 30 amino acids, 2) its internalization by cells is protein independent, and 3) it is capable of cargo delivery. However, many new CPPs do not strictly follow this definition because a peptide can be called a CPP if it demonstrates the ability to cross biological membranes. Using peptides as a shuttle for the cellular delivery of nucleic acids represents an innovative and alternative way to overcome the hurdles faced in this delivery. The sequences of commonly used CPPs are summarized in Table 14.2. The mechanisms underlying the internalization of CPPs are still poorly understood and are the subject of controversial discussions. For the arginine- or lysine-rich CPP-cargo conjugates, it is generally believed that these conjugates first interact with the membrane-associated proteoglycans, and this step is followed by internalization via endocytosis. The precise mechanism of the internalization is unclear and strongly depends on the nature of the CPP, the conjugated cargo, the cell lines, the transfection conditions, and other factors [103, 104]. There are two major strategies to conjugate a cargo with CPP: 1) via a covalent linkage formed by either chemical conjugation or the expression of a fusion protein with CPP and 2) via a noncovalent complex. In addition to conjugating a CPP simply with nucleic acids, more complex systems involving conjugation with polymers are being developed to produce nanoparticles with appropriate zeta potential and size. For example, many attempts focus on the combination of peptides with PEI [105], cationic liposomes [106], and dendrimers [107]. One large advantage of peptide-based vectors over other nonviral vectors is the potential of overcoming various barriers in the delivery simply by just employing a single-fusion protein with various functional segments. Cationic peptides with repeated lysine and/or arginine residues are capable of condensing nucleic acids efficiently into small and compact particles. The net positive charge of the particles can interact with negative charged biological membrane and facilitate the delivery of nucleic acids.

14.7 VIRAL VECTORS

Viral vectors are the major vehicles that are used in the delivery of therapeutic nucleic acids. They have already shown great promise in many clinical trials because of the high transfection efficiency. Viruses are naturally evolved vehicles that deliver their genes efficiently into host cells. Although the differences between virus families are very significant from their origin to the host cell they infected, they all consist of two or three components: genetic material that existed in the form of DNA or RNA that can express its genes by using the host cellular machinery, a protein coat that can protect their genetic material, and in some types of virus an envelope of lipids surrounds the protein coat that help virus actively bind to the host cells. The information in virus genomes can be classified into two parts, *cis*-acting and *trans*-acting elements. The *Cis*-acting sequences exert their functions at the nucleotide level, such as the regulation of transcription, translation, and replication, whereas the *trans*-acting elements contain protein-coding genes that guide the production of the enzymes and structural proteins for the assembly of new virion. Therefore, the artificial viral genomes, also referred to as viral vectors, can be constructed by replacing part or all of the protein-coding genes with heterologous sequences. Commonly used virus vectors in nucleic acid delivery include retrovirus, lentivirus, adenovirus, and adeno-associated virus. The characteristics of these viruses are outlined in Table 14.3.

Retroviruses are small, enveloped, and single-stranded RNA viruses. Their insert capacity of the heterologous gene

TABLE 14.2 Classic CPP Sequences

Name	Origin	Sequence	References
Tat 48-60	HIV-1 transactivator (Tat)	GRKKRRQRRRPPQ	[111]
Penetratin (pAntp)	Antennapedia *Drosophila melanogaster*	RQIKIWFQNRRMKWK	[112]
Transportan	Galanin and Mastoparan	GWTLNSAGYLLGKINLKALAALAKKIL	[111]
Oligoarginine	From t Arg residues in Tat	$(R)_n$, $n = 6–12$	[113, 114]
MAP	Model amphipatic peptides	KLALKLALKALKAALKA	[115]
MPG	HIV-1 gp 41and NLS SV40	GALFLGFLGAAGSTMGAWSQPKKKRKV	[116]

TABLE 14.3 Characteristics of Various Viral Vectors

Key Feature	Retrovirus	Lentivirus	Adenovirus	Adeno-Associated Virus
Genome	ssRNA	ssRNA	dsDNA	ssDNA
Insert capability (kb)	9.0	9.0	7.5	4.5
Stable integration	Stable	Stable	Transient	Stable
Infection in nondividing cell	No	Yes	Yes	Yes
Insertional mutagenesis	Yes	Yes	No	No
Titer	Moderate	Low	High	High
Duration of transgene expression	Months to years	Months to years	Weeks to months	Months to years
Immunogenicity	Maybe high-risk concern in systemic circulation	Low	High	Moderate to low

ssDNA = single-stranded DNA; ssRNA = single-stranded RNA.

is about 8–10 kb. They have the ability to integrate transgenes into the host genome with the help of an enzyme called reverse transcriptase. In principle, the insertion of a heterologous gene into the chromosomal DNA of the host cell may cause mutations. Whether the mutation is harmful or innocent depends on the sequence of heterologous gene and the site of insertion. For retroviruses, they can insert their genome randomly into any site of the chromosomal DNA of the host without any preference, which may cause insertion mutagenesis. Lentiviruses are a subgroup of retroviruses. Both of them can integrate their genome into chromosomal DNA of the host cell in a stable fashion. However, unlike other retroviruses that can only infect dividing cells, they can integrate into genome of nondividing cells as well as dividing cells.

Adenoviruses are nonenveloped viruses with double-stranded linear DNA, which can infect both dividing and nondividing cells. As opposed to retroviruses, they do not integrate into the host cell chromosomes. Therefore, adenoviruses only permit transient expression of the target gene, although their genome maybe maintained as an episome after a proper modification [108]. The advantages of adenovirus over retrovirus are easy production with high titers and high DNA insert capacity. The primary drawback of adenoviruses is the strong immune response resulted from multiple administrations. The viral genome and capsid are both regarded as important stimuli in provoking the immediate immune responses [109].

Adeno-associated viruses (AAVs) are derived from nonpathogenic arboviruses, which are one of the smallest mammalian DNA viruses and contain a single-stranded DNA [110]. Similar to adenoviruses, AAVs can infect both dividing and quiescent cells. But their life cycle is unique, which consists of a productive phase and a latent phase. The productive phase of naturally occurring AAV requires regulatory proteins from other helper viruses, such as adenoviruses. Therefore, trans-acting factors from AAVs as well as an adenovirus are required in the construction of the cellular production systems for AAV vector. In the latent phase, AAV cargo can integrate specifically into the chromosome 19 on the host cell genome, which is a unique attraction for gene therapy application. In general, although viral vectors can produce higher efficiency compared with nonviral systems, safety concerns, including the risk of insertional mutagenesis and innate or adaptive immune responses to vector particles, are the main challenges for the application of AAVs in clinical trials.

14.8 CONCLUSION AND FUTURE PERSPECTIVES

As the development of small-molecule drugs becomes more and more difficult and complex, and the underlying mechanisms of many incurable diseases involving gene deficits have been elucidated, the development of nucleic acids therapeutics represents a very promising strategy not only to speed up the process of developing new therapies but also to provide a high probability of curing the incurable diseases. However, unlike traditional drugs that are generally apolar with small molecular weight, the unique features of nucleic acids, such as their large molecular weight, negative charge, and susceptibility to nucleases, make nucleic acids unfavorable candidates for therapy. To fully realize the potential of nucleic acids in various therapies, many strategies and delivery systems have been developed in the past two decades to compensate for these adverse features of nucleic acids and to overcome the barriers that exist between the administration and the site of action of the nucleic acids. The chemical modification of the structure of nucleic acids represents a very effective strategy to reduce the toxicity and enhance the resistance of nucleic acids to nucleases, and this method has already provided promising results in many clinical trials. In contrast to viral vectors, nonviral delivery systems, such as lipid and polymer materials, result in a lower immune response and are much easier to manufacture; however, the transfection efficiency of these nonviral system is relatively low, particularly for *in vivo* application. Although significant progress has been made in preclinical studies, the major issues associated with the therapeutic use of nucleic acids, including inefficient delivery to the target site, immunogenicity, and toxicity, have not been fully resolved. Therefore, more efforts and collaborations among biology, medicine, chemistry, and pharmaceutical sciences need to be done in the long run to realize the full therapeutic potential of nucleic acids.

ASSESSMENT QUESTIONS

14.1. Please describe the main types of nucleic acids therapeutics and their mechanisms.

14.2. What are the advantages and potentials of nucleic acids therapeutics over traditional small-molecule drugs?

14.3. What are the main challenges and barriers for nucleic acids delivery?

14.4. Please list some common strategies to overcome these challenges.

14.5. Please describe some nonviral carriers and their features used in nucleic acids therapeutics delivery.

REFERENCES

1. Zhu, L., Mahato, R.I. (2010). Lipid and polymeric carrier-mediated nucleic acid delivery. *Expert Opinion on Drug Delivery, 7(10)*, 1209–1226.
2. Keefe, A.D., Pai, S., Ellington, A. (2010). Aptamers as therapeutics. *Nature Reviews Drug Discovery, 9(7)*, 537–550.
3. Fattal, E., Bochot, A. (2006). Ocular delivery of nucleic acids: Antisense oligonucleotides, aptamers and siRNA. *Advanced Drug Delivery Reviews, 58(11)*, 1203–1223.
4. Mastrobattista, E., Hennink, W.E., Schiffelers, R.M. (2007). Delivery of nucleic acids. *Pharmaceutical Research, 24(8)*, 1561–1563.
5. Uherek, C., Wels, W. (2000). DNA-carrier proteins for targeted gene delivery. *Advanced Drug Delivery Reviews, 44(2–3)*, 153–166.
6. Kim, S.W. and Lee, M. (2005). Biomaterials for delivery and targeting of proteins and nucleic acids, in R.I. Mahato (eds.), *Biomaterials for Delivery and Targeting of Proteins and Nucleic Acids*, CRC Press, Boca Raton, FL, pp. 615–642.
7. Crooke, S.T. (1999). Molecular mechanisms of action of antisense drugs. *Biochimica et Biophysica Acta, 1489(1)*, 31–44.
8. Mahato, R.I., Cheng, K., Guntaka, R.V. (2005). Modulation of gene expression by antisense and antigene oligodeoxynucleotides and small interfering RNA. *Expert Opinions on Drug Delivery, 2(1)*, 3–28.
9. Zamore, P.D., et al. (2000). RNAi: Double-stranded RNA directs the ATP-dependent cleavage of mRNA at 21 to 23 nucleotide intervals. *Cell, 101(1)*, 25–33.
10. Schwarz, D.S., et al. (2003). Asymmetry in the assembly of the RNAi enzyme complex. *Cell, 115(2)*, 199–208.
11. Liu, J., et al. (2004). Argonaute2 is the catalytic engine of mammalian RNAi. *Science, 305(5689)*, 1437–1441.
12. Ireson, C.R., Kelland, L.R. (2006). Discovery and development of anticancer aptamers. *Molecular Cancer Therapy, 5(12)*, 2957–2962.
13. Bock, L.C., et al. (1992). Selection of single-stranded DNA molecules that bind and inhibit human thrombin. *Nature, 355(6360)*, 564–566.
14. Chen, C.K. (2007). Complex SELEX against target mixture: Stochastic computer model, simulation, and analysis. *Computer Methods and Programs in Biomedicine, 87(3)*, 189–200.
15. Shamah, S.M., Healy, J.M., Cload, S.T. (2008). Complex target SELEX. *Accounts of Chemical Research, 41(1)*, 130–138.
16. Phillips, J.A., et al. (2008). Applications of aptamers in cancer cell biology. *Analytica Chimica Acta, 621(2)*, 101–108.
17. Guerrier-Takada, C., et al. (1983). The RNA moiety of ribonuclease P is the catalytic subunit of the enzyme. *Cell, 35(3 Pt 2)*, 849–857.
18. Scanlon, K.J. (2004). Anti-genes: siRNA, ribozymes and antisense. *Current Pharmaceutical Biotechnology, 5(5)*, 415–420.
19. Yao, Y., et al. (2009). Antisense makes sense in engineered regenerative medicine. *Pharmaceutical Research, 26(2)*, 263–275.
20. Cordeiro, M.F., et al. (1999). Molecular therapy in ocular wound healing. *British Journal of Ophthalmology, 83(11)*, 1219–1224.
21. Long, M.B., et al. (2003). Ribozyme-mediated revision of RNA and DNA. *Journal of Clinical Investigation, 112(3)*, 312–318.
22. Mosser, D.M., Edwards, J.P. (2008). Exploring the full spectrum of macrophage activation. *Nature Reviews Immunology, 8(12)*, 958–969.
23. Alexis, F., et al. (2008). Factors affecting the clearance and biodistribution of polymeric nanoparticles. *Molecular Pharmacology, 5(4)*, 505–515.
24. Brenner, B.M., Deen, W.M., Robertson, C.R. (1976). Determinants of glomerular filtration rate. *Annual Review of Physiology, 38*, 11–19.
25. Geary, R.S., et al. (2001). Pharmacokinetic properties of 2′-*O*-(2-methoxyethyl)-modified oligonucleotide analogs in rats. *Journal of Pharmacology and Experimental Therapeutics, 296(3)*, 890–897.
26. Mehta, D., Malik, A.B. (2006). Signaling mechanisms regulating endothelial permeability. *Physiological Reviews, 86(1)*, 279–367.
27. Rippe, B., et al. (2002). Transendothelial transport: The vesicle controversy. *Journal of Vascular Research, 39(5)*, 375–390.
28. Scherphof, G.L. (1991). In vivo behavior of liposomes: Interaction with themononuclear phagocyte system and

implications for drug targeting, in R.L. Juliano (ed.), *Targeted Drug Delivery: Handbook of Experimental Pharmacology*, Springer-Verlag, Berlin, Germany, pp. 285–327.

29. Jang, S.H., et al. (2003). Drug delivery and transport to solid tumors. *Pharmaceutical Research, 20(9)*, 1337–1350.
30. Greish, K. (2007). Enhanced permeability and retention of macromolecular drugs in solid tumors: A royal gate for targeted anticancer nanomedicines. *Journal of Drug Targeting, 15(7–8)*, 457–464.
31. Juliano, R.L. (2007). Biological barriers to nanocarrier-mediated delivery of therapeutic and imaging agents, in C.M.a.M.C. A. Niemeyer (ed.), *Nanobiotechnology II*, Wiley-VCH, Weinheim, Germany.
32. Khalil, I.A., et al. (2006). Uptake pathways and subsequent intracellular trafficking in nonviral gene delivery. *Pharmacological Reviews, 58(1)*, 32–45.
33. Eckstein, F. (2000). Phosphorothioate oligodeoxynucleotides: What is their origin and what is unique about them? *Antisense Nucleic Acid Drug Development, 10(2)*, 117–121.
34. Stein, C.A., et al. (1988). Physicochemical properties of phosphorothioate oligodeoxynucleotides. *Nucleic Acids Research, 16(8)*, 3209–3221.
35. Corey, D.R. (2007). RNA learns from antisense. *Nature Chemical Biology, 3(1)*, 8–11.
36. Grillone, L.R., Lanz, R. (2001). Fomivirsen. *Drugs Today (Barc), 37(4)*, 245–255.
37. Morrissey, D.V., et al. (2005). Activity of stabilized short interfering RNA in a mouse model of hepatitis B virus replication. *Hepatology, 41(6)*, 1349–1356.
38. Morrissey, D.V., et al. (2005). Potent and persistent in vivo anti-HBV activity of chemically modified siRNAs. *Nature Biotechnology, 23(8)*, 1002–1007.
39. Soutschek, J., et al. (2004). Therapeutic silencing of an endogenous gene by systemic administration of modified siRNAs. *Nature, 432(7014)*, 173–178.
40. Hall, A.H., et al. (2004). RNA interference using boranophosphate siRNAs: Structure-activity relationships. *Nucleic Acids Research, 32(20)*, 5991–6000.
41. Crooke, R.M., et al. (2005). An apolipoprotein B antisense oligonucleotide lowers LDL cholesterol in hyperlipidemic mice without causing hepatic steatosis. *The Journal of Lipid Research, 46(5)*, 872–884.
42. Kawasaki, A.M., et al. (1993). Uniformly modified 2′-deoxy-2′-fluoro phosphorothioate oligonucleotides as nuclease-resistant antisense compounds with high affinity and specificity for RNA targets. *Journal of Medicinal Chemistry, 36(7)*, 831–841.
43. Rusckowski, M., et al. (2000). Biodistribution and metabolism of a mixed backbone oligonucleotide (GEM 231) following single and multiple dose administration in mice. *Antisense Nucleic Acid Drug Devevelopment, 10(5)*, 333–345.
44. Zhang, H., et al. (2000). Reduction of liver Fas expression by an antisense oligonucleotide protects mice from fulminant hepatitis. *Nature Biotechnology, 18(8)*, 862–867.
45. Allerson, C.R., et al. (2005). Fully 2′-modified oligonucleotide duplexes with improved in vitro potency and stability compared to unmodified small interfering RNA. *Journal of Medicinal Chemistry, 48(4)*, 901–904.
46. Jackson, A.L., et al. (2006). Position-specific chemical modification of siRNAs reduces "off-target" transcript silencing. *RNA, 12(7)*, 1197–1205.
47. Snove, O., Jr., Rossi, J.J. (2006). Chemical modifications rescue off-target effects of RNAi. *ACS Chemical Biology, 1 (5)*, 274–276.
48. Braasch, D.A., Corey, D.R. (2001). Locked nucleic acid (LNA): Fine-tuning the recognition of DNA and RNA. *Chemistry & Biology, 8(1)*, 1–7.
49. Kumar, R., et al. (1998). The first analogues of LNA (locked nucleic acids): Phosphorothioate-LNA and 2′-thio-LNA. *Bioorganic & Medicinal Chemistry Letters, 8(16)*, 2219–2222.
50. Kaur, H., et al. (2006). Thermodynamic, counterion, and hydration effects for the incorporation of locked nucleic acid nucleotides into DNA duplexes. *Biochemistry, 45(23)*, 7347–7355.
51. Obad, S., et al. (2011). Silencing of microRNA families by seed-targeting tiny LNAs. *Nature Genetics, 43(4)*, 371–378.
52. Swayze, E.E., et al. (2007). Antisense oligonucleotides containing locked nucleic acid improve potency but cause significant hepatotoxicity in animals. *Nucleic Acids Research, 35(2)*, 687–700.
53. Obika, S., et al. (1997). Synthesis of 2′-O,4′-C-methyleneuridine and -cytidine. Novel bicyclic nucleosides having a fixed C3,-endo sugar puckering. *Tetrahedron Letters, 38(50)*, 8735–8738.
54. http://www.santaris.com/product-pipeline.
55. Albertshofer, K., et al. (2005). Structure-activity relationship study on a simple cationic peptide motif for cellular delivery of antisense peptide nucleic acid. *Journal of Medicinal Chemistry, 48(21)*, 6741–6749.
56. Maier, M.A., et al. (2006). Evaluation of basic amphipathic peptides for cellular delivery of antisense peptide nucleic acids. *Journal of Medicinal Chemistry, 49(8)*, 2534–2542.
57. Iversen, P.L. (2001). Phosphorodiamidate morpholino oligomers: Favorable properties for sequence-specific gene inactivation. *Current Opinion in Molecular Therapeutics, 3(3)*, 235–238.
58. Gryaznov, S.M. (2010). Oligonucleotide n3'-->p5' phosphoramidates and thio-phoshoramidates as potential therapeutic agents. *Chemistry & Biodiversity, 7(3)*, 477–493.
59. Kolb, G., et al. (2005). Hexitol nucleic acid-containing aptamers are efficient ligands of HIV-1 TAR RNA. *Biochemistry, 44(8)*, 2926–2933.
60. Wolff, J.A., et al. (1990). Direct gene transfer into mouse muscle in vivo. *Science, 247(4949 Pt 1)*, 1465–1468.
61. Liu, F., Song, Y., Liu, D. (1999). Hydrodynamics-based transfection in animals by systemic administration of plasmid DNA. *Gene Therapy, 6(7)*, 1258–1266.
62. Klein, R.M., et al. (1992). High-velocity microprojectiles for delivering nucleic acids into living cells. *1987. Biotechnology, 24*, 384–386.

63. Titomirov, A.V., Sukharev, S., Kistanova, E. (1991). In vivo electroporation and stable transformation of skin cells of newborn mice by plasmid DNA. *Biochimica et Biophysica Acta, 1088(1)*, 131–134.
64. Endoh, M., et al. (2002). Fetal gene transfer by intrauterine injection with microbubble-enhanced ultrasound. *Molecular Therapy, 5(5 Pt 1)*, 501–508.
65. Luten, J., et al. (2008). Biodegradable polymers as non-viral carriers for plasmid DNA delivery. *Journal of Controlled Release, 126*(2), 97–110.
66. Satija, J., Gupta, U., Jain, N.K. (2007). Pharmaceutical and biomedical potential of surface engineered dendrimers. *Critical Reviews in Therapeutic Drug Carrier Systems, 24(3)*, 257–306.
67. Ruoslahti, E. (2004). Vascular zip codes in angiogenesis and metastasis. *Biochemical Society Transactions, 32(Pt 3)*, 397–402.
68. Holliger, P., Hudson, P.J. (2005). Engineered antibody fragments and the rise of single domains. *Nature Biotechnology, 23(9)*, 1126–1136.
69. McNamara, J.O., 2nd, et al. (2006). Cell type-specific delivery of siRNAs with aptamer-siRNA chimeras. *Nature Biotechnology, 24(8)*, 1005–1015.
70. Pun, S.H., Davis, M.E. (2002). Development of a nonviral gene delivery vehicle for systemic application. *Bioconjugate Chemistry, 13(3)*, 630–639.
71. Collard, W.T., et al. (2000). Biodistribution, metabolism, and in vivo gene expression of low molecular weight glycopeptide polyethylene glycol peptide DNA co-condensates. *Journal of Pharmaceutical Sciences, 89(4)*, 499–512.
72. Hatakeyama, H., Akita, H., Harashima, H. (2011). A multifunctional envelope type nano device (MEND) for gene delivery to tumours based on the EPR effect: A strategy for overcoming the PEG dilemma. *Advanced Drug Delivery Reviews, 63(3)*, 152–160.
73. Mishra, S., Webster, P., Davis, M.E. (2004). PEGylation significantly affects cellular uptake and intracellular trafficking of non-viral gene delivery particles. *European Journal of Cell Biology, 83(3)*, 97–111.
74. Oh, Y.K., Park, T.G. (2009). siRNA delivery systems for cancer treatment. *Advanced Drug Delivery Reviews, 61(10)*, 850–862.
75. Zhu, L., Mahato, R.I. (2010). Lipid and polymeric carrier-mediated nucleic acid delivery. *Expert Opinion on Drug Delivery, 7(10)*, 1209–1226.
76. Zelphati, O., Szoka, Jr., F.C. (1996). Mechanism of oligonucleotide release from cationic liposomes. *Proceedings of the National Academy of Sciences USA, 93(21)*, 11493–11498.
77. Opanasopit, P., Nishikawa, M., Hashida, M. (2002). Factors affecting drug and gene delivery: Effects of interaction with blood components. *Critical Reviews in Therapeutic Drug Carrier Systems, 19(3)*, 191–233.
78. Liu, F., et al. (1997). Factors controlling the efficiency of cationic lipid-mediated transfection in vivo via intravenous administration. *Gene Therapy, 4(6)*, 517–523.
79. Barron, L.G., Gagne, L., Szoka, Jr., F.C. (1999). Lipoplex-mediated gene delivery to the lung occurs within 60 minutes of intravenous administration. *Human Gene Therapy, 10(10)*, 1683–1694.
80. Meyer, O., et al. (1998). Cationic liposomes coated with polyethylene glycol as carriers for oligonucleotides. *The Journal of Biological Chemistry, 273(25)*, 15621–15627.
81. Foged, C., Nielsen, H.M., Frokjaer, S. (2007). Liposomes for phospholipase A2 triggered siRNA release: Preparation and in vitro test. *International Journal of Pharmaceutics, 331*(2), 160–166.
82. Boussif, O., et al. (1995). A versatile vector for gene and oligonucleotide transfer into cells in culture and in vivo: Polyethylenimine. *Proceedings of the National Academy of Sciences USA, 92(16)*, 7297–7301.
83. Akhtar, S., Benter, I.F. (2007). Nonviral delivery of synthetic siRNAs in vivo. *Journal of Clinical Investigation, 117(12)*, 3623–3632.
84. von Harpe, A., et al. (2000). Characterization of commercially available and synthesized polyethylenimines for gene delivery. *Journal of Controlled Release, 69*(2), 309–322.
85. Ogris, M., et al. (1998). The size of DNA/transferrin-PEI complexes is an important factor for gene expression in cultured cells. *Gene Therapy, 5(10)*, 1425–1433.
86. Neu, M., Fischer, D., Kissel, T. (2005). Recent advances in rational gene transfer vector design based on poly(ethylene imine) and its derivatives. *The Journal of Gene Medicine, 7(8)*, 992–1009.
87. Intra, J., Salem, A.K. (2008). Characterization of the transgene expression generated by branched and linear polyethylenimine-plasmid DNA nanoparticles in vitro and after intraperitoneal injection in vivo. *Journal of Controlled Release, 130*(2), 129–138.
88. Al-Dosari, M.S., Gao, X. (2009). Nonviral gene delivery: Principle, limitations, and recent progress. *AAPS Journal, 11(4)*, 671–681.
89. Lee, M.K., et al. (2005). The use of chitosan as a condensing agent to enhance emulsion-mediated gene transfer. *Biomaterials, 26(14)*, 2147–2156.
90. Liu, X., et al. (2007). The influence of polymeric properties on chitosan/siRNA nanoparticle formulation and gene silencing. *Biomaterials, 28(6)*, 1280–1288.
91. Katas, H., Alpar, H.O. (2006). Development and characterisation of chitosan nanoparticles for siRNA delivery. *Journal of Controlled Release, 115*(2), 216–225.
92. MacLaughlin, F.C., et al. (1998). Chitosan and depolymerized chitosan oligomers as condensing carriers for in vivo plasmid delivery. *Journal of Controlled Release, 56(1–3)*, 259–272.
93. Borchard, G. (2001). Chitosans for gene delivery. *Advanced Drug Delivery Reviews, 52*(2), 145–150.
94. Dufes, C., Uchegbu, I.F., Schatzlein, A.G. (2005). Dendrimers in gene delivery. *Advanced Drug Delivery Reviews, 57(15)*, 2177–2202.

95. Zinselmeyer, B.H., et al. (2002). The lower-generation polypropylenimine dendrimers are effective gene-transfer agents. *Pharmaceutical Research*, *19(7)*, 960–967.
96. Davis, M.E., et al. (2004). Self-assembling nucleic acid delivery vehicles via linear, water-soluble, cyclodextrin-containing polymers. *Current Medicinal Chemistry*, *11(2)*, 179–197.
97. Davis, M.E., et al. (2010). Evidence of RNAi in humans from systemically administered siRNA via targeted nanoparticles. *Nature*, *464(7291)*, 1067–1070.
98. Gonzalez, H., Hwang, S.J., Davis, M.E. (1999). New class of polymers for the delivery of macromolecular therapeutics. *Bioconjugate Chemistry*, *10(6)*, 1068–1074.
99. Pun, S.H., et al. (2004). Cyclodextrin-modified polyethylenimine polymers for gene delivery. *Bioconjugate Chemistry*, *15(4)*, 831–840.
100. Bellocq, N.C., et al. (2003). Transferrin-containing, cyclodextrin polymer-based particles for tumor-targeted gene delivery. *Bioconjugate Chemistry*, *14(6)*, 1122–1132.
101. Frankel, A.D., Pabo, C.O. (1988). Cellular uptake of the tat protein from human immunodeficiency virus. *Cell*, *55(6)*, 1189–1193.
102. Langel, U.E. (2002). *Cell-Penetrating Peptides: Processes and Applications*, CRC Press, Boca Raton, FL.
103. Maiolo, J.R., Ferrer, M., Ottinger, E.A. (2005). Effects of cargo molecules on the cellular uptake of arginine-rich cell-penetrating peptides. *Biochimica et Biophysica Acta*, *1712(2)*, 161–172.
104. Mano, M., et al. (2005). On the mechanisms of the internalization of S4(13)-PV cell-penetrating peptide. *Biochemical Journal*, *390(Pt 2)*, 603–612.
105. Kilk, K., et al. (2005). Evaluation of transportan 10 in PEI mediated plasmid delivery assay. *Journal of Controlled Release*, *103(2)*, 511–523.
106. Torchilin, V.P., et al. (2003). Cell transfection in vitro and in vivo with nontoxic TAT peptide-liposome-DNA complexes. *Proceedings of the National Academy of Sciences USA*, *100(4)*, 1972–1977.
107. Bayele, H.K., et al. (2005). Versatile peptide dendrimers for nucleic acid delivery. *Journal of Pharmaceutical Sciences*, *94(2)*, 446–457.
108. Volpers, C., Kochanek, S. (2004). Adenoviral vectors for gene transfer and therapy. *The Journal of Gene Medicine*, *6 Suppl 1*, S164–S171.
109. McCaffrey, A.P., et al. (2008). The host response to adenovirus, helper-dependent adenovirus, and adeno-associated virus in mouse liver. *Molecular Therapy*, *16(5)*, 931–941.
110. Coura Rdos, S., Nardi, N.B. (2007). The state of the art of adeno-associated virus-based vectors in gene therapy. *Virology Journal*, *4*, 99.
111. Vives, E., Brodin, P., Lebleu, B. (1997). A truncated HIV-1 Tat protein basic domain rapidly translocates through the plasma membrane and accumulates in the cell nucleus. *The Journal of Biological Chemistry*, *272(25)*, 16010–16017.
112. Derossi, D., et al. (1994). The third helix of the Antennapedia homeodomain translocates through biological membranes. *The Journal of Biological Chemistry*, *269(14)*, 10444–10450.
113. Futaki, S., et al. (2001). Arginine-rich peptides. An abundant source of membrane-permeable peptides having potential as carriers for intracellular protein delivery. *The Journal of Biological Chemistry*, *276(8)*, 5836–5840.
114. Mitchell, D.J., et al. (2000). Polyarginine enters cells more efficiently than other polycationic homopolymers. *Journal of Peptide Research*, *56(5)*, 318–325.
115. Oehlke, J., et al. (1998). Cellular uptake of an alpha-helical amphipathic model peptide with the potential to deliver polar compounds into the cell interior non-endocytically. *Biochimica et Biophysica Acta*, *1414(1–2)*, 127–139.
116. Morris, M.C., et al. (1997). A new peptide vector for efficient delivery of oligonucleotides into mammalian cells. *Nucleic Acids Research*, *25(14)*, 2730–2736.

15

DELIVERY OF VACCINES

Hari R. Desu, Rubi Mahato, and Laura A. Thoma

LIST OF ABBREVIATIONS

Abbreviation	Acronym
APC	Antigen-presenting cell
CpG	Cytosine-phosphate-guanine
EDTA	Ethylenediaminetetraacetic acid
HBcAg	Hepatitis B core antigen
HBsAg	Hepatitis B surface antigen
HPV	Human papilloma virus
IFN	Interferon
Ig	Immunoglobulin
IL	Interleukin
MHC	Major histocompatibility complex
PAMAM	Poly(amidoamine)
PE	Phosphatidyl ethanolamine
PEG	Poly(ethylene glycol)
PEI	Poly(ethylenimine)
PGA	Poly(glycolic acid)
PLA	Poly (lactic acid)
PLGA	Poly(D,L-lactic acid-glycolic acid)
RES	Reticuloendothelial system
TAP	ATP-transporter assisted antigen processing
TGF-β	Transforming growth factor-β
T_H	T-helper cell
TLR	Toll-like receptor
Tm	Phase transition temperature

Note: The "vaccine" and "antigen" terms impart the same meaning, but are used as is required in different sections for better understanding of the topic sections.

15.1 CHAPTER OBJECTIVES

- To outline fundamental immunization mechanisms and different types of vaccines.
- To understand physicochemical features of vaccine delivery systems.
- To discuss delivery systems for vaccines.
- To learn different administration routes of vaccines.

15.2 INTRODUCTION

Vaccines are biological products that enhance or induce immunity to a particular disease. Despite their great success in disease control, current vaccines still face challenges for inducing a strong and long-lasting immune response without compromising safety and tolerability. Ongoing research on new-generation vaccines focuses on exploring novel vaccine delivery systems (carriers) that mimic pathogen-associated molecular patterns of microbes and induce strong immune responses. These biosynthetic or synthetic polymer fabricated vaccine delivery systems have been engineered for overcoming weak immunogenicity of antigens. Certain polymers

Advanced Drug Delivery, First Edition. Edited by Ashim K. Mitra, Chi H. Lee, and Kun Cheng.

possess inherent immunogenic properties and function as immune adjuvants for enhancing immune responses. In addition, vaccine delivery systems can be either surface modified with antigen-presenting cell (APC) (e.g., macrophage, dendritic cell, and B cell) receptor ligands or co-encapsulated with adjuvants for enhancing immunity. It is now well recognized that polymer material properties and physicochemical (design) features of delivery systems dictate immunogenic properties. Key design features that mimic pathogens, such as size, shape, and geometry play a significant role in the engineering of various soluble and colloidal vaccine formulations for guiding the nature (humoral versus cellular) and pace (rapid vs delayed) of immune responses. The design features of vaccine carriers can be harnessed for their direct interaction with APCs in the secondary lymph organs and peripheral tissues, and induce a durable immunogenic response. In this chapter, we will review various delivery systems, such as micelles, liposomes, emulsions, nanoparticles, dendrimers, and virus-like particles, for vaccines or adjuvants.

15.3 IMMUNOLOGICAL MECHANISMS

Immunological mechanisms per se are considered to co-evolve with microorganisms, which are capable of using immune machinery to their advantage. These immunological mechanisms have been divided into innate and adaptive components with specific functions and roles. As illustrated in Figure 15.1a and b, host innate and adaptive immune responses constantly monitor and ward off microbial infections. The innate immune system constitutes the first line of host defense and plays a critical role in early recognition of pathogens and triggering of nonspecific proinflammatory responses. On the other hand, an adaptive immune system displays a delayed, but strong, pathogen-specific immune response that eliminates pathogens.

15.3.1 Innate Immunity

It is believed that the innate immune system evolved before the adaptive immune system and exists in all multicellular organisms [1]. Innate immunity is mediated by germ-line-encoded receptors, whose specificity is limited. The innate immune receptors may not be able to recognize all antigens, but they recognize highly conserved structures of microorganisms [2]. These structures are referred to as pathogen-associated patterns (PAMPs), and the receptors that evolved to recognize PAMPs are pattern-recognition receptors. The pattern-recognition receptors are expressed on immune effector cells, such as macrophages, dendritic cells, and B cells. Some examples of PAMPs are bacterial lipopolysaccharides, peptidoglycans, lipotechoic acids, mannans, bacterial DNA, double-stranded RNA, and glucans [1].

The innate immune system's ability to recognize and limit microbes early during infection is based on complement activation, phagocytosis, autophagy, and immune activation by different families of pattern-recognition receptors [3–5]. An important feature of the innate immune system is that a single class of pathogen can be sensed by different pattern-recognition receptors. These pattern-recognition receptors can be divided into secreted, endocytic, and signaling receptors [6]. The secretory pattern-recognition receptors (e.g., mannan binding lectins) function as opsonins binding to microbial cell walls (e.g., bacteria, yeast, viruses, and parasites), which trigger recognition by a complement activation system and phagocytes for complete destruction of pathogens. Endocytic pattern-recognition receptors (e.g., macrophage mannose receptors), which occur on the surface of phagocytes, mediate recognition, uptake, and delivery of pathogens into lysosomes. Furthermore, pathogens are processed via major histocompatibility complex (MHC) for pathogen destruction and elicitation of pathogenic antigen-specific immune responses. Signaling pattern-recognition receptors (e.g., Toll-like receptors) located intracellularly or at the cell surface of immune effector cells recognize PAMPs and activate signal-transduction pathways resulting in expression and synthesis of proflammatory cytokines, chemokines, and interferons [7–9]. The proinflammatory cytokines and chemokines in turn participate in acute recruitment and activation of immune effector cells, such as neutrophils, macrophages, dendritic cells, and natural killer cells to infection sites. Particularly, neutrophils and natural killer cells are critical innate effector cells protecting the host by killing pathogenic microbes and infected cells, respectively [8]. Interferons play a significant role in eliciting innate antiviral defenses [10].

15.3.2 Connecting Innate and Adaptive Immune Responses

An innate immune system signals the presence of infection through a multitude of signaling mechanisms, which control activation of adaptive immune responses. After recognition of PAMPs as "danger signals" by Toll-like receptors (TLRs), immature dendritic cells capture (beginning of adaptive immunity) and internalize antigens, and then they undergo activation and maturation processes to become mature dendritic cells. During activation, dendritic cells lose their phagocytic and tissue adhesion capabilities, increase their expression of lymphoid chemokines, and reorganize their cytoskeleton to attain mobility toward secondary lymph organs (e.g., lymph nodes) [11]. The maturation phenomenon upregulates surface expression of co-stimulatory (e.g., CD80 and CD86) and MHC molecules in dendritic cells. The expression of lymphoid chemokines and co-stimulatory molecules are under the control of innate immune system. In the presence of infection, TLRs induce co-stimulatory molecules on antigen-presenting cells. Meanwhile, internalized antigens undergo degradation into peptides, which bind to MHC molecules inside the endoplasmic reticulum. As shown in Figure 15.2a and b, the MHC-antigenic peptide complex translocates to dendritic cell surface for presenting to lymph node-resident T cells, leading to the initiation of adaptive immune responses [12–14].

15.3.3 Adaptive Immunity

In contrast to innate immunity, adaptive (acquired) immunity displays immunological memory against mutating pathogens and imparts long-lasting protection. Adaptive immune recognition relies on a somatic and diverse repertoire of antigen-specific T-cell receptors (e.g., $CD4^+$ and $CD8^+$ receptors) and B-cell receptors. The generation and maintenance of B- (humoral) and $CD8^+$ T-cell (cellular) responses is provided by $CD4^+$ T-helper (T_H) cells [15, 16]. Antigenic receptors bind to antigens regardless of their origin—microbial, environmental, or self.

*15.3.3.1 **Humoral Immunity*** Humoral immunity leads to the production of antigen-specific antibodies. A multitude of immunological mechanisms is involved in the generation of antibodies (refer to Figure 15.1a). The dendritic cells with MHC-II antigenic peptides on their cell surface migrate to lymph nodes and interact with naïve $CD4^+$ T cells resulting in their activation and differentiation into T_H cells (refer to Figure 15.1a). The activation of naïve $CD4^+$ T cells is the result of two distinct signals [17, 18]: 1) ligation of naïve $CD4^+$ T-cell receptors with antigen-specific MHC-II antigenic peptide complex on dendritic cells and 2) activation of co-stimulatory molecules (CD80 and CD86) on dendritic cells. In the presence of cytokines secreted by dendritic cells, naïve $CD4^+$

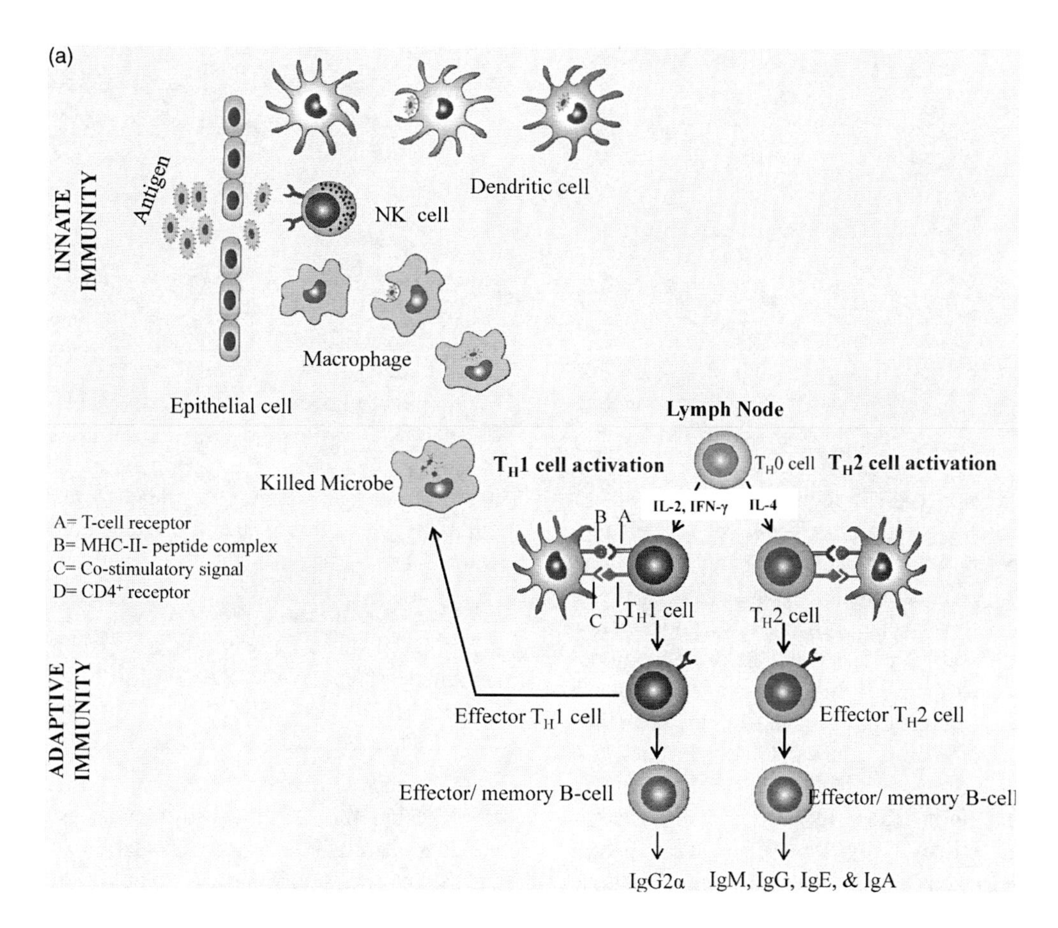

FIGURE 15.1 (a) During a bacterial infection, immature dendritic cells capture vaccine antigens and migrate from infection sites to afferent lymph nodes to become mature dendritic cells. During dendritic cell maturation, ingested antigen undergoes degradation in acidic endosomes to produce small peptides. As a result of an exchange mechanism in the endoplasmic reticulum, antigenic-peptide fragments bound to MHC molecules are translocated to the dendritic cell surface. These mature dendritic cells differentiate naïve T cells into T_H1 and T_H2 cells, which further differentiate naïve B cells to plasma (effector) and memory B cells. Distinct classes of cytokines trigger antibody production as well as class switching of antibodies in plasma B cells. (b) Demonstrates cellular immune mechanism. Specific internalized antigens, such as viruses, virus-like antigens, intracellular pathogens, and soluble proteins are retained inside dendritic cell endosomes. The internalized antigens escape endosomes and cross into cytosol. Now, the effector cytotoxic T cells cause lysis of pathogen loaded cells through distinct cell-death mechanisms. (See color figure in color plate section.)

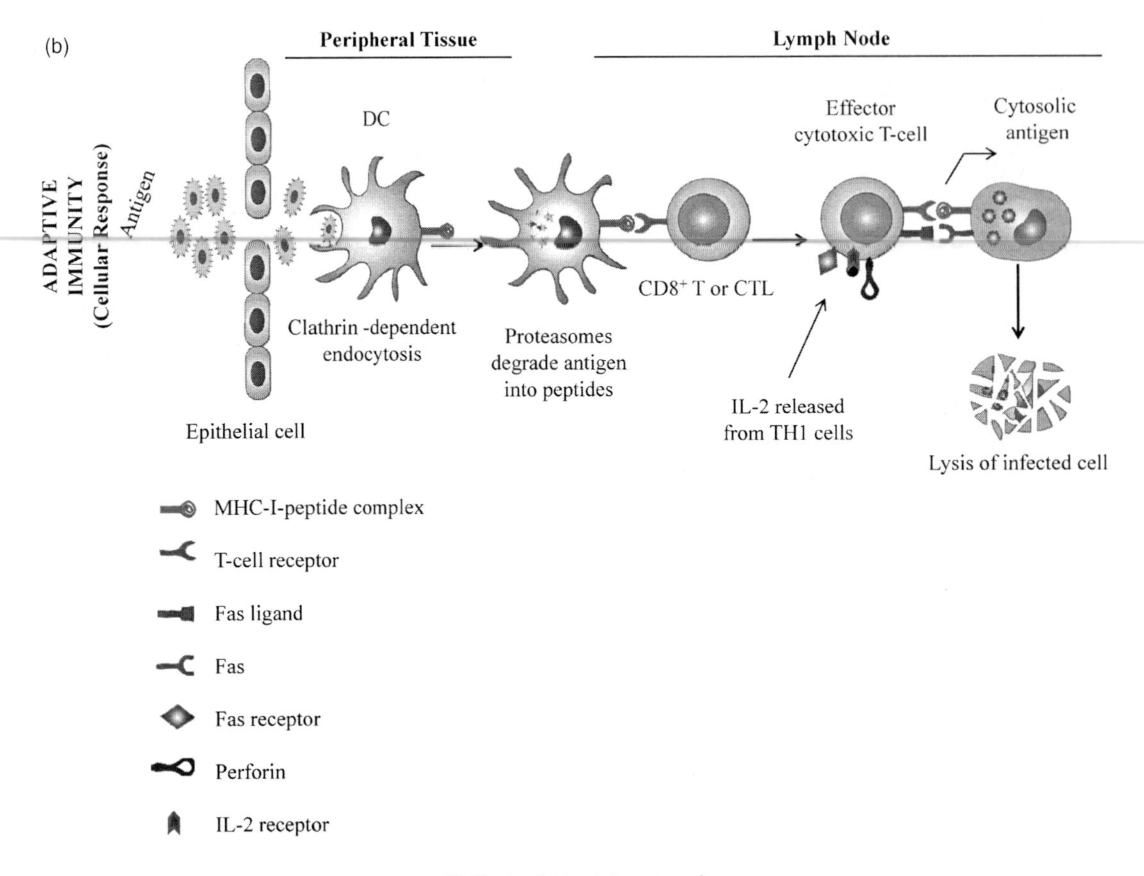

FIGURE 15.1 *(Continued)*

T cells differentiate first into T_H0 cells and then into distinct classes of T_H cells [19–22]. Cytokines, such as interleukin (IL)-6, IL-12, and interferon-γ (IFN-γ) generally induce T_H1 cells, whereas cytokines IL-4 and IL-10 induce T_H2 cells, and IL-17 induce T_H17 cells.

During microbial infection, naïve B cells transform as immunocompetent B cells inside the lymphoid follicles (B-cell zone) of lymph nodes. Similar to dendritic cells, immunocompetent B cells internalize antigens, undergo activation, and migrate from B-cell zone to T-cell zone of lymph nodes, where B cells present MHC-II antigen peptide complex to T-cell receptors of T_H cells. Like T_H cells, immunocompetent B cells require multiple extracellular signals for activation [23]: 1) signal provided by antigen-binding B-cell receptor (BCR), a surface bound immunoglobulin (Ig); 2) signal provided by either T_H1 or T_H2 cell; and 3) cytokine secretion by T_H cells. The T_H cells help activate immunocompetent B cells to proliferate and differentiate into plasma (effector) and memory cells. Distinct classes of cytokines secreted by T_H1 and T_H2 cells trigger different classes of antibody production in plasma B cells [24, 25].

Postinfection, T-cell-dependent B-cell responses do not provide immune protection for at least 5–7 days; this response is too delayed to control blood-borne infections against virus and bacteria. To compensate this limitation, B cells (marginal zone) undergo rapid antibody production in response to a microbial pathogen-associated molecular pattern [26]. Table 15.1 describes the functional role of Igs in response to antigen exposure. Furthermore, antibodies can either inactivate antigens directly or lead to antigen destruction indirectly through enhanced complement activation and phagocytosis [27].

15.3.3.2 Cellular Immunity Cytotoxic T cells ($CD8^+$ T cells; CTL) are another class of effector T cells of the immune system, with the ability to lyse target cells (Figure 15.1b). The MHC-I-restricted cytolytic T-lymphocyte (CTL) responses:

(1) Generate direct killing of virus infected cells, tumor cells, allografted cells, or parasites.
(2) Can facilitate cross-presentation of antigens where antigens from donor cells could be transferred to host APCs and subsequently be implicated in immune responses to viruses, tumor antigens, and transplantation antigens. The cross-presentation is essential for raising immunity against organisms that otherwise fail to infect APCs (e.g., Epstein-Barr virus) or tumor cells that by themselves are poor APCs.
(3) Can nullify viral challenge, even if not predisposed to the antibodies of a viral challenge. An effector CTL

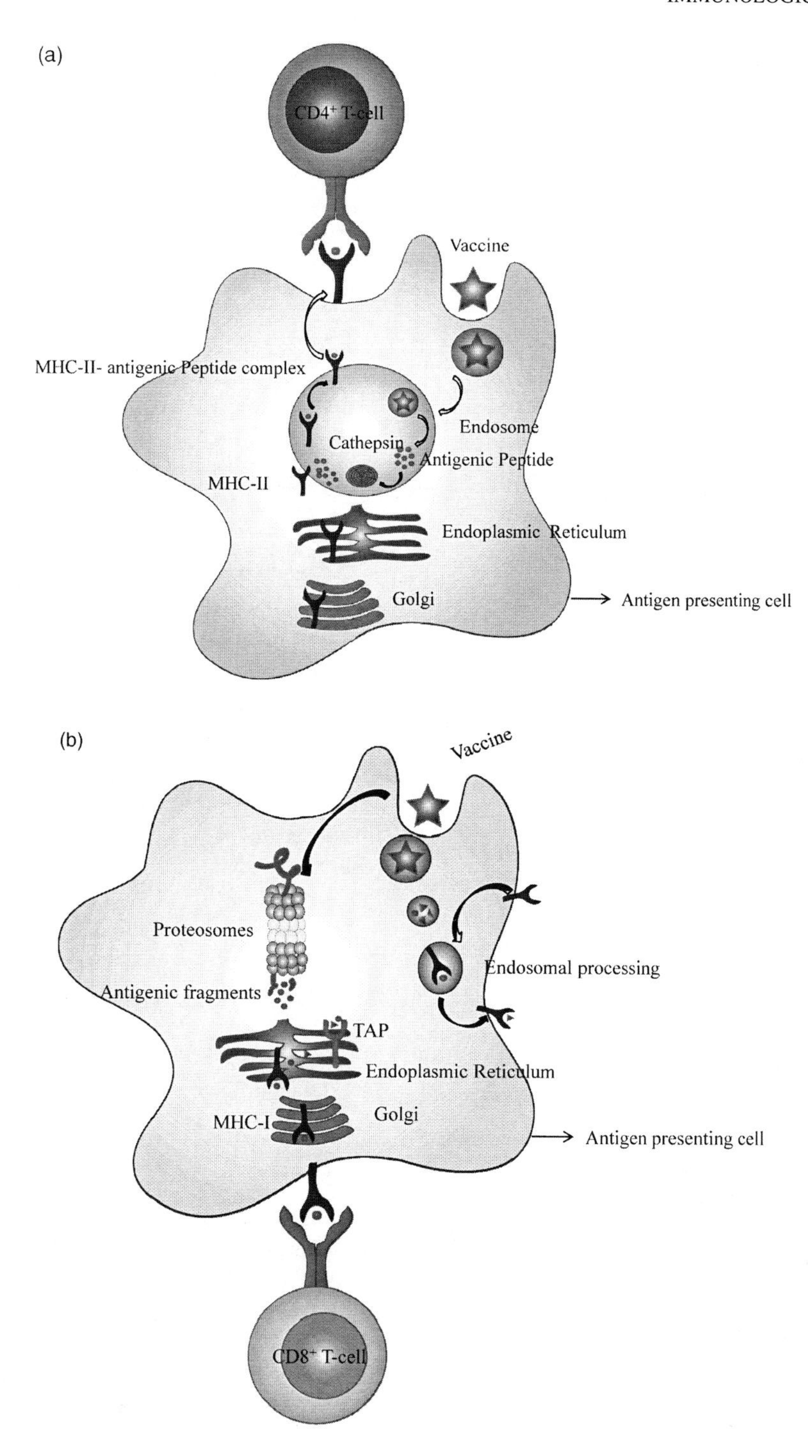

FIGURE 15.2 (a) APC phagocytosed antigens or antigen carriers enter acidic endosomes, where proteases degrade antigens into small peptides. In the endoplasmic reticulum, MHC-II molecules bind to an invariant protein, which directs the transportation of MHC-II-invariant protein from endoplasmic reticulum into endosomes. Inside the endosomes, invariant protein cleaves leaving a peptide fragment termed as CLIP, which still binds to MHC-II molecules. CLIP fragment exchanges with antigenic peptide and binds to MHC-II molecules. The MHC-II-antigenic peptide is translocated to cell surface to present to $CD4^+$ T cells. In general, the MHC-II pathway leads to humoral immunity. (b) APC phagocytosed antigens or antigen carriers can escape from endosomes and slowly hydrolyze in the cytoplasm, releasing encapsulated antigenic proteins. Released proteins are degraded by proteasomes into smaller peptides, which are then transported by TAP into the endoplasmic reticulum, where they bind MHC-I molecules. The MHC-I-antigenic peptides migrate to the cell surface. Multiple forms of exogenous (e.g., apoptotic cells and necrotic cells) and endogenous antigens (self- or virus-derived proteins) access the MHC-I pathway. Alternatively, antigens might be processed into peptides within endosomes, where they can access MHC-I molecules.

TABLE 15.1 Classes of Antibodies and Their Functional Role in Immune Responses

Antibody	Serum Composition	Serum Half-Life	Functional Role
IgM	20% of serum immunoglobulins	9–11 days	• First immunoglobulin secreted during primary immune responses • Potent activator of complement system
IgG	70% of serum immunoglobulins	25–35 days	• Predominant serum immunoglobulin during primary immune responses • Opsonizes antigens for phagocytosis and activates complement system
IgE	<1% of serum immunoglobulins	2–3 days	• Triggers secretion of inflammatory mediators • Mediates allergic reactions
IgA	<10% of serum immunoglobulins	≈5 days	• Secreted in large quantities across mucosal surfaces • Protects mucosa from colonization by bacteria and microorganisms
IgD	<1% of serum immunoglobulins	—	• No major role identified

kills an infected cell when it recognizes antigenic-peptide fragments bound to MHC-I molecule on the infected cell surface (e.g., dendritic cell or macrophage) (refer to Figure 15.2b).

After MHC-I-antigen-peptide recognition, CTLs undergo activation, proliferation, and differentiation promoted by cytokines (e.g., IL-15). As a result, CTLs become polarized and form unique lysosomal granules containing lytic proteins. The lysis of target cells via CTL is mediated by two different mechanisms: exocytosis of lytic proteins (perforins and granzymes) and/or receptor-ligand binding of Fas/APO molecules. Perforin-mediated killing results in necrosis of targeted cells, whereas Fas/APO pathways mediate apoptotic cell death [28].

15.4 TYPES OF VACCINES

Vaccines can be whole cells or subunits (e.g., proteins or polysaccharides) derived from cells. These vaccines are natural, synthetic, or recombinant in origin. Vaccines designed for induction of humoral or cellular immunity can be formulated in a soluble or particulate form. The next sections describe various types of vaccines used in commercial vaccine products or investigational studies.

15.4.1 Live Vaccines

Live vaccines are derived from disease-causing (wild) microbes, which are attenuated for administration into humans. These vaccines retain the ability to replicate and produce immunity, but they do not cause illness. Live, attenuated vaccines produce immunity in most recipients with a single dose, except those administered via oral route. The recipients who do not respond to first dose of an injected live, attenuated vaccine (e.g., measles, mumps, rubella vaccine) require a booster dose to provide strong immune protection [29].

15.4.2 Inactivated Antigen Vaccines

Inactivated vaccines are made of dead whole-cell microbes or fractions (proteins or polysaccharides) derived from pathogen subunits. These vaccines are produced by growing viruses or bacteria in culture media, followed by inactivation with heat, chemicals (usually formalin), or radiation. In general, the first dose of inactivated vaccines "primes" the immune system, and a strong immune response develops after additional doses. The immune response to an inactivated vaccine is mainly humoral rather than cellular [30].

Polysaccharide vaccines (e.g., Typhim Vi, a typhoid vaccine; Sanofi-Aventis, Bridgewater, NJ) are inactivated subunit vaccines composed of sugar molecules from the cell walls of bacteria. Pure polysaccharide vaccine typically elicits a T-cell-independent humoral response. However, the induced IgM antibodies are less immunogenic [31]. This problem can be overcome by conjugating polysaccharide to a protein. Such vaccines are termed as conjugate vaccines. For instance, the meningococcal conjugate is composed of capsular polysaccharide (polyribosylribitol phosphate), which is conjugated to an outer membrane protein complex (OMPC) of *Neisseria meningitides*. As a result of conjugation, the immune response shifts from T-cell-independent to T-cell-dependent antibody production, leading to enhanced immunity in infants [32].

Protein-based vaccines include toxoids (inactivated bacterial toxin) or subunits derived from microbes. The administration of protein vaccines produces a targeted response, which eliminates the risk of infection observed with live, attenuated vaccines or even inactivated vaccines where inactivation is incomplete. For example, anthrax (Biothrax; Emergent Biosolutions, Rockville, MD), Japanese encephalitis vaccine (IXIARO; Novartis Vaccines and Diagnostics, Inc., Cambridge, MA), and diphtheria and tetanus toxoids contain inactivated and purified proteins derived from a bacteria or virus.

15.4.3 Recombinant Vaccines

Recombinant vaccines are produced by genetic engineering technology. For example, human papillomavirus (HPV) and hepatitis B vaccines are produced by the insertion of a segment of the respective viral gene into gene of a yeast, *Saccharomyces cerevisiae* [33, 34]. The genetically modified yeast produces a pure HPV capsid protein or a hepatitis B surface protein, which are used as vaccines to induce immune responses against these viruses. Various recombinant strategies have been designed to use harmless viruses, bacteria, and yeast cells as immunization vectors.

15.4.3.1 Viral Vectors In approaches using viruses as immunization vectors, complementary DNAs (cDNAs) encoding whole or fraction of a gene from a microbe are inserted into a viral genome. The resulting recombinant viruses are introduced into the body, leading to the expression of selected antigens to stimulate the immune system [35]. An ideal viral vector should have the following characteristics: safe, efficient presentation of antigens to the immune system, genetic stability, ease of scalability and purification, and stability in the final formulation. However, viral vectors may cause potential safety issues, such as viral gene integration into host genome, or may revert to wild-type viruses, which results in fatal illness. Table 15.2 [36–42] demonstrates the characteristics of various viral vectors used for designing recombinant vaccines.

15.4.3.2 Bacterial Vectors In addition to viral vectors, attenuated bacteria have been used as vaccine vectors for the mucosal delivery of DNA vaccines [43]. For example, Bacillus Calmette–Guérin, *Listeria monocytogenes*, and

TABLE 15.2 Characteristics of Viral Vectors Used for Design of Recombinant Vaccines

Vector	Replication	Safety Concerns	Investigation Studies	References
DNA Viruses				
Adenovirus (ADV)	A foreign gene of 3–4 kb can be inserted into viral genome; stable recombinant gene	• Inflammatory responses generated by vectors. • Weakened efficacy of vectored-immunogen in the presence of anti-vector immunity.	Adenoviral vector encoding suppressor, p53 gene was approved in China for squamous cell head and neck cancer, malaria, and HIV	[36]
Adeno-associated virus (AAV)	A foreign gene of 5 kb can be inserted into viral genome	• Recombinant virus is safe and well tolerated. • Primary-booster dose regimens using AAV may hamper the clinical efficacy of recombinant viral gene.	HIV	[37]
Pox virus	Viral genome is large and stable to carry large amounts of foreign genes	• Preexisting immunity was attributed to those who had been immunized against smallpox. • A recombinant gene has low preexisting immunity.	Malaria and HIV	[38, 39]
RNA Viruses				
Vesicular stomatitis virus (VSV)	A foreign gene of 4.5 kb can be inserted into viral genome	• Low preexisting immunity exists against viral vector. • Neuropathy was observed.	HIV	[40]
Measles virus	Multiple foreign gene insertion sites (cloning) into viral genome	• Presence of antibody and cellular immunity against measles virus does not preclude a substantial boost by vaccination with recombinant vaccine.	HIV	[41]
Alpha virus	Multiple foreign gene insertion sites (cloning) into viral genome; can target dendritic cells and induce innate immune responses	• Because the alpha virus is zoonotic (mosquitoes) in certain geographical regions, preexisting immunity occurs. • Primary immunization with alpha viral vectored immunogen may hamper the efficacy of booster immunization with the same vector.	HIV	[42]

Salmonella typhi have been tested as vectors because of their established safety in humans and their capacity to accommodate large fragments of foreign DNA. After phagocytosis by APCs, recombinant bacteria survive inside the cells and release recombinant DNA into cytosol. The bacterial DNA integrates with APC nucleus and expresses the encoded antigen, which can be presented in association with MHC molecules to $CD4^+$ or $CD8^+$ T cells to elicit humoral or cellular immune responses, respectively.

15.4.3.3 Nucleic Acids Nucleic acids consisting of either DNA or RNA can be used for translation into antigenic proteins by host cells, and thus represent as candidates for the development of vaccines [35]. As a result of the absence of a coating, naked nucleic acids are not subjected to neutralizing antibody reactions that hinder the clinical efficacy of some vaccines. However, immunization with naked nucleic acids resulted in weak immune responses. Different approaches including genetic engineering have been explored to overcome the challenge of poor immune responses. For example, DNA fusion gene vaccine (Figure 15.3) can incorporate multiple genes either within the same vaccine vector or in separate vectors encoding a range of co-stimulatory molecules to enhance immune responses. Also, the fusion gene vaccine can be designed to program $CD8^+$ T cells for killing tumor cells or help B cells produce antibodies [44].

Self-replicating or replicon-based genetic vaccines also are designed to overcome inadequate immune responses of naked nucleic acids [45, 46]. Such vaccines can be generated by replacing genes for viral structural proteins with a specific antigen. Replication takes place in the cytoplasm of host cell and, therefore, is independent of the host's replication system. Despite the low antigen expression levels, an increase in immunogenicity was observed because of the abundant production of double-stranded RNA (dsRNA), a requisite intermediate of RNA replication. The dsRNA triggers host cell production of IFNs leading to infected cell death by apoptosis. The antigen-loaded dead cells trigger danger signals, leading to induction of adaptive immune responses [47].

15.5 PHYSICOCHEMICAL PROPERTIES OF VACCINE DELIVERY SYSTEMS

Many vaccine delivery systems are particulate systems to which antigens can be associated with carriers for extended periods. The biomaterials used for fabrication of delivery systems (e.g., micelles, emulsions, liposomes, virosomes, virus-like particles, polymeric nanoparticles, and dendrimers) are engineered for the induction of a specific immune response. Most of the prophylactic vaccines are based on the induction of long-lived, T-cell-dependent IgG production, whereas therapeutic vaccines (e.g., cancer and chronic infections) rely on the induction of T-cell-dependent humoral and cellular responses. For the successful induction of an immune response, upstream immune processes, including APC uptake, MHC pathways, lymphatic trafficking, cytokine presence, and strength of APC interactions with T cells, are

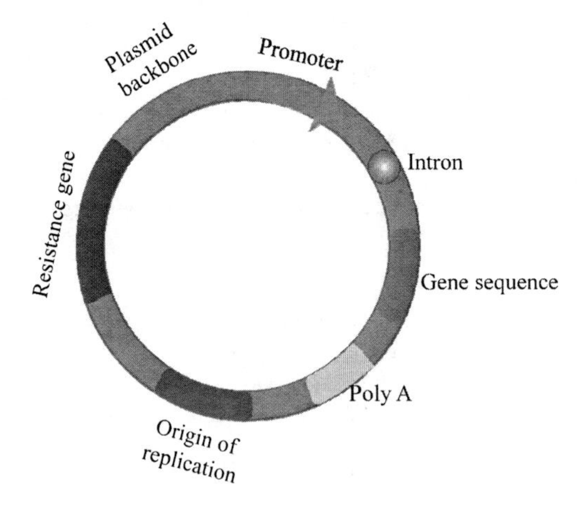

FIGURE 15.3 DNA fusion gene vaccine design. A DNA fusion gene vaccine has two main structures: plasmid backbone and transcriptional unit. The transcriptional unit contains the promoter and an insert or gene encoding the antigen of interest followed by a transcript termination/polyadenylation sequence. (a) The plasmid backbone (e.g., pVax1, pUC, and Pbr322) contains an origin of replication for amplification of the plasmid in bacteria, as well as an antibiotic resistance gene, conferring resistance to antibiotic, for example, to enable selective growth of the plasmid in bacteria. (b) Viral promoters, such as cytomegalovirus (CMV), simian virus (SV) 40, and sarcoma virus are often used to drive the expression of transgenic antigen in a number of mammal cells. Nonviral promoters, such as MHC-II promoter, chimeric, and other synthetic promoters, are also considered. (c) Transgene facilitates the possibility of encoding multiple proteins in a single gene construct because not only can an antigen be added, but also the sequences encoding adjuvant can be added to enhance vaccine potency. (d) Polyadenylation sequence (poly A) is an essential aspect of gene expression, playing an important role in messenger RNA (mRNA) stability and translation. Most vectors contain SV40 or bovine growth hormone poly A signal.

critical. To a large extent, the initiation and strength of upstream immune processes depend on the physicochemical features of a vaccine or its delivery system that mimic targeted microbes. These features include size, charge, hydrophobicity, and geometry.

15.6 VACCINE DELIVERY SYSTEMS

Particulate carriers have been used and widely investigated for vaccine/adjuvant delivery to lymph nodes and peripheral tissue-resident APCs for immunostimulation and immunosuppression (e.g., autoimmune disorders, allergic responses, and graft transplantation) purposes. The particulate vaccine carrier offers unique advantages over soluble form of vaccines, which include the following [48, 49]:

(1) Efficient up-take of vaccine by APCs
(2) Protects vaccine from proteolytic degradation
(3) Enhanced tissue-permeation or active-targeting of vaccine
(4) Controlled pharmacokinetic and tissue distribution kinetics of vaccine
(5) Controlled polymer degradation *in vivo* to sustain the release of encapsulated vaccine and prolong immune response
(6) Restricted entry of encapsulated vaccine to systemic circulation
(7) Co-delivery of vaccine and adjuvant to enhance immunity
(8) Encapsulates potent adjuvants and limit the magnitude of adverse immunogenic reactions
(9) Functionalization with peptides, proteins, antibodies, and other targeting polymers via noncovalent or covalent reactions
(10) Cross-presents vaccine to induce CTL responses

In addition, biodegradable and biocompatible vaccine carriers can be administered through multiple routes [50]. In detail, the next sections describe the various particulates that have been used as vaccine or adjuvant delivery systems.

15.6.1 Micelles

Micelles are aggregates of amphiphilic molecules (e.g., surfactants) dispersed in an aqueous medium (Figure 15.4a).

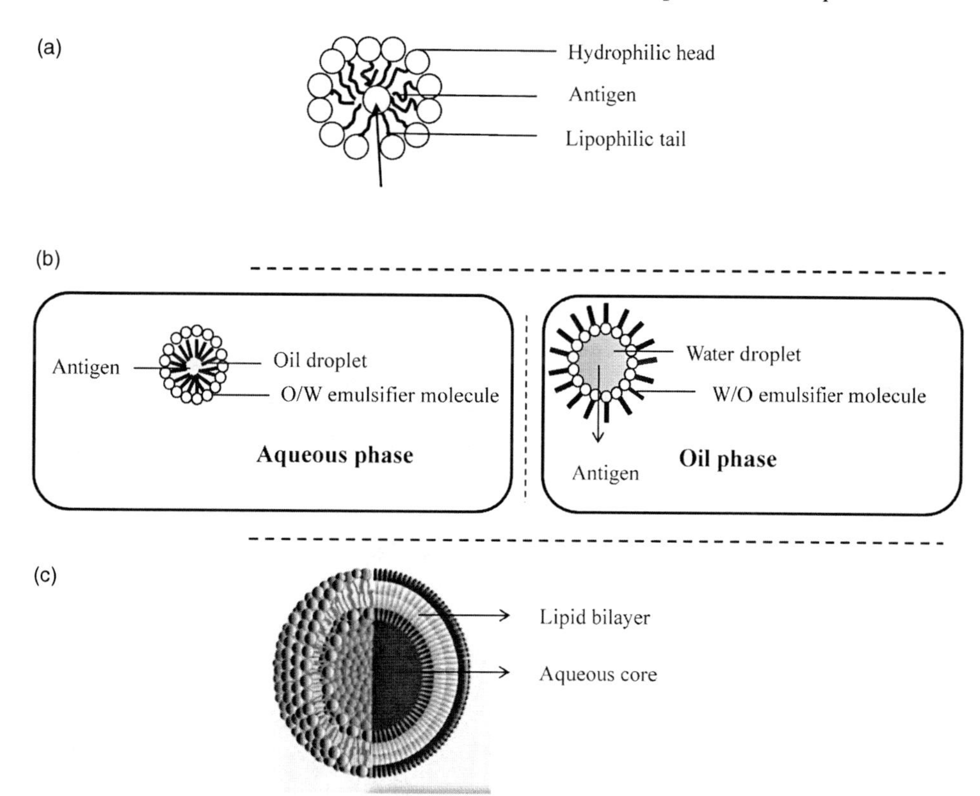

FIGURE 15.4 Various vaccine delivery systems include: (a) micelles, (b) emulsions, (c) liposomes (Reprinted with permission from Ref. 51), (d) virosomes, (e) virus-like particles, (f) polymeric nanoparticles, and (g) dendrimers. (Left: A G5 PPI (generation 5 poly (propyleneimine) dendrimer; generations ("shells") are indicated. Right: MAP dendron (basic MAP core based on lysine as the only monomer, indicating core structure and generation dependent increase of amino group numbers, leading to increased crowding of amino groups in shells of higher generation). Reprinted with permission from Ref. 54.

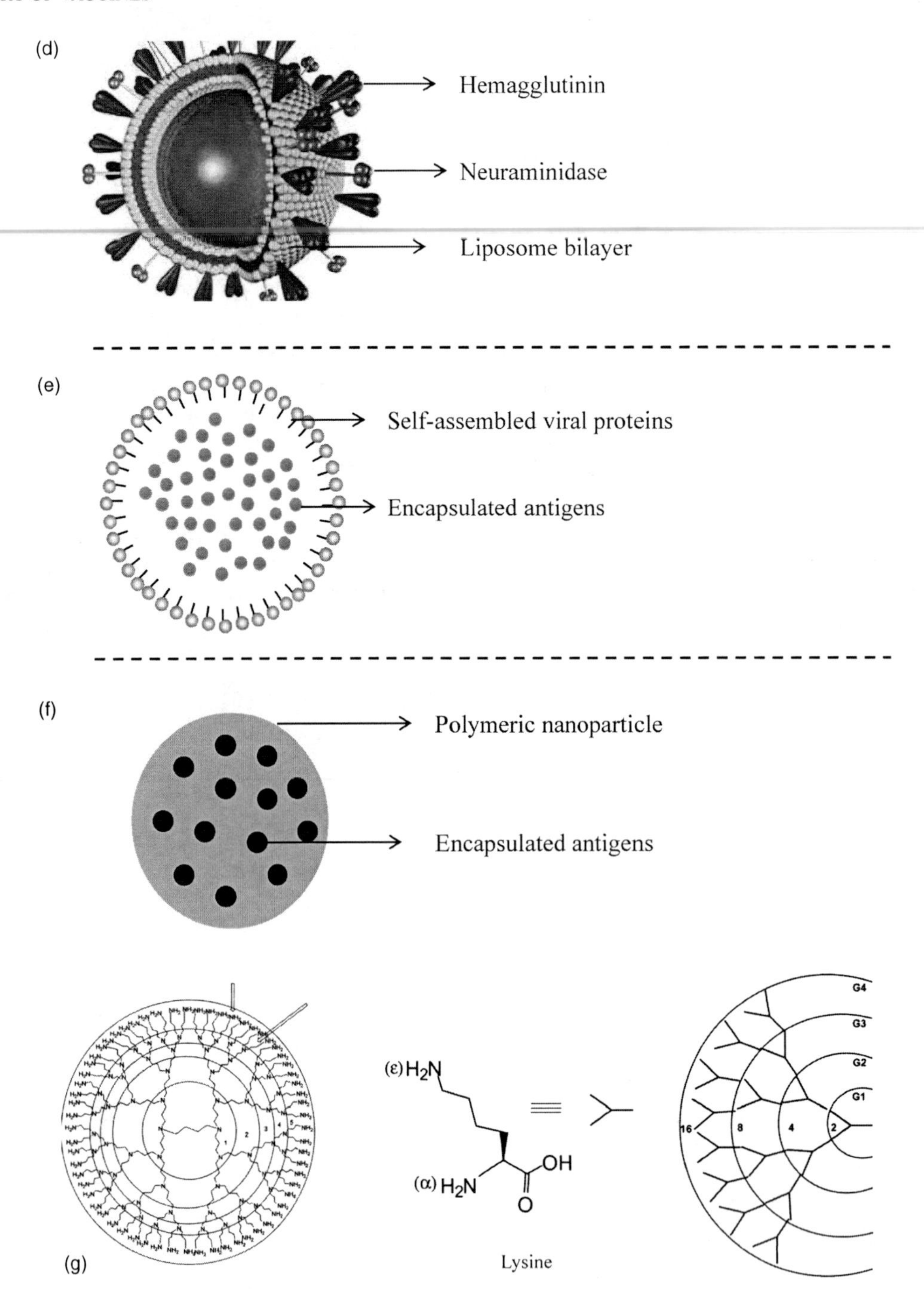

FIGURE 15.4 *(Continued)*

The narrow size distribution (10–60 nm) of micelles prevents their uptake by the reticuloendothelial system (RES). The hydrophobic fragments of amphiphilic molecules form the core of a micelle, which can be used to incorporate lipophilic vaccines. The outer layer of micelles is formed by hydrophilic fragments of the amphiphilic molecules. On the other hand, reverse micelles can be used for encapsulating hydrophilic vaccines inside the hydrophilic core of micelles. The small size of micelles enables them to accumulate in pathological areas with leaky vasculature, contributing to enhanced permeation. In addition to surfactants (e.g., polysorbates and pluronics), polymeric micelles (e.g., amphiphilic and double-hydrophilic block co-polymers) are being investigated as vaccine carriers. Amphiphilic polymer micelles usually have a low critical micelle concentration (CMC), which makes them stable *in vivo*. Charge can be imparted to block or graft co-polymers to control dendritic cell maturation and direct the nature of immune response (cellular vs humoral) [52, 53]. Cationic carriers with block or graft co-polymer architecture (e.g., polyethylene glycol [PEG]-*b*-poly(L-lysine), PEG-*b*-polyspermine, and PEG-g-polyethylene imine [PEI]) can be used for the delivery of negatively charged vaccines [53].

15.6.2 Emulsions

Emulsions are liquid disperse systems consisting of two immiscible phases (aqueous and oleaginous phases) emulsified by an emulsifier [55] (Figure 15.4b). Nanosized (20–200 nm) emulsion imparts kinetic stability against chemical, thermal, and pressure-triggered creaming and sedimentation processes. Nanoemulsions offer unique advantages: 1) offer versatile delivery of hydrophilic and lipophilic vaccines, 2) act as vaccine adjuvant to enhance immunity, and 3) sustain the release of vaccines after lipolysis of the oil phase. In general, lipophilic vaccines or adjuvants are incorporated into oil in water (O/W) emulsion, whereas hydrophilic vaccines are included in W/O emulsion. Shi et al. [56] developed an emulsion-based vaccine to co-deliver gastric cancer-specific antigen, MG7 and immunostimulatory CpG motif [57]. Mice immunized with co-encapsulated emulsion showed significant inhibition of tumor growth after challenging with MG-7 expressing cancer cells. Co-delivery of MG7 antigen and CpG motif augmented MG7-specific immunity compared with a nanoemulsion-containing antigen alone. Ge et al. developed a W/O nanoemulsion encapsulating melanoma-associated antigens (MAGE-1) for targeting melanoma. Following vaccination with nanoemulsion vaccine, mice responded with increased production of MAGE-1 specific antibodies as well as inhibition of tumor growth [58].

Because of their large interfacial area and heterogeneous nature, emulsions are generally unstable. It therefore requires the optimization of formulation and process variables for the preparation of a stable emulsion. Long- and medium-chain triglycerides alone or in combination are considered for developing emulsions. Long-chain triglycerides include soybean oil, safflower oil, sesame oil, and castor oil, whereas medium-chain triglycerides include Miglyol 810 and 812. The solubility and stability of active ingredients govern the selection of lipid phase. Medium-chain triglycerides possess good solubilizing and oxidative stability properties compared with long-chain triglycerides.

Emulsifiers reduce the interfacial tension between oil and aqueous phase, and thus produce a stable colloidal dispersion. Being biocompatible and nontoxic, egg and soy lecithins have been used in injectable emulsions. Other potential emulsifiers in injectable emulsions include PEGylated phospholipids (e.g., PEGylated phosphatidylethanolamine) and nonionic surfactants (e.g., Pluronic F68; BASF Corporation, Florham Park, NJ). The aqueous phase includes inactive ingredients, such as antioxidants, preservatives, tonicity modifiers, and pH-adjusting (buffering) agents. Antioxidants, which have a higher redox potential than active ingredients or excipients, prevent the oxidation of drug product ingredients. Antioxidants that impart protection in the aqueous phase include sodium metabisulfite, ascorbic acid, thioglycerol, and cysteine. Oil-soluble antioxidants include α-tocopherol, propyl gallate, ascorbyl palmitate, and butylated hydroxytoluene. Antimicrobial agents such as benzalkonium chloride, benzyl alcohol, parabens, and sodium benzoate are added to aqueous phase to prevent microbial growth. Complexing agents, such as ethylenediaminetetraacetic acid (EDTA) are incorporated to form inactive complexes with metals (chelates), which in their free-form initiate oxidation reactions. Tonicity can be achieved with glycerol and sorbitol. A slightly alkaline pH is preferred because sterilization reduces the pH of emulsion because of the production of free fatty acids.

15.6.3 Liposomes

Liposomes are unilamellar or multilamellar vesicles composed of phospholipids (Figure 15.4c). Liposomes possess unique properties resulting from the amphipathic character of lipids, which make them suitable for vaccine delivery. Numerous liposome formulations have been approved for the treatment of cancer and systemic fungal infections, whereas many liposome-based formulations are being developed as therapeutic vaccines against malaria, HIV, hepatitis A, and cancer [59–61]. Because lipids possess intrinsic adjuvant property, conventional liposomes can be used as adjuvants to enhance innate immunity. Liposome compositions can be varied to direct the encapsulated antigens to MHC-I or II pathways, and elicit cellular and humoral immune responses, respectively.

In general, water-soluble antigens are entrapped inside the liposomes, whereas lipophilic antigens are incorporated into lipid bilayers. However, water-soluble antigens exhibit low entrapment efficiency because of the porous nature of lipid bilayers, and these antigens necessitate the optimization of lipid composition and manufacturing process or even alter antigenic properties without changing immunogenic responses. For example, Baca-Estrada et al. incorporated a full-length glycoprotein-containing lipophilic membrane anchor into large unilamellar vesicles and observed higher glycoprotein incorporation efficiency than a truncated form lacking the lipophilic membrane anchor [50]. Along with antigen encapsulation, it may be necessary to improve delivery to target cells (e.g., dendritic cells) for the induction of long-lasting immunity. For this purpose, the lipid bilayer of liposomes can be manipulated to attach targeting moieties, such as PEG, peptides, and proteins [59]. Various types of phospholipid vesicles have been designed for delivery to

APCs in peripheral tissues and lymph nodes. Some of them include stealth, cationic, pH-sensitive liposomes, and fusogenic liposomes.

15.6.4 Virosomes

Virosomes are unilamellar phospholipid vesicles of approximately 150 nm in size. The virosomes mimic influenza virus envelopes devoid of genetic information (Figure 15.4d) [55]. During the production process, viral antigens, such as neuraminidase and hemagglutinin are integrated into liposome bilayer [62]. The hemagglutinin glycoprotein mediates virosome binding to the dendritic cell receptor and facilitates internalization [63]. Inside the dendritic cell endosomes, low pH causes conformational changes in hemagglutinin, resulting in the fusion of virosomes with endosome membranes. Within the endosome, virus antigen is proteolyzed to antigenic peptides, which are presented in the context of both MHC-I and MHC-II pathways for induction of cellular and humoral immune responses [64, 65]. Inflexal (Crucell, Leiden, The Netherlands) and Epaxal (Crucell) are virosome based vaccines. Inflexal, approved in Europe for prophylaxis of flu, consists of a mixture of three monovalent virosome pools, each formed with one influenza strain specific hemagglutinin and neuraminidase glycoproteins. Epaxal is a hepatitis A vaccine that was approved in Europe. The Epaxal vaccine has formalin-inactivated hepatitis A virions of RG-SB strain attached to the phospholipids of virosomes. Virosomes enable immunostimulation without inducing nonspecific inflammatory responses.

15.6.5 Virus-Like Particles

The viral capsid proteins, which self-assemble into noninfectious virus-like particles, have emerged as vaccine carriers (Figure 15.4e). For example, human papillomavirus vaccines (e.g., GARDASIL (Merck, Whitehouse Station, NJ) and CERVARIX (GlaxoSmithKline, Research Triangle Park, NC)) are prepared from major HPV capsid proteins. The virus-like particles lack viral genome and do not replicate. Virus-like particles taken up by dendritic cells via macropinocytosis and endocytosis induce strong cellular and humoral responses [66].

Because of the tendency of hepatitis B surface antigen (HBsAg) to form self-assembled virus-like particles, gp120 protein was co-expressed with the carrier protein HBsAg. These virus-like particles have gp120 at the lipid–water interface while displaying conformational epitopes to elicit immunity. The gp120-HBsAg virus-like particles showed enhanced vaccine potency through the induction of neutralizing antibodies with fewer doses than native gp120. Other carrier proteins investigated to form virus-like particles include retrovirus gag protein, bovine papilloma virus L1 protein, and VSV virions.

15.6.6 Polymeric Nanoparticles

Nanoparticles containing encapsulated or surface-engrafted antigens have drawn attention as vaccine delivery systems to enhance immunity and minimize immunization frequency (Figure 15.4f). Polymeric nanoparticles are colloidal carriers ranging in the size from 10 to 1000 nm. These nanoparticles can be nanocapsules or nanospheres, with the former particles being the vesicles composed of polymeric shell and an inner core, whereas the latter are composed of polymeric matrix. Polymeric nanoparticles offer distinct advantages, such as vaccine protection from proteolytic degradation, sustained release of vaccine, and restricted entry of vaccine to systemic circulation. Various synthetic or natural polymers are used for the fabrication of nanoparticles. Some of the synthetic polymers include aliphatic polyesters, such as poly (lactic acid) (PLA), poly(glycolic acid) (PGA), poly(D,L-lactic-co-glycolic acid) (PLGA), poly(e-caprolactone) (PCL), poly(hydroxybutyrate) (PHB), polyorthoesters (POEs), polyanhydrides, poly(aliphatic acids), and polyions, whereas natural polymers include alginate, chitosan, and gelatin.

One of the widely investigated polymers for vaccine delivery is PLGA co-polymer. Several studies have shown that PLGA nanoparticles can be used to deliver antigens and adjuvants for the induction and enhancement of antigen-specific immune responses [67, 68]. Because the size of PLGA nanoparticles (200–500 nm) is comparable with that of pathogens, nanoparticles become natural targets for dendritic cells. After recognition and uptake by dendritic cells, the encapsulated antigens can be processed as follows: 1) PLGA nanoparticles can be hydrolyzed in endo-lysosomes, where encapsulated antigenic proteins are degraded by lysosomal proteases into antigenic peptides, which bind to MHC-II molecules and present to $CD4^+$ T cells [69], and 2) some of the endosome internalized nanoparticles undergo slow hydrolysis to release encapsulated antigens into cytosol. The released antigens are degraded by proteasomes into peptides, which are transported via TAP mechanism into endoplasmic reticulum to bind to MHC-I molecules forming MHC-I-antigenic-peptide complexes. These complexes migrate to the cell surface for presenting to $CD8^+$ T cells and elicit cellular immune responses [70–73].

In aqueous medium, PLGA undergoes bulk erosion, where diffusion of water within the polymer matrix is faster than the rate of hydrolytic ester bond cleavage of the polymer chain. PLGA degradation continues until a critical molecular weight is reached, at which the degradation products become small enough to be solubilized. After PLGA degradation, the polymer structure becomes porous enough for the release of encapsulated substances. This bulk-erosion model hinders the early release of antigens, allowing dendritic cells to internalize antigen-encapsulated nanoparticles. The rate of PLGA degradation depends on the molecular weight, hydrophilicity, and crystallinity of the polymer [74]. The smaller the molecular weight of polymer, the higher the degradation rate (because of acid-triggered degradation of relatively high amount of carboxylic groups at the end of polymer chain) of the polymer. Glycolic acid is more hydrophilic than lactic acid, and therefore a high ratio of glycolic acid-to-lactic acid increases the hydrophilicity of the polymer and, subsequently, the degradation rate. L-lactic acid is crystalline and exhibits a slow hydrolytic degradation rate, but D,L-lactic acid is amorphous and shows a faster degradation rate. The PLGA co-polymer can exhibit fast degradation rate because of the amorphous nature of lactic and glycolic acid chains [75]. The degradation rate of PLGA can be manipulated by varying the proportion of crystalline and amorphous ratios of individual polymers. Also, PLGA co-polymers could be modified as higher-order (e.g., tri-block) block co-polymers or with PEG derivatives [67]. The PEGylation phenomenon causes steric repulsion between particles, which subsequently improves the stability of nanoparticles. In some instances, targeting can be increased through surface modification of PLGA nanoparticles using ligands, such as peptides, proteins, and antibodies. The interaction between surface modified PLGA nanoparticles and dendritic cells improves the specificity of nanoparticles for dendritic cell receptors, which results in enhanced uptake of nanoparticles through receptor-mediated endocytosis [76].

The co-delivery of antigen and adjuvant in PLGA nanoparticles has been demonstrated to induce the activation of both $CD4^+$ and $CD8^+$ T-cell-dependent immunogenic responses. For example, immunization with PLGA nanoparticles containing HBcAg antigen and MPLA adjuvant induced a stronger HBcAg-specific cellular response than those induced by HBcAg alone or HBcAg mixed with MPLA [77]. In another study, co-delivery of OVA and 7-acyl lipid A in PLGA nanoparticles promoted OVA-specific IFN-γ secretion by $CD4^+$ and $CD8^+$ T cells [71].

In addition to synthetic polymers, natural biodegradable polymers remain attractive because of their abundance, biocompatibility, and biodegradability. Proteins and polysaccharides have been investigated widely as vaccine carriers. Compared with proteins, polysaccharides are less immunogenic and can be modified readily by simple chemical reactions for vaccine delivery. Some of the examples of polysaccharides include chitosan, alginic acid, and dextran, whereas protein's example include gelatin.

15.6.7 Dendrimers

Dendrimers are hyper-branched polymers designed for the delivery of various therapeutic agents. Several dendrimers, such as poly (amidoamine) (PAMAM), polypropyleneimine (PPI), and multiple-antigen peptides (MAPs), have been investigated for vaccine delivery. The basic structure of a dendrimer has three components: a core, branches, and end groups, from the center toward the periphery. The branching pattern defines the dendrimer generation with generation 1 being the dendrimer containing only one layer of branching points, and whose addition represents an increase in dendrimer generation. For example, fifth-generation PAMAM dendrimer or G5-PAMAM contains five branching shells. In general, PAMAM and PPI dendrimers possess symmetric spherical structure, whereas the MAP dendrimer has a tree-like (dendron) structure. In higher generation dendrimers ($G > G3$), the core region is shielded off from the surrounding solution by an outer shell (Figure 15.4g). As a consequence of intense branching in the dendrimer structure, higher-generation dendrimers become globular in structure, whereas several functional groups can be displayed on the surface [54].

Dendrimers can be synthesized by two methods: 1) the divergent method, where the dendrimer is synthesized from the core and out towards the surface, and 2) the convergent method, where the dendrimer is synthesized from the surface and inward by joining two or more dendron fragments at the core. Because the interior of dendrimer is largely restricted from exposure to the outside environment, the biological properties of dendrimer are governed by surface groups. Based on the surface charge, dendrimers can be classified into cationic, anionic, and neutral. A positively charged higher generation dendrimer ($G > G6$) with an amine terminal group interacts with the cell membrane causing cell lysis *in vitro* as well as *in vivo*. Also, cationic dendrimers result in inflammation and activation of the complement system. Negatively charged dendrimers with carboxyl end groups do not interact with cellular surfaces and, therefore, do not produce significant cytotoxicity. The neutral dendrimer's end groups can be polar or nonpolar. The polar groups (e.g., PEG) are relatively nontoxic, whereas nonpolar lipid end groups can interact with hydrophobic domains of cells causing cytotoxicity. The cytotoxic characteristic of the dendrimers may help target bacterial cells to produce cellular immune response.

Because of their well-defined, multivalent, derivatizable, and stable structure, dendrimers can be used as vaccine antigen delivery systems or as vaccine adjuvants. Among derivatized dendrimers, MAP carriers are the most investigated dendrimers for immunological purposes. The basic structure of MAP dendrimer consists of solely lysine, whose two amino groups (α and ε) function as branching points for logarithmic growth. Tetrameric and octameric MAP cores are preferred, as these dendrimers possess favorable immunogenicity and stable attached-peptide structures for immunostimulation [78]. Other peptide-based dendrimers used for controlled display of antigens include sequential oligopeptide carriers (SOCs) of peptide antigens. The SOCs restrict conformational freedom of peptide antigens but present them in a better spatial manner [79].

Nonpeptide dendrimers used as vaccine or adjuvant carriers include PAMAM dendrimers. A G7 PAMAM administered with influenza antigens stimulated antibody production [80]. At physiological pH, hemagglutinin antigens are anionic and bind to cationic amino groups of PAMAM dendrimers. The adjuvant activity of PAMAM dendrimers correlated well with the number of amino groups. The cationic PAMAM dendrimers can be used for nonviral delivery of negatively charged DNA vaccines [81].

15.7 ADJUVANTS (IMMUNOPOTENTIATORS)

Alums are the only U.S. Food and Drug Administration approved adjuvants to date. Many experimental adjuvants have advanced to clinical trials; some have demonstrated potency, but most have proven too toxic for clinical use. Recent investigations have led to a greater understanding of adjuvants at the molecular level. Adjuvants that mimic pathogens are effective because of their activation of pattern recognition receptors. These adjuvants, also termed as immunopotentiators, induce innate responses targeting antigen-presenting cells. In addition, adjuvants can stimulate APCs to produce cytokines that play a key role in priming and polarization of adaptive immune responses [82].

Bacteria-derived substances constitute a potential source of adjuvants. *N*-Acetyl-muramyl-L-alanyl-D-isoglutamine derived from the cell walls of bacteria mediates the activation of TLRs of an innate immune system. In saline, *N*-acetyl-muramyl-L-alanyl-D-isoglutamine enhances humoral immunity, whereas in liposomes, it induces cellular immunity [83, 84]. Monophosphoryl lipid A of Gram-negative bacteria when combined with Fluarix (GSK) emulsion demonstrated higher $CD4^+$ T-cell responses [85]. Like lipopolysaccharides, monophosphoryl lipid A interacts with TLR4 on APCs resulting in the release of proinflammatory cytokines. The CpG motifs present in bacterial nucleic acids produce strong humoral (IgG2a) and cellular responses [86]. The CpG motifs interact with TLR9, leading to the production of inflammatory cytokines and co-stimulatory molecules. Many adjuvants mediate their immunostimulation via induction of cytokines and chemokines. Different cytokines have been co-delivered with antigens for the induction of strong immune responses [87]. However, all cytokines face limitation of their short half-life.

Both vaccine delivery systems and adjuvants exhibit their own immune induction mechanisms. In fact, some adjuvants exhibit both innate and adaptive immune features, and contribute to a synergistic immune response. Combinations of delivery systems and adjuvants are being developed either to enhance or modulate the immune response. Many new vaccine candidates for the prevention of challenging diseases (e.g., cancer and HIV) contain adjuvant combinations (e.g., AS04 and AS01) intended for generation of T_H1 activated cellular immune response [88].

15.8 ROUTE OF ADMINISTRATION AND DEVICES

Several devices are available for oral, intranasal (IN), intramuscular (IM), subcutaneous (SC), intradermal (ID), and transdermal delivery of vaccines. Novel vaccine devices are being developed: 1) to improve safety, 2) for ease of administration, 3) for administration of small doses of antigens, and 4) to meet dose requirements of new routes of administration. Table 15.3 shows the U.S.-approved vaccines administered by different routes.

15.8.1 Oral Route

The primary reason for oral vaccination is that the gastrointestinal mucosa is susceptible to common microbial infections. Examples include gastrointestinal infections caused by *Vibrio cholera* and *Escherichia coli*; respiratory infections caused by *Mycoplasma pneumonia* and influenza virus; and genital infections caused by HIV, herpes simplex virus, chlamydia, and *Neisseria gonorrhea* [89]. The mucosal-associated lymphoid tissue represents a compartmentalized immunological system, which functions independently of the systemic immune apparatus [90]. Vaccines invoke both humoral and cellular responses, with the former one predominantly mediated by sIgA antibodies produced from mucosal cells and muco-epithelial cells [91]. Consistent with compartmentalization, mucosal immune cells activated at one site (inductive site) disseminate immunity to remote mucosal tissues (effector sites) rather than to systemic sites. The mucosal compartmentalization thus determines the choice of vaccination route for inducing effective responses at the desired sites. In gastrointestinal infections, oral immunization results in substantial secretion of sIgA antibodies in the small intestine [92]. In infections (respiratory or enteric infections, such as *Shigella* or *Salmonella typhi*) where mucosa is permeable to the transudation of serum antibodies, a parenteral route of administration seems a viable option. Nasal immunization induces a humoral response in the upper airway mucosa and regional secretions (saliva and nasal) [93, 94].

About half a dozen mucosal vaccines have been approved for human use. The oral polio vaccine (OPV) elicits local sIgA response in the intestinal mucosa to block poliovirus entry and produces serum antibodies against poliomyelitis to prevent the spread of virus to nervous system. But the risk of reversion of OPV viral strains towards neurovirulence led to the replacement with inactivated polio vaccine [95]. Rotavirus is the most common cause of severe diarrhea in children resulting in 600,000 deaths worldwide every year. Rotarix (GSK) and Rotateq (Merck, Whitehouse Station, NJ) are oral, live attenuated vaccines that induce high titers of serum IgA levels and correlate well with intestinal

TABLE 15.3 List of Vaccines Licensed for Immunization in the United States

Product Name (Trade Name)	Nature (Formulation)	Disease	Immunity	Admn. Route
Live, Attenuated Vaccines				
BCG (Mycobax; Connaught Laboratories Ltd., Ontario Canada)	Lyophilized (suspension)	Tuberculosis	$CD8^+$	PC
Influenza A virus (H5N1) (no trade name)	Liquid suspension	Influenza	IgG	IM
Influenza vaccine (FluMist; MedImmune, Inc.)	Intranasal spray solution	Influenza	IgG, IgA, $CD8^+$	IN
Measles, mumps, rubella, and varicella (ProQuad; Merck)	Lyophilized (solution)	MMR and chickenpox	IgG	SC
Rotavirus pentavalent (ROTARIX; GSK)	Lyophilized (suspension)	Gastritis	IgG	Oral
Rubella virus (Meruvax II; Merck)	Lyophilized (solution)	German measles	IgG	SC
Smallpox (vaccinia) (ACAM2000; Acambis plc, Bridgewater, NJ)	Lyophilized (solution)	Smallpox	$CD8^+$	PC (scarification)
Typhoid, Ty21a (Vivotif; Crucell)	Lyophilized (suspension)	Typhoid fever	IgG	Oral
Varicella virus (Varivax; Merck) or Zoster (Zostavax; Merck)	Lyophilized (suspension)	Chickenpox	IgG	SC
Yellow fever (YF-Vax; Sanofi-Pasteur, Inc., Swiftwater, PA)	Lyophilized (suspension)	Yellow fever	IgG	SC
Nonlive or Inactivated Vaccines				
Hepatitis A (VAQTA; Merck)	Whole virus/liquid suspension	Hepatitis A	IgG	IM
Rabies (Imovax; Sanofi-Pasteur, Inc.)	Killed rabies virus/lyophilized (suspension)	Rabies	IgG	IM
Typhoid Vi polysaccharide (TYPHIM Vi; Sanofi-Pasteur, Inc.)	Polysaccharide (solution)	Typhoid fever	IgG	IM
Anthrax (Biothrax; Emergent biosolutions, Inc.)	Inactivated proteins (liquid suspension)	Anthrax	IgG	IM
Human papillomavirus, recombinant (GARDASIL; Merck)	HPV proteins (liquid suspension)	Vulvar, vaginal, anal cancers	IgG	IM
Japanese encephalitis virus (IXIARO; Novartis Vaccines and Diagnostics, Inc.)	Inactivated proteins (liquid suspension)	Japanese encephalitis	IgG	IM
DAPTACEL, IPOL, Hib Conjugate (Pentacel; Sanofi-Pasteur Inc.)	DT toxoids, inactivated pertussis protein, poliovirus protein, haemophilus-tetanus toxoid conjugate/lyophilized (suspension)	Diphtheria, tetanus, and pertussis, polio, meningitis	IgG	IM
Haemophilus b (Hib) conjugate (PedvaxHIB; Merck)	Meningococcal protein conjugate (liquid suspension)	Meningitis	IgG	IM
Meningococcal (Menveo; Novartis Vaccines and Diagnostics, Inc.)	Oligosaccharide diphtheria CRM_{197} conjugate/lyophilized (solution)	Meningitis	IgG	IM
Pneumococcal 13-valent conjugate (Prevnar 13; Wyeth, Madison, NJ)	Diphtheria CRM_{197} protein conjugate (liquid suspension)	Pneumonia	IgG	IM

Information regarding product/trade name, disease, formulation, and route of administration was retrieved from www.FDA.gov.
DPT = diphtheria, pertussis, tetanus; Hib = *Haemophilus influenza* b; PC = percutaneous; lyophilized preparations after reconstitution form either solution or suspension for administration.

IgA antibodies conferring protection from gastroenteritis in children [96].

15.8.2 Intranasal Route

The nasal mucosa provides a convenient surface for vaccine deposition and induction of systemic and local mucosal immunity. Recently, a live influenza vaccine delivered by intranasal spray (FluMist; MedImmune, Gaithersburg, MD) was approved in the United States. Unlike injectable vaccines against influenza, intranasal vaccines induce a high titer of locally produced sIgA to confer protection of the upper respiratory tract, and serum IgG antibodies to impart protection of the lower respiratory tract [97]. A distinct advantage of intranasal delivery is that the absorption through nasal mucosa can be achieved in 24–48 h, providing rapid protection against airborne pathogens that enter the body through respiratory tract. Another key benefit of intranasal vaccines is their potential to induce both cellular and humoral immunity.

Advances in dry powder formulation and nano-technology-based processes have made possible for new intranasal vaccine delivery systems [98]. Dry powder enhances the stability of a vaccine and reduces the cold-chain requirements or the addition of preservatives. The Becton Dickinson (BD) and Aktiv-Dry developed dry powder inhalers that could be adapted for intranasal vaccine delivery. An intranasal delivery system, VersiDoser (Mystic Pharmaceuticals, Inc., Cedar Park, TX.) is simple, self-administrable, disposable, and capable of precise aseptic delivery of formulations for maximum deposition in nasal mucosa. VersiDoser uses a proprietary aseptic form-fill seal unit-dose manufacturing technology to produce and fill blisters with a liquid vaccine. VersiDoser unit-dose blisters deliver dose volumes ranging from 15 to 500 μL.

15.8.3 Intramuscular/Subcutaneous Route

Most vaccines are delivered through IM or SC routes to optimize immunogenicity of vaccines and minimize their adverse reactions. Various factors including the nature of antigen, adjuvant, formulation, dose, and type of immune response affect the route of administration. Abundant musculature, presence of APCs, and fast onset of immune response are the primary reasons for IM administration of vaccines. With alum adjuvanted vaccines (e.g., hepatitis, diphtheria, tetanus, and pertussis vaccines), the IM route is strongly preferred because SC administration leads to an increased incidence of local reactions, such as irritation, inflammation, granuloma formation, and necrosis [99]. However, because of the fat layers in muscle tissues, some of the IM vaccination sites do not contain APCs necessary to initiate immunity. As a result, the vaccine may take longer time to reach blood circulation, leading to a delay in vaccine processing and presentation to T and B cells. Through the SC route, vaccine formulations can drain directly from injection site to peripheral lymph nodes, where immune cells reside [100]. Solution-based vaccines drain through lymphatic endothelial gaps into lymph nodes, whereas suspensions in the size range of 0.1 to 1 μm are phagocytized by peripheral tissue-resident dendritic cells [101]. Because of the poor vasculature, SC vaccination may slow mobilization and processing of vaccine formulations, leading to low sero-conversion rates and a rapid decay of antibody response.

Needle syringe is the most common device for IM and SC delivery of vaccines. A wide-bore needle ensures that the vaccine is dissipated over a wider area, thus reducing the risk of localized redness and swelling. Various IM and SC injection devices have been developed to address problems, such as needle-associated injuries, reconstitution errors, and shipping issues [102]. For example, disposable syringe-jet injectors are used for IM delivery of liquid vaccine formulations. The jet injectors consist of a reusable hand piece containing a propulsion system and a disposable vaccine containing a needle-free syringe or cartridge (prefilled or end-user filled). The most widely used disposable syringe jet injector is Biojector (Bioject Medical Technologies, Inc., Tigard, OR) for the administration of IM vaccines. Other disposable syringe-jet injector devices in clinical trials include Zetaject (Bioject Medical Technologies, Inc.), PharmaJet (PharmaJet, Golden, CO), and LectraJet M3RA (D'Antonio Consultants International, Inc., Tully, NY).

15.8.4 Intradermal Route

Intradermal delivery has been used as the route of choice for only a very limited number of vaccines, such as Bacillus Calmette–Guérin, and in at least some countries for post-exposure rabies vaccination. The renewed interest in intradermal delivery has been driven largely by the perception that intradermal route might offer several clinical, immunological, safety, and logistic advantages. Some of the potential benefits include improved immunogenicity, dose sparing, increased availability of "limited" antigens, and avoidance of adjuvants.

Various intradermal devices include needle-syringe, microneedles, and jet injector devices. The intradermal needle-syringe devices are available as prefilled or end-user-filled devices. The Soluvia device (Beckton, Dickinson and Company, Franklin Lakes, NJ), referred to as the "microinjection system" is a prefilled syringe with a single 30-gauge needle to deliver 100–200 μL of fluid. The device is also designed to protect the needle after injection, reducing the risk of injury and preventing reuse. Microneedles are micron-scale needles designed to deliver vaccines to the epidermis and dermis. Microneedle-based intradermal devices are needle free with a small package volume of components [103]. Because of their micron-sized height, microneedles do not stimulate underlying nociceptors and have been shown to be painless in multiple human studies [104]. Potential benefits include the reduction of sharps, dose sparing, and reduction of cold chain volumes.

15.8.5 Transdermal Route

Transdermal delivery offers attractive opportunities to improve vaccine administration. Vaccine delivery via skin is attractive because it targets epidermal Langerhans and dermal dendritic cells that may generate a strong immune response at much lower doses than deep injections

[105]. The ease of self-administering vaccine patches by patients could facilitate compliance with routine, seasonal, and pandemic vaccination needs. Adequate immunity via skin may be achieved by increasing skin permeability to antigens.

Some of the transdermal physical (e.g., electroporation, cavitation ultrasound, and microneedles) and chemical (e.g., permeation enhancers) methods have been shown to enhance immunity [106–109]. As conventional injectable approaches of DNA vaccines failed to achieve a strong immune response, it is believed that physical delivery approaches (e.g., electroporation and sonophoresis) are needed to deliver DNA vaccines to target cells [44]. Electroporation uses brief electrical pulses to create transient "pores" in the cell membrane, thus allowing large molecules, such as DNA or RNA, to enter the cell cytoplasm [110]. After the cessation of electric field, these pores would close, and molecules would be trapped inside the cytoplasm without causing cell death. In addition to increased permeability of target cells, electroporation may also enhance immunity through increased protein expression, secretion of inflammatory cytokines and chemokines, and recruitment of APCs to the electroporation site.

15.9 CONCLUSION

An ideal vaccine requires the ability to induce rapid and sustained immune responses. For many existing vaccines, a strong and long-lasting immune response against a pathogenic antigen requires large and multiple doses, which pose limitations in terms of storage and transportation. To overcome these challenges, new biomaterials are being developed to design vaccine delivery systems for a targeted immune response with a minimal dose. Also, vaccine delivery systems can be co-encapsulated or surface modified with adjuvants for enhancing immune responses. Along with particle engineering, the route of administration has also become a key factor in improving vaccine delivery. Therefore, a combination of polymer chemistry, molecular immunology, lymphatic physiology, and device engineering will help design successful vaccine delivery systems for many chronic diseases.

ASSESSMENT QUESTIONS

15.1. An animal in a herd acquired immunity from another animal and remained immune to the disease for a brief period. Such immunity is called:

- **a.** Herd immunity
- **b.** Intrinsic immunity
- **c.** Passive immunization
- **d.** Active immunization

15.2. Which of the following immune responses is a rapid and nonspecific immune response?

- **a.** Adaptive immune response
- **b.** Innate immune response
- **c.** Both A and B
- **d.** None of the above

15.3. Which class of antibody has the longest serum half-life and opsonizes antigens for phagocytosis?

- **a.** Immunoglobulin A (IgA)
- **b.** Immunoglobulin G (IgG)
- **c.** Immunoglobulin M (IgM)
- **d.** Immunoglobulin E (IgE)

15.4. A woman visits a clinic for symptoms of a viral infection (fever). To confirm the diagnosis, the physician draws a blood sample and tests her antibody titer level against viral particles. An initial blood sample shows a low titer of antibody, but the blood sample drawn a week later shows high antibody titers. This situation is an example of:

- **a.** A cellular response to viral infection
- **b.** An inflammatory response to viral infection
- **c.** A secondary immune response to viral infection
- **d.** A primary immune response to viral infection

15.5. A parent brings an 8-year-old wounded child to a clinic. If no information of the child's vaccination history is available, then what should the physician recommend?

- **a.** An antiseptic cleanup of the wound area
- **b.** Tetanus toxoid (Td)
- **c.** Tetanus immunoglobulin (TIG)
- **d.** Both TIG and Td at separate sites

15.6. $CD8^{+}$ T cells specifically recognize antigens in which form?

- **a.** Bound to MHC class II molecules on the surface of dendritic cells
- **b.** Bound to MHC class I molecules on the surface of a body cell
- **c.** Bound to both MHC class I and II molecules on the surface of a body cell
- **d.** None of the above

15.7. In the antiviral immunity, which immune cell recognizes and kills viral infected cells?

- **a.** B cells
- **b.** Cytotoxic T cells
- **c.** Antibodies
- **d.** Interferons

15.8. Which of the following is a valid statement about live attenuated vaccines?

a. Attenuated vaccines often require multiple doses.

b. Live, attenuated vaccines require a low dose to elicit an immune response.

c. Inactivated vaccines require a low dose to elicit a strong immune response.

d. Killed, inactivated vaccines produce lifelong immunity in one or two doses.

15.9. Which of the following vaccines is approved for intranasal delivery in the United States?

a. Yellow fever vaccine

b. Influenza vaccine

c. Polio vaccine

d. MMR vaccine

15.10. Which of the following polio vaccines is approved in the United States?

a. Four doses of IPV plus a booster at 18 years of age.

b. Four doses of IPV.

c. Two doses of OPV and two doses of IPV.

d. Polio vaccination is not recommended in the United States.

15.11. Which of the following vaccines has both a polysaccharide and a protein conjugated vaccine on the U.S. market?

a. Hemophilus influenza type B vaccine and meningococcal vaccine

b. Pneumococcal and meningococcal vaccine

c. Polio vaccine and smallpox vaccine

d. Japanese encephalitis vaccine and anthrax vaccine

15.12. Which of the following is a recombinant vaccine produced from yeast cells?

a. MMR vaccine

b. Smallpox vaccine

c. Hepatitis B vaccine

d. Bacillus Calmette–Guérin vaccine

15.13. The most common adverse reaction to an inactivated vaccine is:

a. Rash

b. Injection site reactions

c. Severe headache

d. Rhinorrhea

15.14. Which of the following vaccines also is available as live, attenuated bacterial vaccine in the United States?

a. Polio vaccine

b. DTaP

c. Varicella vaccine

d. Bacillus Calmette–Guérin vaccine

15.15. If a second dose of a vaccine were given too soon, then the correct course of action would be:

a. Continue with the next dose as scheduled

b. Reduce the next dose

c. Do not count the dose and repeat it after the minimal time period has passed since the incorrect dose

d. Avoid the next dose

15.16. The only vaccine recommended at birth is:

a. IPV

b. MMR vaccine

c. Hepatitis B vaccine

d. DTaP vaccine

15.17. Which of the following enzymes is responsible for transcription of DNA from mRNA during the synthesis of complementary DNA?

a. RNA polymerase

b. Reverse transcriptase

c. DNA transferase

d. Glutaminase

Directions for questions 18–20: The questions and incomplete statements in this section can be answered correctly or completed by one or more of the suggested answers. Choose the correct answer, a–d:

a. If II only is correct

b. If I and II are correct

c. If II and III are correct

d. If I, II, and III are correct

15.18. Which of the following statements best describes a vaccine adjuvant?

I. Adjuvants activate naïve T cells into T-helper cells or regulatory T cells.

II. Adjuvants enhance the immune response of vaccine antigens.

III. Adjuvants act as preservatives in vaccine formulations.

15.19. Which of the following statements is relevant to particulate vaccine delivery systems?

I. Vaccine delivery systems allow the slow release of antigens.

II. M59, an oil-in-water emulsion, is considered a particulate vaccine delivery system.
III. Particulate vaccine delivery systems are taken up by APCs and elicit adaptive immune responses.

15.20. Which of the following statements is relevant to immunopotentiators?

I. Immunopotentiators act as ligands for pattern recognition receptors expressed on antigen-presenting cells (APCs) .
II. CpG motifs present in bacterial nucleic acids elicit strong immune responses.
III. Particle size plays a key role in the elicitation of immune responses.

Directions for questions 21–24: The questions and incomplete statements in this section can be correctly answered or completed by one or more of the suggested answers. Choose the correct answer, a–d:

a. If II only is correct
b. If I and II are correct
c. If II and III are correct
d. If I, II, and III are correct

15.21. An immunologist is working on the compatibility of a new alum adjuvanted vaccine formulation with various routes of administration. The immunologist observed mucosal tolerance and possible local reactions. In such a situation, what would be a potential route of administration?

I. Oral route
II. Intramuscular route
III. Subcutaneous route

15.22. Which of the following statements are valid?

I. Langerhans cells are key antigen-presenting cells in intranasal delivery of vaccine antigens.
II. Mucosal associated lymphoid tissue represents a compartmentalized immunological system, which functions independently of systemic immune apparatus.
III. As a result of reversion of virus strains toward neurovirulence, oral polio vaccine (OPV/Sabin) was replaced with injectable inactivated (Salk) polio vaccine.

15.23. A chemist is evaluating various formulation approaches for an IM administered vaccine. In his observations, the vaccine antigen exhibited degradation in aqueous medium. Which of the following formulations would help overcome the stability issues?

I. Liquid suspension
II. Dry powder
III. Lyophilized powder

15.24. Which of the following statements are valid for the intranasal influenza vaccine (FluMist)?

I. FluMist contains no preservatives.
II. FluMist is available as 0.2-mL, prefilled, single-use intranasal spray.
III. FluMist contains a live, attenuated influenza virus.

REFERENCES

1. Medzhitov, R., Janeway, C.A. (2000). Innate immunity. *New England Journal of Medicine*, *343*, 338–343.
2. Janeway, C.A. (1989). Approaching the asymptote? Evolution and revolution in immunology. *Cold Spring Harbor Symposia on Quantitative Biology*, *54*, 1–13.
3. Janeway, C.A., Jr., Medzhitov, R. (2002). Innate immune recognition. *Annual Review of Immunology*, *20*, 197–216.
4. Meylan, E., Tschopp, J., Karin, M. (2006). Intracellular pattern recognition receptors in the host response. *Nature*, *442(7098)*, 39–44.
5. Muruve, D.A., et al. (2008). The inflammasome recognizes cytosolic microbial and host DNA and triggers an innate immune response. *Nature*, *452(7183)*, 103–107.
6. Mogensen, T.H. (2009). Pathogen recognition and inflammatory signaling in innate immune defenses. *Clinical Microbiological Reviews*, *22(2)*, 240–273.
7. Barton, G.M., Medzhitov, R. (2002). Control of adaptive immune responses by Toll-like receptors. *Current Opinion in Immunology*, *14(3)*, 380–383.
8. Iwasaki, A., Medzhitov, R. (2004). Toll-like receptor control of the adaptive immune responses. *Nature Immunology*, *5*, 987–995.
9. Miettinen, M., et al. (2001). IFNs activate Toll-like receptor gene expression in viral infections. *Gene Immunology*, *2*, 349–355.
10. Isaacs, A., Lindemann, J. (1957). Virus interference I. The interferon. *Proceedings of the Royal Society London B*, *147*, 258–267.
11. Winzler, C., et al. (1997). Checkpoints and functional stages in DC maturation. *Advances in Experimental Medicine and Biology*, *417*, 59–64.
12. Turley, S.J., et al. (2000). Transport of peptide-MHC class II complexes in developing dendritic cells. *Science*, *288(5465)*, 522–527.
13. Mellman, I., Steinman, R.M. (2001). Dendritic cells: Specialized and regulated antigen processing machines. *Cell*, *106(3)*, 255–258.
14. Steinman, R.M. (2001). Dendritic cells and the control of immunity: Enhancing the efficiency of antigen presentation. *Mount Sinai Journal of Medicine*, *68(3)*, 160–166.

15. Bennett, S.R., et al. (1998). Help for cytotoxic-T-cell responses is mediated by CD40 signalling. *Nature, 393 (6684)*, 478–480.
16. Bottomly, K. (1989). Subsets of CD4 T cells and B cell activation. *Seminars in Immunology, 1(1)*, 21–31.
17. Murray, J.S., et al. (1989). MHC control of CD4+ T cell subset activation. *The Journal of Experimental Medicine, 170(6)*, 2135–2140.
18. Miceli, M.C., Parnes, J.R. (1991). The roles of CD4 and CD8 in T cell activation. *Seminars in Immunology, 3(3)*, 133–141.
19. Constant, S.L., Bottomly, K. (1997). Induction of Th1 and Th2 $CD4^+$ T cell responses: The alternative approaches. *Annual Review of Immunology, 15*, 297–322.
20. Janeway, C. A., Jr. (1989). The priming of helper T cells. *Seminars in Immunology, 1(1)*, 13–20.
21. Palmer, E.M., van Seventer, G. A. (1997). Human T helper cell differentiation is regulated by the combined action of cytokines and accessory cell-dependent costimulatory signals. *Journal of Immunolology, 158(6)*, 2654–2662.
22. Nakamura, T., et al. (1997). Polarization of IL-4- and IFN-gamma-producing CD4+ T cells following activation of naive CD4+ T cells. *Journal of Immunolology, 158(3)*, 1085–1094.
23. Bottomly, K., Janeway, Jr., C.A. (1989). Antigen presentation by B cells. *Nature, 337(6202)*, 24.
24. Brinkmann, V., Heusser, C.H. (1993). T cell-dependent differentiation of human B cells into IgM, IgG, IgA, or IgE plasma cells: High rate of antibody production by IgE plasma cells, but limited clonal expansion of IgE precursors. *Cellular Immunology, 152(2)*, 323–332.
25. Croft, M., Swain, S.L. (1991). B cell response to T helper cell subsets. *II. Both the stage of T cell differentiation and the cytokines secreted determine the extent and nature of helper activity. Journal of Immunolology, 147(11)*, 3679–3689.
26. Fagarasan, S., Honjo, T. (2000). T-Independent immune response: New aspects of B cell biology. *Science, 290 (5489)*, 89–92.
27. Burton, D.R. (2002). Antibodies, viruses and vaccines. *Nature Reviews Immunology, 2(9)*, 706–713.
28. Groscurth, P., Filgueira, L. (1998). Killing mechanisms of cytotoxic T lymphocytes. *News in Physiological Sciences, 13*, 17–21.
29. Davidkin, I., et al. (2000). Duration of rubella immunity induced by two-dose measles, mumps and rubella (MMR) vaccination. *A 15-year follow-up in Finland. Vaccine, 18(27)*, 3106–3112.
30. Baxter, D. (2007). Active and passive immunity, vaccine types, excipients and licensing. *Occupational Medicine (London), 57(8)*, 552–556.
31. Ivanoff, B., Levine, M.M., Lambert, P.H. (1994). Vaccination against typhoid fever: Present status. *Bulletin of the World Health Organization, 72(6)*, 957–971.
32. Frasch, C.E. (1989). Vaccines for prevention of meningococcal disease. *Clinical Microbiology Reviews, 2* Suppl, S134–S138.
33. Stephenne, J. (1990). Development and production aspects of a recombinant yeast-derived hepatitis B vaccine. *Vaccine, 8 Suppl, S69–S73; discussion* S79–S80.
34. Inglis, S., Shaw, A., Koenig, S. (2006). Chapter 11: HPV vaccines: Commercial research & development. *Vaccine, 24 Suppl 3, S3/* 99–S105.
35. Restifo, N.P. et al. (2000). The promise of nucleic acid vaccines. *Gene Therapy, 7(2)*, 89–92.
36. Keefer, M.C., et al. (2012). A phase I double blind, placebo-controlled, randomized study of a multigenic HIV-1 adenovirus subtype 35 vector vaccine in healthy uninfected adults. *PLoS One, 7(8)*, e41936.
37. Shoji, M., et al. (2012). Immunogenic comparison of chimeric adenovirus 5/35 vector carrying optimized human immunodeficiency virus clade C genes and various promoters. *PLoS One, 7(1)*, e30302.
38. Gomez, C.E., et al. (2012). Removal of vaccinia virus genes that block interferon type I and II pathways improves adaptive and memory responses of the HIV/AIDS vaccine candidate NYVAC-C in mice. *Journal of Virology, 86(9)*, 5026–5038.
39. Vijayan, A., et al. (2012). Adjuvant-like effect of vaccinia virus 14K protein: A case study with malaria vaccine based on the circumsporozoite protein. *Journal of Immunology, 188 (12)*, 6407–6417.
40. Mendenhall, A., et al. (2012). Packaging HIV- or FIV-based lentivector expression Constructs and transduction of VSV-G pseudotyped viral particles. *Journal of Visualized Experiments, 2012(62)*, e3171.
41. Liniger, M., et al. (2009). Recombinant measles viruses expressing single or multiple antigens of human immunodeficiency virus (HIV-1) induce cellular and humoral immune responses. *Vaccine, 27(25–26)*, 3299–3305.
42. Wecker, M., et al. (2012). Phase I safety and immunogenicity evaluations of an alphavirus replicon HIV-1 subtype C gag vaccine (AVX101) in healthy HIV-1 uninfected adults. *Clinical and Vaccine Immunology, 19(10)*, 1651–1660.
43. Shata, M.T., et al. (2000). Recent advances with recombinant bacterial vaccine vectors. *Molecular Medicine Today, 6(2)*, 66–71.
44. Rice, J., Ottensmeier, C.H., Stevenson, F.K. (2008). DNA vaccines: Precision tools for activating effective immunity against cancer. *Nature Reviews Cancer, 8(2)*, 108–120.
45. Leitner, W.W., Ying, H., Restifo, N.P. (1999). DNA and RNA-based vaccines: Principles, progress and prospects. *Vaccine, 18(9–10)*, 765–777.
46. Ying, H., et al. (1999). Cancer therapy using a self-replicating RNA vaccine. *Nature Medicine, 5(7)*, 823–827.
47. Berglund, P., et al. (1998). Enhancing immune responses using suicidal DNA vaccines. *Nature Biotechnology, 16(6)*, 562–565.
48. Bachmann, M.F., Jennings, G.T. (2010). Vaccine delivery: A matter of size, geometry, kinetics and molecular patterns. *Nature Reviews Immunology, 10(11)*. 787–796.

49. Reddy, S.T., et al. (2007). Exploiting lymphatic transport and complement activation in nanoparticle vaccines. *Nature Biotechnology, 25(10)*, 1159–1164.
50. Baca-Estrada, M.E., et al. (2000). Vaccine delivery: Lipid-based delivery systems. *Nature Biotechnology, 83(1–2)*, 91–104.
51. Chandrawati, R., Caruso, F. (2012). Biomimetic liposome and polymersome-based multicompartmentalized assemblies. *Langmuir, 28(39)*, 13798–13807.
52. Boudier, A., et al. (2009). The control of dendritic cell maturation by pH-sensitive polyion complex micelles. *Biomaterials, 30(2)*, 233–241.
53. Caputo, A., et al. (2002). Micellar-type complexes of tailor-made synthetic block copolymers containing the HIV-1 tat DNA for vaccine application. *Vaccine, 20(17–18)*, 2303–2317.
54. Heegaard, P.M.H., Boas, U., Sorensen, N.S. (2010). Dendrimers for vaccine and immunostimulatory uses: A review. *Bioconjugate Chemistry, 21*, 405–418.
55. Everett, D.H. *Definitions, Terminology and Symbols in Colloid and Surface Chemistry*, International Union of Pure and Applied Chemistry, Washington, DC, 1972, pp. 1–78.
56. Shi, R., et al. (2005). Enhanced immune response to gastric cancer specific antigen Peptide by coencapsulation with CpG oligodeoxynucleotides in nanoemulsion. *Cancer Biology & Therapy, 4(2)*, 218–224.
57. Xu, L., Jin, B.Q., Fan, D.M. (2003). Selection and identification of mimic epitopes for gastric cancer-associated antigen MG7 Ag. *Molecular Cancer Therapeutics, 2(3)*, 301–306.
58. Ge, W., et al. (2006). MAGE-1/Heat shock protein 70/ MAGE-3 fusion protein vaccine in nanoemulsion enhances cellular and humoral immune responses to MAGE-1 or MAGE-3 in vivo. *Cancer Immunology, Immunotherapy, 55(7)*, 841–849.
59. Torchillin, V.P. (2005). Recent advances with liposomes as pharmaceutical carriers. *Nature Reviews Drug Discovery, 4 (February)*, 145–160.
60. Chikh, G., Schutze-Redelmeier, M.P. (2002). Liposomal delivery of CTL epitopes to dendritic cells. *Bioscience Reports, 22(2)*, 339–353.
61. Alving, C.R. (1992). Immunologic aspects of liposomes: Presentation and processing of liposomal protein and phospholipid antigens. *Biochimica et Biophysica Acta, 1113(3–4)*, 307–322.
62. Mischler, R., Metcalfe, I.C. (2002). Inflexal V, a trivalent virosome subunit influenza vaccine production. *Vaccine, 20 Suppl 5*, B17–23.
63. Moser, C., et al. (2007). Influenza virosomes as a combined vaccine carrier and adjuvant system for prophylactic and therapeutic immunizations. *Expert Review of Vaccines, 6 (5)*, 711–721.
64. Arkema, A., et al. (2000). Induction of cytotoxic T lymphocyte activity by fusion-active peptide-containing virosomes. *Vaccine, 18(14)*, 1327–1333.
65. Huckriede, A., et al. (2005). The virosome concept for influenza vaccines. *Vaccine, 23 Suppl 1*, S26–S38.
66. Marsac, D., et al. (2002). Enhanced presentation of major histocompatibility complex class I-restricted human immunodeficiency virus type 1 (HIV-1) Gag-specific epitopes after DNA immunization with vectors coding for vesicular stomatitis virus glycoprotein-pseudotyped HIV-1 Gag particles. *Journal of Virology, 76*, 7544–7553.
67. Mundargi, R.C., et al. (2008). Nano/micro technologies for delivering macromolecular therapeutics using poly(D, L-lactide-co-glycolide) and its derivatives. *Journal of Controlled Release, 125(3)*, 193–209.
68. Hamdy, S., et al. (2007). Enhanced antigen-specific primary CD4+ and CD8+ responses by codelivery of ovalbumin and toll-like receptor ligand monophosphoryl lipid A in poly(D, L-lactic-co-glycolic acid) nanoparticles. *Journal of Biomedical Materials Research Part A, 81(3)*, 652–662.
69. Trombetta, E.S., Mellman, I. (2005). Cell biology of antigen processing in vitro and in vivo. *Annual Review of Immunology, 23*, 975–1028.
70. Davis, I.D., et al. (2004). Recombinant NY-ESO-1 protein with ISCOMATRIX adjuvant induces broad integrated antibody and CD4(+) and CD8(+) T cell responses in humans. *Proceedings of the National Academy of Sciences U S A, 101 (29)*, 10697–10702.
71. Panyam, J., et al. (2002). Rapid endo-lysosomal escape of poly(DL-lactide-co-glycolide) nanoparticles: Implications for drug and gene delivery. *FASEB Journal, 16(10)*, 1217–1226.
72. Pack, D.W., et al. (2005). Design and development of polymers for gene delivery. *Nature Reviews Drug Discovery, 4(7)*, 581–593.
73. Shen, L., et al. (2004). Important role of cathepsin S in generating peptides for TAP-independent MHC class I cross-presentation in vivo. *Immunity, 21(2)*, 155–165.
74. Cutright, D.E., et al. (1974). Degradation rates of polymers and copolymers of polylactic and polyglycolic acids. *Oral Surgery, Oral Medicine, Oral Pathology, Oral Radiology, and Endodontology 37(1)*, 142–152.
75. Miller, R.A., Brady, J.M., Cutright, D.E. (1977). Degradation rates of oral resorbable implants (polylactates and polyglycolates): Rate modification with changes in PLA/PGA copolymer ratios. *Journal of Biomedical Materials Research, 11(5)*, 711–719.
76. Reddy, S.T., Swartz, M.A., Hubbell, J.A. (2006). Targeting dendritic cells with biomaterials: Developing the next generation of vaccines. *Trends in Immunology, 27(12)*, 573–579.
77. Chong, C.S., et al. (2005). Enhancement of T helper type 1 immune responses against hepatitis B virus core antigen by PLGA nanoparticle vaccine delivery. *Journal of Controlled Release, 102(1)*, 85–99.
78. Veprek, P., Jezek, J. (1999). Peptide and glycopeptide dendrimers. Part II. *Journal of Peptide Science, 5*, 203–220.

79. Kargakis, M., et al. (2007). A palmitoyl-tailored sequential oligopeptide carrier for engineering immunogenic conjugates. *Vaccine, 25*, 6708–6712.
80. Wright, D.C. (1998). Adjuvant properties of poly(amidoamine) dendrimers. U.S. Patent 08/597,938.
81. Ruponen, M., et al. (2003). Extracellular and intracellular barriers in non-viral gene delivery. *Journal of Controlled Release, 93*, 213–217.
82. O'Hagan, D.T., Rappuoli, R. (2004). Novel approaches to vaccine delivery. *Pharmaceutical Research, 21(9)*, 1519–1530.
83. Audibert, F., et al. (1976). Distinctive adjuvanticity of synthetic analogs of mycobacterial water-soluble components. *Cellular Immunology, 21(2)*, 243–249.
84. Parant, M.A., et al. (1980). Immunostimulant activities of a lipophilic muramyl dipeptide derivative and of desmuramyl peptidolipid analogs. *Infection and Immunity, 27(3)*, 826–831.
85. Giannini, S.L., et al. (2006). Enhanced humoral and memory B cellular immunity using HPV16/18 L1 VLP vaccine formulated with the MPL/aluminium salt combination (AS04) compared to aluminium salt only. *Vaccine, 24(33–34)*, 5937–5949.
86. Weiner, G.J., et al. (1997). Immunostimulatory oligodeoxynucleotides containing the CpG motif are effective as immune adjuvants in tumor antigen immunization. *Proceedings of the National Academy of Sciences U S A, 94(20)*, 10833–10837.
87. van der Meide, P.H., et al. (2002). Stimulation of both humoral and cellular immune responses to HIV-1 gp120 by interleukin-12 in Rhesus macaques. *Vaccine, 20(17–18)*, 2296–2302.
88. Garcon, N., Chomez, P., Van Mechelen, M. (2007). GlaxoSmithKline Adjuvant Systems in vaccines: Concepts, achievements and perspectives. *Expert Review of Vaccines, 6(5)*, 723–739.
89. Holmgren, J., Czerkinsky, C. (2005). Mucosal immunity and vaccines. *Nature Medicine, 11(4 Suppl)*, S45–S53.
90. Mowat, A.M. (2003). Anatomical basis of tolerance and immunity to intestinal antigens. *Nature Reviews Immunology, 3(4)*, 331–341.
91. Goodrich, M.E., McGee, D.W. (1998). Regulation of mucosal B cell immunoglobulin secretion by intestinal epithelial cell-derived cytokines. *Cytokine, 10(12)*, 948–955.
92. Kozlowski, P.A., et al. (1997). Comparison of the oral, rectal, and vaginal immunization routes for induction of antibodies in rectal and genital tract secretions of women. *Infection and Immunity, 65(4)*, 1387–1394.
93. Johansson, E.L., et al. (2004). Comparison of different routes of vaccination for eliciting antibody responses in the human stomach. *Vaccine, 22(8)*, 984–990.
94. Johansson, E.L., et al. (2001). Nasal and vaginal vaccinations have differential effects on antibody responses in vaginal and cervical secretions in humans. *Infection and Immunity, 69(12)*, 7481–7486.
95. Zhaori, G., Sun, M., Ogra, P.L. (1988). Characteristics of the immune response to poliovirus virion polypeptides after immunization with live or inactivated polio vaccines. *The Journal of Infectious Diseases, 158(1)*, 160–165.
96. Gray, J. (2011). Rotavirus vaccines: Safety, efficacy and public health impact. *Journal of Internal Medicine, 270(3)*, 206–214.
97. Cox, R.J., Brokstad, K.A., Ogra, P. (2004). Influenza virus: Immunity and vaccination strategies. Comparison of the immune response to inactivated and live, attenuated influenza vaccines. *Scandinavian Journal of Immunology, 59(1)*, 1–15.
98. Suman, J.D. (2003). Nasal drug delivery. *Expert Opinion on Biological Therapy, 3(3)*, 519–523.
99. Zuckerman, J.N. (2000). The importance of injecting vaccines into muscle. Different patients need different needle sizes. *British Medical Journal, 321(7271)*, 1237–1238.
100. Oussoren, C., Storm, G. (2001). Liposomes to target the lymphatics by subcutaneous administration. *Advanced Drug Delivery Reviews, 50(1–2)*, 143–156.
101. Higuchi, M., et al. (1999). Transport of colloidal particles in lymphatics and vasculature after subcutaneous injection. *Journal of Applied Physiology, 86(4)*, 1381–1387.
102. Williams, J., et al. (2000). Hepatitis A vaccine administration: Comparison between jet-injector and needle injection. *Vaccine, 18(18)*, 1939–1943.
103. Sachdeva, V., Banga, A.K. (2011). Microneedles and their applications. *Recent Patents on Drug Delivery & Formulation, 5(2)*, 95–132.
104. Gill, H.S., et al. (2008). Effect of microneedle design on pain in human volunteers. *The Clinical Journal of Pain, 24(7)*, 585–594.
105. Glenn, G.M., Kenney, R.T. (2006). Mass vaccination: Solutions in the skin. *Current Topics in Microbiology and Immunology, 304*, 247–268.
106. Zhao, Y.L., et al. (2006). Induction of cytotoxic T-lymphocytes by electroporation-enhanced needle-free skin immunization. *Vaccine, 24(9)*, 1282–1290.
107. Tezel, A., et al. (2005). Low-frequency ultrasound as a transcutaneous immunization adjuvant. *Vaccine, 23(29)*, 3800–3807.
108. Bramson, J., et al. (2003). Enabling topical immunization via microporation: a novel method for pain-free and needle-free delivery of adenovirus-based vaccines. *Gene Therapy, 10(3)*, 251–260.
109. Williams, A.C., Barry, B.W. (2004). Penetration enhancers. *Advanced Drug Delivery Reviews, 56(5)*, 603–618.
110. Zhang, L., Widera, G., Rabussay, D. (2004). Enhancement of the effectiveness of electroporation-augmented cutaneous DNA vaccination by a particulate adjuvant. *Bioelectrochemistry, 63(1–2)*, 369–373.

PART III

TRANSLATIONAL RESEARCH OF ADVANCED DRUG DELIVERY

16

REGULATORY CONSIDERATIONS AND CLINICAL ISSUES IN ADVANCED DRUG DELIVERY

Mei-Ling Chen

16.1 CHAPTER OBJECTIVES

- To outline fundamental concepts, rationale, and principles for advanced drug delivery systems.
- To provide regulatory background and general statutory requirements for pharmaceutical products.
- To examine potential issues in clinical pharmacology and biopharmaceutics for different dosage forms and drug products with advanced delivery systems.
- To illustrate regulatory concerns and considerations for assuring the efficacy, safety, and quality of these products.

16.2 INTRODUCTION

16.2.1 Drug Development

The development of a new drug from its discovery to regulatory assessment and postapproval marketing involves a series of activities that are complex and resource intensive. Modern drug discovery and development occurs primarily in the laboratories of the pharmaceutical industry and in academic and government research centers. However, the success rate is small with thousands of drugs screened in early laboratory and animal studies before a few can be considered suitable for studies in humans. In general, drug development entails a number of nonclinical (animal) and clinical (human) studies. The clinical studies move through three discrete phases. Phase 1 studies focus on safety coupled with pharmacokinetic and pharmacodynamic studies in small numbers of usually healthy subjects. Phase 2 studies continue with patients to explore efficacy (sometimes termed "proof of concept" studies). Phase 3 studies involve more trials in a larger number of patients to further confirm efficacy and assess safety. Many additional studies may be performed in association with these primary studies to assess drug–drug interaction, bioavailability and bioequivalence, subpopulation effects, and others that may be useful to practitioners, patients, and consumers in better understanding of how to use the new drug optimally. Figure 16.1 displays the flowchart for drug development and regulatory approval process. Although development of many drugs follows the sequences defined in Phases 1–3, this is not always the case. Depending on the intended indications, safety profile, therapeutic need, and other factors, modifications to the general sequence may occur on an investigational drug.

16.2.2 Regulatory Background

Regulation of drug products by the U.S. Food and Drug Administration (FDA) dates back more than 100 years to the passage of the Pure Food and Drugs Act in 1906. This law was enacted because of widespread concern about the

Advanced Drug Delivery, First Edition. Edited by Ashim K. Mitra, Chi H. Lee, and Kun Cheng.

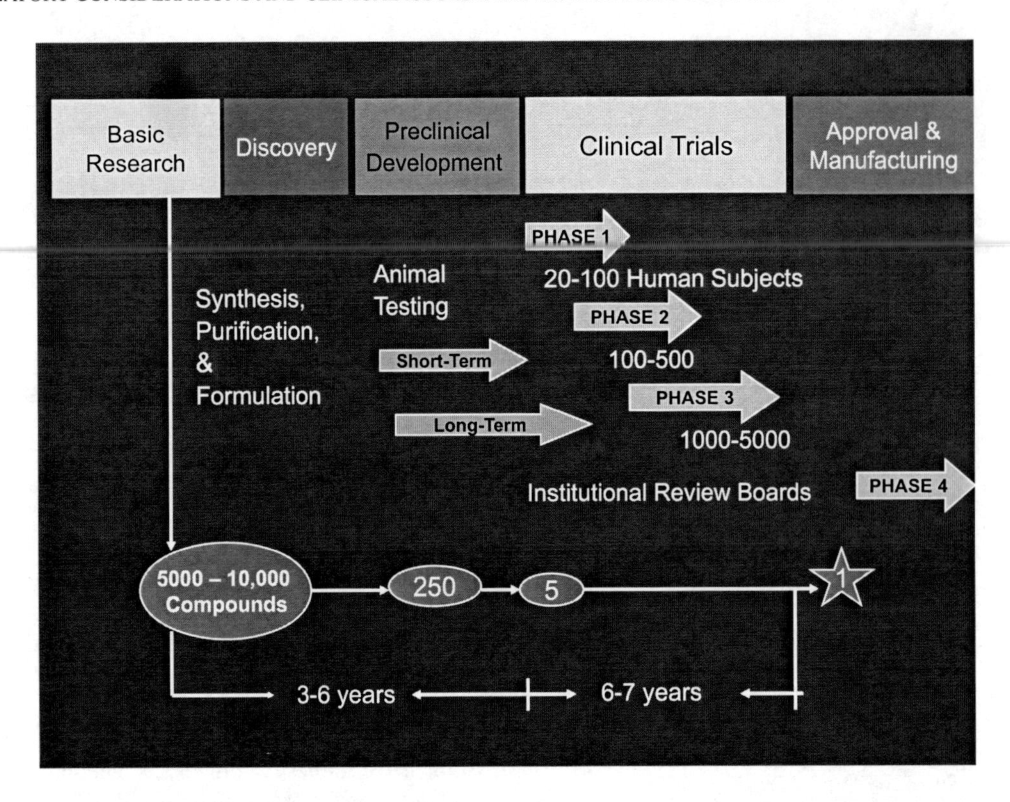

FIGURE 16.1 The flowchart for drug development and regulatory approval process.

quality of medicines in the United States at that time. It created an important concept that drugs marketed should not be adulterated and should not be misbranded, i.e., should not make unsubstantiated claims or otherwise present misleading information. Another landmark drug regulation was the Federal Food, Drug, and Cosmetic Act (FD&C Act), which was enacted in 1938 in response to a tragedy caused by sulfanilamide elixir. Using the excipient, diethylene glycol, to solubilize a sulfa drug (sulfanilamide), the elixir became a potent nephrotoxin that killed over 100 children and adults. It was marketed without provision of any kind of information to the FDA. In response, the 1938 FD&C Act established a safety standard that requires performance of adequate tests using reasonable methods to demonstrate the safety of a drug product before its marketing. Many amendments have been made to the FD&C Act since 1938. The most significant was the Kefauver-Harris Amendment that was enacted in 1962 as a result of a thalidomide tragedy in Europe. In addition to the mandate of safety demonstration, this Amendment required all drug manufacturers to establish the effectiveness of their products for the claimed indications before marketing. In 1984, the Drug Price Competition and Patent Term Restoration Act (also known as the Hatch-Waxman Amendment) created an abbreviated process for regulatory approval of generic versions of pioneer drug products. The Hatch-Waxman Amendment requires manufacturers of generic drugs to demonstrate that their products are, among other things, bioequivalent to the pioneer drug products.

Current federal law requires that a new drug be the subject of an approved marketing application before it is transported or distributed across state lines. The primary goals of a new drug application (NDA) are to provide adequate safety, efficacy, and quality information for regulatory approval of the drug and drug product under consideration. To support the labeled indications, an NDA is generally composed of the following six technical sections: 1) nonclinical (preclinical) pharmacology and toxicology; 2) human pharmacokinetics and bioavailability; 3) clinical; 4) biostatistics; 5) chemistry, manufacturing, and controls (CMC); and 6) microbiology. In contrast, for an abbreviated new drug application (ANDA), sponsors of generic drug products only need to include information on 1) bioequivalence; 2) CMC; and 3) microbiology. The 1984 Hatch-Waxman Amendment deems drug products as *therapeutic equivalents* if they are pharmaceutical equivalents and can be expected to have the same clinical effect and safety profile when administered to patients under the conditions specified in the labeling [1]. Accordingly, a major premise underlying the current law is that evidence of pharmaceutical equivalence and bioequivalence provides the assurance of therapeutic equivalence, hence, interchangeability between a generic drug product and its innovator product [1].

Under U.S. regulations, pharmaceutically equivalent products should contain the same amount of active ingredient in the same dosage form, have the same route of administration, identical in strength or concentration, and meet the same compendial or other applicable standards (i.e., strength, quality, purity, and identity). However, they may differ in characteristics such as shape, scoring configuration, release mechanisms, packaging, excipients (including colors, flavors, and preservatives), expiration time, and within certain limits, labeling [1]. On the other hand, bioequivalence is defined as "the absence of a significant difference in the rate and extent to which the active ingredient or active moiety in pharmaceutical equivalents or pharmaceutical alternatives becomes available at the site of drug action when administered at the same molar dose under similar conditions in an appropriately designed study" [1]. The FDA requires drug applicants to conduct bioequivalence testing using the most accurate, sensitive, and reproducible approach. Hence, comparative pharmacokinetic studies are generally used for systemically absorbed drug products, while pharmacodynamic studies and clinical trials are often employed for locally acting drug products. To evaluate bioequivalence using pharmacokinetic studies, the rate of absorption is commonly assessed by peak concentration (C_{max}) and time-to-peak concentration (T_{max}) obtained from the plasma concentration-time profile, whereas the extent of absorption is determined by the area-under-the-curve to the last quantifiable drug concentration (AUCt) and to time infinity (AUC_{∞}) [1]. Two drug products are bioequivalent if the 90% confidence interval of the geometric mean ratio of the test to reference product meets the 80–125% limit for C_{max} and AUCs [2]. No statistical tests are applied to T_{max} values, but they should be similar between products in comparison [1].

16.2.3 Advanced Drug Delivery Systems

Conventional drug delivery systems are often referred to simple dosage forms such as solutions and immediate-release, solid, oral dosage forms. Over the decades, continual advances in pharmaceutical science and technology have led to the development of more sophisticated dosage forms and drug delivery systems. In addition to controlling the rate or duration of drug release, a modern drug delivery system may be designed to deliver a drug to the target site of action [3], avoid drug uptake by the macrophages *in vivo* [4], or respond to the biofeedback mechanism such as the glucose levels in hyperglycemic patients [5]. As such, drug delivery systems play a vital role in the overall scheme of rational drug design for optimized therapy. The complexity of modern drug delivery systems, however, has presented many challenges to the pharmaceutical and regulatory scientists in establishing product quality and performance.

This chapter aims to 1) discuss some of the potential challenges in clinical pharmacology and biopharmaceutics for advanced drug delivery systems currently available, and 2) provide regulatory considerations for assuring safety, efficacy, and quality of these drug products. Note that the chapter focuses primarily on small-molecule drugs and not on biotechnology or biological products. The FDA regulates biological and biotechnology products under the provisions of the Public Health Service Act (PHS Act), which include different regulations from those in the FD&C Act for small-molecule drug products.

16.3 MODIFIED-RELEASE ORAL DOSAGE FORM

Modified-release dosage forms can be referred to those dosage forms whose drug-release properties are chosen to accomplish therapeutic or convenience objectives not offered by conventional dosage forms (such as solutions or immediate-release, solid oral dosage form). Traditionally, modified-release dosage forms are composed of two categories of drug products, delayed- and extended (or called controlled)-release drug products [6]. As defined by the United States Pharmacopeia (USP), delayed-release drug products are those that release drugs at a time later than immediately after administration and thus exhibit a lag time in quantifiable plasma concentrations. Coatings (e.g., enteric coatings) are typically incorporated into solid oral dosage forms to delay the release of medication until the drug product has passed through the acidic medium of the stomach. As for extended-release dosage forms, they release the drug slowly and maintain plasma levels for a longer period of time as compared with conventional dosage forms so that a reduction in dosing frequency is allowed. In addition to the delayed- and prolonged-release characteristics, newer modified-release drug products may exhibit pulsatile-release, chrono-release, or targeted delivery. Although the pattern of drug release may be characterized by a rhythmic pulsation for pulsatile-release products, chrono-release products release the drug at a predetermined time, for example, in the morning after administration at bedtime. Some of the orally administered modified-release drug products may also include combinations of immediate-release, delayed-release, and/or extended-release components (see Table 16.1). Each of these products may exhibit its unique mechanism for drug release to achieve different goals of therapeutic outcome.

16.3.1 Regulatory Concerns for Dose-Dumping

A major regulatory concern for extended-release dosage forms lies in the possibility of dose-dumping as a result of product failure or interaction between the drug product and environmental factors. Dose-dumping tends to occur for

TABLE 16.1 Examples of Multiphasic Modified Release Oral Dosage Forms

Drug	Trade Name	Dosage Form	Formulation
Amoxicillin	Moxatag™ (Shionogi Inc., Florham Park, NJ)	Tablets, extended-release	Three components: one immediate-release and two delayed-release
Amphetamine + dextroamphetamine (mixed salts)	Adderall XR® (Shire Pharmaceuticals, Wayne, PA)	Capsules, extended-release	Two types of beads: one fast-release and another slow-release
Methylphenidate hydrochloride	Concerta® (Janssen Pharmaceuticals Inc., Titusville, NJ)	Tablets, extended-release	Immediate-release + extended-release
Nifedipine	Adalat® CC (Bayer Healthcare Pharmaceuticals, Montville, NJ)	Tablets, extended-release	Slow-release coat and fast-release core
Zolpidem tartrate	Ambien CR® (Sanofi-Aventis, Bridgewater, NJ)	Tablets, extended-release	Two layers: one immediate-release and another slow-release

extended-release drug products because of their inherent design with a large amount of drugs loaded into the matrix or reservoir of the dosage form. Potential environmental factors that may cause premature and exaggerated release of a drug from these dosage forms may include food and alcohol. An example of significant food-induced dose-dumping is from Theo-24, an oral, once-a-day, extended-release formulation of theophylline [7]. This phenomenon was illustrated by a pharmacokinetic study where eight healthy volunteers received, in a crossover manner, single doses of a theophylline reference solution and Theo-24 under both fasting and fed conditions. A fatty breakfast with bacon and eggs was consumed by the participants in the fed study. The food-induced dose-dumping resulted in an average of 2.3 times higher serum levels of theophylline than after a fasting dose, which caused toxic effects in six of the eight subjects. Another example of dose-dumping came from the market withdrawal of Palladone XL (Purdue Pharma, Stamford, CT; hydromorphone extended-release capsules) [8]. Palladone XL has a matrix system in design, which is prone to dose-dumping when the patient drinks alcohol while taking the medicine. Palladone XL was pulled off the market as a result of the concern over the potentially fatal interaction between this narcotic and alcohol on the basis of a pharmacokinetic study in healthy volunteers [9]. The study demonstrated that co-ingestion of this product with 240 mL of 40% (80 proof) alcohol resulted in an average peak concentration of approximately six times greater than when taken with water (one subject in this study experienced a 16-fold increase). In certain subjects, 240 mL of 4% alcohol resulted in almost twice the peak plasma concentration than when the drug was ingested with water [9].

It should be noted that the FDA requires the NDA sponsor of an extended-release drug product to conduct *in vivo* bioavailability study with which the extended-release claim can be made for the product only when all of the following conditions are met [10]:

(a) The drug product meets the extended-release claims made for it.

(b) The bioavailability profile established for the drug product rules out the occurrence of any dose dumping.

(c) The drug product's steady-state performance is equivalent to a currently marketed noncontrolled release or controlled-release drug product that contains the same active drug ingredient or therapeutic moiety.

(d) The drug product's formulation provides consistent pharmacokinetic performance between individual dosage units.

16.3.2 Bioequivalence Assessment

For delayed-release dosage forms, the use of enteric coating is intended for protection of an acid-labile drug from degradation by the acidic medium present in the stomach. A major bioequivalence issue rests on the variation of these coating materials available on the market because they may possess a comparable protective function with different onset times for coating breakdown and drug release. It has been speculated that variation in the quality of enteric coatings may account, in part, for the observed difference in clinical effectiveness between formulations [11, 12].

From the bioequivalence standpoint, various product designs are possible to attain the same C_{max} and AUC for an extended-release dosage form. This can simply be achieved by altering the type of polymer, drug/polymer ratio, excipients, compression pressure, and/or temperature [13]. The resulting formulations, however, may yield a set of concentration-time profiles that vary widely in T_{max} and/or shape of the profile. Despite the established bioequivalence limit (80–125%) for C_{max} and AUC based on a confidence interval approach, statistical comparison of T_{max} or shape of the curve is not performed as a result of the lack of appropriate methods. The question is that to what extent a discrepancy in the plasma profiles will translate into a significant difference in clinical outcomes.

It is acknowledged that C_{max} and AUC are generally sufficient for evaluating bioequivalence. Nevertheless, there are concerns for some special situations where an additional measure(s) may be needed to assure bioequivalence. For instance, an early drug exposure may be necessary to warrant a rapid onset of an analgesic effect or to avoid reflex tachycardia of an antihypertensive agent. In this regard, to ensure a better control of drug input for such products, both the U.S. FDA and Health Canada have added a *partial AUC* (pAUC) metric (calculated up to an early time point) as the early exposure measure for bioequivalence determination [5, 14]. The pAUC metrics have also been shown to be useful for evaluation of multiphasic modified-release drug products [15, 16]. As an example, although the immediate-release formulation of zolpidem (Ambien; Sanofi-Aventis, Bridgewater, NJ) is indicated for short-term treatment of insomnia characterized by difficulties with sleep initiation, the extended-release formulation (Ambien CR) offers additional benefits of treating difficulties associated with sleep maintenance and producing no residual effects after wake-up. In this case, the $AUC_{0-1.5h}$ and $AUC_{1.5h-t}$ metrics have been recommended by the FDA for evaluation of zolpidem bioavailability responsible for the sleep onset and sleep maintenance phases, respectively [16]. The truncation points for these pAUCs were determined based on the pharmacokinetic/pharmacodynamic characteristics inherent in the reference formulation [17, 18].

16.4 SUSTAINED-RELEASE PARENTERAL DOSAGE FORMS

Parenteral dosage forms can be used for delivery of small molecules, proteins, peptides, and biologics. This route of administration is particularly convenient for protein and peptide therapeutics in that they possess poor permeability across the gastrointestinal (GI) membrane and suffer from a high level of physical and/or chemical instability in the GI tract [19]. However, there are disadvantages for parenteral drug delivery. In addition to the pain associated with the injections, some proteins and peptides have short half-lives and require frequent injections to achieve desired therapeutic effects [19]. To overcome these limitations, considerable efforts have been made to develop sustained-release delivery systems for parenteral products. In general, conventional long-acting parenteral products consist of lipophilic drugs in either aqueous solvents (as suspensions) or vegetable oils. Recent novel approaches for sustained-release injectable drug delivery may include the use of polymer-based systems, implantable systems, or a combination of targeted delivery with controlled-release strategy [19–21].

The polymer-based, sustained-release products for parenteral administration can be exemplified by micro/nanospheres and *in situ* depot-forming systems. Microspheres and/or nanospheres are prepared from polymeric materials with varying co-polymer ratios, molecular weights, and micro/nanosphere sizes. The polymers can be formulated for drug release up to several weeks, months, or years, depending on the physicochemical properties of the polymer and the specific drug encapsulated. Table 16.2 lists some micro/nanosphere products currently marketed in the United States. Examples of *in situ* depot-forming systems may include Lantus (Sanofi-Aventis; insulin glargine injection—rDNA injection) and Eligard (Sanofi-Aventis; leuprolide acetate for injectable suspension). Although Lantus is given once a day, Eligard provides sustained release of the drug over 1–6 months [22].

Implants represent another type of dosage form that can be inserted subcutaneously or placed in a specific body site for sustained-release of small-molecule drugs, proteins, peptides, and biologics. Few implant products are available, perhaps as a result of the invasive nature of this dosage form.

TABLE 16.2 Examples of Micro-/Nanosphere Products Marketed in the United States

Drug	Trade Name	Route of Administration	Dosing Frequency	Indication
Leuprolide	Lupron Depot® (Abbott, Abbott Park, IL)	Intramuscular injection	Every 1–3 months	Prostate cancer, endometriosis
Minocycline	Arestin® (Orapharma, Long Beach, CA)	Subgingival injection	Every 3 months	Periodontitis
Naltrexone	Vivitrol® (Alkermes, Dublin 4, Ireland)	Intramuscular injection	Every 4 weeks	Alcohol dependence
Octreotide	Sandostatin® LAR (Norvatis Pharmaceuticals, Basal, Switzland)	Intramuscular injection	Monthly	Acromegaly
Paliperidone	Invega® Sustenna® (Janssen Pharmaceuticals Inc., Titusville, NJ)	Intramuscular injection	Monthly	Schizophrenia
Risperidone	Risperdal® Consta® (Janssen Pharmaceuticals Inc., Titusville, NJ)	Intramuscular injection	Every 2 weeks	Schizophrenia, bipolar disorder
Somatropin	Nutropin® Depot (Genetech, South San Francisco, CA)	Subcutaneous injection	Every 1–2 months	Growth deficiencies
Triptorelin	Trelstar™ Depot (Watson Labs., Parsippany, NJ)	Intramuscular injection	Every 4–24 weeks	Prostate cancer

Minor surgical procedures are required for insertion of implantable systems. Conversely, the surgically retrievable feature of these systems may be an advantage if early termination of the treatment is warranted in case of adverse events. Some implants, such as Zoladex (AstraZeneca, London, U.K.; goserelin acetate implant), have biodegradable polymers and thus exhibit an initial burst of the drug [22]. Other implants such as Supprelin LA (Endo Pharmaceuticals, Inc., Chadds Ford, PA; histrelin acetate) include non-biodegradable polymers and will have to be surgically removed by the end of use [22]. While both Zoladex and Supprelin LA can be inserted subcutaneously, Gliadel Wafer (Eisai Inc., Woodcliff Lake, NJ; polifeprosan 20 with carmustine) is implanted in the resection cavity of patients with recurrent glioblastoma multiforme [22].

16.4.1 Formulation, Processing, and Performance

Many sustained-release parenteral products use the biodegradable polymers such as poly(lactic-*co*-glycolic acid) (PLGA). A regulatory concern with the use of PLGA polymers for protein and peptide delivery relates to both drug and product stability. Proteins and peptides can be degraded in the presence of acidic pH as a result of PLGA degradation during manufacturing, storage, and release [23]. The proteins or peptides may also be deactivated as a result of adsorption to the polymer surface. Another problem with the polymeric-based delivery system is its limited control on release kinetics [23]. Several factors can influence the drug release from micro/nanospheres, including intrinsic polymer properties, polymer hydrophilicity and molecular weight, core solubility, and microsphere structure [21]. In many cases, a significant initial burst was observed followed by incomplete release after subcutaneous or intramuscular injection of these dosage forms [22].

A regulatory issue with the initial burst effect lies in the lack of information/data to indicate whether such an effect has any safety or efficacy implication. Moreover, a question has often been raised concerning the appropriate metrics used for assessment of bioavailability and bioequivalence in the presence of the burst [24, 25]. Traditionally, peak concentration (C_{max}) and peak time (T_{max}) from plasma/serum profiles have been used as an indicator for rate of drug absorption. However, if the initial burst is not relevant for clinical efficacy or safety, it may not be appropriate to use C_{max} and/or T_{max} for bioavailability/bioequivalence evaluation. Under these circumstances, as an alternative, the systemic exposure concept currently recommended by the FDA for oral solid dosage forms may be applicable [6]. Defined relative to the total, peak, and early portions of the plasma profile, systemic exposure can be expressed as total exposure, peak exposure, and early exposure, respectively [6]. The total exposure to a drug is readily expressed by total AUC and the peak exposure by C_{max}. The early exposure can be measured by the partial AUC calculated to an early time point specified on the basis of the pharmacokinetic/pharmacodynamic or pharmacokinetic/clinical response relationship [6].

To ensure adequate product quality and performance, a number of critical variables should be considered during the development and manufacturing of polymeric-based, sustained-release delivery systems. These may include the choice of polymers (hydrophilicity or lipophilicity, molecular weight, co-polymer ratio, and crystallinity), drug loading efficiency, interfacial properties, method of manufacture and scale-up, particle size, stability, and sterility [24, 25]. Several factors can affect the drug loading efficiency of these products, e.g., characteristics of polymers/co-polymers used, preparation methods, and sphere size [26–29]. In terms of stability, various aspects of stability need to be considered for a sustained-release, parenteral dosage form, including shelf-life stability, product stability, *in vivo* product stability, and *in vivo* integrity of a targeted product. Also, issues of syringeability and injectability cannot be overemphasized for micro/nanospheres and hydrogel depot products. A major problem of poor injectability is the clogging of needles. Yet, the use of a large needle size may cause pain upon injection. Microsphere and/or nanosphere products should be manufactured by an aseptic process because terminal sterilization (such as heat sterilization and gamma irradiation) can lead to the degradation of micro/nanospheres and loss of polymer molecular weight [30]. In view of the complexity in the manufacturing process for these products, an appropriate quality control strategy should be designed for the development program.

16.4.2 *In Vitro* Release Testing and *In Vitro–In Vivo* Correlation (IVIVC)

It is well known that *in vitro* release and dissolution testing play multiple roles in several dosage forms [5, 31–36]. For example, during the drug development stage, it is mostly used to guide the selection of appropriate formulations for *in vivo* studies. It is also used as a preliminary test for detection of possible bio*in*equivalence between products before and after manufacturing or formulation changes. As a quality control tool, *in vitro* release and/or dissolution testing is often employed to set specifications for batch release. Furthermore, *in vitro* release and/or dissolution testing, if correlated with *in vivo* data, can serve as a surrogate for *in vivo* bioequivalence studies.

From a regulatory perspective, two types of *in vitro* release testing are generally required for evaluation of sustained-release, parenteral products, i.e., 1) a long-term release test, and 2) an accelerated, short-term release test [24, 25]. The former is preferably conducted during the early stages of drug development, which is carried out under the experimental conditions that simulate the *in vivo* environment. The *in vitro* release testing of sustained-release parenteral products is mainly used for quality control purposes. However, best efforts should be made to correlate a short-term (accelerated) release test with *in vivo* performance using biorelevant media and maintaining the release mechanism as observed in the long-term test. Monitoring of drug stability is essential during the *in vitro* release testing of polymer-based, sustained-release, parenteral products, especially for proteins and peptides.

Conduct of *in vivo* pharmacokinetic studies or bioavailability/bioequivalence studies for a sustained-release, parenteral dosage form is inevitably time-consuming and resource-intensive. Hence, it is advantageous to develop an appropriate *in vitro* release test method that is capable of predicting *in vivo* performance of these products. The establishment of the *in vitro–in vivo* correlation (IVIVC) is particularly useful for biowaivers of sustained-release parenteral products in the presence of scale-up and postapproval changes (SUPAC). Most FDA guidance documents have described the role and methods for development of IVIVC in oral solid dosage forms [5, 30, 31–36]. It should be noted that similar scientific principles can be applied for sustained-release, parenteral dosage forms. General issues associated with the development of IVIVC in these dosage forms have been discussed elsewhere [24, 25, 37].

16.4.3 Safety Concerns

Several safety concerns have been expressed with respect to polymer-based, sustained-release drug delivery systems, including biocompatibility and biodegradability of the polymer, impurity, sterility, residual solvents, as well as initial burst of the product [24, 25]. In addition, a key challenge for protein therapeutics in parenteral dosage forms is that proteins can degrade by both physical and chemical degradation pathways. A notable end product from physical degradation is protein aggregates, which may have an impact on bioprocessing, formulation, quality, and immunogenicity of protein therapeutics [38]. Not only the size or amount of aggregates present but also the physical characteristics of the aggregates will play a role in immunogenicity [39]. The hypothesis is that multimers consisting of natively formed proteins may be efficient at eliciting a humoral antibody response that is independent of T cells. Moreover, these antibodies may be efficient in interacting with properly folded protein, resulting in neutralization of potency of the administered therapeutic, alteration of pharmacokinetics, or neutralization of endogenous protein activity. Hence, aggregates, particularly large molecular weight aggregates and particulates, pose a clear risk to the safety and efficacy of therapeutic protein products and are considered a critical quality attribute. Aggregates, including protein particles, should be characterized, quantified, and controlled in therapeutic protein products at release and on stability.

It is known that immunogencity is a major issue for protein therapeutics [40]. Apart from protein aggregation, many factors can contribute to the generation of an immune response including patient characteristics, disease state, the therapy itself, and product-related factors. Product-related factors, such as the molecule design, the expression system, posttranslational modifications (*in vitro* and *in vivo*), impurities, contaminants, formulation and excipients, as well as container and closure, are all implicated. The clinical effect of patient immune responses to therapeutic proteins can range from no effect at all to extreme harmful effects to patient health. Because of the varied immune responses, clinicians often rely on the information posted in the package labeling that contains immunogenicity rates observed during clinical trials. Hence, it is important to develop valid and sensitive immune assays during the product development. In this aspect, the FDA has issued a guidance for industry on the assay development for immunogenicity testing of therapeutic proteins [41].

16.5 LIPID-BASED ORAL DOSAGE FORMS

Most lipid-based oral dosage forms use lipid vehicles or excipients to solubilize a lipophilic drug and improve its bioavailability. In the case of hydrophilic drugs, they are generally solubilized in the water-in-oil emulsions or microemulsions, and phase inversion takes place later *in vivo* [42]. A variety of lipid-based oral dosage forms can be made depending on the methods used to incorporate an active drug into lipid vehicles. These may include oils, surfactant dispersions, emulsions, microemulsions, self-emulsifying drug delivery systems (SEDDSs), self-microemulsifying drug delivery systems (SMEDDSs), self-nanoemulsifying drug delivery systems (SNEDDSs), and solid-lipid nanoparticles (SLNs) [43–50]. As such, the lipid-based dosage forms encompass a wide range of compositions and exhibit a broad character and functionality.

The unique physicochemical characteristics of these dosage forms have posed a number of challenges to pharmaceutical scientists in all stages of drug development. Although lipid excipients can solubilize drugs within the dosage form matrix, they can also be digested and dispersed in the GI tract. Therefore, a key formulation issue is whether the drug would remain in solubilized form *in vivo* in the presence of changing phases of the formulation after it is administered [50]. The ability of a formulation to maintain solubilization and prevent precipitation on dispersion and digestion may largely depend on 1) the nature of lipid (chain length) and particle size, 2) relative proportions of lipid versus surfactant, and 3) impact of lipid *and* surfactant digestion on the properties of solubilization [51–53].

Apart from the formulation challenges, lipid-based formulations can be transported by serum lipoproteins

TABLE 16.3 Lipid Excipients/Surfactants that Interact with Enzymes/Transporters *In Vivo* or *In Vitro*

Lipid Excipient or Surfactant	Example	Remark
Polyoxyethylated/pegylated		
Polyoxyl 35 castor oil	Cremophor	CYP3A and P-gp inhibitors
PEG-15-hydroxystearate	Solutol HS-15	CYP3A and P-gp inhibitors
Medium chain glycerol and PEG esters	Labrasol, Softigen 767, Acconon	P-gp inhibitor
Polysorbates	Tween 80, Tween 20	CYP3A and P-gp inhibitors
Sucrose esters	Sucrose monolaurate	P-gp inhibitor
Tocopherol esters	Vitamin E-TPGS*	P-gp inhibitor
Polymers	Pluronic block copolymers	CYP3A and P-gp inhibitors

*TPGS: d-alpha-tocopheryl polyethylene glycol 1000 succinate.

that are involved in the intrinsic lipid pathway through the vascular and extravascular body fluids to the cells [54, 55]. Lipoprotein levels can be influenced by disease states, diet or fat content, and co-administered compounds. In addition, the content and composition of circulating lipoproteins may change with age and gender [56]. The binding of lipoproteins may affect the efficacy and/or safety profile of a drug, especially when the drug is given to a patient with abnormal lipid metabolism secondary to the disease state [54, 55].

In view of all the complicating factors discussed above, regulatory concerns have been expressed for lipid-based dosage forms in many areas related to product quality and product performance. Some of these concerns (discussed below) may include the use of lipid excipients, availability of suitable *in vitro* dissolution/release testing, and bioequivalence issues between products before and after a change in manufacturing or formulation.

16.5.1 Lipid Excipients

Historically, excipients are considered to be inert substances used mainly as diluents, fillers, binders, lubricants, coatings, solvents, or dyes, in the manufacture of drug products. Over the years, however, advances in pharmaceutical science have facilitated the availability of a wide range of novel excipients. In some cases, known and/or unknown interactions can occur between an excipient and an active ingredient, an inactive ingredient(s), biological surroundings, or even a container closure system. As such, the FDA has generally required nonclinical (animal) and clinical (human) studies to demonstrate the safety of a new excipient before use [57]. However, such studies are not necessary for *generally recognized as safe* (GRAS) substances [58]. In addition, the FDA maintains a guide on inactive ingredients, i.e., *Inactive Ingredient Guide* (IIG), for excipients that have been approved for marketing [59]. Excipients play an integral part in a drug product, and thus, they are reviewed and approved as a "component" of the drug product in the FDA.

Several lipid excipients and/or surfactants present in pharmaceutical formulations have been found to inhibit cytochrome P450 (CYP) 3A metabolism or P-glycoprotein (P-gp) transport (Table 16.3) [60]. CYP3A isozymes are major enzymes responsible for phase I metabolism, whereas P-gp is an efflux transporter expressed along the GI tract, in the liver, kidney, blood-brain barrier, and placenta [61, 62]. Incidentally, many hydrophobic drugs in lipid formulations are primarily metabolized by CYP3A or serve as the substrate and/or inhibitor of P-gp [63, 64]. The interplay between the lipid excipients/surfactants and the enzymes/transporters has raised regulatory concerns about the predictability of drug absorption and bioavailability of lipid-based dosage forms. Hence, conduct of *in vitro* and *in vivo* studies are encouraged to elucidate these potential interactions during the pharmaceutical development.

16.5.2 *In Vitro* Dissolution or Release Testing

From a regulatory perspective, *in vitro* dissolution and/or release testing is important for assuring product quality and product performance. Although general approaches may be available for conducting *in vitro* dissolution and/or release testing of solid oral dosage forms, there is no standardized methodology for lipid-based oral formulations because of the unique characteristics of these products. Except for simple formulations, it is challenging to develop an appropriate *in vitro* dissolution/release method for predicting *in vivo* performance of lipid-based products, and thus, most *in vitro* dissolution/release testing has currently been developed for quality control only. In the case of simple lipid formulations, some modifications to the conventional dissolution media may be able to reflect physiological conditions and serve the purposes of assessing drug bioavailability and/or food effect on drug absorption [65–74]. For gelatin capsules, the USP two-tier dissolution testing has been employed to prevent gelatin crosslinking [75]. However, conventional *in vitro* dissolution or release testing is limited in predicting *in vivo* behavior of a complex lipid-based formulation in view of the fact that dissolution of the drug and GI processing of the lipid vehicle (including digestion and dispersion) are intrinsically linked to each other. Ideally, the *in vitro* dissolution/release testing for lipid formulations should incorporate the dynamics of lipid digestion, formation of various intermediate colloidal products, and solubilization of the drug under examination [76–78]. Further research is needed to establish a general protocol for developing appropriate *in vitro* dissolution or release testing based on the characteristics of each lipid-based formulation under study.

16.5.3 Bioequivalence Issues

It may be challenging to determine bioequivalence and/or therapeutic equivalence of complex lipid-based formulations given their unique formulation characteristics as well as the potential interactions among the drug, lipid excipients, surfactants, and/or physiological environment. Indeed, this can be illustrated by the cases of cyclosporine where a difference in the makeup of the lipid formulations has resulted in differential bioavailability between the products. Both Neoral and Sandimmune are lipid-based cyclosporine oral solutions from the innovator (Novartis Pharmaceuticals, Basel, Switzerland). However, for a given trough concentration, cyclosporine exposure was shown to be greater with Neoral than with Sandimmune [22]. Hence, these two products are not bioequivalent and cannot be used interchangeably without physician supervision. Furthermore, a generic cyclosporine solution (SangCya; Novartis) had been withdrawn from the market [79] as a result of the finding of a lower bioavailability compared with the reference product (Neoral oral solution) when administered with apple juice. A *post hoc* analysis revealed that Neoral formed a microemulsion while SangCya formed microdispersion upon mixing with apple juice. In contrast, however, these two products were found bioequivalent when mixed with chocolate milk [60].

16.6 TRANSDERMAL DELIVERY SYSTEMS

Transdermal delivery represents an excellent alternative to oral route of administration, bypassing the GI tract to obviate GI irritation or avoid first-pass metabolism in the gut and/or liver. Transdermal systems are noninvasive and thus have advantages over hypodermic injections that are painful to patients. In addition, as it is convenient to apply patches on the skin, transdermal drug delivery enhances patient compliance. Although transdermal delivery is an ideal route of administration, the stratum corneum constitutes an effective barrier to drug absorption through the skin. Only a small number of drug substances with unique characteristics can penetrate the skin successfully.

Table 16.4 shows some characteristics of drugs that are delivered by a transdermal route of administration. Typically, these drugs possess high lipophilicity, low molecular weight (less than 500 Daltons), and are effective at low dose.

The major products currently marketed for transdermal absorption are the transdermal therapeutic systems (TTSs), also known as patches. It is important to know the fundamental differences between the two types of patches available on the market, the reservoir system and the matrix (drug-in-adhesive) system. The reservoir systems have the drug stored in a reservoir that may be enclosed on the one side with an impermeable backing and on the other side with an adhesive to contact with the skin. Some product designs have the drug dissolved in a liquid- or gel-based reservoir and permit the use of a liquid chemical enhancer, such as ethanol. The reservoir systems generally have four layers: an impermeable backing membrane, a drug reservoir, a semipermeable membrane, and an

TABLE 16.4 Some Characteristics of Drugs for Transdermal Delivery

Drug	Mol. Wt. (Daltons)	Trade Name	Daily Dose	Application
Clonidine	230	Catapress-TTS® (Boehringer-Ingelheim, Ingelheim, Germany)	0.1–0.3 mg	Weekly
Estradiol	272	Alora® (Watson Labs., Parsippany, NJ)	0.014–0.1 mg	Twice weekly
		Climara® (Bayer Healthcare Pharmaceuticals, Montville, NJ)		
		Estraderm® (Norvatis Pharmaceuticals, Basal, Switzland)		
		Menostar® (Bayer Healthcare Pharmaceuticals, Montville, NJ)		
		Vivelle® (Norvatis Pharmaceuticals, Basal, Switzland)		
		Vivella-Dot® (Norvatis Pharmaceuticals, Basal, Switzland)		
Ethinyl estradiol	296	Ortho-Evra® (Janssen Pharmaceuticals Inc., Titusville, NJ)	0.75 mg (EE)	Weekly
+ Norelgestromin	328		6 mg (NGMN)	
Fentanyl	337	Duragesic TDS® (Janssen Pharmaceuticals Inc., Titusville, NJ)	0.6 mg	Once every 3 days
Lidocaine	234	Lidoderm® (Teikoku Pharma, San Jose, CA)	—	Daily
Nicotine	162	Nicoderm-CQ® (Alza Corporation, Mountain View, CA)	7–21 mg	Daily
Nitroglycerin	227	Nitro-Dur® (Merck Sharp & Dohme, Whitehouse Station, NJ)	1.4–11.2 mg	Daily for 12–14 hours
		Minitran® (Medicis Pharmaceutical Corp., Scottsdale, AZ)		
Scopolamine	303	Transderm-Scop® (Norvatis Pharmaceuticals, Basal, Switzland)	0.33 mg	Once every 3 days
Testosterone	288	Androderm® (Watson Labs., Parsippany, NJ)	2.5–5 mg	Daily

adhesive layer. In contrast, the matrix system may have three layers, which incorporates the drug in a solid polymer matrix and eliminates the semipermeable membrane, or have only two layers by directly incorporating the drug into the adhesive [80].

Most of the commercially available transdermal patches contain drug substances that are capable of crossing the skin at a therapeutic rate with little or no penetration enhancers. However, newer transdermal delivery systems have increased skin permeability and driving forces for transport of small-molecule drugs, with the use of chemical enhancers and iontophoresis. The continual advances in novel penetration enhancement technology, such as cavitational ultrasound and electroporation, will make future transdermal systems available for targeted delivery of macromolecules (including proteins and DNA) and even virus-based/other vaccines [80].

16.6.1 Dose-Dumping and Residual Drug Issues

An important regulatory concern for transdermal delivery systems may be dose-dumping as a result of product failure, which can be serious particularly for highly potent drugs. Although both reservoir and matrix systems can provide comparable plasma profiles of a drug, these transdermal delivery systems may have very different risks with respect to dose-dumping [81]. For reservoir systems, as the entire load of the active ingredient is in the reservoir, the reservoir must be completely sealed to avoid dose-dumping. In contrast, for the matrix system, the drug is incorporated directly into the adhesive or polymeric layer, thereby mitigating the risk of drug leakage and dose-dumping. For transdermal products containing controlled substances, development of a product with a tamper-resistant feature is highly recommended to prevent drug abuse.

During the manufacturing process of transdermal delivery systems, a surplus of drug is generally needed to achieve the desirable release rate and/or maintain the appropriate systemic level of the drug throughout the application period. It has been estimated that currently marketed transdermal drug delivery systems and topical patches may retain 10–95% of the initial total amount of drug after the intended use period. This has raised a potential safety issue not only to the patient, but also to others including family members, caregivers, and children. In fact, over the years, reported adverse events resulting from various quality problems pertaining to these products have led to several product recalls, withdrawals, and public health advisories. In view of all the concerns, the FDA has recently issued a guidance document on the topic of residual drugs in transdermal and related drug delivery systems [82]. It is noted that the choice of formulation, design, and system components can provide potential pathways to optimize drug delivery and minimize residual drug in the transdermal delivery systems. Examples may include the use of penetration enhancers, use of self-depleting solvent systems, and judicious choice of adhesive layer. Other factors that should be considered may encompass the type and concentration of excipients, drug load, adhesive thickness, and the composition and thickness of the backing layer. In essence, a scientific risk-based approach should be taken to minimize the amount of residual drug to the lowest possible level in a transdermal system after use [82, 83].

16.6.2 Adhesion Performance

Poor skin adhesion is another regulatory concern for some of the transdermal delivery systems and topical patches [84]. To function properly, transdermal drug delivery systems must rely on maintenance of good adhesion over the application period, which may last many hours to several days or weeks. Reduction in the surface area of contact as a result of patch lift or even falling off diminishes drug delivery from the patch. In addition, patches that fail to adhere for their prescribed time period must be replaced, thereby increasing the cost to the patient. Adhesive performance is a critical factor that determines drug delivery, therapeutic effect, and patient compliance for transdermal delivery systems.

Many clinical trials use placebo patches to determine the adhesion performance of a new patch product [22]. This practice may not be realistic in that the presence of drug and/or excipients may affect the adhesion properties of the patches. Alternatively, the *in vivo* adhesion performance of medicated patches may be assessed in a pharmacokinetic study or a separate adhesion study based on subjective observations [85]. The adhesion performance may be evaluated using a scoring system based on patch lift (Table 16.5).

Adhesion is scored from 0 to 4 in which 0 indicates that the patch had 90% adherence throughout the application period and 4 indicates that the patch fell off the skin. As most *in vivo* studies are costly and time-consuming, it is important to develop appropriate *in vitro* adhesion testing methods that are correlated with the *in vivo* performance. Currently, consistent methodology to test the adhesion properties of transdermal patches does not exist although several *in vitro*

TABLE 16.5 A scoring System for Evaluation of Patch Adhesion

Score	Percentage Adhered	Remark
0	≥90%	Essentially no lift off the skin
1	≥75% to <90%	Some edges only lifting off the skin
2	≥50% to <75%	Less than half of the patch lifting off the skin
3	>0% to <50%	Adhered but not detached (more than half of the patch lifting off the skin without falling off)
4	0%	Patch detached (patch completely off the skin)

adhesion test methods are available for industrial pressure-sensitive tapes [84]. More research and investigations are needed in this area.

16.6.3 Skin Irritation and Sensitization

Skin irritation may be caused by chemical irritants and manifested as itching, rash, or perspiration. In contrast to irritation, skin sensitization is a response of the adaptive immune system, in which there is a delayed T-cell-mediated allergic reaction to chemically modified skin proteins [86]. Transdermal products have properties that may lead to skin irritation and/or sensitization. The delivery system or the system in conjunction with the drug substance may cause these reactions [87]. During the development of new transdermal products, dermatologic adverse events are evaluated primarily with animal studies [88] and safety assessment in the context of large clinical trials generally associated with the submission of NDAs [89]. Separate skin irritation and sensitization studies can also be used for this purpose, which are often designed to detect irritation and sensitization under conditions of maximal stress [89]. For ANDAs, comparative skin irritation and sensitization studies are generally conducted for transdermal products in healthy volunteers [85, 90]. Continuous same-site exposure is recommended to provide maximal provocative exposure. The study may consist of two phases, a 21-day induction phase followed by a challenge phase, with a rest period of 2–3 weeks between the phases [85, 90]. For potent drugs such as fentanyl, because of safety concerns, generic versions of fentanyl patches have been evaluated for skin irritation and sensitization by testing a vehicle patch versus a positive control patch that produces mild irritation (e.g., 0.1% sodium lauryl sulfate or lower concentration) [85]. The vehicle patch has the same inactive ingredients in the same concentrations as the proposed product. Skin irritation can be scored on a scale that describes the amount of erythema, edema, and other features indicative of irritation (Table 16.6) [90].

TABLE 16.6 An Example Scoring System for the Skin Irritation Test

Scale 1: Dermal Response Skin Appearance	Score
No evidence of irritation	0
Minimal erythema, barely perceptible	1
Definite erythema, readily visible; minimal edema or minimal papular response	2
Erythema and papules	3
Definite edema	4
Erythema, edema, and papules	5
Vesicular eruption	6
Strong reaction spreading beyond the application site	7

Scale 2: Other Effects Observation	Score (Numeric Equivalent)
Slightly glazed appearance	A (0)
Marked glazed appearance	B (1)
Glazing with peeling and cracking	C (2)
Glazing with fissures	F (3)
Film of dried serous exudates covering all or part of the patch site	G (3)
Small petechial erosions and/or scabs	H (3)

16.7 RESPIRATORY DRUG DELIVERY SYSTEMS

For decades, respiratory drug delivery systems have been considered the most complex dosage forms in the pharmaceutical formulary although they have been used for a variety of therapeutic benefits. Delivery of drugs directly into the lungs by inhalation is common for bronchodilators and corticosteroids in the treatment of asthma and chronic obstructive pulmonary disease (COPD) [91]. This route of drug delivery is also used for local action in patients with various respiratory conditions, including antibiotics, antivirals, and mucoactive agents. In addition, several systemically acting drugs (such as peptides, proteins, and vaccines) are currently being developed for pulmonary delivery [92].

The complexity of respiratory delivery systems can be attributed to a number of factors that govern the lung deposition of drugs, including 1) physicochemical properties of the droplets or particles being delivered, 2) physiological and anatomical features of the lungs, and 3) mechanical aspects of aerosol dispersion usually associated with the delivery device [93]. The aerodynamic properties (such as particle diameter, shape, and density) are the most important physicochemical characteristics that impact on the performance of aerosols. However, the particle size of aerosols may change as they travel through the high-humidity environment of the lungs, which in turn will alter their lung deposition. Most lung deposition models are constructed based on the influence of particle size on aerosol deposition [94, 95]. Yet, breathing parameters (e.g., tidal volume and breathing frequency) can also influence lung deposition, which may vary with age, gender, and disease state [96]. Depending on the sites of deposition in the airways, the drug can be cleared through mucociliary transport (into the GI tract), absorption (into the systemic circulation), and cell-mediated translocation (to lymphatics and then blood circulation). Indeed, the intricate nature of the clearance mechanism in the lungs and the interaction with the aerosol particles complicates the pharmacokinetic profiles of drugs delivered by pulmonary route of administration.

It is to be noted that although many respiratory delivery systems have drug and device in combination, their

TABLE 16.7 Examples of DPI Formulations Currently Marketed in the United States

Trade Name	Drug(s)	Dosage Form	Product	Remark/Indication
Foradil® Aerolizer (Norvatis Pharmaceuticals, Basal, Switzland)	Formoterol fumate	Capsule	Unit dose	Long-acting beta2-adrenergic agonist (LABA) for asthma
Advair® Diskus (Glaxo Group Limited, Greenford, UK)	Fluticasone propionate + Salmeterol xinafoate	Blister	Multiple unit dose	FP—LABA; SX—corticosteroid
Pulmicort® Turbuhaler® (AstraZeneca, London, UK)	Budesonide	Reservoir	Multi-dose	Corticosteroid
Asmanex® Twisthaler® (Schering, Berlin-Wedding, Germany)	Mometasone furoate	Reservoir	Multi-dose	Corticosteroid

applications to the FDA are only reviewed and approved by the drug center. The device in the delivery system is considered a "component" of the drug product. The following subsections provide current regulatory considerations for respiratory drug delivery systems, including both drug and device.

16.7.1 Device and Formulation Design

Pressurized metered-dose inhalers (pMDIs) are the most common type of inhalers. Chloroflurocarbon (CFC) propellants have been widely used in pMDIs for many years. However, CFC propellants were banned in the late 1980s as a result of the finding that they played a significant role in ozone depletion [97]. To date, most CFC-containing pMDIs have been reformulated with ozone-friendly propellants, e.g., hydrofluoralkanes (HFAs). An issue with the use of HFA propellants lies in their poor solubility for several excipients that are commonly incorporated into CFC-containing formulations, and thus, manufacturers have to seek other excipients when reformulating. The basic components of a pMDI are the canister, metering valve, and a mouthpiece/actuator combination [92]. The canister must be capable of withstanding the high internal pressure generated by the propellant and provide an inert surface (with appropriate coatings) that will resist physical and chemical changes to the contents. Historic problems to the metering valve may include sealing issue (as a result of propellant characteristics) and dose variation (as a result of drainage from the metering chamber at rest; i.e., loss of prime). The "loss of prime" issue is the reason why pMDIs are recommended to be operated for one or two noninhaled shots prior to use. Quantifying the loss of prime is required by several health authorities.

Dry powder inhalers (DPIs) are an alternative to pMDIs, which depend on effective dispersion of particles in a respirable size range (typically 5–10 μm) and rely on the force of patient inhalation to entrain powder from the device. Compared with pMDIs, lung deposition from DPIs is generally higher and less variable, and some DPIs have the advantage of delivering larger doses. DPIs do not contain propellants, and most are breath-actuated (passive), circumventing the problem of poor coordination between actuation and inhalation in pMDIs. Table 16.7 shows some examples of DPI formulations currently on the market. Most DPI formulations consist of a micronized drug, which must be blended with larger carrier particles to enhance flow, prevent aggregation, and aid in dispersion. Therefore, excipients can comprise >99% of the formulation and should be chosen carefully to optimize product performance.

Unlike MDIs and DPIs, nebulizers use compressed air or ultrasonic power to break up solutions or suspensions into small aerosol droplets that can be directly inhaled from the device mouthpiece. Misuse of the device is a major issue for nebulizers. This problem may be avoided using facemasks with a tight seal around the mouth and nose [92].

16.7.2 *In Vitro* Assessment

The primary goals of *in vitro* tests for nasal and inhaled products are to ensure that the product discharges an accurate amount of drug, and the drug product is stable within the labeled shelf life. *In vitro* tests can be very useful to guide preclinical development of these products. In the presence of a minor change in formulation or manufacturing, *in vitro* testing can also be employed to detect possible bio*in*equivalence between the products before and after change. Given the complexity of respiratory delivery devices and the special requirement of lung deposition for therapeutic effects, it is crucial to have appropriate *in vitro* test methods in place to ensure product quality and performance.

A number of *in vitro* test methods can be used for assessment of nasal and inhaled products [98, 99]. In principle, the key parameters to be assessed for these products include 1) a delivered or emitted dose, 2) aerodynamic particle size distribution (APSD), 3) spray pattern and plume geometry, and 4) impurities and/or microbial contaminants in formulations and devices during storage or use. In addition, it is essential to evaluate product performance in terms of physical and chemical compatibilities between drug

TABLE 16.8 Examples of *In Vitro* Tests for MDI and DPI Drug Products

- Appearance and color
- Identification of the drug substance in the drug product
- Microbial limits
- Water or moisture content
- Dehydrated alcohol content (if used as a co-solvent in the formulation)
- Net content (fill) weight
- Drug content (assay) of the entire container
- Impurities and degradation products
- Dose content uniformity (for individual container, among containers, and among batches)
- Dose content uniformity through container life
- Particle size distribution
- Microscopic evaluation
- Spray pattern and plume geometry
- Leak rate
- Pressure testing
- Valve delivery
- Leachables

and device component. Table 16.8 provides a list of *in vitro* tests from the FDA guidance for MDI or DPI products [98]. Several methods are available for determination of particle size and size distribution. However, the FDA guidance has recommended the use of cascade impaction for particle sizing of pMDIs and DPIs. It is further advised that manufacturers specify the conditions of use for a cascade impactor to minimize distortion and ensure the reproducibility of the data [98].

16.7.3 *In Vivo* Assessment

Pharmacokinetic studies are generally used to assess the bioavailability and bioequivalence of systemically absorbed drug products in that drug levels measured in the systemic circulation are relevant to the clinical efficacy and safety of these products. For nasal and inhalation products, however, drugs may be deposited at the local site of action (lungs) or in the upper airways. If deposited in the upper airways, the drug will be swallowed and entered into the GI tract. Therefore, the drug present in the systemic circulation via nasal or oral inhalation may come from two different sources, i.e., absorption from the lungs and absorption from the GI tract (and possibly the oropharyngeal cavity). If a drug has little or negligible oral absorption, pharmacokinetic data may reflect pulmonary drug delivery. However, if drug absorption occurs in both the lungs and GI tract, which is probably the case for most inhaled drugs, pharmacokinetic studies cannot be used to assess pulmonary bioavailability. Under such circumstances, activated charcoal may be used to prevent GI absorption, allowing for the use of systemic drug levels for measurement of pulmonary bioavailability [92]. Gamma scintigraphy is another approach that has been employed to quantify pulmonary drug delivery for these products [92].

The U.S. regulation allows waivers of *in vivo* bioavailability/bioequivalence testing in certain drug products for which bioavailability/bioequivalence may be self-evident [100]. As such, the *in vivo* bioequivalence testing is not needed for nasal solutions. However, such testing is required for suspension-based nasal sprays as a result of the lack of a suitable method for particle size determination in suspension formulations [101]. Moreover, *in vivo* testing cannot be exempted for nasal solutions in metered dose devices because they are drug–device combination products. In addition to the *in vivo* testing, generic sponsors of nasal aerosols and nasal sprays must conduct various *in vitro* tests to provide evidence of equivalent performance between the test and reference products. These *in vitro* tests for bioequivalence comparisons are shown in Table 16.9.

In general, bioequivalence based on pharmacokinetic measures suggests that equivalence in rate and extent of systemic exposure equates to similarity in clinical effectiveness and safety. Although this assumption may be valid for most drugs with systemic action, it cannot be applied to nasal and inhalation products that are locally acting. Bioequivalence determination for the metered products is further complicated by the fact that drug delivery is dependent on the metering device that is an integral part of the drug product. Because of the complexity of these dosage forms, establishment of bioequivalence for metered nasal and inhalation products in the United States has been based on an "aggregate weight of evidence" approach [101]. This approach uses the following criteria for documentation of bioequivalence: 1) *in vitro* studies between test and reference products to support equivalent performance of metering device, 2) pharmacokinetic studies to establish equivalence in systemic exposure, and 3) pharmacodynamic or clinical endpoint studies to demonstrate equivalence in local action [101, 102]. Additional information on the conduct of bioequivalence studies using pharmacodynamic and/or clinical endpoints can be found in guidelines issued by Health Canada [103–105].

TABLE 16.9 *In Vitro* Tests to Support Bioequivalence of Nasal Aerosols and Nasal Sprays

- Single actuation content through container life
- Droplet size distribution by laser diffraction
- Drug in small particles/droplets, or particle/droplet size distribution by cascade impactor
- Drug particle size distribution by microscopy
- Spray pattern
- Plume geometry
- Priming and repriming

16.8 DRUG-ELUTING STENTS

Drug-eluting stents are an improvement for bare-metal stents in reducing restenosis as a result of neointimal hyperplasia associated with bare-metal stenting [106, 107]. In many cases, a drug is incorporated into a polymeric coating and released at the intended site of action for the intended duration. The chemical, physical, and mechanical attributes of the polymer coating are important for stent deployment, biocompatibility, and stability. There are two kinds of stents—metal stents and bioresorbable (or biodegradable) stents—that can be used for several applications, including coronary, urethral, tracheal, and other systems. As a combination product, applications of drug-eluting stents are reviewed in the FDA by both CDRH and CDER. However, the FDA Office of Combination Products assigns the jurisdiction for regulatory responsibility to a lead center (drug or device) based on the primary mode of action for the product. The regulatory assessment of a drug-eluting stent encompasses the comprehensive evaluation of individual components (drug, polymer, and stent) as well as the finished drug–device combination product [108].

16.8.1 Safety Considerations

The FDA has determined that drug-eluting stents can pose a significant risk [109]. Hence, the development of a new drug-eluting stent calls for a thorough exploration of safety on all of the relevant components [108]. For example, in selecting the polymer or other carriers, considerations should be given to the following: 1) the ability to control drug elution, 2) the compatibility of the polymer with arterial tissue, and 3) the ability of the polymer to conform to the stent platform without significant delamination upon stent delivery and deployment [108]. All relevant components in the combination product, including drug substance, delivery system, and finished drug-eluting stent, should be carefully characterized [108]. The drug substance can be evaluated in terms of chemistry, mechanism of action, and safety profile. Both *in vitro* and animal testing can be performed to reveal any toxicity that may result from the drug and the exposure levels at which toxicity occurs. Developmental animal studies are encouraged to provide an understanding of the local and systemic exposure to the drug. If stent implantation results in significant systemic exposure, data from human safety studies, specifically single- and multiple-dose escalation studies, are necessary. Similarly, for a finished drug-eluting stent and its delivery system, they may be characterized through engineering studies, biocompatibility evaluation, animal studies, and complete CMC information [108]. Evaluation of the finished product should include a pharmacokinetic study on systemic exposure in humans and clinical information associated with stenting outcomes. In the event that a significant systemic drug exposure occurs after stent implantation, additional studies should be carried out to examine potential factors that may affect exposure, e.g., concomitant drugs and/or co-morbidities such as renal or hepatic failure [108].

16.8.2 Drug-Release Profiles

The release profile of a drug from an erodible polymer carrier of biodegradable stents often shows a slow diffusion phase (with or without a burst effect), followed by erosion or degradation of the polymer. Conversely, the elution of drugs from nonerodible coatings of metallic stents exhibits a biphasic profile that has an initial burst followed by a very slow release of the drug. The characteristics of consistent elution throughout the intended duration of action are crucial in maintaining the therapeutic benefit of a drug-eluting stent.

A major regulatory concern for drug-eluting stents has been the development of an appropriate *in vitro* release testing method and setting meaningful release specifications that are relevant from an *in vivo* standpoint. The FDA is encouraging drug sponsors to develop an *in vitro* release method that is indicative of drug bioavailability while having the ability of ejecting bad batches that are deemed inadequate for release to the market. In the cases where the measurable plasma levels reflect *in vivo* elution of drug from the stent, and the *in vitro* release conditions yields *in vitro* elution rates that mimic those observed *in vivo*, the *in vitro* release specifications should be set based on the *in vitro* elution rate. If plasma levels are too low to be measured, animal models may be used to determine the elution characteristics of a drug-eluting stent. With animal models, the stent could be explanted at different time intervals and the drug amount remaining on the stent (or in the adjacent tissues) could be measured. Alternatively, it may be possible to monitor the *in vivo* drug release from the stent using X-ray computer technologies. The clinical performance of a drug-eluting stent is another important consideration for setting the elution specification. If there is a correlation between elution rates and clinical data, specifications for elution rate can be set in such a way that only batches with acceptable efficacy (and/or safety) profiles will be released to the market.

16.9 NANOTECHNOLOGY-DERIVED DRUG DELIVERY SYSTEMS

Drug delivery systems derived from nanotechnology represent a promising approach in pharmaceutical development that may achieve desirable "drug" properties by altering the pharmacokinetic and toxicological profiles of the molecule [110]. Drug delivery systems derived from nanotechnology can be available in a variety of platforms and dosage forms for different indications. Nanotechnology such as nanocrystal/nanomill technology has often been used to reduce the particle size of a drug, thereby increasing the dissolution rate and perhaps absorption of the drug. Many nanotechnology-derived delivery systems are designed to encapsulate a drug in carriers (e.g., liposomes, dendrimers, nanoemulsions, micelles, and metal colloids), which allows for targeted delivery, avoiding systemic toxicity and improving efficacy of the drug, or enhances the bioavailability of the drug that exhibits poor solubility/permeability or is prone to metabolism/degradation *in vivo*. Other nanotechnology-derived delivery systems may involve covalent conjugation of a drug with carriers (e.g., polymers and antibodies) to facilitate targeted drug delivery and provide favorable clinical outcomes. Several drug products with nanoscale materials have been approved by the FDA (Table 16.10).

Because of the small size and extremely high ratios of surface area to volume, nanoscale materials have unique physicochemical properties and biological activities that are distinctly different from those in the bulk forms. There is ample evidence that physicochemical properties, e.g., particle size and surface chemistry, can dramatically affect nanomaterial behavior in the biological system and impact the safety and efficacy of these products [111–113]. In reference to nanoparticles within the range of 1–100 nm, an area of safety and environmental concern is nanotoxicity. Assessing nanomaterial toxicity is top priority for regulatory authorities, which is currently under active investigation. It appears that all classes of nanoparticles have extensive tissue retention although the state of nanomaterials, once deposited in tissue, is largely unknown. Many nanoparticles accumulate in the reticuloendothelial system (RES), but those with hydrodynamic radii of less than 5–6 nm, such as metal oxides and dendrimers, can be eliminated from the kidney. From the regulatory perspective, there is an urgent need for better characterization, standardization, manufacturing controls, quality assurance, and safety assessment for pharmaceuticals containing nanoscale materials.

TABLE 16.10 Examples of Approved Nanomaterial-Containing Drug Products in the United States

Platform	Trade Name	Drug	Dosage Form	Indication
Liposomes	AmBisome® (Astellas Pharma, BangKok, Thailand)	Amphotericin B	Injection	Fungal infections
	DaunoXome® (Galen, Craigavon, UK)	Daunorubicin	Injection	Antineoplastic
	DepoCyt® (Pacira Pharmaceuticals, Parsipanny, NJ)	Cytarabine	Injection	Lymphomatous meningitis
	Doxil® (Alza Corporation, Mountain View, CA)	Doxorubicin	Injection	Antineoplastic
Micelles	Amphotec® (Alkopharma USA Inc., Irvine, CA)	Amphotericin B	Injection	Fungal infection
	Estrasorb® (Medicis Pharmaceutical Corp., Scottsdale, AZ)	Estradiol	Emulsion	Vasomotor symptoms
	Taxotere® (Sanofi-Aventis, Bridgewater, NJ)	Docetaxel	Injection	Antineoplastic
Nanocrystals	Emend® (Merck & Company, Inc., Whitehouse Station, NJ)	Aprepitant	Capsules	Antiemetic
	Tricor® (Abbvie Inc., North Chicago, IL)	Fenofibrate	Tablets	Hypercholesterolemia, hypertriglyceridemia
	Triglide (Skyepharma AG, London, UK)	Fenofibrate	Tablets	Hypercholesterolemia, mixed dyslipidemia
	Megace® ES (Par Pharmaceuticals, Woodcliff, NJ)	Megestrol acetate	Oral suspension	Anorexia, cachexia
	Rapamune® (Wyeth Pharmaceuticals, Madison, NJ)	Sirolimus	Oral solution and tablets	Immunosuppressant
Nanoparticles	Abraxane® (Abraxis BioScience, Los Angeles, CA)	Paclitaxel	For injectable suspension	Metastatic breast cancer
Nanotubes	Somatuline® Depot (Ipsen Pharma, Paris, France)	Lanreotide	Injection	Acromegaly
Superparamagnetic ion oxide	Feraheme (AMAG Pharmaceuticals Inc., Lexington, MA)	Ferumoxytol	Injection	Iron deficiency anemia
	Feridex (AMAG Pharmaceuticals Inc., Lexington, MA)	Ferumoxides	Injection	MRI contrast agent
	GastroMARK™ (AMAG Pharmaceuticals Inc., Lexington, MA)	Ferumoxsil	Oral suspension	MRI contrast agent

16.9.1 Product Quality Assessment

Quality assessment for any drug product can be tailored into three important areas: 1) physicochemical characterization, 2) quality control, and 3) manufacturing. In the case of small molecules, the standard CMC data for these drug products may comprise, but not be limited to, structure, composition, crystal structure, stability, quality, purity, and strength, as well as the synthetic methods and manufacturing. Apart from the standard tests for small molecules, additional physicochemical characterization is absolutely necessary for nanomaterial-containing drug products as a result of their small size and large surface area. Typically, these characterization tests should include measurement of particle size, size distribution, shape or architecture, surface chemistry (such as charge, coating, and density), and aggregation (or agglomeration) state [114]. Traditional analytical methodology used for small molecules can be adapted for characterization of nanomaterials. However, some of these methods may be limited and advanced methods must be developed for better characterization of nanomaterial-containing drug products [111]. For instance, dendrimers are known to have interference with a standard endotoxin test. In lieu of conventional optical microscopy, electron microscopy may be more appropriate for nanoparticle size or shape measurement. Size characterization is often complicated by the polydispersity of nanoscale materials, and thus use of multiple methods such as transmission electron microscopy (TEM) and dynamic light scattering (DLS) has been recommended. The DLS technique measures the hydrodynamic size of nanoparticles and is suitable for use in biological fluids. Characterization of nanomaterial-containing formulations (e.g., cream and gel) may be difficult when nanomaterials share a similar size or basic composition with the bulk matrix. In this case, chemical analysis (e.g., X-ray and confocal Raman analysis) can be applied in place of traditional light scattering [114].

It is noteworthy that the physicochemical properties of nanomaterials may vary with the environment and conditions used in their characterization [114]. For example, particle size distribution at physiological pH and ionic strength may be different from those in the water or dry state. As such, it is critical to carry out the characterization studies in physiological conditions. In addition, these studies should be conducted with the final form of nanomaterials to which the end-user will be exposed. As protein binding tends to occur with nanomaterials in the blood, the understanding of protein-bound size may be more relevant to the nanomaterial disposition *in vivo* [114].

16.9.2 Product Safety Assessment

Market approval of a new drug product, regardless of whether it contains nanomaterials, must be subject to rigorous preclinical evaluation for safety and efficacy. Preclinical evaluation may include a series of studies in animals on pharmacology (including major organs), toxicology (including repeated-dose, genetic, reproductive, and developmental), mutagenicity, and pharmacokinetics (including absorption, distribution, metabolism, and excretion). In this context, the FDA and International Conference on Harmonization (ICH) have published several guidance documents that delineate the design and timeline of these preclinical studies [112].

Concerns for drug products with nanomaterials stem mostly from the observations that these tiny materials not only affect the physicochemical properties of the molecules but also increase the uptake and interaction with biological systems. The combination of these effects can yield serious adverse reactions in living cells that would not otherwise be possible with the same material in larger form. As such, regulatory assessment for safety of nanomaterial-containing drug products has been focused on biodistribution, clearance, metabolism, and toxicity. Depending on the formulation of nanoscale materials, there may be more or less requirements for preclinical studies. As an example, fewer studies are required for a reformulated product from a previously approved drug to a nanoscale material if the latter was made by simple milling of the drug [112, 114]. The key studies for regulatory evaluation of these reformulated products are the bridging studies on pharmacokinetics and toxicology, which should be designed to compare the previously approved formulation with the newly developed nanomaterial formulation. The requirement for preclinical data may be modified based on the results of these bridging studies [112, 114]. In addition, tissue distribution studies are important for both small-molecule- and nanomaterial-containing drug products. If the nanomaterials have the potential to be opsonized *in vivo*, it is pertinent to perform long-term biodistribution studies [114].

16.9.3 Bioavailability and Bioequivalence

The pharmacokinetic approach is commonly used for assessment of bioavailability and bioequivalence of systemically absorbed drug products. This can apply to both bulk materials and some nano-formulations of existing drugs (e.g., nanocrystals). However, for many nanotechnology-derived delivery systems, the active ingredient may be encapsulated in the carriers or conjugated with carriers (also ligands). If the nanoscale material product is designed for targeted delivery to tissues or organs, measurement of drug concentrations in the systemic circulation may not be appropriate for bioavailability or bioequivalence evaluation because blood levels cannot reflect drug availability at the site of action.

16.9.4 Liposomes

Liposomes have been widely used as an example of nanotechnology-derived drug delivery systems although they are

TABLE 16.11 Classification of Liposomes

Classification Scheme	Example	Remark
Size and lamellarity	Small unilamellar vesicles (SUVs)	25–100 nm
	Large unilamellar vesicles (MUVs)	>100 nm
	Multilamellar vesicles (MLVs)	>500 nm
	Giant vesicles	>1000 nm
Coating	Plain liposomes	Most conventional liposomes; have short blood circulation time; accumulate in MPS (RES)
	Stealth liposomes	Carry polymer coatings; avoid MPS uptake; prolong blood circulation time
	Immunoliposomes	Antibodies attached to the surface; enhance binding at the target site
	Cationic liposomes	Coated with a positive charge; promote cellular internalization
Uptake by MPS or RES*	MPS-avoiding	Circulate in bloodstream for days; extravasate in tissues
	MPS-targeting	Relatively short duration in systemic circulation

*MPS: mononclear phagocytic system; RES: reticuloendothelial system.

larger particulate carriers compared with most other nanoscale material platforms. Liposomes are tiny vesicles composed of one or more bilayers of amphipathic lipid molecules enclosing one or more aqueous compartments [115]. The number of aqueous compartments is usually equal to the number of lipid bilayers. As a delivery system, the drug is added during the formation process. Hydrophilic compounds are usually incorporated into the aqueous compartment while hydrophobic compounds are in the lipid bilayers [116]. Depending on the classification scheme, several types of liposomes can be available (Table 16.11). They may be classified based on liposome size, lamellarity, coatings, or uptake by the mononuclear phagocytic system (MPS, also called RES). The size of liposomes may range from 25 nm to 1 μm, available as either unilamellar or multilamellar vesicles. Unlike plain liposomes, stealth liposomes have polymer coatings such as polyethylene glycol (PEG) that can create steric hindrance to phagocytosis. Immunoliposomes have antibodies attached to the liposome surface that enhance their bindings at the target site. Similarly, cationic liposomes coated with a positive charge can interact with the negatively charged DNA and promote cellular internalization of genetic materials. Of particular relevance to *in vivo* performance may be the classification scheme based on pharmacological behavior of liposomes toward MPS (or RES). Most conventional liposomes such as AmBisome (Astellas Pharma, Bangkok, Thailand) are plain liposomes, which can be easily taken up by the macrophages in MPS and thus have a relatively short residence time in the blood. In contrast, stealth liposomes such as Doxil (ALZA Corporation, Mountain View, CA) are designed to avoid the MPS uptake, thereby circulating in the bloodstream for a long period of time [117]. The prolongation of residence time in the blood increases the chances for Doxil to extravasate into the inflamed tissues or tumor cells, a mechanism known as the enhanced permeability and retention (EPR) effect [116].

16.9.4.1 Challenges in Chemistry, Manufacturing, and Controls Liposome drug products are unique in that their compositions and physicochemical properties are critical to product quality and clinical performance. Critical factors for manufacturing of liposome drug products may encompass a wide range of variables, including drug substance, structural lipid matrix, particle size distribution, and liposome surface properties (such as coating and charge). Unlike conventional dosage forms, the physicochemical properties are deemed critical to establishing the identity of a liposome drug product. As such, the FDA has required physicochemical characterization tests for liposome drug products to ensure batch-to-batch product quality although not all of the characterization tests have to be included in the specification for batch release [115]. Some of the unique physicochemical properties of liposome drug products are shown in Table 16.12 [115].

TABLE 16.12 Some Physicochemical Properties of Liposome Drug Products

- Morphology of the liposome (including lamellarity)
- Surface characteristics
- Liposomal integrity (ability of liposome product to retain the drug substance inside the liposome)
- Net charge
- Drug product viscosity
- Entrapment parameters such as efficiency and capacity
- Particle size (mean and distribution profile) defined on the basis of volume or number
- Phase transition temperature
- *In vitro* release of the drug substance from the drug product
- Leakage rate of drug substance from the liposome on stability
- Osmotic properties related to liposome volume changes in response to changes in salt concentration
- Spectroscopic data (e.g., phosphorus nuclear magnetic resonance)

Liposomal dosage forms are extremely sensitive to changes in manufacturing conditions, such as shear force, temperature, and effect of scale [115]. Nonetheless, product failure *in vivo* can be difficult to detect using *in vitro* testing of the finished liposomal product. Accordingly, it is pertinent to establish rigorous critical process controls to ensure the quality of these drug products. Because of the complexity of liposomal delivery systems, the FDA has advised that any changes in significant manufacturing parameters be evaluated in terms of their effect on product characteristics. In some cases, *in vivo* studies may be warranted, even if the physicochemical characteristics are unchanged [115].

16.9.4.2 Biopharmaceutics and Therapeutic Equivalence Issues Development of an *in vitro* release test is essential for liposomal drug delivery systems to ensure product quality and process controls. However, it is difficult to develop an appropriate *in vitro* release test correlated to the *in vivo* performance of a liposome product. Ideally, an *in vitro* release test may be developed depending on the mechanism of drug release from the liposome product. The conventional dissolution method may be adequate for *in vitro* release testing if a liposome product is intended for systemic drug delivery. However, if a liposome product is designed for targeted delivery, it may be more appropriate to adopt a cell-based model for *in vitro* release.

Several drug applications submitted for liposomes are based on an approved drug product in the conventional dosage form given by the same route of administration to improve the therapeutic index of the drug [118]. As both old and new formulations possess the same active moiety, the FDA has required study data that compare product performance in terms of pharmacokinetic profiles [115]. The pharmacokinetic information is useful in determining the dose-(concentration)-response relationship, which allows for establishment of a dosage/dosing regimen for the new liposome drug product under study. The *in vivo* integrity of liposomes can also be evaluated using a single-dose pharmacokinetic study. The liposome product can be considered stable *in vivo* if the drug remains in the circulation substantially in the encapsulated form and the ratio of unencapsulated to encapsulated drug is relatively constant over the time course of the study [115]. In such circumstances, measurement of total drug concentration may be adequate. Conversely, if the product is unstable *in vivo*, separate measurement of the encapsulated and unencapsulated drug is necessary to allow for proper interpretation of the pharmacokinetic data.

Assessment of bioavailability and bioequivalence is challenging for most liposomal drug products because of the lack of knowledge on their precise disposition *in vivo*. To determine bioavailability and/or bioequivalence using a pharmacokinetic approach, one must be able to address the following two questions: 1) when and where the drug is released from the formulation *in vivo* and 2) if the drug is available at the site of action. However, neither of the two questions can be answered with certainty for most liposomal products on the market with the exception of Doxil (doxorubicin HCl liposome injection). For Doxil, the liposome-encapsulated drug can circulate in the bloodstream for a prolonged period of time, permitting the use of blood sampling for pharmacokinetic studies. Additionally, the characteristics of this liposome drug product have been extensively studied since its introduction in 1995. Therefore, the FDA advises generic sponsors to demonstrate "sameness" in composition, drug-loading process, and liposome characteristics before they initiate *in vivo* bioequivalence studies [119]. Basically, the test (generic) and reference (innovator) products should have equivalent liposome characteristics, which includes composition, state of encapsulated drug, internal environment of liposome, liposome size distribution, number of lamellar layers, grafted PEG at the liposome surface, electrical surface potential or charge, and *in vitro* leakage rates [119]. This example illustrates the importance of scrutinizing the "pharmaceutical equivalence" of a complex drug product, by means of the state-of-the-art methodology, to support *in vivo* bioequivalence studies so that therapeutic equivalence can be ensured between generic and innovator drug products.

16.10 NUCLEIC ACID THERAPEUTICS

In recent decades, there has been growing interest and remarkable revolution in the field of nucleic acid-based therapy, such as antisense oligonucleotides, RNA interference (RNAi), peptide nucleic acids, nucleic acid-based nanoparticles, and DNA-modified gene therapy. Although antisense oligonucleotides were discovered earlier than RNAi technology, the latter may be gaining more momentum in the development of therapeutic agents for a number of diseases [120, 121]. RNAi is a mechanism of gene-silencing produced by small RNAs, which may include endogenous microRNA (miRNA) and exogenous small interfering RNA (siRNA) or short hairpin RNA (shRNA) [122]. Although miRNAs can function as tumor suppressors or oncogenes, siRNA and shRNA have been extensively used to silence cancer-related targets [123].

Despite the numerous RNAi therapeutics reported in preclinical development, several hurdles must be overcome for RNAi therapies to move from the bench to the clinic. In general, challenges in the development of RNAi therapeutics may include 1) efficient target delivery, 2) induction of innate immune response, 3) potential off-target effects and unwanted cytotoxicity, and 4) understanding of molecular mechanism and pharmacokinetics of RNAi therapeutics [123, 124]. For regulatory filing, documentation of the molecular mechanism and pharmacokinetics is necessary. Nucleic-acid-based therapy is still in its infancy at this time. However, detailed information on the efficient delivery of nucleic acid therapeutics can be found in Chapter 14 of this book.

ASSESSMENT QUESTIONS

16.1. Which of the following regulations establishes a safety standard for drug products marketed in the United States?

a. Pure Food and Drugs Act of 1906
b. Federal Food, Drug, and Cosmetic Act of 1938
c. Kefauver-Harris Amendments of 1962
d. Hatch-Waxman Amendments of 1984

16.2. Which of the following regulations requires drug manufacturers to establish the effectiveness of their drug products before marketing in the United States?

a. Pure Food and Drugs Act of 1906
b. Federal Food, Drug, and Cosmetic Act of 1938
c. Kefauver-Harris Amendments of 1962
d. Hatch-Waxman Amendments of 1984

16.3. Which of the following methods is most frequently used for determination of bioequivalence of systemically absorbed drug products?

a. Comparative pharmacodynamic studies
b. Comparative clinical trials
c. Comparative pharmacokinetic studies
d. Comparative *in vitro* dissolution or release studies

16.4. Which of the following may increase the potential of dose-dumping in an orally administered extended-release drug product?

a. Grape fruit juice
b. High fat meal
c. Alcohol
d. B and C
e. All of the above

16.5. Despite its wide use for polymer-based, sustained-release, parenteral products, PLGA [poly(lactic-co-glycolic acid)] may have the following disadvantages:

a. Proteins/peptides may be degraded in the acidic environment of PLGA
b. Control of drug release from PLGA is limited, and it may produce a significant initial burst followed by incomplete release of the drug
c. Loss of polymer molecular weight may occur if aseptic process is used for the parenteral product
d. A and B only
e. All of the above

16.6. As with most common excipients, lipid excipients are inert substances that will not interact with any enzymes or transporters *in vivo*.

a. True
b. False

16.7. Which of the following factors may not influence serum levels of lipoproteins that are involved in the transport of lipid-based formulations *in vivo*?

a. Age and gender
b. Body surface area
c. Diet or fat content
d. Disease state.

16.8. Which of the following may be a regulatory concern and should be taken into consideration when developing a transdermal drug delivery system?

a. Dose dumping
b. Skin irritation and sensitization
c. Adhesion problem
d. Amount of residual drugs in the transdermal system
e. All of the above

16.9. Which of the following may affect lung deposition of the drug from a respiratory delivery system?

a. Physicochemical properties of the particles being delivered
b. Physiological and anatomical features of the lungs
c. Mechanical aspects of aerosol dispersion in the delivery device
d. A and B
e. All of the above

16.10. Discuss the types of studies used by the U.S. FDA for evaluation of bioequivalence in metered nasal and inhalation products.

16.11. In addition to the standard tests on chemistry, manufacturing, and controls for small molecules, special tests are needed for characterization of nanomaterial-containing drug products to assure product quality and performance. Please describe those tests typically used and explain why they are important for these drug products.

REFERENCES

1. U.S. Department of Health and Human Services, Food and Drug Administration, Center for Drug Evaluation and Research, Office of Pharmaceutical Science, Office of Generic Drugs. *Electronic Orange Book: Approved*

Drug Products with Therapeutic Equivalence Evaluations. 2011.

2. Schuirmann, D.J. (1987). A comparison of the two one-sided tests procedure and the power approach for assessing the equivalence of average bioavailability. *Journal of Pharmacokinetics and Biopharmaceutics*, *15*, 657–680.
3. Nugent, L., Jain, R. (1984). Extravascular diffusion in normal and neoplastic tissues. *Cancer Research*, *44*, 238–244.
4. Minko, T., et al. (2006). New generation of liposomal drugs for cancer. *Anti-Cancer Agents in Medicinal Chemistry*, *6*, 537–552.
5. Fischei-Ghodsian, F., et al. (1988). Enzymatically controlled drug delivery. *Proceeding of National Academy of Sciences of USA*, *5*, 2403–2406.
6. U.S. Department of Health and Human Services, Food and Drug Administration, Center for Drug Evaluation and Research. *Guidance for Industry: Bioavailability and Bioequivalence Studies for Orally Administered Drug Products—General Considerations.* March 2003.
7. Hendeles, L., et al. (1985). Food-induced "dose-dumping" from a once-a-day theophylline product as a cause of theophylline toxicity. *Chest*, *87*, 758–765.
8. Murray, S., Wooltorton, E. (2005). Alcohol-associated rapid release of a long-acting opioid. *Canadian Medical Association Journal*, *173*(*7*), 756.
9. Meyer, R. Clinical relevance of alcohol-induced dose dumping. FDA Advisory Committee for Pharmaceutical Science Meeting, Rockville, Maryland. October 25–262005.
10. U.S. Food and Drug Administration, Title 21 Code of Federal Regulations (CFR) Part 320.25(f), Office of Federal Register, National Archives and Records Administration, U.S. Government Printing Office, Washington, DC, 2011.
11. Farinha, A., et al. (1999). Bioequivalence evaluation of two omeprazole enteric-coated formulations in humans. *European Journal of Pharmaceutical Sciences*, *7*, 311–315.
12. Elkoshi, Z., et al. (2002). Multiple-dose studies can be a more sensitive assessment for bioequivalence than single-dose studies—The case with omeprazole. *Clinical Drug Investigation*, *22*, 585–592.
13. Brayden, D.J. (2003). Controlled release technologies for drug delivery. *Drug Discovery Today*, *8*, 976–978.
14. Health Canada, Health Products and Food Branch. *Draft Guidance Document—Comparative Bioavailability Standards: Formulations Used for Systemic Effects.* January 25, 2010.
15. Chen, M.-L., et al. (2011). Using partical area for evaluation of bioavailability and bioequivalence. *Pharmaceutical Research*, *28*, 1939–1947.
16. U.S. Department of Health and Human Services, Food and Drug Administration, Center for Drug Evaluation and Research. *Individual Product Bioequivalence Recommendation—Zolpidem (Draft guidance).* August 2009.
17. Hindmarch, I., Legangneux, E., Stanley, N. (2007). A randomized double-blind, placebo-controlled, 10-way crossover study shows that a new zolpidem modified-release formulation improves sleep maintenance compared to standard zolpidem. *Sleep*, *27*, A55.
18. Roth, T., et al. (2006). Efficacy and safety of zolpidem-modified release: A double-blind, placebo-controlled study in adults with primary insomnia. *Sleep Medicine*, *7*, 397–406.
19. Kumar, T.R.K., Soppimath, K., Nachaegari, S.K. (2006). Novel delivery technologies for protein and peptide therapeutics. *Current Pharmaceutical Biotechnology*, *7*, 261–276.
20. Rhee, Y. -S, et al. (2010). Sustained-release injectable drug delivery—A review of current and future systems. *Pharmaceutical Technology—Drug Delivery*, S6–S13.
21. Shi, Y., Li, L.C. (2005). Current advances in sustained-release systems for parenteral drug delivery. *Expert Opinion on Drug Delivery*, *2*(*6*), 1039–1058.
22. *Physicians' Desk Reference*. Physicians' Desk Reference, Inc. 2011.
23. Berkland, C., et al. (2007). Macromolecule release from monodisperse PLG microspheres: Control of release rates and investigation of release mechanism. *Journal of Pharmaceutical Sciences*, *96*(*5*), 1176–1191.
24. Burgess, D.J., et al. (2002). Assuring quality and performance of sustained- and controlled-release parenterals: Workshop report. *Journal of American Association of Pharmaceutical Scientists*, *4*(*2*).
25. Burgess, D.J., et al. (2004). EUFEPS Workshop Report: Assuring quality and performance of sustained- and controlled-release parenterals. *European Journal of Pharmaceutical Sciences*, *21*, 679–690.
26. Kim, S., et al. (2010). Overcoming the barriers in micellar drug delivery: Loading efficiency, *in vivo* stability, and micelle-cell interaction. *Expert Opinion in Drug Delivery*, *7*(*1*), 49–62.
27. Ito, F., et al. (2010). Control of drug loading efficiency and drug release behavior in preparation of hydrophilic drug-containing monodisperse PLGA microspheres. *Journal of Material Science: Materials in Medicine*, *21*(*5*), 1563–1571.
28. Dawes, G.J.S., et al. (2009). Size effect of PLGA spheres on drug loading efficiency and release profiles. *Journal of Material Science: Materials in Medicine*, *20*, 1089–1094.
29. Ito, F., Fujimori, H., Makino, K. (2008). Factors affecting the loading efficiency of water-soluble drugs in PLGA microspheres. *Colloids Surfaces B. Biointerfaces.* *61*(*1*), 25–29.
30. Kumar, R., Palmieri Jr., M.J. (2010). Points to consider when establishing drug product specification for parenteral microspheres. *Journal of American Association of Pharmaceutical Scientists*, *12*(*1*), 27–32.
31. U.S. Department of Health and Human Services, Food and Drug Administration, Center for Drug Evaluation and Research. *Guidance for Industry: Immediate Release Solid Oral Dosage Forms. Scale-Up and Postapproval Changes: Chemistry, Manufacturing and Controls, In Vitro Dissolution Testing, and In Vivo Bioequivalence Documentation.* November 1995.

32. U.S. Department of Health and Human Services, Food and Drug Administration, Center for Drug Evaluation and Research. *Guidance for Industry: Nonsterile Semisolid Dosage Forms. Scale-Up and Postapproval Changes: Chemistry, Manufacturing and Controls, In Vitro Release Testing, and In Vivo Bioequivalence Documentation.* May 1997.

33. U.S. Department of Health and Human Services, Food and Drug Administration, Center for Drug Evaluation and Research. *Guidance for Industry: Dissolution Testing of Immediate Release Solid Oral Dosage Forms.* August 1997.

34. U.S. Department of Health and Human Services, Food and Drug Administration, Center for Drug Evaluation and Research. *Guidance for Industry: Modified Release Solid Oral Dosage Forms. Scale-Up and Postapproval Changes: Chemistry, Manufacturing and Controls, In Vitro Dissolution Testing, and In Vivo Bioequivalence Documentation.* September 1997.

35. U.S. Department of Health and Human Services, Food and Drug Administration, Center for Drug Evaluation and Research. *Guidance for Industry: Extended Release Oral Dosage Forms: Development, Evaluation and Application of In Vitro/In Vivo Correlation.* September 1997.

36. U.S. Department of Health and Human Services, Food and Drug Administration, Center for Drug Evaluation and Research. *Guidance for Industry: Waiver of In Vivo Bioavailability and Bioequivalence Studies for Immediate-Release Solid Oral Dosage Forms Based on a Biopharmaceutics Classification System.* August 2000.

37. Burgess, D.J. *Injectable Dispersed Systems—Formulation, Processing, and Performance.* Taylor & Francis Group, Boca Raton, FL, 2005, pp. 166–179.

38. Shire, S.J., Cromwell, M., Liu, J. Concluding summary: Proceedings of the AAPS Biotec Open Forum on "Aggregation of Protein Therapeutics". (2006). *Journal of American Association of Pharmaceutical Scientists, 8(4)*, B729–B730.

39. Rosenberg, A.S. Effect of protein aggregates: An immunologic perspective. (2006). Journal of American Association of Pharmaceutical Scientists, *8(3)*, B501–B507.

40. Van de Weert, M., Moller, E.H. *Immunogenicity of Biopharmaceuticals: Causes, Methods to Reduce Immunogenicity, and Biosimilars.* Springer, New York, NY, 2008, Volume 8, pp. 97–111.

41. U.S. Department of Health and Human Services, Food and Drug Administration, Center for Drug Evaluation and Research. Center for Biologic Evaluation and Research. *Draft Guidance for Industry: Assay Development for Immunogenicity Testing of Therapeutic Proteins.* December 2009.

42. New, R.R.C., Kirby, C.J. (1997). Solubilization of hydrophilic drugs in oily formulations. *Advanced Drug Delivery Reviews, 25*, 59–69.

43. Charman, W.N. (2000). Lipids, lipophilic drugs, and oral drug delivery—Some emerging concepts. *Journal of Pharmaceutical Sciences, 89*, 967–978.

44. Pouton, C.W. (2000). Lipid formulations for oral administration of drugs: Non-emulsifying, self-emulsifying and 'self-microemulsifying' drug delivery systems. *European Journal of Pharmaceutical Sciences, 11(2)*, S93–S98.

45. Constantinides, P.P. (2005). Lipid microemulsions for improving drug dissolution and oral absorption: Physical and biopharmaceutical aspects. *Pharmaceutical Research, 12(11)*, 1561–1572.

46. Hauss, D.J. Oral lipid-based formulations—Enhancing bioavailability of poorly water-soluble drugs. In Series: Drugs and the Pharmaceutical Sciences, vol. 170, Informa Healthcare, London, UK, 2007.

47. Pouton, C.W., Porter, C.J. (2008). Formulation of lipid-based delivery systems for oral administration: Materials, methods and strategies. *Advanced Drug Delivery Reviews, 60(6)*, 625–637.

48. Porter, C.J., et al. (2008). Enhancing intestinal drug solubilisation using lipid-based delivery systems. *Advanced Drug Delivery Reviews, 60(6)*, 673–691.

49. Nielsen, F.S., Gibault, E., Ljusberg-Wahren, H., Arleth, L., Pedersen, J.S., Müllertz, A. (2007). Characterization of prototype self-nanoemulsifying formulations of lipophilic compounds. *Journal of Pharmaceutical Scienecs, 96(4)*, 876–892.

50. Bummer, P.M. (2004). Physical chemical considerations of lipid-based oral drug delivery—Solid lipid nanoparticles. *Critical Review in Therapeutic Drug Carrier System, 21*, 1–19.

51. Porter, C.J., Wasan, K.M., Con Constantinides, P. (2008). Lipid-based systems for the enhanced delivery of poorly water soluble drugs. *Advanced Drug Delivery Reviews, 60(6)*, 615–616.

52. Pouton, C.W., Porter, C.J. (2008). Formulation of lipid-based delivery systems for oral administration: Materials, methods and strategies. *Advanced Drug Delivery Reviews, 60(6)*, 625–637.

53. Porter, C.J., et al. (2008). Enhancing intestinal drug solubilisation using lipid-based delivery systems. *Advanced Drug Delivery Reviews, 60(6)*, 673–691.

54. Wasan, K.M., Cassidy, S.M. (1998). Role of plasma lipoproteins in modifying the biological activity of hydrophobic drugs. *Journal of Pharmaceutical Sciences, 87*, 411–424.

55. Wasan, K.M., et al. (2002). Role of plasma lipoproteins in modifying the toxic effects of water-insoluble drugs: Studies with cyclosporine A, *Journal of American Association of Pharmaceutical Scientists, 4*, E30.

56. Jolliffe, C.J., Janssen, I. (2006). Distribution of lipoproteins by age and gender in adolescents. *Circulations, 114*, 1056–1062.

57. U.S. Department of Health and Human Services, Food and Drug Administration, Center for Drug Evaluation and Research, Center for Biologics Evaluation and Research. *Guidance for Industry: Nonclinical Studies for the Safety Evaluation of Pharmaceutical Excipients.* May 2005.

58. U.S. Food and Drug Administration, Title 21, Code of Federal Regulations, Part 182 184, 186. Office of the Federal Register, National Archives and Records Administration. 2007.

59. U.S. Food and Drug Administration, Center for Drug Evaluation and Research. *Inactive Ingredient Guide.* January 2011.

60. Chen, M.-L. (2008). Lipid excipients and delivery systems for pharmaceutical development: A regulatory perspective. *Advanced Drug Delivery Reviews*, *60*, 768–777.

61. Hunter, J., Hirst, B.H. (1997). Intestinal secretion of drugs. The role of P-glycoprotein and related drug efflux systems in limiting oral drug absorption. *Advanced Drug Delivery Reviews*, *25*, 129–157.

62. Ueda, K., Yoshida, A., Amachi, T. (1999). Recent progress in P-glycoprotein research. *Anticancer Drug Design*, *14*, 115–121.

63. Wu, C.-Y., Benet, L.Z. (2005). Predicting drug disposition via application of BCS: Transport/absorption/elimination interplay and development of a biopharmaceutics drug disposition classification system. *Pharmaceutical Research*, *22*, 11–23.

64. Hardman, J.G., et al. *Goodman & Gilman's The Pharmacological Basis of Therapeutics*. McGraw-Hill, Health Professions Division, New York, NY, 1996, pp. 11, 12.

65. Charman, W.N. (2000). Lipids, lipophilic drugs, and oral drug delivery—Some emerging concepts. *Journal of Pharmaceutical Science*, *89*, 967–978.

66. Porter, C.J., Charman, W.N. (2001). *In vitro* assessment of oral lipid based formulation. *Advanced Drug Delivery Reviews*, *50*, S127–S147.

67. Wasan, K.M. (2001). Formulation and physiological and biopharmaceutical issues in the development of oral lipid-based drug delivery systems, *Drug Development and Industrial Pharmacy*, *27*, 267–276.

68. Ilardia-Arana, D., Kristensen, H.G., Mullertz, A. (2006) Biorelevant dissolution media: Aggregation of amphiphiles and solubility of estradiol, *Journal of Pharmaceutical Sciences*, *95*, 248–255.

69. Sunesen, V.H., et al. (2005). *In vivo-in vitro* correlation for a poorly soluble drug, danazol, using the flow-through dissolution method with biorelevant dissolution media. *European Journal of Pharmaceutical Sciences*, *24*, 305–313.

70. Pedersen, B.L., et al. (2000). Dissolution of hydrocortisone in human and simulated intestinal fluids. *Pharmaceutical Research*, *17*, 183–189.

71. Dressman, J.B., Reppas, C. (2000). *In vitro-in vivo* correlations for lipophilic, poorly water-soluble drugs. *European Journal of Pharmaceutical Sciences*, *11*, S73–S80.

72. Charman, W.N., et al. (1997). Physicochemical and physiological mechanisms for the effects of food on drug absorption: The role of lipids and pH. *Journal of Pharmaceutical Sciences*, *86*, 269–282.

73. Lindahl, A., et al. (1997). Characterization of fluids from the stomach and proximal jejunum in men and women. *Pharmaceutical Research*, *14*, 497–502.

74. Naylor, L.J., et al. (1995). Dissolution of steroids in bile salt solutions is modified by the presence of lecithin. *European Journal of Pharmaceutics and Biopharmaceutics*, *41*, 346–353.

75. Gray, V.A. Two-tier dissolution testing. *Dissolution Technology*. May, 1998.

76. Zangenberg, N.H., et al. (2001). A dynamic in vitro lipolysis model. I. Controlling the rate of lipolysis by continuous addition of calcium. *European Journal of Pharmaceutical Sciences*, *14*, 115–122.

77. Zangenberg, N.H., et al. (2001) A dynamic in vitro lipolysis model. II. Evaluation of the model. *European Journal of Pharmaceutical Sciences*, *14*, 237–244.

78. Fatouros, D.G., et al. (2008) In vitro–in vivo correlations of self-emulsifying drug delivery systems combining the dynamic lipolysis model and neuro-fuzzy networks. *European Journal of Pharmaceutics and Biopharmaceutics*, *69(3)*, 887–898.

79. Henney, J.E. (2000). Nationwide recall of SangCya oral solution. *Journal of the American Medical Association*, *284*, 1234.

80. Prausnitz, M.R., Langer, R. (2008). Transdermal drug delivery. *Nature Biotechnology*, *26(11)*, 1261–1268.

81. Raw, A.S., Lionberger, R., Yu, L.X. (2011). Pharmaceutical equivalence by design for generic drugs: Modified-release products. *Pharmaceutical Research*, *28*, 1445–1453.

82. U.S. Department of Health and Human Services, Food and Drug Administration, Center for Drug Evaluation and Research. *Draft Guidance for Industry: Residual Drug in Transdermal and Related Drug Delivery Systems*. August 2010.

83. U.S. Department of Health and Human Services, Food and Drug Administration, Center for Drug Evaluation and Research, Center for Biologics Evaluation and Research. *Guidance for Industry: Q8 (R2) Pharmaceutical Development*. November 2009.

84. Wokovich, A.M., et al. (2006). Transdermal drug delivery system (TDDS) adhesion as a critical safety, efficacy and quality attribute. *European Journal of Pharmaceutics and Biopharamceutics*, *64(1)*, 1–8.

85. U.S. Department of Health and Human Services, Food and Drug Administration, Center for Drug Evaluation and Research. *Individual Product Bioequivalence Recommendation—Fentanyl Extended Release Transdermal (Draft Guidance)*. February 2010.

86. Frosch, P., Menné, T., Lepoittevin, J.-P. *Contact Dermatitis*. Springer, Heidelberg, Germany, 2006, pp. 11–44.

87. Holdiness, M.R. (1989). A review of contact dermatitis associated with transdermal therapeutic systems. *Contact Dermatitis*, *20(1)*, 3–9.

88. Basketter, D., Darlenski, R., Fluhr, J.W. (2008). Skin irritation and sensitization: Mechanisms and new approaches for risk assessment. *Skin Pharmacology and Physiology*, *21*, 191–202.

89. U.S. Department of Health and Human Services, Food and Drug Administration, Center for Drug Evaluation and Research. *Guidance for Industry—Acne Vulgaris: Developing Drugs for Treatment*. September 2005.

90. U.S. Department of Health and Human Services, Food and Drug Administration, Center for Drug Evaluation and Research. *Individual Product Bioequivalence Recommendation—Lidocaine Patches/Topical (Draft Guidance)*. December 2007.

91. Op't Holt, T.B. (2007). Inhaled beta agonists. *Respiratory Care*, *52*, 820–832.

92. Newman, S. *Respiratory Drug Delivery—Essential Theory & Practice*, Respiratory Drug Delivery Online, Virginia, 2009, pp. 357–365.
93. Banker, G.S., Rhodes, C.T. *Modern Pharmaceutics*, Marcel Dekker, Inc.New York, NY, 2002, pp. 479–499.
94. Weibel, E.R. (1963). *Morphometry of the Human Lung*, Academic Press, New York, NY.
95. Horsfield, K., Woldenberg, M.J. (1986). Branchin ratio and growth of tree-like structures. *Respiratory Physiology, 63*, 97–107.
96. Martonen, T.B., et al. (1992). Use of analytically defined estimates of aerosol respirable fraction to predict lower lung deposition. *Pharmaceutical Research, 9*, 1634–1639.
97. Molina, M.J., Rowland, F.S. (1974). Stratospheric sink for chlorofluoromethanes: Chlorine atoms catalyzed destruction of ozone. *Nature, 249*, 1810.
98. U.S. Department of Health and Human Services, Food and Drug Administration,Center for Drug Evaluation and Research. *Guidance for Industry: Metered Dose Inhaler (MDI) and Dry Powder Inhaler (DPI) Drug Products—Chemistry, Manufacturing, and Controls Documentation.* November 1998.
99. Lee, S.L., Adams, W.P., Li, B.V., Conner, D.P., Chowdhury, B.A., Yu, L.X. (2009). In vitro considerations to support bioequivalence of locally acting drugs in dry powder inhalers for lung diseases. *Journal of American Association of Pharmaceutical Scientists, 11*, 414–423.
100. U.S. Food and Drug Administration, Title 21 Code of Federal Regulations (CFR) Part 320.22, Office of Federal Register, National Archives and Records Administration, U.S. Government Printing Office, Washington, DC, 2011.
101. U.S. Department of Health and Human Services, Food and Drug Administration, Center for Drug Evaluation and Research. *Guidance for Industry: Bioavailability and Bioequivalence Studies for Nasal Aerosols and Nasal Sprays for Local Action.* April 2003.
102. Shargel, L., Kanfer, I. *Generic Drug Development—Specialty Dosage Forms.* Informa Healthcare, London, UK, 2010, pp. 189–217.
103. Health Canada, Therapeutic Products Programme. Guidance to Establish Equivalence or Relative Potency of Safety and Efficacy of a Second Entry Short-acting Beta2-agonist Metered Dose Inhaler. April 16, 1999.
104. Health Canada, Health Products and Food Branch. Draft Guidance Document: Submission Requirements for Subsequent Market Entry Inhaled Corticosteroid Products for Use in the Treatment of Asthma. August 2, 2007.
105. Health Canada, Health Products and Food Branch. Draft Guidance Document: Submission Requirements for Subsequent Market Entry Steroid Nasal Products for Use in the Treatment of Allergic Rhinitis. August 2, 2007.
106. Moses, J.W., et al. (2003). Sirolimus-eluting stents versus standard stents in patients with stenosis in native coronary artery. *New England Journal of Medicine, 349*, 1315–1323.
107. Stone, G.W., et al. (2004). One-year clinical results with the slow-release, polymer-based, paclitaxel-eluting TAXUS stent: The TAXUS-IV trial. *Circulation, 109*, 1942–1947.
108. U.S. Department of Health and Human Services, Food and Drug Administration, Center for Drug Evaluation and Research. *Guidance for Industry: Coronary Drug-Eluting Stents: Nonclinical and Clinical Studies.* March 2008.
109. U.S. Food and Drug Administration, Title 21 Code of Federal Regulations (CFR) Part 812.3(m), Office of Federal Register, National Archives and Records Administration, U.S. Government Printing Office, Washington, DC, 2011.
110. Devalapally, H., Chakilam, A., Amiji, M.M. (2007). Role of nanotechnology in pharmaceutical product development. *Journal of Pharmaceutical Science. 96*, 2547–2565.
111. Hall, J.B., et al. (2007). Characterization of nanoparticles for therapeutics. *Nanomedicine, 2*, 789–803.
112. Zolnik, B.S., Sadrieh, N. (2009). Regulatory perspective on the importance of ADME assessment of nanoscale material containing drugs. *Advanced Drug Delivery Reviews, 61*, 422–427.
113. Nel, A., et al. (2006). Toxic potential of materials at the nanolevel. *Science, 311*, 622–627.
114. McNeil, S.E. Characterization of nanoparticles intended for drug delivery. Methods in Molecular Biology, vol. 697 Springer Science-Business Media, LLC. Philadelphia, PA, 2011, pp. 17–31.
115. U.S. Department of Health and Human Services, Food and Drug Administration, Center for Drug Evaluation and Research. *Draft Guidance for Industry: Liposome Drug Products - Chemistry, Manufacturing and Controls; Human Pharmacokinetics and Bioavailability; and Labeling Documentation.* August 2002.
116. Allen, T.M., Cullis, P.R. (2004). Drug delivery systems: Entering the mainstream. *Science, 303*, 1818–1822.
117. Product Information. Doxil® doxorubicin HCl liposome injection. Ortho Biotech Products L.P., New Jersey. 2001.
118. Burgess, D.J. *Injectable Dispersed Systems—Formulation, Processing, and Performance*, Taylor & Francis Group, Boca Raton, FL, 2005, pp. 621–644.
119. U.S. Department of Health and Human Services, Food and Drug Administration, Center for Drug Evaluation and Research. *Individual Product Bioequivalence Recommendation—Doxorubicin Hydrochloride (Draft guidance).* February 2010.
120. Dias, N., Stein, C.A. (2002). Antisense oligonucleotides: Basic concepts and mechanisms. *Molecular Cancer Therapeutics, 1*, 347–355.
121. Cheng, K., Mahato, R.I. (2011). Biological and therapeutic applications of small RNAs. *Pharmaceutical Research, 28*, 2961–2965.
122. Fire, A., et al. (1998). Potent and specific genetic interference by double-stranded RNA in *Caenorhabditis elegans. Nature, 391*, 806–811.
123. Wang, Z., et al. (2011). RNA interference and cancer therapy. *Pharmaceutical Research, 28*, 2983–2995.
124. Singh, S., Narang, A.S., Mahato, R.I. (2011). Subcelluar fate and off-target effects of siRNA, shRNA, and miRNA. *Pharmaceutical Research, 28*, 2996–3015.

17

ADVANCED DRUG DELIVERY IN CANCER THERAPY

Wanyi Tai and Kun Cheng

17.1 CHAPTER OBJECTIVES

- To provide the basic concepts related to cancer and tumor microenvironment.
- To classify drug delivery systems into three major categories based on their delivery mechanisms.
- To summarize the most advanced drug delivery systems that are under cancer clinical trials.
- To describe the advantages and limitations of different drug delivery systems in cancer therapy.

17.2 INTRODUCTION

Cancer is a leading cause of death worldwide that has accounted for approximately 13% of all human deaths in 2008 (7.6 million) [1]. GLOBOCAN 2008 estimated that there were approximately 12.7 million cancer cases in 2008. Because the human population is continually growing and aging, the incidence of cancer is becoming even more common, and approximately 12 million cancer-related deaths are estimated in 2030 (World Health Organization). Moreover, environmental factors, which are the major causes of cancer, are likely to contribute to increased cancer mortality in the future because people are becoming more subjected to tobacco, poor diet, obesity, infection, radiation, and environmental pollutants [2]. The global burden of cancer continues to increase in both economically developing and developed countries.

Characterized by uncontrollable and abnormal cell growth in the body, cancer is a large class of very difficult diseases to treat. Cancers are primarily caused by genetic mutations that alter cell growth and mediate invasion and metastasis. These genetic mutations often either upregulate oncogenes or downregulate tumor-suppressor genes. Compared with normal cells, cancer cells have many unique biological characteristics that can be exploited as therapeutic targets. For example, overexpressed receptors in cancer cells could be targeted by monoclonal antibodies for cancer therapy or targeted drug delivery, whereas overactivated proteases could be employed to activate prodrugs specifically at tumor sites. Moreover, solid tumors develop a tumor microenvironment that is favorable for targeted drug delivery. The microenvironment is characterized by large fenestration, lack of smooth muscle layers, and ineffective lymphatic drainage, and therefore, it helps to accumulate nanoscale particles and macromolecules in tumor tissues rather than in normal tissues. This passive targeting phenomenon is termed the enhanced permeability and retention (EPR) effect. Both active targeting and passive targeting therapies have been used extensively in translational research of advanced drug delivery in cancer therapy. In this chapter, the biological characteristics of cancer including angiogenesis, the tumor microenvironment, and metastasis will be elucidated. Recent advances in drug delivery systems for translational research will be summarized for the following three active drug delivery systems: nanoparticles, bioconjugates, and gel systems. The drug delivery systems

Advanced Drug Delivery, First Edition. Edited by Ashim K. Mitra, Chi H. Lee, and Kun Cheng.

described in this chapter focus mainly on those already in the market or under clinical evaluations.

17.3 BIOLOGICAL CHARACTERISTICS OF CANCER

17.3.1 Molecular Characteristics

Cancers have unique molecular characteristics that make their cells different from normal cells and unique to each other. All of the unique molecular characteristics are related to genomic instability and mutations, which drive the process of cancer development directly. The molecular characteristics of cancers can be classified into two phenotypes: the overexpression of oncogenes and the down-regulation of tumor suppressor genes. This section is mainly focused on oncogenes because overexpressed oncogenes are the most popular target for cancer drug therapy. Oncogenes and their pathways, such as sonic hedgehog, Wnt, transforming growth factor β (TGFβ), and Hippo signal pathways, are overexpressed or activated in cancer cells, but they are used mainly as targets for cancer therapy rather than for targeted drug delivery. In this section, two types of oncogenes, oncogenic receptors and oncogenic enzymes, will be discussed in detail.

The overexpression of cell signaling receptors is one of the most common oncogenic alterations in cancer. When the receptors are overexpressed, the downstream signaling pathways are hyperactivated, and tumors are generated with unlimited proliferation potential and an unstable genotype. Human epidermal growth factor receptor 2 (HER2) is a well-known oncogenic receptor that is overexpressed in many cancers. Approximately 25% of all breast cancer cases are associated with HER2 overexpression [3]. The expression level of HER2 in breast cancer cells is generally 10–100-fold higher than in normal tissues [4]. The overexpression of HER2 significantly promotes the formation of HER2 hetero dimers, which activates the HER2 signaling cascades, including the phosphoinositide phospholipase C γ (PLCγ), phosphatidylinositol 3 kinase (PI3K), and mitogen-activated protein kinase (MAPK) pathways. As an oncogenic membrane receptor, overexpressed HER2 is a reasonable target for cancer therapy and targeted drug delivery. Several HER2 specific antibodies and antibody–drug conjugates have been developed in clinical research [3]. Besides HER2, the prostate-specific membrane antigen (PSMA) in prostate cancer, CD33 in relapsed acute myeloid leukemia, epidermal growth factor receptor (EGFR) in lung cancer, and mesothelin in pancreatic cancer are also commonly altered molecular characteristics of cancers.

Oncogenic enzymes, including kinases and digestive enzymes, have been found to be overexpressed in many human cancers. Kinases represent one of the largest enzyme families, and more than 500 kinases are encoded in the human genome [5, 6]. Kinases regulate most of the important intracellular signal transduction pathways and directly control cell proliferation and biological responses to environmental stimuli. Numerous kinases, especially the key components of signal transduction pathways, are attractive targets for cancer chemotherapy. These kinases include the PI3K family, AGC kinase family, CMGC kinase family, Abelson cytoplasmic tyrosine kinase (Abl), aurora kinase, and cyclin-dependent kinase (CDK) [7–9]. Small-molecule drugs, rather than antibodies, are the most successful inhibitors to modulate kinase activities because of their high penetration ability, potency, and selectivity. Digestive enzymes are another type of enzyme overexpressed in many human cancers. For example, matrix metalloproteinase (MMP) is a zinc-dependent endopeptidase that degrades all types of extracellular matrix proteins. Degradation of the extracellular matrix is crucial for malignant tumor growth, angiogenesis, invasion, and metastasis. Elevated MMP expression has been detected in the serum and tumor tissues of patients with advanced cancer. Prostate-specific antigen (PSA) and PSMA are two enzymes commonly overexpressed in prostate cancer. PSA is a small proteinase produced by the prostate gland. Elevated levels of PSA have been associated with prostate cancer. Consequently, PSA testing is considered the most effective assay for the early detection of prostate cancer [10]. PSMA is a zinc metalloenzyme that localizes in the cell membrane. It catalyzes the hydrolysis of *N*-acetylaspartylglutamate (NAAG) to glutamate and *N*-acetylaspartate. Although PSMA is expressed in many tissues, it is strongly expressed in human prostate cancer. PSMA is expressed 100-fold greater in prostate cancer than in most other tissues and 8–12-fold above noncancerous prostate tissue [11]. Digestive enzymes in cancer tissues are usually exploited to activate prodrugs by cleaving the peptide linker of the prodrug. After cleavage, the parent drug is released and elicits its therapeutic effect at the tumor site where the digestive enzyme is overexpressed. Several of these prodrugs are under preclinical or clinical evaluations [12–15].

17.3.2 Tumor Angiogenesis

Angiogenesis is the physiological process involving the formation of new blood vessels from preexisting vessels. Angiogenesis is important in embryogenesis, development, wound healing, tumor growth, and metastasis. In tumors, angiogenesis is essentially required for the transition of tumor cells from a dormant state to a malignant state. When a solid tumor is smaller than 2 mm in diameter, oxygen and nutrients can diffuse easily from a nearby blood supply into its center [16]. However, neoangiogenesis is required to form an independent blood supply within solid tumors larger than 2 mm in diameter. Tumors easily become hypoxic when they outgrow the existing blood supply. As a result, tumor angiogenesis is initiated by the hypoxic microenvironment that switches the balance between anti-antiogenic and proantiogenic factors in favor of angiogenesis [17]. Hypoxia promotes the production of proangiogeneic factors such as vascular endothelial growth factor (VEGF), platelet-derived growth factor (PDGF), basic fibroblastic growth factor (bFGF), nitric oxide synthase, and TGF-α and -β. Among them, VEGF is the most important growth factor for regulating tumor angiogenesis [18]. Proangiogenic factors diffuse across the extratumoral matrix and activate preexisting vascular endothelial cells, which migrate toward the solid tumor and form new vessel lumen [19]. Other precursor cells such as bone-marrow-derived endothelial progenitor cells (EPCs), tissue-derived EPCs, and hematopoietic stem cells also contribute to the formation of the tumor-associated endothelial cells [20]. The establishment of neovasculature inside the tumors shifts them from having a nonangiogenic to an angiogenic phenotype. This process, also termed the "angiogenic switch," is a hallmark of cancer progression [21].

The tumor vasculature is structurally and functionally abnormal compared with normal vessels in healthy tissues (Figure 17.1). Tumor vessels are unevenly distributed, heterogeneous, chaotic, irregularly branched, tortuous, leaky, thin walled, and pericyte depleted [22]. In contrast to quiescent endothelial cells, activated tumor endothelial cells can lose their polarity and detach from the basement membrane. Because of its wide junctions and multiple fenestrations that range from 10 to 1000 nm, the tumor vasculature is often leaky [23]. Macromolecules or particles ranging from 20 to 200 nm tend to extravasate and accumulate inside the interstitial space, which has been called the EPR effect [24]. In addition, abnormal tumor vessels also function poorly. Because of the chaotic network and uneven distribution of abnormal tumor vessels, the blood flow is chaotic and even stagnant in some areas. The blood flow direction is also unpredictable, and in a given vessel, blood can flow in both directions [25]. Moreover, because of the leakiness of tumor vessels, the escaping fluid increases the interstitial fluid pressure.

17.3.3 Tumor Microenvironment

Tumor hypoxia occurs when a portion of tumor cells undergoes oxygen deprivation because of a disordered vasculature. As tumors grow rapidly, high levels of cell proliferation consume oxygen and nutrients at an accelerated rate, which leads to a significantly lower concentration of oxygen in the tumor hypoxic zone than in healthy tissues. Hypoxic tumor cells are relatively quiescent, which renders them resistant to chemotherapy and radiotherapy. Tumor cells in the hypoxic zone are thought to be susceptible to additional genetic mutations that make them resistant to traditional therapy, ultimately contributing to relapse and treatment failure [26]. In clinics, hypoxia has been demonstrated to correlate

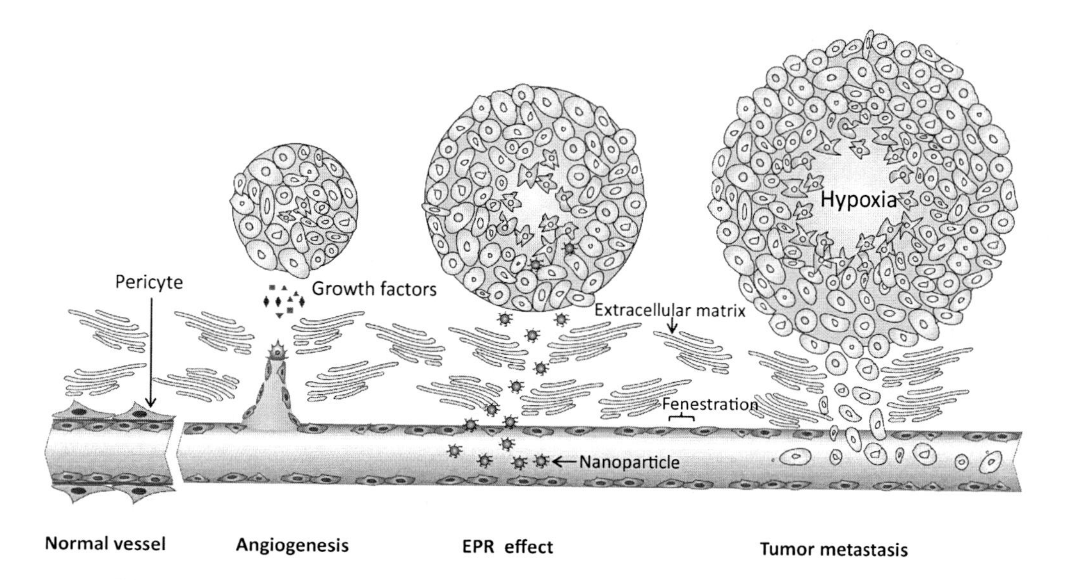

FIGURE 17.1 Tumor microenvironment. The tumor vasculature is structurally different from normal vessels in healthy tissues. In normal vessels, endothelial cells are well aligned along the vessel wall, which is surrounded by pericytes. The walls of tumor vessels have fenestrations and they are not protected by pericytes. The abnormal structure of tumor vasculature leads to the accumulation of macromolecules or particles in tumor tissue, which is called the EPR effect. Tumor cells secrete endothelial growth factors and induce the angiogenesis. Tumor cells also metastasize to other organs through tumor vessels. (See color figure in color plate section.)

positively with cancer progression and therapeutic relapse [27]. Tumor hypoxia has therefore been considered to be a potential therapeutic target for cancer. Hypoxic cytotoxins selectively kill the oxygen-deficient tumor cells and have demonstrated potent anticancer activities in several preclinical and clinical studies [28, 29].

As a consequence of anaerobic metabolism and poor perfusion, solid tumors exhibit lower external pH than normal tissues. The external pH of a solid tumor is acidic and in the range of 6.0–7.0, whereas the pH in normal tissues and blood is approximately 7.4 [30]. According to the Warburg effect, tumor cells predominantly produce energy by aerobic glycolysis unlike normal cells, which undergo mitochondrial oxidative phosphorylation [31]. Most tumor cells undergo the high rate of glycolysis that generates lactic acids by lactic acid fermentation. Moreover, both hypoxia and genetic mutations promote the expression of lactate dehydrogenase A and decrease the activation of pyruvate dehydrogenase, both of which drive the accumulation of lactatic acid. To favor metabolic flux and avoid cytotoxicity, lactate is then exported from the cytoplasm with one proton by monocarboxylate transporters [32]. The acidification of the extracellular space is also exacerbated by the overexpression of carbonic anhydrase IX in hypoxic tumor cells. Carbonic anhydrase IX converts CO_2 into a proton and bicarbonate. The bicarbonate anion is subsequently taken up into the cytoplasm by the anion Cl^-/bicarbonate exchanger, whereas the proton is kept and contributes to the acidification [33]. This acidic microenvironment is common in solid tumors but rare in healthy tissues, and therefore, it provides a potential strategy for stimuli-responsive nanomedicines. The low pH-cleavable PEG-lipid has been used in liposomes and micelles to increase drug half-life without compromising cellular uptake [34].

Interstitial hypertension is another general characteristic of solid tumors. This phenomenon occurs when interstitial fluid pressure in solid tumors is elevated because of the high permeability of the blood vessels. In normal tissues, the pressure in healthy blood vessels is higher than the fluid pressure in the interstitial space. However, in tumors, the fluid escapes from the blood vessels and accumulates in the tumor tissues, leading to a slightly higher pressure in the interstitial space than that in the blood vessel [35]. Interstitial hypertension has been recognized as a significant cause of poor radiotherapy and chemotherapy drug delivery. Interstitial tumor hypertension reduces drug diffusion and penetration but increases drug efflux, which leads to a poor uptake of anticancer drugs, especially large therapeutic agents [36].

17.3.4 Cancer Metastasis

As one of the most important hallmarks of malignancy, cancer metastasis is the process by which malignant tumor cells spread from the original site to other nonadjacent organs. A primary tumor generally develops from a single genetically damaged cancer stem cell, which presents the malignant phenotype. The cancer stem cell undergoes unlimited proliferation to produce excessive cancer cells and to form the primary tumor in the local area. In some cases, primary tumors can progress into malignant cancers, which are often caused by genetic mutations in the tumor cells. The metastatic process can be classified into several basic steps: local invasion, intravasation, survival in circulation, distant organ infiltration, and colonization [37]. Local invasion starts with activation of metastasis initiation genes that allow primary tumor cells to invade the surrounding tissues. These genes increase cell motility, elevate the expression of proteases to degrade extracellular matrices, and promote angiogenesis. Metastasis genes drive cancer cells to invade through the basement membrane, penetrate blood vessels, and enter the circulation. Circulating tumor cells are subjected to additional mechanical stresses, including the shear stress from the circulation system. The number of cells that survive in such a microenvironment is very small, and the circulating tumor cells are at a concentration of approximately 0 to 214 cells/mL of blood [38]. However, these cells always display a more aggressive phenotype. Distant organ infiltration and colonization by circulating tumor cells involves a reverse procedure of intravasation. Because the microenvironment of each organ is different, circulating tumor cells need to infiltrate through different barriers, survive in that specific microenvironment, and finally overtake that tissue. Different types of tumor cells can colonize into the same distant organs, but some tumor cells prefer to metastasize to restricted sites. For example, prostate cancer mostly metastasizes to the bone, whereas ocular melanoma metastasis is confined largely to the liver. Colorectal and pancreatic cancer cells often colonize in the liver and lung. Breast and lung carcinoma usually spread to the bone, liver, brain and adrenal gland [37]. It still remains unclear which genes contribute to the organ-specific metastasis.

17.4 DRUG DELIVERY TO CANCER CELLS BY NANOSCALE CARRIERS

Drug delivery by nanoscale carriers is a very promising strategy to deliver both hydrophobic and hydrophilic drugs. These nanoscale carriers include all cluster, sphere, rod and fiber structures in the range of 10–1000 nm. The most commonly used nanoscale carriers in translational cancer research are the liposome, nanoparticle, polymeric micelle, and dendrimer.

17.4.1 Liposome

Liposomes are artificially prepared nanoscale vesicles consisting of aqueous cores and lipid bilayers. Both natural and synthetic phospholipids with variable chain lengths have been used widely in the preparation of liposomes. Other co-lipids, such as cholesterol, are commonly added into liposomes to increase their stability. Compared with other nanoscale carriers, the liposome is biologically compatible and weakly immunogenic. Moreover, liposomes can encapsulate a wide variety of drugs with different lipophilicities and sizes, including small molecule drugs, proteins, small-interfering RNAs (siRNAs), and plasmids. Lipophilic drugs are entrapped in the bilayer of the liposome, whereas hydrophilic drugs are encapsulated in the aqueous core. Drugs with moderate lipophilicity and hydrophilicity are located in both compartments [39]. The unique structure and properties of the liposome make it a promising drug delivery system for cancer therapy. Significant progress in translational research has been made since its first introduction into drug delivery in the 1970s [40]. As of 2010, 11 liposome formulations had been launched into the market, and dozens of other formulations are undergoing various preclinical and clinical trials [41, 42]. Seventeen of them were applied in cancer therapy, including the conventional liposome, stealth liposome, and targeted liposome, as listed in Table 17.1 [43–59].

The conventional liposome is the first generation of liposomes to be used in therapeutic applications. Generally, the conventional liposome is only composed of neutral and/or charged lipids plus co-lipids. It is also the most popular liposome formulation in translational research. To date, 2 conventional liposome formulations have been approved by the U.S. Food and Drug Administration (FDA) for cancer therapy, and 11 others are in clinical trials. DaunoXome (Galen Limited, Craigavon, U.K.) was the first liposome to reach the market. It is also the leading first-line treatment for advanced Kaposi's sarcoma associated with HIV. DaunoXome is composed of DSPC/cholesterol and encapsulates daunorubicin as the anticancer agent [43]. This liposome formulation is relatively stable and available as a ready-to-inject liquid formulation. However, Myocet (Sopherion

TABLE 17.1 Liposome Formulations that Have Been Approved by the FDA or Under Clinical Evaluations

Product Name	Active Agent	Type	Application	Trial Phase	Company	Reference
DaunoXome	Daunorubicin	Conventional	Kaposi's sarcoma	Approved	NeXStar Pharmaceuticals, Boulder, Co	[43]
Myocet	Doxorubicin	Conventional	Breast cancer	Approved	Elan Pharmaceuticals, Dublin Ireland	[44]
LEP-ETU	Paclitaxel	Conventional	Ovarian, breast, and lung cancer	Phase III	NeoPharm Inc., Lake Bluff, IL	[50]
LEM-ETU	Mitoxantrone	Conventional	Several cancer types	Phase II	NeoPharm Inc.	[51]
LE-SN38	SN-38	Conventional	Metastatic colorectal cancer	Phase II	NeoPharm Inc.	[52]
Aroplatin	NDDP	Conventional	Colorectal cancer	Phase II	Antigenics Inc., Lexington, MA	[45]
MBT-0206	Paclitaxel	Conventional	Breast cancer	Phase I	MediGene AG, Martinsried, Germany	[46]
OSI-211	Lurtotecan	Conventional	Ovarian, head, and lung cancer	Phase II	Enzon Corp., Piscataway Township, NJ	[47]
Marqibo	Vincristine	Conventional	Non-Hodgkin's lymphoma	Phase II	Inex Pharma, Vancouver, Canada	[48]
INX-0125	Vinorelbine	Conventional	Advanced solid tumor	Phase I	Inex Pharma	[49]
INX-0076	Topotecan	Conventional	Solid tumor	Phase I	Inex Pharma	[42]
SPI-007	Cisplatin	Stealth	Head and neck cancer, lung cancer	Phase I/II	Sequus Pharmaceuticals, Menlo Park, CA	[54]
DOXIL	Doxorubicin	Stealth	Kaposi's sarcoma	Approved	Sequus Pharma	[53]
Lipoplatin	Cisplatin	Stealth	NSCLC	Phase III completed	Regulon Inc., Mountain View, CA	[55]
CKD602	CKD602	Stealth	Refractory solid tumor	Phase I	Alza Corp., Mountain View, CA	[56]
MCC-465	Doxorubicin	Targeted	Metastatic stomach cancer	Phase I	Mitsubishi Pharma, Warren, NJ	[58]
Anti-EGFR ILs-dox	Doxorubicin	Targeted	Advanced solid tumor	Phase I	University of Basel, Basel, Switzerland	[59]

Therapeutics, Princeton, NJ), another approved conventional liposome, is supplied in three separate components: empty liposome in citric buffer, doxorubicin powder, and sodium carbonate solution [44]. Prior to administration, the three components are mixed, thus providing a consistent drug entrapment and good stability in the final liposome formulation. The lipid composition and the entrapped drug are the major differences between the approved and emerging liposome formulations [42, 45]. For example, MBT-0206 is prepared using the lipids of DOPE/DO-trimethylammoniumpropane, whereas OSI-211 is composed of hydrogenated soy phosphatidylcholine (HSPC) and cholesterol [46, 47]. The same lipid-based formulation can also be used to encapsulate different anticancer drugs. INEX Pharmaceuticals has successfully used the same DSPPC/cholesterol/sphingosine formulation for three different anticancer drugs (vincristine, vinorelbine, and topetecan) [42, 48, 49]. Another successful liposome composition is DOPE/cholesterol/cardiolipin, which has three formulations in clinical trials, including LEM-ETU, LEP-ETU, and LE-SN38 [50–52]. The co-lipid cardiolipin is thought to play an important role in drug entrapment. This negatively charged diphosphatidylglycerol lipid can form an electrostatic interaction with the entrapped drug, such as mitoxantrone in LEM-ETU and paclitaxel in LEP-ETU, leading to a higher loading capability than other liposome formulations [50, 51].

The stealth liposome is a second-generation liposome, and its surface is modified with polyethylene glycol (PEG). Compared with the conventional liposome, the stealth liposome escapes the uptake by the mononuclear phagocyte system (MPS) and avoids lysis by the complement system, which dramatically prolongs blood circulation time and improves biodistribution. Moreover, the PEGylated liposome exhibits good stability with minimized vesicle aggregation. Doxil (ALZA Corporation, Mountain View, CA) is the only stealth liposome that has been approved by the FDA for cancer therapy [53–56]. It is composed of HSPC, cholesterol, and methoxy PEG (mPEG)-distearoyl-phosphatidyl-ethanolamine (DSPE) at a molar ratio of 55:40:5. The most important characteristic of the stealth liposome is its long-circulation property. The blood circulation time is positively correlated with the amount and length of the grafted PEG. Typically, 5–10% (molar ratio) of PEGylation of the lipid is enough to maintain long-term circulation and prevent premature leakage. Moreover, the long-chain PEG has better pharmacokinetic profiles than short-chain polymers. However, the stealth property of the stealth liposome is not always helpful in the drug delivery process. When the stealth liposome accumulates in tumor tissues by a passive targeting effect, the hydrophilic PEG on the liposome surface prevents the integration of the liposomal lipids into the tumor cell membrane. As a result, the liposome could be localized predominantly in the extracellular space without actually entering the cells. This major drawback in cellular uptake can be overcome by attaching a tumor-specific ligand to the PEG, which is named the targeted liposome.

Targeted liposomes are prepared by coupling targeting ligands to the PEG-end of stealth liposomes via a stable or cleavable linker. Targeted liposomes cannot increase the drug accumulation in tumors compared with stealth liposomes, but they exhibit higher selectivity and cellular uptake [57]. The targeting ligands include monoclonal antibodies (mAbs) or their fragments (Fab and scFv), peptides, aptamers, small molecules, and natural receptor ligands. The antibody-modified liposome, also called the immunoliposome, is the most actively studied category in liposomal drug delivery systems. MCC-465 is a doxorubicin-encapsulated PEG immunoliposome, and its phase I clinical trial in metastatic stomach cancer has been completed. MCC-465 is tagged with the Fab fragment of human mAb GAH, which binds to 90% of stomach cancers but not to normal tissues. MCC-465 is well tolerated in humans at a dose up to 32.5 mg dox/m^2 and shows similar pharmacokinetic profiles as the stealth liposome Doxil [58]. The doxorubicin-loaded anti-EGFR immunoliposome (Anti-EGFR ILs-dox) is another example that is under clinical evaluation. When modified with the Fab' fragment of the monoclonal antibody C225 (cetuximab), the PEGlyated liposome can selectively deliver doxorubicin to various solid tumors with overexpressed EGFR [59]. Several other targeted liposomes that target HER2, CD19, and CD22 have also entered into the preclinical stage [60–62].

17.4.2 Polymeric Micelle

A polymeric micelle is a nanosized system that is composed of bi-block co-polymers. The bi-block co-polymer always contains a hydrophilic and a hydrophobic block. The hydrophobic parts of the co-polymer spontaneously self-assemble into an inner core in aqueous buffer, whereas the hydrophilic chains arrange outside to form a hydrophilic shell. The diameter of this core-shell structure is in the range of 20–100 nm, which is sufficient to be accumulated in tumors by the EPR effect. The therapeutic agent is incorporated in the inner core by either physical entrapment or chemical conjugation.

Several drug-incorporating polymeric micelles are under clinical evaluation, including paclitaxel-incorporating micelle NK105, doxorubicin-incorporating micelle NK911, SN-38-incorporating micelle NK012, cisplatin-incorporating micelle NC-6004, and others (Table 17.2) [63–67]. NK105 and NK012 have similar compositions and structures [63, 68]. The co-polymer consists of PEG, which constitutes the hydrophilic outer shell of the micelle, and a poly(glutamic acid)–drug conjugate, which forms the hydrophobic core of the micelle. The driving force of micelle formation in NK105, NK911, and NK012 is the

TABLE 17.2 Polymeric Micelles in Translational Cancer Research

Product	Polymer	Drug	Mechanism of Micelle Formation	Indication	Trial Phase	Company	Reference
NK012	PEG-poly(Glu)	SN-38	Hydrophobic	Breast cancer	Phase II	Nippon Kayaku, Tokyo, Japan	[63]
NK105	PEG-poly(Asp)	Paclitaxel	Hydrophobic	Stomach cancer	Phase II	NanoCarrier, Chiba, Japan	[68]
NK911	PEG-poly(Asp)	Doxorubicin	Hydrophobic	Solid tumors	Phase I	Nippon Kayaku	[64]
NC-6004	PEG-poly(Glu)	Cisplatin	Chelation	Various solid tumors	Phase II	NanoCarrier	[65]
Genexol-PM	PEG-poly(di-lactide)	Paclitaxel	Hydrophobic	Various cancers	Phase II	Samyang, Seoul, Korea	[66]
SP1049C	Pluronic polymer	Doxorubicin	Hydrophobic	Adenocarcinoma	Phase III	Supratek, Montréal, Canada	[67]

hydrophobic interaction between the poly(glutamic acid) blocks [63, 64, 68]. The cisplatin-incorporating micelle NC6004 is different from NK015 and NK012. In the inner core of NC6004, platinum (II) atoms are chelated by carboxylates in the side chain of poly(glutamic acid) [65]. The polymer–metal complexes crosslink with different chains of the co-polymer to form a solid and stable core of the micelle [69]. This cisplatin-incorporating micelle exhibits remarkable stability at high dilutions compared with typical micelles prepared with amphiphilic co-polymers [70].

17.4.3 Other Nanoparticles

Since the discovery of the EPR effect, nanoparticle-mediated cancer therapy has been a very active area in translational research of cancer therapy. Besides liposomes and polymeric micelles, other nanoparticles have also been used for targeted drug delivery through either passive or active tumor targeting. For example, metal nanoparticles have emerged in the field of nanotechnology and present many unique benefits for drug delivery. Gold nanoparticles might be one of the most common metal nanoparticles that have been employed to deliver anticancer drugs to tumors. Gold nanoparticles have large surface areas, which allows for efficient loading of anticancer drugs and tumor-targeting ligands on nanoparticles' surfaces. Moreover, gold nanoparticles can be excited by infrared light and can kill tumor cells by thermal enhancement. Another type of nanoparticle is the albumin nanoparticle that is developed by American BioSciences Inc. (Blauvelt, NY). The preparation of albumin nanoparticles is relatively simple. Drug molecules are mixed with albumin in an aqueous solution and are passed through a jet under high pressure to form the albumin nanoparticles in the size range of 100–200 nm [71]. The albumin paclitaxel nanoparticle, Abraxane (Abraxis Bioscience, Los Angeles, CA), was approved by the FDA in 2005 for treating metastatic breast cancer [71].

17.5 DRUG DELIVERY TO CANCER CELLS BY BIOCONJUGATES

17.5.1 Antibody–Drug Conjugate

Antibody–drug conjugates are constructed by conjugating a recombinant antibody covalently to a cytotoxic chemical via a synthetic linker. Antibody–drug conjugates are considered a successful combination of biologicals and small molecules, which creates the highly potent targeting agents. Cytotoxic chemicals provide the pharmacological potency, whereas highly specific antibodies serve as the targeting agent, which also includes a carrier that increases the half-life and biocompatibility of the conjugate. The antibody–drug conjugate is one of the most popular bioconjugates in translational research. Currently more than 15 antibody–drug conjugates are undergoing clinical trials [72]. As listed in Table 17.3 [73–95], they have different targets, cytotoxic chemicals, and chemical linkers.

In cancer therapy, tumor-associated antigens are mainly selected as targets for antibody–drug conjugates. The antigens are either expressed in all tumors or in a specific type of tumor, and they should be well characterized in preclinical and clinical evaluations. The antigen must have high expression levels in cancer cells but low or no expression in normal tissues. The elevated expression level not only provides increased selectivity for the antibody–drug conjugate but also guarantees that a sufficient amount of drug can be delivered into the tumor cells. Another critical property of the antigen is its ability to be internalized after binding of antibody–drug conjugates to tumor cells. The internalization is directly related to the therapeutic effect of antibody–drug conjugates. Depending on the chemical linker, internalization generally triggers the release of cytotoxic agents from the conjugate to elicit therapeutic effects. Internalization of antibody–drug conjugates is crucial to reduce the toxicity that is associated with the premature release of drug dose in

TABLE 17.3 Antibody–Drug Conjugates in Cancer Clinical Trials

Product Name	Target	Active Agent	Linkers	Application	Trial Phase	Company	References
Mylotarg	CD33	Calicheamycin	Hydrazone + disulfide	Acute myelogenous leukemia	Withdrawn 2010	Pfizer, New York, NY	[73]
SGN35	CD30	Monomethyl auristatin E	Val-Cit	Hodgkin lymphoma	Approved	Seattle Genetics, Bothell, WA	[74]
CMC-544	CD22	Calicheamycin	Hydrazone + disulfide	Non-Hodgkin lymphoma	Phase III terminated	Pfizer	[75, 76]
T-DMI	HER2	DM1	Thioether	Breast cancer	Phase III	Roche, Laboratory, Nutley, NJ	[77, 78]
CDX-011	GPNMB	Monome thyl auristatin E	Val-Cit	Breast cancer	Phase II	Celldex, Roseland, NJ	[79]
IMGN901	CD56	DM1	Disulfide	Small lung cancer	Phase II	ImmunoGen, Waltham, MA	[80]
IMGN242	CanAg	DM4	Disulfide	Gastric cancer	Phase II	ImmunoGen	[81]
HuC242-DM1	CamAg	DM1	Disulfide	Various cancers	Phase I	ImmunoGen	[82]
AVE9633	CD33	DM4	Disulfide	Acute myelogenous leukemia	Phase I	Sanofi-Aventis, Bridgewater, NJ	[83]
IMMU-110	CD74	Doxorubicin	Hydrazone	Multiple myeloma	Phase I	Immunomedics, Morris Plains, NJ	[84]
SGN-75	CD70	Monomethyl auristatin F	Val-Cit	Various cancers	Phase I	Seattle Genetics	[85]
IMGN388	Integrin	DM4	Disulfide	Various cancers	Phase I	ImmunoGen	[86]
SAR3419	CD19	DM4	Disulfide	Non-Hodgkin lymphoma	Phase I	Sanofi-Aventis	[87, 88]
AGS-16M8F	AGS-16	Monomethyl auristatin F	Thioether	Renal and liver cancer	Phase I	Agensys, Santa Monica, CA	[89]
ASG-5ME	SLC44A4	Monomethyl auristatin E	Val-Cit	Various epithelial tumor	Phase I	Seattle Genetics	[90]
B1B015	Cripto protein	DM4	Disulfide	Various cancers	Phase I	Biogenidec, Cambridge, MA	[91]
BT-062	CD138	DM4	Disulfide	Multiple myeloma	Phase I	Biotest, Singapore	[92]
PSMA ADC	PSMA	Monomethyl auristatin E	Val-Cit	Prostate cancer	Phase I	Progenics, Tarrytown, NY	[93]
MEDI-547	EphA2	Monomethyl auristatin F	Thioether	Various tumors	Phase I terminated	MedImmune, Gaithersburg, MD	[94]
MDX-1203	CD70	Duocarmycin	Val-Cit	Various cancers	Phase I	Bristol-Myers Squibb, New York, NY	[95]

extracellular compartments [72]. A wide variety of tumor-associated antigens has been applied to antibody–drug conjugate in clinical trials. These antigens include CD33 for acute myeloid leukemia (AML), CD30 for Hodgkin disease, HER2, PSMA, CanAg, and EGFR for solid carcinomas, and integrin for endothelial cells. A summary of these well-identified antigens and an introduction of some new potential targets have been extensively reviewed by Teicher [96].

The cytotoxic agents used in antibody–drug conjugates are numerically rare and restricted to four major families of compounds: calicheamycin, maytansinoids (DM1 and DM4), auristatins (MMAE and MMAF), and duocarmycin (Figure 17.2). The common feature of these cytotoxic agents is the high cytotoxic potency. The IC_{50} of the cytotoxic agents is generally as low as 10^{-9} to 10^{-11} M. These highly toxic drugs have very low therapeutic windows and cannot be used as a single agent for cancer therapy [97]. The high toxicity of chemical drugs is essential to enhance the potency of the antibody–drug conjugates. Theoretically, the number of antigens/targets per tumor cell is limited (10^3 to 10^6). Therefore, only thousands of antibody–drug molecules can be internalized to release the active parent drugs. The drug payload of antibody–drug conjugates is

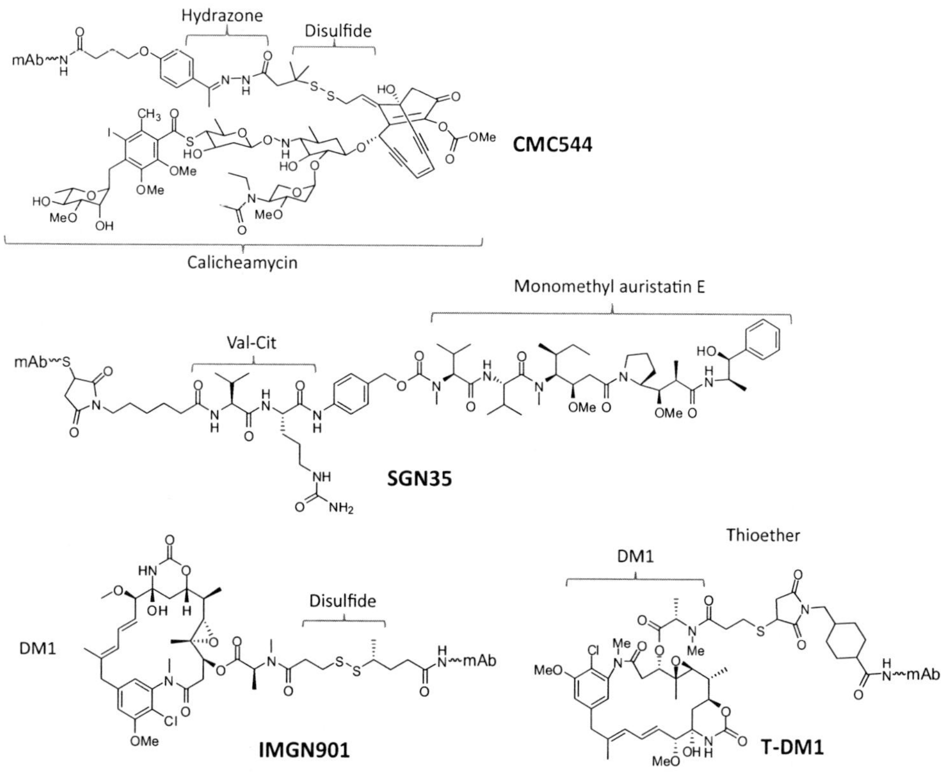

FIGURE 17.2 Structures of CMC544, SGN35, IMGN901, and T-DM1.

generally low, and each antibody molecule only conjugates with 1–3 cytotoxic molecules. The information described previously indicates that the chemical agent must be sufficiently potent that several thousands of them can eradicate the tumor cells efficiently. The first-generation antibody–drug conjugate SNG-15, in which the antibody BR96 is conjugated with the low potent drug doxorubicin (IC_{50}: $\sim 10^{-7}$ M), was significantly hampered by the low potency of the chemical. Very limited antitumor activity was observed in the phase I and II clinical trials even at a dose of approximately 700 mg/m^2 [98, 99]. By contrast, a new generation antibody–drug conjugates showed clinical activity at a dose of 3.6 mg/kg for Trastuzumab-DM1, a dose of 1.8 mg/kg for SGN-35 (Brentuximab-vedotin), and a dose of 1.3–1.8 mg/kg for MDX-1203 [74, 75, 77].

The chemical linker is also a key component of antibody–drug conjugates. A successful linker should be stable in circulation, but it should be labile when antibody–drug conjugates enter the tumor microenvironment or tumor cells. A wide variety of chemical linkers has been investigated in preclinical and clinical studies. For example, CMC-544 (inotuzumab ozogamicin) and IMMU-110 have an acid-labile hydrazone linker, which is stable at physiological pH ($\sim$7.4), but it is cleavable in the intracellular compartment of the lysosome because of its low pH (5.0–6.0) [76, 84]. This linker has been successfully applied in Mylotarg (Pfizer, New York, NY [73]. Disulfide bond-based linkers have also been used in antibody–drug conjugates [80–83, 86, 87, 91]. Disulfide bonds exhibit moderate stability in the plasma but break down quickly in the cytoplasm because of the reductive intracellular environment [78]. BT-062 and SAR3419 are two typical antibody–drug conjugates that use disulfide bond-based chemical linkers [88, 92]. Noncleavable thioether linkers have been proven recently to be superior to disulfide bonds in a preclinical study [78]. This is probably because the thioether linker has a higher degree of stability *in vivo*, which results in increased pharmacokinetic exposure and better toxicity tolerance compared with disulfide bonds. After internalization/endocytosis, the thioether-linked antibody undergoes lysosomal degradation to release chemical drugs. Several thioether based antibody–drug conjugates (T-DM1, AGS-16M8F, and MEDI-547) are currently in clinical trials [78, 89, 94]. More recently, peptide linkers have been developed to release chemical drug selectively after cleavage by a lysosomal protease (cathepsin B). Among them, the valine-citrulline (val-cit) dipeptide linker is the most commonly used peptide linker in antibody–drug conjugates. It has been employed in SGN-35 (brentuximab-vedotin), CDX-011 (glembatumumab-vedotin), SGN-75, ASG-5ME, PSMA ADC, and MDX-1203 [74, 79, 85, 90, 93, 95].

17.5.2 Peptide–Drug Conjugate

Beside antibodies and their fragments, peptides represent another class of attractive ligands for tumor targeting. Peptide ligands have a molecular weight less than 5 kDa and therefore exhibit excellent tumor penetration as well as a higher drug payload compared with antibody ligands. Because of its simple structure, a peptide–drug conjugate could be easily prepared by organic synthesis. The conjugation sites of peptide ligands are always well defined, and therefore pure chemical entities can be used in cancer therapy. In the case of antibody–drug conjugates, drug molecules are always attached to antibodies by nonspecific conjugation, leading to a complicated mixture of antibody–drug conjugates. The conjugation site and numbers of drug may vary dramatically between different antibody molecules and different preparation batches. Several peptide–drug conjugates have entered clinical trials (Table 17.4 [100–110]).

In translational research, peptide–drug conjugates have been used successfully for peptide receptor radiation therapy (PRRT). Regulatory peptide receptors are overexpressed in numerous human cancers [111] and can be used as molecular targets for tumor diagnosis and therapeutic use. Currently, the somatostatin receptor and gastrin-releasing peptide (GRP) receptor have been established for tumor targeting in PRRT. The peptide tracers for somatostatin receptor and GRP receptors are radiolabeled octreotide analogs and bombesin analogs, respectively. These peptide ligands are usually characterized by binding affinities in the low nanomolar range and nonimmunogenicity. An octreotide (Sandostatin; Novartis Pharmaceuticals, Basel, Switzerland) is an octapeptide that mimics natural somatostatin pharmacologically. Four radiolabeled octreotides are in clinical use. For example, ^{111}In-DTPA-octreotide (Octreoscan; Mallinckrodt, Inc., Hazelwood, MO) is used to image somatostatin receptor-expressing tumors noninvasively [100]. As shown recently, Gallium-68 labeled octreotides (68Ga-DOTATOC) have high resolution and sensitivity in detecting small tumors or tumors with a low density of the receptor [101]. Octreotides can also be labeled with a radionuclide to treat neuroendocrine tumors. DOTA chelated ^{90}Y (such as ^{90}Y-SMT-487 and ^{90}Y-DOTALAN) and ^{177}Lu (such as ^{177}Lu-DOTATATE) are commonly used in the clinic [102–104]. The major difference between them lies in the somatostatin-receptor subtype affinity profiles [112]. Bombesin is a 14-mer peptide that shows high affinity for the GRP receptor. Two ^{99m}Tc-labeled bombesins are being used clinically. ^{99m}TC-BN and ^{99m}Tc-N3S-X-BN(2-14) are used primarily to identify breast and prostate primary cancer and metastases [105, 106, 113]. ^{68}Ga and ^{111}In labeled bombesins are also under preclinical evaluation [114, 115].

TABLE 17.4 Peptide–Drug Conjugates in Translational Cancer Research

Product Name	Peptide	Radionuclide/ Drug	Target	Application	Trial Phase	Company	References
Octreoscan	Octreotide	^{111}In	Somatostatin receptor	Nuclear imaging	Approved	Covidien, Doblin, Ireland	[100]
68Ga-DOTATOC	Octreotide	^{68}Ga	Somatostatin receptor	Nuclear imaging	Phase I	European Institute of Oncology, Milan, Italy	[101]
^{90}Y-SMT-487	Octreotide	^{90}Y	Somatostatin receptor	Radiotherapy	Phase II	Novartis, Basel, Switzerland	[102]
90Y-DOTALAN	Larreotide	^{90}Y	Somatostatin receptor	Radiotherapy	Phase I	University of Vienna, Vienna, Austria	[103]
^{177}Lu-DOTATATE	Octreotate	^{177}Lu	Somatostatin receptor	Radiotherapy	Phase III	Excel Diagnostics and Nuclear, Oncology Center, Houston, TX	[104]
^{99m}TC-BN	Bombesin	^{99m}Tc	GRP receptors	Nuclear imaging	Phase I	University "La Sapienza"	[105]
^{99m}Tc-N_3S-X-BN(2-14)	Bombesin	^{99m}Tc	GRP receptors	Nuclear imaging	Preclinical	—	[106]
ANG1005	Angiopep-2	Paclitaxel	Brain cancer	Chemotherapy	Phase I	AngioChem, Montréal, Canada	[107, 108]
SF1226	RGD	LY294002	Various cancers	Chemotherapy	Phase I	Semafore Pharmaceuticals, Indianapolis, IN	[109, 110]

Besides regulatory peptides, a wide range of radiolabeled peptides is under preclinical development. Peptide ligands such as RGD peptide, neurotensin, and Tat penetrating peptide offer promising radioligand candidates for various cancers in future radiation therapy [116].

Moreover, peptides have been used to guide chemical drugs to various tumors. ANG1005 and SF1226 are the two examples in clinical evaluations. ANG1005 is a peptide–drug conjugate engineered to deliver paclitaxel across the blood–brain barrier (BBB) for glioma therapy. The peptide Angiopep-2 is a ligand that binds to the low density lipoprotein receptor-related protein (LRP) receptor at BBB. The binding of Angiopep-2 with the LRP receptor results in crossing the BBB by receptor-mediated transport. ANG1005 is composed of Angiopep-2 linked to three molecules of paclitaxel with a cleavable succinyl ester linkage [107]. After conjugation, Angiopep-2 dramatically increases the uptake capacity of paclitaxel into the brain. The *in vivo* uptake of ANG1005 into the brain and brain tumors is 4-fold to 54-fold higher than that of paclitaxel. Moreover, ANG1005 bypasses P-gp and resides in the brain much longer even after capillary deletion and vascular washout [108]. Phase I clinical trials of ANG1005 were started in 2008. SF1126 is a novel RGD-conjugated LY294002 prodrug. LY294002 is a pan phosphoinositide 3-kinase (PI3K) inhibitor that shows *in vitro* and *in vivo* antitumor effects. However, LY294002 is not a valuable drug candidate because of its poor water solubility and short plasma half-life. The RGD (Arg-Gly-Asp) peptide was conjugated to LY294002 to increase its solubility and targetability to integrins in the tumor compartment [109]. Recent data from a phase I clinical trial reveal that SF1126 was well tolerated up to 1110 mg/m^2 given intravenously twice a week. Clinical activity was also observed in 19/33 ($\sim$58%) patients with multiple solid tumors. No significant toxicity or effect on glucose level were reported [110].

17.5.3 Polymer–Drug Conjugate

The first attempt to attach drugs to water-soluble polymers was achieved in the middle 1970s [117]. Since then, polymer–drug conjugates have been studied extensively, and dozens of polymer–drug conjugates have entered clinical evaluation; several of them have been approved by the FDA for cancer therapy [118]. Conjugating with polymer carriers modulates not only the pharmacokinetics but also the water solubility and toxicity of the cytotoxic chemical. Active targeting can also be achieved when a tumor-homing ligand is introduced to the same polymer carrier. Based on the types of drugs, polymer–drug conjugates can be categorized into two groups: polymer-conjugated chemical drugs and polymer-conjugated proteins.

Synthesis of polymer-conjugated chemical drugs is an active area in cancer therapy. To date, one of the polymer-conjugated chemical drugs has been approved by the FDA, and nine of them are undergoing clinical trials (Table 17.5 [119–131]). Among them, the poly(L-glutamic acid)-paclitaxel conjugate (CT-2103, Xyotax; Cell Therapeutics, Inc., Seattle, WA; and Opaxio; Cell Therapeutics, Inc.), in which paclitaxel is conjugated to the carboxyl group of poly (L-glutamic acid) via an ester bond, has advanced into phase III clinical trials and been granted fast track designation by the FDA. CT-2103 shows high water solubility (>20 mg/kg) and a significantly improved pharmacokinetics profile compared with paclitaxel [132]. Preclinical studies revealed that CT-2103 could also penetrate into tumors and distribute into the necrotic zone of tumors several days after injection [133]. The tumor-penetration property of the polymer–drug conjugate is probably achieved through several routes: 1) diffusion of the intact polymer–drug conjugate; 2) diffusion of small fragments of CT-2103 such as paclitaxel, Glu-paclitaxel, or Glu-Glu-paclitaxel; and 3) redistribution through the migration of macrophages because CT-2103 can be captured by macrophages [107]. In the phase I study, the maximal tolerated dose of CT2103 was up to 233 mg/m^2 with a 3-week schedule and 177 mg/m^2 with a 2-week schedule [134]. Moreover, the plasma half-life was approximately 185 h and the area under concentration (AUC) of CT-2103 was about 50 times higher than that of free paclitaxel [119]. CT2103 advanced into phase II trials for androgen-independent prostate cancer and phase III trials for non-small cell lung carcinoma (NSCLC). Besides polyglutamic acid based polymer–drug conjugates (CT2103, CT2106), various chemical drugs have been conjugated with *N*-(2-hydroxyprpyl)-methacrylamide co-polymer (HPMA), PEG, cyclodextrin-based polymer, and carboxymethyldextran [107, 120–131, 135].

Polymer–conjugated proteins, namely polymer–protein conjugates, have become a fast-growing field in cancer therapy. Nine of them have been approved by the FDA, and all of them use PEG as the drug carrier [118]. PEGylation of proteins results in reduced immunogenicity and enhanced circulation time compared with native proteins. After covalent conjugation, the long, flexible, and hydrophilic PEG provides a steric shield for therapeutic proteins, which reduces the opportunity to be recognized by the immune system. Moreover, PEG can increase the size of the native proteins dramatically, thereby enhancing the circulation half-life. Taking Oncaspar (Sigma-Tau Pharmaceuticals, Inc., Gaithersburg, MD) as an example, 5-kDa PEG increases the half-life of L-asparaginase from 20 h to approximately 357 h. PEG-INTRON, a 12-kDa PEG-conjugated interferon α-2b, has a half-life of 48–72 h, which is 6–10 times longer than that of the native protein. The PEG polymer along with its associated water molecules surrounds the protein drug and protects it from enzyme degradation, renal filtration, and immune response, thereby amplifying dramatically the therapeutic benefits and limiting the adverse effects.

TABLE 17.5 Polymer–Drug Conjugates in Cancer Clinical Trials

Product Name	Polymer	Drug	Molecular Weight	Indication	Trial Phase	Company	Reference
CT-2103	Poly(Glu)	Paclitaxel	~80 kDa	Various cancers	Approved	Cell Therapeutics	[119]
PK 1	HMAP	Doxorubicin	~30 kDa	Lung and breast cancer	Phase II	Pfizer	[120]
PK 2	HMAP-galactosamine	Doxorubicin	~25 kDa	Hepatocellular carcinoma	Phase II	Pfizer	[121]
PNU 166148	HMAP	Camptothecin	~18 kDa	Various cancers	Phase I terminated	Pfizer	[122]
PNU 166945	HMAP	Paclitaxel	25–35 kDa	Various cancers	Phase I terminated	Pfizer	[123]
AP5346	HMAP	Oxaliplatin	~25 kDa	Various cancers	Phase II	Access Pharmaceuticals, Dallas, TX	[124]
AP5280	HMAP	Carboplatin	22 kDa	Various cancers	Phase I	Access Pharmaceuticals	[125]
Pegamotecan	PEG	Camptothecin	40 kDa	Solid tumors	Phase I terminated	Enzon	[126]
EZN-2208	PEG	SN-38	40 kDa	Solid tumors	Phase I	Enzon	[127]
IT-101	Cyclodextrin-based polymer	Camptothecin	85 ± 23 kDa	Solid tumors	Phase I	Insert Therapeutics, Pasadena, CA	[128]
DE-310	Carboxymethyl-dextran	Exatecan	~340 kDa	Solid tumors	Phase I	Daii chi Pharmaceuticals, Tokyo, Japan	[129]
CT-2106	Poly(Glu)	Camptothecin	~50 kDa	Various cancers	Phase I	Cell Therapeutics	[130]
AD-70	Dextran	Doxorubicin	~70 kDa	Various cancers	Phase I	Alpha Therapeutics, Rochester Hills, MI	[131]

However, PEGylation may also decrease the activities and stability of a protein drug. Steric hindrance of the PEG chains could reduce the binding affinity between proteins and its antigens. Additionally, chemical modification of protein drug might cause conformational change of the protein, which always leads to activity loss and protein aggregation. However, the quality of PEG-protein conjugates could be well controlled once the standard PEGylation method is established.

17.5.4 Other Conjugates

Antibody–drug conjugates, peptide–drug conjugates, and polymer–drug conjugates have emerged as the leading strategies in translational research. Attention should also be paid to other bioconjugation approaches that have unique potentials. The albumin–drug conjugate is one of these examples. Accounting for 60% of human plasma protein, albumin has a molecular weight of approximately 67 kDa and is ready to be conjugated with various drugs. The molecular weight of albumin–drug conjugates is approximately 67–70 kDa, which could easily overcome rapid renal clearance from the circulation. Human plasma albumin exhibits an average half-life of 20 days. Because of the long half-life of albumin in the body, conjugating a therapeutic drug to albumin is an attractive method to improve the pharmacokinetic profiles of the drug. Albumin and its drug conjugates can easily accumulate in solid tumors because of the passive tumor targeting via the EPR effect. Studies showed that 3–25% of radiolabeled albumin could be found in tumors [136]. Clinically, two albumin–drug conjugates are under clinic evaluation: methotrexate-albumin conjugate (MTX-HSA) and an albumin-conjugated prodrug (DOXO-EMCH). MTX-HSA is the first albumin–drug conjugate that has been evaluated in clinic trials. The conjugate site of MTX-HSA is not chemically clear, and the drug-load of ~1.3 molecules per albumin showed the best antitumor activity [137, 138]. To define the albumin–drug conjugate more clearly, extensive studies have been performed to improve the bioconjugate methods that control precisely the coupling sites and drug-loading ratio. In contrast to MTX-HSA, DOXO-EMCH is an albumin-coupling prodrug that is ready to be conjugated with circulating albumin in a few minutes after administration [139]. It is an acid-sensitive doxorubicin prodrug with a maximal tolerated dose (MTD) 4.5 times higher than free doxorubicin. DOXO-EMCH dramatically improves the therapeutic effect of doxorubicin in preclinical and clinic studies. DOXO-EMCH has been announced recently to initiate its phase II study in 2011. A summary of this conjugate has been extensively reviewed by Kratz [71].

17.6 DRUG DELIVERY TO CANCER BY GEL SYSTERMS

Gel system is another promising platform for drug delivery. Based on its composition, gel system can be classified into hydrogel and organogel. Both of them are semisolid systems in which liquid medium (either aqueous or organic solvent) is chelated in a three-dimensional network. Although the solid network material only accounts for 0.1 to 15% of the weight, the gel system shows the solid appearance and rheological behavior. Therapeutic agents could be encapsulated in the organic or aqueous medium and efficiently released into circulation or target site through passive diffusion, matrix swelling, or chemical reaction of the drug/matrix [140]. The typical mesh size of the gel network ranges from 5 to 100 nm, which is large enough to allow passive diffusion of most therapeutic agents including antibodies [141].

Although introduced several decades ago, the gel system is still not successful in translational research. Several gel systems, such as the Resiquimod gel (3M Pharmaceuticals, St. Paul, MN), bexarotene gel, and PEP005 gel, have entered clinical trials [142, 143]. However, all of these gel systems are traditional and administrated only by transdermal route. Nanogel, especially nanohydrogel, is a new generation gel system for drug delivery. It has gained lots of attention as a promising drug delivery system because of its unique potentials by combining the advantages of gel systems and nanoparticles [140]. Nanogel exhibits the physiological property which resembles tissues. Moreover, the nanoscale diameter enables nanogel to accumulate passively in tumors and enhance therapeutic activity dramatically by the EPR effect. Because of its nanosize, nanogel could also be administrated by various routes rather than the transdermal route. Several hydrogel nanoparticles have shown the therapeutic potentials in preclinical studies [140]. However, none of them have been tested in clinical trials.

17.7 CONCLUSION AND FUTURE PERSPECIVES

Advanced drug delivery systems modify drug release, distribution, absorption, and elimination, which could significantly improve the efficiency and safety of cancer therapeutics. In this chapter, three drug delivery systems were discussed: nanoscale delivery systems, bioconjugate systems, and gel systems. As a well-defined drug delivery platform, nanoscale systems are favorable for cancer therapy because of the EPR effect. Targeting ligands can be conjugated to the surfaces of nanoparticles to enhance active targeting and cellular uptake. Bioconjugation is a relatively new and complicated system. Antibody–drug conjugates are the realization of the "magic bullet" theory and will probably emerge as a new standard therapy for cancer. Although traditional gel systems are commonly used for topical diseases, nanohydrogel is emerging as a new system for cancer therapy.

It has become more and more difficult to develop new chemical agents for cancer therapy. Instead, development of advanced drug delivery systems for existing anticancer agents has emerged as one of the most promising but challenging fields in pharmaceutical sciences. Many of the advanced drug delivery systems for cancer therapy have successfully transferred from the laboratory bench to market. However, it is important to mention that the development and manufacturing of advanced drug delivery systems are complicated, which may limit the enthusiasm of small companies to invest in this technology.

ASSESSMENT QUESTIONS

17.1. List the biological characteristics that make cancer different from other diseases.

17.2. Describe the enhanced permeability and retention (EPR) effect and how it is related to tumor angiogenesis.

17.3. What are the three major types of liposomes? Explain the difference among them.

17.4. Why are highly potent cytotoxic chemicals more suitable for use in the antibody–drug conjugate strategy?

17.5. ANG1005 is a peptide–drug conjugate that can penetrate the blood–brain barrier (BBB). Provide an explanation for how it works.

REFERENCES

1. Jemal, A., et al. (2011). Global cancer statistics. *CA A Cancer Journal for Clinicians*, *61*(2), 69–90.
2. Anand, P., et al. (2008). Cancer is a preventable disease that requires major lifestyle changes. *Pharmaceutical Research*, *25*(9), 2097–2116.
3. Tai, W., Mahato, R., Cheng, K. (2010). The role of HER2 in cancer therapy and targeted drug delivery. *Journal of Controlled Release*, *146*(3), 264–275.
4. Venter, D.J., et al. (1987). Overexpression of the c-erbB-2 oncoprotein in human breast carcinomas: Immunohistological assessment correlates with gene amplification. *Lancet*, *2*(8550), 69–72.

5. Blume-Jensen, P., Hunter, T. (2001). Oncogenic kinase signalling. *Nature, 411(6835)*, 355–365.
6. Manning, G., et al. (2002). The protein kinase complement of the human genome. *Science, 298(5600)*, 1912–1934.
7. Cohen, P. (2002). Protein kinases–the major drug targets of the twenty-first century? *Nature Reviews Drug Discovery, 1(4)*, 309–315.
8. Vieth, M., et al. (2004). Kinomics-structural biology and chemogenomics of kinase inhibitors and targets. *Biochimica et Biophysica Acta, 1697(1–2)*, 243–257.
9. Garcia-Echeverria, C., Fabbro, D. (2004). Therapeutically targeted anticancer agents: Inhibitors of receptor tyrosine kinases. *Mini Reviews in Medicinal Chemistry, 4(3)*, 273–283.
10. Balk, S.P., Ko, Y.J., Bubley, G.J. (2003). Biology of prostate-specific antigen. *Journal of Clinical Oncology, 21(2)*, 383–391.
11. O'Keefe, D.S., Bacich, D.J., Heston, W.D. (2004). Comparative analysis of prostate-specific membrane antigen (PSMA) versus a prostate-specific membrane antigen-like gene. *Prostate, 58(2)*, 200–210.
12. Garsky, V.M., et al. (2001). The synthesis of a prodrug of doxorubicin designed to provide reduced systemic toxicity and greater target efficacy. *Journal of Medicinal Chemistry, 44(24)*, 4216–4224.
13. Denmeade, S.R., et al. (2003). Prostate-specific antigen-activated thapsigargin prodrug as targeted therapy for prostate cancer. *Journal of the National Cancer Institute, 95(13)*, 990–1000.
14. Denmeade, S., et al. (2009) *A Thapsigargin Prodrug Produces Sustained Growth Inhibition and Substantial Regression of Human Breast Cancers In Vivo with Minimal Host Toxicity*. Thirty-Second Annual CTRC-AACR San Antonio Breast Cancer Symposium.
15. Van Valckenborgh, E., et al. (2005). Targeting an MMP-9-activated prodrug to multiple myeloma-diseased bone marrow: A proof of principle in the 5T33MM mouse model. *Leukemia, 19(9)*, 1628–1633.
16. Acker, H., Pietruschka, F., Deutscher, J. (1990). Endothelial cell mitogen released from HT29 tumour cells grown in monolayer or multicellular spheroid culture. *British Journal of Cancer, 62(3)*, 376–377.
17. Carmeliet, P. (2000). Mechanisms of angiogenesis and arteriogenesis. *Nature Medicine, 6(4)*, 389–395.
18. Eichholz, A., Merchant, S., Gaya, A.M. (2010). Anti-angiogenesis therapies: Their potential in cancer management. *OncoTargets and Therapy, 3*, 69–82.
19. Hoeben, A., et al. (2004). Vascular endothelial growth factor and angiogenesis. *Pharmacological Reviews, 56(4)*, 549–580.
20. Furuya, M., Yonemitsu, Y., Aoki, I. (2009). III. Angiogenesis: Complexity of tumor vasculature and microenvironment. *Current Pharmaceutical Design, 15(16)*, 1854–1867.
21. Abdollahi, A., et al. (2007). Transcriptional network governing the angiogenic switch in human pancreatic cancer. *Proceedings of the National Academy of Sciences U S A, 104(31)*, 12890–12895.
22. Nagy, J.A., et al. (2009). Why are tumour blood vessels abnormal and why is it important to know? *British Journal of Cancer, 100(6)*, 865–869.
23. Torchilin, V.P. (2000). Drug targeting. *British Journal of Cancer, 11 Suppl 2*, S81–S91.
24. Matsumura, Y., Maeda, H. (1986). A new concept for macromolecular therapeutics in cancer chemotherapy: Mechanism of tumoritropic accumulation of proteins and the antitumor agent smancs. *Cancer Research, 46(12 Pt 1)*, 6387–6392.
25. Jain, R.K. (1988). Determinants of tumor blood flow: A review. *Cancer Research, 48(10)*, 2641–2658.
26. Blancher, C., et al. (2001). Effects of ras and von Hippel-Lindau (VHL) gene mutations on hypoxia-inducible factor (HIF)-1alpha, HIF-2alpha, and vascular endothelial growth factor expression and their regulation by the phosphatidylinositol 3′-kinase/Akt signaling pathway. *Cancer Research, 61(19)*, 7349–7355.
27. Vaupel, P., Mayer, A. (2007). Hypoxia in cancer: Significance and impact on clinical outcome. *Cancer and Metastasis Reviews, 26(2)*, 225–239.
28. Ahn, G.O., Brown, M. (2007). Targeting tumors with hypoxia-activated cytotoxins. *Frontiers in Bioscience, 12*, 3483–3501.
29. McKeown, S.R., Cowen, R.L., Williams, K.J. (2007). Bioreductive drugs: From concept to clinic. *Clinical Oncology: A Journal of the Royal College of Radiologists, 19(6)*, 427–442.
30. Cardone, R.A., Casavola, V., Reshkin, S.J. (2005). The role of disturbed pH dynamics and the Na+/H+ exchanger in metastasis. *Nature Reviews Cancer, 5(10)*, 786–795.
31. Kim, J.W., Dang, C.V. (2006). Cancer's molecular sweet tooth and the Warburg effect. *Cancer Research, 66(18)*, 8927–8930.
32. Feron, O. (2009). Pyruvate into lactate and back: From the Warburg effect to symbiotic energy fuel exchange in cancer cells. *Radiotherapy & Oncology, 92(3)*, 329–333.
33. Brahimi-Horn, M.C., Pouyssegur, J. (2007). Oxygen, a source of life and stress. *FEBS Letters, 581(19)*, 3582–3591.
34. Sawant, R.M., et al. (2006). "SMART" drug delivery systems: Double-targeted pH-responsive pharmaceutical nanocarriers. *Bioconjugate Chemistry, 17(4)*, 943–949.
35. Carmeliet, P., Jain, R.K. (2011). Principles and mechanisms of vessel normalization for cancer and other angiogenic diseases. *Nature Reviews Drug Discovery, 10(6)*, 417–427.
36. Baxter, L.T., Jain, R.K. (1991). Transport of fluid and macromolecules in tumors. IV. A microscopic model of the perivascular distribution. *Microvascular Research, 41(2)*, 252–272.
37. Nguyen, D.X., Bos, P.D., Massague, J. (2009). Metastasis: From dissemination to organ-specific colonization. *Nature Reviews Cancer, 9(4)*, 274–284.
38. Balasubramanian, P., et al. (2009). Confocal images of circulating tumor cells obtained using a methodology and technology that removes normal cells. *Molecular Pharmacology, 6(5)*, 1402–1408.

39. Mishra, G.P., et al. (2011). Recent applications of liposomes in ophthalmic drug delivery. *Journal of Drug Delivery, 2011*, 863734.

40. Gregoriadis, G. (1991). Overview of liposomes. *Journal of Antimicrobial Chemotherapy, 28 Suppl B*, 39–48.

41. Zhang, L., et al. (2008). Nanoparticles in medicine: Therapeutic applications and developments. *Clinical Pharmacology & Therapeutics, 83(5)*, 761–769.

42. Immordino, M.L., Dosio, F., Cattel, L. (2006). Stealth liposomes: Review of the basic science, rationale, and clinical applications, existing and potential. *International Journal of Nanomedicine, 1(3)*, 297–315.

43. Offidani, M., et al. (2003). High-dose daunorubicin as liposomal compound (Daunoxome) in elderly patients with acute lymphoblastic leukemia. *The Hematology Journal, 4(1)*, 47–53.

44. Mrozek, E., et al. (2005). Phase I trial of liposomal encapsulated doxorubicin (Myocet; D-99) and weekly docetaxel in advanced breast cancer patients. *Ann Oncol, 16(7)*, 1087–1093.

45. Dragovich, T., et al. (2004). A phase II trial of aroplatin (L-NDDP), a liposomal DACH platinum, in patients with metastatic colorectal cancer (CRC): A preliminary report. *Gastrointestinal Cancers Symposium, 2004.*

46. Eichhorn, M.E., et al. (2006). Paclitaxel encapsulated in cationic lipid complexes (MBT-0206) impairs functional tumor vascular properties as detected by dynamic contrast enhanced magnetic resonance imaging. *Cancer Biology & Therapy, 5(1)*, 89–96.

47. Seiden, M.V., et al. (2004). A phase II study of liposomal lurtotecan (OSI-211) in patients with topotecan resistant ovarian cancer. *Gynecologic Oncology, 93(1)*, 229–232.

48. Hwu, P. et al. (2007). A pharmacokinetic comparison of the Marqibo 3 and 5 vial injection kits in metatastic melanoma patients. *2007 ASCO Annual Meeting Proceedings Part I*, vol. 25, p. 18s.

49. Eisenhardt, M.L., Yuan, Z.-N., Leone, R., Lam, K., Martyn, A.H., Klimuk, S.K., Hope, M.J., Cullis, P.R., Semple, S.C. (2004). Pharmacokinetics, anti-tumor activity and tolerability of INX-0125, a liposomal formulation of vinorelbine, in mice. *Proceedings of the American Association for Cancer Research*, vol. 45.

50. Zhang, J.A., et al. (2005). Development and characterization of a novel Cremophor EL free liposome-based paclitaxel (LEP-ETU) formulation. *European Journal of Pharmaceutics and Biopharmaceutics, 59(1)*, 177–187.

51. Ugwu, S., et al. (2005). Preparation, characterization, and stability of liposome-based formulations of mitoxantrone. *Drug Development and Industrial Pharmacy, 31(2)*, 223–229.

52. Xuan, T., Zhang, J.A., Ahmad, I. (2006). HPLC method for determination of SN-38 content and SN-38 entrapment efficiency in a novel liposome-based formulation, LE-SN38. *Journal of Pharmaceutical and Biomedical Analysis, 41(2)*, 582–588.

53. Soundararajan, A., et al. (2009). [(186)Re]Liposomal doxorubicin (Doxil): In vitro stability, pharmacokinetics, imaging and biodistribution in a head and neck squamous cell carcinoma xenograft model. *Nuclear Medicine and Biology, 36(5)*, 515–524.

54. Newman, M.S., et al. (1999). Comparative pharmacokinetics, tissue distribution, and therapeutic effectiveness of cisplatin encapsulated in long-circulating, pegylated liposomes (SPI-077) in tumor-bearing mice. *Cancer Chemotherapy and Pharmacology, 43(1)*, 1–7.

55. Fantini, M., et al. (2011). Lipoplatin treatment in lung and breast cancer. *Chemotherapy Research and Practice, 2011*, 125192.

56. Zamboni, W.C., et al. (2009). Phase I and pharmacokinetic study of pegylated liposomal CKD-602 in patients with advanced malignancies. *Clinical Cancer Research, 15(4)*, 1466–1472.

57. Kirpotin, D.B., et al. (2006). Antibody targeting of long-circulating lipidic nanoparticles does not increase tumor localization but does increase internalization in animal models. *Cancer Research, 66(13)*, 6732–6740.

58. Matsumura, Y., et al. (2004). Phase I and pharmacokinetic study of MCC-465, a doxorubicin (DXR) encapsulated in PEG immunoliposome, in patients with metastatic stomach cancer. *Annals of Oncology, 15(3)*, 517–525.

59. Mamot, C., et al. (2011). A phase I study of doxorubicin-loaded anti-EGFR immunoliposomes in patients with advanced solid tumors. *2011 ASCO Annual Meeting, No. 3029.*

60. Park, J.W., et al. (2002). Anti-HER2 immunoliposomes: Enhanced efficacy attributable to targeted delivery. *Clinical Cancer Research, 8(4)*, 1172–1181.

61. Harata, M., et al. (2004). CD19-targeting liposomes containing imatinib efficiently kill Philadelphia chromosome-positive acute lymphoblastic leukemia cells. *Blood, 104(5)*, 1442–1449.

62. Tuscano, J.M., et al. (2010). Efficacy, biodistribution, and pharmacokinetics of CD22-targeted pegylated liposomal doxorubicin in a B-cell non-Hodgkin's lymphoma xenograft mouse model. *Clinical Cancer Research, 16(10)*, 2760–2768.

63. Sumitomo, M., et al. (2008). Novel SN-38-incorporated polymeric micelle, NK012, strongly suppresses renal cancer progression. *Cancer Research, 68(6)*, 1631–1635.

64. Nakanishi, T., et al. (2001). Development of the polymer micelle carrier system for doxorubicin. *Journal of Controlled Release, 74(1–3)*, 295–302.

65. Wilson, R.H., Plummer, R., Adam, J., Eatock, M.M., Boddy, A.V., Griffin, M., Miller, R., Matsumura, Y., Shimizu, T., Calvert, H. (2008). Phase I and pharmacokinetic study of NC-6004, a new platinum entity of cisplatin-conjugated polymer forming micelles. *2008 ASCO Annual Meeting.*

66. Kim, T.Y., et al. (2004). Phase I and pharmacokinetic study of Genexol-PM, a cremophor-free, polymeric micelle-formulated paclitaxel, in patients with advanced malignancies. *Clinical Cancer Research, 10(11)*, 3708–3716.

67. Valle, J.W., et al. (2011). A phase 2 study of SP1049C, doxorubicin in P-glycoprotein-targeting pluronics, in patients with advanced adenocarcinoma of the esophagus and gastroesophageal junction. *Investigative New Drugs, 29(5)*, 1029–1037.

68. Kato, K., et al. (2011). Phase II study of NK105, a paclitaxel-incorporating micellar nanoparticle, for previously treated advanced or recurrent gastric cancer. *Investigative New Drugs, 30(4)*, 1621–1627.
69. Matsumura, Y. (2008). Poly (amino acid) micelle nanocarriers in preclinical and clinical studies. *Advanced Drug Delivery Reviews, 60(8)*, 899–914.
70. Nishiyama, N., et al. (2003). Novel cisplatin-incorporated polymeric micelles can eradicate solid tumors in mice. *Cancer Research, 63(24)*, 8977–8983.
71. Kratz, F., Albumin as a drug carrier: Design of prodrugs, drug conjugates and nanoparticles. *Journal of Controlled Release*, 2008. *132(3)*, 171–183.
72. Beck, A., et al. (2010). The next generation of antibody-drug conjugates comes of age. *Discovery Medicine, 10(53)*, 329–339.
73. Bross, P.F., et al. (2001). Approval summary: Gemtuzumab ozogamicin in relapsed acute myeloid leukemia. *Clinical Cancer Research, 7(6)*, 1490–1496.
74. Younes, A., et al. (2010). Brentuximab vedotin (SGN-35) for relapsed CD30-positive lymphomas. *New England Journal of Medicine, 363(19)*, 1812–1821.
75. Ogura, M., et al. (2010). Phase I study of inotuzumab ozogamicin (CMC-544) in Japanese patients with follicular lymphoma pretreated with rituximab-based therapy. *Cancer Science, 101(8)*, 1840–1845.
76. DiJoseph, J.F., et al. (2004). Potent and specific antitumor efficacy of CMC-544, a CD22-targeted immunoconjugate of calicheamicin, against systemically disseminated B-cell lymphoma. *Clinical Cancer Research, 10(24)*, 8620–8629.
77. Burris, H.A., Vukelja, S., Rugo, H.S., Vogel, C., Borson, R., Tan-Chiu, E., Birkner, M., Holden, S.N., Klencke, B., O'Shaughnessy, J. (2008). A phase II study of trastuzumab-DM1 (T-DM1), a HER2 antibody-drug conjugate (ADC), in patients (pts) with HER2+ metastatic breast cancer (MBC). *2008 Breast Cancer Symposium, No. 155.*
78. Lewis Phillips, G.D., et al. (2008). Targeting HER2-positive breast cancer with trastuzumab-DM1, an antibody-cytotoxic drug conjugate. *Cancer Research, 68(22)*, 9280–9290.
79. Keir, C.H., Vahdat, L.T. (2012). The use of an antibody drug conjugate, glembatumumab vedotin (CDX-011), for the treatment of breast cancer. *Expert Opinion on Biological Therapy, 12(2)*, 259–263.
80. Berdeja, J.G., Ailawadhi, S., Weitman, S.D., Zildjian, S., O'Leary, J. J., O'Keeffe, J., Guild, R., Whiteman, K., Chanan-Khan, A.A.A. (2011). Phase I study of lorvotuzumab mertansine (LM, IMGN901) in combination with lenalidomide (Len) and dexamethasone (Dex) in patients with CD56-positive relapsed or relapsed/refractory multiple myeloma (MM). *2011 ASCO Annual Meeting*, Sarah Cannon Research Institute, Nashville, TN.
81. Qin, A., Watermill, J., Mastico, R.A., Lutz, R.J., O'Keeffe, J., Zildjian, S., Mita, A.C., Phan, A.T., Tolcher, A.W. (2008). The pharmacokinetics and pharmacodynamics of IMGN242 (huC242-DM4) in patients with CanAg-expressing solid tumors. *2008 ASCO Annual Meeting.*
82. Xie, H., et al. (2004). Pharmacokinetics and biodistribution of the antitumor immunoconjugate, cantuzumab mertansine (huC242-DM1), and its two components in mice. *Journal of Pharmacology and Experimental Therapeutics, 308(3)*, 1073–1082.
83. Lapusan, S., et al. (2011). Phase I studies of AVE9633, an anti-CD33 antibody-maytansinoid conjugate, in adult patients with relapsed/refractory acute myeloid leukemia. *Investigative New Drugs, 30(3)*, 1121–1131.
84. Sapra, P., et al. (2005). Anti-CD74 antibody-doxorubicin conjugate, IMMU-110, in a human multiple myeloma xenograft and in monkeys. *Clinical Cancer Research, 11(14)*, 5257–5264.
85. Thompson, J. A., Forero-Torres, A., Heath, E.I., Ansell, S.M., Pal, S.K., Infante, J.R., De Vos, S., Hamlin, P.A., Zhao, B., Klussman, K., Whiting, N.C. (2011). The effect of SGN-75, a novel antibody–drug conjugate (ADC), in treatment of patients with renal cell carcinoma (RCC) or non-Hodgkin lymphoma (NHL): A phase I study. *2011 ASCO Annual Meeting.*
86. Thompson, D.S., Patnaik, A., Bendell, J.C., Papadopoulos, K., Infante, J.R., Mastico, R.A., Johnson, D., Qin, A., O'Leary, J.J., Tolcher, A.W. (2010). A phase I dose-escalation study of IMGN388 in patients with solid tumors. *2010 ASCO Annual Meeting*, Tennessee Oncology, PLLC, Nashville, TN.
87. Blanc, V., et al. (2011). SAR3419: An anti-CD19-Maytansinoid Immunoconjugate for the treatment of B-cell malignancies. *Clinical Cancer Research, 17(20)*, 6448–6458.
88. Al-Katib, A.M., et al. (2009). Superior antitumor activity of SAR3419 to rituximab in xenograft models for non-Hodgkin's lymphoma. *Clinical Cancer Research, 15(12)*, 4038–4045.
89. Gudas, J.M., Torgov, M., An, Z., Jia, X.C., Morrison, K.J., Morrison, R.K., Kanner, S.B., Raitano, A.B., Jakobovits, A. (2010). AGS-16M8F: A novel antibody drug conjugate (ADC) for treating renal and liver cancers. *2010 Genitourinary Cancers Symposium.*
90. Gudas, J.M., An, Z., Morrison, R.K., Morrison, K.J., Duniho, S.M., Moser, R., Smith, L., Senter, P., Benjamin, D., Jakobovits, A., Agensys, Inc., Santa Monica, CA. (2010). ASG-5ME: A novel antibody-drug conjugate (ADC) therapy for prostate, pancreatic, and gastric cancers. *2010 Genitourinary Cancers Symposium.*
91. Kelly, R.K., et al. (2011). An antibody-cytotoxic conjugate, BIIB015, is a new targeted therapy for Cripto positive tumours. *European Journal of Cancer, 47(11)*, 1736–1746.
92. Jagannath, S. (2011). BT062, an antibody-drug conjugate directed against CD138, shows clinical activity in patients with relapsed or relapsed/refractory multiple myeloma. *American Society of Hematology Annual Meeting.*
93. Wang, X., et al. (2011). In vitro and in vivo responses of advanced prostate tumors to PSMA ADC, an auristatin-conjugated antibody to prostate-specific membrane antigen. *Molecular Cancer Therapeutics, 10(9)*, 1728–1739.
94. Lee, J.W., et al. (2010). EphA2 targeted chemotherapy using an antibody drug conjugate in endometrial carcinoma. *Clinical Cancer Research, 16(9)*, 2562–2570.

95. Derwin, D., Passmore, D., Sung, J., Tengco, D., Lee, B., Aguilar, B., Chen, T., Zhang, Q., Sufi, B., Cong, C., Gangwar, S., Salles, A., Huber, M., Stevens, A., Rao, C., Deshpande, S., Rangan, V. (2010). Activation of antibody drug conjugate MDX-1203 by human carboxylesterase 2. *AACR Annual Meeting 2010.*
96. Teicher, B.A. (2009). Antibody-drug conjugate targets. *Current Cancer Drug Targets, 9(8)*, 982–1004.
97. Hughes, B. (2010). Antibody-drug conjugates for cancer: Poised to deliver? *Nature Reviews Drug Discovery, 9(9)*, 665–667.
98. Sugarman, S., Murray, J., Saleh, M., LoBuglio, A.F., Jones, D., Daniel, C., LeBherz, D., Brewer, H., Healey, D., Kelley, S. A phase I study of BR96-doxorubicin (BR96-Dox) in patients with advanced carcinoma expressing the Lewis(Y) antigen. *1995 ASCO Annual Meeting, No. 1532.*
99. Tolcher, A., Sugarman, S., Gelmon, K., Cohen, R., Saleh, M., Isaacs, C., Young, L., Healey, D., Slichenmyer, W. (1998). Phase II randomized study of BMS-182248-1 (BR96-doxorubicin immunoconjugate) versus single-agent doxorubicin in patients with metastatic breast cancer. *1998 ASCO Annual Meeting, No. 438.*
100. Guidoccio, F., et al. (2011). Current role of 111In-DTPA-octreotide scintigraphy in diagnosis of thymic masses. *Tumori, 97(2)*, 191–195.
101. Kowalski, J., et al. (2003). Evaluation of positron emission tomography imaging using [68Ga]-DOTA-D Phe(1)-Tyr(3)-Octreotide in comparison to [111In]-DTPAOC SPECT. First results in patients with neuroendocrine tumors. *Molecular Imaging and Biology, 5(1)*, 42–48.
102. Bushnell, D., et al. (2003). Evaluating the clinical effectiveness of 90Y-SMT 487 in patients with neuroendocrine tumors. *Journal of Nuclear Medicine, 44(10)*, 1556–1560.
103. McStay, M.K., et al. (2005). Large-volume liver metastases from neuroendocrine tumors: Hepatic intraarterial 90Y-DOTA-lanreotide as effective palliative therapy. *Radiology, 237(2)*, 718–726.
104. Sierra, M.L., et al. (2009). Lymphocytic toxicity in patients after peptide-receptor radionuclide therapy (PRRT) with 177Lu-DOTATATE and 90Y-DOTATOC. *Cancer Biotherapy and Radiopharmaceuticals, 24(6)*, 659–665.
105. Scopinaro, F., et al. (2005). Fast cancer uptake of 99mTc-labelled bombesin (99mTc BN1). *In Vivo, 19(6)*, 1071–1076.
106. Fragogeorgi, E.A., et al. (2009). Spacer site modifications for the improvement of the in vitro and in vivo binding properties of (99m)Tc-N(3)S-X-bombesin[2-14] derivatives. *Bioconjugate Chemistry, 20(5)*, 856–867.
107. Regina, A., et al. (2008). Antitumour activity of ANG1005, a conjugate between paclitaxel and the new brain delivery vector Angiopep-2. *British Journal of Pharmacology, 155(2)*, 185–197.
108. Thomas, F.C., et al. (2009). Uptake of ANG1005, a novel paclitaxel derivative, through the blood-brain barrier into brain and experimental brain metastases of breast cancer. *Pharmaceutical Research, 26(11)*, 2486–2494.
109. Garlich, J.R., et al. (2008). A vascular targeted pan phosphoinositide 3-kinase inhibitor prodrug, SF1126, with antitumor and antiangiogenic activity. *Cancer Research, 68(1)*, 206–215.
110. Mahadevan, D., Chiorean, E.G., Harris, W., Von Hoff, D. D., Younger, A., Rensvold, D.M., Cordova, F., Qi, W., Shelton, C.F., Becker, M.D., Garlich, J.R., Ramanathan, R.K. (2011). *Phase I evaluation of SF1126, a vascular targeted PI3K inhibitor, administered twice weekly IV in patients with refractory solid tumors. 2011 ASCO Annual Meeting, No. 3015.*
111. Reubi, J.C. (2003). Peptide receptors as molecular targets for cancer diagnosis and therapy. *Endocrine Reviews, 24(4)*, 389–427.
112. Reubi, J.C., et al. (2000). Affinity profiles for human somatostatin receptor subtypes SST1-SST5 of somatostatin radiotracers selected for scintigraphic and radiotherapeutic use. *European Journal of Nuclear Medicine and Molecular Imaging, 27(3)*, 273–282.
113. Reubi, J.C., Macke, H.R., Krenning, E.P. (2005). Candidates for peptide receptor radiotherapy today and in the future. *Journal of Nuclear Medicine, 46 Suppl 1*, 67S–75S.
114. Breeman, W.A., et al. (2002). Preclinical comparison of (111) In-labeled DTPA- or DOTA-bombesin analogs for receptor-targeted scintigraphy and radionuclide therapy. *Journal of Nuclear Medicine, 43(12)*, 1650–1656.
115. Dimitrakopoulou-Strauss, A., et al. (2007). 68Ga-labeled bombesin studies in patients with gastrointestinal stromal tumors: Comparison with 18F-FDG. *Journal of Nuclear Medicine, 48(8)*, 1245–1250.
116. Ferro-Flores, G., et al. (2010). Peptides for in vivo target-specific cancer imaging. *Mini Reviews in Medicinal Chemistry, 10(1)*, 87–97.
117. Ringsdorf, H. (1975). Structure and properties of pharmacologically active polymers. *Journal of Polymer Science Symposium, 51*, 135–153.
118. Alconcel, S.N.S., Baas, A.S., Maynard, H.D. (2011). FDA-approved poly(ethylene glycol)-protein conjugate drugs. *Polymer Chemistry, 2(7)*, 1442–1448.
119. Todd, R., Sludden, J., Boddy, A.V., Griffin, M.J., Robson, L., Cassidy, J., Bissett, D., Main, M., Brannan, M.D., Elliott, S., Fishwick, K., Verrill, M., Calver, H. (2001). Phase I and pharmacological study of CT-2103, a poly (L-glutamic acid)-paclitaxel conjugate. *2001 ASCO Annual Meeting*, p. 439.
120. Duncan, R., Coatsworth, J.K., Burtles, S. (1998). Preclinical toxicology of a novel polymeric antitumour agent: HPMA copolymer-doxorubicin (PK1). *Human & Experimental Toxicology, 17(2)*, 93–104.
121. Hopewel, J.W., et al. (2001). Preclinical evaluation of the cardiotoxicity of PK2: A novel HPMA copolymer-doxorubicin-galactosamine conjugate antitumour agent. *Human & Experimental Toxicology, 20(9)*, 461–470.
122. Bissett, D., et al. (2004). Phase I and pharmacokinetic (PK) study of MAG-CPT (PNU 166148): a polymeric derivative of camptothecin (CPT). *British Journal of Cancer, 91(1)*, 50–55.

123. Meerum Terwogt, J.M., et al. (2001). Phase I clinical and pharmacokinetic study of PNU166945, a novel water-soluble polymer-conjugated prodrug of paclitaxel. *Anticancer Drugs, 12(4)*, 315–323.
124. Rice, J.R., et al. (2006). Preclinical efficacy and pharmacokinetics of AP5346, a novel diaminocyclohexane-platinum tumor-targeting drug delivery system. *Clinical Cancer Research, 12(7 Pt 1)*, 2248–2254.
125. Rademaker-Lakhai, J.M., et al. (2004). A Phase I and pharmacological study of the platinum polymer AP5280 given as an intravenous infusion once every 3 weeks in patients with solid tumors. *Clinical Cancer Research, 10(10)*, 3386–3395.
126. Scott, L.C., et al. (2009). A phase II study of pegylated-camptothecin (pegamotecan) in the treatment of locally advanced and metastatic gastric and gastro-oesophageal junction adenocarcinoma. *Cancer Chemotherapy and Pharmacology, 63(2)*, 363–370.
127. Sapra, P., et al. (2009). Marked therapeutic efficacy of a novel polyethylene glycol-SN38 conjugate, EZN-2208, in xenograft models of B-cell non-Hodgkin's lymphoma. *Haematologica, 94(10)*, 1456–1459.
128. Schluep, T., et al. (2006). Pharmacokinetics and biodistribution of the camptothecin-polymer conjugate IT-101 in rats and tumor-bearing mice. *Cancer Chemotherapy and Pharmacology, 57(5)*, 654–662.
129. Wente, M.N., et al. (2005). DE-310, a macromolecular prodrug of the topoisomerase-I-inhibitor exatecan (DX-8951), in patients with operable solid tumors. *Investigative New Drugs, 23(4)*, 339–347.
130. Homsi, J., et al. (2007). Phase I trial of poly-L-glutamate camptothecin (CT-2106) administered weekly in patients with advanced solid malignancies. *Clinical Cancer Research, 13(19)*, 5855–5861.
131. Danhauser-Riedl, S., et al. (1993). Phase I clinical and pharmacokinetic trial of dextran conjugated doxorubicin (AD-70, DOX-OXD). *Investigative New Drugs, 11(2–3)*, 187–195.
132. Li, C., et al. (1998). Complete regression of well-established tumors using a novel water-soluble poly(L-glutamic acid)-paclitaxel conjugate. *Cancer Research, 58 (11)*, 2404–2409.
133. Li, C., et al. (2000). Biodistribution of paclitaxel and poly(L-glutamic acid)-paclitaxel conjugate in mice with ovarian OCa-1 tumor. *Cancer Chemotherapy and Pharmacology, 46(5)*, 416–422.
134. Boddy, A.V., et al. (2005). A phase I and pharmacokinetic study of paclitaxel poliglumex (XYOTAX), investigating both 3-weekly and 2-weekly schedules. *Clinical Cancer Research, 11(21)*, 7834–7840.
135. Sanchis, J., et al. (2010). Polymer-drug conjugates for novel molecular targets. *Nanomedicine (London), 5(6)*, 915–935.
136. Kratz, F., Beyer, U. (1998). Serum proteins as drug carriers of anticancer agents: A review. *Drug Delivery, 5(4)*, 281–299.
137. Stehle, G., et al. (1997). The loading rate determines tumor targeting properties of methotrexate-albumin conjugates in rats. *Anticancer Drugs, 8(7)*, 677–685.
138. Stehle, G., et al. (1997). Pharmacokinetics of methotrexate-albumin conjugates in tumor-bearing rats. *Anticancer Drugs, 8(9)*, 835–844.
139. Kratz, F., et al. (2002). Probing the cysteine-34 position of endogenous serum albumin with thiol-binding doxorubicin derivatives. Improved efficacy of an acid-sensitive doxorubicin derivative with specific albumin-binding properties compared to that of the parent compound. *Journal of Medicinal Chemistry, 45(25)*, 5523–5533.
140. Hamidi, M., Azadi, A., Rafiei, P. (2008). Hydrogel nanoparticles in drug delivery. *Advanced Drug Delivery Reviews, 60(15)*, 1638–1649.
141. Cruise, G.M., Scharp, D.S., Hubbell, J.A. (1998). Characterization of permeability and network structure of interfacially photopolymerized poly(ethylene glycol) diacrylate hydrogels. *Biomaterials, 19(14)*, 1287–1294.
142. Szeimies, R.M., et al. (2008). A phase II dose-ranging study of topical resiquimod to treat actinic keratosis. *British Journal of Dermatology, 159(1)*, 205–210.
143. Siller, G., et al. (2009). PEP005 (ingenol mebutate) gel, a novel agent for the treatment of actinic keratosis: Results of a randomized, double-blind, vehicle-controlled, multicentre, phase IIa study. *Australasian Journal of Dermatology, 50(1)*, 16–22.

18

ADVANCED DELIVERY IN CARDIOVASCULAR DISEASES

Gayathri Acharya, Wuchen Wang, Divya Teja Vavilala, Mridul Mukherji, and Chi H. Lee

18.1 CHAPTER OBJECTIVES

- To summarize the basic anatomy and physiology of cardiovascular systems and heart valves.
- To understand cardiovascular diseases and treatments.
- To understand the mechanism of heart valve dysfunction and the limitations of conventional treatment options available.
- To outline the potential problems associated with bioprosthetic heart valve replacement therapy.
- To address the application of tissue engineering technologies on the development of synthetic heart valves and the implications of tissue engineering in heart valve diseases.

18.2 CARDIOVASCULAR SYSTEM

The heart is a vital organ that regulates blood flow, which is pumped through or out of the heart in one direction aided by heart valves. The heart with a weight of about 300 grams accomplishes a total of 3 billion beats, propels 250 million liters of blood during a lifetime of 70 years, and produces 100,000 Joules of work daily.

Biomedical advancements, particularly in the last few decades, have drastically changed the therapeutic management of cardiovascular diseases. Yet, cardiovascular diseases remain the number one cause of death globally and, in many countries, account for up to 50% of all deaths. According to the World Health Organization (WHO), cardiovascular diseases caused more than 17 million deaths in the world in 2008, representing 30% of all global deaths. The WHO has projected that more than 23 million people will die every year from cardiovascular diseases by 2030; thus, it will remain the leading cause of death worldwide. Therefore, a better understanding of cardiovascular diseases would lead to improved diagnosis, medications, and surgical procedures. This progress, combined with lifestyle and dietary changes, can significantly reduce the percentage of people dying of cardiovascular diseases in the future.

18.2.1 Architecture of the Cardiovascular Systems

18.2.1.1 Heart Anatomy The heart and the circulation system are the main components of the cardiovascular system. A fully developed and mature heart is slightly larger than the size of an adult fist. It is located in front of the lungs in a cavity on the left side of the chest and consists of four compartments or chambers (Figure 18.1). The upper chambers are called the right- and left-atriums, while the lower chambers are termed the right- and left-ventricles. The atriums and ventricles are separated by layers of muscles, called the septum. The heart also has four valves, and they ensure orderly unidirectional blood flow.

Blood is pumped by the heart via the circulation system into organs, tissues, and cells. The flow of deoxygenated blood from the right atrium into the right ventricle is regulated by the tricuspid valve, while the flow of the

Advanced Drug Delivery, First Edition. Edited by Ashim K. Mitra, Chi H. Lee, and Kun Cheng.

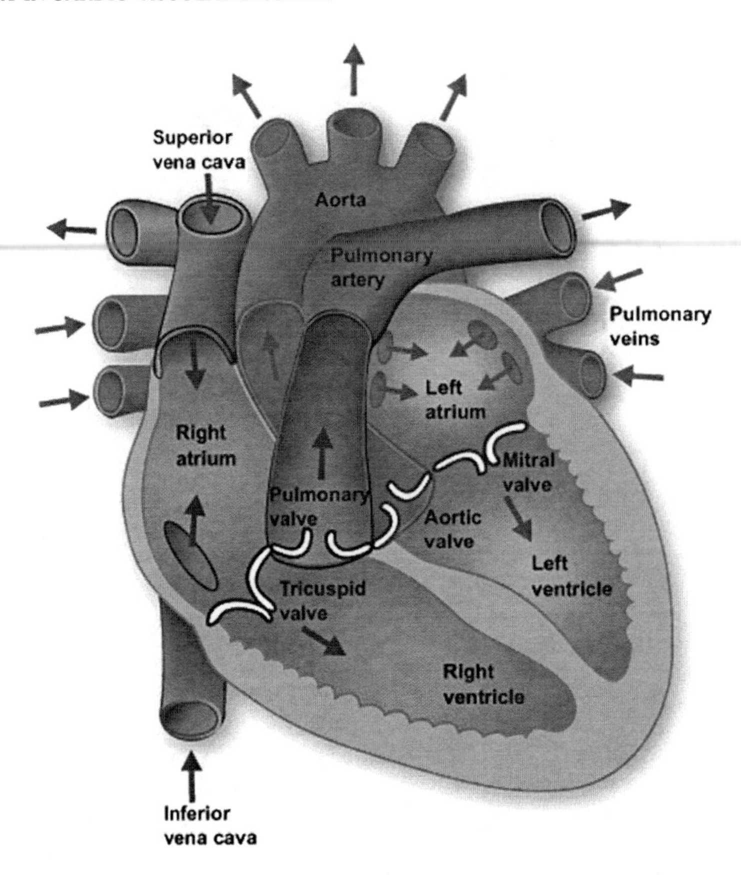

FIGURE 18.1 A cross-section of human heart showing internal chambers and valves. The right chambers, in blue, contain deoxygenated blood. The left heart chambers, in blue, contain oxygenated blood. Reproduced with permission from the Texas Heart Institute. (See color figure in color plate section.)

same deoxygenated blood from the right ventricle into the pulmonary arteries for oxygenation in lungs is regulated by the pulmonary valve. The oxygenated blood from the lungs comes back into the left atrium and flows into the left ventricle via the mitral valve. The oxygenated blood from the left ventricle flows into the aorta via the aortic valve. As the left ventricle generates enough force to push blood through the aortic valve into the entire body, it is the strongest and largest chamber in the heart. In contrast, the right ventricle is around half as thick as the left ventricle because the right ventricle only needs enough force to push blood through the pulmonary valve into the nearby lungs.

18.2.1.2 Circulation System The heart is connected to the vascular system, allowing it to circulate the blood throughout the body. The flow of blood within this vascular system is called blood circulation. Two major circulation systems constitute the cardiovascular system: the systemic and pulmonary circulation systems. The systemic circulation is regulated by the left ventricle that pumps oxygenated blood to the whole body via the aorta, whereas the systemic circulation returns the deoxygenated blood to the right atrium by veins. In contrast, the pulmonary circulation system is regulated by the right ventricle, which pumps deoxygenated blood to the lungs via the pulmonary artery and then returns the oxygenated blood to the left atrium via the pulmonary veins.

The systemic circulation transports oxygen and nutrients via blood to the cells and removes metabolic waste products and carbon dioxide from those cells, which is essential for survival. A complex network of 20 major arteries carry blood from the heart to the rest of the body. When these arteries reach tissues, they branch into smaller vessels called arterioles. Arterioles further branch into capillaries that deliver oxygen and nutrients to cells. Upon delivery, the capillaries pick up metabolic waste products and carbon dioxide from cells and transfer the blood back via the wider vessels called venules. Venules eventually join to form veins, which deliver the blood back to the heart's right atrium for oxygenation from the lungs. Thus, in systemic circulation, arteries carry oxygenated blood away from the heart, while veins carry deoxygenated blood back to the heart. However, the roles are reversed in the pulmonary circulation, in which the pulmonary artery carries deoxygenated blood into the lungs while the pulmonary vein transports oxygenated blood back to the heart from the lungs.

The coronary circulation system is a part of the systemic circulation and is designed to supply blood to the heart muscles [1]. The base of the aorta near the left ventricle bifurcates into two coronary arteries. These coronary arteries further branch into smaller arteries, which supply oxygenated blood to the heart muscles. The right coronary artery predominantly supplies blood to the right side of the heart, while the left coronary artery supplies blood to the left side of the heart.

18.2.1.3 Cardiac Cycle and Heartbeat A heartbeat consists of a two-part pumping process that takes about a second. The heart muscles, called the myocardium, generate an electrical impulse causing the heart to contract in two phases. This electrical impulse originates in the sinoatrial (SA) node, which is located at the top of the right atrium (Figure 18.1). The SA node is also known as the natural pacemaker of the heart. The electrical impulse originates in the SA node when blood collects in the right and left atria, causing them to contract. This contraction pushes blood into the resting right and left ventricles through the tricuspid and mitral valves, respectively. This longer phase of the two-part pumping process is called *diastole*. The second part of the pumping process begins when the electrical impulses from the SA node travel to the atrioventricular (AV) node, which is located on the septum near the tricuspid valve. The AV node propagates the signal through the muscle fibers of the ventricles causing them to contract, which is called the *systole*. At this point the ventricles are full of blood and the closed tricuspid and mitral valves prevent a back flow, and the aortic and pulmonary valves are pushed open. While the oxygen-rich blood flows from the left ventricle to the whole body, the right ventricle pushes blood into the lungs for oxygenation. Once blood is pushed into the aorta and pulmonary artery, the aortic and pulmonary valves close and the empty ventricles relax. A lower pressure resulting from empty ventricles allows the tricuspid and mitral valves to open and the start of a new cycle of contractions. This diastole-systole cycle, which occurs about 60–80 times a minute, is continuously repeated throughout the life of humans.

18.2.2 Diseases of the Cardiovascular System

18.2.2.1 Angina and Heart Attack The coronary artery diseases occur when fatty plaques deposit inside the coronary arteries, which is known as atherosclerosis [2, 3]. When the buildup is ample enough to restrict, but not stop, the flow of blood in the coronary arteries, oxygen supply to the heart muscles is reduced. This results in discomfort or pain in the chest, commonly known as angina, which is not a disease but a symptom of a coronary artery disease. However, when the size of the atherosclerotic buildup is large enough to block the flow of blood in the coronary arteries, the result is death of the heart muscle cells, causing myocardial infarction (MI) or acute myocardial infarction (AMI), commonly known as a heart attack. The coronary artery diseases, whose symptoms are both angina and heart attack, are the most common heart diseases [4, 5].

18.2.2.2 Congestive Heart Failure The most common causes of congestive heart failure are coronary artery disease, cardiomyopathy, high blood pressure, and diabetes. Congestive heart failure develops when the heart's pumping power is lower than normal; thus, it cannot pump enough blood throughout the body [6]. The ventricles, which are the main pumps in the heart, often are responsible for insufficient blood flow. The flow of blood throughout the body becomes slow when the heart is unable to pump blood as effectively as usual. Subsequently, blood begins to back up in the veins, causing congestion in the chest. One of the most common symptoms of congestive heart failure is water retention in the body, which occurs as a result of the reduced blood flow to the kidney. This water retention commonly causes swelling in the legs and ankles, known as edema. Medications that improve the heart's pumping action include the β-blockers or diuretics, which help remove salt and fluid from the body and, thus, are used for the treatment of congestive heart failure.

18.2.2.3 Atherosclerosis Cholesterol is a naturally occurring fatty substance that plays an important role in the formation of cell membrane and hormones [3]. Cholesterol is present in the bloodstream and cells throughout the body. However, an excess amount of cholesterol poses potential health risks. As cholesterol does not dissolve in blood, it is transported by two types of lipoproteins called the low-density lipoproteins (LDLs) and the high-density lipoproteins (HDLs). The cholesterol contained in the LDL (LDL–C) is known as the bad cholesterol because its excess amount in the bloodstream tends to build up in the arterial wall and forms plaques. This plaque formation obstructs and hardens the arteries, leading to a condition known as atherosclerosis [3]. This can lead to coronary artery diseases or congestive heart failure. The HDL-bound cholesterol is known as the good cholesterol because it is carried back to the liver where it is removed from the body.

18.2.2.4 Hypertension The pressure of blood on the vessels of the circulation system is called blood pressure, which pushes the blood from the heart through the circulation system (aorta, arterioles, and finally capillaries) into tissues and cells. Blood pressure normally means systemic arterial blood pressure, which is around 120/80 mm/Hg in healthy individuals. Systolic blood pressure, the first value (120 mm/Hg), is the pressure in the arteriole system when the heart's ventricles are contracting. This pushes the blood from the heart into the body generating the blood pressure.

Thus, the pressure in the arterial system is higher in systolic blood pressure, which represents ventricle contraction. Diastolic blood pressure, the second value (80 mm/Hg), is the lower pressure in the arteriole system when the ventricles of the heart are relaxing.

Several factors, such as family history, lifestyle, obesity, renal diseases, pregnancy, cardiovascular disorders, alcoholism, exercise, salt consumption, and stress, can cause arterioles to narrow [7]. When this happens, the heart has to work harder to push blood though the smaller arterial openings, producing high blood pressure or hypertension. It is estimated that one in every six people worldwide suffers from hypertension, which is one of the leading causes of cardiovascular diseases [7].

18.2.3 Major Drug Classes Used to Treat Cardiovascular Diseases

18.2.3.1 Renin-Angiotensin System This system plays a critical role in the pathophysiology of myocardial infarction, congestive heart failure, and hypertension by controlling arterial blood pressure [8–10]. When the kidneys sense a decreased blood flow (renal hypoperfusion), they secrete a protease called renin. The substrate of renin is angiotensinogen, an abundant glycoprotein primarily synthesized in the liver, which also circulates in plasma. Renin cleaves the decapeptide angiotensin I from the amino terminus of angiotensinogen (Figure 18.2). The angiotensin-converting enzyme (ACE) removes the carboxy-terminal dipeptide from angiotensin I to produce the octapeptide angiotensin II. Thus, angiotensin II, the most active angiotensin peptide, is produced from angiotensinogen in two proteolytic steps catalyzed by renin and ACE. Angiotensin II is a ligand for two specific hepta-spanning G-protein–coupled receptors (GPCRs), Angiotensin I and II Receptors (AT_1 and AT_2). Most biological activities of angiotensin II are mediated by the AT_1 receptor. The binding of angiotensin II to the AT_1 receptor causes blood vessels to contract, leading to an increase in blood pressure [11].

18.2.3.2 Angiotensin Converting Enzyme (ACE) Inhibitors As ACE catalyzes the conversion of angiotensin I

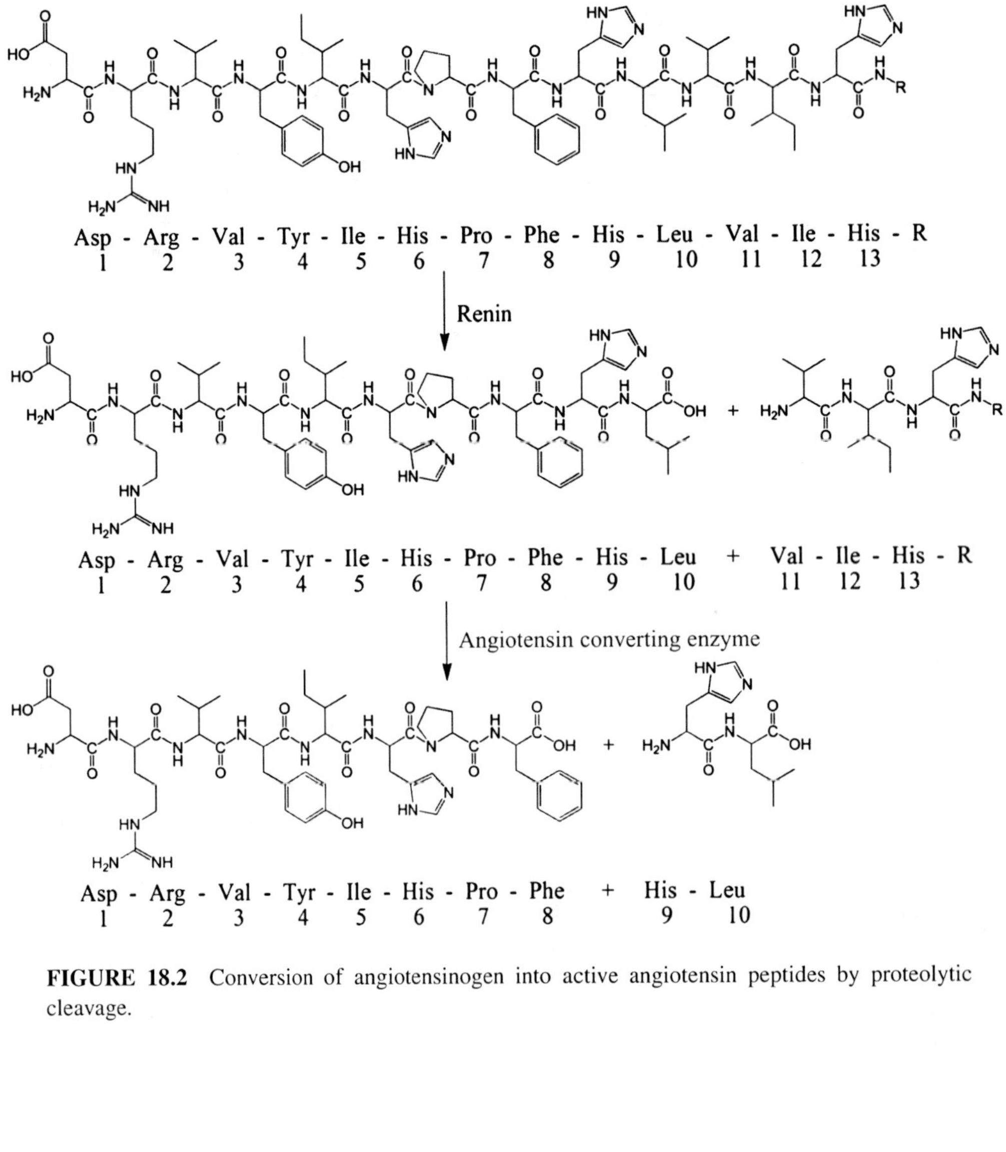

Asp - Arg - Val - Tyr - Ile - His - Pro - Phe - His - Leu - Val - Ile - His - R
1 2 3 4 5 6 7 8 9 10 11 12 13

Renin

Asp - Arg - Val - Tyr - Ile - His - Pro - Phe - His - Leu + Val - Ile - His - R
1 2 3 4 5 6 7 8 9 10 11 12 13

Angiotensin converting enzyme

Asp - Arg - Val - Tyr - Ile - His - Pro - Phe + His - Leu
1 2 3 4 5 6 7 8 9 10

FIGURE 18.2 Conversion of angiotensinogen into active angiotensin peptides by proteolytic cleavage.

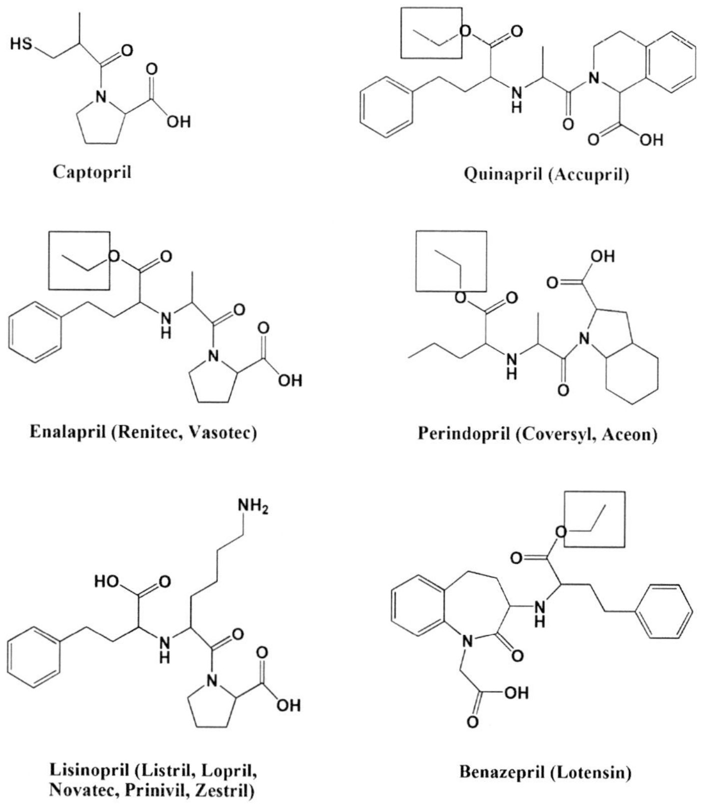

Captopril

Quinapril (Accupril)

Enalapril (Renitec, Vasotec)

Perindopril (Coversyl, Aceon)

Lisinopril (Listril, Lopril, Novatec, Prinivil, Zestril)

Benazepril (Lotensin)

FIGURE 18.3 Chemical structures of selected angiotensin-converting enzyme (ACE) inhibitors. ACE inhibitors such as captopril and lisinopril are active drugs. Other ACE inhibitors such as benazepril, enalapril, perindopril, and quinapril are relatively inactive prodrugs until converted into their corresponding diacids. The part of structures drawn in rectangular boxes are removed by cellular esterases and replaced with a hydrogen atom to form the active drug. The brand names of the drugs are in parentheses.

into angiotensin II (which binds to the AT_1 receptor and raises the blood pressure), inhibitors of ACE are useful in treating hypertension [12, 13]. The orally active ACE inhibitors (Figure 18.3) are developed based on the analysis of the dipeptide cleaved from the angiotensin I during the formation of angiotensin II by ACE. This approach has led to the synthesis of a series of carboxy-alkanoyl derivatives that are potent competitive inhibitors of ACE and are administered as active drugs or as prodrugs. For example, compounds such as captopril, lisinopril, and enalaprilat are active molecules, whereas benazepril, enalapril, fosinopril, moexipril, perindopril, quinapril, ramipril, and trandolapril are inactive until they are converted into their corresponding di-acid forms (Figure 18.3).

18.2.3.3 ***Angiotensin II Receptor Blockers (ARBs)*** The binding of angiotensin II to the AT_1 receptor ultimately leads to hypertension that can be blocked by angiotensin II analogs. These analogs compete for the binding site at the AT_1 receptor with angiotensin II [14, 15]. Based on the structure-activity relationships of angiotensin II binding at the AT_1 receptor, potent peptides-based angiotensin II receptor antagonists were developed. However, these antagonists were of no clinical use as a result of the lack of oral bioavailability. Later, a potent, orally active, and selective nonpeptide AT_1-receptor antagonist *losartan* was developed [16]. Since then, several additional AT_1-receptor antagonists, mostly either biphenylmethyl derivatives or a thienylmethylacrylic acid derivative (Figure 18.4), have been approved by the FDA [17, 18].

18.2.3.4 ***Diuretics*** These drugs are commonly known as water pills, which help remove excess water and salt from blood in the form of urine (Figure 18.5) [19–21]. A reduction in the fluid flowing into the blood vessels decreases the pressure on the arterial walls. The diuretics are classified into three types: thiazide, loop, and potassium-sparing diuretics. Each type works on a different part of the kidneys and has a different therapeutic usage. Although all diuretics remove excess fluid, only thiazide diuretics (e.g., Esidrix and Zaroxolyn) are used to treat hypertension, whereas the loop diuretics (e.g., Lasix and Bumex) and the potassium-sparing

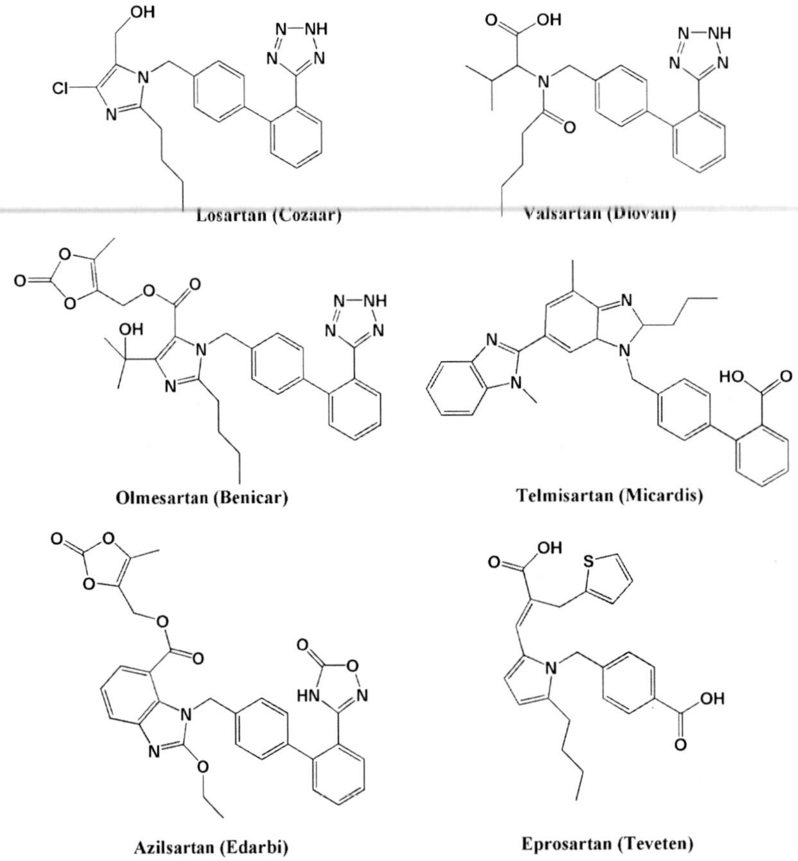

Losartan (Cozaar)

Valsartan (Diovan)

Olmesartan (Benicar)

Telmisartan (Micardis)

Azilsartan (Edarbi)

Eprosartan (Teveten)

FIGURE 18.4 Chemical structures of selected FDA-approved angiotensin II-receptor antagonists (ARBs). The brand names of the drugs are in parentheses.

diuretics (e.g., Aldactone) are used to treat patients with congestive heart failure [22].

18.2.3.5 ***Nitrovasodilators*** These agents are also known as organic nitrates. Nitrovasodilators are prodrugs, which are absorbed by the kidneys, liver, intestinal mucosa, lungs, and vascular tissues after oral administration [23]. Upon absorption, these drugs are rapidly converted to generate nitric oxide (NO), which causes vasodilation by relaxing the vascular smooth muscles in the bronchi and gastrointestinal (GI) tract.

Five nitrovasodilators are clinically used to treat angina: amyl nitrite, nitroglycerin, isosorbide dinitrate, erythrityl tetranitrate, and pentaerythritol tetranitrate. All nitrovasodilator drugs are nitrate esters ($C—O—NO_2$) and are characterized by a sequence of carbon–oxygen–nitrogen bonds (Figure 18.6). Although the number of nitrate esters in the clinically used nitrovasodilator drugs can range from 2 to >6, no correlation has been observed between the number of nitrate ester groups and their potency. However, a relationship has been observed between the lipophilicity and the potency of drugs [24]. In general, the higher the lipophilicity, the more potent the vasodilatory effect of the compound.

As a result of the presence of susceptible C—O bonds, nitrovasodilators are prone to hydrolysis. Therefore, an exposure of these drugs to moisture should be minimized during the compounding process to reduce the loss of active ingredient. The low-molecular-mass organic nitrates (e.g., nitroglycerin) are oily liquids with moderate volatility, and in a pure form (without an inert carrier such as lactose), they are explosive. In contrast, the high-molecular-mass nitrate esters (e.g., isosorbide dinitrate and isosorbide mononitrate) are solids. As a result of the small size and nonpolar characteristics, these drugs are highly vaporizable, which makes them very useful in emergency situations where rapid absorption and action is essential.

18.2.3.6 ***Calcium Channel Blockers*** The voltage-gated calcium channels open in response to electrical impulses,

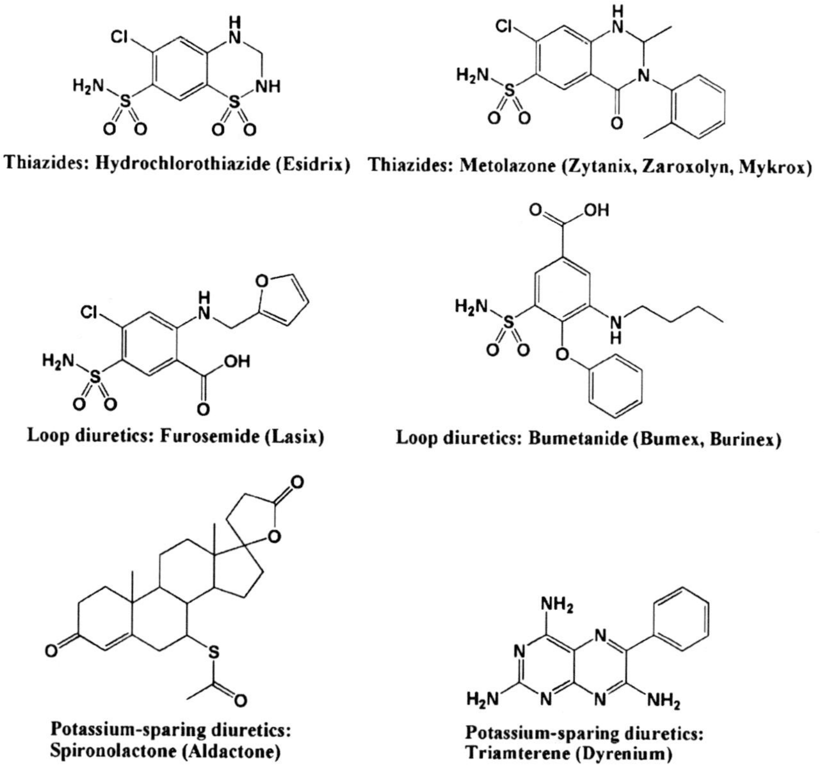

Thiazides: Hydrochlorothiazide (Esidrix) Thiazides: Metolazone (Zytanix, Zaroxolyn, Mykrox)

Loop diuretics: Furosemide (Lasix) Loop diuretics: Bumetanide (Bumex, Burinex)

Potassium-sparing diuretics: Spironolactone (Aldactone)

Potassium-sparing diuretics: Triamterene (Dyrenium)

FIGURE 18.5 Chemical structures of selected thiazides, loop, and potassium-sparing diuretics. The brand names of the drugs are in parentheses.

allowing for an influx of calcium cations (Ca^{2+}) into the muscles from either the sarcoplasmic reticulum (a special type of smooth endoplasmic reticulum that stores calcium ions) or the extracellular space. An increase in the cytosolic calcium ion concentration activates the myosin light-chain kinase, which then initiates muscle contraction by the sliding filament mechanism (i.e., the ripping of myosin and actin filaments over each other). Thus, the contraction of heart muscle cells, like that of any other muscle cells, is regulated by calcium levels, which are manipulated by the calcium ion flow through the voltage-gated calcium channels.

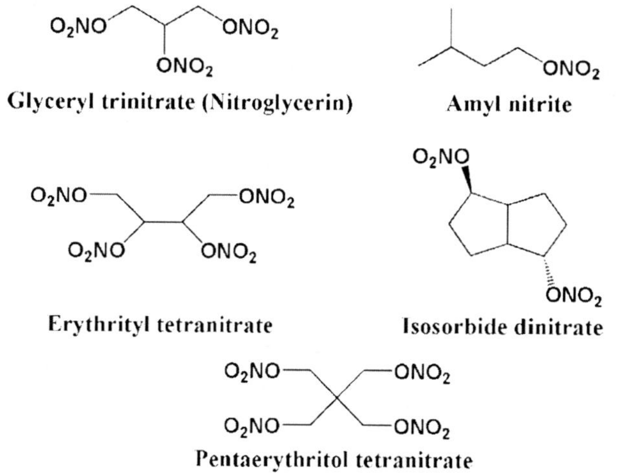

Glyceryl trinitrate (Nitroglycerin) Amyl nitrite

Erythrityl tetranitrate Isosorbide dinitrate

Pentaerythritol tetranitrate

FIGURE 18.6 Chemical structures of five nitrovasodilator drugs that are clinically used for angina. The brand names of the drugs are in parentheses.

The calcium channel antagonists (aka calcium channel blockers) block the calcium channel function in the heart and blood vessel walls, leading to relaxation of the vascular smooth muscles. The calcium channel blockers bind to the $\alpha 1$ subunit of the L-type or long-lasting calcium channels, which are widespread in the vascular smooth muscles of the heart and blood vessel walls [25]. There are five major classes of calcium channel blockers with diverse chemical structures (Figure 18.7): phenylalkylamines, benzothiazepines, dihydropyridines, benzimidazole-substituted tetralines, and diarylaminopropylamine. The phenylalkylamines, benzothiazepines, and dihydropyridines are selective calcium channel blockers, while the benzimidazole-substituted tetralines and diarylaminopropylamine are nonselective calcium channel blockers. Calcium channel antagonists are used to treat angina, hypertension, and abnormal heart rhythms [26]. These drugs are also used to treat pulmonary hypertension and cardiomyopathy.

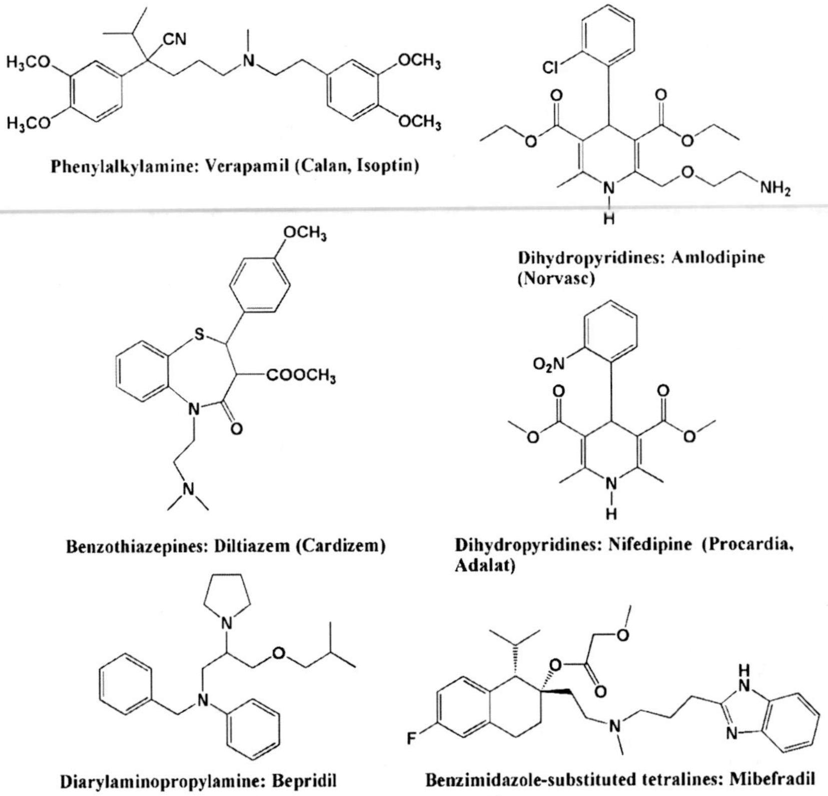

Phenylalkylamine: Verapamil (Calan, Isoptin)

Dihydropyridines: Amlodipine (Norvasc)

Benzothiazepines: Diltiazem (Cardizem)

Dihydropyridines: Nifedipine (Procardia, Adalat)

Diarylaminopropylamine: Bepridil

Benzimidazole-substituted tetralines: Mibefradil

FIGURE 18.7 Chemical structures of the five major classes of calcium channel blockers. The phenylalkylamines, benzothiazepines, and dihydropyridines are selective calcium channel blockers, while benzimidazole-substituted tetralines and diarylaminopropylamine are nonselective calcium channel blockers. Dihydropyridines are identified by the suffix "-dipine."

18.2.3.7 Alpha Blockers The receptors for the adrenergic catecholamines (epinephrine or adrenaline and norepinephrine or noradrenaline) are hepta-spanning GPCRs. There are three main types of adrenergic GPCR receptors: $\alpha 1$, $\alpha 2$, and β. The alpha blockers antagonize the binding of adrenergic agents (especially norepinephrine and epinephrine to some extent) to alpha adrenergic receptors ($\alpha 1$ and $\alpha 2$) found in the prostate, baroreceptors (a special blood pressure sensor), and blood vessels. Because blood vessels including both arteries and veins are innervated by the sympathetic adrenergic nerves, alpha blockers inhibit norepinephrine-mediated tightening of blood vessel walls. This allows arteries and veins to remain relaxed and open, increasing blood flow and lowering blood pressure.

With the exception of phenoxybenzamine, which is an irreversible alkylating agent that covalently binds to alpha receptors, most of these agents are competitive antagonists of alpha adrenergic receptors (Figure 18.8) [27]. Alpha blockers are classified into four chemically diverse classes: β-haloethylamine alkylating agents, piperazinyl quinazolines, imidazolines, and indole derivatives. Functionally, the alpha-blockers are classified into three groups: nonselective, $\alpha 1$- selective, and $\alpha 2$-selective adrenergic blockers. Some drugs (e.g., carvedilol and labetalol) block both alpha and beta adrenergic receptors. These drugs (aka alpha-adrenergic blocking agents or adrenergic blocking agents or alpha-adrenergic antagonists or alpha-blocking agents) are used to treat pathological conditions such as hypertension, benign prostatic hyperplasia, and Raynaud's disease [28, 29]. As alpha blockers attenuate the relaxation of other muscles, they are also prescribed to improve urine flow in patients with prostate problems. In general, the $\alpha 2$-selective adrenergic blockers are not used for the treatment of cardiovascular diseases.

18.2.3.8 Beta Blockers The beta adrenergic GPCR receptor is further divided into three types: β_1, β_2, and β_3 receptors. The beta adrenergic receptors regulate a number of important functions depending on their location in the body. The β_1 receptors are present in the heart, kidneys, and eyes; the β_2 receptors are present in the liver, gastrointestinal tract, lungs, uterus, skeletal muscle, and vascular smooth muscle, while the β_3 adrenergic receptors are found in adipose tissue. Binding of epinephrine to β_1 receptors

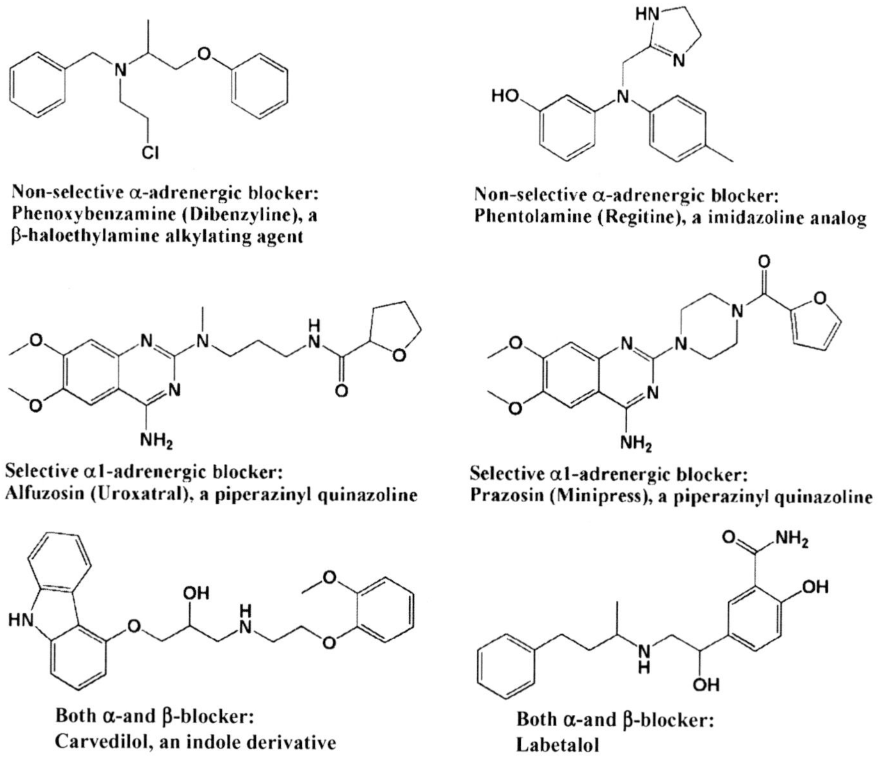

Non-selective α-adrenergic blocker: Phenoxybenzamine (Dibenzyline), a β-haloethylamine alkylating agent

Non-selective α-adrenergic blocker: Phentolamine (Regitine), a imidazoline analog

Selective α1-adrenergic blocker: Alfuzosin (Uroxatral), a piperazinyl quinazoline

Selective α1-adrenergic blocker: Prazosin (Minipress), a piperazinyl quinazoline

Both α-and β-blocker: Carvedilol, an indole derivative

Both α-and β-blocker: Labetalol

FIGURE 18.8 Chemical structures of selected alpha blockers. Almost all these agents are competitive antagonists of the alpha adrenergic receptor except for phenoxybenzamine, an irreversible alkylating agent that binds covalently to alpha receptors. The brand names of the drugs are in parentheses.

induces chronotropic (increased heart rate) and inotropic (increased strength of muscular contraction) effects on the heart. Although a stimulation of β_1 receptors by epinephrine binding in kidney results in renin release, activation of β_2 receptors induces tremors in skeletal muscle, smooth muscle relaxation, and glycogenolysis in the muscles and liver.

Beta blockers mainly antagonize binding of adrenergic catecholamines to β_1 and β_2 receptors (Figure 18.9) . Thus, beta blockers reduce blood pressure by dilating blood vessels. They also reduce physical exertion on the heart rate and the force of contraction by blocking the effects of norepinephrine and epinephrine [30]. Based on their functions, beta blockers can be classified into three groups: β_1-selective, β_2-selective, and nonselective beta blockers. Beta blockers are also known as beta antagonists, beta-adrenergic antagonists, or beta-adrenergic blocking agents. These drugs are mainly used for cardiac arrhythmias and cardio protection after heart attack [31, 32]. They are also used for hypertension, myocardial infarction, angina, tremors, and migraines [33].

18.2.3.9 Statins The main cause of atherosclerosis and conditions associated with atherosclerosis, such as the coronary artery disease, is a result of the presence of high levels of cholesterol in the blood [34, 35]. Statins are the most effective medication for regulating the levels of LDL cholesterol, the bad cholesterol in the blood [36, 37]. Statins lower cholesterol levels by competitively inhibiting 3-hydroxy-3-methylglutaryl coenzyme A (HMG-CoA) reductase (Figure 18.10), an enzyme that catalyzes an early rate-limiting reaction in cholesterol biosynthesis.

Mevastatin, lovastatin, simvastatin, and pravastatin (Figure 18.11) are fungal metabolites, and each contains a hexahydronaphthalene ring. Lovastatin has a methyl group at carbon 3, which is absent in mevastatin. Some statins like simvastatin and lovastatin are converted in the liver into their active hydroxy-acid forms because they are lactone prodrugs and thus less water soluble than other statins. Fluvastatin, rosuvastatin, and atorvastatin are synthetic compounds (Figure 18.11). The critical side chain in statins, a mevalonic acid-like hydroxy acid group, forms a six-membered analog of an intermediate compound in the HMG-CoA reductase catalyzed reaction. This hydroxyl acid side chain binds to HMG-CoA reductase and competitively inhibits the enzyme, leading to reduced cholesterol biosynthesis [38].

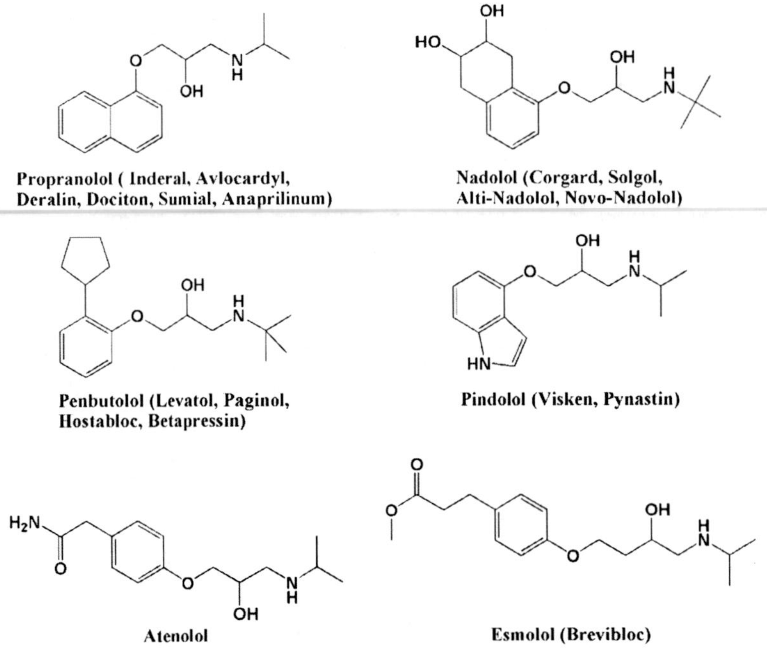

Propranolol (Inderal, Avlocardyl, Deralin, Dociton, Sumial, Anaprilinum)

Nadolol (Corgard, Solgol, Alti-Nadolol, Novo-Nadolol)

Penbutolol (Levatol, Paginol, Hostabloc, Betapressin)

Pindolol (Visken, Pynastin)

Atenolol

Esmolol (Brevibloc)

FIGURE 18.9 Chemical structures of selected beta blockers. There are two main classes of beta adrenergic receptor antagonists: nonselective and β1 selective. The brand names of the drugs are in parentheses.

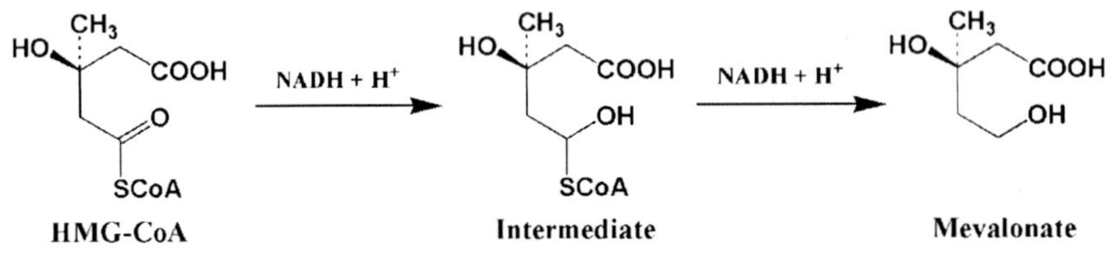

HMG-CoA → ($NADH + H^+$) → Intermediate → ($NADH + H^+$) → Mevalonate

FIGURE 18.10 Scheme showing 3-hydroxy-3-methylglutaryl coenzyme A (HMG-CoA) reductase catalyzed formation of mevalonate, an early rate-limiting reaction in cholesterol biosynthesis.

18.3 THE FUNCTION OF HEART VALVES

The mammalian heart has four chambers, two atria in the upper position and two ventricles in the lower position of the heart [39]. The mammalian heart also has four valves, two atrioventricular valves and two semilunar valves. The mitral valve and tricuspid valve are two atrioventricular valves. The mitral valve has two leaflets (also known as cusps) and regulates blood flow between the left atrium and the left ventricle. Similarly, the tricuspid valve has three cusps and regulates blood flow between the right atrium and the right ventricle.

Aortic and pulmonary valves are two semilunar valves, which are located between the ventricles and respective arteries and pump oxygenated blood into the lungs and all the other organs in the body. The aortic valve has three leaflets, which regulate blood flow between the left ventricle and the aorta. In a rare genetic disorder, the aortic valve is bicuspid where the valves are fused by birth to form two valves. During the beginning of systole, pressure in the left ventricle increases above that of the aorta; as a result, blood pushes the aortic valve and enters into the aorta. At the end of systole, the pressure in the left ventricle drops and pressure in the aorta increases, forcing the aortic valve to close. The pulmonary valve is located between the right ventricle and the pulmonary artery, and its structure and functioning are similar to the aortic valves. Unlike atrioventricular valves, which have connective tissues for running the cuspal cycle, the working function of semilunar valves simply depends on the pressure gradient [40].

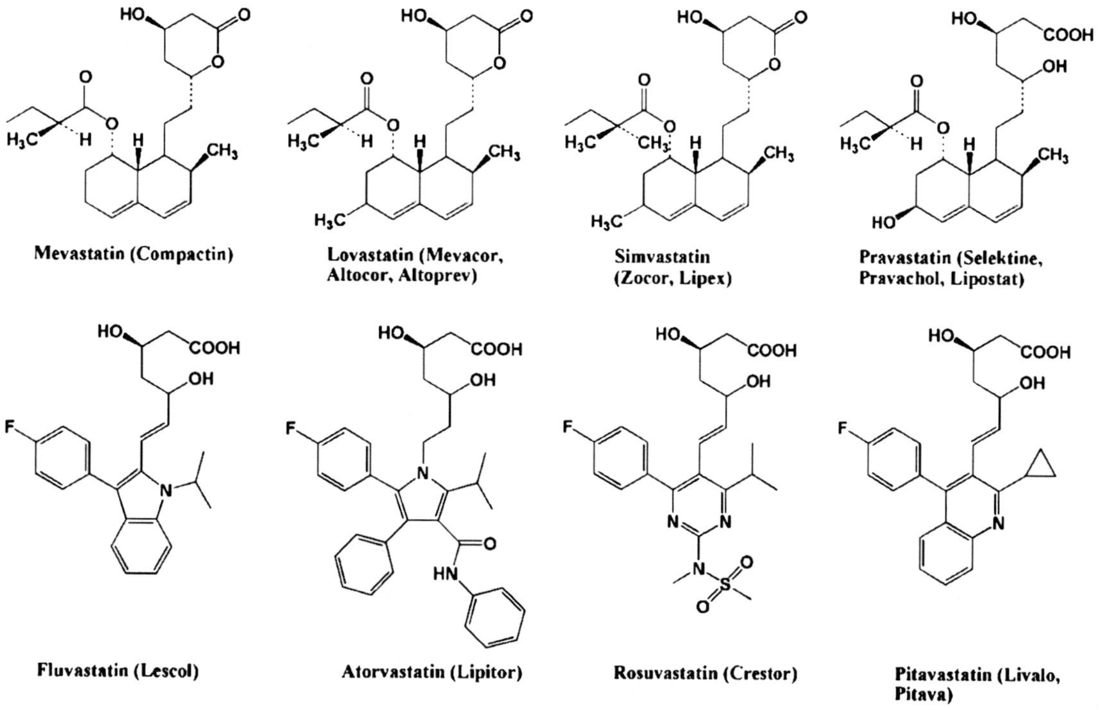

Mevastatin (Compactin) | Lovastatin (Mevacor, Altocor, Altoprev) | Simvastatin (Zocor, Lipex) | Pravastatin (Selektine, Pravachol, Lipostat)

Fluvastatin (Lescol) | Atorvastatin (Lipitor) | Rosuvastatin (Crestor) | Pitavastatin (Livalo, Pitava)

FIGURE 18.11 Chemical structures of selected FDA-approved statin drugs.

18.4 THE STRUCTURE OF HEART VALVES

Both semilunar valves (i.e., aortic and pulmonary valves) comprise three anatomical components: leaflets, aorta walls, and sinuses [41]. Leaflets or cusps are bulgy flap-like structures, serving as the load-bearing component of the valve. Leaflets of the heart valve open with forward blood flow and then close briskly upon minimal back-pressure. The unique architecture of the leaflets and their excellent structure enable the heart valve to function effectively [42]. The ventricularis on the inflow surface is composed of mostly collagenous tissue with elastin fibers radially aligned, providing mechanical strength to the leaflet tissue. The centrally located spongiosa is composed of glycosoaminoglycans.

Two general types of cells constitute the semilunar valves: a covering layer of endothelium (present in most of the cardiovascular system) and interstitial cells with features of both smooth muscle cells and fibroblasts called myofibroblasts. Valve interstitial cells (VICs) possess the ability to produce extracellular matrix components, maintaining both the mechanical and contractile properties of the leaflets [43]. The myofibroblasts construct, repair, and remodel the highly specialized and functionally designed extracellular matrix.

The aortic artery portion of the valve is referred to as the wall portion of the valve. The aortic wall behind each leaflet expands to form a pouch-like structure called the sinus. The *sinuses* are essential in initiating *valve* closing and cushion leaflets from being constrained against the aortic *wall* during valve opening. Each sinus is differentiated regionally based on the orifices of the coronary arteries, supplying fresh blood to the valves. Two of the three sinuses containing orifices are called left and right coronary based on position, and the sinus without an orifice is called the noncoronary. Similarly, the pulmonary valve is differentiated into right, left, and anterior/nonfaced. The fibrosa, beneath the surface of the sinus, is composed of predominantly crimped, densely packed collagen fibers.

18.5 HEART VALVE DYSFUNCTION

Heart diseases are the major cause of human mortality in the world and heart valve dysfunction contributes to most of them. Aortic or pulmonary valve stenosis, the most common case of heart valve dysfunction, is characterized by diminished blood flow from the ventricle due to abnormal opening of the valve in heart or lung, respectively. Incomplete closing of the valve mostly due to abnormalities in the valve root leads to valve leakage (regurgitation), which causes blood to flow in a reverse direction. Valvular dysfunction is mainly caused by the combination of stenosis and regurgitation.

18.5.1 Causes

The major causes for heart valve dysfunction are occasionally unknown, but some common causes are as follows [44]:

- Bicuspid aortic valve disease is a congenital aortic valve dysfunction, where only two leaflets are developed instead of the normal three leaflets. Bicuspid valves are generally stiff and leaky as a result of the absence of the third leaflet.
- Infective endocarditis occurs when bacteria enters the bloodstream and manifests in the heart valve, leading to valve stenosis and scarring.
- Rheumatic fever is an inflammatory disease usually caused by untreated bacterial infection, especially streptococcus bacteria. Antibodies produced to fight the germs react with the heart valve, causing inflammation and scarring.
- Myxomatous degeneration is the most common cause of mitral valve insufficiency, attributing to weakening of the connective tissue.
- Dilation of the aorta is related to enlargement of the aorta resulting from weakness in the wall tissue.

18.5.2 Treatment: Valve Replacement Therapies

Heart valve dysfunction is treated through valve replacement therapies. In the early stages of valve degeneration, antibodies are used to prevent further infections and attenuate symptoms. Valve replacement therapies with autograft (i.e., Ross procedure) and allograft/xenograft with artificial valves (i.e., mechanical and bioprosthetic heart valves) are the most common treatment options available for valve dysfunction [45, 46]. The transplant types are categorized based on their source as follows:

- Autograft—within one individual from one site to another
- Isograft—between genetically identical individuals (i.e., identical twins)
- Homograft/allograft—between different individuals of the same species
- Heterograft/xenograft—between members of different species
- Autotropic—transplanted in correct anatomical location
- Heterotropic—transplanted to different anatomical location

18.5.2.1 Autograft Approach: Ross Procedure In the Ross procedure, the malfunctioning aortic valve is replaced with a healthy pulmonary valve from the same individual and a pulmonary autograft is used to replace the pulmonary valve [46]. The procedure is most suitable for patients who have a long life expectancy and no other major illnesses. The Ross procedure is effective for most male patients and ideal for women of childbearing age because it eliminates the need for anticoagulant therapy (i.e., Coumadin), which can lead to birth defects.

The main advantages of the Ross procedure involve biocompatible valve growth, no anticoagulant therapy needed, free of damage as a result of calcification, and favorable hemodynamics [47]. As a new valve is created from the patient's own tissue, the valve is already alive and healthy, free of rejection from the body, and does not need to be frozen or treated with chemicals.

18.5.2.2 Allograft and Xenograft Approach: Artificial Heart Valve Replacement

Mechanical Valves Mechanical heart valves (Figure 18.12) with artificial leaflets sewn into a metal frame made from durable materials are proven to be biocompatible and safe for human use. They are highly durable with a life of about 20–30 years, but they require continuous use of anticoagulants, such as Coumadin and Heparin, to prevent blood clotting on the valve.

Biological leaflets are also used to be sewn into a metal frame. This tissue is typically harvested from the *pericardial sac* of either bovine (cows) or equine (horses) as a result of its superior durability. The tissue is sterilized so that the biological markers are removed, eliminating a response from the host's immune system. The leaflets are flexible and physically durable and usually do not require the patient to take blood thinners for the rest of his or her life.

Based on frame structure, they are classified into stent framed and not framed, whereas based on the mechanism involved in valve operation, they are classified into caged

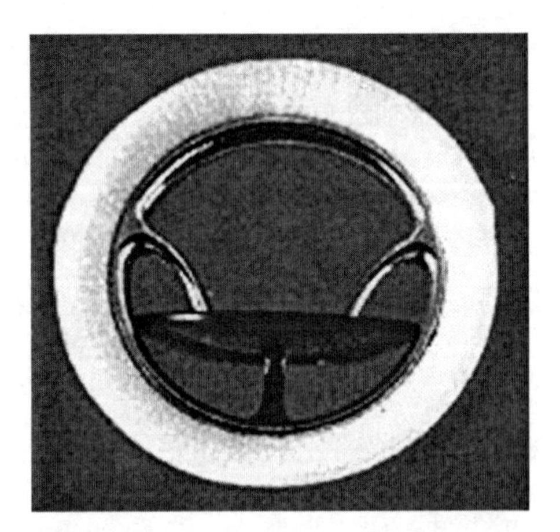

FIGURE 18.12 A mechanical valve made entirely of artificial components. This is a tilting disc valve made of pyrolitic carbon, stainless steel, and dacron.

ball valve, tri-leaflet valve, bi-leaflet valve, and tilting disc valve.

- Percutaneous implantation
- Stent framed
- Not framed
- Sternotomy/thoracotomy implantation
- Ball and cage
- Tilting disk
- Bi-leaflet
- Tri-leaflet

The key advantages and disadvantages of mechanical heart valves are as follows:

Advantage:

- Mechanical heart valves are very durable because they are made of strong materials like carbon, titanium, Teflon, polyester, and dacron. Subsequently, the patient risk for future valve replacement or reoperations is lowered.

Disadvantages:

- Blood thinners needed to prevent a risk of blood clots forming on the valve are the most common drug therapy for mechanical valve replacement patients.
- Mechanical heart valve replacements often produce a clicking noise in some patients.

Bioprosthetic Heart Valves Bioprosthetic heart valves (BHVs) are either xenografts from a porcine or bovine aortic valve or allografts from human cadavers. These materials were modified with several chemical procedures to make them suitable for implantation in the human heart. BHVs are generally fixed with low concentrations of glutaraldehyde and anti-calcification agents before implantation [45]. BHVs have a lifespan of 10–15 years and are used in patients who cannot take blood thinners especially over 75 years of age. BHVs closely resemble natural valves in functional and hemodynamic properties and have good thrombo-resistance properties.

Major causes for BHV failure are wear and tear, fatigue, and degenerative calcification [48]. Abnormal conditions of BHV also include calcification, thromboembolism, endocarditis, and infection [49]. Damage to the valve leads to structural dysfunction that progresses toward tissue deterioration and finally valve failure.

The key advantages and disadvantages of BHV replacements are as follows:

Advantages:

- Bioprosthetic valves used in heart valve replacement therapy generally offer immunity and biocompatible functional properties (e.g., hemodynamics and resistance to thrombosis) that are more similar to those of native valves.
- Patients do not need to use anticoagulants after surgery.
- They do not produce a clicking noise.

Disadvantages:

- Bioposthetic heart valves are liable to calcification and not as durable as mechanical valves, requiring another operation later in life.
- Pig valves last between 10 and 15 years, while cow valves can last beyond 20 years in some cases.
- Xenograft is associated with immune rejection to foreign material by the human body.

18.6 BIOPROSTHETIC HEART VALVE FAILURE

18.6.1 Calcification

Pathological deposition of calcium phosphate on the surface of valve tissue that leads to thickening, stiffening, tearing, and narrowing of the valve opening is known as valvular calcification. Calcification is the most common valvular disease among patients older than 65 years [50]. The intensity of valve calcification is directly correlated with the extent of disease progression [51]. Narrowing and tearing of the valve reduces blood flow to the outside of the heart, causing chest pain or heart attack.

Valvular calcification is the most common process of BHV failure [48, 52, 53]. Although valve calcification is similar to bone calcification, two components of the valve, cusps and aortic wall, show different binding properties to minerals as a result of different structural properties and thickness. As there are similarities in the development of disease in blood vessels (i.e., aortic atherosclerosis) and heart valve leaflets (i.e., aortic valve sclerosis), particularly the early accumulation of lipids, they are known to be different manifestations of the same disease [54]. If it can be demonstrated that the risk factors for both valve sclerosis and aortic atherosclerosis are independently associated with aortic valve abnormalities in the general population and that the modifications of structure are early changes that are common to both disease processes, then there could be a benefit of novel therapies suitable for the treatment of both pathologies [55].

18.6.1.1 Causes The overall progress of calcification takes place in three steps: initiation, nucleation, and proliferation. Initially, cell death resulting from mechanical stress together with other risk factors causes formation of apoptotic bodies [56]. In normal valves, these apoptotic bodies are removed by phagocytosis and the failure in clearance of these apoptotic bodies leads to calcium accumulation as a result of enhanced membrane permeability [56, 57]. The rate of net calcium uptake increased as the amount of bound mineral increased and tended to approach a plateau, which is indicative of the presence of a rate-limiting step involving the calcium ion that does not participate in the calcium exchange reaction.

A matrix made of collagen and lipid acts as a nucleation site for crystal formation [56]. Pathologically lipids activate valve endothelium and VICs, resulting in their osteogenic phenotypes and synthesizing extracellular bone matrix proteins. These proteins were mineralized by deposition of hydroxyapatite, which stimulates the calcification process [58, 59]. Glutaraldehyde crosslink fixation of BHV further induces cell death, and cells eventually become highly permeable to intracellular calcium deposition, facilitating nucleation of crystals [60].

Once calcium deposition or nucleate formation establishes, valve cells stop expressing calcium-associated proteins and endothelial regulators, which serve as potent natural calcification inhibitors [59]. Matrix Gla protein, fetuin, and osteopontin are calcium-associated proteins that basically act through chelating and inhibition of apatite crystal growth [61], and the absence of them induces crystal growth and proliferation as a result of deposition of calcium phosphate on bone-like matrix of collagen [57].

The overall rates of heart valve calcification are dependent on mechanical damage, chemical crosslinking imposed on the heart valve, and exposed cellular components. Several potential genetic and cellular factors, such as sex, age, hormone status, shear material, protein adsorption, and thrombus, may contribute to valve calcification [62–64].

18.6.1.2 Involved Variables As shown in Table 18.1, various physicochemical/formulation variables are involved in BHV calcification. The selected variables and rationales behind each environmental/structural condition are as follows: 1) biochemical conditions of the physiological fluid (calcium binding proteins including noncollagenous proteins, CRP, ICAM, NOS, and lipoproteins), which have individual variance and can be experimentally determined; 2) physicodynamic conditions of the physiological fluid (fluid rate/volume, fluid pH, dynamic stress), which are computed by *in silico* or computer-based models and cannot be manipulated directly in a real situation; and 3) physicochemical conditions of heart valves (composition: collagen/elastin/GAG ratios, surface property: surface uniformity, surface pH, mechanical property: cyclic loading, crosslinking agents), which are adjustable during the heart valve substitute development process.

Physiological Variables As calcified degeneration involves deposition of calcium phosphates and associated minerals, its process is usually affected by interaction between tissues and proteins [65]. It is also postulated that for pathological calcification to occur, the coordinate and regulatory expression of all involved components is required [57, 66].

In heart valve substitute replacements, special interest has been placed on the binding property of the collagen or elastin fibrils to calcium and extracellular proteins. A heart valve is composed of an aortic wall, which is made of collagen (90%) and elastin (10%), and cusp (i.e., leaflets), which is made of mainly collagen (99%) and elastin (<1%) [67]. Calcium is deposited in the vessel wall or collagen in heart valves as hydroxyapatite, the major calcium constituents in bone [68]. The low content of elastin in the early perinatal aorta makes it less prone to calcification because elastin has a high affinity to calcium and extracellular proteins [69, 70]. When porcine aortic walls were implanted subcutaneously in the rats for up to 8 weeks, the total extracted amount of proteins from the control aortic walls was significantly greater than those from ethanol (i.e., anticalcification agent) treated aortic walls (1.63 ± 0.1 vs. 1.41 ± 0.08 μg/mg in the aortic wall after 8 weeks of implantation), indicating that the substrate affinity of tissues to protein was significantly reduced in the less calcified tissues [64, 71]. This finding further suggests that there is a close link between the extracted amounts of proteins and calcium from porcine aortic walls.

The role of various proteins like calcium-associated proteins (CAPs), inflammatory proteins, and the neuronal calcium sensor protein family, which are found at higher concentrations during the calcification process of a heart valve substitute and other events pertaining to cardiac pathology including atherosclerosis, needs to be examined (Table 18.2). CAP includes noncollagenous proteins (NCPs), such as osteopontin, osteoprotegerin, and bone sialoprotein II; extracellular matrix (ECM) glycoprotein; and proteins containing gamma-carboxyglutamate [61].

Osteopontin (OPN), an Non Collagenous Proteins (NCP), produced a high degree of apatite formation when it was covalently bound to certain substrates *in vitro*, implying that osteopontin bound to type I collagen may induce apatite formation *in vivo* [62]. OPN that is expressed in a tissue-specific manner, is a strong inhibitor of crystal formation and growth *in vitro*, and acts as an inhibitor to normal and pathological conditions related to calcification or atherosclerosis [63]. Ongoing debate seems to continue regarding its effects on crystal adhesion to tubular epithelial cells and subsequently on calcification [72].

Vitamin K-dependent (VKD) proteins present in blood are an important factor to bone mineralization, arterial calcification, apoptosis, phagocytosis, growth control, chemotaxis, and signal transduction [73]. VKD proteins regulate blood coagulation as well as bone growth and calcification through the synthesis of at least two proteins involved in calcium and bone metabolism, namely,

TABLE 18.1 Physiological/Pathological Variables Involved with Bioprosthetic Heart Valve Substitute Calcification

Class	Variable	Condition	Description	References
Animal/heart cell lines	Rat	8 weeks vs. 12 weeks old rat vs. mouse	Differences in the calcification rate as a result of varying host responses (age or species) should be investigated	[3, 10, 36, 38, 57, 63]
	Mouse	Apo knock-out mice	Normal vs. pathological status (genetically transgenic mice: LDL (>130 mg/dL), CRP (>0.44 mg/dL))	[28, 39]
	Heart cell lines	Cytokine-induced ICAM expression	Porcine aortic valve interstitial cells (PAVICs), normal vs. pathological status (5–6 times increase in ICAM expression)	[68]
Biochemical conditions of physiological fluid	Protein profiles	Heart cell lines, rat model	Proteomics: time-dependent expression profiles of 96 proteins will be examined, and their patterns, surface interaction, and binding profiles with calcium will be established	[23, 24]
	CRP/ICAM	0–5000 ng/mL, 0–500 μg/mL	The plasma concentrations of ICAM and CRP in healthy individuals are about 550 ng/mL and 1.0 μg/mL, respectively. Under the conditions of tissue damage and infection, the level can raise to several times higher	[23, 24]
	Lipoprotein	LDL (>130 mg/dL)	In normal individuals, LDL concentration is on average (130 mg/dL), which can be much greater in an at-risk population. Lacidipine treatment at 3 or 10 mg/kg	[25, 26]
Physico-dynamic conditions of fluids	Fluid rate	Flow rate: 100–1200 mL/min	Normal fluid rate vs. abnormal condition (with a slower rate) will be examined with blood flow: 100–1200 mL/min; heart (250), kidney (1100), muscle (1200)	[29, 30]
	Fluid pH	6.8–7.6	A balance between bicarbonate and carbon dioxide determines blood pH. Normal vascular pH is 7.4. Blood pH of below 6.9 or above 7.9 is usually considered fatal	[29, 31]
Physico-chemical conditions of heart valves	Collagen/elastin/GAG concentration	Collagen/elastin 90:10, 50:50, and 20:80 GAG (1%)	Collagen-elastin matrix (CEM) with different ratios of collagen and elastin as well as glycosaminoglycan was developed as a heart valve scaffold	[32]
	Mechanical property of heart valves	Cyclic loading	Mechanical properties of CEM under fluid pressure and cyclic loading were examined for their contribution to tissue calcification	[33, 34]
	Surface property of heart valves	Uniformity, contact angle, pH: 7.4, 5.0, and 3.4	Contact angle assesses adhesion, surface treatments, and polymer film modification. Surface pH can be modified ranging from 3.4 (acidic) to 7.4 (neutral)	[35]
	Crosslinking agent	Glutaraldehyde 0.1–0.6%	The amount of glutaraldehyde in bovine pericardium rat implants has a quantitative relationship with calcific deposits	[36, 37]

osteocalcin and matrix Gla-protein (MGP) [74, 75]. Osteocalcin was present at low levels in all calcified cardiovascular tissues (4.5–175.7-ng osteocalcin/mg protein) with trace levels present in noncalcified tissue. Osteocalcin is accounted for a small proportion of the total protein-bound gamma-carboxyglutamic acid (Gla) (0.01–0.05%) [76]. It was also reported that Sox9 was expressed in the developing heart valves [77]. Sox9 is a transcription factor required for both early and late stages of cartilage formation as well as precursor cell expansion and extracellular matrix organization during mouse heart valve development.

The synthesis and structure of glycosaminoglycans, proteoglycans, and hyaluronans were exquisitely regulated, and the signaling pathways controlling these processes should provide tissue-specific opportunities for concomitant prevention of atherosclerosis and calcific aortic valve disease

TABLE 18.2 The Positive and Negative Reactants in Plasma Involved in Heart Valve Substitute Calcification

	Positive Reactant	Negative Reactant
Calcium binding proteins	C-reactive protein/ICAM	Albumin
	Serum amyloid A protein	Transthyretin
	Fibronectin	High-density
Lipoprotein	α1-acid glycoprotein	Low-density
Lipoprotein	Globulin	
	ITGA	
Noncollagenous proteins	Osteonectin, osteocalcin	Osteopontin
	Bone morphogenic protein	
Inflammatory proteins	E-selectin	
	Integrin	
	IL-1, 6, 8, 10, 18	
Proteinase inhibitors	α1-antitrypsin	Inter α-antitrypsin
	α1-antichymotrypsin	
	α1-macroglobulin	
	Antithrombin	
Coagulation/ fibrinolysis proteins	Fibrinogen	
	Prothrombin	
	Factor VIII	
	Plasminogen	
Complement proteins	C1s	Properdin
	B	
	C2, C3, C4, C5	
	C1INH	

Source: Refs. 23, 24, 27, and 28.

[78]. The exact function of those proteins, whether they play a permissive or regulatory role in the BHV calcification process, is yet to be clearly elucidated.

Endothelial Regulation Endothelial regulation is yet another factor affecting calcification. Reduced nitric oxide production by endothelial nitric oxide synthase causes enhanced leucocyte adhesion, platelet aggregation, and inflammation, which are early signs of calcification and atherosclerosis [79]. In hypercholesterolemic rabbits, the expression of endothelial nitric oxide synthase decreased [80], and the absence of this enzyme in mice causes abnormal congenital aortic valve development [81]. Therefore, nitric oxide regulation is likely to play an integral role in the pathogenesis of calcific aortic valve diseases. The report that nitric oxide donors act as an inhibitor against valve calcification [82] adds to the evidence of involvement of endothelial regulation in heart valve calcification.

In normal valves, superoxide levels were relatively low and distributed homogeneously throughout the valve, whereas in stenotic valves, superoxide levels were increased twofold near the calcified regions of the valve ($p < 0.05$) [83]. Oxidative stress in calcific aortic valves seems associated with increased levels of superoxide and hydrogen peroxide by inhibition of nitric oxide synthases (NOS), which is indicative of uncoupling of the enzyme [84]. As total superoxide dismutase (SOD) activity and expression of all three SOD isoforms were significantly lowered, antioxidant activities were reduced in calcified regions of the aortic valve.

It was also shown that the activity of inhibitors, such as chondromodulin-I, an anti-angiogenic factor, decreased in aged mice with calcific valve disease [85], contributing to both pathologic angiogenesis and dystrophic calcification of heart valves. The complexity of the active calcific process is different from that of atherosclerosis in blood vessels and seems to be potentiated by genetic and clinical factors [86], implying there are numerous potential targets in the endothelial regulation process for prevention of calcific valve progression.

18.6.2 Heart Valve Fatigue

Damage to the structural proteins accelerates the process of valve deterioration, leading to bioprosthetic heart valve (BHV) failure. Mechanical forces affected the biosynthetic activity of cells in tissue matrices by modulate cell physiology [87]. As primarily passive structures of heart valves are driven by forces exerted by the surrounding blood and heart, the biomechanics of BHV should be examined from multidimensional perspectives including physiological, surgical, and medical aspects. As BHVs are an inert tissue and exhibit complex mechanical behaviors, hemodynamic stress is known as one of the important factors that determine the biocompatibility and performance of implantable systems [88, 89].

Among structural components of the heart valve (i.e., collagen, elastin, and GAG), collagen is the main component of connective tissue and contributes to the strength and stiffness of the heart valve. It also reduces stress and stabilizes valve motion. Fatigue leads to tissue deterioration resulting from damage to the collagen type I and loss of GAG proteins [90, 91]. A decrease in the extensibility of tissue as a function of the number of cycles may be attributable to the capability of collagen fibers to undergo larger changes in orientation and crimp with cyclic loading [92]. Biaxial mechanical outcomes indicated a decreasing radial extensibility that can be explained by stiffening of the effective collagen fiber network as well as a decrease in the splay of the collagen fibers [89]. These findings along with the subsequent study [93] suggested that the loss in flexural rigidity with fatigue may be a result of not only loss of collagen stiffness but also of fiber debonding and degradation of the amorphous extracellular matrix.

Elastin forms a matrix that surrounds collagen and links the collagen fiber bundles, enabling collagen to extend in diastole and contract in systole, thus, maintaining its rest geometry. GAGs are important structural components of the connective tissues, cushioning shock during valve cycles. The loss of GAGs during fatigue leads to increased interfibrillar calcification and inadequate material stability. These findings could lead to the development of chemical/physical endurable technologies that minimize hemodynamic stress and reduce fatigue-induced damage on BHV.

18.7 TISSUE ENGINEERING IN HEART VALVES

18.7.1 Introduction of Tissue-Engineered Scaffolds

Tissue engineering is the construction of tissue from its cellular components, which combine most of the characteristics of a natural healthy tissue. The term "tissue engineering" was introduced by Dr. Fung in 1987 and denotes an emerging multidisciplinary field involving biology, medicine, and engineering techniques to create new organs and body parts out of your own cells or someone with a similar biological makeup [94]. Tissue engineering is vastly applied to heart valve therapy because of its nonthrombogenicity, infection resistance capability, and cellular viability, allowing for the growth and remodeling of the tissue-engineered heart valves and eliminating repetitive replacement procedures in a growing recipient.

Cells are often implanted or seeded into an artificial structure (i.e., scaffolds) capable of supporting three-dimensional tissue formation. Scaffolds usually serve to recapitulate the *in vivo* milieu, allowing cells to influence their own microenvironments. Scaffolds can be used for one of the following purposes [95, 96]:

- Allow cell attachment and migration
- Deliver and retain cells and biochemical factors
- Enable diffusion of vital cell nutrients and expressed products
- Exert certain mechanical and biological influences to modify the behavior of the cell phase

The traditional approach of seeding or implanting a three-dimensional, biodegradable scaffolding with cells has not been as successful as expected as a result of the complexity and difficulty in duplicating cell structures. Some innovative approaches with endothelialized networks containing a vascular geometry or bioartificial constructs seemed to be promising in engrafting and maintaining essential functionalities [97, 98], but they were still considered far from bearing fruit. As an alternative approach, individual tissue modules were created from specialized cells and then embedded in tiny cubes like Legos, so that 3D structures could be built in such a way that they form the right organs, such as myofibers for muscles, lobules for livers, and nephrons for kidneys [99]. This technique was used to build tubes that could function as capillaries, potentially helping to provide an immediate blood supply and nutrients to scaffolds.

Among various cardiovascular applications of tissue-engineering techniques, three potential approaches to the field of tissue-engineered heart valves are 1) cell seeding of polymeric scaffolds, 2) cell seeding of acellularized xenogeneic valves and subsequent implantation, and 3) *in vivo* repopulation of acellularized donor valves with the recipients' own endothelial cells and fibroblasts [100–102]. The main challenges in tissue-engineered heart valves as a blood-contacting implantable device are ease of structural deterioration, ease of *in vivo* thrombosis of the implanted tissue-engineered valves, and the maintenance of *in vivo* growth potential for the congenital heart surgery application [103, 104].

18.7.2 Synthetic Scaffolds for Heart Valves

The field of cardiovascular tissue engineering encompasses the production of bioartificial, tissue-engineered heart valves and vessels. However, all manufactured tissues are symmetric and isotropic; i.e., they do not resemble the helical assembly of the cardiac muscle bands; instead, they display a uniform microstructure [105]. The macro- and microstructure of the heart are highly asymmetric and anisotropic. The ingenious interplay of muscle fibers and myocardial sheets in the native heart muscle explains the increase of thickness of the left ventricular wall at a rate of 35–40% during systole, while the single myofiber only increases its thickness at a rate of 8%. To achieve this functionality, the heart muscle has to rely on a dense network of vessels. The plain construct seems unable to develop the vortex forces and the orchestrated sheer stress, which is necessary for the effective production of cardiac work.

Tissue-engineered synthetic scaffolds (Figure 18.13) are usually polymeric matrices made of polyglycolic acid,

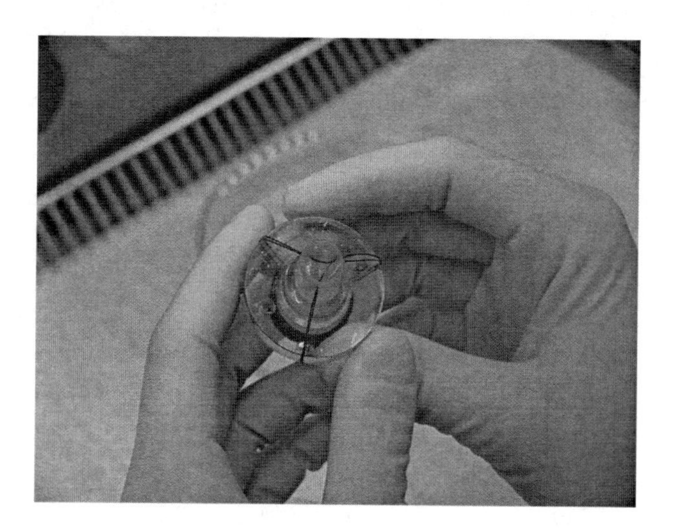

FIGURE 18.13 Tissue-engineered heart valve.

polyglycolic acid, and polylactic acid [106–108]. These polymers are biocompatible, biodegradable, well characterized, and FDA approved for human implantation. Synthetic polymers are processed into tissue-engineered heart valves in two structural stages: a primary structure where the polymer exists in a basic form and a secondary structure where these basic forms are transformed into more complex and structurally complete scaffolds [109].

Several fabricating processes are available for the valve structure (or tertiary structure) of the tissue-engineered heart valves. The common method used the sewing technique for the leaflets of neotissue into position, thus, forming a complete valve. The surgical procedure in the sewing method is technically demanding and time consuming. As a simplified method, scaffolds were produced by bonding an assembly of nonwoven mesh through needle punching the textiles together [110]. The most recent and advanced methodology uses stereolithography to create the tertiary structure of a heart valve, in which the heart valve matrix is recreated from models derived via X-ray computed tomography. These models subsequently used the thermal processing technique to generate the heart valve scaffolds [111].

The use of a synthetic scaffold has major merits in two folds. First, it means that those in need of a surgery or implantation don't have to wait for a cadaver. Stem cells even serve as a means to produce new one. Second, the use of a fully synthetic scaffold means that the patient's own cells rather than animal's create the new organ. As a result, the body recognizes the new organ as its own and does not attempt to reject it, removing the need for immunosuppressive drugs. The major disadvantages of synthetic scaffolds are occasional incidences of cell necrosis and apoptosis.

18.7.3 Natural and Acellularized Scaffolds for Heart Valves

Natural scaffold is composed of either intact animal tissue or pure structural components, such as collagen and elastin, and maintains the architecture and biological information of the native tissue. Although cryopreserved homografts have been successful, allowing for a satisfactory quality of life to the operated patients, valve substitutes seemed to have some drawbacks in humans as a result of limited availability and structural modifications with time. The structural change has been related mostly to the absence of a number of viable cells great enough to allow for an active remodeling and turnover of the extracellular matrix [112].

To overcome these problems, valvular substitutes were devised to be repopulated by homologous differentiated or undifferentiated cells (multipotent or stem cells) grown on a scaffold obtained by acellularization of a native extracellular matrix (ECM) (human, porcine) or on biodegradable synthetic polymers [113]. Although a completely artificial scaffold has stringent requirements related to design, composition, and biomechanical performance with time, a natural scaffold retains mechanical and structural properties, such as tensile strength resulting from extracellular matrix proteins, GAGs, and growth factors [101].

An acellularized scaffold does not require prior cell seeding as it has the probability of repopulation with endogenous circulating cells. Natural valve leaflets contain a higher calcium amount than the neighboring sinuses and wall tissues, which is correlated with increased leaflet degenerative calcification clinically. As a result of reduced calcium content and the absence of viable cellular components including apoptotic cells, mineral deposition sites, and nucleation, an acellularized scaffold has reduced antigenicity and calcification [114]. A recent study on acellularized scaffolds implanted in the sheep model has displayed lowered calcification as compared with the natural cryopreserved valves [115].

Acellular biological tissues, bovine pericardia (BP), have been generated for tissue-engineering applications [116]. Acellular BP was treated with acetic acid, which increased the pore size and porosity of the scaffolds and subsequently conjugated with RGD polypeptides. RGD-modified acellular scaffolds served as the best one for the attachment of human mesenchymal stem cells (hMSCs) and the fastest one for their proliferation among various testing conditions in 10-day *in vitro* cell line studies. Seeded cells reside deep into the scaffold, adding evidence for the potential application of modified acellular BP to tissue-engineered heart valves.

18.7.4 Future Tissue Engineering in Heart Valves

Future tissue engineering will be most keenly felt in the fields of advanced electronic and computer sciences. Software development is one of the most socially transforming technologies to date, which can be applicable to tissue engineering. The evolutionary paths of medicine and electronics are correlated, with electronic innovation enabling new medical devices, while medical innovation yields new capabilities of electronics.

Much of the motivation for nanotechnology comes from the fact that the scale of engineering is shrinking on numerous areas. For instance, a microchip provides solutions to medical designers for electroporation and related challenges in tissue-engineering devices including artificial heart valves [117]. Microscale electroporation in biological cells involves rapid structural rearrangement and formation of pores in the lipid bilayer in response to an externally applied electric field [118]. Advent of the implantable chip may allow an entire organ to be constructed on a single microchip, in which the microscopic structure of the system is interchanneled and organized. Similarly, an implantable chip equipped with a noninvasive sensor could be designed for assessment of blood pressure and functionality of heart valves and remotely monitored patient's blood status and health conditions.

Other technologies, such as particle leaching, soft lithography and bioprinting, enhanced pores, microfluidic channels, and stem cell approach [119–127], will greatly contribute to the therapeutic potential of tissue engineering in cardiovascular applications. With the advancement of tissue engineering, the artificial heart could be created to test new drugs or therapies for cardiovascular diseases. If engineered hearts are easily and economically produced, numerous experiments can be made without sacrificing animals or getting help from human volunteers.

ASSESSMENT QUESTIONS

18.1. What are the main cardiovascular diseases?

18.2. What are the main cardiovascular drug classes?

18.3. Describe briefly how the renin-angiotensin system regulates blood pressure.

18.4. What is the characteristic sequence of chemical bonds present in all nitrovasodilator drugs?

18.5. Which enzyme is inhibited by statins?

18.6. Which type of calcium channel is inhibited by the calcium channel blockers/antagonists?

18.7. Angiotensin II binds to which receptor to control arterial blood pressure?

18.8. What is the mechanism of action of organic nitrates or nitric oxide?

18.9. Why are the low-molecular-mass organic nitrates such as nitroglycerin administered with an inert carrier such as lactose?

18.10. What are the most effective drugs for the reduction of LDL levels?

18.11. How do the cholesterol-lowering drugs such as statins work? What is their target and mechanism of action?

18.12. Why are some statins like lovastatin and simvastatin less water soluble than other statins?

18.13. Which enzyme converts angiotensin I into angiotensin II?

18.14. When was the first clinically used angiotensin II receptor blocker (ARB) developed?

18.15. What are the two main components of the cardiovascular system?

18.16. How many compartments or chambers are present in a fully developed and mature heart?

18.17. What are the two major circulation systems that constitute the cardiovascular system?

18.18. What is the type of blood carried by the pulmonary artery and the pulmonary vein?

18.19. The mammalian heart has four valves; what are they and where are they located?

18.20. Describe how differences in the structure between the two types of heart valves (type I: aortic and pulmonary; type II: tricuspid and mitral) relate to heart function?

Type I: thinner leaflets, no chordae tendinae, closed during filling of ventricles

Type II: thicker leaflets, chordae tendinae connect valve to inside of ventricle wall to prevent inversion during contraction of ventricles

18.21. You have been asked to design a new artificial valve graft as an implantable device.

a. Discuss the conditions and constraints of this design, the material requirements, and your choice of material.

b. What would you conduct to assess biocompatibility? What information do the results of each test provide (in general terms)?

c. For the above tests, what can't you determine at each stage of the testing (or what problems are there that require further, more complicated testing)?

18.22. Define the different types of grafts that are possible based on the relationship of the donor and the recipient. Explain the basis of compatibility for natural tissue implants and the difference in the degree of compatibility among various graft types.

18.23. As a result of the shortage of organ donors, many options have been considered for heart transplants. Give an example of an allograph and a xenograph in the area of heart transplants. What three types of testing would need to be completed before an allograft transplant? Why would a xenograft be less likely to be accepted by the recipient's immune system?

18.24. Discuss the relative advantages/disadvantages of heart valve replacement by porcine xenograft and by a metal valve design, respectively. Your discussion should include the issues of calcification as well as other failure mechanisms (including physiological function).

18.25. What three types of testing would need to be completed before an allograft transplant? Why would a xenograft be less likely to be accepted by the recipient's immune system?

18.26. What are major courses of bioprothetic heart valve failure?

18.27. What are major steps for tissue calcification?

18.28. Discuss the application of tissue-engineering techniques to the development of synthetic heart valves.

18.29. What factors are mainly involved with a blood-contacting implant? What implant properties may influence these factors and in what way?

18.30. You are asked to evaluate biomaterials: ceramics, titanium, and PVC (polyvinylchloride). Which may have the least potential of causing cancer? What testing would you do to assess the carcinogenic potential of these materials? Are there any limitations in each test?

REFERENCES

1. Spaan, J., et al. (2008). Coronary structure and perfusion in health and disease. *Philosophical transactions. Series A, Mathematical, Physical, and Engineering Sciences*, *366* (*1878*), 3137–3153.
2. Libby, P., Ridker, P.M., Hansson, G.K. (2011). Progress and challenges in translating the biology of atherosclerosis. *Nature*, *473*(*7347*), 317–325.
3. Weber, C., Noels, H. (2011). Atherosclerosis: current pathogenesis and therapeutic options. *Nature Medicine*, *17*(*11*), 1410–1422.
4. Chaitman, B.R., Laddu, A.A. (2012). Stable angina pectoris: antianginal therapies and future directions. *Nature Reviews Cardiology*, *9*(*1*), 40–52.
5. Cannon, R.O. (2005). Mechanisms, management and future directions for reperfusion injury after acute myocardial infarction. *Nature Clinical Practice Cardiovascular Medicine*, *2*(2), 88–94.
6. Landmesser, U., Drexler, H. (2005). Chronic heart failure: an overview of conventional treatment versus novel approaches. *Nature Clinical Practice Cardiovascular Medicine*, *2*(*12*), 628–638.
7. Ruilope, L.M. (2012). Current challenges in the clinical management of hypertension. *Nature Clinical Practice Cardiovascular*, (*5*), 267–275.
8. Harrison-Bernard, L.M. (2009). The renal renin-angiotensin system. *Advances in Physiology Education*, *33*(*4*), 270–274.
9. Mirzoyev, Z., Anavekar, N.S., Chen, H.H. (2005). Renal and humoral pathophysiological actions of angiotensin II in congestive heart failure. *Drugs Today (Barc)*, *41*(2), 129–139.
10. Dai, W., Kloner, R.A. (2011). Potential role of renin-angiotensin system blockade for preventing myocardial ischemia/reperfusion injury and remodeling after myocardial infarction. *Journal of Postgraduate Medicine*, *123*(2), 49–55.
11. Mehta, P.K., Griendling, K.K. (2007). Angiotensin II cell signaling: physiological and pathological effects in the cardiovascular system. *American Journal of Physiology - Cell Physiology*, *292*(*1*), C82–C97.
12. Nantel, P., Rene de Cotret, P. (2010). The evolution of angiotensin blockade in the management of cardiovascular disease. *Canadian Journal of Cardiology*, *26*, 7E–13E.
13. Gerc, V., Buksa, M. (2010). Advantages of renin-angiotensin system blockade in the treatment of cardiovascular diseases. *Medical Archives*, *64*(*5*), 295–299.
14. Dasgupta, C., Zhang, L. (2011). Angiotensin II receptors and drug discovery in cardiovascular disease. *Drug Discovery Today*, *16*(*1–2*), 22–34.
15. Timmermans, P.B., et al. (1993). Angiotensin II receptors and angiotensin II receptor antagonists. *Pharmacological Reviews*, *45*(2), 205–251.
16. Pitt, B., et al. (1997). Randomised trial of losartan versus captopril in patients over 65 with heart failure (Evaluation of Losartan in the Elderly Study, ELITE). *Lancet*, *349*(*9054*), 747–752.
17. Naik, P., et al. (2010). Angiotensin II receptor type 1 (AT1) selective nonpeptidic antagonists--a perspective. *Bioorganic & Medicinal Chemistry*, *18*(*24*), 8418–8456.
18. Brunner, H.R., et al. (1993). Angiotensin II antagonists. *Clinical and Experimental Hypertension*, *15*(*6*), 1221–1238.
19. Sarafidis, P.A., Georgianos, P.I., Lasaridis, A.N. (2010). Diuretics in clinical practice. Part I: mechanisms of action, pharmacological effects and clinical indications of diuretic compounds. *Expert Opinion on Drug Safety*, *9*(2), 243–257.
20. Sarafidis, P.A., Georgianos, P.I., Lasaridis, A.N. (2010). Diuretics in clinical practice. Part II: electrolyte and acid-base disorders complicating diuretic therapy. *Expert Opinion on Drug Safety*, *9*(2), 259–273.
21. Ernst, M.E., Moser, M. (2009). Use of diuretics in patients with hypertension. *New England Journal of Medicine*, *361* (22), 2153–2164.
22. Paul, S. (2002). Balancing diuretic therapy in heart failure: loop diuretics, thiazides, and aldosterone antagonists. *Journal of Congestive Heart Failure and Circulatory Support*, *8*(*6*), 307–312.
23. Mayer, B., Beretta, M. (2008). The enigma of nitroglycerin bioactivation and nitrate tolerance: news, views and troubles. *British Journal of Pharmacology*, *155*(2), 170–184.
24. Morley, D., Keefer, L.K. (1993). Nitric oxide/nucleophile complexes: a unique class of nitric oxide-based vasodilators. *Journal of Cardiovascular Pharmacology*, *22*(7), S3–S9.
25. Triggle, D.J. (2006). L-type calcium channels. *Current Pharmaceutical Design*, *12*(*4*), 443–457.
26. Nadar, S., Blann, A.D., Lip, G.Y. (2004). Antihypertensive therapy and endothelial function. *Current Pharmaceutical Design*, *10*(29), 3607–3614.

27. Du, L., Li, M. (2010). Modeling the interactions between alpha(1)-adrenergic receptors and their antagonists. *Current Computer-Aided Drug Design, 6(3)*, 165–178.
28. Heran, B.S., Galm, B.P., Wright, J.M. (2009). Blood pressure lowering efficacy of alpha blockers for primary hypertension. *Cochrane Database of Systematic Review, 4*, CD004643.
29. Djavan, B., et al. (2010). Benign prostatic hyperplasia: current clinical practice. *Primary Care, 37(3)*, 583–597.
30. Cruickshank, J.M. (2010). Beta-blockers and heart failure. *Indian Heart Journal, 62(2)*, 101–110.
31. Frishman, W.H. (2008). Beta-Adrenergic blockers: a 50-year historical perspective. *American Journal of Therapy, 15(6)*, 565–576.
32. Zicha, S., et al. (2006). Beta-blockers as antiarrhythmic agents. *Handbook of Experimental Pharmacology, 171*, 235–266.
33. Aronow, W.S. (2010). Current role of beta-blockers in the treatment of hypertension. *Expert Opinion on Pharmacotherapy, 11(16)*, 2599–2607.
34. Sadowitz, B., Maier, K.G., Gahtan, V. (2010). Basic science review: Statin therapy—Part I: The pleiotropic effects of statins in cardiovascular disease. *Vascular and Endovascular Surgery, 44(4)*, 241–251.
35. Sadowitz, B., et al. (2010). Statin therapy—Part II: Clinical considerations for cardiovascular disease. *Vascular and Endovascular Surgery, 44(6)*, 421–433.
36. Law, M.R., Wald, N.J., Rudnicka, A.R. (2003). Quantifying effect of statins on low density lipoprotein cholesterol, ischaemic heart disease, and stroke: Systematic review and meta-analysis. *BMJ, 326(7404)*, 1423.
37. Gotto, A.M., Jr., (2006). Statins, cardiovascular disease, and drug safety. *The American Journal of Cardiology, 97(8A)*, 3C–5C.
38. Tang, W.H., Francis, G.S. (2010). Statin treatment for patients with heart failure. *Nature Reviews Cardiology, 7(5)*, 249–255.
39. Avraham, R. *The Circulatory System*. Chelsea House Publishers, Philadelphia, PA, 2000.
40. Davis, G.P., Park, E. *The Heart: The Living Pump*. U.S. News Books, Washington, DC, 1981.
41. Chilnick, L.D. *Heart Disease: An Essential Guide for the Newly Diagnosed*. Perseus Books Group, Philadelphia, PA, 2008.
42. Breuer, C.K., et al. (2004). Application of tissue-engineering principles toward the development of a semilunar heart valve substitute. *Tissue Engineering, 10(11–12)*, 1725–1736.
43. Taylor, P.M., et al. (2003). The cardiac valve interstitial cell. *The International Journal of Biochemistry & Cell Biology, 35(2)*, 113–118.
44. Tsiaras, A. *The InVision Guide to a Healthy Heart*. HarperCollins, New York, NY, 2005.
45. Butany, J., et al. (2003). Biological replacement heart valves. Identification and evaluation. *Cardiovascular Pathology, 12 (3)*, 119–139.
46. Ross, D.N. (1962). Homograft replacement of the aortic valve. *Lancet, 2(7254)*, 487.
47. Yacoub, M.H., et al. (2006). An evaluation of the Ross operation in adults. *Journal of Heart Valve Disease, 15(4)*, 531–539.
48. Lee, C.H., et al. (1998). Inhibition of aortic wall calcification in bioprosthetic heart valves by ethanol pretreatment: Biochemical and biophysical mechanisms. *Journal of Biomedical Materials Research, 42(1)*, 30–37.
49. Zakir, R.M., Al-Dehneh, A., Dabu, L., Kapila, R., Saric, M. (2004). Mitral bioprosthetic valve endocarditis caused by an unusual microorganism, Gemella morbillorum, in an intravenous drug user. *Journal of Clinical Microbiology, 42(10)*, 4893–4896.
50. Stewart, B.F., et al. (1997). Clinical factors associated with calcific aortic valve disease. Cardiovascular Health Study. *Journal of the American College of Cardiology, 29(3)*, 630–634.
51. Davies, S.W., Gershlick, A.H., Balcon, R. (1991). Progression of valvar aortic stenosis: A long-term retrospective study. *European Heart Journal, 12(1)*, 10–14.
52. O'Keefe, J.H., Jr., et al. (1991). Degenerative aortic stenosis. One effect of the graying of America. *Postgraduate Medicine, 89(2)*, 143–146151–144.
53. Schoen, F.J., Levy, R.J. (2005). Calcification of tissue heart valve substitutes: Progress toward understanding and prevention. *Annals of Thoracic Surgery, 79(3)*, 1072–1080.
54. Agmon, Y., et al. (2001). Aortic valve sclerosis and aortic atherosclerosis: Different manifestations of the same disease? Insights from a population-based study. *Journal of the American College of Cardiology, 38(3)*, 827–834.
55. Ballinger, M.L., et al. (2004). Regulation of glycosaminoglycan structure and atherogenesis. *Cellular and Molecular Life Sciences, 61(11)*, 1296–1306.
56. Farzaneh-Far, A., et al. (2001). Vascular and valvar calcification: Recent advances. *Heart, 85(1)*, 13–17.
57. Speer, M.Y., Giachelli, C.M. (2004). Regulation of cardiovascular calcification. *Cardiovascular Pathology, 13(2)*, 63–70.
58. Akat, K., Borggrefe, M., Kaden, J.J. (2009). Aortic valve calcification: Basic science to clinical practice. *Heart, 95(8)*, 616–623.
59. Rajamannan, N.M. (2010). Mechanisms of aortic valve calcification: The LDL-density-radius theory: a translation from cell signaling to physiology. *American Journal of Physiology - Heart and Circulatory Physiology, 298(1)*, H5–15.
60. Weska, R.F., et al. (2010). Natural and prosthetic heart valve calcification: Morphology and chemical composition characterization. *Artificial Organs, 34(4)*, 311–318.
61. Miller, J.D., et al. (2008). Dysregulation of antioxidant mechanisms contributes to increased oxidative stress in calcific aortic valvular stenosis in humans. *Journal of the American College of Cardiology, 52(10)*, 843–850.
62. Ito, S., Saito, T., Amano, K. (2004). *In vitro* apatite induction by osteopontin: Interfacial energy for hydroxyapatite nucleation on osteopontin. *Journal of Biomedical Materials Research Part A, 69(1)*, 11–16.

63. Matsui, Y., et al. (2003). Osteopontin deficiency attenuates atherosclerosis in female apolipoprotein E-deficient mice. *Arteriosclerosis, Thrombosis, and Vascular Biology, 23(6)*, 1029–1034.
64. Warrier, B., et al. (2005). The functional role of C-reactive protein in aortic wall calcification. *Cardiology, 104*(2), 57–64.
65. Mahnken, A.H., et al. (2007). MDCT detection of mitral valve calcification: Prevalence and clinical relevance compared with echocardiography. *American Journal of Roentgenology, 188*(5), 1264–1269.
66. Shi, S.R., et al. (1999). Calcium-induced modification of protein conformation demonstrated by immunohistochemistry: What is the signal? *Journal of Histochemistry and Cytochemistry, 47(4)*, 463–470.
67. Scott, M.J., Vesely, I. (1996). Morphology of porcine aortic valve cusp elastin. *Journal of Heart Valve Disease, 5(5)*, 464–471.
68. Schmid, K., et al. (1980). Chemical and physicochemical studies on the mineral deposits of the human atherosclerotic aorta. *Atherosclerosis, 37*(2), 199–210.
69. Gerrity, R.G., Cliff, W.J. (1975). The aortic tunica media of the developing rat. I. Quantitative stereologic and biochemical analysis. *Lab Investigation, 32(5)*, 585–600.
70. Singla, A., Lee, C.H. (2003). Inhibition of CEM calcification by the sequential pretreatment with ethanol and EDTA. *Journal of Biomedical Materials Research Part A, 64(4)*, 706–713.
71. Shen, M., et al. (1996). Proteins and bioprosthetic calcification in the rat model. *Journal of Heart Valve Disease, 5(1)*, 50–57.
72. Kleinman, J.G., Wesson, J.A., Hughes, J. (2004). Osteopontin and calcium stone formation. *Nephron Physiology, 98*(2), 43–47.
73. Berkner, K.L., Runge, K.W. (2004). The physiology of vitamin K nutriture and vitamin K-dependent protein function in atherosclerosis. *Journal of Thrombosis and* Haemostasis, *2(12)*, 2118–2132.
74. Schurgers, L.J., et al. (2001). Role of vitamin K and vitamin K-dependent proteins in vascular calcification. *Zeitschrift für Kardiologie, 90(3)*, 57–63.
75. Shanahan, C.M., et al. (1998). The role of Gla proteins in vascular calcification. *Critical Reviews in Eukaryotic Gene Expression, 8(3–4)*, 357–375.
76. Levy, R.J., et al. (1983). Biologic determinants of dystrophic calcification and osteocalcin deposition in glutaraldehyde-preserved porcine aortic valve leaflets implanted subcutaneously in rats. *American Journal of Pathology, 113* (2), 143–155.
77. Lincoln, J., et al. (2007). Sox9 is required for precursor cell expansion and extracellular matrix organization during mouse heart valve development. *Developmental Biology, 305(1)*, 120–132.
78. Grande-Allen, K.J., et al. (2007). Glycosaminoglycan synthesis and structure as targets for the prevention of calcific aortic valve disease. *Cardiovascular Research, 76(1)*, 19–28.
79. Chenevard, R., et al. (2006). Persistent endothelial dysfunction in calcified aortic stenosis beyond valve replacement surgery. *Heart, 92(12)*, 1862–1863.
80. Rajamannan, N.M., et al. (2005). Atorvastatin inhibits calcification and enhances nitric oxide synthase production in the hypercholesterolaemic aortic valve. *Heart, 91(6)*, 806–810.
81. Lee, T.C., et al. (2000). Abnormal aortic valve development in mice lacking endothelial nitric oxide synthase. *Circulation, 101(20)*, 2345–2348.
82. Kanno, Y., et al. (2008). Nitric oxide regulates vascular calcification by interfering with TGF- signalling. *Cardiovascular Research, 77(1)*, 221–230.
83. Bosse, Y., Mathieu, P., Pibarot, P. (2008). Genomics: The next step to elucidate the etiology of calcific aortic valve stenosis. *Journal of the American College of Cardiology, 51(14)*, 1327–1336.
84. Lindroos, M., et al. (1994). Factors associated with calcific aortic valve degeneration in the elderly. *European Heart Journal, 15*(7), 865–870.
85. Otto, C.M., et al. (1994). Characterization of the early lesion of 'degenerative' valvular aortic stenosis. Histological and immunohistochemical studies. *Circulation, 90*(2), 844–853.
86. Messika-Zeitoun, D., et al. (2007). Aortic valve calcification: Determinants and progression in the population. *Arteriosclerosis, Thrombosis, and Vascular Biology, 27(3)*, 642–648.
87. Armstrong, E.J., Bischoff, J. (2004). Heart valve development: Endothelial cell signaling and differentiation. *Circulation Research, 95(5)*, 459–470.
88. Robicsek, F., Thubrikar, M.J., Fokin, A.A. (2002). Cause of degenerative disease of the trileaflet aortic valve: Review of subject and presentation of a new theory. *Annals of Thoracic Surgery, 73(4)*, 1346–1354.
89. Sacks, M.S. (2001). The biomechanical effects of fatigue on the porcine bioprosthetic heart valve. *Journal of Long-Term Effects of Medical Implants, 11(3–4)*, 231–247.
90. Broom, N.D. (1977). The stress/strain and fatigue behaviour of glutaraldehyde preserved heart-valve tissue. *Journal of Biomechanics, 10(11/12)*, 707–724.
91. Vyavahare, N., et al. (1999). Mechanisms of bioprosthetic heart valve failure: Fatigue causes collagen denaturation and glycosaminoglycan loss. *Journal of Biomedical Materials Research, 46(1)*, 44–50.
92. Sacks, M.S., Yoganathan, A.P. (2007). Heart valve function: A biomechanical perspective. *Philosophical Transactions of the Royal Society of London—Series B: Biological Sciences, 362(1484)*, 1369–1391.
93. McClure, R.S., et al. (2010). Late outcomes for aortic valve replacement with the Carpentier-Edwards pericardial bioprosthesis: Up to 17-year follow-up in 1,000 patients. *Annals of Thoracic Surgery, 89(5)*, 1410–1416.
94. Vesely, I. (2005). Heart valve tissue engineering. *Circulation Research, 97(8)*, 743–755.
95. Ma, P.X. (2004). Scaffolds for tissue fabrication. *Materials Today, 5(5)*, 30–40.

96. Mikos, A., Temenoff, J. (2000). Formation of highly porous biodegradable scaffolds for tissue engineering. *Electronic Journal of Biotechnology, 3(2)*, 114–119.
97. Levenberg, S., et al. (2005). Engineering vascularized skeletal muscle tissue. *Nature Biotechnology, 23(7)*, 879–884.
98. Shin, M., et al. (2004). Endothelialized networks with a vascular geometry in microfabricated poly(dimethyl siloxane). *Biomedical Microdevices, 6(4)*, 269–278.
99. Du, Y., et al. (2008). Directed assembly of cell-laden microgels for fabrication of 3D tissue constructs. *Proceedings of the National Academy of Science of the USA, 105(28)*, 9522–9527.
100. Korossis, S.A., et al. (2002). Tissue engineering of cardiac valve prostheses II: Biomechanical characterization of decellularized porcine aortic heart valves. *Journal of Heart Valve Disease, 11(4)*, 463–471.
101. Mendelson, K., Schoen, F.J. (2006). Heart valve tissue engineering: Concepts, approaches, progress, and challenges. *Annals of Biomedical Engineering, 34(12)*, 1799–1819.
102. Rieder, E., et al. (2005). Tissue engineering of heart valves: Decellularized porcine and human valve scaffolds differ importantly in residual potential to attract monocytic cells. *Circulation, 111(21)*, 2792–2797.
103. Schenke-Layland, K., et al. (2003). Complete dynamic repopulation of decellularized heart valves by application of defined physical signals-an *in vitro* study. *Cardiovascular Research, 60(3)*, 497–509.
104. Sodian, R., et al. (2000). Fabrication of a trileaflet heart valve scaffold from a polyhydroxyalkanoate biopolyester for use in tissue engineering. *Tissue Engineering, 6(2)*, 183–188.
105. Bloor, D., et al. *The Encyclopedia of Advanced Materials. 4 Vol. Set*. Pergamon Press, Oxford, UK, 1994.
106. Hoerstrup, S.P., et al. (2000). Functional living trileaflet heart valves grown *in vitro*. *Circulation, 102(19)*, 44–49.
107. Shinoka, T., et al. (1996). Tissue-engineered heart valves. Autologous valve leaflet replacement study in a lamb model. *Circulation, 94(9)*, 164–168.
108. Sodian, R., et al. (2000). Tissue engineering of heart valves: In vitro experiences. *Annals of Thoracic Surgery, 70(1)*, 140–144.
109. Fong, P., et al. (2006). The use of polymer based scaffolds in tissue-engineered heart valves. *Progress in Pediatric Cardiology, 21(2)*, 193–199.
110. Sutherland, F.W., et al. (2005). From stem cells to viable autologous semilunar heart valve. *Circulation, 111(21)*, 2783–2791.
111. Sodian, R., et al. (2002). Application of stereolithography for scaffold fabrication for tissue engineered heart valves. *Journal of the American Society of Artificial Internal Organs, 48(1)*, 12–16.
112. Holmes, T.C., et al. (2000). Extensive neurite outgrowth and active synapse formation on self-assembling peptide scaffolds. *Proceedings of the National Academy of Science of the USA, 97(12)*, 6728–6733.
113. Semino, C.E., et al. (2004). Entrapment of migrating hippocampal neural cells in three-dimensional peptide nanofiber scaffold. *Tissue Engineering, 10(3–4)*, 643–655.
114. Oray, B.N., et al. (2009). Novel propylene oxide-treated bovine pericardium as soft tissue repair material and potential scaffold for tissue engineering. *Surgical Technology International, 18(47)*, 54.
115. Hopkins, R.A., et al. (2009). Decellularization reduces calcification while improving both durability and 1-year functional results of pulmonary homograft valves in juvenile sheep. *Journal of Thoracic Cardiovascular Surgery, 137(4)*, 907–913, 913e901-904.
116. Dong, X., et al. (2009). RGD-modified acellular bovine pericardium as a bioprosthetic scaffold for tissue engineering. *Journal of Materials Science: Materials in Medicine, 20(11)*, 2327–2336.
117. Li, P.C., Harrison, D.J. (1997). Transport, manipulation, and reaction of biological cells on-chip using electrokinetic effects. *Analytical Chemistry, 69(8)*, 1564–1568.
118. Joshi, R.P., et al. (2001). Self-consistent simulations of electroporation dynamics in biological cells subjected to ultrashort electrical pulses. *Physical Review E Statistical Nonlinear Soft Matter Physics, 64(1 Pt 1)*, 011913.
119. Caplan, A.I. (2007). Adult mesenchymal stem cells for tissue engineering versus regenerative medicine. *Journal of Cellular Physiology, 213(2)*, 341–347.
120. Jamieson, W.R., et al. (1995). Structural deterioration in Carpentier-Edwards standard and supraannular porcine bioprostheses. *Annals of Thoracic Surgery, 60(2)*, S241–247.
121. Jethi, R.K., Inlow, C.W., Wadkins, C.L. (1970). Studies of the mechanism of biological calcification. I. Kinetic properties of the *in vitro* calcification of collagen-containing matrix. *Calcified Tissue Research, 6(2)*, 81–92.
122. Lee, W., et al. (2010). On-demand three-dimensional freeform fabrication of multi-layered hydrogel scaffold with fluidic channels. *Biotechnology and Bioengineering, 105(6)*, 1178–1186.
123. Liu, B., et al. (2010). Modularly assembled porous cell-laden hydrogels. *Biomaterials, 31(18)*, 4918–4925.
124. Liu Tsang, et al. (2007). Fabrication of 3D hepatic tissues by additive photopatterning of cellular hydrogels. *The Journal of the Federation of American Societies for Experimental Biology, 21(3)*, 790–801.
125. Otto, C.M., et al. (1999). Association of aortic-valve sclerosis with cardiovascular mortality and morbidity in the elderly. *New England Journal of Medicine, 341(3)*, 142–147.
126. Stachowiak, A.N., et al. (2005). Bioactive hydrogels with an ordered cellular structure combine interconnected macroporosity and robust mechanical properties. *Advanced Materials, 14(4)*, 399–403.
127. Yue, Z., et al. (2010). Preparation of three-dimensional interconnected macroporous cellulosic hydrogels for soft tissue engineering. *Biomaterials, 31(32)*, 8141–8152.

19

RECENT ADVANCES IN OCULAR DRUG DELIVERY

Varun Khurana, Deep Kwatra, Vibhuti Agrahari, and Ashim K. Mitra

19.1 CHAPTER OBJECTIVES

- To outline fundamental concepts, rationale, and principles for recent advances in ocular drug delivery.
- To provide understanding of general barriers faced when delivering drugs to the eye.
- To compare the advantages and disadvantages of different drug delivery routes used to achieve enhanced ocular drug delivery.
- To compare the advantages and disadvantages of different advanced drug delivery systems used for ocular drug delivery.

19.2 INTRODUCTION

Achieving sufficient ocular bioavailability is the foremost challenge for ophthalmic drug delivery scientists. The presence of the blood–ocular barriers, which consists of the blood–aqueous barrier (BAB) and blood–retinal barrier (BRB), present the most significant obstacle in achieving this goal. Diseases such as age-related macular degeneration (AMD), diabetic retinopathy, and cytomegalovirus (CMV) retinitis have therapies available, but their success depends on the level of drug molecules achieved in the posterior segment of the eye. Although topical drug delivery through eye drops is a very widely used drug delivery method, the delivery of therapeutic agents to the anterior segment by this method is obstructed by factors such as tear turnover, solution drainage, and limited precorneal residence time. Moreover, anatomical barriers prevent actives from reaching the deep ocular tissues after topical administration [1].

To achieve the relevant levels of the therapeutic molecules in the ocular tissues, two major approaches have been taken by ocular drug delivery scientists. The first approach has involved the search for better, noninvasive, and therapeutically more efficient routes for ocular drug delivery. The second approach has involved the advancement of conventional drug delivery strategies resulting in a novel drug delivery system or devices capable of more controlled and targeted therapy. In this chapter, we will describe various advances made in drug delivery routes and drug delivery systems for ocular drugs along with concerns associated with such methods.

19.3 BARRIERS TO OCULAR DRUG DELIVERY

A drug administered either topically or systemically has to cross multiple barriers before it reaches the intended site within the eye. These barriers can be classified broadly as anatomical barriers as well as physiological barriers.

19.3.1 Anatomical Barriers

After topical administration, absorption can be through either the corneal or the noncorneal route. The cornea is composed of five layers: epithelium, Bowman's membrane, stroma, descement's membrane, and endothelium. The corneal

Advanced Drug Delivery, First Edition. Edited by Ashim K. Mitra, Chi H. Lee, and Kun Cheng.

epithelium is considered the chief barrier to most topically administered drugs. Its five to six layers of columnar cells, and significantly tight junctions impart a very high paracellular resistance of 12–16 kΩ cm. Because hydrophilic drugs have to infuse through intercellular spaces, the epithelium acts as a major barrier to them. Lipophilic drugs, in contrast, can transport easily through the epithelium via transcellular transport. Bowman's membrane is a cellular layer composed of arbitrarily arranged collagen fibrils. The stroma is composed of multiple layers of hexagonally arranged collagen fibers with aquatic porous channels. Hence, this layer can easily allow hydrophilic drugs to permeate, whereas it forms a significant barrier for lipophilic drugs. Thus, for a drug to reach into the eye, it should have optimum lipophilicity to infuse through the corneal epithelium as well as sufficient hydrophilicity to permeate across stroma. The remaining layers are leaky and do not act as significant barriers. The anatomy of the eye along with the common delivery routes has been summarized in Figure 19.1.

The noncorneal route involves the movement of drugs across the conjunctiva and sclera to reach the vitreous humor. This route is important especially for large and hydrophilic molecules such as peptides, proteins, and small interfering RNAs (siRNAs) [3]. The permeability of conjunctiva is higher than the cornea for hydrophilic molecules as it does not express tight junction proteins as highly as corneal epithelium. Still, this route is not considered a major pathway for drug delivery as the limbal area has a high blood supply. These blood vessels remove a significant fraction of absorbed dose from the target site into the systemic circulation [4]. Only a small fraction of the dose enters the sclera, then moves into the uveal tract, and finally reaches the vitreous.

19.3.2 Physiological Constraints

Topically administered drugs show poor bioavailability because of additional precorneal factors such as solution drainage, tear dilution, tear turnover, and increased lacrimation [5]. Rapid clearance from the precorneal area reduces contact time between the tissue and the drug, in turn decreasing the time for the drug to permeate, which leads to reduced bioavailability. The average tear volume is 7–9 μL with a turnover rate of 16% per minute [6]. After topical application, lacrimation is increased significantly leading to substantial dilution of the administered drug. This in turn decreases the drug concentration in the precorneal space, thereby reducing drug absorption. A large portion of the administered dose is also lost through nasolacrimal drainage and spillage. All these factors can act synergistically, lowering the drug entry into the eye.

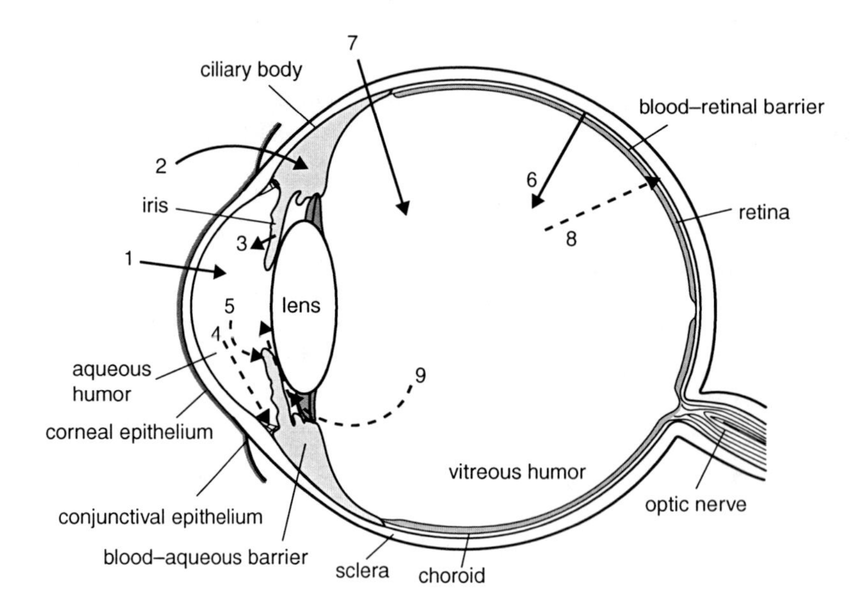

FIGURE 19.1 Schematic presentation of the ocular structure with the routes of drug kinetics illustrated. The numbers refer to the following processes: 1) transcorneal permeation from the lacrimal fluid into the anterior chamber, 2) noncorneal drug permeation across the conjunctiva and sclera into the anterior uvea, 3) drug distribution from the bloodstream via blood–aqueous barrier into the anterior chamber, 4) elimination of drug from the anterior chamber by the aqueous humor turnover to the trabecular meshwork and Sclemm's canal, 5) drug elimination from the aqueous humor into the systemic circulation across the blood–aqueous barrier, 6) drug distribution from the blood into the posterior eye across the blood–retina barrier, 7) intravitreal drug administration, 8) drug elimination from the vitreous via posterior route across the blood–retina barrier, and 9) drug elimination from the vitreous via anterior route to the posterior chamber. Adapted from Ref. 2.

19.3.3 Drug and Dosage Form Related Factors Affecting Bioavailability

The ocular bioavailability of an administered dosage form can also be altered by the physicochemical properties of the drug molecule. The rate of absorption is dependent on the physical properties of the drug molecule (solubility, lipophilicity, degree of ionization, and molecular weight) and on the structure of the tissue.

19.3.3.1 ***Solubility*** Solubility is dependent on the p*K*a of the drug and on the pH of the solution (which further determines the ratio of ionized to unionized molecules). As only the unionized molecules can permeate across the biological membrane, pH and p*K*a also are critical parameters.

19.3.3.2 ***Lipophilicity*** Lipophilicity and corneal permeability have a sigmoidal relationship [7]. As mentioned, it is easier for a lipophilic drug to permeate through the corneal epithelium. The lipophilicity of a molecule is measured using a partition coefficient that is defined as the ratio of unionized solute concentration in octanol and water (Equations (19.1) and (19.2)).

$$\text{Partition coefficient } (P) = \frac{[\text{Solute}]_{\text{octanol}}}{[\text{Solute}]_{\text{water}}^{\text{unionized}}} \tag{19.1}$$

$$\text{Log}\, P = \log\left(\frac{[\text{Solute}]_{\text{octanol}}}{[\text{Solute}]_{\text{water}}^{\text{unionized}}}\right) \tag{19.2}$$

The log P value ranging from 2 to 4 results in optimum corneal permeation [8]. But again, as mentioned, the hydrophilicity of the inner layer of the cornea (stroma) requires higher hydrophilicity for optimal permeation. Thus, for a drug to have optimal permeation across the cornea, it must be unionized, with optimum aqueous solubility as well as lipophilicity.

19.3.3.3 ***Molecular Weight and Size*** Because the major pathway for the permeation of hydrophilic drugs is a paracellular route, molecular weight and particularly size play an important role in determining the permeability characteristics. Because the tight junctions present on the apical cell layers of the corneal epithelium have a diameter of 2 nm, only molecules with less than 500 Dalton molecular weight are allowed to permeate [9]. The paracellular permeability is further limited by the pore density ($4.3 \times 10^6/\text{cm}^2$) of the corneal epithelium. Permeability across the stroma is not supposed to be dependent on the partition coefficient, but it is a function of molecular size and radius [10]. Nonetheless, as mentioned, it still is a rate-limiting factor for highly lipophilic compounds.

19.4 ADVANCES IN OCULAR DRUG DELIVERY

Now with a better understanding of the problems faced by ocular drug delivery, scientists are using various approaches for achieving the sufficient drug concentration in the desired ocular tissues. Two major approaches have been used in this regard. The first is the use of novel routes of drug delivery that somehow bypass the barriers. The second approach is to develop novel formulations that overcome the barriers through innovative drug delivery techniques.

19.4.1 Drug Delivery Through Novel Routes

Conventional routes for ocular drug delivery involve administering drugs topically or through systemic routes. As discussed, these routes of drug delivery face several barriers that limit their success in achieving the desired drug concentrations at the target tissue. Advancements in drug design, drug formulation, and pharmaceutics have overcome many of these flaws. But scientists have experimented with alternative routes of drug delivery that overcome the barriers presented by more conventional routes.

19.4.1.1 ***Intravitreal Injection*** Intravitreal injections (IVIs), as the name suggests, deliver therapeutic agents directly into the vitreous humor through pars plana. They overcome the inaccessibility of the vitreous humor through the cornea and limit the drug loss through scleral blood flow. Drugs introduced through this route are administered as a solution, suspension, or depot formulation. Once equilibrium is reached within the vitreous, the drug concentration declines following first-order kinetics, either through the retina or to the anterior chamber through the aqueous humor [11]. This rate of decline within the vitreous humor is dependent on the molecular weight of the drug. Large-molecular-weight drugs have longer half-lives as high as several weeks compared with less than 3 days for small-molecular-weight compounds [12].

Although it is a highly efficient method for delivering drugs into the posterior segment, it suffers from major limitations. After repetitive dosing (which is common in most retinal diseases), damage to the eye may occur in the form of retinal detachment, cataract, hyperemia, and endophthalmitis [13]. This problem can be overcome by the use of sustained-release drug delivery systems that help by avoiding frequent administration, thus, allowing for better patient compliance.

19.4.1.2 ***Subconjunctival Route*** In this route, the drug is delivered beneath the conjunctiva membrane that lines the inner surface of eyelid, thus circumventing the cornea and conjunctiva. It is much less invasive route when compared with intravitreal injections [14]. As it bypasses the rate-limiting barrier for the hydrophilic drugs, it allows more of the drug to pass through the sclera and enter into the vitreous humor. Delivery of sustained-release systems such as nanoparticles by this route allows the formation of a depot and thus aids in minimizing the dosing frequency [15]. Subconjunctival administration of Avastin (Genentech, South San Francisco, CA) (bevacizumab: a recombinant monoclonal antibody against vascular endothelial growth factor [VEGF]) proved to be effective in reducing the degree of corneal neovascularization [16]. Other publications have shown that delivery of nanoparticles as well as proteins such as insulin through this route gives higher bioavailability and greater sustenance of the drug [17–19].

19.4.1.3 Retrobulbar Route The retrobulbar injection is given through the eyelid and the orbital fascia, and it places the drug into retrobulbar space. This route is used primarily for administrating the drug to the back of the globe such as antibiotics, corticosteroids, and especially anesthesia. It is a delicate procedure because there is a risk of damaging the optic nerve. This can be prevented by limiting the insertion of a needle to less than 1.5 cm behind the globe [13, 20]. This route has been found to be effective in uveitis by infusion of triamcinolone [21]. This route is used primarily for the delivery of anesthetic agents as it has been shown to result in minor or no change in intraocular pressure, although in certain orbital diseases, the reverse is also possible [22–24].

19.4.1.4 Peribulbar Route The peribulbar route for drug delivery involves injections above and/or below the globe. This is the route of choice especially for the delivery of anesthesia in case of cataract surgery as it has a reduced risk of injury to the intraorbital structure compared with the retrobulbar route as the anesthetic is deposited outside the muscle cone [25]. A study conducted by Rizzo et al. showed that this form of administering anesthesia is a safer and more effective alternative to classic techniques of regional ocular anesthesia [26]. Several reports suggest that the chance of retrobulbar hemorrhage recurrence with peribulbar blocks is very low. Although it is a safer method, reports of elevated intraocular pressure as well as bleeding within or outside the muscle cone after peribulbar injection do exist [22, 27, 28].

19.4.1.5 Sub-Tenon Route Sub-Tenon injections are administered into a cavity between Tenon's capsule and sclera. This approach uses a blunt cannula for administration of the drug. Preoperative deep sedation is also not a requirement for this procedure [29]. Because of reduced complications and nonreliance on sharp needles, the sub-Tenon route is believed to be a better route for delivering anesthesia compared with retrobulbar and peribulbar [30]. Injecting steroids through the sub-Tenon route has been shown to be an effective treatment of uveitis and cystoid macular edema complicating uveitis [31]. Triamcinolone acetonide administered through this route is effective against pain and scleral inflammation in nonnecrotizing scleritis [32]. Previously published reports suggest that sub-Tenon delivery of Triamcinolone acetonide results in a low risk of endopthalmitis as compared with intravitreal injections. Although alterations in blood pressure and glucose levels have been reported, its association with drug or delivery route remains unclear [33–35]. Certain reports claim this route to be the safest and most effective way to achieve local ocular anesthesia.

19.4.1.6 Intracameral Route The intracameral route involved the delivery of the drug to the anterior chamber of the eye by injection. Drugs administered through this route are mainly for anterior segment ailments as there is limited accessibility of therapeutic agent to the posterior segment. It is generally employed in cataract surgery [13]. A clinical report suggested that dexamethasone when administered intracamerally is effective in decreasing the postoperative inflammation in glaucomatous and nonglaucomatous patients [36]. In patient with neovascular glaucoma, intracamerally administered bevacizumab has been shown to reduce the aqueous VEGF levels [37]. It is a cost-effective and more efficient method of delivering antibiotics compared with most commonly applied topical antibiotics and antifungal agents [38–40]. This route is preferred to prevent the occurrence of endophthalmitis after cataract surgery [41, 42].

19.5 CONTROLED DRUG DELIVERY

As discussed previously in the chapter, there are multiple barriers to ocular drug delivery. In addition to the progress made in identifying and perfecting various delivery routes to the eye, a lot of progress has been made in generating novel delivery systems. These novel delivery systems are designed with an aim to overcome the ocular barriers, achieve higher targetability, as well as to sustain the drug for the longer periods of time.

19.5.1 Iontophoresis

The noninvasive technique of iontophoresis has been investigated for many years, which enhances the transfer of ionized drug molecule into the tissue by the application of small electric current [43, 44]. The drug is applied using two electrodes: One electrode has the same charge of the drug, and the other electrode is placed elsewhere on the body to complete the circuit and serves as ground electrode [45]. Migration and electro-osmosis are the two mechanisms that help in the movement of drug across the membrane [43]. Iontophoresis has been used in the ophthalmic drug delivery of many antibacterial, antiviral, antifungal, steroids, as well as antimetabolites and even genes for many years. It is a less invasive technique compared with intraocular injections and has an advantage over topical administration in terms of higher bioavailability of the drug molecule [45]. It is used most often for transscleral delivery of drugs to treat posterior chamber eye diseases. It can be used for sustained delivery based on the type of probe used.

19.5.1.1 ***Iontophoretic Device*** The basic components of an electorphoretic device include electrodes, a power source (battery or AC voltage), a timer, and an ampere meter for measuring the output of current [46].

19.5.1.2 ***Probes for Iontophoresis***

(1) *Eyegate Applicator (Eyegate Pharmaceuticals, Inc., Waltham, MA):* The reusable, battery-powered generator and a disposable applicator (made of soft silicone rubber) are the main components of this iontophoretic device. It also consists of two silicone tubes. One tube is used for infusion of drug into the applicator while other tube acts as a drainage tube. There are no signs of vision obstruction in this treatment as the drug solution does not cover the corneal surface, which makes it more patient compatible [46].
(2) *OcuPhor (Iomed, Inc., Salt Lake City, UT):* The main components of this system are a drug applicator, a electrode, and an electric iontophoresis drug controller. A therapeutic level of drugs has been achieved in the anterior and posterior tissues, including the retina and choroids using this device [46].
(3) *Hydrogels:* These are the polymer masses consisting of hydrophilic groups, such as –OH, –COOH, $-CONH_2$, $-SO_3H$, or –COOR. They were synthesized using hydroxyethyl methacrylate (HEMA), which is crosslinked with ethylene glycol dimethacrylate (EGDMA) at different water concentrations (53–80%) and EGDMA contents (0.5–4.0%) in the monomer mixture. Most suitable combination for studies is prepared from HEMA, 2% (v/v) EGDMA, and 75% water. High levels of drug (gentamicin sulfate) were achieved in the posterior segment of rabbit eye by transscleral and transconjunctival iontophoresis using hydrogel probe [46].

19.5.2 Implants

Implants control the release kinetics of drugs from polymeric delivery systems by using various polymer and polymeric membranes. This is an invasive technique in which implants are placed at the pars plana of the eye [43, 47–49].

19.5.2.1 ***Classification of Implants***

Nonbiodegradable Solid Implants As the name suggests, these are made up of nonbiodegradable polymeric material and are needed to be surgically removed after a certain period of time. The most commonly used polymers are polyvinyl alcohol (PVA)-ethylene vinyl acetate (EVA), and polysulfone capillary fiber (PCF). The advantage of PVA-EVA polymeric device that makes it superior from others is that it does not produce an initial burst of drug [50, 51]. PCF is impermeable to water and allows permeation for lipophilic as well as hydrophilic compounds. This polymer has an advantage of having macrovoids in its outer membrane, which provides greater surface area for drug diffusion and release [50].

Examples of non-biodegradable implants are as follows:

(1) *Vitrasert (Bausch & Lomb, Incorporated, Rochester, NY)*: This is a nonbiodegradable control release ganciclovir PVA and EVA implant that is approved by FDA. It is used for the prevention and treatment of CMV retinitis associated with AIDS and controls the progression of disease for 8 months. The disadvantages associated with this implants are occasional endophthalmitis and increased rate of retinal detachments [46].
(2) *Retisert (Bausch & Lomb, Incorporated):* This is used for the treatment of chronic uveitis and is the first marketed silicone laminated fluocinolone acetonide PVA implant that can sustain the drug for up to 3 years. The side effects associated with this implant are cataract and increased intraocular pressure [46].

19.5.2.2 ***Biodegradable Solid Implants*** As the name suggests, these are made up of biodegradable polymeric material and thus get degraded over time; they need not be surgically removed. The most commonly used polymers are PLA, poly(glycolic acid) (PGA), and poly(lactic-co-glycolic acid) (PLGA), and polycaprolactone (PCL). PLA, PGA, and PLGA polymers undergo bulk erosion of encapsulated drug rather than surface erosion, which is limited to the matrix surface of polymers [50, 52]. PCL degradation produces small polymeric fragments on cleavage of an ester bond, which undergoes phagocytosis after getting diffused from matrix [50]. 1,3-Bis carboxyphenoxypropane (PCPP) with sebacic acid (SA) is the most commonly used biodegradable polyanhydride polymer. These polymers have good biocompatibility and undergo surface erosion [50, 53]. Examples of biodegradable implants include Surodex (Oculex Pharmaceuticals, Inc., Sunnyvale, CA) and Posurdex (Posurdex, Allergan, Irvine, CA), which are the biodegradable PLGA implants with $60\,\mu g$ dexamethasone and $700\,\mu g$ dexamethasone, respectively. Surodex and Posurdex are designed for the treatment of intraocular inflammation and macular edema, respectively [46].

19.5.3 Gelifying Systems

These systems include various phase-changing polymers to achieve sustained drug delivery. After administration, the

TABLE 19.1 Application of Implants [47]

Disease	Drug	Implant	Drug Release
Proliferative vitroretinopathy (PVR)	Daunomycin	PCF	21 days
	Dexamethasone	PVA-EVA	More than 3 months
	Fluorouracil	PLGA	Almost 3 weeks
CMV retinitis	Ganciclovir	PVA-EVA	More than 80 days
	Ganciclovir	PLA/PLGA (75/25)	More than 3 months (eye) More than 5 months (choroid)
Endophthalmitis	Ciprofloxacin	PLA or PLGA	Up to 4 weeks
Uveitis	Cyclosporin A	PVA-EVA	More than 6 months
Choroidal neovascular membranes (CNVM)	Triamcinolone acetonide	PVA	At least 35 days

polymer changes into a semisolid or solid matrix, which is responsible for the sustained release of the drug. This change in polymer phase is induced by temperature, ion concentration, or pH [43]. Fluids showing viscoelastic nature are generally preferred as they maintain high viscosity under of low shear conditions and vice versa. Examples of gelifying systems include hyaluronic acid, polyacrylic acid, and chitosan [50].

19.5.3.1 ***Hyaluronic Acid (HA)*** HA is a biological polymer of high molecular weight with linear polysaccharides in its extracellular matrix. Sodium hyaluronate (SH) shows high water-binding capacity, nonirritancy, increased viscosity, pseudoplastic behavior, which makes it an attractive ophthalmic drug-delivery vehicle. On administration of 0.2% and 0.75% SH solutions in an albino rabbit eye, a twofold to threefold increase in the absorption of 1% pilocarpine hydrochloride solution was been observed. The retention potential of a drug at the ocular surface is influenced directly by the molecular weight of the HA polymer [50]. HA has also been employed as a gelling material to prolong drug release of 5-fluorouracil or dexamethasone [54].

19.5.3.2 ***Polyacrylic Acid (PAA) Derivatives*** These are categorized into carbopols and polycarbophils. They differ in terms of crosslinking and type of crosslinking agent used like allyl sucrose for carbopols and divinyl glycol for polycarbophils. A more constant drug release is observed in the case of PAA formulation of betaxolol compared with 0.5% solution of betaxolol in rabbits. An increase in the uptake of gentamicin has been observed when it is formulated with polycarbophil in comparison with its aqueous control formulation [50]. One of the earliest ophthalmic gels available in the market using this technology was Pilopine HS (Alcon Laboratories, Inc., Fort Worth, TX). Various other commercially available products are Zirgan (Sirion Therapeutics, Inc., Tampa, FL), a carbomer-based ophthalmic gel formulation of ganciclovir; AzaSite (Inspire Pharmaceuticals, Durham, NC), azithromycin formulation of polycarbophil; and Nyogel 0.1% (Novartis Opthalmics, Hampshire, U.K.), a carbomer-containing timolol once daily gel [54].

19.5.3.3 ***Chitosan*** Chitosan has various favorable biological properties such as biodegradability, nontoxicity, and biocompatibility. It is a polycationic biopolymer with pseudoplastic and viscoelastic properties. Chitosan formulation shows prolonged drug residence on ocular tissues by increasing the viscosity of solution and also because of its mucoadhesive properties [50]. The bioavailability of indomethacin has been improved dramatically in the cornea as well as in the aqueous humor after topical ocular instillation of polycaprolactone nanoparticles coated with chitosan [51]. De Campos et al. [52] investigated the potential of chitosan nanoparticles loaded with cyclosporine A for the specific delivery of drugs to the ocular mucosa. These chitosan-based formulations have the ability to deliver drug on external ocular tissues without compromising inner ocular structures and systemic drug exposure while simultaneously sustaining the drug release.

19.5.4 Hydrogels

Hydrogels are the polymeric networks that are hydrophilic in nature and can imbibe large quantities of water and biological fluids in a swollen crosslinked gel system for drug delivery. They have the ability to retain hydrophobic and hydrophilic agents, small molecules, and macromolecules after carrying out modifications in their permeation and diffusion characteristics. They can be biodegradeable or nonbiodegradeable and are also biocompatible. Polysaccharides have been used widely in the formation of hydrogel and are considered advantageous over synthetic polymers. Some examples of polysaccharides are alginate, dextran, gellan, carrageenan, pullulan, xanthan, and hyaluronic acid [53]. PNIPAAm hydrogel has a lower critical solution temperature (LCST) or transition temperature at $\sim$32°C. It is widely known as thermosensitive material. The introduction of the polyethylene glycol diacrylate (PEG-DA) to

PNIPAAm improves the thermoresponsive characteristics of hydrogel and has homogeneous pores. PNIPAAm–PEG-DA hydrogels have been used for the encapsulation and delivery of protein (anti-VEGF agent) to the posterior segment of eye. This hydrogel has the ability to encapsulate protein to a greater extent and release the protein in a sustained and controlled fashion. It can be injected in a liquid form to the juxtascleral region or vitreous cavity, and on exposure to body temperature, it forms gel readily and releases the protein [55]. Singh et al. evaluated stimuli-sensitive hydrogels (comprising of polyacrylic acid as gelling agents, hydroxyl ethyl cellulose as viscolizer, and sodium chloride as isotonic agent). These hydrogels formulated using timolol maleate (as a model drug) showed prolonged reduction in intraocular pressure of albino rabbits eye along with a decreased frequency of administration compared with the marketed conventional dosage forms [56].

19.5.5 Particulate Formulations

The particulate formulations consist of microscopic delivery systems that can control the release of drugs as well as enhance its permeation through a barrier. These properties of the formulations allow them to overcome the difficulties in delivering the drug to the posterior of segment of eye by topical administration. Because of the size and targetability of these formulations, these can also be used for targeting systemically administered drugs to the ocular tissues. These formulations are used not only to facilitate drug efficacy but also to rarefy adverse effects [57]. The most commonly used particulate formulations are described in the following sections.

19.5.5.1 Microspheres Microspheres are 1 to 100 μm in size and are formulated using biodegradable and biocompatible polymers that are approved by the U.S. Food and Drug Administration (FDA), such as polylactide and PLGA. Controlled, sustained drug release, subcellular size, and biocompatibility are the various advantages that are offered with the use of microparticles. These systems are usually administered by a less invasive procedure than surgical implantation, i.e., intravitreal injection. Using this strategy, sustained drug release from the formulation has been observed for weeks or even months. Microspheres of PKC412 are given as periocluar injection to treat choroidal neovascularization. PKC412 acts as an inhibitor of protein kinase C and receptors for VEGF, and it suppresses choroidal neovascularization after penetrating the sclera [43]. Rafat et al. reported the effective delivery of a transactivator of transcription-enhanced green fluorescent protein fusion (Tat-EGFP) using PEG-PLA microparticles to the outer segment of the retina. These microparticles exhibit high *in vitro* and *in vivo* stability leading to sustained ocular drug delivery [58].

19.5.5.2 Nanoparticles Nanoparticles are formulated using biodegradeable polymers: natural or synthetic polymers, lipids, phospholipids, and even metals. They usually have diameter less than 1 μm. For efficient drug delivery to ocular tissues, the drug molecule can be encapsulated or attached to the surface of nanoparticles. PLAs, polycyanoacrylate; poly(D,L-lactides); and natural polymers like chitosan, gelatine, sodium alginate, and albumin are various biodegradeable polymers that are employed for the formulation of nanoparticles. Nanoparticles administered by intravitreal injection show their presence for (up to) 4 months in the retinal pigment epithelium (RPE). The presence of polystyrene nanospheres (nonbiodegradable) is observed in neuroretina and RPE of rabbits for 2 months after intravitreal injection. For disease like CMV retinitis, albumin nanoparticles are considered safe and effective drug delivery systems (DDS). These nanoparticles demonstrate biodegradeable, nontoxic, and nonantigenic properties [59–61]. The topical delivery of gatifloxacin for microbial keratitis has been improved using chitosan/sodium alginate nanoparticles that act as submicroscopic reservoirs for ocular drug delivery [62, 63]. Kao et al. reported that pilocarpine-loaded chitosan/carbopol nanoparticles showed best slow release profile that lasted up to 24 h when compared with other formulations of pilocarpine, i.e., solution, gel, or liposomes [62, 64].

19.5.5.3 Liposomes These are biodegradable and amphiphilic DDS that are formulated using phospholipids and cholesterol. Lipid composition, size, surface charge, method of preparation, etc. are the various properties that can be modified according to their use. Liposome-encapsulated phosphodiester (16-mer oligothymidylate) (pdT16) oligonucleotides have been used for CMV retinitis. The administration of these liposomes results in the sustained release of therapeutic agents into the vitreous and retina-choroid instead of nontargeted tissues (sclera and lens) [59, 65, 66]. Afouna et al. [67] reported improved transcorneal permeation and long-lasting intraocular pressure, decreasing the effect of demeclocycline by employing its liposomal formulation. The *in vitro* transcorneal permeability and intraocular distribution of GCV was increased 3.9-fold, and it was decreased 2- to 10-fold, respectively, by employing its liposomal formulations [68].

19.5.5.4 Niosomes These DDS are bilayered structures and can entrap both hydrophilic and lipophilic drugs. They have low toxicity and are chemically stable. Niosomes are also used in their modified form, i.e., discosomes (12–16 μm), in ophthalmology. Discosomes contain non-ionic surfactant, i.e., Solulan C24 (Lubrizol Corporation, Wickliffe, OH). They fit better in the cul-de-sac of the eye and do not get drained into systemic pool because of their large size. High entrapment efficiency of timolol maleate has been observed in discosomes than niosomes by Vyas et al. [59, 66, 69, 70]. Kaur et al. [71] reported that ocular absorption kinetics of timolol maleate (TM) can be improved using bioadhesive niosomal delivery system. In aqueous humor, the concentration of TM (from niosomes) was 1.7 times the TM solution. Also, the area under concentration (AUC) for niosomal formulation of TM was 2.34 times that of the TM solution.

19.5.5.5 ***Dendrimers*** These DDS consist of an inner core surrounded by a series of branches. They have the ability to display multiple copies of surface groups for biological recognition processes and are easy to prepare and functionalize. These properties make them attractive system for drug delivery. Drug release through this DDS can be improved by using bioadhesive polymers, such as poly(acrylic) acids. This modification will help in optimizing contact with the absorbing area, which will ultimately result in a prolonged residence time and decrease dosage frequency. Polyamidoamine (PAMAM) dendrimers are used to overcome problems like blurred vision and the formation of a veil in corneal area, leading to a loss of eyesight associated with bioadhesive polymers [59, 72–75]. Marano et al. [76] used a dendrimer-based approach for the delivery of anti-VEGF oligonucleotide (ODN-1) to treat choroidal neovascularization in rats.

19.5.6 Transporter Targeted Strategy

To improve ocular bioavailability, chemical modification of a drug molecule has been employed as a traditional approach. Transporter targeted modification of a drug is usually employed to improve actively the bioavailability of the therapeutic. Membrane transporters are the membrane-bound proteins that help in the translocation of nutrients across the biological membranes. These transporter systems are classified into two categories: efflux transporter and influx transporter. These transporters belong to adenosine triphosphate (ATP) binding cassette superfamily and solute carrier (SLC) superfamily, respectively. An efflux transporter (depending on their polarization) acts as a hindrance for entry of a drug molecule into the cell, whereas an influx transporter (depending on their polarization) facilitates entry of a drug molecule into the cell [77]. Additional information on influx and efflux transporters is provided in Table 19.2 [80–89] and Table 19.3 [90–106]. The drug molecules are modified in such a way that they can evade the efflux transporters and simultaneously become the target for influx transporters. Amino acid, vitamin, and peptide-conjugated prodrugs of acyclovir and gancyclovir have been generated that were able to both evade efflux and increase permeability across the rabbit cornea [78–80].

19.6 MACROMOLECULAR DRUG DELIVERY

Recently, the delivery of macromolecules such as proteins and peptide offers a promising approach toward ocular diseases. These macromolecules are instilled into the eye for local/topical use. The barriers associated with small molecular delivery become even more significant when macromolecules are delivered. Therapeutic delivery of macromolecule possesses limitations such as large size, charge, hydrophilic nature, membrane permeability, and high susceptibility to metabolic inactivation.

TABLE 19.2 Influx Transporter-Targeted Prodrug Strategy for Ocular Drug Delivery

Membrane Influx Transporter	Tissue/Cell Line	Inference	References
Glucose transporter (GLUT1)	Human retinal pigment epithelial (HRPE) cells	Uptake of Glu-dopamine prodrug via GLUT1	[77, 81]
Amino acid transporter (B0,+)	Cornea	L-aspartate ACV showed four times higher transcorneal permeability as compared with ACV	[77, 82]
Oligopeptide transporter (OPT)	Retina	Gly-Val-, Val-Val-, and Tyr-Val-GCV showed two time higher permeability as compared to GCV	[77, 83]
Sodium-dependent multivitamin transporter (SMVT)	Retina	Biotin-GCV showed higher permeability into retina-choroid and slower elimination from vitreous as compared to GCV	[77, 80]
B(0,+)	Cornea	Gamma-glutamate-ACV (EACV) showed higher aqueous solubility as compared with ACV	[77, 84]
OPT	Cornea	Gly-Val-, Val-Val-, and Tyr-Val-GCV are recognized by OPT transporter, which resulted in higher AUC and C_{max} of GCV	[77, 85, 86]
B(0,+)	Cornea	Phenylalanine-ACV and EACV showed competitive inhibition with L-arginine (substrate of B(0,+))	[77, 87]
OPT	Cornea	L-valine ACV showed three times higher transcorneal permeability as compared with ACV	[77, 88]
OPT	rPCEC cells and cornea	Val-quinidine and Val-Val-quinidine were found to be substrates for peptide transporters	[77, 89]

TABLE 19.3 Expression/Tissue Distribution and Substrates of ABC Family Efflux Transporters

Efflux Transporter	Expression/Tissue Distribution	Selected Ocular Drugs/Substrates*	References
P-glycoprotein (P-gp or MDR1)	Human choroid/RPE tissue, porcine choroid-RPE tissue, D407, h1RPE, rat retinal vessels, and TR-iBRB	Miconazole, azelastin, ketotifen, timolol, cyclosporine, etc.	[90–101]
Multidrug resistance protein (MRP)	Primary human RPE cells, ARPE-19, and porcine choroid-RPE tissue	Cyclosporine, fluorescein, etc.	[90, 91, 93, 96, 102]
MRP1			
MRP2	D407	Cyclosporine	[90, 91, 96]
MRP3	D407, mouse retinal vascular endothelial cell	—	[90, 91, 96, 103]
MRP4	ARPE-19, D407, primary human RPE, bRPE, mouse retinal vascular endothelial cell	Ganciclovir, zidovudine, etc.	[90, 91, 96, 103]
MRP5	Human RPE cells, mouse RPE, ARPE-19, D407	5-Fluorouracil	[90, 91, 96, 104, 105]
MRP6	Mouse retinal vascular endothelial cell	—	[90, 91, 96, 103]
MRP7	Mouse retinal vascular endothelial cell	—	[91, 103]
MRP8		5-Fluorouracil	[91]
Breast cancer resistance protein (BCRP)	Mouse retinal vessels, TR-iBRB, D407	Cyclosporine, triamcinolone, zidovudine, etc.	[90, 91, 96, 106]

*Information regarding selected ocular drug/substrates is solely based on Ref. 91. For additional information, check the cross-references of Ref. 91.

19.6.1 Challenges for Delivery of Macromolecule

The ocular absorption of peptides is limited by an ocular enzyme called peptidase. Endopeptidases (plasmin and collagenase) and exopeptidases (aminopeptidases) are present in ocular fluids and tissues. Usually, endopeptidase levels are low except in the case of an inflamed or injured eye [107, 108]. To achieve therapeutic levels of macromolecules, peptidase activity should be inhibited [2].

The systemic absorption of protein and polypeptide occurs through mucus membrane of conjunctiva and nasolacrimal system. The systemic delivery of protein and polypeptide therapeutic agent through ocular route has the following advantages [109]:

(1) Rapid absorption through the vasculature.
(2) Prolong drug administration can be achieved by designing specific formulation.
(3) The drug can avoid first pass metabolism.

The systemic delivery of topically instilled peptides drugs to the eye is found to be superior to the parenteral route when the drug is potent and the required doses are low. Results from the prior studies suggest that small polypeptides such as thyrotropin-releasing hormone (TRH) (MW-300), enkephalins (MW-600), luteinizing hormone-releasing hormone (LHRH) (MW-1200), and glucagon (MW3500) showed significant absorption through the eyes [110, 111]. Polypeptides with higher molecular weight such as β-endorphin (MW-5000) and insulin (MW-6000) are absorbed to a much lesser extent. However, the absorption of high molecular weight compounds can be improved by simultaneous use of permeation and absorption enhancers [112]. A list of macromolecules commonly administered through ocular route is provided in Table 19.4.

19.6.2 Permeation Enhancers

Research studies have shown that the bioavailability of insulin can be improved via ocular delivery with co-administration of permeation enhancers in the following descending order: polyoxyethylene-9-lauryl ether > sodium deoxycholate > sodium glycocholate > sodium taurocholate [120]. The permeability of several peptides such as enkephalin [126], TRH, LHRH, glucagon, and insulin [110] toward systemic absorption via the ocular route has been increased by the use of permeation enhancer. Some penetration enhancers like cytoskeletal modulators [110], EDTA, bile salts, and cytochalasin B [127] have also been used to enhance the ocular permeability of hydrophilic micromolecules and macromolecules. Among several penetration enhancers, cytochalasin B shows the potential to increase corneal permeability with minimum membrane damage.

19.7 STEM-CELL-BASED DRUG DELIVERY SYSTEM

Degenerative diseases of the eye or damage or loss to retina are a major complication associated with aging and diabetes.

TABLE 19.4 Macromolecule/Protein and Peptide Delivery Through Ocular Route

Macromolecules (Polypeptides and Protein Drugs)	Therapeutic Application of Macromolecules	Species	References
Adrenocorticotropic hormone (ACTH)	Antiallergic, anti-inflammatory	Rabbit	[113]
Endorphin	Analgesic	Rabbit	[114]
Calcitonin	Paget's disease, hypercalcemia	Rabbit	[115]
Glucagon	Hypoglycemic crisis	Rabbit, rat, human	[116]
Immunoglobulin G protein	Chorio-retinal disorders	Rabbit	[117]
Insulin	Diabetes mellitus	Rabbit, rat, human	[118, 119]
Leu-enkephalin	Analgesic	Rabbit	[120]
Met-enkephalin	Immunostimulant	Rabbit	[121]
Oxytocin	Induce uterine contractions	Rabbit	[122]
Somatostatin	Attenuate miotic responses	Rabbit	[123]
TRH	Diagnosis of thyroid cancer	—	[124]
Vasopressin	Diabetes insipidus	Rabbit	[122]
Vasoactive intestinal peptide (VIP)	Secretion of insulin	Rat	[125]

Retinal dystrophies such as retinitis pigmentosa, Stargardt disease, Best disease, Leber congenital amaurosis, and so on share the loss of photoreceptors after the loss of retinal ganglionic cells (RGCs). Currently, there is a requirement for a direct approach for repairing damaged RPE. Novel treatments are developed by using neuroprotective and regenerative strategies that include stem cell therapy as a potential in the treatment of retinal degenerative diseases. Stem cells have potentially been used for both neuroprotection and cell replacement [128, 129]. Stem cells are known as cells with self-renewal capability and the ability differentiate into a wide variety of cell types. These cells have self-healing potential that helps to restore brain, visual, and motor functions for many incurable conditions [129–131]. The capacities of SC to proliferate indefinitely and differentiate into variety of cell types makes it a potential approach for cell replacement therapy, repair and replace non-functioning neuro-retinal cells. The survival of SC is governed by the production of variety of neuro-tropic factors. The desired property required for donor cells includes migration, integration, cell differentiation and to form synapses for a neuro-retinal cell replacement strategy. Stem cell therapy began in 1945, when researchers discovered that bone marrow transplantation into irradiated mice produced hematopoiesis. In 1961, hematopoietic stem cells were first identified and their role in the migration and differentiation into the multiple cell types was documented [129].

19.7.1 Types of Stem Cells

The different types of stem cells are as follows [130]:

(1) Retinal progenitor cells
(2) Embryonic stem cells
(3) Induced pluripotent stem cells
(4) Mesenchymal stem cells (MSCs)
(5) Bone marrow

19.7.2 Stem Cell Delivery to the Eye

Several methods have been used for the delivery of stem cells in to the eye such as subretinal intravitreal and intravenous routes. Subretinal transplantation of stem cells is advantageous because the cells are placed in the close proximity with retina. In the intravitreal method, the transplanted stem cells are placed adjacent to the retina. This method is simple for inner retinal therapies. The transplanted stem cells move from the vitreous cavity into the retina; however, the inner limiting membrane represents a critical barrier to migration. Approximately 1% of intravitreally transplanted cells usually migrate across the retina. Other techniques to deliver stem cells to the eye include injection of donor cells into the optic nerve, the optic tract [132], and intravenous delivery [133]. The likely mechanism by which the stem cell reaches the retina is regulated by chemokines that are upregulated by the degenerating retina. The benefits of systemic administration of stem cells are that the cells can exert their effect over the entire retina, and if needed, multiple administrations can be easily performed. However, the possibility of systemic diffusion and the lack of targeting following intravenous administration make this route less attractive [134]. Several groups have described the use of human embryonic stem cells (hESCs) to generate a monolayer of RPE-like cells. These hESC-derived cells express the markers that are specific to RPE cells including bestrophin, CRALBP, and RPE65. hESC has been shown to be functionally more similar to mature adult RPE than existing RPE cell lines such as APRE-19 and fetal RPE cells. In animal studies, the use of hESC-RPE has been shown to improve both visual performance as well as photoreceptor rescue [135–137]. In RPE injury, genetic manipulation of HSCs to express RPE65 promotes neuro-epithelial cell differentiation, retinal repair, and recovery of visual function in an animal model [131]. Glaucoma is characterized by a progressive loss of retinal ganglion cells (RGCs). Although treatments for this condition involve a decrease in intraocular pressure, still some patients suffer from progressive vision loss regardless of therapy. In a rat model of glaucoma, the use of intravitreal MSCs upholds the survival of RGCs [138]. The recent discoveries show that using stem cells is a promising approach with encouraging results. However, further elucidation of the biology and immunology of such approaches is needed before the full potential can be realized.

19.8 CONCLUSION

Drug delivery to the eye faces many challenges because of multiple barriers, both physiological and formulation based. Ophthalmologists and ocular drug delivery scientists have made advances to overcome these barriers. As a result, much progress has been made in identifying novel routes of ocular drug delivery that are less invasive, cause fewer side effects, and enhance ocular bioavailability. Additionally, novel drug delivery systems have been developed that can overcome the ocular barriers and both sustain and target the drugs at the desired site.

ASSESSMENT QUESTIONS

19.1. What is the value of the paracellular resistance imparted by the corneal epithelium?

- **a.** 12 to 16 Ω cm
- **b.** 12 to 16 kΩ cm
- **c.** 1 to 5 Ω cm
- **d.** 20 to 50 kΩ cm

19.2. What are the major physiological barriers when delivering drugs to the eye?

- **a.** Solution drainage
- **b.** Tear dilution
- **c.** Increased tear turnover and lacrimation rate
- **d.** All of the above

19.3. What physical properties of drug molecules decide their eventual ocular bioavailability?

- **a.** Solubility
- **b.** Lipophilicity
- **c.** Molecular weight
- **d.** All of the above

19.4. What are the advantages of systemic delivery of proteins and polypeptide therapeutic agents through the ocular route?

- **a.** Topical administration of protein and polypeptides via ocular route
- **b.** Systemic absorption is fast
- **c.** Prolong drug administration can be achieved by designing specific formulation
- **d.** The drug can bypass the hepatic circulation thus avoiding first pass metabolism.
- **e.** All of the above

19.5. Write a brief note on implants.

19.6. What are the different types of stem cells?

19.7. What are the disadvantages of the intravitreal route for ocular drug delivery?

19.8. Describe membrane transporters that play a role in ocular drug delivery in brief detail.

19.9. Describe the ideal characteristics of drug delivery systems in brief detail.

REFERENCES

1. Duvvuri, S., Gandhi, M.D., Mitra, A.K. (2003). Effect of P-glycoprotein on the ocular disposition of a model substrate, quinidine. *Current Eye Research*, *27(6)*, 345–353.
2. Urtti, A. (2006). Challenges and obstacles of ocular pharmacokinetics and drug delivery. *Advanced Drug Delivery Reviews*, *58(11)*, 1131–1135.
3. Ahmed, I., Patton, T.F. (1985). Importance of the noncorneal absorption route in topical ophthalmic drug delivery. *Investigative Ophthalmology & Visual Science*, *26(4)*, 584–587.
4. Barar, J., Javadzadeh, A.R., Omidi, Y. (2008). Ocular novel drug delivery: Impacts of membranes and barriers. *Expert Opinions on Drug Delivery*, *5(5)*, 567–581.
5. Lee, V.H., Robinson, J.R. (1986). Topical ocular drug delivery: Recent developments and future challenges. *Journal of Ocular Pharmacology and Therapeutics*, *2(1)*, 67–108.
6. Hughes, P.M.a.M.A.K., Overview of ocular drug delivery and iatrogenic ocular cytopathologies, in A.K. Mitra (ed.), *Ophthalmic Drug Delivery Systems*, Marcel Dekker, Inc., New York, 1993, pp. 1–27.
7. Wang, W., Sasaki, H., Chien, D.S., Lee, V.H. (1991). Lipophilicity influence on conjunctival drug penetration in the pigmented rabbit: A comparison with corneal penetration. *Current Eye Research*, *10(6)*, 571–579.
8. Schoenwald, R.D., Ward, R.L. (1978). Relationship between steroid permeability across excised rabbit cornea and octanol-water partition coefficients. *Journal of Pharmaceutical Sciences*, *67(6)*, 786–788.

9. Aronow, W.S. (1979). Indications for surgical treatment of stable angina pectoris. *Archives of Internal Medicine, 139(6)*, 690–692.
10. Prausnitz, M.R., Noonan, J.S. (1998). Permeability of cornea, sclera, and conjunctiva: A literature analysis for drug delivery to the eye. *Journal of Pharmaceutical Sciences, 87(12)*, 1479–1488.
11. Maurice, D. (2001). Review: Practical issues in intravitreal drug delivery. *Journal of Ocular Pharmacology and Therapeutics, 17(4)*, 393–401.
12. Marmor, M.F., Negi, A., Maurice, D.M. (1985). Kinetics of macromolecules injected into the subretinal space. *Experimental Eye Research, 40(5)*, 687–696.
13. Raghava, S., Hammond, M., Kompella, U.B. (2004). Periocular routes for retinal drug delivery. *Expert Opinions in Drug Delivery, 1(1)*, 99–114.
14. Hosoya, K., Lee, V.H., Kim, K.J. (2005). Roles of the conjunctiva in ocular drug delivery: A review of conjunctival transport mechanisms and their regulation. *European Journal of Pharmaceutics and Biopharmaceutics, 60(2)*, 227–240.
15. Ghate, D., Edelhauser, H.F. (2008). Barriers to glaucoma drug delivery. *Journal of Glaucoma, 17(2)*, 147–156.
16. Erdurmus, M., Totan, Y. (2007). Subconjunctival bevacizumab for corneal neovascularization. *Graefe's Archive for Clinical and Experimental Ophthalmology, 245(10)*, 1577–1579.
17. Misra, G.P., Singh, R.S., Aleman, T.S., Jacobson, S.G., Gardner, T.W., Lowe, T.L. (2009). Subconjunctivally implantable hydrogels with degradable and thermoresponsive properties for sustained release of insulin to the retina. *Biomaterials, 30(33)*, 6541–6547.
18. Anderson, O.A., Bainbridge, J.W., Shima, D.T. (2010). Delivery of anti-angiogenic molecular therapies for retinal disease. *Drug Discovery Today, 15(7–8)*, 272–282.
19. Carrasquillo, K.G., Ricker, J.A., Rigas, I.K., Miller, J.W., Gragoudas, E.S., Adamis, A.P. (2003). Controlled delivery of the anti-VEGF aptamer EYE001 with poly(lactic-co-glycolic)acid microspheres. *Investigative Ophthalmology & Visual Science, 44(1)*, 290–299.
20. Wadhwa, S., Paliwal, R., Paliwal, S.R., Vyas, S.P. (2009). Nanocarriers in ocular drug delivery: An update review. *Current Pharmaceutical Design, 15(23)*, 2724–2750.
21. Okada, A.A., Wakabayashi, T., Morimura, Y., Kawahara, S., Kojima, E., Asano, Y., Hida, T. (2003). Trans-Tenon's retrobulbar triamcinolone infusion for the treatment of uveitis. *British Journal of Ophthalmology, 87(8)*, 968–971.
22. Nassr, M.A., Morris, C.L., Netland, P.A., Karcioglu, Z.A. (2009). Intraocular pressure change in orbital disease. *Survey of Ophthalmology, 54(5)*, 519–544.
23. Netland, P.A., Siegner, S.W., Harris, A. (1997). Color Doppler ultrasound measurements after topical and retrobulbar epinephrine in primate eyes. *Investigative Ophthalmology & Visual Science, 38(12)*, 2655–2661.
24. Yung, C.W., Moorthy, R.S., Lindley, D., Ringle, M., Nunery, W.R. (1994). Efficacy of lateral canthotomy and cantholysis in orbital hemorrhage. *Ophthalmic Plastic & Reconstructive Surgery, 10(2)*, 137–141.
25. Janoria, K.G., Gunda, S., Boddu, S.H., Mitra, A.K. (2007). Novel approaches to retinal drug delivery. *Expert Opinions on Drug Delivery, 4(4)*, 371–388.
26. Rizzo, L., Marini, M., Rosati, C., Calamai, I., Nesi, M., Salvini, R., Mazzini, C., Campana, F., Brizzi, E. (2005). Peribulbar anesthesia: A percutaneous single injection technique with a small volume of anesthetic. *Anesthesia & Analgesia, 100(1)*, 94–96.
27. Gock, G., Francis, I.C., Mulligan, S. (2000). Traumatic intramuscular orbital haemorrhage. *Clinical & Experimental Ophthalmology, 28(5)*, 391–392.
28. Ahmad, S., A. Ahmad, H.T. Benzon. (1993). Clinical experience with the peribulbar block for ophthalmologic surgery. *Regional Anesthesia, 18(3)*, 184–188.
29. Li, H.K., Abouleish, A., Grady, J., Groeschel, W., Gill, K.S. (2000). Sub-Tenon's injection for local anesthesia in posterior segment surgery. *Ophthalmology, 107(1)*, 41–46; discussion 46–47.
30. Faure, C., Faure, L., Billotte, C. (2009). Globe perforation following no-needle sub-Tenon anesthesia. *Journal of Cataract & Refractive Surgery, 35(8)*, 1471–1472.
31. Lafranco Dafflon, M., Tran, V.T., Guex-Crosier, Y., Herbort, C.P. (1999). Posterior sub-Tenon's steroid injections for the treatment of posterior ocular inflammation: Indications, efficacy and side effects. *Graefe's Archive for Clinical and Experimental Ophthalmology, 237(4)*, 289–295.
32. Johnson, K.S., Chu, D.S. (2010). Evaluation of sub-Tenon triamcinolone acetonide injections in the treatment of scleritis. *American Journal of Ophthalmology, 149(1)*, 77–81.
33. Toda, J., Fukushima, H., Kato, S. (2009). Systemic complications of posterior subtenon injection of triamcinolone acetonide in type 2 diabetes patients. *Diabetes Research and Clinical Practice, 84(2)*, e38–e40.
34. Moshfeghi, D.M., Kaiser, P.K., Scott, I.U., Sears, J.E., Benz, M., Sinesterra, J.P., Kaiser, R.S., Bakri, S.J., Maturi, R.K., Belmont, J., Beer, P.M., Murray, T.G., Quiroz-Mercado, H., Mieler, W.F. (2003). Acute endophthalmitis following intravitreal triamcinolone acetonide injection. *American Journal of Ophthalmology, 136(5)*, 791–796.
35. Benz, M.S., Murray, T.G., Dubovy, S.R., Katz, R.S., Eifrig, C.W. (2003). Endophthalmitis caused by Mycobacterium chelonae abscessus after intravitreal injection of triamcinolone. *Archives of Ophthalmology, 121(2)*, 271–273.
36. Chang, D.T., Herceg, M.C., Bilonick, R.A., Camejo, L., Schuman, J.S., Noecker, R.J. (2009). Intracameral dexamethasone reduces inflammation on the first postoperative day after cataract surgery in eyes with and without glaucoma. *Clinical Ophthalmology, 3*, 345–355.
37. Grover, S., Gupta, S., Sharma, R., Brar, V.S., Chalam, K.V. (2009). Intracameral bevacizumab effectively reduces aqueous vascular endothelial growth factor concentrations in neovascular glaucoma. *British Journal of Ophthalmology, 93(2)*, 273–274.

38. Sharifi, E., Porco, T.C., Naseri, A. (2009). Cost-effectiveness analysis of intracameral cefuroxime use for prophylaxis of endophthalmitis after cataract surgery. *Ophthalmology, 116(10)*, 1887–1896 e1.

39. Yu-Wai-Man, P., Morgan, S.J., Hildreth, A.J., Steel, D.H., Allen, D. (2008). Efficacy of intracameral and subconjunctival cefuroxime in preventing endophthalmitis after cataract surgery. *Journal of Cataract & Refractive Surgery, 34(3)*, 447–451.

40. Shen, Y.C., Wang, C.Y., Tsai, H.Y., Lee, H.N. (2010). Intracameral voriconazole injection in the treatment of fungal endophthalmitis resulting from keratitis. *American Journal of Ophthalmology, 149(6)*, 916–921.

41. Lane, S.S., Osher, R.H., Masket, S., Belani, S. (2008). Evaluation of the safety of prophylactic intracameral moxifloxacin in cataract surgery. *Journal of Cataract & Refractive Surgery, 34(9)*, 1451–1459.

42. Espiritu, C.R., Caparas, V.L., Bolinao, J.G. (2007). Safety of prophylactic intracameral moxifloxacin 0.5% ophthalmic solution in cataract surgery patients. *Journal of Cataract & Refractive Surgery, 33(1)*, 63–68.

43. Del Amo, E.M., Urtti, A. (2008). Current and future ophthalmic drug delivery systems. A shift to the posterior segment. *Drug Discovery Today, 13(3–4)*, 135–143.

44. Bejjani, R.A., Andrieu, C., Bloquel, C., Berdugo, M., Ben-Ezra, D., Behar-Cohen, F. (2007). Electrically assisted ocular gene therapy. *Survey of Ophthalmology, 52(2)*, 196–208.

45. Eljarrat-Binstock, E., Domb, A.J. (2006). Iontophoresis: A non-invasive ocular drug delivery. *Journal of Controlled Release, 110(3)*, 479–489.

46. Myles, M.E., Neumann, D.M., Hill, J.M. (2005). Recent progress in ocular drug delivery for posterior segment disease: Emphasis on transscleral iontophoresis. *Advanced Drug Delivery Reviews, 57(14)*, 2063–2079.

47. Bourges, J.L., Bloquel, C., Thomas, A., Froussart, F., Bochot, A., Azan, F., Gurny, R., BenEzra, D., Behar-Cohen, F. (2006). Intraocular implants for extended drug delivery: Therapeutic applications. *Advanced Drug Delivery Reviews, 58(11)*, 1182–1202.

48. Jaffe, G.J., Martin, D., Callanan, D., Pearson, P.A., Levy, B., Comstock, T. (2006). Fluocinolone acetonide implant (Retisert) for noninfectious posterior uveitis: Thirty-four-week results of a multicenter randomized clinical study. *Ophthalmology, 113(6)*, 1020–1027.

49. Yasukawa, T., Ogura, Y., Sakurai, E., Tabata, Y., Kimura, H. (2005). Intraocular sustained drug delivery using implantable polymeric devices. *Advanced Drug Delivery Reviews, 57(14)*, 2033–2046.

50. Kaur, I.P., Smitha, R. (2002). Penetration enhancers and ocular bioadhesives: Two new avenues for ophthalmic drug delivery. *Drug Development and Industrial Pharmacy, 28(4)*, 353–369.

51. Calvo, P., Vila-Jato, J.L., Alonso, M.J. (1997). Evaluation of cationic polymer-coated nanocapsules as ocular drug carriers. *International Journal of Pharmaceutics, 153(1)*, 41–50.

52. De Campos, A.M., Sanchez, A., Alonso, M.J. (2001). Chitosan nanoparticles: A new vehicle for the improvement of the delivery of drugs to the ocular surface. Application to cyclosporin A. *International Journal of Pharmaceutics, 224 (1–2)*, 159–168.

53. Coviello, T., Matricardi, P., Marianecci, C., Alhaique, F. (2007). Polysaccharide hydrogels for modified release formulations. *Journal of Controlled Release, 119(1)*, 5–24.

54. Weiner, A.L., Gilger, B.C. (2010). Advancements in ocular drug delivery. *Veterinary Ophthalmology, 13(6)*, 395–406.

55. Kang Derwent, J.J., Mieler, W.F. (2008). Thermoresponsive hydrogels as a new ocular drug delivery platform to the posterior segment of the eye. *Transactions of the American Ophthalmological Society, 106*, 206–213; discussion 213–24.

56. Singh, V., Bushetti, S.S., Appala, R., Shareef, A., Imam, S.S., Singh, M. (2010). Stimuli-sensitive hydrogels: A novel ophthalmic drug delivery system. *Indian Journal of Ophthalmology, 58(6)*, 477–481.

57. Yasukawa, T., Ogura, Y., Tabata, Y., Kimura, H., Wiedemann, P., Honda, Y. (2004). Drug delivery systems for vitreoretinal diseases. *Progress in Retinal and Eye Research, 23(3)*, 253–281.

58. Rafat, M., Cleroux, C.A., Fong, W.G., Baker, A.N., Leonard, B.C., O'Connor, M.D., Tsilfidis, C. (2010). PEG-PLA microparticles for encapsulation and delivery of Tat-EGFP to retinal cells. *Biomaterials, 31(12)*, 3414–3421.

59. Sahoo, S.K., Dilnawaz, F., Krishnakumar, S. (2008). Nanotechnology in ocular drug delivery. *Drug Discovery Today, 13 (3–4)*, 144–151.

60. Irache, J.M., Merodio, M., Arnedo, A., Camapanero, M.A., Mirshahi, M., Espuelas, S. (2005). Albumin nanoparticles for the intravitreal delivery of anticytomegaloviral drugs. *Mini Reviews in Medicinal Chemistry, 5(3)*, 293–305.

61. Sakurai, E., Ozeki, H., Kunou, N., Ogura, Y. (2001). Effect of particle size of polymeric nanospheres on intravitreal kinetics. *Ophthalmic Research, 33(1)*, 31–36.

62. Diebold, Y., Calonge, M. (2010). Applications of nanoparticles in ophthalmology. *Progress in Retinal and Eye Research, 29(6)*, 596–609.

63. Motwani, S.K., Chopra, S., Talegaonkar, S., Kohli, K., Ahmad, F.J., Khar, R.K. (2008). Chitosan-sodium alginate nanoparticles as submicroscopic reservoirs for ocular delivery: Formulation, optimisation and in vitro characterisation. *European Journal of Pharmaceutics and Biopharmaceutics, 68(3)*, 513–525.

64. Kao, H.J., Lin, H.R., Lo, Y.L., Yu, S.P. (2006). Characterization of pilocarpine-loaded chitosan/Carbopol nanoparticles. *Journal of Pharmacy and Pharmacology, 58(2)*, 179–186.

65. Bochot, A., Fattal, E., Boutet, V., Deverre, J.R., Jeanny, J. C., Chacun, H., Couvreur, P. (2002). Intravitreal delivery of oligonucleotides by sterically stabilized liposomes. *Investigative Ophthalmology & Visual Science, 43(1)*, 253–259.

66. Vyas, S.P., Mysore, N., Jaitely, V., Venkatesan, N. (1998). Discoidal niosome based controlled ocular delivery of timolol maleate. *Pharmazie, 53(7)*, 466–469.

67. Afouna, M.I., Khattab, I.S., Reddy, I.K. (2005). Preparation and characterization of demeclocycline liposomal

formulations and assessment of their intraocular pressure-lowering effects. *Cutaneous and Ocular Toxicology*, *24*(2), 111–124.

68. Shen, Y., Tu, J. (2007). Preparation and ocular pharmacokinetics of ganciclovir liposomes. *AAPS Journal*, *9*(*3*), E371–E377.
69. Aggarwal, D., Garg, A., Kaur, I.P. (2004). Development of a topical niosomal preparation of acetazolamide: Preparation and evaluation. *Journal of Pharmacy and Pharmacology*, *56*(*12*), 1509–1517.
70. Kaur, I.P., Garg, A., Singla, A.K., Aggarwal, D. (2004). Vesicular systems in ocular drug delivery: An overview. *International Journal of Pharmaceutics*, *269*(*1*), 1–14.
71. Kaur, I.P., Aggarwal, D., Singh, H., Kakkar, S. (2010). Improved ocular absorption kinetics of timolol maleate loaded into a bioadhesive niosomal delivery system. *Graefe's Archive for Clinical and Experimental Ophthalmology*, *248*(*10*), 1467–1472.
72. Quintana, A., Raczka, E., Piehler, L., Lee, I., Myc, A., Majoros, I., Patri, A.K., Thomas, T., Mule, J., Baker, J.R. Jr. (2002). Design and function of a dendrimer-based therapeutic nanodevice targeted to tumor cells through the folate receptor. *Pharmaceutical Research*, *19*(*9*), 1310–1316.
73. Padilla De Jesus, O.L., Ihre, H.R., Gagne, L., Frechet, J.M., Szoka, F.C. Jr. (2002). Polyester dendritic systems for drug delivery applications: In vitro and in vivo evaluation. *Bioconjugate Chemistry*, *13*(*3*), 453–461.
74. Ihre, H.R., Padilla De Jesus, O.L., Szoka, F.C., Jr., Frechet, J.M. (2002). Polyester dendritic systems for drug delivery applications: Design, synthesis, and characterization. *Bioconjugate Chemistry*, *13*(*3*), 443–52.
75. Patton, T.F., Robinson, J.R. (1975). Ocular evaluation of polyvinyl alcohol vehicle in rabbits. *Journal of Pharmaceutical Sciences*, *64*(*8*), 1312–1316.
76. Marano, R.J., Toth, I., Wimmer, N., Brankov, M., Rakoczy, P. E. (2005). Dendrimer delivery of an anti-VEGF oligonucleotide into the eye: A long-term study into inhibition of laser-induced CNV, distribution, uptake and toxicity. *Gene Therapy*, *12*(*21*), 1544–1550.
77. Gaudana, R., Ananthula, H.K., Parenky, A., Mitra, A.K. (2010). Ocular drug delivery. *AAPS Journal*, *12*(*3*), 348–360.
78. Katragadda, S., Gunda, S., Hariharan, S., Mitra, A.K. (2008). Ocular pharmacokinetics of acyclovir amino acid ester prodrugs in the anterior chamber: Evaluation of their utility in treating ocular HSV infections. *International Journal of Pharmaceutics*, *359*(*1–2*), 15–24.
79. Janoria, K.G., Boddu, S.H., Natesan, S., Mitra, A.K. (2010). Vitreal pharmacokinetics of peptide-transporter-targeted prodrugs of ganciclovir in conscious animals. *Journal of Ocular Pharmacology and Therapeutics*, *26*(*3*), 265–271.
80. Janoria, K.G., Boddu, S.H., Wang, Z., Paturi, D.K., Samanta, S., Pal, D., Mitra, A.K. (2009). Vitreal pharmacokinetics of biotinylated ganciclovir: Role of sodium-dependent multivitamin transporter expressed on retina. *Journal of Ocular Pharmacology and Therapeutics*, *25*(*1*), 39–49.
81. Dalpiaz, A., Filosa, R., de Caprariis, P., Conte, G., Bortolotti, F., Biondi, C., Scatturin, A., Prasad, P.D., Pavan, B. (2007). Molecular mechanism involved in the transport of a prodrug dopamine glycosyl conjugate. *International Journal of Pharmaceutics*, *336*(*1*), 133–139.
82. Majumdar, S., Hingorani, T., Srirangam, R., Gadepalli, R.S., Rimoldi, J.M., Repka, M.A. (2009). Transcorneal permeation of L- and D-aspartate ester prodrugs of acyclovir: Delineation of passive diffusion versus transporter involvement. *Pharmaceutical Research*, *26*(*5*), 1261–1269.
83. Kansara, V., Hao, Y., Mitra, A.K. (2007). Dipeptide monoester ganciclovir prodrugs for transscleral drug delivery: Targeting the oligopeptide transporter on rabbit retina. *Journal of Ocular Pharmacology and Therapeutics*, *23*(*4*), 321–334.
84. Anand, B.S., Katragadda, S., Nashed, Y.E., Mitra, A.K. (2004). Amino acid prodrugs of acyclovir as possible antiviral agents against ocular HSV-1 infections: Interactions with the neutral and cationic amino acid transporter on the corneal epithelium. *Current Eye Research*, *29*(*2–3*), 153–166.
85. Gunda, S., Hariharan, S., Mitra, A.K. (2006). Corneal absorption and anterior chamber pharmacokinetics of dipeptide monoester prodrugs of ganciclovir (GCV): *In vivo* comparative evaluation of these prodrugs with Val-GCV and GCV in rabbits. *Journal of Ocular Pharmacology and Therapeutics*, *22*(*6*), 465–476.
86. Majumdar, S., Nashed, Y.E., Patel, K., Jain, R., Itahashi, M., Neumann, D.M., Hill, J.M., Mitra, A.K. (2005). Dipeptide monoester ganciclovir prodrugs for treating HSV-1-induced corneal epithelial and stromal keratitis: *In vitro* and *in vivo* evaluations. *Journal of Ocular Pharmacology and Therapeutics*, *21*(*6*), 463–474.
87. Jain-Vakkalagadda, B., Pal, D., Gunda, S., Nashed, Y., Ganapathy, V., Mitra, A.K. (2004). Identification of a Na^+-dependent cationic and neutral amino acid transporter, B(0,+), in human and rabbit cornea. *Molecular Pharmacology*, *1*(*5*), 338–346.
88. Anand, B.S., Mitra, A.K. (2002). Mechanism of corneal permeation of L-valyl ester of acyclovir: Targeting the oligopeptide transporter on the rabbit cornea. *Pharmaceutical Research*, *19*(*8*), 1194–1202.
89. Katragadda, S., Talluri, R.S., Mitra, A.K. (2006). Modulation of P-glycoprotein-mediated efflux by prodrug derivatization: An approach involving peptide transporter-mediated influx across rabbit cornea. *Journal of Ocular Pharmacology and Therapeutics*, *22*(2), 110–120.
90. Mannermaa, E., Vellonen, K.S., Ryhanen, T., Kokkonen, K., Ranta, V.P., Kaarniranta, K., Urtti, A. (2009). Efflux protein expression in human retinal pigment epithelium cell lines. *Pharmaceutical Research*, *26*(*7*), 1785–1791.
91. Mannermaa, E., Vellonen, K.S., Urtti, A. (2006). Drug transport in corneal epithelium and blood-retina barrier: Emerging role of transporters in ocular pharmacokinetics. *Advanced Drug Delivery Reviews*, *58*(*11*), 1136–1163.
92. Constable, P.A., Lawrenson, J.G., Dolman, D.E., Arden, G.B., Abbott, N.J. (2006). P-Glycoprotein expression in

human retinal pigment epithelium cell lines. *Experimental Eye Research*, *83(1)*, 24–30.

93. Steuer, H., Jaworski, A., Elger, B., Kaussmann, M., Keldenich, J., Schneider, H., Stoll, D., Schlosshauer, B. (2005). Functional characterization and comparison of the outer blood-retina barrier and the blood-brain barrier. *Investigative Ophthalmology & Visual Science*, *46(3)*, 1047–1053.
94. Hosoya, K., Tomi, M. (2005). Advances in the cell biology of transport via the inner blood-retinal barrier: Establishment of cell lines and transport functions. *Biological & Pharmaceutical Bulletin*, *28(1)*, 1–8.
95. Shen, J., Cross, S.T., Tang-Liu, D.D., Welty, D.F. (2003). Evaluation of an immortalized retinal endothelial cell line as an in vitro model for drug transport studies across the blood-retinal barrier. *Pharmaceutical Research*, *20(9)*, 1357–1363.
96. Schinkel, A.H., Jonker, J.W. (2003). Mammalian drug efflux transporters of the ATP binding cassette (ABC) family: An overview. *Advanced Drug Delivery Reviews*, *55(1)*, 3–29.
97. Kennedy, B.G., Mangini, N.J. (2002). P-glycoprotein expression in human retinal pigment epithelium. *Molecular Vision*, *8*, 422–430.
98. Greenwood, J. (1992). Characterization of a rat retinal endothelial cell culture and the expression of P-glycoprotein in brain and retinal endothelium *in vitro*. *Journal of Neuroimmunology*, *39(1–2)*, 123–132.
99. BenEzra, D., Maftzir, G. (1990). Ocular penetration of cyclosporin A. The rabbit eye. *Investigative Ophthalmology & Visual Science*, *31(7)*, 1362–1366.
100. BenEzra, D., Maftzir, G., de Courten, C., Timonen, P. (1990). Ocular penetration of cyclosporin A. III: The human eye. *British Journal of Ophthalmology*, *74(6)*, 350–352.
101. BenEzra, D., Maftzir, G. (1990). Ocular penetration of cyclosporine A in the rat eye. *Archives of Ophthalmology*, *108(4)*, 584–587.
102. Aukunuru, J.V., Sunkara, G., Bandi, N., Thoreson, W.B., Kompella, U.B. (2001). Expression of multidrug resistance-associated protein (MRP) in human retinal pigment epithelial cells and its interaction with BAPSG, a novel aldose reductase inhibitor. *Pharmaceutical Research*, *18 (5)*, 565–572.
103. Tachikawa, M., Toki, H., Tomi, M., Hosoya, K. (2008). Gene expression profiles of ATP-binding cassette transporter A and C subfamilies in mouse retinal vascular endothelial cells. *Microvascular Research*, *75(1)*, 68–72.
104. Stojic, J., Stohr, H., Weber, B.H. (2007). Three novel ABCC5 splice variants in human retina and their role as regulators of ABCC5 gene expression. *BMC Molecular Biology*, *8*, 42.
105. Cai, H., Del Priore, L.V. (2006). Bruch membrane aging alters the gene expression profile of human retinal pigment epithelium. *Current Eye Research*, *31(2)*, 181–189.
106. Asashima, T., Hori, S., Ohtsuki, S., Tachikawa, M., Watanabe, M., Mukai, C., Kitagaki, S., Miyakoshi, N., Terasaki, T. (2006). ATP-binding cassette transporter G2 mediates the efflux of phototoxins on the luminal membrane of retinal capillary endothelial cells. *Pharmaceutical Research*, *23(6)*, 1235–1242.
107. Lee, V.H., Carson, L.W., Kashi, S.D., Stratford, R.E., Jr. (1986). Metabolic and permeation barriers to the ocular absorption of topically applied enkephalins in albino rabbits. *Journal of Ocular Pharmacology*, *2(4)*, 345–352.
108. Hayasaka, S., Hayasaka, I. (1979). Cathepsin B and collagenolytic cathepsin in the aqueous humor of patients with Behcet's disease. *Albrecht Von Graefes Archive for Clinical and Experimental Ophthalmology*, *210(2)*, 103–107.
109. Christie, C.D., Hanzal, R.F. (1931). Insulin absorption by the conjunctival membranes in rabbits. *Journal of Clinical Investigation*, *10(4)*, 787–793.
110. Chiou, G.C. and C.Y. Chuang. (1989). Improvement of systemic absorption of insulin through eyes with absorption enhancers. *Journal of Pharmaceutical Sciences*, *78(10)*, 815–818.
111. Chiou, G.C., Chuang, C.Y. (1988). Systemic delivery of polypeptides with molecular weights of between 300 and 3500 through the eyes. *Journal of Ocular Pharmacology*, *4(2)*, 165–177.
112. Harris, D., Robinson, J.R. (1990). Bioadhesive polymers in peptide drug delivery. *Biomaterials*, *11(9)*, 652–658.
113. Chiou, G.C., Shen, Z.F., Li, B.H. (1992). Effects of permeation enhancers BL-9 and Brij-78 on absorption of four peptide eyedrops in rabbits. *Zhongguo Yao Li Xue Bao*, *13(3)*, 201–205.
114. Rohde, B.H., Chiou, G.C. (1991). Effect of permeation enhancers on beta-endorphin systemic uptake after topical application to the eye. *Ophthalmic Research*, *23(5)*, 265–271.
115. Li, B.H., Chiou, G.C. (1992). Systemic administration of calcitonin through ocular route. *Life Sciences*, *50(5)*, 349–354.
116. Chiou, G.C., Shen, Z.F., Zheng, Y.Q. (1990). Adjustment of blood sugar levels with insulin and glucagon eyedrops in normal and diabetic rabbits. *Journal of Ocular Pharmacology*, *6(3)*, 233–241.
117. Geroski, D.H., Edelhauser, H.F. (2000). Drug delivery for posterior segment eye disease. *Investigative Ophthalmology & Visual Science*, *41(5)*, 961–964.
118. Chiou, G.C., Chuang, C.Y., Chang, M.S. (1989). Systemic delivery of insulin through eyes to lower the glucose concentration. *Journal of Ocular Pharmacology*, *5(1)*, 81–91.
119. Chiou, G.C., Li, B.H. (1993). Chronic systemic delivery of insulin through the ocular route. *Journal of Ocular Pharmacology*, *9(1)*, 85–90.
120. Chiou, G.C., Chuang, C.Y., Chang, M.S. (1988). Systemic delivery of enkephalin peptide through eyes. *Life Sciences*, *43(6)*, 509–514.
121. Chiou, G.C., Shen, Z.F., Zheng, Y.Q., Li, B.H. (1992). Enhancement of systemic delivery of met-enkephalin and leu-enkephalin eyedrops with permeation enhancers. *Methods & Findings in Experimental & Clinical Pharmacology*, *14(5)*, 361–366.
122. Chiou, G.C., Shen, Z.F., Zheng, Y.Q. (1991). Systemic absorption of oxytocin and vasopressin through eyes in rabbits. *Journal of Ocular Pharmacology*, *7(4)*, 351–359.

123. Wegewitz, U., Gohring, I., Spranger, J. (2005). Novel approaches in the treatment of angiogenic eye disease. *Current Pharmaceutical Design*, *11(18)*, 2311–2330.

124. Sasaki, H., Ichikawa, M., Yamamura, K., Nishida, K., Nakamura, J. (1997). Ocular membrane permeability of hydrophilic drugs for ocular peptide delivery. *Journal of Pharmacy and Pharmacology*, *49(2)*, 135–139.

125. Camelo, S., Lajavardi, L., Bochot, A., Goldenberg, B., Naud, M.C., Fattal, E., Behar-Cohen, F., de Kozak, Y. (2007). Ocular and systemic bio-distribution of rhodamine-conjugated liposomes loaded with VIP injected into the vitreous of Lewis rats. *Molecular Vision*, *13*, 2263–2274.

126. Binder, M., Tamm, C. (1973). The cytochalasans: A new class of biologically active microbial metabolites. *Angewandte Chemie International Edition*, *12(5)*, 370–380.

127. Berman, M., Manseau, E., Law, M., Aiken, D. (1983). Ulceration is correlated with degradation of fibrin and fibronectin at the corneal surface. *Investigative Ophthalmology & Visual Science*, *24(10)*, 1358–1366.

128. Dahlmann-Noor, A., Vijay, S., Jayaram, H., Limb, A., Khaw, P.T. (2010). Current approaches and future prospects for stem cell rescue and regeneration of the retina and optic nerve. *Canadian Journal of Ophthalmology*, *45(4)*, 333–341.

129. Mooney, I., LaMotte, J. (2008). A review of the potential to restore vision with stem cells. *Clinical and Experimental Optometry*, *91(1)*, 78–84.

130. Huang, Y., Enzmann, V., Ildstad, S.T. (2011). Stem cell-based therapeutic applications in retinal degenerative diseases. *Stem Cell Reviews*, *7(2)*, 434–445.

131. Sengupta, N., Caballero, S., Sullivan, S.M., Chang, L.J., Afzal, A., Li Calzi, S., Kielczewski, J.L., Prabarakan, S., Ellis, E.A., Moldovan, L., Moldovan, N.I., Boulton, M.E., Grant, M.B., Scott, E.W., Harris, J.R. (2009). Regulation of adult hematopoietic stem cells fate for enhanced tissue-specific repair. *Molecular Therapy*, *17(9)*, 1594–1604.

132. Zwart, I., Hill, A.J., Al-Allaf, F., Shah, M., Girdlestone, J., Sanusi, A.B., Mehmet, H., Navarrete, R., Navarrete, C., Jen, L.S. (2009). Umbilical cord blood mesenchymal stromal cells are neuroprotective and promote regeneration in a rat optic tract model. *Experimental Neurology*, *216(2)*, 439–448.

133. Wang, S., Lu, B., Girman, S., Duan, J., McFarland, T., Zhang, Q.S., Grompe, M., Adamus, G., Appukuttan, B., Lund, R. (2010). Non-invasive stem cell therapy in a rat model for retinal degeneration and vascular pathology. *PLoS One*, *5(2)*, e9200.

134. Ong, J.M., da Cruz, L. (2012). A review and update on the current status of stem cell therapy and the retina. *British Medical Bulletin*, *102*, 133–146.

135. Lu, B., Malcuit, C., Wang, S., Girman, S., Francis, P., Lemieux, L., Lanza, R., Lund, R. (2009). Long-term safety and function of RPE from human embryonic stem cells in preclinical models of macular degeneration. *Stem Cells*, *27(9)*, 2126–2135.

136. Vugler, A., Carr, A.J., Lawrence, J., Chen, L.L., Burrell, K., Wright, A., Lundh, P., Semo, M., Ahmado, A., Gias, C., da Cruz, L., Moore, H., Andrews, P., Walsh, J., Coffey, P. (2008). Elucidating the phenomenon of HESC-derived RPE: anatomy of cell genesis, expansion and retinal transplantation. *Experimental Neurology*, *214(2)*, 347–361.

137. Lund, R.D., Wang, S., Klimanskaya, I., Holmes, T., Ramos-Kelsey, R., Lu, B., Girman, S., Bischoff, N., Sauve, Y., Lanza, R. (2006). Human embryonic stem cell-derived cells rescue visual function in dystrophic RCS rats. *Cloning Stem Cells*, *8(3)*, 189–199.

138. Johnson, T.V., Bull, N.D., Hunt, D.P., Marina, N., Tomarev, S.I., Martin, K.R. (2010). Neuroprotective effects of intravitreal mesenchymal stem cell transplantation in experimental glaucoma. *Investigative Ophthalmology & Visual Science*, *51(4)*, 2051–2059.

20

ADVANCED DRUG DELIVERY AGAINST STD

CHI H. LEE

20.1 CHAPTER OBJECTIVES

- To provide physiological issues and pertinent regulatory aspects related to the subject of sexually transmitted diseases (STDs).
- To provide a thorough and critical overview of current aspects, developments, and new trends in advanced formulations and vaginal drug delivery for anti-STD microbicides.

20.2 INTRODUCTION

The vaginal route has been clinically used for site-specific delivery as well as for systemic delivery of therapeutically effective drugs. Formulations available for intravaginal delivery are gels, diaphragm, rings, films, and nano- and microparticles. Currently, most prescription and over-the-counter medications are intended for local activity against the pathological vagina conditions, such as hypertrophy of clitorisis, ectopic ureter, transverse vaginal septum, and candidasis, and prevent unwanted pregnancy [1]. However, given the recent epidemic of AIDS and other sexually transmitted diseases (STDs), including trichomonas, neisseria gonorrhea, genital herpes simplex, and chlamydia, the potential usage and the market growth opportunities of the vaginal formulations containing microbicides and vaccines will be further expanded.

This chapter will describe current research trends in advanced nanotechnology for intravaginal formulations against sexually transmitted infection (STI) including AIDS and human papillomavirus (HPV)-induced cervical cancer. The special emphasis is placed on the development and evaluation of nanotechnology-based formulations loaded with multiple drugs against HIV. The basic information on the physiology of the human vagina, its characteristics of absorption, permeability, and transport mechanisms of exogenous and pharmaceutical compounds, was also addressed.

20.3 PHYSIOLOGY OF VAGINA

20.3.1 General Anatomy

The morphology and anatomy of the vagina have been extensively compiled [2]. The vagina is a canal extending from the vulva to the cervix, and the anterior portion of the vagina in an adult averages 6 to 7 cm in length while the posterior wall is approximately 7.5 to 8.5 cm. Physiologically, the vagina serves a few functions, acting primarily as a conduit for the passage of seminal fluid, as an excretory duct for menstrual discharge, and as the lower part of the birth canal [3].

The vagina is characterized by an exceptional elasticity, having the greatest resiliency at parturition. The vaginal wall itself consists of three layers: the epithelial layer, the muscular coat, and the tunica adventitia. It is a noncornified,

Advanced Drug Delivery, First Edition. Edited by Ashim K. Mitra, Chi H. Lee, and Kun Cheng.

stratified squamous epithelium that is subject to changes with aging. The epithelium atrophies from birth to puberty, at which time hormonal activity increases the thickness and resistance of this layer. In the subepithelial layer, there rests a network of elastic fibers around the lamina propria and collagenous fibers around the tunica adventitia, creating a connection to the muscular coat.

Changes in the cytology of the vaginal epithelium occur with the cyclical stages in women. The epithelium is thickest in the proliferative stage, peaking at ovulation and then diminishing with the secretory phase. The muscular coat of the vagina is composed of smooth muscle and elastic fibers. A spiral arrangement of these fibers provides support to withstand stretching without rupturing the vagina. The tunica adventitia is formed of loose connective tissue that is attached to the muscular coat. Fluctuations in the volume of the vaginal lumen occur as a result of alterations in the tension of this layer. The vagina is encompassed by a vascular supply of arteries, veins, lymph capillaries, as well as sensory and autonomous nerves.

20.3.2 Cellular Structure

The epithelium (i.e., the first layer of three vaginal wall layers) of the vaginal mucosa is found to have five different layers of cells: the basal, parabasal, intermediate, transitional, and superficial cellular layers [4]. The cellular types that make up these various layers renew continuously as they are stimulated by hormonal action and intracellular communication. The basal cells are typically columnar or squamous in shape with microvilli present on the surface of the cell membrane. Parabasal cells are similar to the basal cells in size and structure, but they have a greater formation of surface microvilli and interdigitations. Their polygonal shapes are formed by adapting to spaces left free from neighboring cells. The cells of the intermediate layer possess microvilli and are of the largest cell type. The transitional cells that follow show noticeable signs of involution and surface characteristics of diminishing and thinning microvilli and intracellular junctions (desmosomes). Superficial cells, as indicated by their nomenclature, are the cells of the outermost layer during the follicular phase of the cycle.

The vaginal epithelium contains a network of intercellular channels that continuously undergo development, reaching a maximum during the ovulatory and luteal phases. The channels present in the transitional and superficial layers do not change with the cycle as do those in the basal, parabasal, and intermediate layers. These channels provide a supply of nutrients and transport metabolites to and from the layers of the epithelium. As the vagina is absent of secretory glands, lubrication is provided via these channels. Intercellular junctions, including desmosomes and tight junctions, were also identified. Desmosomes are most prominent in the intermediate layer and progressively become less toward the superficial layer, which significantly influences the desquamation of vaginal cells.

As the vaginal epithelium is affected by ovarian hormones, a cyclical variation including proliferation, differentiation, and desquamation occurs. During the follicular phase, known as the time period between the end of menstruation and the day of ovulation, mitosis develops in the cells of the basal and parabasal layers, increasing the number of layers and the thickness of the epithelium. The desquamating layers increase until ovulation, after which the layers diminish and are sloughed away through the vaginal lumen. During the luteal phase, the period after ovulation, the transitional cells become superficial as a result of the absence of the normal superficial layer.

20.3.3 Vaginal Fluids and Enzymes

The vaginal epithelium varies in degree of stratification depending on the pre- or postmenstrual cycle [6, 7]. The tissue and mucus of vaginal and cervical area are vastly different, and the cellular basis of these alterations is related to hormone status. Despite the paucity of glands, the vaginal epithelium is usually kept moist by a surface film. This film, known as vaginal fluid, consists of cervical mucus and exfoliated cells from the vagina itself. Transudation from the blood vessels through the intercellular channels to the lumen can also contribute to the chemical composition [4]. The fluid can contain carbohydrates, amino acids, aliphatic acids, proteins, and immunoglobulins [8]. Nonserum proteins in human vaginal secretions have also been identified [9, 10]. The vaginal fluid in mature, healthy women typically has a pH in the range of 4 to 5 [11]. This acidic environment is produced by the presence of lactobacilli, which convert carbohydrates into lactic acid.

The cervical mucus, a principal component of the vaginal fluid, is produced by glandular units within the cervical canal and has a pH in the range of 6.5 to 9. In a normal woman, the mucus is produced by the cervix at the rate of 20–60 mg/day. During the mid-cycle, the rate increases to 700 mg/day [12], and the mucus becomes a less viscous and microstructurally more expanded in texture, which facilitates the penetration of sperms [13].

The cervical mucus changes in composition and physical characteristics with the menstrual cycle, facilitating sperm migration during ovulation [14]. At the time of ovulation, the vaginal fluid increases in volume. This is a result of the augmented amount of cervical secretions. The mucus produced at ovulation has increased spinnbarkeit (fibrosity), ferning (crystallization of the mucus when dried on a slide), pH, and mucin content [15]. The appearance of a fernlike pattern (i.e., ferning: fern phenomenon) in a dried specimen of cervical mucus is an indication of the presence of estrogen. Alterations of the epithelial surfaces of the vagina stem from various etiologies, but postmenopausally they lead to vaginal drying [16, 17] or blood flow change [18]. Additionally, there is a decrease in the viscosity, cellularity, and albumin concentration.

The variety of enzymes found in the vagina is an important concern for the development of vaginal delivery systems, particularly with proteases and their effect on protein and peptide candidates [19]. The outer cell layers of the vagina contain varying amounts of β-glucuronidase, acid phosphatase, α-naphthylesterase, diphosphopyridine nucleotide-diaphorase (DPND), phosphoamidase, and succinic dehydrogenase [11]. Enzymatic activity has been shown in the basal cell layers as well, containing β-glucuronidase, succinic dehydrogenase, DPND, acid phosphatase, and α-naphthylesterase.

In addition to enzymes, the vaginal lumen is a nonsterile area inhabited by a variety of microorganisms, mainly the species *Lactobacillus, Bateroides*, and *Staphylococcus epidermidis*, as well as by a potentially pathogenic aerobe [20]. The existence of these microbes and their metabolites may also have a detrimental effect on the intravaginal stability of a vaginal drug delivery device.

20.3.4 The Role of Cervical Mucus

The vaginal mucosa consists of an epithelium having its surface coated with a layer of mucus [21]. The mucus is a heterogeneous secretion that provides a protective barrier to pathogen entrance, to lubricate and enhance wetability, to prevent desiccation, and to retard enzymatic degradation. The mucins in the mucus layer covering the three epitheilial regions provide a chemical and physical barrier and non-immune protection of cervical cavity by

(1) Acting as a lubricant
(2) Serving as a selective permeability barrier against other exogenous insults
(3) Assisting in clearing some microorganisms, fungi, and viruses
(4) Concentrating antimicrobial molecules onto mucosal surfaces
(5) Assisting the use of mucoadhesive, retentive dosage forms

To understand the nature of mucus, it is necessary to understand the structure of glycoprotein, the principal biochemical component of the mucus subunit [22]. Glycoprotein, which has a molecular weight of 320 to 4500 Da, is bound to other subunits through disulfide bonds and probably interacts with other subunits through ionic bonds and entanglements, especially with sialic acids located at the terminal ends of the oligosaccharide chain [23].

Biochemical characterizations of mucins demonstrate that these highly glycosylated glycoproteins are >50% by weight carbohydrate and that the carbohydrates are almost exclusively O-linked to serine and threonine [24]. The carbohydrates can be either simple or complex, and the five commonly found monosaccarides are *N*-acetylgalactosamine, *N*-acetylglucosamine, galactose, fucose, and sialic acid [25, 26]. Backbone proteins contain high percentages of serine, threonine, alanine, glycine, and proline [24, 27].

In addition to glycoproteins, the cervical mucus also contains a wide range of substances, including plasma proteins, enzymes, amino acids, cholesterol, lipids, and inorganic ions, with concentrations known to fluctuate during the cycle [28]. It has been proposed that entanglement of the macromolecules with the specific lectin-like regions contributes to the properties of the cervical mucus [29, 30]. The relationship between the intrinsic viscosity and the molecular weight of the whole mucins and their subunits and T-domains suggested that they are flexible linear macromolecules behaving like a stiff random coil [31].

The hostility of the thickened cervical mucus to sperm penetration has been used as a means to achieve contraception, and low-dose oral contraceptives depend largely on this condition for their effectiveness of fertility control [32, 33]. Sequential oral contraceptives do not affect mucus, and, like estrogen, may even increase sperm penetration.

20.3.5 Viscosity of the Cervical Mucus

Alterations in the biochemical properties of mucus are known to be responsible for changes in rheological behavior and receptivity of mucus to various exogenous compounds [34]. The liquefaction can be regulated by mechanical disruption, systemic carrier dilution, or chemicals, such as mucolytic agents. The effect of the alterations in the physical and physiological properties of cervical mucus on the change in drug permeability through the cervical mucosa was studied [35]. As marked changes occur in the plasma membrane during epididymal maturation and capacitation, analysis of the nature of compounds at a biochemical level was important for understanding the changes in permeation rate in response to the viscosity of mucus [36]. The increased ionic strength and consistency of the periovulatory mucus yielded better permeability to the exogenous compound, and an increased charge favors a higher degree of hydration [37].

The viscosity of mucus was affected by binding between calcium and the mucus, which probably arises from an ionic interaction with the sialic acid in the mucin [29]. These variations are indicated by changes in the pH, viscoelastic properties, water, and protein content of cervical mucus [38]. Calcium is needed in establishing an intercellular contact and the assembly of a tight junction in the cervical epithelium [39]. Changes in extracellular calcium affect the permeability of tight junctions and play a role in regulating the production of cervical mucus [40]. Prostaglandin concentrations in the cervix affect the viscosity of cervical mucus, which in turn affects the cervical softening [41]. The effect of dithiothreitol (DTT) on the viscosity was also reported [42]. Thus, the physical and physiological properties of cervical mucus may reflect alterations in the macromolecular composition or concentration of its components upon exposure to exogenous substrates or hormone replacement therapy [43]. For example, an administration of mestranol (or ethinyl estradiol), in combination with norethisterone or its acetate, strongly influenced the biophysical properties of the cervical mucus and sperm migration [44].

When a purified glycoprotein was treated with various proteolytic enzymes, which degraded [thepurified] glycoprotein, the charge of cervical mucus increased to confer a rigidity by the mutual repulsion of negative charges and to strengthen the coherence and consistency of the secretion [45, 46]. It appears that the menstrual cyclic changes in mucus viscoelasticity in an individual can be accounted for by the changes in mucin concentration [47]. This seems to result from a decrease in the amount of proteins in both the follicular and luteal phases but from an increase in the ovulatory phase [48]. In addition, mucus compositional difference may occur among the individuals, as indicated by the different correlation seen in the viscoelasticity and the mucin concentration [49].

As a result of the viscoelasticity of the mucus, most intravaginal formulations are associated with drawbacks of low retention to the vaginal epithelium, leakage, and messiness, thereby leading to poor patient compliance. To address these challenges, delivery systems with thixotropical properties through thermosensitive or pH-sensitive regulations have been intensively studied using various bioadhesive polymers [50].

20.3.6 Transporters in Vagina Cells

Various transporters in cells serve as a physiological barrier against drug permeation. A human cervical adenocarcinoma cell line, HeLa cell (i.e., a human cervical adenocarcinoma cell line), was used to determine whether there are any transporters involved with drug uptake by vaginal mucosa [51]. The changes in intracellular pH (pH_{in}) and monocarboxylate transporter (MCT)-mediated uptake rates of L-lactic acid by HeLa cells were evaluated under the conditions, whose $[Ca^{2+}]_{in}$ concentrations were altered by various calcium modulators, such as EGTA-AM (a chelator), nifedipine (a Ca^{2+} channel antagonist), and A23187 (an ionophore). The effects of the extracellular sodium concentration on the L-lactic acid uptake by HeLa cells were also evaluated to determine the involvement of Na^+-H^+ exchanger (NHE)-regulated pH changes in the MCT-mediated drug uptake process [52, 53].

The treatment of HeLa cells with A23187 at concentrations of 50 and 100 μM enhanced $[Ca^{2+}]_{in}$ by 100% and 200% of the control, respectively. EGTA/AM (50 μM) or nifedipine (100 μM) did not cause any significant changes in the $[Ca^{2+}]_{in}$ levels, whereas EGTA/AM (100 μM) and nifedipine (200 μM) reduced the $[Ca^{2+}]_{in}$ levels by 30% and 25%, respectively, as compared with the control. A23187 at a concentration of 100 μM in the incubation medium lowered pH_{in} (pH 5) and subsequently the uptake rate of lactic acid by 50% (0.47 ± 0.03 μmol/mg protein/min) of the control. The results of this study demonstrated that there was a close correlation between the $[Ca^{2+}]_{in}$ level and pH_{in} and that NHEs were involved with the MCT-mediated uptake process of lactic acid in HeLa cells. An understanding of the role of $[Ca^{2+}]_{in}$ in the MCT-mediated transport process in vagina cells would provide an efficient strategy to improve the systemic delivery of monocarboxylate substrates through the vagina/cervical mucosa.

20.4 STD AND PREVENTION STRATEGIES

20.4.1 General Facts About STDs

Sexually transmitted diseases (STDs) are infections that can be transferred from one person to another through sexual intercourse. There are more than 15 million cases of sexually transmitted diseases reported annually in the United States, almost half of them among people ages 15 to 24 (as reported by the Centers for Disease Control and Prevention). The most common STDs in the United States are chlamydia, gonorrhea, syphilis, genital herpes, human papillomavirus, hepatitis B, trichomoniasis, and bacterial vaginosis [54]. However, as AIDS is not yet curable, numerous studies on STDs have mainly dealt with prevention of HIV.

Some STDs can lead to cervical cancer or pelvic inflammatory disease, which can cause infertility, while others may even be fatal. STDs can be prevented by various microbicides [55] or some contraceptive devices, such as condoms, but a more efficient and effective means for preventing women from contracting an STD is still under development.

20.4.2 AIDS (HIV: Human Immunodeficiency Virus)

20.4.2.1 Route of HIV Infection Most women acquiring HIV today are primarily infected by mucosal exposure to virus through sexual contact. Many cell types share common epitopes with this protein, even though CD4 lymphocytes play a crucial role. HIV primarily infects cells with a CD4 cell-surface receptor by the adsorption of glycoproteins on its surface followed by fusion of the viral envelope with the cell membrane and the release of the HIV capsid into the cell [56, 57]. As shown in Figure 20.1, entry to the cell begins through interaction of the trimeric envelope complex (gp160

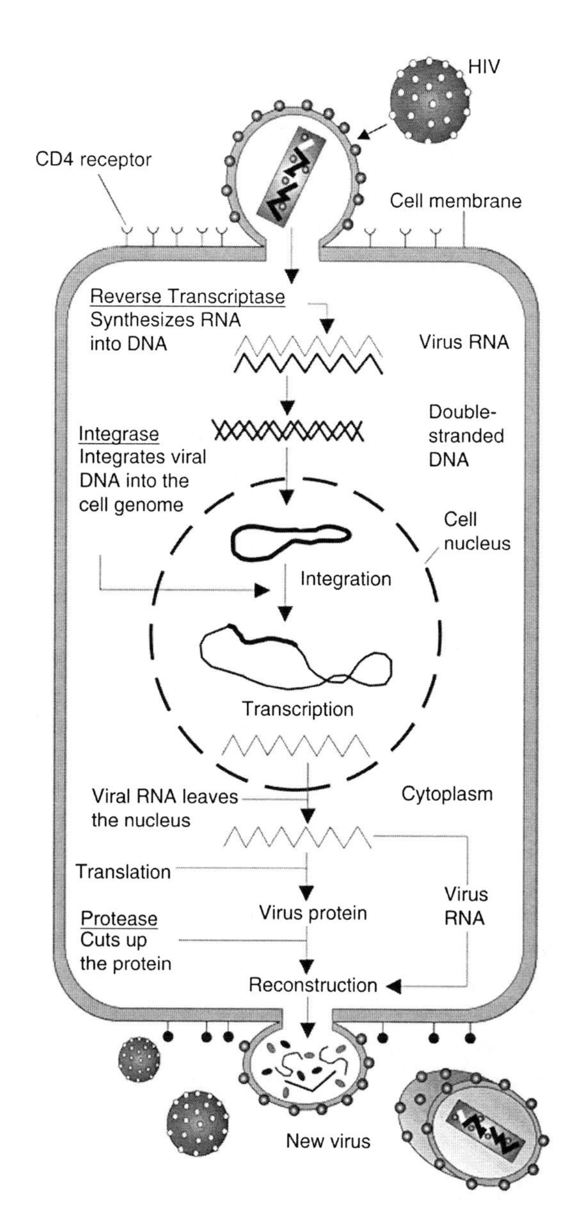

FIGURE 20.1 HIV replication cycle. *Source*: Wikipedia http://en.wikipedia.org/wiki/HIV.

spike) and both CD4 and a chemokine receptor (generally either CCR5 or CXCR4, but others are known to interact) on the cell surface [58, 59].

In macrophages and in some other cells lacking CD4 receptors, such as fibroblasts, an Fc receptor site or complement receptor site may be used for entry of HIV. The virions can infect numerous cellular targets and disseminate into the whole organism. These variants then replicate more aggressively with heightened virulence that causes rapid T-cell depletion, immune system collapse, and opportunistic infections that mark the advent of AIDS [60]. CD4 + T-cell count (T-helper lymphocytes with CD4 cell-surface marker) is widely used as a measure of global immune competence and provides a predictor of the immediate risk, whose number below 350 can be a sign of an unhealthy immune system. More detailed information can be obtainable from http://en.wikipedia.org/wiki/HIV.

20.4.3 Microbicides Against HIV

There is growing interest in development of microbicides used topically by women within the vagina to prevent infection by HIV, and more than 50 are under development [61]. Antiretroviral drugs against HIV are broadly classified by the phase of the retrovirus lifecycle that the drug inhibits. As shown in Table 20.1, there are five groups of antiretroviral drugs to treat HIV. Each of these groups attacks HIV in a different way. It was recommended to patients that they adapt highly active antiretroviral therapy (HAART), the combination of at least three antiretroviral drugs that attack different parts of HIV or stop the virus from entering blood cells, leading to a slower reproduction pace of the virus.

As only a few of those new entities that have proceeded through phase III showed any significant decrease in the rate of HIV transmission [63], advanced novel entities have been intensively tested to find more efficient antiretroviral drugs. Most candidate entities are subjected to three clinical trial phases as described in Table 20.2 to be deemed as new microbicides. For instance, one of the efficient strategies to overcome the initial activation step of 29,39-dideoxynucleoside (ddN) [66] is the synthesis of the acyclic nucleoside phosphonates (ANPs) by replacing the phosphate group with a metabolically stable phosphonate. Tenofovir, 9-[2-(phosphonomethoxy)propyl]adenine (PMPA) is one of the ANPs and is a nucleotide reverse transcriptase inhibitor (NtRTI) that inhibits HIV reverse transcriptase. It was proven to be active against HIV and simian immunodeficiency virus (SIV) in clinical studies [67]. The EC_{50} of tenofovir ([R]-PMPA) ranged between 0.4 and 7.0 μM, and its CC_{50} was >50 μM.

It is not clear when the current candidate HIV vaccines, many of which are primarily targeted to simulate systemic immunity at the mucosal surfaces of the reproductive tract and thereby prevent primary mucosal infection [68], will come to fruition. Women may need help from microbicides or barrier devices for self-protection until an arrival of the first generation of vaccines. This uncertainty provides a rationale to pursue female-controlled vaginal delivery systems made of a mucoadhesive polymer containing microbicides as a means for blocking HIV entry into the vaginal mucosa.

The major challenges on delivering multiple combinations of microbicides are a lack of 1) delivery vehicles that allow for a localized and controlled delivery of multiple microbicides, 2) an *in vitro* system that closely mimics the physicodynamic conditions of the vagina, and 3) an advanced networking classifier for an accurate prediction

TABLE 20.1 Antiretroviral Drugs to Treat HIV

Antiretroviral Class	Abbreviation	Approved Year	Mechanism to Work
Nucleoside/nucleotide reverse transcriptase inhibitors	NRTIs, nucleoside analogues, nukes	1987	NRTIs interfere with the action of an HIV protein called reverse transcriptase, which the virus needs to make new copies of itself
Non-nucleoside reverse transcriptase inhibitors	NNRTIs, non-nucleosides, non-nukes	1997	NNRTIs also stop HIV from replicating within cells by inhibiting the reverse transcriptase protein
Protease inhibitors	PIs	1995	PIs inhibit protease, which is another protein involved in the HIV replication process
Fusion or entry inhibitors		2003	Fusion or entry inhibitors prevent HIV from binding to or entering human immune cells
Integrase inhibitors		2007	Integrase inhibitors interfere with the integrase enzyme, which HIV needs to insert its genetic material into human cells

Source: Ref. 62.

of *in vitro/in vivo* efficacy relationships against HIV. These three challenges should be addressed to make substantive progress toward development and evaluation of an efficient nanoscience-based formulation against HIV.

20.4.4 Immunization Against HIV: Antibody/Vaccination

As mucosal secretory IgA is considered to have an integral role in the prevention of human immunodeficiency virus type 1 (HIV-1) transmission through sexual intercourse, substances that induce an HIV-1-specific IgA antibody in the genital tract could become promising candidates for a prophylactic vaccine against HIV-1 infection [69]. To develop an HIV vaccine, according to the conventional vaccine approach, neutralizing antibodies should be induced against HIV envelope proteins or other engineered fragments of HIV [70]. However, HIV envelope protein antigens do not confer a robust immune response and a proper strategy to induce a long-term immune response in the vaginal mucosa is still lacking [71]. The problem associated with conjugating a mucosal adjuvant with HIV antigen proteins to enhance antibody neutralization response is that they would trigger an inflammatory response, activating CD4+ T cells, thereby enhancing the gateway for HIV transmission [72].

Monoclonal synthetic antibodies against HIV and STD pathogens can be applied directly to genital skin and epithelia for protection [65, 73]. This process may closely mimic the normal function of antibodies in the mucosal immune system. To date, the results of studies performed indicate that monoclonal antibodies delivered through the vagina may help prevent sexual transmission of genital herpes and HIV [74, 75]. Rheologically structured vehicle (RSV) gels were developed as delivery systems for vaginal

TABLE 20.2 Clinical Trial Phases Applicable to Microbicides

Phase Stage	Number of Participants	Length of Treatment	Objective
Phase I	10–100	1 to 2 weeks	To assess local and systemic safety and acceptability and to determine dose and formulation. May run into a phase II trial (called phase I/II)
Phase II	50–200	2 to 6 months	To assess safety and acceptability over a longer time
Phase II/IIb	50–500	6 months to 2 years	To screen for products reaching a minimum level of effectiveness. Smaller, less costly than phase III, but numbers of participants and length of follow-up indicate whether a subsequent larger trial would be worthwhile. If so, participants continue from one trial to the next, and additional participants are recruited (called phase II/III)
Phase III	1000–30,000	1 to 2 years	To evaluate effectiveness in preventing HIV infection and other STIs and to assess long-term safety and acceptability. Some phase III trials will involve multiple products, which will require more participants than those testing only one product

Note: Phases I/II, II/IIb, and II/III are variants of study designs or studies that move from one clinical trial phase to the next. Number of participants and length of treatment and follow-up vary.

Sources: Ref. 208. Adapted from Stone [64], Fleming [27], Mauck et al. [65], and the Alliance for Microbicide Development [3].

mucosal vaccination with an HIV-1 envelope glycoprotein (CN54gp140) [76]. Vaginal administration of RSV to rabbits induced specific serum IgG, and IgG and IgA in genital tract secretions, which support RSVs as a viable delivery modality for vaginal immunization.

A novel approach of repeated mucosal immunization by delivering an HIV-1 envelope glycoprotein (gp) in a gel formulated for intravaginal delivery was attempted [77]. Rabbits were immunized over one to three 19-day cycles of intravaginal dosing with soluble recombinant trimeric HIV-1 clade C gp140 administered in Carbopol gel. A single immunization cycle induced an immunoglobulin G (IgG) antibody detected in the serum and female genital tract, and titers were boosted on further immunization. Vaccine-induced serum antibodies neutralized the infectivity of a pseudovirus carrying a heterologous clade C envelope, proving that the concept that repeated exposure of the female genital tract to HIV envelope can induce a mucosally detectable antibody. The application of antiretrovirals to prevent HIV infection also supported the concept of pre-exposure prophylaxis [78].

It was reported that vaccine delivery through the vaginal route still produced a cytotoxic T lymphocyte activity, even though it failed to induce antibodies. A human simian virus 1 (HSV) vaccine was tested as an aqueous solution or carbopol gel intranasally, vaginally, and subcutaneously in guinea pigs [79]. The animals were challenged 3–5 weeks later with only the subcutaneous response producing IgG and IgA. The nasal and vaginal routes showed that the vaccine could be taking up elicit antibodies, slightly reducing the severity of the disease, but showing no superiority to the subcutaneous route.

In another study, rats were immunized with a synthetic peptide from human immunodeficiency virus envelope glycoprotein and were shown to have greater IgG and IgA response with an enhancer, lysophosphatidyl glycerol [80]. The serum antibodies from subcutaneous and intravaginal delivery were able to recognize the glycoprotein (HIV 1 gp120), but no neutralizing activity against the virus was seen. An antigen delivery system of lysophosphatidylcholine and degradable starch microspheres demonstrated potential intravaginal delivery to sheep [80]. If the vagina is capable of mounting an immune response, antibodies in genital secretions may be able to reduce the transmission of HIV.

20.4.5 Small Interfering RNAs (siRNAs) as a Topical Microbicide

The feasibility of using siRNAs as a topical microbicide was previously demonstrated [81]. The RNAi pathway is mediated through a small, noncoding, double-stranded RNA species termed small interfering RNAs (siRNAs). The siRNA binds to homologous target mRNA, including mRNA cleavage and subsequent protein degradation. RNA interference (RNAi) has been a promising tool to silence gene expression selectively and holds a great potential for the treatment of genetic disorders, viral disease, and cancer [82–84].

The previous studies demonstrated the feasibility of using siRNAs as part of a microbicide to prevent sexually transmitted diseases, such as HIV-1 and HSV-2 [81]. siRNAs that target either HSV-2-specific viral genes or host-encoded viral entry receptors were used to prevent transmission in a mouse model of vaginal HSV-2 infection [85, 86]. Vaginally applied siRNAs were observed in epithelial cells and deep in the lamina propria, and the level of siRNA uptake was sufficient to protect mice from a lethal HSV-2 infection [85, 86].

In addition, the short half-life of siRNA would result in a transient suppression of target gene expression, necessitating a steady long-term delivery system [87–89]. Nanoparticles designed for sustained release of siRNA and applied to vaginal tissue were detected in the epithelium and lamina propria and cervix, yielding silencing of the endogenous gene for 14 days without causing cellular infiltration or epithelial disruption [90].

Even though receptor-mediated siRNA delivery may represent a viable strategy for microbicide development, the major obstacles of *in vivo* application of siRNA to their clinical use are less target selectivity and a lower intracellular delivery rate [91]. Administered siRNAs must make contact with the appropriate cell types and, following internalization, gain access to the cytosol where the RNAi machinery resides, achieving maximized silencing, while minimizing any undesirable off-target effects. Off-target could occur if the siRNA contains sufficient homology to nontargeted mRNA in the open reading frame. Algorithms are a very effective way to identify active sequences and to exclude siRNA that share a degree of homology with no-targeted mRNAs [81]. Also, employing low concentrations of siRNA can reduce the off-target effects [92]. Another effective strategy for inhibiting the HIV transmission rate and reducing the off-target effects is targeting multiple genes, like viral and endogenous genes involved in viral replication [93].

Although lipid-complexed siRNAs showed a promising result without inflammatory infiltrates and induction of interferon-related genes in vaginal tissue, the subsequent studies found lipid-related toxicity using additional criteria [90]. Another drawback of using siRNA as a microbicide was associated with the activation of immune responses via toll-like receptors and retinoic acid inducible gene-I, which was originally believed to be not involved [94]. The immune responses can be avoided by using chemical-modified siRNA. Therefore, a careful and cautious optimization process of siRNA formulation including proper carriers for vaginal delivery should be thoroughly investigated.

20.4.6 Cervical Cancer (HPV; Human Papilloma Virus)

Cervical cancer is the second most common form of cancer among women worldwide and the leading cause of death from cancer among women in developing countries. In a single year, cervical cancer accounted for an estimated 274,000 global deaths and at least 493,000 new cases are identified with 83% of these in developing countries [95, 96].

Cervical cancer is developed from cervical intraepithelial neoplasia, also known as cervical dysplasia, which is characterized by abnormal malignance cells in the cervix. Human papilloma virus (HPV) oncogenes (E6 and E7) that are the predominant etiological factor in the development of cervical cancer would be an ideal target for the treatment of cervical cancer [97].

In June 2006, a cervical cancer vaccine was approved by the Food and Drug Administration (FDA) for girls and women between the ages of 9 and 26. Although this vaccine (Gardasil; Merck, Whitehouse Station, NJ) has been shown to protect against the HPV and 100% effective in trials, it is estimated that it will only reduce total cervical cancer incidence by 50%, and will likely take about 15 years for complete prevention, depending on vaccine strategies and uptake rates [98]. Clearly, there is a huge gap in the current prevention arsenal, and even if we currently had full vaccine coverage, alternative therapies against sexually transmitted HPV would be of great potential benefit.

To address these obstacles, an efficient intravaginal nanocarrier for siRNA that can efficiently silence the target mRNA (HPV E6 and E7) would be a viable option [99]. HPV 16 accounts for approximately 50% of cervical cancer onset [100]. As HPV E6 and E7 are transcribed as a single bicistronical transcript (16E6E7) from the same promoter, p97, and a common early polyadenylation site, a single siRNA species can be used to knock down the expression of both E6 and E7 [101–104].

20.5 VAGINAL DELIVERY SYSTEMS AGAINST STDs

20.5.1 Formulation Types

Intravaginal delivery systems have been widely used for prevention against the STD epidemic. As shown in Table 20.3, three types of dosage forms (i.e., physical, chemical, and immunological barriers) can be used as a female-controlled drug delivery system against unwanted pregnancy and the STD epidemic. Among them, the combinations of physical and chemical barriers or physical and immunological barriers seem to be suitable approaches for female-controlled formulations against HIV.

As with highly active antiretroviral therapy (HAART) for HIV/AIDS treatment, there is a growing consensus that vaginal application of microbicides will benefit from being administered in various combinations, with each compound having a different mechanism of action against sexual transmission of HIV. To find a proper topical carrier for HAART remains a major challenge.

TABLE 20.3 Types of Intravagainal Formulations

Type	Example
Physical	Condom, diaphragm, foams, suppository, gel, film
Chemical	Spermicide/microbicides
Immunological	Mucosal immunity or immune factors (vaccine)

Sources: Refs. 105 and 106.

20.5.2 pH Regulation of Vaginal Device Against STDs

During women's reproductive years, the vaginal bacteria flora maintains acidic pH in the vagina that reduces any type of infection by lowering the viral activities related with various disease onset. This acidic pH is maintained by Doiderlein's bacillus, which produces lactic acid by acting on glycogen contained in desquamated vaginal epithelial cells. Lactobacillus, which is hydrogen peroxide producing a biological product, may play an integral role in maintaining a low vaginal pH and resisting infection.

The vaginal environment is complicated, and these complications can affect the performance of intravaginal systems. The flow properties of intravaginal formulations and their rheological characteristics have been controlled by environmental factors including vaginal fluid rate and pH [107]. The formulation will be initially exposed to acidic pH (i.e., normal healthy vagina pH 4.5) and later to the neutral pH of a male partner's semen (pH. 7.0), as shown in Table 20.4, subsequently affecting its resident time at the vaginal cavity and microbicidal efficacy.

The major challenge in vaginal drug delivery is the limited contact time resulting from numerous protective mechanisms of the vagina, thereby resulting in a short duration of action and low therapeutic efficacy [21, 111]. To remain in the cervix, the formulation should have enough adhesiveness not to slip out of the vagina or flow down the back of cervix [112]. Therefore, various formulations with proper rheological properties have been developed to address those obstacles in the vaginal delivery of microbicides against STDs.

TABLE 20.4 pH of Various Reproductive Fluids

Body Fluid	pH	Reference
Semen	6.9	[108]
Mucus	6–9	[48]
Sialic acid of mucus	2.6	[109]
Vaginal secretion*	3.0–5.5	[110]

20.5.3 Gel Formulations Against HIV

Numerous anionic polymers demonstrated their efficacy as a drug carrier in targeting the entry processes of HIV [113]. Most intravaginal formulations that have been evaluated in the current clinical trials are conventional semi-solid aqueous gels, employing bioadhesive polymers. Bioadhesion is thought to involve an initial interaction of the hydrogel with the mucosal surface, which requires a matching of the polarity between the tissue surface and the polymer surface [114] and, subsequently, an inter-penetration of the mucosal surface by the polymer chains of the hydrogel. The bioadhesive properties of delivery systems, such as gels and hydrogels, could provide controlled release profiles of loaded compounds with intimate contact with and prolonged residence time in the vagina.

Carbopol 934 polymer could be a good bioadhesive candidate for clinical application in the intravaginal delivery of spermicidal agents [44] or microbicides [115]. A Carbopol gel (5% w/w) was tested for the intravaginal administration of SPL7013, which binds and blocks HIV-1 thereby preventing AIDS [115]. The molecular condom having a thixotropical property is developed as an anti-HIV vaginal gel [116]. The semen-triggered vaginal microbicide delivery vehicle was designed to release anti-HIV bioactives upon contact with semen during sexual intercourse. The system contains nanoscale particles and explores the use of bioresponsive drug delivery by customizing the physiological and physicodynamical requirements essential for intravaginal application.

As lactobacilli produce lactic acid and hydrogen peroxide that inactivate numerous pathogens [117, 118], a polyacrylic acid polymeric gel (BufferGel; ReProtect, LLC, Baltimore, MD), provides microbicidal efficacy through maintaining the natural acidity of the vagina [64]. A microemulsion-based gel formulation for phenyl phosphate derivative of zidovudine was developed against HIV, exerting its effectiveness against HIV in multiple intravaginal applications and not causing any side effects in the vaginal epithelium in the rabbit model [119].

A gel comprising a synthetic carbomer, a lactate buffer system, and naphthalene sulfonate as an antiviral agent (PRO 2000 Gel; Indevus Pharmaceuticals, Lexington, MA) was in a stage of the clinical test for the prevention of STIs and HIV [120, 121]. In February 2009, one Pro 2000 trial suggested that it might reduce the risk of getting HIV by 30%, but the small size of the trial meant the findings were not statistically significant.

C31G cream (Savvy; Cellegy Pharmaceuticals, Inc., San Francisco, CA) was prepared based on hydroxyethylcellulose that also acts as a surface-active microbicide. This cream contains a broad-spectrum antimicrobial agent, namely cetyl betaine and myristamine oxide, that had activity against bacteria, fungi, yeasts, and enveloped viruses [122], showing its efficacy in preventing HIV-1 and HIV-2 transmission in phase III clinical trials [64, 123].

Recently, a dendrimer-based gel formulation, SPL7013 Gel (VivaGel®; Starpharma Ltd., Melbourne, Victoria, Australia) was designed to prevent the transmission of STIs including HIV and genital herpes and it was demonstrated that 3% Gel was safe and well tolerated in sexually abstinent women when administered vaginally, twice daily for 14 days. Among these gel formulations, the five products entering phase III clinical trials are as follows: *BufferGel*, *Carraguard*, *PRO 2000*, C31G, and cellulose sulfate; if successful, some of these five products are likely to reach the market.

20.5.4 Gel Formulations for Tenofovir

Despite its antiviral potency, tenofovir, 9-[2-(phosphonomethoxy)propyl]adenine (PMPA) is known by the brand name Viread (Bristol-Myers Squibb, New York, NY) has limited oral bioavailability in animals, presumably as a result of the presence of two negative charges on the phosphonyl group [124]. Tenofovir and other anti-retroviral have been incorporated into gels or creams that are applied to the vagina [125–127] or the rectum [128]. Several studies on monkeys have shown that tenofovir was significantly effective at pre-exposure prophylaxis (PrEP) [129]. Monkeys that received tenofovir for up to 2 days before SIV exposure could avoid the infection. PrEP seems to be working to some degree in humans [130].

Various clinical trials have focused on determining whether tenofovir can prevent infection in uninfected people. A gel formulation containing tenofovir disoproxil fumarate (tenofovir DF; Viread) has been developed for vaginal use [131], and a multicenter phase II trial was conducted in 2005 (website access: http://www.clinicaltrials.gov/ct/show/NCT00111943). The ongoing study, known as MTN-007, is the second early phase trial evaluating the rectal safety of the vaginal product. In an ongoing, large-scale effectiveness trial called VOICE (Vaginal and Oral Interventions to Control the Epidemic), the MTN is testing daily use of tenofovir gel in African women, with results expected in 2013 (Microbicides Trial Network). It was demonstrated by another group that such prophylactic methods could successfully reduce the transmission of HIV by at least 39% using vaginal gel containing tenofovir administered before and after coitus [132].

20.5.5 Gel Formulations for Carrageenan

Carrageenan (CGN), a sulfated polysaccharide polymer acting as an excipient, consists of alternating 3-linked-β-D-galactopyranose and 4-linked-α-D-galactopyranose units [133]. All CGNs (κ-, ι-, and λ-) are highly flexible molecules that, at higher concentrations, wind around each other to form double-helical zones and act as an absorption inhibitor by coating the vagina. Gel formation in κ- and λ-carrageen involves helix formation on cooling from a hot solution together with gel-inducing and gel-strengthening K^+ or Ca^{2+} cations, respectively. Carraguard is a gel-like delivery system comprising CGN [134].

The pharmacological efficacies of CGN as a microbicide have been widely demonstrated. An *in vitro* test with PC-515 (3% λ-CGN, Population Council) resulted in high microbicidal efficiency of CGN against HIV infection [135]. It was found that CGN formulation blocks cell trafficking of macrophages from the vagina that helps to prevent sexual transmission of HIV and that blocking does not result from cytotoxicity [136, 137]. NCI, Laboratory of Cellular Oncology, recently reported that CGN can also block HPV infection through a second, postattachment heparan sulfate-independent effect [138].

CGN is generally recognized as a safe compound by the FDA. Most women found λ-CGN-containing products including PC-515 and PC-503 to be pleasant or neutral in feel and smell and considered extra lubrication to be an advantage [139]. Vaginal use of CGN did not cause significant adverse effects in sexually abstinent low-risk women [140]. Moreover, as CGN has a different microbicidal activity from tenofovir, a combination of CGN and tenofovir would be a promising candidate for combination therapy against HIV.

20.5.6 Vagina Ring: Material and Structures

Vaginal rings inserted and positioned around the cervix provide a means of delivering a pharmacologically active agent to the systemic circulation at a controlled release rate [141]. Compared with the conventional semi-solid gels, the vaginal rings provided an extended sustained release profile of microbicides to the target site [142]. Vaginal rings have been safe and effective for the delivery of estradiol and have been found to be more comfortable than a pessary [143].

Silicone elastomers are widely used for medical application as a result of its excellent biocompatibility of polydimethylsiloxane systems [144]. A smaller silicone elastomeric vaginal ring was developed for application to nonhuman primates, such as pig-tailed and Chinese rhesus macaques. The data suggested that the 25*5-mm ring showed optimal fit in both macaque species and that there was no tissue irritation or significant induction of markers or signs of physical discomfort during the 8-week study period. This study could be used to guide the design mucosal delivery of candidate microbicides from vaginal rings [145].

The frequent occurrence of bleeding irregularities prompted the redesign of the vaginal ring to a new generation of sandwich-type vaginal rings, in which the drug-dispersed silicone polymer matrix is coated with a nonmedicated silicone polymeric membrane. The overcoat design was intended to reduce the initial burst release of drug frequently observed in the first treatment cycle of vaginal rings for contraception. The studies on the effect of the overcoat on the release rate of d norgestrel revealed that the addition of an overcoat minimized or eliminated the burst release of drug and shifted the non-zero-order drug release profile to the constant zero-order release rate profile.

The dual-segment polyurethane vaginal rings to enable simultaneously sustained release of multiple drugs with the contrasting hydrophilicity, such as dapivirine and tenofovir, were developed [146]. The production processes include solvent casting and hot-melt extrusion before joining drug-loaded rods together to form dual-segment vaginal rings. In this formulation, dapivirine and tenofovir are amorphous and crystalline within their individual polymeric segments. These rings are stable mechanically, which is comparable with ordinary vaginal rings. *In vitro* release of tenofovir from the vaginal ring was sustained over 30 days while dapivirine exhibited linear release over the time period. These results suggest that multisegment polyurethane vaginal rings are a promising formulation for the contrasting hydrophilic drugs, such as dapivirine and tenofovir. However, multisegment polyurethane vaginal rings have their drawbacks, requiring a more sophisticated manufacturing scheme than what is required for single-segment vaginal rings.

20.5.7 Types of Vaginal Rings

The vaginal ring containing Dapivirine, which is a potent non-nucleoside reverse transcriptase inhibitor also known as TMC120, was tested as an intravaginal microbicide delivery system for prevention of the transmission of STIs and HIV [147, 148]. The product manufactured by the Silver Spring nonprofit organization is a silicone ring similar to one used in contraceptive devices, such as NuvaRing, releasing Dapivirine into the vagina over a month, after which it is replaced. A vaginal ring against STI would be removed once a month during the menstrual period and could be used for a year. A clinical trial demonstrated that a dapivirine incorporated vaginal ring is very safe and well tolerated over the course of 28 days of continuous use [149].

The insert vaginal ring (InVR) provides an alternative to deliver the hydrophilic and/or macromolecular drugs, including peptides, proteins, and antibodies with high efficacy [150]. InVR achieved the sustained release of a BSA protein used as a model compound beyond 4 weeks. This device takes advantage of a variety of matrices inserted in the ring compartment including silicone rods, compressed tablets, and lyophilized gels. Moreover, every device of InVR can contain over 1 mg of the monoclonal antibody

2F5, offering a better inhibition effect against the transmission of HIV [150].

Vaginal rings made of biosoluble Acacia gum or non-biodegradable hydrogel of 2-hydroxyethyl methacrylate and sodium methacrylate showed the sustained release of loaded drugs for up to 28 days. Another advantage of this ring is its ability to simultaneously contain the combination of several antiviral drugs including TMC120, PMPA, 30f-azido-30 deoxythymidine, and betulonic acid, which provide synergistic effects to inhibit multiple sites in the lifecycle of HIV. In addition, Boc-lysinated betulonic acid showed more than 90% inhibition of HIV-1 infection in H9 cells with little toxicity [151].

Formulations of microbicides into vaginal rings represent a very promising strategy for prevention of HIV. A vaginal ring that contains both contraceptives and an antiretroviral drug is also under development with support from the U.S. Agency for International Development. Although several vaginal rings are already on the market, the microbicide-loaded vaginal rings still need to be improved to offer better adherence and acceptability to achieve the best clinical effect.

20.5.8 Micro- and Nanoparticles Against HIV

Various attempts have been presented to deliver intravaginally microbicides or spermicides loaded in microparticulate systems in a semisolid form having sufficient bioadhesiveness [152–154]. The selection of nanocarriers that are efficient, biocompatible, and that can be tailored to specific infection processes is integral. Nanoparticles can be made with a variety of biodegradable and biocompatible polymers, such as PLGA, PSA, and PLA, and these can release a wide range of low-molecular-weight drugs [155]. Silver or gold nanoparticles are effective in reducing the infectivity of the AIDS virus and kill the causative organisms of other sexually transmitted diseases [156, 157]. The direct conjugation of silver nanoparticles with proteins served as efficient microbicide delivery systems for preventing STIs and HIV transmission [158, 159].

PSC-RANTES, a CCR5 chemokine receptor inhibitor, was encapsulated into PLGA nanoparticles to protect the active agent from the vaginal environment and facilitate penetration of the drug into the vaginal and ectocervical tissue, allowing the drug to reach HIV target cells [160, 161]. It was shown that encapsulated PSC-RANTES was uptaken into the tissue fivefold greater than nonencapsulated PSC-RANTES and that the PSC-RANTES-loaded PLGA nanoparticles were mostly detected in the basal layer of the cervical epithelium [162]. Intravaginal immunization against HSV-2 infection using biodegradable calcium phosphate nanoparticles as an adjuvant resulted in higher mucosal levels of IgG and IgA as compared with intranasal immunization, providing optimal protection against HSV-2 infection in mice [115].

The most widely used systems for delivering siRNA are liposomal carriers, but there are serious concerns in vaginal application against HIV, such as some cationic lipids are known to be cytotoxic and unstable at high ionic conditions. *In vivo* studies on the efficiency of SiRNA-loaded PLGA nanoparticles resulted in effective and sustained gene silencing throughout the female reproductive tract with negligible side effects for at least 14 days [90].

Mucus-penetrating particles (MPPs) were densely coated with neutral hydrophilic surfaces created by polymers such as low-molecular-weight PEG to prevent mucin fibers from forming hydrophobic bonds with the particles [163]. MPPs provided sustained microbicide delivery for more than 24 hours and delivered hydrophobic microbicides more uniformly to the entire vaginal epithelium than application via gels or other vaginal formulations [164].

Bioadhesive microparticles, used in the nasal and oral [drug] delivery of drugs, have a potential for further development of an intravaginal delivery system. The mucoadhesive benzyl ester of hyaluronic acid has been used in preparing microspheres for the intravaginal delivery of salmon calcitonin to rats [165]. Replens (Lil' Drug Store Products, Inc., Cedar Rapids, IA), which has been marketed as a bioadhesive moisturizer and which remains in the vagina for 2–3 days, consists of a bioadhesive crosslinked polycarbophil [166].

Nanospheres were also tested for intravaginal delivery against HIV. Polystyrene nanospheres containing lectin were examined for HIV-1 capturing abilities for their intravaginal application [167]. Intravaginal immunization of Concanavalin A-immobilized polystyrene nanospheres (Con A-NS) effectively induced vaginal anti-HIV-1 IgA antibodies in mice [168] or macaques [107], promoting an effective immunization response. To date, few studies have been successful in exploiting nanoparticle-based microbicidal delivery to the vagina.

20.6 DRUG RELEASE AND EFFICACY STUDIES OF VAGINAL FORMULATIONS

20.6.1 Prototype Formulations

Intravaginal formulation (IVF), which is designed for topical application to the vaginal cavity, must exhibit acceptable mechanical characteristics, such as ease of application, low hardness, and an extended retention period at the site of application. Moreover, the flow properties of topical pharmaceutical preparations and their rheological characteristics need to be controlled. The reversible thixotropic property of polymer allows solutions to flow onto the cervical cavity permitting an intimate surface contact before the formation of a nonocclusive gel on pH change. Thixotropy involves a progressive increase in viscosity, and thus of shear stress, as a result of pH change produced on subjecting the system to continuous exposure to neutral or alkaline fluids, followed by the recovery of the rheological properties after a prolonged rest period [169]. IVF made of carbopol as a polymer base and containing sodium dodecyl sulfate (SDS) or Nonoxynol-9 (N-9) along with EDTA as microbicidal agents is one of the promising candidates [105, 106]. This system has dual goals: 1) a barrier against STD pathogen to reduce the STD epidemic including AIDS and HPV-induced cervical cancer, and 2) a barrier against sperm to prevent unwanted pregnancy.

Nonoxynol-9 (N-9) has been a leading agent as a spermicide/microbicide and has been widely used as a major ingredient of over-the-counter products for fertility control. Even though the efficiency of N-9 as a spermicidal agent has been expansively demonstrated, the activity of N-9 in the presence of cervical mucosa was found to be not as effective as *in vitro* [170]. Recently, it was also reported that N-9 may even increase human immunodeficiency virus type 1 (HIV-1) transmission, showing that multiple N-9 use can promote HIV-1 transmission through interleukin-1-mediated NF-kappaB activation, which leads to chemokine-induced recruitment of HIV-1 host cells and increased HIV-1 replication in infected cells [171]. Sodium dodecyl sulfate (SDS) is an alkyl sulfate with antimicrobial activity and is widely used in hygiene products. Other agents, such as C31 G, which is a mixture of two amphoteric surfactants of a C14 alkylamine oxid and a C16 alkyl betaine that shows broad-spectrum antimicrobial and spermicidal activity, can be used as a substitute for N-9 [172].

Nanoparticles (NPs) made of Eudragit S-100 (ES), which is anionic co-polymers composed of methacrylic acid and methyl methacrylate, was developed for dual delivery of microbicides [173]. An ES-based nanoparticle which is able to contain both hydrophilic (i.e., tenofovir) and lipophilic compounds (i.e., estrogen), can be fabricated by a modified emulsion solvent diffusion method. As the vagina is acidic under normal conditions and semen from the male partner is neutral, pH-dependent conformational changes of NP upon exposure to semen has a great advantage in achieving high mucoadhesiveness and pharmacological efficacy of intravaginally delivered formulations.

20.6.2 Experimental Setup: Preparation of Simulated Vaginal System (SVS): Cervical Membrane (SCM) and Artificial Vaginal Fluid (AVF)

To better appreciate the extent of the rheological interaction of cervical mucosa with microbicidal agents, artificial vaginal fluid (AVF), simulating the cervical membrane (SCM) and a simulated vaginal system (SVS), were prepared. Previous studies elucidated the difficulties encountered with the existing methods, such as pipetting or swabbing, of obtaining a known weight or volume of vaginal secretion. A direct or indirect swab analysis proved inadequate for collection of fluids in a homogenized form. When secretion was collected with a calibrated pipette, it was often difficult to expel the collected volume from the pipette [174]. AVF is based on previous reports on composition of AVF [175, 176]. AVF is free from uneven homogenization and independent of differences in viscosity and density of secretion. The composition of the IVF, which consists of 0.01-M Tris buffer, supplemented with 100-mM glucose, 1.17-mM $CaCl_2$, and 1.03-mM $MgCl_2$ (pH 7.4), was designed to duplicate normal human vagina conditions including the electrolyte, nitrogenous, and pH status [110, 177].

For the evaluation of the drug release profiles from IVF, an *in vitro* "Simulated Vaginal System" (SVS), which closely mimics the physicodynamic conditions of the vagina by being internally coated with the rabbit vaginal mucosa and subsequently equilibrated with vaginal fluid simulant (VFS) can be used. Compared with Katz diffusion cells (Figure 20.2), it has advantages of capability of not only incorporating external variables but also of monitoring and regulating those variables during experiments. As shown in Figure 20.3, the dialysis membrane (3.5-kDa cut-off) with a diameter and a length of 2.5 and 20 cm, respectively, was internally coated with the rabbit vaginal mucosa. The bottom of the dialysis membrane was closed with a clipper, and the dialysis membrane was filled with AVF [178].

SCM is developed to investigate rheological change including viscosity, bioadhesive strength, shear stress, and tension strength in a simulated vaginal environment. The assessment of these factors in vaginal fluid usually lacks the physicochemical properties of the vaginal environment. SCM can provide better approximation of the vaginal environment under *in vitro* conditions, providing a rigidity to load IVF and serving as a matrix base for evaluation of any changes in viscosity and rheology of cervical mucosa upon contact with microbicides. SCM is mainly composed of

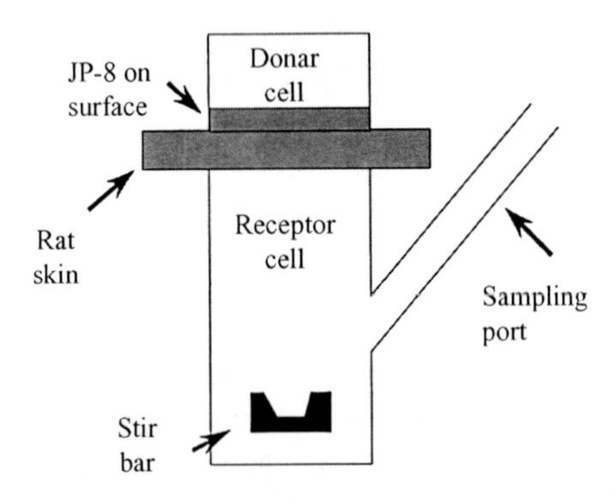

FIGURE 20.2 Kershary-Chien diffusion cell with the receptor solution (JP-8 stands for the vaginal formualtions).

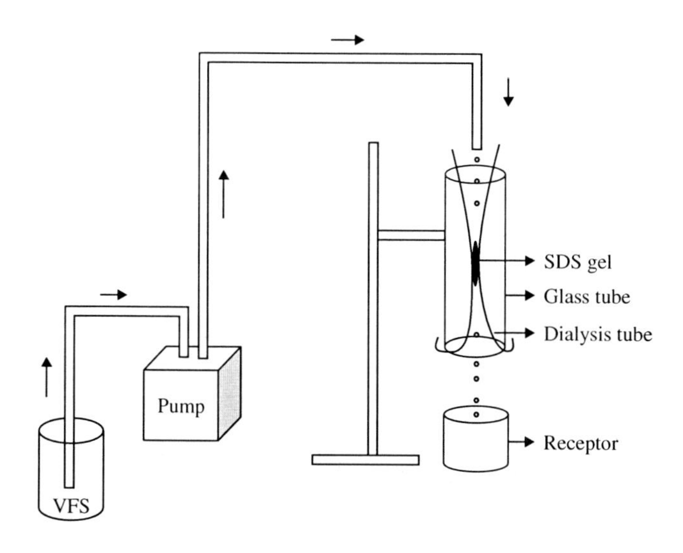

FIGURE 20.3 Simulated vaginal system (SVS) [5].

collagen (90%), cholesterol and phospholipid (9%), and elastin (1%) [179]. Collagen mainly provides rigidity, whereas cholesterol appears to maintain the bilayer in an intermediate fluid state by regulating mobility of phospholipid fatty acid acyl chains. The cholesterol/phospholipid molar ratio is a determinant of membrane fluidity and deformability [180]. SCM still lacks physiological and physical characteristics of the cervical membrane, but it partially simulates an *in vivo* situation by providing interactive properties with microbicides.

20.6.2.1 Rationale for the Selection of Biological Variables The effects of formulation variables on the onset and duration of effective concentrations should be examined to identify the most efficient formulation composition. The sex-specific biological variables involved in pharmacological efficacy of IVF are categorized as follows (Table 20.5) : 1) biological variables (vaginal fluid pH, vaginal fluid secretion speed, protein binding, rotation/vibration speed of movement), which are computed by the model and cannot be manipulated directly in a real situation; 2) extrinsic variables (inserting position and inserting time before intercourse), which can be manipulated externally by customers; and 3) formulation variables (IVF loading weight, loading doses in IVF), which are adjustable during the formulation development process. The insertion position refers to the distance between the loading site of IVF and the bottom of the tube (i. e., orifice).

Variables that are not taken into consideration in an *in vitro* experiment are studies on the diffusion process, transporter-mediated and genetic factors involved processes, which will also significantly affect the outcome of pharmacological efficacy of systemically active drugs (i.e., as compared with topically effective model compounds). The effects of selected variables in various combinations on pharmacological efficacy of model compounds loaded in IVF will be studied using the SVS (Figure 20.3).

20.6.2.2* In Vitro *Drug Release Study from IVF using the Simulated Vaginal System (SVS) The release profiles of two model compounds from IVF will be performed under the same conditions to define the impact of physicodynamic properties (i.e., hydrophilic vs. hydrophobic) of each compound on the release rate and pharmacological efficacy. The sampling time will be prefixed, and discontinuity will be smoothed out using a time-step function. Drug release studies were performed using either Katz diffusion cells or SVS.

The rabbit vaginal mucosa attached inside the dialysis membrane was equilibrated with AVF for 30 minutes, and AVF was removed from the membrane by opening the clipper. The soaked dialysis membrane was inserted into a modified glass tube with a diameter and a length of 2.5 and

TABLE 20.5 Factors Affecting the Drug Release Profile and Efficacy of the Intravaginal System

Variable	Condition	Description
Microbicides concentration in IVS	~100 μM, ~3%	The concentration of microbicide at the application site to achieve the minimum effective concentration required for HIV or HPV inhibition within 2 min of initial application will be determined
Loading weight of IVS	1.5, 3.0, 4.5 g	The loading weight of IVS will evaluate the volume effects on the rate of drug release from IDS
Flow rate of VFS	3, 4, 5 mL/h	The flow rate of VFS will reflect the physiological secretion rate (30–60 mg/day) of vaginal mucus at the different phases of the menstrual cycle
pH of VFS	4.0, 5.5, 7.4	Normal pH range of vaginal secretion is 3.0–5.5. Menstrual and cervical secretions and semen act as alkalizing agents to increase vaginal pH
Speed of rotation	0, 2.5, 5 rpm	The dynamic movement was added on the system by shaking and rotating from vertical to horizontal position at various speeds
Site of application	7.5, 10, 15 cm	The loaded position of IVS will determine the time required to achieve the effective microbicidal concentration at the application site

Source: Ref. 181.

15 cm, respectively. The bottom of the dialysis membrane was opened and tied to the glass tube. The top of the dialysis membrane remained open without being tied to the glass tube. NP containing various concentrations of loaded compounds were loaded into the dialysis tube at 7.5 cm (along with 10 and 15 cm) above the bottom of the tube.

The glass tube was vibrated and shaken at a programmed speed controlled by a motor (0–5 rpm). AVF was dropped on top of the dialysis tube at a predetermined flow rate (3–5 mL/h), which was controlled by a pump. The perfused VFS was collected into a receptor beaker placed under the glass tube or the inserted tampon-type plug (i.e., as used in *in vivo* application), and the amount of released microbicides was determined. Once the tubing or mucosa is soaked with AVFS, it becomes mucoadhesive and closely adheres to each other, and it can hold IVF. SVS has major advantages over other *in vitro* apparatus, simulating the physicodynamic conditions of the vagina and precisely reflecting changes in physiological variables, which may occur during intercourse.

The modified Higuchi equation $Q = (2A \times DC_s t)^n$ can be used to examine the release profile of loaded compounds from IVF, in which Q is the percentage of drug released from IVF at time t (in hours), n is the diffusion exponent, A is the total concentration of drug in the system, D is the diffusion coefficient of the drug in the system, and C_s is the solubility of the drug in the physiological buffer [181, 182]. Diffusion in multicomponent mixtures is usually approximated by defining one single diffusion coefficient for each solute, where the diffusion coefficient rates the concentration gradient of the solute to its flux (Fick's law). Measurements of the diffusion coefficient are typically used to predict and model the kinetics of several *in vivo*, medical, and pharmaceutical applications.

From the above equation, the following equation could be derived: $\ln M_t/M_\infty = n \times \ln(2AC_sD) + n \times \ln t$, in which M_t/M_∞ is the percentage of the total drug released from IVF at time t (in hours), n is the diffusion exponent, and K $(n \times \ln(2AC_sD))$ is the constant apparent release rate (% h^{-1}) [183]. The values of n and K derived from the release profiles of loaded compounds from IVF under various combinations of variables were compared, and the contribution proportion of each variable on the release profiles was examined.

For the analysis of formulation efficacy, the computer model will be needed as an advanced networking classifier based on *in vitro/in vivo* relationships. The computer model can properly predict changes in drug release profiles and microbicidal efficacy as a function of the formulation and physiological variables [5]. The model-based predictions may allow each customer to ensure a self-controllable regimen, which further guarantees NP as the efficient intravaginal barrier against HIV.

20.6.3 Evaluation of Cellular Uptake of Candidate Nanoparticles

Normal vaginal epithelial cell line, VK2/E6E7 (ATCC), can be used for evaluation of the cellular uptake profiles of ES nanoparticles. The properties of IVF or nanoparticles being uptaken by vagina epithelium has huge advantages in that IVF can be used for systemic delivery of compounds as well as vaccine delivery. The schematic uptake profile of nanoparticles is depicted in Figure 20.4. VK2/E6E7 were harvested with keratonized serum-free medium (K-SFM) (Gibco, Carlsbad, CA) containing bovine pituitary extract (BPE) (50 μg/mL), human recombinant epidermal growth factor (EGF) (0.1 ng/mL), $CaCl_2$ (0.4 mM), penicillin (100 U/mL), and streptomycin (100 μg/mL). They were incubated at 37°C under 5% CO_2 and 95% humidity. Cells were incubated with phosphate buffer (pH 6.5) containing nile red-loaded ES nanoparticles (equivalent to 0.5-mg/mL nile red) for 1 hour. Nile red solution (0.5 mg/mL) was used as a control. The cells were fixed with 2% paraformaldehyde, and the cellular uptake profiles of ES nanoparticles was examined using a Nikon TE-2000U scanning fluorescence confocal

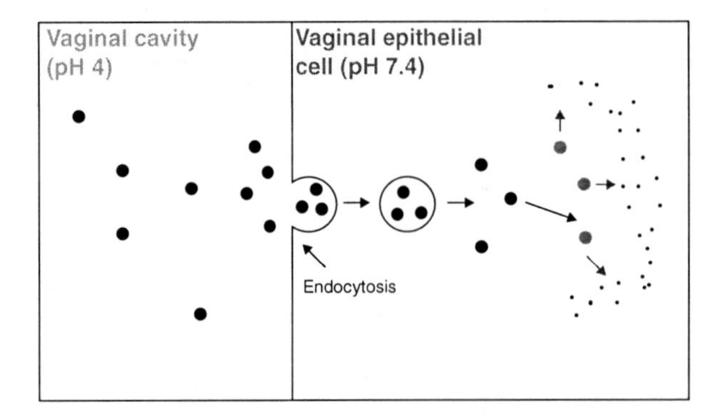

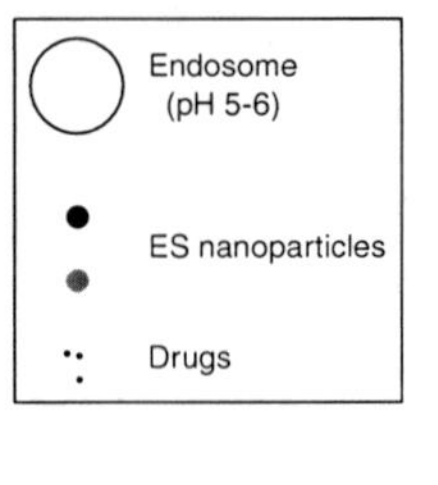

FIGURE 20.4 Hypothetical presentation of ES NP delivery to vaginal epithelial cells. Endosome and lysosome's pH is 5–6.5, at which ES NP is not dissolved. Cytosol pH is pH 7.3–7.5, where the drug is released. Therefore, the drug will be released only at cytosol [173].

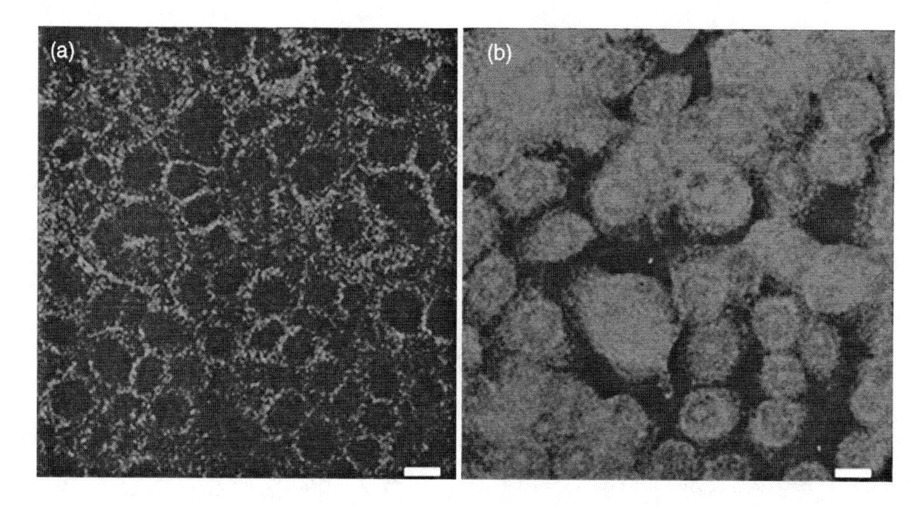

FIGURE 20.5 Cellular uptake profiles of ES nanoparticles in vaginal cells. (a) Nile red solution. Nile red bound on the cell membrane but not crossing the membrane. (b) Nile red-loaded ES nanoparticles. Vaginal cells internalized ES nanoparticles containing nile red and nile red distributed in entire cells, implying that nile red was released from ES nanoparticles in cytosol. Scale bar = 10 μm [173]. (See color figure in color plate section.)

microscope (Nikon Inc., Melville, NY). The digital images were processed using Image-J software (National Institute of Mental Health, Bethesda, MD).

The uptake study of ES nanoparticles incorporated with nile red was performed on vaginal cells [173]. Nile red, which was not formulated with ES nanoparticles, bound on cell membranes and no nile red was found inside the cells (Figure 20.5a), indicating that nile red is not able to penetrate the cells. The ES nanoparticles containing nile red, however, stained at most part of the cells (Figure 20.5b), indicating that ES nanoparticles were internalized into vaginal cells and released as nile red. The results of this study clearly supported that ES nanoparticles can be used for not only for the systemic but also for the combinatorial delivery of both hydrophilic and hydrophobic compounds.

20.6.3.1 Permeability and Pharmacokinetic Evaluation The permeation profiles of those compounds used for systemic pharmacological activities including estrogen and microbicides via vaginal route are affected by physicodynamic and physiology conditions of the vaginal membrane. Drug transport across the vaginal membrane may occur through three primary pathways: the transcellular route, by which diffusion occurs through the cell as a result of a concentration gradient; the intercellular route, where diffusion through spacing between cells; or by a vesicular or receptor-mediated transport [19, 21].

Vaginal permeation studies using the rabbit as an animal model show constancy in the histological, biochemical, and physiological properties and produce a minimal variability in the permeability of the vaginal membrane [184–187]. For vaginal absorption, the apparent permeability coefficient P_{app} of exogenous compounds is related to the first-order rate constant for the disappearance of drug from the vaginal lumen (k_v) [188–191]. The associated equations for permeability and pharmacokinetic profiles of exogenous compounds via a vaginal route are described in detail in the chapter titled "Vaginal Route" in the *Encyclopedia of Pharmaceutical Technology* [192].

20.7 TESTING OF BIOCOMPATIBILITY OF THE VAGINAL SYSTEMS

20.7.1 Cell Culture Models for Microbicide Evaluation

Cell culture models, which can provide various aspects of reproductory organs, can be used to elucidate the effects of IVF on vagina homeostasis. Cell culture models have efficiently demonstrated the biocompatibility and potential cytotoxicity of implantable formulations because any inflammation in a clinical situation would have been randomly distributed throughout the reproductory track without being noticed [193–195].

The epithelial lining of the vagina and ectocervix consist of multiple layers of stratified squamous epithelial cells that are in a nonsterile environment. The endocervical epithelium consists of a single layer of columnar type cells that forms a sterile passage into the upper genital tract. The epithelial cell lines maintain differentiation characteristics of their tissues of origin, demonstrating that columnar epithelial cells of the human endocervix produce more cytokines than do stratified squamous epithelial cells of the ectocervix and vagina [171, 196]. Epithelial cells in the human genital reproductive tract play important and diverse roles in immune defense, and epithelial cell differentiation pathways, along with regulatory factors at different anatomical sites in the tissue environment, affect the defense functions of the vagina. This diversity of the reproductory organ should be considered in the selection processes of the cell line models.

Various cell lines were examined for the study of pathology in ovarian tissue, the cervix, and the vagina. Two plain model cell lines, Hela, an estrogen receptor negative cell line, and NIH: OVACAR-3, an estrogen receptor positive cell line, from ATCC (Manassas, VA), were tested based on their previous usage for assessment of transporters and related mechanisms. Three-dimentional ectocervico-vaginal tissue cells, EpiVagina (MatTek Co., Ashland, MA), that expressed phenotypic markers of the vagina and demonstrated similar histological, ultrastructural, and protein expression characteristics to native vaginal/ectocervical tissue [197], were also used for the evaluation of any changes in cervical morphology upon exposure to external stimuli.

As Hela and NIH:OVACAR-3 cell lines are derived from adenocarcinoma and a stable transfectant could be developed in them, the cell line from normal human vaginal epithelia immortalized by expression of human papillomavirus-16/E6E7 has been tested. This cell line expressed phenotypes resembling those of normal vaginal epithelial cells for more than one year in continuous culture (>200 population doublings). Moreover, the morphological and immunocytochemical characteristics of this cell line are similar to normal vaginal cells, being equipped with tight junctions and involucrin. The VK2 cell line provides the basis for valid, reproducible *in vitro* models for studies on vaginal physiology and infections, and for evaluation of pharmacological agents loaded in intravaginal formulations. The major characteristics of each cell are described in Table 20.6.

20.7.2 Cell Culture Studies

Tissue culture studies will be performed for assessment of biocompatibility and side effects of intravaginal formulations (IVFs). The results of cell line studies showed variances as a result of usage of different cell lines, cell types, and the materials, so proper cell lines should be used to study specific aspects and sensitivities to stimuli [198]. The tissue culture measures early, acute reactions between IVF and host cells, such as

- Cell survivability
- Cell reproduction
- Metabolic activity
- Effective activity—locomotion, phagocytosis, and change in cell shape or size
- Cell damage—mutation and neoplasm formation

The major disadvantages of a tissue culture are [199] 1) lack of systemic pathways within culture, 2) cannot give results in remote tissues or organs, 3) no systemic feedback loops to provide a physiological response, 4) no local circulation (i.e., cell death can occur as a result of a lack of nutrients for cells located at a distance from the nutrient supply, 5) lower metabolism rates than are observed *in vivo*, and 6) some physiological processes do not occur *in vitro* (e.g., fracture healing of bone).

20.7.3 Tests for Carcinogenicity

Most chemical carcinogens are mutagens; thus, the following carcinogenicity tests can be conducted to check whether vaginal formulations have any potential to produce carcinogenicity.

I. Agar diffusion test (the antibiotic sensitivity of compound or material) [200]
II. MTT test (3-(4,5)-dimethyldiazol-2-yl-2,5-diphenyltetrazoliumbromide test (DNA quantity)). Cells will be used to assess the toxicity of metals as well as the organic compounds that may require bioactivation to be toxic [201].

TABLE 20.6 Characteristics of Cervico/Vagina Cell Lines

Name	HeLa	VK2/E6E7	Vaginal Tissue
Type	Human cervical adenocarcinoma (epithelial)	Human vagina (epithelial)	
Subculture ratio	1:2–1:6	1:3–1:5	
Growth media	Minimum essential medium FBS	Keratinocyte-SFM EGF, BPE, and $CaCl_2$	
Tight junctions	−	+	+
Involucrin	−	+	+
Estrogen receptor	+	+	+
Cytokine 19	+	+	+
Cytokine 10,13,16	−	+	+
Cytokine 8,18	+	+	−
Secretary protein	+	+	+

Source: Refs. 171, 172, and 196.

III. Ames test. Method of tissue culture for detecting carcinogenic materials: Culture of mutated bacterial cells, which require histidine to reproduce, are exposed to the material being tested. Only cells that mutate back to the histidine independent state can multiply. Thus, if cells multiply and do not die out, it can be determined that the material causes mutagenesis [202].

Problem with In Vitro Tests for Carcinogenicity High doses of the material, which are used to improve the statistical response and lower the test cost, may lead to problems of extrapolating to behavior at lower, normal doses. Thus, necessary precautions, such as 1) use multiple cell strains, 2) use a range of material dose, and 3) establishment of both positive and negative controls, are needed for assessment of any carcinogenicity from IVF.

20.7.4 *In Vivo* Study with the Animal Model

The rabbit is a proper *in vivo* model for the evaluation of efficacy and biocompatibility of vaginal formulations and their components. As the rabbit vaginal irritation (RVI) model is the most widely used preclinical model for assessment of inflammation and irritation of intravaginal delivery systems, it has major advantages over other animal models in that not only pharmacological efficacy of vaginal formulations but also toxicity at tissues expressed by protein and DNA levels of biomarkers, such as ICAM and NF-kB, upon exposure to vaginal formulations, will be simultaneously investigated at various time points.

The rabbit vagina is about 13–14 cm in length of which the upper and middle portions of the vagina (about 10 cm) are lined by a simple columnar epithelium similar to its endocervix. As a result of a simple columnar epithelium, inflammatory responses of the whole part of the vaginal mucosa to each external compound are expected to be similar. The sensitivity of the rabbit vaginal mucous membrane was previously compared with that of the rat upon exposure to microbicides, such as nonoxynol-9 (N-9) [203]. Both rabbit and rat showed an N-9 concentration-dependent response, but the concentration of N-9 needed to produce irritation activity was smaller in the rabbit than in the rat, revealing that the irritation level produced in the rabbit as a result of 5% concentration of N-9 was equivalent to that produced in the rat by 50% concentration of N-9. Therefore, irritation responses that may not be detectable in the rats can be clearly observable in the rabbits, which would yield a more sensitive, reproducible, and correlated response to the irritation potential of the microbicide on the human vagina. Subsequently, microbicidal agents including Dapivirine against HIV have been tested using a rabbit model [204].

The test vaginal formulations will be uniformly administered at the middle portion of the vaginal lumen, and the cytotoxicity and irritation activity of components will be examined. As the first indication of irritation or inflammation is the histological changes in the epithelial tissue, the vaginal epithelium of the rabbits will be examined on a daily basis for inflammatory responses including edema or redness upon exposure to vaginal formulations [205–207].

20.8 CONCLUSION

Females are considered to be the most vulnerable to sexually transmitted infection because of their social and psychological position in various regions of the world, so the traditional way of protection before sex, such as a condom, may be hard to implement. Therefore, a female-controlled protective method is ideal, with the vaginal formulation being a more convenient way of deployment of medication and alleviation of user compliance.

The conventional STD treatment involves antiviral drug therapy primarily based on the administration of antiviral agents orally for the prophylaxis in a postexposure manner; instead, intravaginal use of microbicides would provide direct prevention for STI including heterosexual transmission of HIV. A formulation containing the combination of the drugs would be developed to attack viruses at different stages of infection and avoid the resistance of the virus to the drug.

From a perspective of formulation itself, the employment of intravaginal devices also renders great promise in preventing sexually transmitted infections in that it avoids repeated deployment in a female-controlled fashion. Numerous polymers and their combinations in various formulation types can be optimized for the most efficient system.

ASSESMENT QUESTIONS

Questions 1–2 are true or false. Write T for true and F for false, respectively, in the left margin preceding the question number.

20.1. Soluble mucins form intermolecular disulfide bridges that provide viscoelastic and lubricating properties.

20.2. Hela is a human cervical adenocarcinoma cell line that is used for studies on the effects and sensitivities to stimuli evoked by intravaginally applied microbicides.

Describe/solve the following question.

20.3. How does pH affect the performance of vaginal formulations?

20.4. Please describe the 1) "thixotropical property" and 2) rationale behind its application to intravaginal formulations.

20.5. A contraceptive tool, product AAA, has a thixotropic property sensitive to its pH changes, maintaining solution form at pH 3.0 and semisolid form at 6.0. Let us assume that product AAA has a very low buffer capacity (β1), while vaginal/cervical mucosa has a buffering system (β2) consisting of glycogen and lactic acid transporters, and a proton exchange system, which maintains mucosa pH at about 4.0 and can be changed up to pH 5.0 upon exposure to exogenous fluid (pH 7.4). And assume that 1) the volume of product AAA and the exogenous fluid are the same, and 2) once the exogenous fluid is administered, product AAA is exposed evenly to the exogenous fluid (pH 7.4) and mucosa fluid. Please derive the equation (in a form of variables) and expected profile for pH changes in product AAA upon exposure to exogenous fluid (pH 7.4).

*You can arbitrarily define all the necessary variables. Clearly specify your rationale behind the equation, and identify all the references (*Int J Pharmaceutics* format) you referred to. Your answers will be graded based on the rationale and on an innovative idea.

REFERENCES

1. Joglekar, A., Rhodes, C.R., Danish, M. (1991). *Drug Development and Industrial Pharmacy*, *17*, 2103–2113.
2. Platzer, W., Poisel, W. Functional anatomy of the human vagina, in E.S.E. Hafez and T.N. Evans (eds.), *The Human Vagina*. North Holland, New York, NY, 1978, pp. 39–53.
3. Kistner, R.W. Physiology of the vagina, in E.S.E. Hafez and T.N. Evans (eds.), *The Human Vagina*. North Holland, New York, NY, 1978, pp. 109–120.
4. Burgos, M.H., Roig de Varnas-Linares, C.E. In E.S.E. Hafez and T.N. Evans (eds.), *The Human Vagina*. North Holland, New York, NY, 1978, pp. 63–93.
5. Wang, Y., Lee, CH. (2004). In vitro release of sodium dodecyl sulfate from a female controlled drug delivery system. *International Journal of Pharmaceutics*, *282(1–2)*, 173–181.
6. King, B.F. (1983). Ultrastructure of the nonhuman primate vaginal mucosa: Epithelial changes during the menstrual cycle and pregnancy. *Journal of Ultrastructure Research*, *82*, 1–18.
7. Sjöberg, I., Cajander, S., Rylander, E. (1988). Morphometric characteristics of the vaginal epithelium during the menstrual cycle. *Gynecologic and Obstetric Investigation*, *26*, 136–144.
8. Averette, H.E., Weinstein, G.D., Frost, P. (1970). *American Journal of Obstetrics and Gynecology*, *108*, 8–17.
9. Wagner, G., Levin, R.J. Vaginal Fluid, in E.S.E. Hafez and T. N. Evans (eds.), *The Human Vagina*. North Holland, New York, NY, 1978, pp. 121–137.
10. Itoh, Y. (1990). Analysis of human vaginal secretions using rabbit anti-human vaginal secretions: detection of non-serum proteins. *Japanese Journal of Legal Medicine*, *44*, 267–271.
11. Itoh, Y., Furuhata, A., Sato, Y. (1991). Immunohistochemical studies on the localization of non-serum proteins detectable in human vaginal secretions. *Japanese Journal of Legal Medicine*, *45*, 26–29.
12. Schmidt, E.H., Beller, F.K. Biochemistry of the vagina, in E. S.E. Hafez and T.N. Evans (eds.), *The Human Vagina*. North Holland, New York, NY, 1978, pp. 139–149.
13. Moghissi, K.S. Composition and function of cervical secretions, In R.O. Greep and E.B. Astwood (eds.), *Handbook of Physiology*, Section 7, Vol. II, Part 2. American Physiological Society, Washington, DC, 1978, pp. 25–48.
14. Cohen, M.S. *Vaginitis and Vaginosis*, B.J. Horowitz and P.-A. Mardh (eds.). Wiley-Liss, New York, NY, 1991, pp. 33–37.
15. Richardson, J.L., Illum, L. (1992). *Advanced Drug Delivery Reviews*, *8*, 341–366.
16. Sparks, R.A., et al. (1977). *Obstetrics & Gynecology*, *84*, 701.
17. Brenner, P.F. (1988). The menopausal syndrome. *Obstetrics & Gynecology*, *72*, 6S–11S.
18. Pelligrino, D.A. et al. (2000). Nitric-oxide-dependent pial arteriolar dilation in the female rat: effects of chronic estrogen depletion and repletion. *Biochemical and Biophysical Research Communications*, *269(1)*, 165–71.
19. Barbo, D.M. (1987). The physiology of menopause. *Clinical Chemistry and Laboratory Medicine*, *71*, 11–22.
20. Masters, W.H., Johnson, V.E. *Human Sexual Response*. Little, Brown, Boston, MA, 1966.
21. Steger, R.W., Hafez, E.S.E. Age-associated changes in the vagina, in E.S.E. Hafez and T.N. Evans (eds.), *The Human Vagina*. North Holland, New York, NY, 1978, pp. 95–106.
22. Brown, W.J. (1978). Microbial ecology of the normal vagina, in E.S.E. Hafez and T.N. Evans (eds.), *The Human Vagina*. North Holland, New York, NY, *1978*, pp. 407–422.
23. Robinson, G.D. (1927). *Journal of Pharmacology and Experimental*, *32*, 81–88.
24. Strous, G.J., Dekker, J. (1992). Mucin-type glycoproteins. *Critical Reviews in Biochemistry and Molecular Biology*, *27*, 57–92.
25. Gipson, I. K., et al. (1992). Char- acteristics of a glycoprotein in the ocular surface glycocalyx. *Investigative Ophthalmology Visual Science*, *33*, 218–227.
26. Gipson, I.K., et al. (1995). Stratified squamous epithelia produce mucin-like glycoproteins. *Tissue and Cell*, *27(4)*, 397–404.
27. Gum, J.R., Jr. (1992). Mucin Genes and the proteins they encode: Structure, diversity, and regulation. *American Journal of Respiratory Cell and Molecular Biology*, *7*, 557–564.
28. Macht, D.D.J. (1928). Concerning the absorption of qunin and oxyquinolin sulphate through the vagina. *Pharmacology and Experimental Therapeutics*, *34*, 137–145.
29. Millman, N., Hartman, C.G., Stavorski, J., Botti, J. (1950). Comparison of vaginal tolerance tests of spermicidal preparations in rabbits. *Proceedings of the National Academy of Sciences of the United States of America*, *9*, 89.
30. Hartman, C.G. (1959). The permeability of the vaginal mucosa. *Annals of the New York Academy of Sciences*, *83*, 313–327.
31. El-Sheikha, A.Z., Hafez, E.S.E. Absorption of drugs and hormones in the vagina, in E.S.E. Hafez and T.N. Evans (eds.), *The Human Vagina*. North Holland, New York, NY, 1978, pp. 179–191.

32. Benzinger, D.P., Edelson, J. (1983). Absorption from the vagina. *Drug Metabolism Reviews*, *14*, 137–168.
33. Rosenzweig, M., Walzer, M. (1943). Absorption of protein from the vagina and uterine cervix. *American Journal of Obstetrics and Gynecology*, *45*, 286–290.
34. Cunningham, F.E., et al. (1994). Pharmacokinetics of intravaginal metronidazole gel. *The Journal of Clinical Pharmacology*, *34*, 1060–1065.
35. Chien, Y.W. Mucosal Drug Delivery, in Y.W. Chien (eds.), *Novel Drug Delivery Systems*. Marcel Dekker, New York, NY, 1992, pp. 197–228.
36. Hwang, S., et al. (1976). Systems approach to vaginal delivery. *Journal of Pharmacy & Pharmaceutical Sciences*, *65*, 1574–1578.
37. Hwang, S., et al. (1977). Systems approach to vaginal delivery of drugs V. *Journal of Pharmacy & Pharmaceutical Sciences*, *66*, 781–784.
38. Bengtsson, L.P. (1954). Absorption of phosphorus-32 from the rabbit vagina under various hormonal conditions. *Nature*, *1954(173)*, 954–955.
39. Yotsuyanagi, T., et al. (1975). Systems approach to vaginal delivery of drugs I. *Journal of Pharmacy & Pharmaceutical Sciences*, *64*, 71.
40. Hwang, S., et al. (1977). Systems approach to vaginal delivery of drugs V. *Journal of Pharmacy & Pharmaceutical Sciences*, *66*, 778–780.
41. Flynn, G.L., et al. Interfacing matrix release and membrane absorption analysis of steroid absorption from a vaginal device in the rabbit doe, in D.R. Paul and F.W. Harris (eds.), *Controlled Release of Polymeric Formulations*. American Chemical Society, Washington, DC, 1976, pp. 87–122.
42. Ho, H.F.H., et al. (1976). Systems approach to vaginal delivery of drugs III. *Journal of Pharmacy & Pharmaceutical Sciences*, *65*, 1578.
43. Corbo, D.C., Liu, J.C., Chien, Y.W. (1990). Characterization of the barrier properties of mucosal membranes. *Journal of Pharmacy & Pharmaceutical Sciences*, *79*, 202–206.
44. Rojanasaku, Y., et al. (1992). The increase of carboxyfluorescein binding to macrophages. *Research in Pharmacy*, *9*, 1029–1034.
45. Sanders, J.M., Matthews, H.B. (1990). Vaginal absorption of polyvinyl alcohol in Fischer 344 rats. *Human & Experimental Toxicology*, *9*, 71–77.
46. Yu, K., Chien, Y.W. (1995). Spermicidal activity structure relationship of oligomers of nonoxynol-9. *International Journal of Pharmacy*, *125*, 81–90.
47. Chien, Y.W., et al. (1975). Controlled drug release from polymeric delivery devices. 3. In vitro-in vivo correlation for intravaginal release of ethynodiol diacetate from silicone devices in rabbits. *Journal of Pharmacy & Pharmaceutical Sciences*, *64*, 1776.
48. Moghissi, K.S.Composition and function of cervical secretion, in R.O. Greep and E.B. Astwood (eds.), *Handbook of Physiology*. American Physiological Society, Washington, DC, 1973, pp. 25–48.
49. Eriksen, G.V., et al. (1998). *Fertility and Sterility*, *70*, 350–354.
50. Morales, P., Roco, M., Vigil, P. (1993). *Human Reprodroduction*, *8*, 78–83.
51. Cheeti, S., Lee, C.H. (2010). The involvement of intracellular calcium in the regulation of mct-mediated drug uptake by hela cells. *Molecular Pharmaceutics*, *7(1)*, 169–176.
52. Maly, K., et al. (2002). Critical role of protein kinase C alpha and calcium in growth factor induced activation of the Na (+)/H(+) exchanger NHE1. *FEBS Letters*, *521(1–3)*, 205–210.
53. Pinto, V., et al. (2008). Oxidative stress and the genomic regulation of aldosterone-stimulated NHE1 activity in SHR renal proximal tubular cells. *Molecular and Cellular Biochemistry*, *310*, 1–2.
54. Brown, T.J., Yen-Moore, A., Trying, S.K., (1999). An overview of sexually transmitted diseases. Part 1. *Journal of the American Academy of Dermatology*, *41(4)*, 511–532.
55. Howett, M.K., et al. (1999). A broad-spectrum microbicide with virucidal activity against sexually transmitted diseases. *Antimicrobial Agents and Chemotherapy*, *43*, 314–321.
56. Koot, M., et al. (1996). Relation between changes in cellular load, evolution of viral phenotype, and the clonal composition of virus populations in the course of human immunodeficiency virus type 1 infection. *Journal of Infectious Diseases*, *173(2)*, 349–54.
57. Cheney, K., McKnight, A. HIV-2 tropism and disease, lentiviruses and macrophages. *Molecular and Cellular Interactions*. Academic Press, New York, NY, 2010.
58. Chan, D., Kim, P. (1998). HIV entry and its inhibition. *Cell*, *93(5)*, 681–684.
59. Wyatt, R., Sodroski, J. (1998). The HIV-1 envelope glycoproteins: fusogens, antigens, and immunogens. *Science*, *280 (5371)*, 1884–1888.
60. Moore, J.P. (1997). Coreceptors: implications for HIV pathogenesis and therapy. *Science*, *276(5309)*, 51–52.
61. Cutler, B., Justman, J. (2008). Vaginal microbicides and the prevention of HIV transmission. *Lancet Infectious Diseases*, *8*, 685–697.
62. Upadhyay, U. Microbicides: New Potential for protection. *The INFO Reports*, No. 3. Baltimore, Johns Hopkins Bloomberg School of Public Health, 2005.
63. Hladik, F., Doncel GF. (2010). Preventing mucosal HIV transmission with topical microbicides: challenges and opportunities. *Antiviral Research*, *88(1)*, S3–S9.
64. Van Damme, L. (2002). Alliance for microbicide development. *Health and Sexuality Microbicides*, 1–8.
65. Murata, L.B., Dodson, M.S. (1999). *Journal of Biological Chemistry*, *274(52)*, 37079–37086.
66. De Clercq, E. (2004). New anti-HIV agents in preclinical and clinical development. *Frontiers in Medicinal Chemistry*, *1 (1)*, 543–579.
67. Margot, N. A., et al. (2002). Genotypic and phenotypic analyses of HIV-1 in antiretroviral-experienced patients treated with tenofovir DF. *Aids*, *16(9)*, 1227–1235.

68. Eiben, G.L., et al. (2003). Cervical cancer vaccines: recent advances in HPV research. *Viral Immunology*, *16*(2), 111–121.
69. Wolf, D.P., et al. (1977). *Fertility and Sterility*, *28*, 53–58.
70. Wegmann, F., Krashias, G., Luhn, K. (2011). A novel strategy for inducing enhanced mucosal HIV-1 antibody responses in an anti-inflammatory environment. *PLoS Medicine*, *6(1)*, e15861.
71. Montefiori, D., et al. (2007). Antibody-based HIV-1 vaccines: Recent developments and future directions. *PLoS Medicine*, *4*, e348.
72. Li, Q., et al. (2009). Glycerol monolaurate prevents mucosal SIV transmission. *Nature*, *458*, 1034–1038.
73. Pigman, W. *The Glycoconjugate*, M.I. Horowitz and W. Pigman (eds.). Academic Press, New York, NY, Vol *1*, 1977.
74. Lee, C.H., Chien, Y.W. Drug delivery, vaginal route. *Encyclopedia of Pharmaceutical Technology*, 2nd edition. 2005, pp. 961–985.
75. Silberberg, A., Meyer, F.A. *Mucus in Health and Disease II*, E. Chantler, J. Elder, and M. Eionstein (eds.). Springer, New York, NY, 1982, pp. 53–74.
76. Sheehan, J.K., Carlstedt, I. (1984). *Biochemical Journal*, *217*, 93–101.
77. Blasco, L. (1977). *Fertility and Sterility*, *28*, 1133.
78. Romanelli, F., Murphy, B. (2010). Systemic preexposure prophylaxis for human immunodeficiency virus infection. *Pharmacotherapy*, *30(10)*, 1021–1030.
79. Lee, C.H., Anderson, M., Chien, Y.W. (1996). *Journal of Pharmacy & Pharmaceutical Sciences*, *85*, 649–654.
80. Vigil, P., et al. (1991). *Human Reproduction*, *6*, 475–479.
81. Katakowski, J.A., Palliser, D. (2011). Optimizing siRNA delivery to the genital mucosa. *Discovery Medicine*, *11* (*57*), 124–132.
82. Capodici, J., Kariko, K., Weissman, D. (2002). Inhibition of HIV-1 infection by small interfering RNA-mediated RNA interference. *The Journal of Immunology*, *169*, 5196–5201.
83. Dasgupta, R., Perrimon, N. (2004). Using RNAi to catch Drosophila genes in a web of interactions: insights into cancer research. *Oncogene*, *23*, 8359–8365.
84. Bitko V., et al. (2005). Inhibition of respiratory viruses by nasally administered siRNA. *Nature Medicine*, *11*, 50–55.
85. Palliser, D., et al. (2006). An siRNA-based microbicide protects mice from lethal herpes simplex virus 2 infection. *Nature*, *439*(*7072*), 89–94.
86. Wu, Y., et al. (2009). Durable protection from Herpes Simplex Virus-2 transmission following intravaginal application of siRNAs targeting both a viral and host gene. *Cell Host & Microbe*, *5*(*1*), 84–94.
87. Butz, K., et al. (2003). siRNA targeting of the viral E6 oncogene efficiently kills human papillomavirus-positive cancer cells. *Oncogene*, *22*, 5938–5945.
88. Jiang, M., Rubbi, C.P., Milner, J. (2004). Gel-based application of siRNA to human epithelial cancer cells induces RNAi-dependent apoptosis. *Oligonucleotides*, *14*, 239–248.
89. Yoshinouchi, M., et al. (2003). In vitro and in vivo growth suppression of human papillomavirus 16-positive cervical cancer cells by E6 siRNA. *Molecular Therapy*, *8*, 762–768.
90. Woodrow, K.A., Cu, Y. (2009). Intravaginal gene silencing using biodegradable polymer nanoparticles densely loaded with small-interfering RNA. *Nat Materials*, *8*(*6*), 526–533.
91. Gu, W., et al. (2007). The development and future of oligonucleotide-based therapies for cervical cancer. *Current Opinion in Molecular Therapeutics*, *9*, 126–131.
92. Vaishnaw, A.K., Gollob, J. (2010). A status report on RNAi therapeutics. *Silence*, *1*(*1*), 14.
93. Mamo, T., et al. (2010). Emerging nanotechnology approaches for HIV/AIDS treatment and prevention. *Nanomedicine*, *5*(2), 269–285.
94. Robbins, M, Judge, A. (2009). siRNA and innate immunity. *Oligonucleotides*, *19*(2), 89–102.
95. Parkin, D.M., et al. (2005). Global cancer statistics, 2002. *A Cancer Journal for Clinicians*, *55*, 74–108.
96. Jemal, A., et al. (2005). Cancer statistics. *A Cancer Journal for Clinicians*, *55*, 10–30.
97. Putral, L.N., et al. (2005). RNA interference against human papillomavirus oncogenes in cervical cancer cells results in increased sensitivity to cisplatin. *Molecular Pharmacology*, *68*, 1311–1319.
98. Wright, T.C., et al. (2006). Chapter 14: HPV vaccine introduction in industrialized countries. *Vaccine*, *24*(*3*), S122–131.
99. Tan, S.J., et al. (2011). Engineering nanocarriers for siRNA delivery. *Small*, *7*(*7*), 841–851.
100. Bosch, F.X., et al. (1995). Prevalence of human papillomavirus in cervical cancer: A worldwide perspective. International biological study on cervical cancer (IBSCC) Study Group. *Journal of the National Cancer Institute*, *87*, 796–802.
101. Fujii, T., et al. (2006). Intratumor injection of small interfering RNA-targeting human papillomavirus 18 E6 and E7 successfully inhibits the growth of cervical cancer. *International Journal of Oncology*, *29*, 541–548.
102. Gu, W., et al. (2006). Inhibition of cervical cancer cell growth in vitro and in vivo with lentiviral-vector delivered short hairpin RNA targeting human papillomavirus E6 and E7 oncogenes. *Cancer Gene Therapy*, *13*, 1023–1032.
103. Hall, A.H., Alexander, K.A. (2003). RNA interference of human papillomavirus type 18 E6 and E7 induces senescence in HeLa cells. *Journal of Virology*, *77*, 6066–6069.
104. Tang, S., et al. (2006). Short-term induction and long-term suppression of HPV16 oncogene silencing by RNA interference in cervical cancer cells. *Oncogene*, *25*, 2094–2104.
105. Krebs, F.C., et al. (1999). Inactivation of human immunodeficiency virus type 1 by nonoxynol-9, C31G, or an alkyl sulfate, sodium dodecyl sufate. *Antiviral Research*, *43*, 157–173.
106. Krebs, F.C., et al. (2000). Sodium dodecyl sulfate and C31G as microbicidal alternatives to nonoxynol-9: Comparative sensitivity of primary human vaginal keratinocytes. *Antimicrobial Agents and Chemotherapy*, *44*, 1954–1960.

107. Lai, B.E., et al. (2008). Dilution of microbicide gels with vaginal fluid and semen simulants: Effect on rheological properties and coating flow. *Journal of Pharmacy & Pharmaceutical Sciences*, *97(2)*, 1030–1038.

108. White, D.R., Aitken, R.J. (1989). Relationship between calcium, cyclic amp, atp, and intracellular ph and the capacity of hamster spermatozoa to express hyperactivated motility. *Gamete Research*, *22*, 163–177.

109. Johnson, P.M., Rainsford, K.D. (1972). The physical properties of mucus. *Biochimica et Biophysica Acta*, *286*, 72.

110. Wagner, G., Levine, R.J. Vaginal fluids, in E.S.E. Hafez and T.N. Evans (eds.), *The Human Vagina*. North Holland, New York, NY, 1978, pp. 109–120.

111. Szeri, A.J., et al. (2008). A model of transluminal flow of anti-HIV microbicide vehicle: Combined elastic squeezing and gravitational sliding. *Physics of Fluids*, *20*, 083101–083110.

112. Bonferoni, M.C., et al. (2006). Chitosan gels for the vaginal delivery of lactic acid: Relevance of formulation parameters to mucoadhesion and release mechanisms. *Journal of American Association of Pharmaceutical Scientists*, *7(5)*, 104.

113. Ndesendo, V.M.K., Pilly, V., Choonara, Y.E. (2008). A review of current intravaginal drug delivery approaches employed for the prophylaxis of HIV/AIDS and prevention of sexually transmitted infections. *Journal of American Association of Pharmaceutical Scientists*, *9(2)*, 505–520.

114. Lundholm, P., et al. (1999). *Vaccine*, *17*, 2036–2042.

115. Jiang, Y.H., et al. (2005). SPL7013 gel as a topical microbicide for prevention of vaginal transmission of SHIV89.6P in macaques. *AIDS Research of Human Retroviruses*, *21(3)*, 207–213.

116. Stone, A. (2002). Microbicides: A new approach to preventing HIV and other sexually transmitted infections. *Nature Reviews*, *1*, 977–985.

117. Smit, A.J. (2004). Medicinal and pharmaceutical uses of seaweed natural products: A review. *Journal of Applied Psychics*, *16(4)*, 245–262.

118. Zacharopoulos, V.R., Phillips, D.M. (1997). Vaginal formulations of carrageenan protect mice from herpes simplex virus infection. *Clinical and Diagnostic Laboratory Immunology*, *4(4)*, 465–468.

119. Lamont, R.F., et al. (2003). The efficacy of vaginal clindamycin for the treatment of abnormal genital tract flora in pregnancy. *Infectious Diseases in Obstetrics and Gynecology*, *11*, 181–189.

120. Balzarini, J., Van Damme, L. (2007). Microbicide drug candidates to prevent HIV infection. *The Lancet*, *369*, 787–797.

121. De Clercq E. (2009). The history of antiretrovirals: Key discoveries over the past 25 years. *Reviews in Medical Virology*, *19*, 287–299.

122. Kristmundsdóttir, T.S., et al. (2000). Development and evaluation of microbicidal hydrogels containing monoglyceride as the active ingredient. *Journal of Pharmacy & Pharmaceutical Sciences*, *88(10)*, 1011–1015.

123. Harrison, P.F., Rosenberg, Z, Bowcut, J. (2003). Topical microbicides for disease prevention: Status and challenges. *Clinical Infectious Diseases*, *26*, 1290–1294.

124. Cundy, K.C., et al. (1998) Pharmacokinetics and bioavailability of the anti-human immunodeficiency virus nucleotide analog 9-[(R)-2-(phosphonomethoxy) propyl]adenine (PMPA) in dogs. *Antimicrobial Agents and Chemotherapy*, *42*, 687–690.

125. Otten, R.A., et al. (2000). Efficacy of postexposure prophylaxis after intravaginal exposure of pig-tailed macaques to a human-derived retrovirus (human immunodeficiency virus type 2). *Journal of Virology*, *74(20)*, 9771–9775.

126. Otten, R.A., et al. (2005). Multiple vaginal exposures to low doses of R5 simian-human immunodeficiency virus: Strategy to study HIV preclinical interventions in nonhuman primates. *Journal of Infectious Diseases*, *191(2)*, 164–173.

127. Veazey, R.S., et al. (2003). Use of a small molecule CCR5 inhibitor in macaques to treat simian immunodeficiency virus infection or prevent simian-human immunodeficiency virus infection. *Journal of Experimental Medicine*, *198(10)*, 1551–1562.

128. D'Cruz, O.J. (2004). Uckun FM. Clinical development of microbicides for the prevention of HIV infection. *Current Pharmaceutical Design*, *10(3)*, 315–336.

129. Mills, E. (2005). Tenofovir trials raise ethical issues. *HIV AIDS Policy Law Review*, *10(2)*, 31–32.

130. Hazra, R., et al. (2005). Tenofovir disoproxil fumarate and an optimized background regimen of antiretroviral agents as salvage therapy for pediatric HIV infection. *Pediatrics*, *116(6)*, e846–e854.

131. Pecora Fulco, P., Kirian, M.A. (2003). Effect of tenofovir on didanosine absorption in patients with HIV. *The Annals of Pharmacotherapy*, *37*, 1325–1328.

132. Karim, Q.A., et al. (2010). Effectiveness and safety of tenofovir gel, an antiretroviral microbicide, for the prevention of HIV infection in women. *Science*, *329(5996)*, 1168–1174.

133. Trius, A., Sebranek, J.G. (1996). Carrageenan and their use in meat products. *Critical Reviews in Food Science and Nutrition*, *36(1–2)*, 69–85.

134. Pearce-Pratt, R., Phillips, D.M. (1996). Sulfated polysaccharides inhibit lymphocyte-to-epithelial transmission of human immunodeficiency virus-1. *Biology of Reproduction*, *54(1)*, 173–182.

135. Chaowanachan, T., et al. (2000). In vitro effect of Carrageenan Microbicide PC-515 and Methyl Cellulose Placebo Gels on COBAS Amplicor and Gen-Probe Chlamydia trachomatis and Neisseria gonorrhoeae, and InPouch TV trichomonas vaginalis tests. *Int Conf AIDS*. *13*: abstract no. WePeA4112.

136. Perotti, M.E., Pirovano, A., Phillips, D.M. (2003). Carrageenan formulation prevents macrophage traffickering from vagina: Implications for microbicide development. *Biology of Reproduction*, *69(3)*, 933–939.

137. Fernandez-Romero, J.A., et al. (2007). Carrageenan/MIV 150 (PC-815), a combination microbicide. *Sexually Transmitted Diseases*, *34*, 9–14.

138. Buck, C.B., et al. (2006). Carrageenan is a potent inhibitor of papillomavirus infection. *Biol Reprod. PLoS Pathogens, 2(7)*, e69.

139. Coggins, C., et al. (2000). Preliminary safety and acceptability of a carrageenan gel for possible use as a vaginal microbicide. *Sexually Transmitted Infections, 76*, 480–483.

140. Milligan, G.N., et al. (2004). Effect of candidate vaginally-applied microbicide compounds on recognition of antigen by CD4+ and CD8+ T lymphocytes1. *Biology of Reproduction, 71(5)*, 1638–1645.

141. Dezarnaulds, G., Fraser, I.S. (2002). Vaginal ring delivery of hormone replacement therapy – a review. *Expert Opinion on Pharmacotherapy*, *4*(2), 201–212.

142. Malcolm, R.K., et al. (2010). Advances in microbicide vaginal rings. *Antiviral Research, 88(1)*, S30–S39.

143. Timmer, C.J., Apter, D., Voortman, G. (1990). Pharmacokinetics of 3-keto-desogestrel and ethinylestradiol released from different types of contraceptive vaginal rings. *Contraception, 42(6)*, 629–642.

144. Rahimi, A.M. (2009). Silicone polymers in controlled drug delivery systems: A review. *Iranian Polymer Journal, 18*, 16.

145. Promadej-Lanier, N., et al. (2009). Development and evaluation of a vaginal ring device for sustained delivery of HIV microbicides to non-human primates. *Journal of Medical Primatology, 38*, 263–271.

146. Johnson, T.J., et al. (2010). Segmented polyurethane intravaginal rings for the sustained combined delivery of antiretroviral agents dapivirine and tenofovir. *European Journal of Pharmaceutical Sciences, 39*, 203–212.

147. Woolfson, A.D., et al. (2010). Freeze-dried, mucoadhesive system for vaginal delivery of the HIV microbicide, dapivirine: Optimisation by an artificial neural network. *International Journal of Pharmacy, 388*, 136–143.

148. Brij, B.S., et al. (2009). Sustained release of microbicides by newly engineered vaginal rings. *AIDS, 23*, 917–922.

149. Nel, A., et al. (2009). Safety and pharmacokinetics of dapivirine delivery from matrix and reservoir intravaginal rings to HIV-negative women. *Journal of Acquired Immune Deficiency Syndromes, 51*, 416–423.

150. Morrow, R.J., et al. (2011). Sustained release of proteins from a modified vaginal ring device. *European Journal of Pharmaceutics and Biopharmaceutics, 77*, 3–10.

151. Saxena, B.B., et al. (2009). Sustained release of microbicides by newly engineered vaginal rings. *AIDS, 23*, 917–922.

152. Kast, C.E., et al. (2002). Design and in vitro evaluation of a novel bioadhesive vaginal drug delivery system for clotrimazole. *Journal of Controlled Release, 81(3)*, 347–354.

153. Maria-Elisa, P., Pirovano, A., Phillips, D.M. (2003). Carageenan formulation prevents macrophage trafficking from vagina: Implications for microbicide development. *Biology of Reproduction, 69(3)*, 933–939.

154. Valenta, C. (2005). The use of mucoadhesive polymers in vaginal delivery. *Advanced Drug Delivery Reviews, 57(11)*, 1692–1712.

155. Kim, P.S., Read, S.W. (2010). Nanotechnology and HIV: Potential applications for treatment and prevention. *Wiley Interdisciplinary Reviews: Nanomedicine and Nanobiotechnology, 2(6)*.

156. Bernstein, D.I., Stanberry, L.R., Sacks, S. (2003). Evaluations of unformulated and formulated dendrimer-based microbicide candidates in mouse and guinea pig models of genital herpes. *Antimicrob. Agents Chemotherapy, 47(12)*, 3784–3788.

157. Seol, Y., Carpenter, A.E., Perkins, T.T. (2006). Gold nanoparticles: enhanced optical trapping and sensitivity coupled with significant heating. *Optics Letters, 31(16)*, 2429–2431.

158. Cho, K., et al. (2005). The study of antimicrobial activity and preservative effects of nanosilver ingredient. *Electrochimica Acta. 51(5)*, 956–960.

159. Pal, S., Tak, Y.K. Song, J.M. (2007). Does the antibacterial activity of silver nanoparticles depend on the shape of the nanoparticle? A study of the gram-negative bacterium Escherichia coli. *Applied and Environmental Microbiology, 73(6)*, 1712–1720.

160. Torchilin, V.P. (2000). Drug targeting. *European Journal of Pharmaceutical Sciences, 11*(2), S81–S91.

161. Lederman, M.M., et al. (2004). Prevention of vaginal SHIV transmission in rhesus macaques through inhibition of CCR5. *Science, 306*, 485–487.

162. Ham, A.S., et al. (2009). Targeted delivery of PSC-RANTES for HIV-1 prevention using biodegradable nanoparticles. *Research in Pharmacy, 26*, 502–511.

163. Wang, Y.Y., et al. (2008). Addressing the PEG mucoadhesivity paradox to engineer nanoparticles that "slip" through the human mucus barrier. *Agnew Chemie International Edition, 47*, 9726–9729.

164. Whaley, K.J., et al. (2010). Novel approaches to vaginal delivery and safety of microbicides: Biopharmaceuticals, nanoparticles, and vaccines. *Antiviral Research, 88(1)*, S55–S66.

165. Friend, D.S. (1982). Plasma membrane diversity in a highly polarized cell. *Journal of Cellular Biology, 93*, 243–249.

166. Yanagimachi, R. Sperm egg fusion. *Current Topics in Membranes and Transport*. Academic Press, New York, NY, 1988, pp. 3–43.

167. Barbara, E., Valeria, F., Fabrizio, E. (2006). Candidate HIV-1 tat vaccine development from basic science to clinical trials. *AIDS, 20(18)*, 2245–2261.

168. Akagi, K., et al. (2003). Mucosal immunization with inactivated HIV-1-capturing nanospheres induces a significant HIV-1-specific vaginal antibody response in mice. *Journal of Medical Virology, 69*(2), 163–172.

169. Eccleston, G.M., et al. (2000). Rheological behavior of nasal sprays in shear and extension. *Drug Development and Industrial Pharmacy, 26*, 975–983.

170. Lee, C. H., et al. (1997). Development of silicone-based barrier devices for controlled release of spermicidal agent. *Journal of Controlled Release, 43*, 283–290.

171. Fichorova RN, Anderson DJ. (1999). Differential expression of immunobiological mediators by immortalized human cervical and vaginal epithelial cells. *Biology of Reproduction, 60* (2), 508–514.

172. Piret, J., et al. (2000). In vitro and in vivo evaluation of sodium lauryl sulfate and dextran sulfate as microbicides against herpes simplex and human immunodeficiency viruses. *Journal of Clinical Microbiology, 38,* 110–119.

173. Yoo, J.W., Giri, N., Lee, C.H. (2011). pH-sensitive Eudragit nanoparticles for mucosal drug delivery. *International Journal of Pharmaceutics, 403,* 262–267.

174. Wilks, M., Thin, R.N. (1982). Quantitative methods for studies on vaginal flora. *Journal of Medical Microbiology, 15,* 141–147.

175. Owen, D. H., Katz, D.F. (1999). A vaginal fluid simulant. *Contraception, 59,* 91–95.

176. Dorr, R.T., et al. (1982). In vitro retinoid binding and release from a collagen sponge material in a simulated intravaginal environment. *Journal of Biomedical Materials Research, 16,* 839–850.

177. Moghissi, K.S. Cervical factor in fertility, in E.E. Wallach and H.A. Zacur (eds.), *Reproductive Medicine and Surgery.* Mosby Book, Chicago, IL, 1995, pp. 376–397.

178. Wang, Y., Lee, C.H. (2002). Characterization of a female controlled drug delivery system for microbicides. *Contraception, 66(4),* 281–287.

179. Coata, G., et al. (1995). Effect of low –dose oral triphasic contraceptives on blood viscosity, coagulation and lipid metabolism. *Contraception, 52,* 151–157.

180. Rotten, D., et al. (1988). Evolution of the elastic fiber network of the human uterine cervix before, during and after pregnancy. A quantitaitve ecvaluation by automated image analysis. *Clinical Physiology & Biochemistry, 6,* 285–292.

181. Higuchi, T. (1963). Mechanisms of sustained action medication: Theoretical analysis of the rate of release of solid drugs dispersed in solid matrices. *Journal of Pharmacy & Pharmaceutical Sciences, 52,* 1145–1149.

182. Toddywala, R., Chien, Y.W. (1990). Evaluation of silicone-based pressure-sensitive adhesives for transdermal drug delivery. I. Effect of penetrant hydrophilicity. *Journal of Controlled Release, 14,* 29–41.

183. Ritger, P.L., Peppas, N. (1987). Bioadhesive intraoral release systems: Design, testing and analysis. *Journal of Controlled Release, 5,* 37–42.

184. Barentsen, R., Peter, H.M. (1997). *European Journal of Obstetrics & Gynecology and Reproductive Biology, 71,* 73–80.

185. Jovov, B., et al. (1994). *American Journal of Physiology, 266,* F775–F784.

186. Gorodeski, G.I., Jin, W., Hopper, U. (1997). Extracellular Ca2+ directly regulates tight junctional permeability in the human cervical cell line CaSki. *American Journal of Physiology, 272,* C511–C524.

187. Platz-Christensen, J.J., et al. (1997). *Prostaglandins, 53,* 253–261.

188. Gonzalez-Estrella, J. A., et al. (1994). *Fertility and Sterility, 62,* 1238–1243.

189. Casper, F., Petri, E. (1999). *International Urogynecology Journal, 10,* 171–176.

190. Odeblad, E. (1968). *Acta Obstertricia et. Gynecologica Scandinavica, 47(8),* 7–19.

191. Moghissi, K.S. Cervical factor in fertility, in E.E. Wallach and H.A. Zacur (eds.), *Reproductive Medicine and Surgery.* Mosby Book, Chicago, IL, 1995, pp. 376–397.

192. Chien, Y.W., Lee, C.H. Drug delivery, vaginal route. *Encyclopedia of Pharmaceutical Technology,* 2nd edition, 2005, pp. 961–985.

193. Tan, X., Pearce-Pratt, R., Phillips, D.M. (1993). Productive infection of a cervical epithelial cell line with human immunodeficiency virus: Implications for sexual transmission. *Journal of Virology, 67(11),* 6447–6452.

194. Devine, P.J., Rajapaksa, K.S., Hoyer, P.B. (2002). In vitro ovarian tissue and organ culture: a review. *Frontiers in Bioscience, 7,* d1979–d1989.

195. Doncel, G.F., Chandra, N., Fichorova, R.N. (2004). Preclinical assessment of the proinflammatory potential of microbicide candidates. *Journal of Acquired Immune Deficiency Syndromes, 37(3),* S174–S180.

196. Fichorova, R.N., Tucker, L.D., Anderson, D.J. (2001). The molecular basis of nonoxynol-9-induced vaginal inflammation and its possible relevance to human immunodeficiency virus type 1 transmission. *Journal of Infectious Diseases, 184* (4), 418–428.

197. Elkeeb, R., Zdanowicz, M., Belmonte, A. (2003). Evaluation of reconstituted human vaginal epithelium as a model for drug delivery of fluconazole gel for treating vulvovaginal candidiasis. The American Association of Pharmaceutical Scientists (AAPS) Annual Meeting and Exposition in Salt Lake City, UT, October 26–30.

198. Cummins, J.E. Jr, Doncel, G.F. (2009). Biomarkers of cervicovaginal inflammation for the assessment of microbicide safety. *Sexually Transmitted Diseases, 36(3),* S84–S91.

199. Krebs, F.C., et al. (2002). Comparative in vitro sensitivities of human immune cell lines, vaginal and cervical epithelial cell lines, and primary cells to candidate microbicides nonoxynol 9, C31G, and sodium dodecyl sulfate. *Antimicrobial Agents and Chemotherapy, 46(7),* 2292–2298.

200. Beyth, N., et al. (2008). Surface antimicrobial activity and biocompatibility of incorporated polyethylenimine nanoparticles. *Biomaterials, 29(31),* 4157–4163.

201. Wan, H., et al. (1994). A study of the reproducibility of the MTT test. *Journal of Materials Science: Materials in Medicine, 5(3),* 154–159.

202. Flamand, N., et al. (2001). Ames test used in a prescreening assay for point mutagenesis assessment. *Toxicology in Vitro, 15(2),* 105–114.

203. Kaminsky, M., et al. (1985). Comparison of the sensitivity of the vaginal mucous membranes of the albino rabbit and laboratory rat to nonoxynol-9. *Food and Chemical Toxicology, 23,* 705–708.

204. Nuttall, J.P., et al. (2008). Concentrations of dapivirine in the rhesus macaque and rabbit following once daily intravaginal administration of a gel formulation of [14C]dapivirine for 7 Days. *Antimicrobial Agents and Chemotherapy*, *52*(*3*), 909–914.

205. Alt, C., et al. (2009). Increased CCL2 expression and macrophage/monocyte migration during microbicide-induced vaginal irritation. *Current HIV Research*, *7*(*6*), 639–649.

206. Macht, D.D. (1918). On the absorption of drugs and poisons through the vagina. *Journal of Pharmacology and Experimental Therapeutics*, *10*, 509–521.

207. Miyake, A., et al. (2004). Induction of HIV-specific antibody response and protection against vaginal SHIV transmission by intranasal immunization with inactivated SHIV-capturing nanospheres in macaques. *Journal of Medical Virology*, *73*(*3*), 368–377.

21

ADVANCED DRUG DELIVERY TO THE BRAIN

NANDA K. MANDAVA, MITESH PATEL, AND ASHIM K. MITRA

21.1 CHAPTER OBJECTIVES

- To provide an overview on challenges for drug delivery across blood–brain interfaces.
- To highlight various direct systemic and central nervous system (CNS) methods used for brain drug delivery.
- To provide expression of various endogenous transporters and receptors expressed on the blood–brain barrier.
- To present various drug delivery approaches with special focus on transporter-targeted drug delivery.

21.2 INTRODUCTION

The treatment of neurodegenerative diseases, brain cancers, and infections requires therapeutic drug concentrations in the brain. Drug delivery to the central nervous system (CNS) poses several challenges for researchers in drug development because of limited access for therapeutic agents. The low brain absorption of therapeutic agents is attributed mainly to two physiological barriers, the blood–brain barrier (BBB), and the blood–cerebrospinal fluid barrier (BCSFB). The BBB is formed by polarized endothelial cells of brain microvasculature and several other cell populations such as astrocytes and pericytes, which support endothelial cells collectively in restricting the entry and exit of nutrients and xenobiotics. The BCSFB is located at the choroid plexus and is formed by epithelial cells which are connected by tight junctions. Stroma and fenestrated blood vessels are present underneath the epithelial cells. These blood vessels lack tight junctions, but tight junctions between epithelial cells restrict the entry of drugs into cerebrospinal fluid (CSF) [1]. Even though the brain is highly vascularized, these barriers separate the brain from the general blood supply. The BBB and BCSFB play an important role in controlling the entry of nutrient and therapeutic agents into brain, thus, maintaining brain homeostasis. Other than cellular tight junctions, various efflux proteins such as P-glycoprotein (P-gp), multidrug resistance protein (MRP), and breast cancer-resistant protein (BCRP) are highly expressed on the BBB and contribute significantly to limit brain absorption of drugs. In this chapter, we have made an attempt to describe various drug delivery methods and a few of the novel approaches explored for enhanced drug delivery to the brain. This chapter mainly emphasizes the physiological approaches that take advantage of specific transporters and receptors expressed on the capillary endothelial cells forming the BBB. This chapter will also serve as a valuable reference to researchers interested in learning the fundamental function of the BBB and those working on improving brain drug delivery via physiological approaches.

Advanced Drug Delivery, First Edition. Edited by Ashim K. Mitra, Chi H. Lee, and Kun Cheng.

21.3 BARRIERS FOR BRAIN DRUG DELIVERY

Several therapeutic agents are unsuccessful in treating CNS disorders resulting from ineffective delivery to the brain. Drug delivery to the brain poses a great challenge even though the brain is highly perfused with blood flow. This is a result of the physiological barriers that separate brain tissue from blood circulation and control transport of several compounds including nutrients. The barriers attributing to the low brain bioavailability of drugs are the BBB and BCSFB. The important functions of these barriers are to impede free diffusion between brain fluids and blood and to provide transport processes for essential nutrients, ions, and metabolic waste products [2]. To deliver drugs to the brain effectively, it is necessary to learn about the morphology of these barriers.

21.3.1 Blood–Brain Barrier

The brain is protected from foreign organisms and toxic substances by the BBB. It is made up of three layers: an inner endothelial cell layer that forms the wall of brain capillaries, a basement membrane, and feet processes of astrocytes and pericytes. Figure 21.1 is the schematic representation of the BBB and other components of the vascular unit and their arrangement. Brain capillaries have a complex morphology, which provides special characteristics to the endothelial cell layer with respect to diffusion of solutes. Brain endothelial cells (BECs) are interconnected by tight junctions (TJs) and occlude paracellular spaces. Moreover, BECs exhibit minimal pinocytotic activity. In addition, these BECs are secluded by astrocytic end feet and pericytes on the brain side, which further restrict the permeability of various drugs.

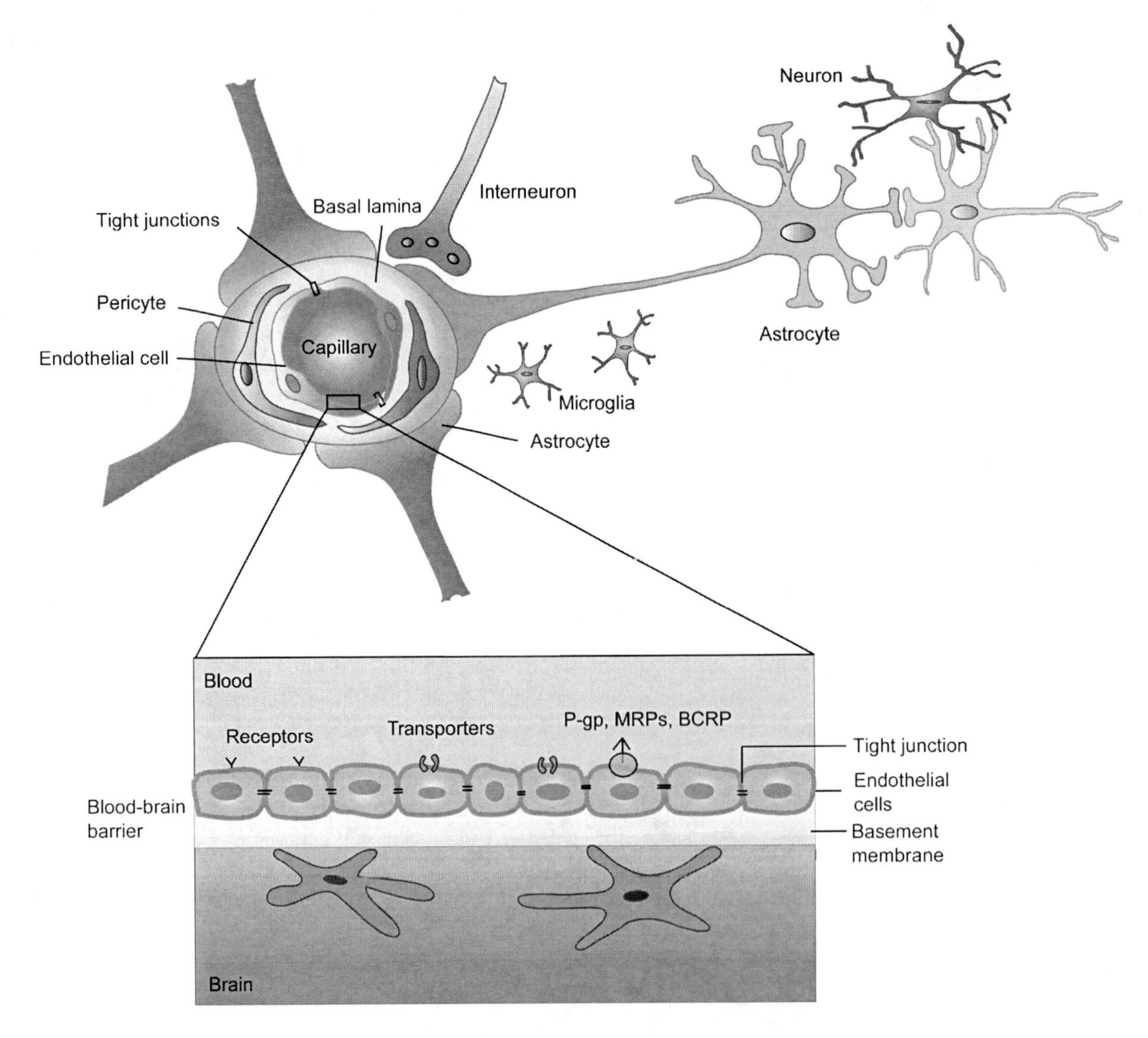

FIGURE 21.1 Schematic representation of the blood–brain barrier. (See color figure in color plate section.)

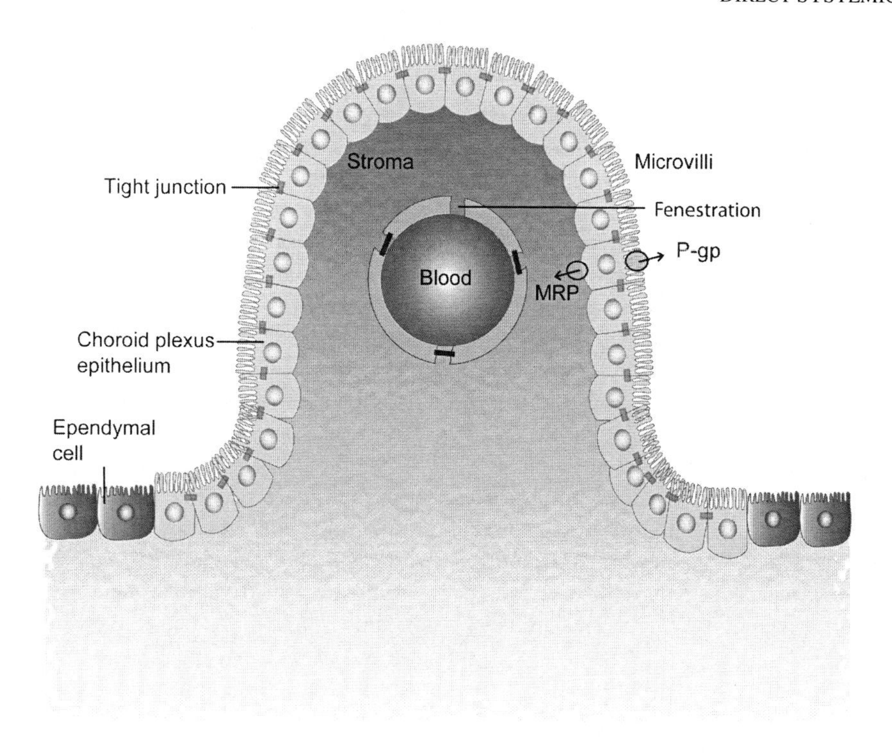

FIGURE 21.2 Schematic representation of the blood–CSF barrier.

Overall the BBB exhibits very high transendothelial electrical resistance (TEER) values, around 1500 $\Omega\,cm^2$, which is very high compared with other tissues that range from 3 to 33 $\Omega\,cm^2$ [3]. Thus, the BBB provides very high resistance to permeability of solutes, drugs, and xenobiotics. As mentioned, other than BECs, other cell populations which constitute BBB include astrocytes and pericytes. Both astrocytes and pericytes help in the differentiation and maintenance of the BBB function. Astrocytes account for 60% of the total non-neuronal cell population, which provide biochemical support for endothelial cells, transport essential nutrients to nervous tissue, and maintain extracellular ion balance. They also play a crucial role in repair and scarring processes after injuries and inflammation [4]. Pericytes secrete growth factors that are important for maturation and remodeling of vascular system. They are involved in transport across the BBB and regulation of vascular permeability [5].

21.3.2 Blood–Cerebrospinal Fluid Barrier

The BCSFB is another barrier that restricts the entry of systemically administered drugs into the CNS. The BCSFB functions in conjunction with the BBB and meninges to safeguard the brain. CSF is secreted from the choroid plexus epithelium (CPE) and circulates through ventricles around the brain and spinal cord [6]. The choroid plexus (CP) is a villous structure floating in cerebrospinal fluid that is attached to the ventricular ependyma. The ependyma is continuous with the epithelial layer of CP composed of a single layer of cells. These CPE cells constitute the BCSFB [7]. Figure 21.2 represents the blood–CSF barrier. Tight junctions are present in the CP epithelium, restricting solute transport. Tight junctions on the BCSFB are distinct and exhibit less restriction to the diffusion of solutes in comparison with the BBB [8]. In addition to TJs, the CP epithelium is fortified with an organic acid transporter system that is responsible for driving organic acids in the CSF to the blood. Hence, a variety of therapeutic organic acids, such as zidovudine, methotrexate, and penicillin, cannot gain access to the brain parenchyma. The arachnoid epithelium serves as another barrier for the transport of drugs to the brain. The arachnoid is one of three meninges, underlying the dura, which covers the entire CNS as a protective sheath and separates extracellular fluids of CNS from the rest of the body [7, 9]. However, low surface area and the avascular nature of the arachnoid makes it a less significant interface for solute exchange from the blood to the CNS [10]. All these barriers form a combination of physical, transport, and metabolic barriers resulting in restricted environment for solute entry into brain.

21.4 DIRECT SYSTEMIC DELIVERY

21.4.1 Intravenous Delivery

Intravenous (IV) is the commonly adapted method for administering high doses of drugs into the general circulation. Drugs administered by this route will have the advantage of avoiding first-pass metabolism and providing good potential for drugs to enter the brain [11]. As discussed, the brain is highly perfused with blood circulation with a total surface area of 20 m^2 [12]. Hence, the IV route serves as a better route for brain drug targeting. However, the presence of barriers and rapid clearance from brain extracellular fluid (ECF) limits drug transport. Moreover, brain absorption of drugs largely depends on the stability of drugs in plasma, permeability across the BBB, and absorption into brain parenchyma. Several researchers attempted to deliver drugs by the IV route using colloidal carriers such as liposomes and nanoparticles, which may sustain drug release and enhance blood circulation time. Steiniger et al. attempted to deliver doxorubicin intravenously using polysorbate 80-coated nanoparticles. A 40% cure rate for glioblastoma in rats was observed [13]. Several drugs, such as loperamide, tubocurarine, and hexapeptide dalagrin, have been delivered successfully to the brain using polysorbate 80-coated nanoparticles intravenously [12].

21.4.2 Intra-Arterial Delivery

The intra-arterial (IA) route has been studied for brain delivery, as it offers advantages such as direct access to brain vasculature before peripheral circulation, and avoids first-pass metabolism. This route has been exploited to deliver especially antitumor agents to treat gliomas. The transport of drugs may follow two pathways: 1) the movement of drugs in capillaries to the CP epithelium, finally reaching CSF, or 2) reaching CSF through white matter from arterial blood following the perivascular pathway [14]. Often, the BBB disrupting agents enhanced the brain absorption of drugs after IA administration. Usually, the bradykinin receptor agonist and hypertonic mannitol are used along with drugs in IA delivery [15]. Rainov et al. delivered replication-deficient adenoviral vectors and cationic liposomeplasmid DNA complexes effectively to brain tumors. The number of transgene-expressing tumor cells was further increased by bradykinin infusion [16].

21.4.3 Transnasal Delivery

Transnasal delivery to the brain is based on the hypothesis that xenobiotics, toxic substances, and viruses enter the brain from the nasal cavity via olfactory neurons, hence this route can be used for brain drug delivery [17]. The intranasal route has been studied extensively by several researchers to deliver small-molecule drugs, therapeutic peptides, viral vectors, and even cells to the brain. This method is the most noninvasive for circumventing the BBB to deliver drugs and therapeutic peptides to the brain. Nasal cavities are divided into three regions: nasal vestibular, respiratory, and olfactory regions. The nasal vestibular region is responsible for filtering out airborne particles and has no significant role in drug absorption. The respiratory region is the largest part of the nasal cavity and is highly vascularized. The respiratory region is responsible for drug absorption into systemic circulation. The drug absorption pathways include paracellular and transcellular pathways, transcytosis, and carrier-mediated transport. The olfactory region (next to the respiratory region) is the major portal for drug absorption to the brain. The intranasal route serves as a better route for brain delivery because of rapid absorption into brain as a result of its high blood flow, porous endothelial membrane, large surface area, and bypassing first-pass metabolism [12]. The intranasal route can be used for both small molecules and macromolecules (therapeutic peptides). Depending on the physicochemical properties of drug molecules and formulation, drug absorption from the olfactory region involves transcellular, paracellular, olfactory or trigeminal neuronal, perivascular, and CSF pathways [18, 19]. Nasal administration of lipophilic small molecules such as progesterone results in higher CSF concentrations than serum concentrations [20]. This clearly demonstrates direct drug absorption from the nasal submucus space to CSF. The olfactory region of the nose consists of olfactory cells that extend up to the cranial cavity. The drug absorption pathway includes diffusion from nasal mucosa, arachnoid, enter olfactory CSF, and then to the CSF compartment of the brain. After nasal administration, drugs may diffuse through mucosa and rapidly get absorbed into CSF, skipping the BBB and achieving rapid CSF levels. However, all CNS acting drugs are not lipophilic and most have molecular weights higher than 400 Da. Hydrophilicity becomes another rate-limiting barrier because of weak partitioning. Small lipophilic drugs or colloidal substances such as gold particles may undergo the transcellular pathway [21]. The transcellular pathway is the most common pathway for lipophilic molecules. Molecular size, degree of ionization, and p*Ka* play an important role in the transcellular pathway. Sometimes drugs permeate through active transport via carrier-mediated transport on nasal mucosa [22]. Another mechanism of transport, the paracellular pathway, refers to transport of drugs between cells by passive diffusion. Usually, polar and charged molecules with molecular weights less than 1000 Da are absorbed by the paracellular pathway [23]. Diffusion is guided by concentration gradient across the epithelium. Sometimes formulation excipients can be used to facilitate passive transport. For example, chitosan opens tight junctions between epithelial cells in nasal mucosa.

In recent years, extensive research has been performed to deliver therapeutic peptides to the brain via the intranasal route. Macromolecules such as proteins, peptides, and DNA have gained considerable attention for the treatment of various brain disorders because of their high specificity and selectivity. Despite their modest advantages, the brain availability of these macromolecules has been a major concern. Intranasal administration of insulin has been proposed for the treatment of Alzheimer's disease (AD). On delineating the mechanism, investigators found that insulin permeated the brain via the olfactory bulb [24]. A similar study demonstrated the transport of insulin-like growth factor-I from the nasal mucosa to the rat brain via olfactory and trigeminal nerves [25]. Significant inhibition in anti-nerve growth factor (anti-NGF) antibodies in AD11 mice was generated after the intranasal administration of NGF [26, 27]. Intranasal administration has been proposed as an excellent alternative route for brain delivery of plasmid DNA encoding therapeutic genes [28]. Intranasal administration generated high systemic bioavailability and brain distribution of plasmid DNA compared with intravenous administration. These reports demonstrate clearly that intranasal administration can be used as an excellent alternative strategy for improving brain delivery of macromolecules.

The administration of NAD+ greatly decreased brain injury in a rat model of transient focal ischemia and profoundly decreased oxidative cell death [29]. Similarly, intranasal administration of gallotannin, a poly (ADP-ribose) glycohydrolase (PARG) inhibitor, showed a marked reduction in the frequency of ischemic brain injury in rats [30]. Olanzapine, when delivered intranasally as mucoadhesive microemulsion formulation, showed better effectiveness of the route of drug delivery into brain [31]. The delivery of buspirone hydrochloride as mucoadhesive formulation using chitosan and hydroxylpropyl beta cyclodextrin showed better brain concentration after intranasal administration in mice [32]. Similarly, intranasal mucoadhesive microemulsion of sumatriptan showed better cerebral concentration and a reduction in migraine headache [33]. Despite the advantages of the intranasal route for brain drug delivery, it has some limitations, such as damage of nasal mucosa on frequent use of this route, rapid clearance of drugs by mucociliary clearance system, interference from nasal congestion, systemic clearance from respiratory region, and partial degradation of drugs/therapeutic proteins [34, 35].

21.5 DIRECT CNS DELIVERY

Various newer approaches have been presented for the direct delivery of drug molecules to the CNS. These approaches have the advantage of delivering a much higher concentration of neurotherapeutics by injecting the drug directly into CSF or parenchymal space, subsequently reducing the drug concentration in the peripheral environment [11]. Several factors that monitor the CSF concentration include drug volume distribution, site of puncture, rate of clearance, drug diffusion, transport pathways, and CSF production rate [36]. Several approaches that have been developed for the direct delivery of drug molecules and peptides into the CNS include intracerebral, intraventricular, and intrathecal (intra-CSF) delivery. Table 21.1 describes the advantages and limitations of all the brain drug delivery methods.

21.5.1 Intracerebral (Intraparenchymal) Delivery

Intracerebral delivery involves direct drug administration into the parenchymal space either as bolus or infusion [37]. Intraparenchymal administration as a bolus dose has certain limitations. Drugs have to diffuse through tightly packed parenchyma. This leads to a reduced diffusion coefficient, and drugs may not traverse to the target site. Very high doses of drugs need to be administered because diffusion phenomenon is concentration dependent [38]. To overcome this problem, the continuous infusion method was employed, which used convection-enhanced delivery (CED) phenomena. CED involves stereotactically guided catheter insertion to brain parenchyma through which infusate is pumped into brain parenchyma and penetrates into interstitial space [39]. The outcome of CED infusion depends on accurate catheter placement and other infusion parameters. Several drugs such as paclitaxel and immunotoxin were delivered effectively by infusion [11].

Another approach attempted for direct controlled parenchymal delivery is intracerabral implants and polymer depots. Implants made up of biodegradable/nonbiodegradable polymers encapsulating small molecule drugs and therapeutic proteins have been studied. These implants protect drugs from degradation and allow controlled local drug release. Drug released from these implants/polymeric depots has to diffuse through brain parenchyma. Various intracerebral implants have been used to deliver small molecules and proteins. For example, an implant containing NGF exhibited better results in patients with quadriplegia [40, 41]. Various neurodegenerative diseases such as Huntington's and Parkinson's diseases can be treated using intracerebral implants [42]. Gliadel (Eisai Inc., Woodcliff Lake, NJ) was the first product approved based on intracranial controlled delivery. Gliadel is a wafer consisting of BCNU (1,3-bis(2-chloroethyl)-1-nitrosourea; carmustine) as a drug and poly(bis(*p*-carboxyphenoxy)propane-sebacic acid) as a polymer. It is approved for the treatment of glioblastome multiforme [43]. It showed drug release over a period of 5 days when placed in the tumor resection cavity. The poor release characteristics of the wafer can be resolved by placement of monolithic depots in an effective way. These monolithic depots are made up of polymers and co-polymers. Monolithic depots increase the active transport to endothelial cells with decreased chances of drug elimination from parenchyma by interstitial fluid flow [44]. The most promisingly used monolithic polymeric depots made up of co-polymer like poly(lactide-co-glycolide) are of recent interest in delivery of drugs and peptides into the CNS across the BBB because of their size, biodegradability, and biocompatibility [11].

TABLE 21.1 Advantages and Limitations of Various Brain Drug Delivery Methods

Brain Drug Delivery Method	Advantages	Limitations
	Systemic delivery	
Intravenous delivery	High doses of drugs can be administered directly into blood circulation Avoids first-pass metabolism	Stability of drug in plasma. Permeation across the BBB is the rate-limiting factor
Intra-arterial delivery	Direct access to brain vasculature before peripheral circulation. Avoids first-pass metabolism	The BBB is the rate-limiting factor for drug absorption
Transnasal delivery	Noninvasive method. Rapid absorption into the brain Large surface area facilitates absorption	The BCSFB is the barrier for drugs absorbed from olfactory region The BBB is the barrier for drugs absorbed from respiratory region
	Direct CNS delivery	
Intracerebral (intraparenchymal) delivery	Bypasses the BBB Direct drug delivery into brain parenchyma	Highly invasive Injection/catheter placement site must be specific Concentrations at the target site depend on the drug diffusion coefficient
Intraventricular delivery (transcranial drug delivery)	Bypasses the BBB Direct administration into ventricles Better suited for ventricular and subarachnoid infections	Highly invasive Drug clearance from CSF into blood circulation If the target site is not close to ventricles, then this approach is not suitable because parenchymal drug diffusion is poor
Intrathecal delivery (intra-CSF drug delivery)	Direct drug delivery to CSF Less invasive than other direct CNS delivery methods Bypasses the BBB Suitable for treating spinal cord infections/disorders	Limited drug diffusion to deep parenchymal tissue Rapid drug clearance from CSF into blood

Osmotic pump devices and vapor pressure-activated implants are also developed for controlled delivery. These implants contain a refillable reservoir and a catheter. The most widely known device is the ALZET osmotic pump (DURECT Corporation, Cupertino, CA), which can deliver dopamine or dopamine agonist for about 4 weeks [45]. The fate of drugs released from these implants is based on the rate of drug transport by diffusion and fluid convection, the rate of elimination from the brain by degradation, and metabolism [45]. Polymer depots have been employed for the sustained delivery of drugs into the cerebrum. Drug release from these polymer depots depends on drug loading, matrix thickness, and polymer selection [46].

21.5.2 Intraventricular Delivery (Transcranial Drug Delivery)

The intraventricular route is direct drug administration into the cerebral ventricle. Intraventricular delivery, like intracerebral delivery, bypasses the BBB. This route of administration is adapted in the treatment of meningioma and metastatic cells in CSF because drug distribution mainly takes place into ventricles and subarachnoid space in the brain [47]. One advantage of intraventricular injection over intracerebral injection is a lack of a connection with interstitial fluid [12]. However, a major disadvantage is that drugs administered by this route may be cleared from CSF into the blood circulation. This occurs because of CSF turnover every 4–5 h and the exit of CSF into the blood [48]. Moreover, there is speculation that drugs administered by the intraventricular route will be distributed more into the blood than the brain [49]. Intraventricular administration may also lead to high drug exposure to ependymal surface and may lead to related toxicities such as subependymal astrogliotic reactions [50, 51]. However, this route has been studied by researchers for brain delivery of drugs and therapeutic proteins. Nutt et al. attempted to deliver glial-derived neurotrophic factor (GDNF) by intracerebroventrical (ICV) injection to treat Parkinson's disease [52]. No therapeutic effect was observed in patients because GDNF did not reach the striatum of the brain [53]. Drug distribution is mainly governed by diffusion across brain tissue. Because the brain parenchyma is tightly packed tissue, drug diffusion decreases exponentially with distance from the administration site [54]. However, slow intraventricular infusion is effective in comparison with intraventricular bolus administration and may also result in sustained drug release into the brain. For example, Murry et al. delivered cytosine arabinoside by intraventricular infusion. The continuous slow infusion of intraventricular of cytosine arabinoside liposomes exhibited 71% better efficacy compared with intrathecal administration in treating neoplastic meningitis and an increase in half life from 0.74 to 156 h [55]. Rocque et al. compared intraventricular baclofen (IVB) with intrathecal baclofen (ITB) for secondary dystonia and performed a comparison of complications. These investigators concluded that IVB is as safe as ITB [56].

21.5.3 Intrathecal Delivery (Intra-CSF Drug Delivery)

Intrathecal administration involves direct drug injection into the cistern magna of the brain. This route is less invasive compared with intracebral, intraventricular routes and bypasses the BBB, resulting in high CSF concentrations [12]. Drugs administered via this route cannot diffuse into deep parenchymal tissues of the brain. Another major limitation is rapid clearance from CSF into the blood at multiple sites along the length of the brain and spinal canal [57]. Because of this reason, the intrathecal route is employed to treat spinal cord diseases but not brain parenchymal diseases [58].

21.6 CHEMICAL AND PHYSIOLOGICAL APPROACHES

The BBB poses one of the most challenging barriers for the transport of therapeutics from the systemic circulation to the brain. The high expression of tight junctions between BECs prevents the diffusion of hydrophilic drug molecules. In addition, efflux proteins such as P-gp, MRPs, and BCRP may also modulate drug transport at the BBB. Several noninvasive strategies have been explored thoroughly in recent years to increase drug permeability across the BBB. These include the following:

- Altering BBB properties by using membrane disrupting agents
- Conjugation of lipids for increasing membrane interaction
- Chemical derivatization of drugs with transporter/receptor targeting moieties
- Using drug delivery systems such as nanoparticles, liposomes, and micelles for efficient drug delivery

21.6.1 Lipidation

One of the major reasons for the poor transport of therapeutic agents across the BBB is their high hydrophilicity. Lipidation is an approach used to increase the permeability of hydrophilic drugs by enhancing their interaction with the absorbing membrane. This approach involves conjugation of small chain fatty acids or lipids to therapeutic drug molecules.

Several lipid prodrugs have been investigated previously for determining their efficacy in enhancing drug transport across the BBB. The brain transport of ketoprofen is highly limited because of its complete ionization at physiological pH, poor lipophilicity, and efflux clearance. 1,3-Diacetyl-2-ketoprofen glyceride (DAKG) lipid prodrug generated a threefold increase in the area under a brain concentration-time curve of ketoprofen relative to ketoprofen alone [59]. The brain uptake clearance obtained with DAKG and ketoprofen alone was 1.60 ± 0.16 and 0.0308 ± 0.0046 mL/min/g. This result indicated clearly that the lipid derivative produced a significant increase in the brain permeability of ketoprofen. Furthermore, *in vitro* metabolism and tissue homogenate studies demonstrated the hydrolytic conversion of DAKG to ketoprofen. DP-155, a lipid prodrug of indomethacin, has been proposed for the chronic treatment of Alzheimer's disease and analgesia [60]. The brain-to-plasma ratio obtained with DP-155 was 3.5 times higher relative to indomethacin. Similar enhancements in brain absorption have been obtained with (+/-)-3′-azido-2′,3′-dideoxy-5′-*O*-(2-bromomyristoyl) thymidine lipid prodrug relative to 3′-azido-2′,3′-dideoxythymidine (AZT). The brain concentration and area under concentration-time profile of lipid prodrug and AZT obtained was 25.7 and 9.8 nmol/g and 2.8 and 1.4 μmol·min/g, respectively [61]. Lipid prodrugs of gamma-amino butyric acid have also been found capable of penetrating through the BBB [62]. Niflumic acid lipid prodrugs exhibited high anti-inflammatory activity at significantly lower concentrations [63].

Although lipid prodrugs have proved to be efficient in increasing the penetration of therapeutic agents across the BBB, it may suffer several limitations such as high plasma protein binding, nonspecific tissue distribution, reduced receptor binding affinity, and intracellular sequestration [64]. Novel lipid-based drug delivery systems including solid lipid nanoparticles and liposomes have become popular for enhancing drug delivery across the BBB.

21.6.2 Modulation of Efflux Proteins

The permeation of chemotherapeutics across the BBB is limited by the presence of several ATP-binding cassette (ABC) efflux transporters, i.e., P-gp, BCRP, and MRPs. The major efflux proteins expressed on the BBB are shown in Figure 21.3 [65, 66]. A high expression of P-gp, MRPs, and BCRP has been reported as one of the major causes for therapeutic failure [67]. P-gp belongs to large ATP-binding cassette superfamily of transport proteins and is encoded by ABCB1 gene [68]. It is a 170-kDa phosphorylated and glycosylated membrane protein composed of two homologous halves, each containing six transmembrane domains (TMDs) separated by a polypeptide linker. MRPs also belong to the ABC superfamily, and several isoforms (MRP1–9) have been identified in the central nervous

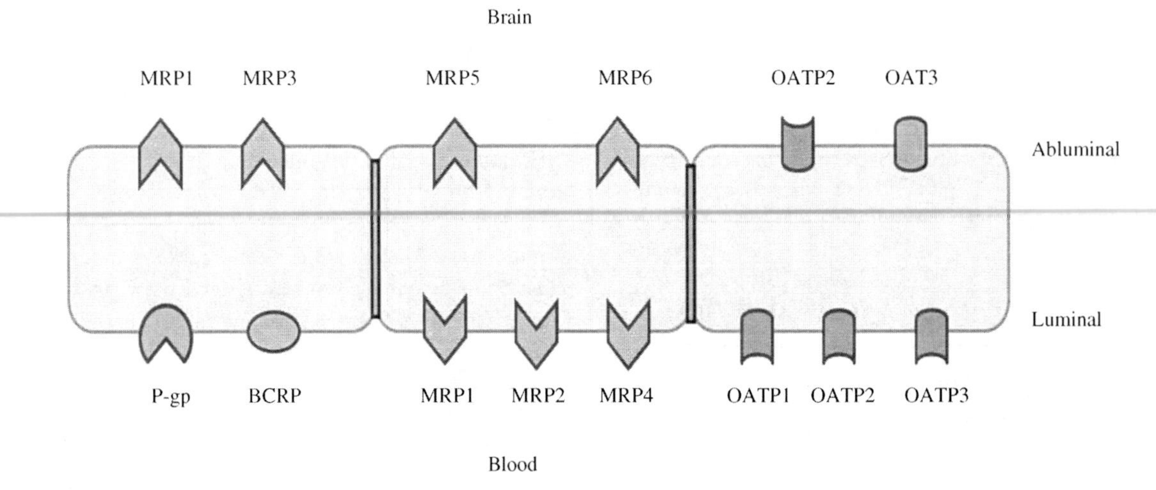

FIGURE 21.3 Schematic representation of expression of efflux proteins on brain capillary endothelial cells.

system [69]. These isoforms differ significantly with respect to substrate specificity, tissue distribution, and physiological function. MRP1 and MRP2 are transporter proteins encoded by the ABCC1 and ABCC2 genes, respectively [70, 71]. These are approximately 190-kDa membrane glycoproteins and consist of three transmembrane domains (TMD_0, TMD_2, and TMD_3) with a cytoplasmic linker located between the first two TMDs [72, 73]. BCRP (ABCG2) is a 75-kDa polytopic membrane protein that belongs to the G subfamily to the ABC superfamily and is encoded by the ABCG2 gene [74].

Efflux proteins expressed on the luminal side of brain capillary endothelial cells prevent the entry of systemically administered drugs into the central nervous system. These are primary active efflux pumps that bind and extrude drug molecules across the concentration gradient by consuming the energy provided from ATP hydrolysis. The transport of protease inhibitors including saquinavir, amprenavir, indinavir, and ritonavir has been reported to be modulated by P-gp and MRPs *in vitro* [75, 76]. Furthermore, it has been found that prolonged exposure of protease inhibitors to BECs resulted in overexpression of P-gp [77–79]. Such upregulation of functionally active P-gp can further limit the brain permeation of chemotherapeutic agents.

Similarly, the transport of several lipophilic anticancer drugs such as vinca alkaloids, doxorubicin, cyclosporin A, and digoxin has been significantly diminished by P-gp at the BBB [80]. Recently, it has been reported that BCRP regulates the transport of chemotherapeutic agents such as prazosin and mitoxantrone across the BBB [81, 82]. Thus, the expression of efflux proteins on the BBB can play a significant role in drug disposition by restricting the absorption of therapeutic agents and causing drug resistance. Various strategies have been proposed to circumvent P-gp mediated drug efflux; however, it remains a major challenge to CNS drug absorption.

21.6.2.1 Inhibition of Efflux Process Drug delivery strategies capable of circumventing drug efflux mediated by ABC transporters will enhance brain absorption. Such strategies will provide better drug efficacy and lower resistance. Several approaches have been developed to inhibit or bypass efflux transporters. One of the most feasible approaches is the coadministration of inhibitors with P-gp or MRPs substrates (therapeutic agents). These inhibitors will terminate the functional activity of efflux proteins, thereby enhancing intracellular accumulation of substrate drug molecules.

The oral and brain bioavailability of various therapeutic agents such as paclitaxel and saquinavir has been drastically improved with co-administration of P-gp inhibitors. Coadministration of SDZ PSC833 generated a 10-fold increase in oral bioavailability of paclitaxel [83]. Similarly, oral bioavailability of paclitaxel increased from 9.3 to 67% on co-administering with cyclosporine [84]. This enhancement in the systemic levels of paclitaxel was attributed to P-gp inhibition by SDZ PSC833 and cyclosporine.

Similar to their influence on oral absorption, P-gp inhibitors have demonstrated a higher potential in enhancing the brain bioavailability of therapeutic drugs. Cyclosporin, PSC833 and GF120918 significantly increased the brain uptake of paclitaxel in mice by 3-, 6.5-, and 5-fold [85]. A 3-fold increase in the brain-to-plasma ratio of saquinavir is achieved with co-administration of mefloquine (P-gp inhibitor) [86]. The oral and brain absorption of saquinavir was significantly increased with co-administration of GF120918 [87]. These results clearly indicate that co-administration of inhibitors could be a viable strategy for enhancing drug permeation across the BBB. However, the major concern in using this approach is the high risk of developing unacceptable systemic toxicities resulting from lack of specificity and high doses required to inhibit P-gp *in vivo*.

21.6.3 Circumvention of Efflux Process

One of most promising approach to improve brain absorption of P-gp or MRPs substrates (therapeutic agents) is by circumventing the efflux process at the BBB. Prodrug approach is one such viable option for improving brain permeation of therapeutic agents (substrates). Prodrugs are chemically derivatized drug molecules and are pharmacologically inactive. For enhancing brain permeation of prodrugs, endogenous transporter substrates such as amino acids, vitamins, or other nutrients moieties are covalently linked to drug molecules. The ligand coupled drug conjugates permeate the BBB by binding and translocating through endogenous (influx) transporters or receptors while evading efflux proteins such as P-gp and MRPs. On reaching cell cytoplasm, the ligand is cleaved by intracellular enzymes and the released drug is available for producing a pharmacological response.

Several influx transporters such as folate, amino acids, glucose, sodium-dependent multivitamin transporter (SMVT), nucleoside transport, and monocarboxylate transporters are expressed on the luminal side of brain capillary endothelial cells [88–93]. Various nutrients and xenobiotics essential for cell growth and proliferation are transported primarily inside the brain through these influx transporters. Thus, the BBB not only functions as an implausible barrier for the translocation of therapeutic molecules but also influxes the nutrient moieties required for cell maintenance. The expression of the endogenous transport system on blood–brain barrier has been shown in Table 21.2 [88–91, 93–97]. Several of these influx transporters on the BBB have been targeted via prodrugs to examine their potential in enhancing the brain permeation of therapeutic drugs.

21.6.3.1 GLUT1 Transporter The massive and continuous need of energy supply required for proper brain functioning and metabolic activity is supplied by glucose. The transport of glucose from systemic circulation into the brain is mediated primarily by a specific transporter known as GLUT1 [98, 99]. A 15- to 3000-fold higher transport value for glucose is reported for GLUT1 [100]. Hence, GLUT1 could serve as a potential target for increasing the brain penetration of poorly permeable therapeutic drugs.

Glucose-conjugated ketoprofen and indomethacin prodrug exhibited a high affinity toward GLUT1 [101]. Glucosyl chlorambucil prodrug generated 160-fold inhibition in [^{14}C]-glucose uptake indicating a higher interaction with GLUT1 [102]. A threefold enhancement in brain concentration was obtained with glucose ibuprofen derivatives [103]. Glucosyl prodrugs have been proposed to have significant potential in enhancing the brain bioavailability of HIV protease inhibitors and antiepileptics [100–102]. However, glucosyl deferiprone derivatives failed to generated higher brain concentrations relative to deferiprone alone [107].

GLUT1 is reported to be expressed on both apical as well as the basolateral side of brain capillary endothelial cells. A fourfold higher expression of GLUT1 is reported on the basolateral membrane relative to the apical membrane [108]. Such a higher expression on the abluminal side might increase the probability of the prodrug to be effluxed back to the systemic circulation. This would limit the accumulation of glucosyl prodrugs inside the brain. An alternative strategy has been proposed for unidirectional transport of glucosyl prodrugs [100]. This strategy involves derivatization of drugs with glucosyl thiamine disulfide bonds. Such modifications significantly increased the brain permeation of naproxen. Conjugation of therapeutic agents at C-6 position of glucose was proposed to have a higher interaction with GLUT1 relative to the C-1 and C-3 positions [109].

21.6.3.2 Amino Acid Transporters Several amino acid transporters responsible for the transport of amino acids

TABLE 21.2 Endogenous Transporter Expressed on Brain Capillary Endothelial Cells

No.	Transporter	Endogenous Substrate	References
1	Amino acid		[90]
	Neutral amino acid (L)	L-leucine, L-isoleucine, L-phenylalanine, L-tryptophan, L-tyrosine, L-isoleucine, L-methionine, and L-valine	
	Cationic amino acid (y^+)	L-Arginine, L-ornithine, and L-lysine	
	Anionic amino acid (x^-)	L-aspartic acid and L-glutamic acid	
2	Glucose (GLUT1)	Glucose	[94]
3	Monocarboxylate (MCT)	Lactic acid, pyruvic acid, γ-hydroxybuytrate (GHB), salicylic acid, benzoic acid, and other carboxylates	[93, 95]
4	Folate	Folic acid and methyltetrahydrofolic acid	[91]
5	SMVT	Biotin, pantothenic acid, lipoic acid, and desthiobiotin	[88]
6	Riboflavin	Riboflavin	[96]
7	Nucleoside	Adenosine	[89]
8	Ascorbic acid (SVCT2)	Ascorbic acid	[97]

from systemic circulation to the brain are reported to be expressed on brain capillary endothelial cells. These endogenous transporters differ significantly in substrate specificity and sodium dependence for the transport of amino acids [90]. These systems are designated as L, y, x, and T depending on the affinity and charge of amino acids they transport.

System L transports large neutral amino acids such as phenylalanine, tyrosine, leucine, isoleucine, methionine, tryptophan valine, and histidine. System y mediates transport of cationic amino acids such as arginine, lysine, and ornithine. System T transports thyroid hormones such as T3 and T4. System x primarily transports negatively charged amino acids such as glutamic and aspartic acid. The uptake of amino acids mediated by systems L, y, and x is sodium independent.

Recently, system L has been widely investigated for transporter targeted delivery of poorly permeable therapeutic agents. Tyrosine phosphonoformate prodrug generated significant inhibition of [^{3}H]-tyrosine uptake in porcine brain microvessel endothelial cells [110]. This result suggests that tyrosine phosphonoformate prodrug has a high affinity toward the large neutral amino acid transport system (LAT1). Tyrosine ester prodrug of nipecotic acid generated a dose-dependent effect on the andiogenic seizures in mice on intraperitoneal administration [106].

Tyrosine ketoprofen prodrug exhibited saturable brain uptake with a K_m value of 22.49 ± 9.18 μM and a V_{max} value of 1.41 ± 0.15 pmol/mg/min [111]. In the presence of a specific LAT1 substrate, 2-aminobicyclo(2,2,1)heptane-2-carboxylic acid, the brain uptake of ketoprofen prodrug significantly reduced to 40%. This result clearly suggests the high affinity of tyrosine ketoprofen prodrug toward LAT1. Phenylalanine prodrugs of valproic acid exhibited higher brain uptake relative to valproic acid [112]. Conjugation of the valproic acid on the *meta*-position of phenylalanine increased LAT1 affinity and brain uptake by 10- and 2-fold relative to *para*-substitution. Thus, LAT1 serves as a potential target in enhancing the brain bioavailability of poorly permeable therapeutic agents.

Similarly, several other nutrient transporters can be used for enhancing the transport of therapeutic agents across the BBB. The blood-to-brain transport of vitamin C is mediated by a specific Na^+-dependent transporter, SVCT2 [97, 113]. Previously, ascorbate and 6-bromine ascorbate prodrugs have been synthesized and examined for their efficacy in enhancing the transport of nipecotic, kynurenic, and diclofenamic acids [114, 115]. These prodrugs were recognized by SVCT2 transporter; however, only the nipecotic acid prodrug exhibited excellent anticonvulsant activity after systemic administration in mice. Biotin saquinavir conjugates generated a potent inhibitory effect on [3H]-biotin uptake in MDCK-MDR1 cells, indicating that biotin saquinavir conjugate was recognized by SMVT [116]. Similarly, biotin-ganciclovir improved the delivery of ganciclovir in human retinal pigmented epithelium cells (ARPE-19) and rabbit retina [117]. These results suggest clearly that SVCT2 and SMVT can be used for improving the brain delivery of poorly permeable by highly potent therapeutic agents.

21.6.4 Receptor-Mediated Endocytosis

In addition to nutrient transporters, the BBB has been reported to express several receptors such as folate, transferrin, low-density lipoproteins, and insulin. These receptors are widely known for their application in the brain delivery of colloidal systems such as nanoparticles and liposomes.

21.6.4.1 Transferrin Receptor The transferrin receptor is one of the most commonly explored receptors because of its high expression on luminal side of brain capillary endothelial cells. It primarily regulates the transport of iron in the form of the iron binding protein transferrin into brain tissues [118]. Previously, transferrin receptors have been used for enhancing the brain delivery of therapeutic agents. Shin et al. investigated the potential of transferrin receptors in enhancing the brain accumulation of human immunoglobulin G3 (IgG3) immunoglobulin antibody. It was observed that the fusion of transferrin to the hinge region of human IgG3 immunoglobulin antibody enhanced the brain uptake of the fusion proteins significantly *in vivo* [119]. Transferrin receptors have also been used for enhancing intracellular accumulation of small chemotherapeutic agents such as adriamycin, paclitaxel, and doxorubicin [120, 121]. Transferrin adriamycin conjugates demonstrated better antitumor efficacy in mice compared with adriamycin alone. Similarly, transferrin doxorubicin conjugates demonstrated higher selectivity and comparable antitumor efficacy to free doxorubicin in breast cancer and leukemic cells [122]. These results suggest that the overexpression of transferrin can be used for enhancing the intracellular accumulation of chemotherapeutic agents in brain tumors.

Recently, transferrin functionalized PEGylated albumin nanoparticles were used to enhance brain transport of AZT. The brain accumulation of AZT obtained with transferrin-functionalized nanoparticles was significantly higher compared with unmodified nanoparticles after intravenous administration in albino rats [123]. The percentage brain accumulation of AZT was 21.1% with transferrin-functionalized nanoparticles and 9.3% with unmodified nanoparticles. These studies demonstrate that the conjugation of transferrin could be a viable strategy for enhancing brain accumulation of therapeutic agents and drug delivery systems. However, high endogenous levels of transferrin (25 μM) can significantly reduce the receptor interaction of transferrin-targeted conjugates [124]. Hence, to maximize receptor interaction while preventing competition with endogenous transferrin, monoclonal antibody OX26 has been widely used for targeting transferrin receptors.

Several studies have demonstrated the suitability of the OX26 monoclonal antibody as a targeting ligand for the brain delivery of therapeutic agents. The conjugation of OX26 antibody generated a 10-fold increase in brain uptake of vasoactive intestinal peptide (VIP) relative to free VIP [125]. Moreover, intravenous injection of OX26 antibody VIP conjugate increased the brain blood flow by 60% in conscious rats relative to free VIP. Human basic fibroblast growth factor (bFGF) OX26 conjugates generated 80% reduction in infarct volume relative to parent neurotrophin in rats with permanent occlusion of middle cerebral artery [126]. Similar improvements in the brain delivery of nerve growth factors, daunomycin, antisense oligonucleotides, and other peptide-based therapeutics has been reported on conjugation with OX26 monoclonal antibody [127–132].

21.6.4.2 Insulin Receptor In addition to transferrin receptors, the luminal side of brain capillary endothelial cells abundantly expresses insulin receptors [133]. It is a 300-kDa integral membrane glycoprotein constituting of two α-subunits and two β-subunits [134]. Unlike transferrin, insulin has never been used as a targeting ligand because of its poor plasma half-life [135]. Monoclonal antibody 83–14 has been used to target human insulin receptor. The brain transport of 83–14 monoclonal antibody in rhesus monkey is 4% which corresponds to 0.04% ID/g, ~100 g/brain after 3 h of injection [136]. This finding suggests that the brain transport of 83–14 is approximately 10-fold greater than anti-human transferrin receptor monoclonal antibody (0.3% brain uptake at 24 h) [137, 138]. Later, both the chimeric and fully humanized form of 83–14 antibody was produced and found effective in enhancing the brain accumulation of conjugated therapeutic agents [139].

21.6.4.3 Low-Density Lipoprotein Receptor-Related Protein 1 and 2 Low-density lipoprotein (LDL) receptor related proteins 1 and 2 are distinct receptors that have been preferentially targeted for enhancing the brain delivery of colloidal systems such as nanoparticles. Apolipoproteins AII, B, CII, E, or J coated poly(butyl cyanoacrylate) nanoparticles loaded with the hexapeptide dalargin produced a pronounced antinociceptive effect when injected in mice [140]. On delineating the mechanism of brain uptake, it was found that these nanoparticles underwent receptor-mediated endocytosis via low-density lipoprotein receptors expressed on the luminal side of brain capillary endothelial cells. The precise transport mechanism is not yet clear; however, it is proposed that the nanoparticles adsorbed apolipoproteins from the bloodstream and therefore could interact with low-density lipoprotein receptors. Recently, a new family of peptides, Angiopeps, has been designed by Demeule et al. [141, 142]. These peptides especially angiopep-2 generated higher transcytosis capacity and brain parenchymal accumulation relative to lactoferrin, transferrin, and avidin. Later, it was found that low-density lipoprotein receptor-related proteins were involved in transcytosis of angiopep-2.

21.6.4.4 Folate Receptor The folate receptor is yet another endogenous influx system that has been differentially targeted for improving the brain permeability of therapeutic drugs. This receptor is reported to be overly expressed in malignant tumors relative to normal tissues [143]. In the brain, an overexpression of high-affinity folate receptors has been observed in choroid plexus tumors [144]. Conjugation of therapeutic agents to a gamma carboxyl group of folic acid results in specific binding of conjugates to folate receptors [145]. Previously, these receptors have been targeted for enhancing the brain uptake of macromolecular drugs. KJ16 antibody folate conjugates generated a 10- to 20-fold increase in T-cell infiltration into brain tumors relative to the KJ16 antibody alone [146]. Conjugation of folic acid produced an 8-fold increase in the uptake of antisense oligodeoxynucleotide in ovarian cancer cells [147]. This result suggests that folate receptors can be targeted preferentially for improving the delivery of nucleic acids to brain tumors. However, the size of folate and macromolecular drug conjugates needs to be considered as it may affect uptake in brain tumors significantly [148].

21.7 CONCLUSION

The BBB presents a formidable barrier for the brain transport of therapeutic agents from systemic circulation. Complex tight junctions and efflux proteins at the luminal side of capillary endothelial cells significantly limit brain permeation of hydrophilic compounds. This inability of therapeutic agents to access brain parenchyma from systemic circulation led to the exploration of several direct methods for brain drug administration. These approaches involve direct injection or infusion of therapeutic compounds into the brain, require skilled labor and are patient incompliant. Moreover, these methods also suffer severe drawbacks such as nonspecificity and poor distribution to brain parenchyma. Lipidation emerged as a promising approach to enhance brain permeation of poorly permeable but highly potent therapeutic agents. However, brain permeation with this indirect approach is significantly compromised because of nonspecific tissue distribution, poor solubility, and high plasma protein binding. Physiological strategies involving the use of transporter or receptor-targeted delivery and circumvention of the efflux process have also been investigated to enhance transport across the BBB. This approach takes advantage of endogenous transporters and receptors highly expressed at the luminal side of brain capillary endothelial cells. With this approach, several promising results have been obtained in enhancing the brain permeation of therapeutic agents such as ketoprofen and valproic acid. Moreover, monoclonal antibodies and ligands targeting specific receptors have been used for transcytosis of therapeutic agents to the CNS. Recent progress in brain drug delivery techniques has definitely provided considerable opportunities to overcome formidable barriers such as the BBB. However, the development of a safe and effective strategy to overcome the BBB is a complex procedure, and continuous efforts need to be dedicated to produce a viable strategy for the treatment of CNS disease. Combination of approaches such as colloidal carriers targeted toward specific receptors/transporters may provide better treatment for CNS diseases. Hence, newer technologies need to be developed to improve drug permeation across the BBB, which may provide uniform and rapid drug exposure to brain tissue.

ASSESSMENT QUESTIONS

21.1. Why is the blood–brain barrier a formidable challenge for brain drug delivery?

21.2. What are various direct systemic delivery modes? Briefly describe them.

21.3. Describe the various drug diffusion pathways involved in transnasal delivery to the brain.

21.4. List various direct CNS delivery modes, and briefly describe their limitations.

21.5. List a few efflux proteins expressed in brain capillary endothelial cells.

21.6. Do efflux proteins require energy to efflux therapeutic agents?

21.7. List a few approaches that can be used to enhance brain permeation of therapeutic agents.

21.8. List a few endogenous transporters expressed on brain capillary endothelial cells.

21.9. Which of the following amino acid transporters are expressed on brain capillary endothelial cells?

- **a.** Neutral amino acid transporter, LAT
- **b.** Anionic amino acid transporter, x^-
- **c.** Basic amino acid transporter, y^+
- **d.** All of the above

21.10. Which of the following receptors are expressed on brain capillary endothelial cells?

- **a.** Insulin
- **b.** Transferin
- **c.** Folate
- **d.** All of the above

21.11. How does the lipidation approach enhance the brain permeation of therapeutic agents?

REFERENCES

1. Scherrmann, J.M. (2002). Drug delivery to brain via the blood-brain barrier. *Vascular Pharmacology, 38(6)*, 349–354.
2. Redzic, Z. (2011). Molecular biology of the blood-brain and the blood-cerebrospinal fluid barriers: Similarities and differences. *Fluids Barriers CNS, 8(1)*, 3.
3. Crone, C., Christensen, O. (1981). Electrical resistance of a capillary endothelium. *The Journal of General Physiology, 77(4)*, 349–371.
4. Sarafian, T.A., Montes, C., Imura, T., Qi, J., Coppola, G., Geschwind, D.H., Sofroniew, M.V. (2010). Disruption of astrocyte STAT3 signaling decreases mitochondrial function and increases oxidative stress in vitro. *PLoS One, 5(3)*, e9532.
5. Allt, G., Lawrenson, J. G. (2001). Pericytes: Cell biology and pathology. *Cells Tissues Organs, 169(1)*, 1–11.
6. Engelhardt, B., Sorokin, L. (2009). The blood-brain and the blood-cerebrospinal fluid barriers: Function and dysfunction. *Seminars in Immunopathology, 31(4)*, 497–511.
7. Abbott, N.J., Patabendige, A.A., Dolman, D.E., Yusof, S.R., Begley, D.J. (2010). Structure and function of the blood-brain barrier. *Neurobiology of Disease, 37(1)*, 13–25.
8. Johanson, C.E., Duncan, J.A., Stopa, E.G., Baird, A. (2005). Enhanced prospects for drug delivery and brain targeting by the choroid plexus-CSF route. *Pharmaceutical Research, 22(7)*, 1011–1037.
9. Abbott, N.J., Ronnback, L., Hansson, E. (2006). Astrocyte-endothelial interactions at the blood-brain barrier. *Nature Reviews Neuroscience, 7(1)*, 41–53.
10. Abbott, N.J. (2005). Dynamics of CNS barriers: Evolution, differentiation, and modulation. *Cellular and Molecular Neurobiology, 25(1)*, 5–23.
11. Huynh, G.H., Deen, D.F., Szoka, F. C., Jr. (2006). Barriers to carrier mediated drug and gene delivery to brain tumors. *Journal of Controlled Release, 110(2)*, 236–259.
12. Alam, M.I., Beg, S., Samad, A., Baboota, S., Kohli, K., Ali, J., Ahuja, A., Akbar, M. (2010). Strategy for effective brain drug delivery. *European Journal of Pharmaceutical Sciences, 40(5)*, 385–403.
13. Steiniger, S.C., Kreuter, J., Khalansky, A.S., Skidan, I.N., Bobruskin, A.I., Smirnova, Z.S., Severin, S.E., Uhl, R., Kock, M., Geiger, K.D., Gelperina, S.E. (2004). Chemotherapy of glioblastoma in rats using doxorubicin-loaded nanoparticles. *International Journal of Cancer, 109(5)*, 759–767.
14. Rautioa, J., Chikhale, P. J. (2004). Drug delivery systems for brain tumor therapy. *Current Pharmaceutical Design, 10(12)*, 1341–1353.
15. Borlongan, C.V., Emerich, D.F. (2003). Facilitation of drug entry into the CNS via transient permeation of blood brain barrier: Laboratory and preliminary clinical evidence from bradykinin receptor agonist, Cereport. *Brain Research Bulletin, 60(3)*, 297–306.
16. Rainov, N.G., Ikeda, K., Qureshi, N.H., Grover, S., Herrlinger, U., Pechan, P., Chiocca, E.A., Breakefield, X.O., Barnett, F.H. (1999). Intraarterial delivery of adenovirus vectors and

liposome-DNA complexes to experimental brain neoplasms. *Human Gene Therapy*, *10(2)*, 311–318.

17. Howe, H.A., Bodian, D. (1941). Second attacks of poliomyelitis: An experimental study. *Journal of Experimental Medicine*, *74(2)*, 145–166.
18. Mistry, A., Stolnik, S., Illum, L. (2009). Nanoparticles for direct nose-to-brain delivery of drugs. *International Journal of Pharmaceutics*, *379(1)*, 146–157.
19. Wu, H., Hu, K., Jiang, X. (2008). From nose to brain: Understanding transport capacity and transport rate of drugs. *Expert Opinions on Drug Delivery*, *5(10)*, 1159–1168.
20. Anand Kumar, T.C., David, G.F., Sankaranarayanan, A., Puri, V., Sundram, K.R. (1982). Pharmacokinetics of progesterone after its administration to ovariectomized rhesus monkeys by injection, infusion, or nasal spraying. *Proceedings of the National Academy of Sciences USA*, *79(13)*, 4185–4189.
21. Gopinath, P.G., Gopinath, G., Kumar, A. (1978). Target site of intranasally sprayed substances and their transport across the nasal mucosa: A new insight into the intranasal route of drug delivery. *Current Therapeutic Research*, *23*, 596–607.
22. Bahadur, S., Pathak, K. (2012). Physicochemical and physiological considerations for efficient nose-to-brain targeting. *Expert Opinions on Drug Delivery*, *9(1)*, 19–31.
23. Kimura, R., Miwa, M., Kato, Y., Yamada, S., Sato, M. (1989). Nasal absorption of tetraethylammonium in rats. *Archives Internationales de Pharmacodynamie et de Therapie*, *302*, 7–17.
24. Dhuria, S.V., Hanson, L.R., Frey, W.H., 2nd. (2010). Intranasal delivery to the central nervous system: Mechanisms and experimental considerations. *Journal of Pharmaceutical Sciences*, *99(4)*, 1654–1673.
25. Thorne, R.G., Pronk, G.J., Padmanabhan, V., Frey, W.H., 2nd. (2004). Delivery of insulin-like growth factor-I to the rat brain and spinal cord along olfactory and trigeminal pathways following intranasal administration. *Neuroscience*, *127(2)*, 481–496.
26. De Rosa, R., Garcia, A. A., Braschi, C., Capsoni, S., Maffei, L., Berardi, N., Cattaneo, A. (2005). Intranasal administration of nerve growth factor (NGF) rescues recognition memory deficits in AD11 anti-NGF transgenic mice. *Proceedings of the National Academy of Sciences USA*, *102(10)*, 3811–3816.
27. Capsoni, S., Giannotta, S., Cattaneo, A. (2002). Nerve growth factor and galantamine ameliorate early signs of neurodegeneration in anti-nerve growth factor mice. *Proceedings of the National Academy of Sciences USA*, *99(19)*, 12432–124337.
28. Han, I.K., Kim, M.Y., Byun, H.M., Hwang, T.S., Kim, J.M., Hwang, K.W., Park, T.G., Jung, W.W., Chun, T., Jeong, G.J., Oh, Y.K. (2007). Enhanced brain targeting efficiency of intranasally administered plasmid DNA: An alternative route for brain gene therapy. *Journal of Molecular Medicine (Berlin)*, *85(1)*, 75–83.
29. Ying, W., Wei, G., Wang, D., Wang, Q., Tang, X., Shi, J., Zhang, P., Lu, H. (2007). Intranasal administration with NAD+ profoundly decreases brain injury in a rat model of transient focal ischemia. *Frontiers in Bioscience*, *12*, 2728–2734.
30. Wei, G., Wang, D., Lu, H., Parmentier, S., Wang, Q., Panter, S.S., Frey, W.H., 2nd, Ying, W. (2007). Intranasal administration of a PARG inhibitor profoundly decreases ischemic brain injury. *Frontiers in Bioscience*, *12*, 4986–4996.
31. Kumar, M., Misra, A., Mishra, A.K., Mishra, P., Pathak, K. (2008). Mucoadhesive nanoemulsion-based intranasal drug delivery system of olanzapine for brain targeting. *Journal of Drug Targeting*, *16(10)*, 806–814.
32. Khan, S., Patil, K., Yeole, P., Gaikwad, R. (2009). Brain targeting studies on buspirone hydrochloride after intranasal administration of mucoadhesive formulation in rats. *Journal of Pharmacy and Pharmacology*, *61(5)*, 669–675.
33. Vyas, T.K., Babbar, A.K., Sharma, R.K., Singh, S., Misra, A. (2006). Preliminary brain-targeting studies on intranasal mucoadhesive microemulsions of sumatriptan. *AAPS PharmSciTech*, *7(1)*, E8.
34. Ali, J., Ali, M., Baboota, S., Sahani, J.K., Ramassamy, C., Dao, Bhavna, L. (2010). Potential of nanoparticulate drug delivery systems by intranasal administration. *Current Pharmaceutical Design*, *16(14)*, 1644–1653.
35. Illum, L. (2000). Transport of drugs from the nasal cavity to the central nervous system. *European Journal of Pharmaceutical Sciences*, *11(1)*, 1–18.
36. Hocking, G., Wildsmith, J.A. (2004). Intrathecal drug spread. *Britain Journal of Anesthesia*, *93(4)*, 568–578.
37. MacKay, J.A., Deen, D.F., Szoka, F.C., Jr. (2005). Distribution in brain of liposomes after convection enhanced delivery; modulation by particle charge, particle diameter, and presence of steric coating. *Brain Research*, *1035(2)*, 139–153.
38. Nicholson, C., Sykova, E. (1998). Extracellular space structure revealed by diffusion analysis. *Trends in Neuroscience*, *21(5)*, 207–215.
39. Gabathuler, R. (2010). Approaches to transport therapeutic drugs across the blood-brain barrier to treat brain diseases. *Neurobiology of Disease*, *37(1)*, 48–57.
40. Haugland, M., Sinkjaer, T. (1999). Interfacing the body's own sensing receptors into neural prosthesis devices. *Technology and Health Care*, *7(6)*, 393–399.
41. Kennedy, P.R., Bakay, R.A. (1998). Restoration of neural output from a paralyzed patient by a direct brain connection. *Neuroreport*, *9(8)*, 1707–1711.
42. Menei, P., Benoit, J.P., Boisdron-Celle, M., Fournier, D., Mercier, P., Guy, G. (1994). Drug targeting into the central nervous system by stereotactic implantation of biodegradable microspheres. *Neurosurgery*, *34(6)*, 1058–1064; discussion 1064.
43. Lawson, H.C., Sampath, P., Bohan, E., Park, M.C., Hussain, N., Olivi, A., Weingart, J., Kleinberg, L., Brem, H. (2007). Interstitial chemotherapy for malignant gliomas: The Johns Hopkins experience. *Journal of Neurooncology*, *83(1)*, 61–70.
44. Brem, H., Gabikian, P. (2001). Biodegradable polymer implants to treat brain tumors. *Journal of Controlled Release*, *74(1–3)*, 63–67.

45. Pathan, S.A., Iqbal, Z., Zaidi, S.M., Talegaonkar, S., Vohra, D., Jain, G.K., Azeem, A., Jain, N., Lalani, J.R., Khar, R.K., Ahmad, F.J. (2009). CNS drug delivery systems: Novel approaches. *Recent Patents on Drug Delivery & Formulation, 3(1)*, 71–89.

46. Brem, H., Piantadosi, S., Burger, P.C., Walker, M., Selker, R., Vick, N.A., Black, K., Sisti, M., Brem, S., Mohr, G., et al. (1995). Placebo-controlled trial of safety and efficacy of intraoperative controlled delivery by biodegradable polymers of chemotherapy for recurrent gliomas. The Polymer-brain Tumor Treatment Group. *Lancet, 345(8956)*, 1008–1012.

47. Groothuis, D.R., Benalcazar, H., Allen, C.V., Wise, R.M., Dills, C., Dobrescu, C., Rothholtz, V., Levy, R.M. (2000). Comparison of cytosine arabinoside delivery to rat brain by intravenous, intrathecal, intraventricular and intraparenchymal routes of administration. *Brain Research, 856(1–2)*, 281–290.

48. Pardridge, W.M. (2007). Brain drug development and brain drug targeting. *Pharmaceutical Research, 24(9)*, 1729–1732.

49. Aird, R.B. (1984). A study of intrathecal, cerebrospinal fluid-to-brain exchange. *Experimental Neurology, 86(2)*, 342–358.

50. Day-Lollini, P.A., Stewart, G.R., Taylor, M.J., Johnson, R.M., Chellman, G.J. (1997). Hyperplastic changes within the leptomeninges of the rat and monkey in response to chronic intracerebroventricular infusion of nerve growth factor. *Experimental Neurology, 145(1)*, 24–37.

51. Yamada, K., Kinoshita, A., Kohmura, E., Sakaguchi, T., Taguchi, J., Kataoka, K., Hayakawa, T. (1991). Basic fibroblast growth factor prevents thalamic degeneration after cortical infarction. *Journal of Cerebral Blood Flow & Metabolism, 11(3)*, 472–478.

52. Nutt, J.G., Burchiel, K.J., Comella, C.L., Jankovic, J., Lang, A.E., Laws, E.R., Jr., Lozano, A.M., Penn, R.D., Simpson, R. K., Jr., Stacy, M., Wooten, G.F. (2003). Randomized, double-blind trial of glial cell line-derived neurotrophic factor (GDNF) in PD. *Neurology, 60(1)*, 69–73.

53. Pardridge, W.M. (2007). Blood-brain barrier delivery. *Drug Discovery Today, 12(1–2)*, 54–61.

54. Fung, L.K., Shin, M., Tyler, B., Brem, H., Saltzman, W.M. (1996). Chemotherapeutic drugs released from polymers: Distribution of 1, 3-bis(2-chloroethyl)-1-nitrosourea in the rat brain. *Pharmaceutical Research, 13(5)*, 671–682.

55. Murry, D.J., Blaney, S.M. (2000). Clinical pharmacology of encapsulated sustained-release cytarabine. *The Annals of Pharmacotherapy, 34(10)*, 1173–1178.

56. Rocque, B.G., Leland Albright, A. (2012). Intraventricular vs intrathecal baclofen for secondary dystonia: A comparison of complications. *Neurosurgery, 70(2 Suppl Operative), 321–325; discussion* 325–326.

57. Soderquist, R.G., Mahoney, M.J. (2010). Central nervous system delivery of large molecules: And new frontiers for intrathecally administered therapeutics. *Expert Opinion on Drug Delivery, 7(3)*, 285–293.

58. Kerr, J.Z., Berg, S., Blaney, S.M. (2001). Intrathecal chemotherapy. *Critical Reviews in Oncology/Hematology, 37(3)*, 227–236.

59. Deguchi, Y., Hayashi, H., Fujii, S., Naito, T., Yokoyama, Y., Yamada, S., Kimura, R. (2000). Improved brain delivery of a nonsteroidal anti-inflammatory drug with a synthetic glyceride ester: A preliminary attempt at a CNS drug delivery system for the therapy of Alzheimer's disease. *Journal of Drug Targeting, 8(6)*, 371–381.

60. Dvir, E., Elman, A., Simmons, D., Shapiro, I., Duvdevani, R., Dahan, A., Hoffman, A., Friedman, J.E. (2007). DP-155, a lecithin derivative of indomethacin, is a novel nonsteroidal antiinflammatory drug for analgesia and Alzheimer's disease therapy. *CNS Drug Reviews, 13(2)*, 260–277.

61. Parang, K., Wiebe, L.I., Knaus, E.E. (1998). Pharmacokinetics and tissue distribution of (+/-)-3′-azido-2′,3′-dideoxy-5′-O-(2-bromomyristoyl)thymidine, a prodrug of 3′-azido-2′, 3′-dideoxythymidine (AZT) in mice. *Journal of Pharmacy and Pharmacology, 50(9)*, 989–996.

62. Hesse, G.W., Jacob, J.N., Shashoua, V.E. (1988). Uptake in brain and neurophysiological activity of two lipid esters of gamma-aminobutyric acid. *Neuropharmacology, 27(6)*, 637–640.

63. el Kihel, L., Bourass, J., Richomme, P., Petit, J.Y., Letourneux, Y. (1996). Synthesis and evaluation of the anti-inflammatory effects of niflumic acid lipophilic prodrugs in brain edema. *Arzneimittelforschung, 46(11)*, 1040–1044.

64. Witt, K.A., Davis, T.P. (2006). CNS drug delivery: Opioid peptides and the blood-brain barrier. *AAPS Journal, 8(1)*, E76–E88.

65. Loscher, W., Potschka, H. (2005). Blood-brain barrier active efflux transporters: ATP-binding cassette gene family. *NeuroRx, 2(1)*, 86–98.

66. Omidi, Y., Barar, J. (2012). Impacts of blood-brain barrier in drug delivery and targeting of brain tumors. *BioImpacts, 2(1)*, 5–22.

67. Leslie, E.M., Deeley, R.G., Cole, S.P. (2005). Multidrug resistance proteins: Role of P-glycoprotein, MRP1, MRP2, and BCRP (ABCG2) in tissue defense. *Toxicology and Applied Pharmacology, 204(3)*, 216–37.

68. Ueda, K., Clark, D.P., Chen, C.J., Roninson, I.B., Gottesman, M.M., Pastan, I. (1987). The human multidrug resistance (mdr1) gene. cDNA cloning and transcription initiation. *The Journal of Biological Chemistry, 262(2)*, 505–508.

69. Dallas, S., Miller, D.S., Bendayan, R. (2006). Multidrug resistance-associated proteins: Expression and function in the central nervous system. *Pharmacological Reviews, 58 (2)*, 140–161.

70. Rosenberg, M.F., Mao, Q., Holzenburg, A., Ford, R.C., Deeley, R.G., Cole, S.P. (2001). The structure of the multidrug resistance protein 1 (MRP1/ABCC1). crystallization and single-particle analysis. *The Journal of Biological Chemistry, 276(19)*, 16076–16082.

71. Mayer, R., Kartenbeck, J., Buchler, M., Jedlitschky, G., Leier, I., Keppler, D. (1995). Expression of the MRP gene-encoded conjugate export pump in liver and its selective absence from the canalicular membrane in transport-deficient mutant hepatocytes. *The Journal of Cell Biology, 131 (1)*, 137–150.

72. Keitel, V., Nies, A.T., Brom, M., Hummel-Eisenbeiss, J., Spring, H., Keppler, D. (2003). A common Dubin-Johnson syndrome mutation impairs protein maturation and transport activity of MRP2 (ABCC2). *American Journal of Physiology Gastrointestinal and Liver Physiology*, *284(1)*, G165–G174.
73. Tran, H.D., Lally, J.F. (1984). Abdominal computed tomography in a man with lung cancer. *Delaware Medical Journal*, *56(4)*, 233–234.
74. Ni, Z., Bikadi, Z., Rosenberg, M.F., Mao, Q. Structure and function of the human breast cancer resistance protein (BCRP/ABCG2). *Current Drug Metabolism*, *11(7)*, 603–617.
75. Park, S., Sinko, P.J. (2005). P-glycoprotein and mutlidrug resistance-associated proteins limit the brain uptake of saquinavir in mice. *Journal of Pharmacology and Experimental Therapeutics*, *312(3)*, 1249–1256.
76. van der Sandt, I.C., Vos, C.M., Nabulsi, L., Blom-Roosemalen, M.C., Voorwinden, H.H., de Boer, A.G., Breimer, D.D. (2001). Assessment of active transport of HIV protease inhibitors in various cell lines and the in vitro blood--brain barrier. *AIDS*, *15(4)*, 483–491.
77. Zastre, J.A., Chan, G.N., Ronaldson, P.T., Ramaswamy, M., Couraud, P.O., Romero, I.A., Weksler, B., Bendayan, M., Bendayan, R. (2009). Up-regulation of P-glycoprotein by HIV protease inhibitors in a human brain microvessel endothelial cell line. *Journal of Neuroscience Research*, *87(4)*, 1023–1036.
78. Perloff,M.D., von Moltke, L.L., Fahey, J.M., Greenblatt, D. J. (2007). Induction of P-glycoprotein expression and activity by ritonavir in bovine brain microvessel endothelial cells. *Journal of Pharmacy and Pharmacology*, *59(7)*, 947–953.
79. Gimenez, F., Fernandez, C., Mabondzo, A. (2004). Transport of HIV protease inhibitors through the blood-brain barrier and interactions with the efflux proteins, P-glycoprotein and multidrug resistance proteins. *Journal of Acquired Immune Deficiency Syndromes*, *36(2)*, 649–658.
80. Tsuji, A. (1998). P-glycoprotein-mediated efflux transport of anticancer drugs at the blood-brain barrier. *Therapeutic Drug Monitoring*, *20(5)*, 588–590.
81. Zhou, L., Schmidt, K., Nelson, F.R., Zelesky, V., Troutman, M.D., Feng, B. (2009). The effect of breast cancer resistance protein and P-glycoprotein on the brain penetration of flavopiridol, imatinib mesylate (Gleevec), prazosin, and 2-methoxy-3-(4-(2-(5-methyl-2-phenyloxazol-4-yl)ethoxy) phenyl)propanoic acid (PF-407288) in mice. *Drug Metabolism and Disposition*, *37(5)*, 946–955.
82. Cisternino, S., Mercier, C., Bourasset, F., Roux, F., Scherrmann, J.M. (2004). Expression, up-regulation, and transport activity of the multidrug-resistance protein Abcg2 at the mouse blood-brain barrier. *Cancer Research*, *64(9)*, 3296–3301.
83. van Asperen, J., van Tellingen, O., Sparreboom, A., Schinkel, A.H., Borst, P., Nooijen, W.J., Beijnen, J.H. (1997). Enhanced oral bioavailability of paclitaxel in mice treated with the P-glycoprotein blocker SDZ PSC 833. *British Journal of Cancer*, *76(9)*, 1181–1183.
84. van Asperen, J., van Tellingen, O., van der Valk, M.A., Rozenhart, M., Beijnen, J.H. (1998). Enhanced oral absorption and decreased elimination of paclitaxel in mice cotreated with cyclosporin A. *Clinical Cancer Research*, *4(10)*, 2293–2297.
85. Kemper, E.M., van Zandbergen, A.E., Cleypool, C., Mos, H.A., Boogerd, W., Beijnen, J.H., van Tellingen, O. (2003). Increased penetration of paclitaxel into the brain by inhibition of P-Glycoprotein. *Clinical Cancer Research*, *9(7)*, 2849–2855.
86. Owen, A., Janneh, O., Hartkoorn, R. C., Chandler, B., Bray, P. G., Martin, P., Ward, S.A., Hart, C.A., Khoo, S.H., Back, D.J. (2005). In vitro synergy and enhanced murine brain penetration of saquinavir coadministered with mefloquine. *Journal of Pharmacology and Experimental Therapeutics*, *314(3)*, 1202–1209.
87. Huisman, M.T., Smit, J.W., Wiltshire, H.R., Beijnen, J.H., Schinkel, A.H. (2003). Assessing safety and efficacy of directed P-glycoprotein inhibition to improve the pharmacokinetic properties of saquinavir coadministered with ritonavir. *Journal of Pharmacology and Experimental Therapeutics*, *304(2)*, 596–602.
88. Park, S., Sinko, P.J. (2005). The blood-brain barrier sodium-dependent multivitamin transporter: A molecular functional in vitro-in situ correlation. *Drug Metabolism and Disposition*, *33(10)*, 1547–1554.
89. Chishty, M., Begley, D.J., Abbott, N.J., Reichel, A. (2003). Functional characterisation of nucleoside transport in rat brain endothelial cells. *Neuroreport*, *14(7)*, 1087–1090.
90. Smith, Q.R. (2000). Transport of glutamate and other amino acids at the blood-brain barrier. *Journal of Nutrition*, *130 (4S Suppl)*, 1016S–1022S.
91. Wu, D., Pardridge, W.M. (1999). Blood-brain barrier transport of reduced folic acid. *Pharmaceutical Research*, *16(3)*, 415–419.
92. Agus, D.B., Gambhir, S.S., Pardridge, W.M., Spielholz, C., Baselga, J., Vera, J.C., Golde, D.W. (1997). Vitamin C crosses the blood-brain barrier in the oxidized form through the glucose transporters. *Journal of Clinical Investigation*, *100(11)*, 2842–2848.
93. Terasaki, T., Takakuwa, S., Moritani, S., Tsuji, A. (1991). Transport of monocarboxylic acids at the blood-brain barrier: Studies with monolayers of primary cultured bovine brain capillary endothelial cells. *Journal of Pharmacology and Experimental Therapeutics*, *258(3)*, 932–937.
94. Cornford, E.M., Hyman, S., Cornford, M.E., Landaw, E.M., Delgado-Escueta, A.V. (1998). Interictal seizure resections show two configurations of endothelial Glut1 glucose transporter in the human blood-brain barrier. *Journal of Cerebral Blood Flow & Metabolism*, *18(1)*, 26–42.
95. Leino, R. L., Gerhart, D. Z., Drewes, L. R. (1999). Monocarboxylate transporter (MCT1) abundance in brains of suckling and adult rats: A quantitative electron microscopic immunogold study. *Brain Research. Developmental Brain Research*, *113(1–2)*, 47–54.

96. Patel, M., Vadlapatla, R.K., Pal, D., Mitra, A.K. (2012). Molecular and functional characterization of riboflavin specific transport system in rat brain capillary endothelial cells. *Brain Research*, *1468*, 1–10.

97. Gess, B., Sevimli, S., Strecker, J.K., Young, P., Schabitz, W.R. (2011). Sodium-dependent vitamin C transporter 2 (SVCT2) expression and activity in brain capillary endothelial cells after transient ischemia in mice. *PLoS One*, *6*(2), e17139.

98. Klepper, J., Voit, T. (2002). Facilitated glucose transporter protein type 1 (GLUT1) deficiency syndrome: Impaired glucose transport into brain-- a review. *European Journal of Pediatrics*, *161(6)*, 295–304.

99. Regina, A., Roux, F., Revest, P. A. (1997). Glucose transport in immortalized rat brain capillary endothelial cells in vitro: Transport activity and GLUT1 expression. *Biochimica et Biophysica Acta*, *1335(1–2)*, 135–143.

100. Fan, W., Wu, Y., Li, X. K., Yao, N., Li, X., Yu, Y.G., Hai, L. (2011). Design, synthesis and biological evaluation of brain-specific glucosyl thiamine disulfide prodrugs of naproxen. *European Journal of Medicinal Chemistry*, *46*(9), 3651–3661.

101. Gynther, M., Ropponen, J., Laine, K., Leppanen, J., Haapakoski, P., Peura, L., Jarvinen, T., Rautio, J. (2009). Glucose promoiety enables glucose transporter mediated brain uptake of ketoprofen and indomethacin prodrugs in rats. *Journal of Medicinal Chemistry*, *52(10)*, 3348–3353.

102. Halmos, T., Santarromana, M., Antonakis, K., Scherman, D. (1996). Synthesis of glucose-chlorambucil derivatives and their recognition by the human GLUT1 glucose transporter. *European Journal of Pharmacology*, *318(2–3)*, 477–484.

103. Chen, Q., Gong, T., Liu, J., Wang, X., Fu, H., Zhang, Z. (2009). Synthesis, in vitro and in vivo characterization of glycosyl derivatives of ibuprofen as novel prodrugs for brain drug delivery. *Journal of Drug Targeting*, *17(4)*, 318–328.

104. Rouquayrol, M., Gaucher, B., Greiner, J., Aubertin, A.M., Vierling, P., Guedj, R. (2001). Synthesis and anti-HIV activity of glucose-containing prodrugs derived from saquinavir, indinavir and nelfinavir. *Carbohydrate Research*, *336(3)*, 161–180.

105. Battaglia, G., La Russa, M., Bruno, V., Arenare, L., Ippolito, R., Copani, A., Bonina, F., Nicoletti, F. (2000). Systemically administered D-glucose conjugates of 7-chlorokynurenic acid are centrally available and exert anticonvulsant activity in rodents. *Brain Research*, *860(1–2)*, 149–156.

106. Bonina, F.P., Arenare, L., Palagiano, F., Saija, A., Nava, F., Trombetta, D., de Caprariis, P. (1999). Synthesis, stability, and pharmacological evaluation of nipecotic acid prodrugs. *Journal of Pharmaceutical Sciences*, *88(5)*, 561–567.

107. Roy, S., Preston, J.E., Hider, R.C., Ma, Y.M. (2010). Glucosylated deferiprone and its brain uptake: Implications for developing glucosylated hydroxypyridinone analogues intended to cross the blood-brain barrier. *Journal of Medicinal Chemistry*, *53(15)*, 5886–5889.

108. Farrell, C.L., Partridge, W.M. (1991). Blood-brain barrier glucose transporter is asymmetrically distributed on brain capillary endothelial lumenal and ablumenal membranes: An electron microscopic immunogold study. *Proceedings of the National Academy of Sciences USA*, *88(13)*, 5779–5783.

109. Fernandez, C., Nieto, O., Fontenla, J.A., Rivas, E., de Ceballos, M.L., Fernandez-Mayoralas, A. (2003). Synthesis of glycosyl derivatives as dopamine prodrugs: Interaction with glucose carrier GLUT-1. *Organic & Biomolecular Chemistry*, *1(5)*, 767–771.

110. Walker, I., Nicholls, D., Irwin, W.J., Freeman, S. (1994). Drug delivery via active transport at the blood-brain barrier: Affinity of a prodrug of phosphonoformate for the large amino acid transporter. *International Journal of Pharmaceutics*, *104*(2), 157–167.

111. Gynther, M., Laine, K., Ropponen, J., Leppanen, J., Mannila, A., Nevalainen, T., Savolainen, J., Jarvinen, T., Rautio, J. (2008). Large neutral amino acid transporter enables brain drug delivery via prodrugs. *Journal of Medicinal Chemistry*, *51*(4), 932–936.

112. Peura, L., Malmioja, K., Laine, K., Leppanen, J., Gynther, M., Isotalo, A., Rautio, J. (2011). Large amino acid transporter 1 (LAT1) prodrugs of valproic acid: New prodrug design ideas for central nervous system delivery. *Molecular Pharmacology*, *8*(5), 1857–1866.

113. Sotiriou, S., Gispert, S., Cheng, J., Wang, Y., Chen, A., Hoogstraten-Miller, S., Miller, G.F., Kwon, O., Levine, M., Guttentag, S.H., Nussbaum, R.L. (2002). Ascorbic-acid transporter Slc23a1 is essential for vitamin C transport into the brain and for perinatal survival. *Nature Medicine*, *8*(5), 514–517.

114. Dalpiaz, A., Pavan, B., Vertuani, S., Vitali, F., Scaglianti, M., Bortolotti, F., Biondi, C., Scatturin, A., Tanganelli, S., Ferraro, L., Marzola, G., Prasad, P., Manfredini, S. (2005). Ascorbic and 6-Br-ascorbic acid conjugates as a tool to increase the therapeutic effects of potentially central active drugs. *European Journal of Pharmaceutical Sciences*, *24*(4), 259–269.

115. Manfredini, S., Pavan, B., Vertuani, S., Scaglianti, M., Compagnone, D., Biondi, C., Scatturin, A., Tanganelli, S., Ferraro, L., Prasad, P., Dalpiaz, A. (2002). Design, synthesis and activity of ascorbic acid prodrugs of nipecotic, kynurenic and diclophenamic acids, liable to increase neurotropic activity. *Journal of Medicinal Chemistry*, *45*(3), 559–562.

116. Luo, S., Kansara, V.S., Zhu, X., Mandava, N.K., Pal, D., Mitra, A.K. (2006). Functional characterization of sodium-dependent multivitamin transporter in MDCK-MDR1 cells and its utilization as a target for drug delivery. *Molecular Pharmacology*, *3*(3), 329–339.

117. Janoria, K.G., Boddu, S.H., Wang, Z., Paturi, D.K., Samanta, S., Pal, D., Mitra, A.K. (2009). Vitreal pharmacokinetics of biotinylated ganciclovir: Role of sodium-dependent multivitamin transporter expressed on retina. *Journal of Ocular Pharmacology and Therapeutics*, *25*(1), 39–49.

118. Jefferies, W.A., Brandon, M.R., Hunt, S.V., Williams, A.F., Gatter, K.C., Mason, D.Y. (1984). Transferrin receptor on endothelium of brain capillaries. *Nature*, *312(5990)*, 162–163.

119. Shin, S.U., Friden, P., Moran, M., Olson, T., Kang, Y.S., Pardridge, W.M., Morrison, S.L. (1995). Transferrin-

antibody fusion proteins are effective in brain targeting. *Proceedings of the National Academy of Sciences USA, 92 (7)*, 2820–2824.

120. Bicamumpaka, C., Page, M. (1998). In vitro cytotoxicity of paclitaxel-transferrin conjugate on H69 cells. *Oncology Reports, 5(6)*, 1381–1383.
121. Singh, M., Atwal, H., Micetich, R. (1998). Transferrin directed delivery of adriamycin to human cells. *Anticancer Research, 18(3A)*, 1423–1427.
122. Kratz, F., Beyer, U., Roth, T., Tarasova, N., Collery, P., Lechenault, F., Cazabat, A., Schumacher, P., Unger, C., Falken, U. (1998). Transferrin conjugates of doxorubicin: Synthesis, characterization, cellular uptake, and in vitro efficacy. *Journal of Pharmaceutical Sciences, 87(3)*, 338–346.
123. Mishra, V., Mahor, S., Rawat, A., Gupta, P.N., Dubey, P., Khatri, K., Vyas, S.P. (2006). Targeted brain delivery of AZT via transferrin anchored pegylated albumin nanoparticles. *Journal of Drug Targeting, 14(1)*, 45–53.
124. Qian, Z.M., Li, H., Sun, H., Ho, K. (2002). Targeted drug delivery via the transferrin receptor-mediated endocytosis pathway. *Pharmacological Reviews, 54(4)*, 561–587.
125. Wu, D., Pardridge, W.M. (1996). Central nervous system pharmacologic effect in conscious rats after intravenous injection of a biotinylated vasoactive intestinal peptide analog coupled to a blood-brain barrier drug delivery system. *Journal of Pharmacology and Experimental Therapeutics, 279(1)*, 77–83.
126. Song, B.W., Vinters, H.V., Wu, D., Pardridge, W.M. (2002). Enhanced neuroprotective effects of basic fibroblast growth factor in regional brain ischemia after conjugation to a blood-brain barrier delivery vector. *Journal of Pharmacology and Experimental Therapeutics, 301*(2), 605–610.
127. Zhang, Y., Pardridge, W.M. (2006). Blood-brain barrier targeting of BDNF improves motor function in rats with middle cerebral artery occlusion. *Brain Research, 1111(1)*, 227–229.
128. Penichet, M.L., Kang, Y.S., Pardridge, W.M., Morrison, S.L., Shin, S.U. (1999). An antibody-avidin fusion protein specific for the transferrin receptor serves as a delivery vehicle for effective brain targeting: Initial applications in anti-HIV antisense drug delivery to the brain. *Journal of Immunology, 163(8)*, 4421–4426.
129. Boado, R.J., Tsukamoto, H., Pardridge, W.M. (1998). Drug delivery of antisense molecules to the brain for treatment of Alzheimer's disease and cerebral AIDS. *Journal of Pharmaceutical Sciences, 87(11)*, 1308–1315.
130. Huwyler, J., Yang, J., Pardridge, W. M. (1997). Receptor mediated delivery of daunomycin using immunoliposomes: Pharmacokinetics and tissue distribution in the rat. *Journal of Pharmacology and Experimental Therapeutics, 282(3)*, 1541–1546.
131. Huwyler, J., Wu, D., Pardridge, W.M. (1996). Brain drug delivery of small molecules using immunoliposomes. *Proceedings of the National Academy of Sciences USA, 93(24)*, 14164–14169.
132. Kordower, J.H., Charles, V., Bayer, R., Bartus, R.T., Putney, S., Walus, L.R., Friden, P.M. (1994). Intravenous administration of a transferrin receptor antibody-nerve growth factor conjugate prevents the degeneration of cholinergic striatal neurons in a model of Huntington disease. *Proceedings of the National Academy of Sciences USA, 91(19)*, 9077–9080.
133. Havrankova, J., Brownstein, M., Roth, J. (1981). Insulin and insulin receptors in rodent brain. *Diabetologia, 20 Suppl*, 268–273.
134. Ullrich, A., Bell, J.R., Chen, E.Y., Herrera, R., Petruzzelli, L. M., Dull, T.J., Gray, A., Coussens, L., Liao, Y.C., Tsubokawa, M., et al. (1985). Human insulin receptor and its relationship to the tyrosine kinase family of oncogenes. *Nature, 313(6005)*, 756–761.
135. Bickel, U., Yoshikawa, T., Pardridge, W. M. (2001). Delivery of peptides and proteins through the blood-brain barrier. *Advanced Drug Delivery Reviews, 46(1–3)*, 247–279.
136. Jones, A.R., Shusta, E.V. (2007). Blood-brain barrier transport of therapeutics via receptor-mediation. *Pharmaceutical Research, 24(9)*, 1759–1771.
137. Friden, P.M., Olson, T.S., Obar, R., Walus, L.R., Putney, S.D. (1996). Characterization, receptor mapping and blood-brain barrier transcytosis of antibodies to the human transferrin receptor. *Journal of Pharmacology and Experimental Therapeutics, 278(3)*, 1491–1498.
138. Pardridge, W.M., Kang, Y.S., Buciak, J.L., Yang, J. (1995). Human insulin receptor monoclonal antibody undergoes high affinity binding to human brain capillaries in vitro and rapid transcytosis through the blood-brain barrier in vivo in the primate. *Pharmaceutical Research, 12(6)*, 807–816.
139. Boado, R.J., Zhang, Y., Wang, Y., Pardridge, W.M. (2008). GDNF fusion protein for targeted-drug delivery across the human blood-brain barrier. *Biotechnology and Bioengineering, 100*(2), 387–396.
140. Kreuter, J., Shamenkov, D., Petrov, V., Ramge, P., Cychutek, K., Koch-Brandt, C., Alyautdin, R. (2002). Apolipoprotein-mediated transport of nanoparticle-bound drugs across the blood-brain barrier. *Journal of Drug Targeting, 10(4)*, 317–325.
141. Demeule, M., Currie, J.C., Bertrand, Y., Che, C., Nguyen, T., Regina, A., Gabathuler, R., Castaigne, J.P., Beliveau, R. (2008). Involvement of the low-density lipoprotein receptor-related protein in the transcytosis of the brain delivery vector angiopep-2. *Journal of Neurochemistry, 106(4)*, 1534–1544.
142. Demeule, M., Regina, A., Che, C., Poirier, J., Nguyen, T., Gabathuler, R., Castaigne, J.P., Beliveau, R. (2008). Identification and design of peptides as a new drug delivery system for the brain. *Journal of Pharmacology and Experimental Therapeutics, 324(3)*, 1064–1072.
143. Weitman, S.D., Frazier, K.M., Kamen, B.A. (1994). The folate receptor in central nervous system malignancies of childhood. *Journal of Neurooncology, 21(2)*, 107–112.
144. Patrick, T.A., Kranz, D.M., van Dyke, T.A., Roy, *E. J.* (1997). Folate receptors as potential therapeutic targets in choroid plexus tumors of SV40 transgenic mice. *Journal of Neurooncology, 32*(2), 111–123.

145. Wang, S., Lee, R.J., Mathias, C.J., Green, M.A., Low, P.S. (1996). Synthesis, purification, and tumor cell uptake of 67Ga-deferoxamine--folate, a potential radiopharmaceutical for tumor imaging. *Bioconjugate Chemistry*, *7(1)*, 56–62.

146. Roy, E.J., Cho, B.K., Rund, L.A., Patrick, T.A., Kranz, D.M. (1998). Targeting T cells against brain tumors with a bi-specific ligand-antibody conjugate. *International Journal of Cancer*, *76*(*5*), 761–766.

147. Li, S., Deshmukh, H.M., Huang, L. (1998). Folate-mediated targeting of antisense oligodeoxynucleotides to ovarian cancer cells. *Pharmaceutical Research*, *15*(*10*), 1540–1545.

148. Kennedy, M.D., Jallad, K.N., Lu, J., Low, P.S., Ben-Amotz, D. (2003). Evaluation of folate conjugate uptake and transport by the choroid plexus of mice. *Pharmaceutical Research*, *20*(*5*), 714–719.

PART IV

FUTURE APPLICATIONS OF ADVANCED DRUG DELIVERY IN EMERGING RESEARCH AREAS

22

CELL-BASED THERAPEUTICS

ZHAOYANG YE, YAN ZHOU, HAIBO CAI, AND WEN-SONG TAN

22.1 CHAPTER OBJECTIVES

- To enlist different potential cell candidates applied for cell-based therapies.
- To understand the rationale of selecting cell candidates for treating different diseases.
- To know the state-of-the-art in translating into clinical applications.
- To understand the pharmaceutical requirements for developing cell-based therapeutics.

22.2 INTRODUCTION

Cell-based therapy represents a novel philosophy that offers prospective hopes for patients with traumatic defects, end-stage organ failure, degenerative disorders, and many other currently incurable clinical issues, such as cancer, central nervous system diseases, diabetic mellitus (DM), and pulmonary hypertension (PH). By definition, cell-based therapy exploits cells as the therapeutic agent, through either administration of exogenous cells into human subjects or stimulating endogenous cells via biological means to cure diseases [1]. Current pharmacological interventions are curative but merely symptomatic, and as such, these treatments produce only temporary clinical benefits, leaving the pathological process causing diseases to continue. In contrast, cell-based therapy treats diseases by directly introducing functioning units of the human body, i.e., live cells, to replace the damaged tissues.

Different cell types have been explored for potential applications in treating different diseases, and some of them—including chondrocytes and β islet cells—have already been advanced successfully to clinical applications. However, with the discovery of stem cells, cell-based therapy is boosted with even more stimulus. Stem cells quickly become the salivant cell sources for cell-based therapeutics because of their self-renewal capacity and pluri/multipotency of differentiation into various tissue lineages. In addition to embryonic stem cells (ESCs), which are pluripotent and have the potential to differentiate to all different cell lineages in the body, stem cells that give rise to cells of different lineages restricted to a single germ layer are designated as multipotent. Multipotent stem cells, or alternatively, adult stem cells, emerge in fetal and early postnatal life when specific gene expression patterns are imprinted. It is generally recognized that adult stem cells are responsible for maintaining cellular homeostasis of tissues by replenishing cells that are lost through maturation and senescence or through injury. However, it is still debatable whether multipotent stem cells reside in all self-renewing organs for a lifetime or are continuously supplied from a central pool of stem cells, which is currently believed to be bone marrow [2]. In contrast, tissue-specific progenitor (unipotent) stem cells arise from multipotent cells and give rise to cells of only specific tissue

Advanced Drug Delivery, First Edition. Edited by Ashim K. Mitra, Chi H. Lee, and Kun Cheng.

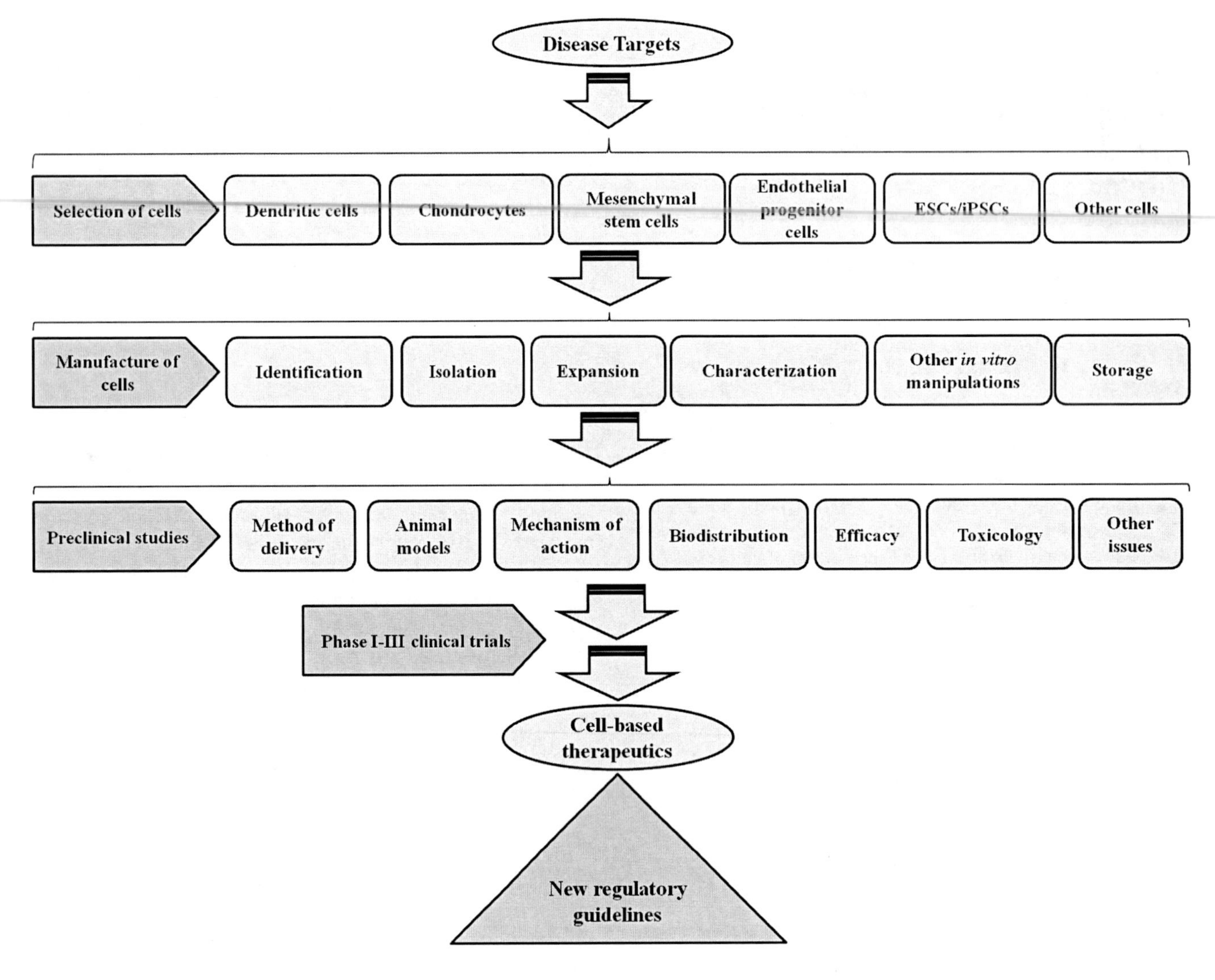

FIGURE 22.1 A flowchart of issues in developing cell-based therapeutics.

types [3]. Currently, many clinical trials have been carried out aimed at assessing the safety of cell products; however, the therapeutic benefits are yet to be established.

In this chapter, various aspects related to the development of cell-based therapeutics are introduced briefly (as schematically shown in Figure 22.1), including different cell sources, mechanism of action, *in vitro* expansion, their applications for treating different diseases, clinical status, pharmaceutical considerations, and regulatory guidelines.

22.3 BONE MARROW TRANSPLANTATION AS A PROTOTYPE OF CELL-BASED THERAPEUTICS

Bone marrow transplantation preceded the emergence of the concept of cell-based therapy. In 1957, Thomas et al. reported on the first clinical study of intravenous infusion of allogenic bone marrow into patients receiving irradiation and chemotherapy [4]. In the next year, Kurnick et al. used autologous bone marrow to restore the hematopoietic function of a patient subjected to chemotherapy [5]. Subsequently, several studies further confirmed the feasibility of bone marrow transplantation, establishing its application in reconstituting bone marrow [6, 7]. Although these early studies resulted only in short-term benefits, late in 1963, Mathe et al. reported on the first case of a long-term (20 months) survival after allogenic bone marrow transplantation [8]. With the understanding of human leukocyte antigen (HLA) immunophenotype, a series of bone marrow transplantation were performed on the patients with immunological deficiency and the long-term (15 years) survival was achieved [9–12]. Nevertheless, the allogenic transplantation leads to immunological rejection reaction eventually and the application of bone marrow transplantation is obviously limited because of the shortage in HLA matching donors. With the discovery of hematopoietic stem cells

(HSCs) and their successful isolation in humans, especially those from fetal cord blood bearing an immune-tolerant property, bone marrow reconstitution can be achieved through the transplantation of HSCs [13, 14]. More recent progress in bone marrow reconstitution involves employing chemicals and/or growth factors (e.g., granulocyte-macrophage colony-stimulating factor [GM-CSF] and granulocyte colony-stimulating factor [G-CSF]) to mobilize HSCs to enrich them in peripheral blood for subsequent transplantation [15, 16]. These early works laid the foundation for successful clinical application of HSCs in treating many diseases as well as cell-based therapy with other cell types [17].

22.4 CELLS—ACTIVE PHARMACEUTICAL INGREDIENTS OF CELL-BASED THERAPEUTICS

Cells play the central role in cell-based therapeutics as the name suggests. Like conventional pharmacological therapy, a rational selection of appropriate cell candidates for certain treatment is highly dependent on the nature of a disease. On the one hand, for certain diseases, different choices of cell candidates can be available. On the other hand, certain cell types, for example, a certain type of stem cells, can be used in treating many different diseases. However, unlike chemical/protein drugs, which can be designed, synthesized, and manufactured in a standardized procedure, the generation of cell products can be challenging. Because of the distinct properties for each cell type, their identification, expansion, *in vitro* maintenance, and storage can be very different. Standard procedures for processing and manufacture of each cell type are still under development. In this section, major cell types currently exploited in cell-based therapy and the principles behind disease-specific applications of these cell types are introduced.

22.4.1 Dendritic Cells

Dendritic cell (DCs) are primary antigen presenting cells in the body and normally function to present antigens to T cells, which then specifically recognize and ultimately eliminate the antigen source. However, DCs can not only induce innate and adaptive immune responses but also maintain immunological tolerance in the steady state [18, 19]. The maturation of DCs plays a key role in reconciling these two apparently incompatible functions. Although mature DCs are immunogenic after antigen challenging, immature DCs can tolerize the immune system [19]. In addition, DC-induced tolerance may also involve the promotion of anergy of T cells that come into contact with DCs, a shift from TH1- to TH2-type responses, apoptosis of the autoreactive T cells, or the induction of regulatory cells including regulatory T cells and natural killer-T cells [19]. DCs may therefore be manipulated *in vitro* or *in vivo* to achieve modulatory effects on immune responses, and thus, they find therapeutic applications in immune-related diseases.

Both compromised and exacerbated immune responses are implicated in different pathological conditions such as malignancy, persistent infection, autoimmunity, and allergy. For example, the hallmark for autoimmune diseases like type I diabetes mellitus (T1DM) and systemic lupus erythematosus is the breakdown in tolerance as a result of stimulatory DCs [20, 21]. However, the suppression of immunoreaction can be very critical in supporting the survival of transplants, for example, islet transplantation [22]. Tolerogenic DCs can be obtained through ultraviolet irradiation, as well as exposure to cytotoxic T lymphocyte antigen-4: immunoglobulin Fc fusion (CTLA-4Ig), transforming growth factor β (TGF-β) or interleukin (IL)-10 [23]. In addition, in immune reactions, the stabilization of the interaction between DCs and naive T cells through co-stimulatory molecules is required, and therefore, downregulation of the co-stimulation capacity in DCs can initiate a tolerogenic outcome [21]. On the contrary, in most tumors, naive T cells cannot be activated by cancer cells on their own, and instead they become anergic or tolerant to the tumor cells [24]. In this case, DCs can be *in vitro* challenged with tumor-associated antigens such as cancer extracts, cancer antigens, RNA of cancer tissues, and cancer cells to present a potent antigenic stimulus to T cells and provoke tumor-specific immune reactions for cancer treatments [25, 26].

22.4.2 Endothelial Progenitor Cells

The precursors of endothelial cells, termed endothelial progenitor cells (EPCs), play important roles in participating in adult neovasculogenesis and vascular homeostasis [27–29]. At the current stage, an explicative definition of the immunophenotype for EPCs is not yet available, but they are considered to express surface antigen markers simultaneously for both HSCs (CD34 or CD133) and endothelial lineage (fetal liver kinase-1 [Flk-1], also known as vascular endothelial growth factor receptor 2 [VEGFR-2] in mouse, and the human homolog of VEGFR-2 is kinase insert domain receptor [KDR]) [30]. Although CD34, CD133, and Flk-1 are often used individually in isolating EPCs, cells expressing all three markers are deemed to be the most potent [31]. After *in vitro* differentiation, EPCs express endothelial-specific markers including CD31, VE-cadherin, and von Willebrand factor (vWF), and they can form capillary-like structures [31]. EPCs can be isolated from bone marrow, peripheral blood, and placental cord blood. However, their frequency is generally low, representing less than 1% of the mononuclear cells. Studies have demonstrated that *in vitro* long-term expansion can be possible without affecting angiogenic potential at the presence of cytokines such as stem cell factor (SCF), thrombopoietin (TPO), and Fms-related tyrosine kinase 3 ligand (Flt-3L), thus generating a sufficient number of cells to meet the clinical needs [32]. Because of the capability of proliferation, mobilization, and giving rise to a functional progeny, EPCs are very suitable for therapeutic purposes of neovascularization and vascular repair in various vascular diseases.

22.4.3 Mesenchymal Stem Cells

The first evidence regarding the presence of nonhematopoietic, mesenchymal stem cells (MSCs) in bone marrow originated from the work by Friedenstein et al., wherein the cells initially were termed colony-forming-unit fibroblasts (CFU-Fs) [33]. In general, MSCs can be harvested from bone marrow with a low frequency ranging from 1/10,000 to 1/100,000 of bone marrow mononuclear cells. Nevertheless, MSCs can now be successfully acquired from a variety of other adult mesenchymal tissues including adipose tissue, dental pulp, synovial membrane, tendon, skeletal muscle, and umbilical cord blood among others. Currently, a full definition of MSCs still lacks of consensus and the *in vivo* authentic identity of MSCs remains largely unknown [34, 35]. However, the minimal criteria for validating of MSCs have been accepted including plastic adherence, expression of certain surface markers (positive for CD73, CD105, and CD90; negative for CD14, CD34, CD19, HLA-DR, and CD45), and the tripotentiality (differentiation into osteoblasts, chondrocytes, and adipocytes *in vitro*).

In recent years, MSCs turn out to be extremely versatile and represent a very promising candidate as cell-based therapeutics. They not only can differentiate into mesodermal lineages, but also they have been demonstrated to transdifferentiate into myoblasts, neural precursors, and cardiomyocytes among other lineages. Importantly, MSCs are found to be immunoprivileged because of the absence of HLA class II surface antigens and can thus be used as allogeneic products [36]. Most strikingly, MSCs can secrete a diverse array of trophic factors, including anti-inflammatory, angiogenic, neurotrophic, immunomodulatory, and antifibrotic factors [37]. Furthermore, the immunosuppressive ability of MSCs is very impressive, possibly through directly interacting with the immune system, particularly with dendritic cells, T cells, and natural killer cells [38]. Hence, in addition to their applications in tissue regeneration, applications in acute graft-versus-host disease (GvHD), liver disease, diabetic foot ulcers, cutaneous wounds, neurological disease, and bone marrow transplantation, among others, have also been actively explored. Moreover, the homing property of MSCs to injured sites as well as tumors makes them an ideal vehicle for delivering therapeutic agents. For example, in conjunction with genetic modification techniques, MSC-based cancer gene therapy has been developed [39].

22.4.4 Hematopoietic Stem Cells

HSCs mainly reside in bone marrow and have the ability to replenish themselves and differentiate into progenitor cells as well as mature blood cells of all hematopoietic lineages. In addition, the transdifferentiation of HSCs into nonhematopoietic tissues including muscle, liver, vasculature, and skin can also be possible, posing the tantalizing possibility of using HSCs in regenerative medicine. However, the phenotype of HSCs is complicated. The most commonly used marker for human HSCs is CD34. CD34 is expressed on approximately 1–4% of mononuclear cells in human bone marrow and <0.1% of mononuclear cells in steady-state human peripheral blood. But the $CD34^-$ phenotype of HSCs is also possible, and these cells are further characterized as $CD38^-$, lack of lineage-specific cell surface antigens (Lin^-), and $CD133^+$ [40]. Hence, the gold standard to validate the potency of HSCs is to test the ability of the stable long-term reconstitution of entire hematopoietic system after implantation into myeloablated recipients, such as immunodeficient NOD/SCID mice. Currently, *in vitro* expansion technology for HSCs is still not satisfactory and usually results in very modest expansion (<4-fold) [41–43]. Moreover, the therapeutic efficacy of HSCs largely relies on the homing property, which can be stimulated by the administration of cytokines and chemokines, such as stromal cell-derived factor-1 (SDF-1), G-CSF, GM-CSF, SCF, and TPO. Like MSCs, HSCs are also amenable to genetic modification, thus providing a very promising strategy for treating genetic diseases through gene correction of HSCs derived from patients [44].

22.4.5 Embryonic Stem Cells and Induced Pluripotent Stem Cells

ESCs are derived from the inner cell mass of the blastocyst. In 1995, the first cell line of ESCs was established from nonhuman primate [45], which was followed by human ESCs in 1998 [46]. ESCs can differentiate into any cell types in an adult organism (pluripotency). In comparison with adult stem cells (e.g., MSCs and HSCs), ESCs can be expanded indefinitely in an undifferentiated state. These cells are weakly immunogenic because they express only moderately major histocompatibility complex (MHC) class I and no MHC class II proteins [47]. Experimentally, to validate the pluripotency of ESCs, inject them into immunocompromised mice and assay them for the formation of a mixed-cell population, known as teratomas, comprising mesoderm, ectoderm, and endoderm lineages. Unfortunately, whereas ESCs are very promising as a cell source for deriving lineage-committed stem/progenitor as well as mature cells for therapeutic uses, isolating ESCs results in the destruction of a fertilized human embryo, which raises serious ethical issues thus limiting their wide applications.

The recently emerged induced pluripotent stem cells (iPSCs), generated by reprogramming somatic cells using retroviral overexpression of four genes *Oct4*, *Sox2*, *c-Myc*, and *Klf4*, share almost same properties as ESCs [48–51]. These cells not only avoid the legal and ethical issues associated with ESCs but also enable the production of patient-specific cell therapeutics by using autologous cells. However, there are two major concerns in the clinical use of iPSCs: the transfection with the proto-oncogene c-Myc and the use of viral vectors that integrate into the genome, posing potentially tumorigenic consequences to the cells. Very recently, the induction of human iPSCs without c-Myc becomes practical using *Oct4*, *Sox2*, and *Klf4* [51] or alternatively, *Oct4*, *Sox2*, *Nanog*, and *Lin28* [50]. In addition, mouse iPSCs have been generated by the transduction of *Oct4*, *Sox2*, *c-Myc*, and *Klf4* avoiding the potential viral integration using either adenoviruses [52] or plasmids [53].

However, one major obstacle that stands in the way of the therapeutic use of both ESCs and iPSCs is the propensity to form teratomas when injected *in vivo*. Hence, developing optimized differentiation protocols for generating target cells *in vitro* with great purity is very crucial. Despite these concerns, on January 23, 2009, a phase I clinical trial for transplantation of human ESCs-derived oligodendrocytes (a cell type in brain and spinal cord) into spinal cord-injured individuals received approval from the U.S. Food and Drug Administration (FDA), marking it the world's first human trials with human ESCs [54].

22.4.6 Other Tissue-Specific Stem/Progenitor Cells

In addition to the popular ESCs and bone marrow stem cells, there are also many other stem/progenitor cells discovered in different tissues, which can be very useful in treating certain tissue-confined diseases. Although the developmental origin of tissue-specific stem/progenitor cells is unknown, their postulated roles can be maintaining the homeostasis of tissues/organs.

Neural stem cells (NSCs) represent one of the most promising cell candidates for cell-based therapy. The term "neural stem cell" is used loosely to describe cells that 1) can generate neural tissue or are derived from the nervous system, 2) demonstrate the capacity of self-renewal, and 3) can give rise to astrocytes, oligodendrocytes, and neurons [55]. NSCs are usually isolated from a region of fetal or adult brain that has been demonstrated to contain dividing cells, for example, the subventricular zone and hippocampus in the adult and other structures in the developing brain. However, it is generally difficult to establish the identity of NSCs because markers that can identify stem cells in their most primitive state are still missing [56]. Like MSCs, NSCs can migrate to injured sites in brain tissue and demonstrate tumor-tropic capacity, thus holding great potential in the treatment of invasive brain tumors, for example, malignant gliomas via NSC-based drug delivery [57].

Another example of tissue-specific stem cells is cardiac stem cells (CSCs) in the adult heart, which are defined by self-renewal property and the capacity to produce differentiated progenies including cardiomyocytes, smooth muscle cells, and endothelial cells. These cells were identified initially as Hoechst effluxing cells (also called side population [SP] cells) in heart tissues [58]. Then, surface markers including c-Kit, Sca-1, and Isl-1 were applied to harvest these cells [59]. However, a completely different strategy has also been developed to generate CSCs through the outgrowth of heart tissue biopsies into self-assembled clusters, so-called "cardiospheres," and these cells were found to express surface antigen markers including c-Kit, Sca-1, CD31, and CD34 [60, 61]. The ability of human CSCs to regenerate myocardium tissue in a rat acute myocardial infarction model has been demonstrated after intramyocardial injection, via differentiation predominantly into cardiomyocytes and, and to a lesser extent into smooth muscle cells and endothelial cells [62]. These cells thus offer an autologous, expandable, and cardiac committed cell source for myocardial regenerative cell therapy.

22.5 TYPICAL EXAMPLES FOR DISEASE-SPECIFIC APPLICATIONS

22.5.1 Vascular Complications

Vascular complications have been associated with many diseases such as PH and DM, where the hallmark is the dysfunction of endothelium. PH is diagnosed when mean pulmonary arterial pressure exceeds the upper limits of normal (>25 mmHg) at rest [63]. Cell-based therapy with EPCs has emerged a novel option for treating PH. Several studies have demonstrated that EPCs can prevent or even reverse monocrotaline-induced PH in rats [64, 65]. However, the mechanism of action in repairing or replacing abnormally remodeled vascular endothelium by EPCs can be mixed. In addition to the capacity of differentiation into endothelial cells, the paracrine and immune modulatory roles of EPCs can be also important in repairing or replacing abnormally remodeled vascular endothelium [66]. EPCs have been demonstrated to release interleukins, growth factors, and chemokines that altogether regulate $CD14^+$ cells, accelerate vascular network formation, and enhance healing processes [67].

Vascular complications associated with DM include macrovascular complications, cardiomyopathy, nephropathy, neuropathy, retinopathy, and prolonged and incomplete wound healing. Notably, studies have shown that DM is associated also with impaired mobilization of adult stem cells from bone marrow and the dysfunction of circulating progenitor cells [68–70]. Hence, cell-based replacement therapy should be very suitable in addressing these pathologic issues. Specifically, both MSCs and EPCs are very promising in these circumstances because of their ability to produce trophic factors (e.g., basic fibroblastic growth factor [bFGF], VEGF, and hypoxia-inducible factor 1-alpha) and differentiate into vascular cells [67]. The transplantation of MSCs for therapeutic neovascularization has proven beneficial in type I diabetic patients with bilateral upper extremity digital gangrene, demonstrating improved arterial perfusion, good healing of all amputation sites, and cessation of pain [71]. The principal mechanisms causing diabetic nephropathy are the arterial damages and the changes to the glomerular ultrastructure, mainly mesangial expansion and glomerular membrane thickening. After infusion, MSCs could engraft into the kidneys and differentiate into endothelial cells and possibly mesangial cells, leading to a significant decrease in mesangial thickening, extracellular matrix deposition, and macrophages infiltration [72]. Another common complication of DM is characterized with prolonged and incomplete wound healing, caused by compromised angiogenesis, diminished cell recruitment, deprivation of growth factors, and impaired formation of collagen matrix. Transplantation of both MSCs and EPCs has been demonstrated to improve wound healing [73, 74], albeit with slightly different mechanisms, where MSCs may differentiate into fibroblasts and keratinocytes, promote neovascularisation, and regenerate appendages and recruit inflammatory cells into wounds. In contrast, EPCs seem to rely mainly on the release of paracrine mediators, such as VEGF, hepatocyte growth factor, G-CSF, and platelet-derived growth factor [PDGF] [75].

22.5.2 Cancer Therapy

The principle for DCs to permit immunotherapy in cancer treatment relies on initiating and expanding tumor-specific $CD4^+$ and $CD8^+$ T cell responses, on *in vitro* manipulation of DCs to present tumor antigens. In fact, DC-based vaccines had been tested clinically early in the mid-1990s, showing some success in treating patients with melanoma, lymphoma, and renal cell carcinoma, but with a low overall clinical response of under 10–15%. This result can possibly be attributed to the quality of DC-based vaccines as well as the harsh immunosuppressive microenvironment in tumors. Thus, the primary purpose in developing cancer vaccines is to overcome this problem by educating DCs with a stronger antigenic signal and providing optimal conditions for their maturation into potent immune stimulatory antigen-presenting cells [76]. The use of gene-modified DCs represents a promising approach by enforcing DCs to present multi-epitope tumor-associated antigens, to express a variety of immune-potentiating molecules (e.g., co-stimulatory molecules, cytokines and chemokines), or to downregulate negative modulators of DC functioning [77]. Nevertheless, DC-based cancer immunotherapy has proven safe and feasible; however, it can be strengthened even more when in combination with other therapeutic strategies.

As mentioned, the tumor tropism of certain stem cells can be exploited for targeted drug delivery to tumors to achieve better therapeutic benefits. Although the exact molecular mechanism of tumor tropism of MSCs is unknown, it is thought to be mediated by high local concentrations of inflammatory chemokines (e.g., monocyte chemoattractant protein-1 [MCP-1]) and growth factors (e.g., SDF-1α) in the tumor microenvironment as MSCs are known to express a large array of chemokine receptors such as CXCR4 [39]. Studies have shown that irradiation, which leads to apoptosis of tumor cells and release of inflammatory signals in the tumor microenvironment, can promote the tropism and engraftment of MSCs at the tumor site [78, 79]. Moreover, MSCs can be also manipulated to facilitate the infiltration toward tumors through genetic modification to overexpress epidermal growth factor receptor (EGFR) [80]. Therefore, MSCs are ideal for the targeted delivery of biological agents to tumors. Several studies have demonstrated that MSCs transduced with oncolytic adenoviruses can deliver specifically an increased viral load to tumors [81, 82]. MSCs have also been engineered to express herpes simplex virus-thymidine kinase followed by administration of the prodrug ganciclovir for targeted cancer suicide gene therapy [83, 84]. Additionally, the pharmacokinetics of many therapeutic proteins such as interferon-beta (IFN-β), interleukin-12 (IL-12), and tumor necrosis factor (TNF)-related apoptosis inducing ligand (TRAIL), can be improved via tumor-specific gene delivery using MSCs, which in turn results in better therapeutic effects and avoids systemic toxicity [39]. Similarly, NSCs have also been exploited extensively in cancer gene therapy for brain tumors [85].

22.5.3 Ischemic Heart Disease

Ischemic heart diseases eventually result in heart failure, which is defined as a progressive disorder initiated by an acute or gradual loss of functional cardiomyocytes, thus leading to diminished cardiac function. Heart transplantation remains the ultimate resort for end-stage heart failure patients, and the success is restricted by the limited availability of organ donors, complications associated with immune suppressive treatments, and a high chance of long-term graft failure. Cell-based therapy is emerging as a new therapy for regenerating or repairing damaged myocardium, which may be attributed to both replacement of cardiac cells and establishment of a vascular network. So far, skeletal myocytes, blood or bone marrow cells, CSCs, ESCs, and iPSCs have been explored both experimentally and clinically as potential cell candidates for cardiovascular regenerative cell therapy [59, 86–88].

Early clinical trials with skeletal myocytes, however, have indicated that their use may be associated with the incidence of arrhythmias, preventing their further applications [89]. Later on, transplantation of bone marrow cells has been demonstrated safe in both acute myocardial infarction and chronic heart diseases, and it can provide modest benefits [90]. In most clinical trials, the mononuclear fraction of bone marrow from patients is separated out, usually via a density gradient centrifugation, and injected back into the patients' hearts without further manipulation. However, in several studies, a selected subpopulation (i.e., MSCs, HSCs, or EPCs) is purified from bone marrow or the mononuclear fraction of peripheral blood. Cells might be administrated through either intracoronary or transendocardial injection [88]. Furthermore, the mechanisms by which transplanted bone-marrow cells elicit therapeutic effects are also mixed and may include cardiomyogenesis through differentiation into cardiomyocytes, induction of angiogenesis, and paracrine effects [87]. However, because studies have also shown that retention rates of implanted cells in myocardium range from 5% to 11% [91, 92], the paracrine effects are implicated to play a very significant role in myocardial regeneration by protecting residual cardiac cells, promoting angiogenesis, recruiting progenitor cells, suppressing inflammation, and/or preventing myocardial fibrosis [87].

Myocardial regeneration with other cell types is still in the very early stage. Because of the propensity of teratoma formation of undifferentiated ESCs, ESCs-derived cardiomyocytes that exhibit similar functional and molecular characteristics to cardiomyocytes obtained from postnatal tissue with theoretically less potential for disorganized growth are used universally. These cells seemed to improve cardiac function and attenuate left ventricular remodeling in post-infarcted rat hearts without teratoma formation [93, 94]. In contrast, adult stem cells, such as HSCs, MSCs and EPCs from peripheral circulation; bone marrow; and other tissues with limited differentiation potential, have been more commonly used in cell-based treatments for ischemic heart disease. However, the clinical efficacies of these purified cell preparations remain to be verified. The recently discovered CSCs attract much interest because of their definitive cardiogenic capability and epitomize an ideal cell source for cardiac regeneration [95–97]. Moreover, *in vivo* stimulation of the proliferation of endogenous CSCs as well as their differentiation into appropriate cell types via administration of pharmacological agents may represent a constructive strategy for regenerating failing heart through viable techniques with much less complexity.

22.5.4 Type I Diabetes Mellitus

Type I diabetes mellitus (TIDM) is a disorder in glucose homeostasis, resulting from an insufficient insulin supply. The disease is developed via T-cell-mediated, progressive, and chronic inflammation against the islets of Langerhans in the pancreas, especially the insulin-producing β cells, eventually destroying them [23]. Currently, the two main strategies of cell-based therapy proposed for treating T1DM are DC-based immunosuppressive therapy [21] and β-cell replacement therapy [23].

In DC-based immunosuppressive therapy, DCs induce anergy through the augmentation of regulatory T cells, such as $Foxp3^+CD25^+CD4^+$ T cells (T_{regs}), and they have been demonstrated to block the development of autoimmunity by diabetogenic T cells in NOD mice [98]. In a series of studies, DCs maintained in a functionally immature state after *in vitro* treatment with nuclear factor-κ light-chain enhancer of activated B-cells (NF-κB) decoys and antisense oligodeoxyribonucleotides (AS-ODN) to the CD40, CD80, and CD86 co-stimulatory molecules are diabetes preventive in the NOD mice [99, 100]. Based on these promising preclinical results, a phase I clinical trial was initiated to assess the safety of this procedure by intradermal or subcutaneous administration at an anatomic site proximal to the pancreas as illustrated schematically in Figure 22.2 [21]. Furthermore, with the use of AS-ODN encapsulated microspheres, direct *in vivo* priming DCs to obviate the need for *in vitro* treatment of DCs is also envisioned [101].

In humans, other than insulin replacement, the only clinically acceptable treatment for TIDM remains islet transplantation with the assistance of pharmacologic immunosuppression, which is limited because of the availability of donor islets. Hence, alternative sources of β cells are sought. Both ESCs/iPSCs and adult stem cells can generate surrogate β cells. ESCs can differentiate into insulin-producing cells spontaneously, albeit at a very low frequency of only ~1% [102]. Currently, different strategies aiming at improving differentiation efficiency are being explored, and the cells generated by these *in vitro* protocols are generally functionally restricted, showing polyhormonal phenotypes and/or poor nutrient-induced insulin secretory responses [103]. A similar situation holds true for iPSCs, although iPSCs offer the feasibility of generating autologous β cells from patients with TIDM [104]. In contrast, the differentiation potential of bone marrow stem cells (i.e., HSCs and MSCs) into insulin-producing cells is debated widely. Several studies demonstrated that MSCs could differentiate into insulin-producing cells releasing insulin in a glucose-dependent manner [105, 106], whereas in other studies, MSCs were believed to prevent β-cell destruction by T cells *in vivo* through their unique immunomodulatory properties rather than repopulating the islets with transdifferentiated β cells [107, 108].

22.5.5 Central Nervous System Diseases

Central nervous system diseases include Alzheimer's disease, Parkinson's disease (PD), Huntington's disease, multiple sclerosis, traumatic brain injury, and stroke. In these

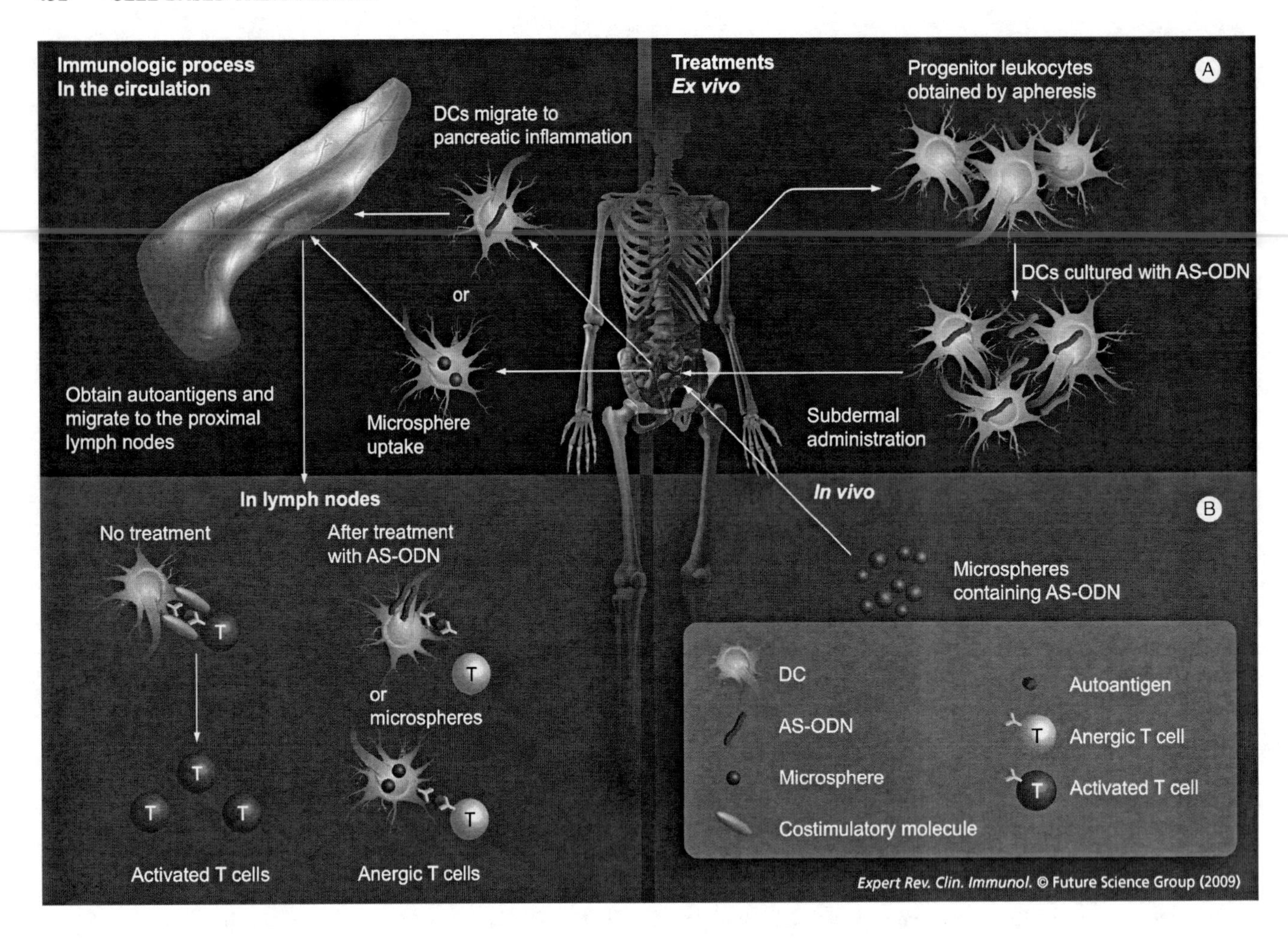

FIGURE 22.2 Using dendritic cells to treat type I diabetes. Reproduced with permission from Ref. 21. (See color figure in color plate section.)

various conditions, neuronal cells are lost either through an acute insult or through a chronic degenerative process. The rationale behind cell-based approaches is to reconstruct neural circuits either by transplanting cells directly into the brain or by stimulating endogenous neural precursor cells to divide and replenish cell populations. Taking PD as an example, it has relatively circumscribed pathology and is characterized by the slow progressive loss of dopaminergic nigrostriatal neurons, which leads to the classic motor triad of bradykinesia, resting tremor, and rigidity. Although treatments based on dopamine replacement are effective to some extent, neuronal degeneration persists. Cell replacement of the lost dopaminergic neurons offers hope to reverse the disease progression, and various cell sources have been investigated in this respect. The transplantation of human fetal tissue/cells, such as fetal ventral mesencephalic tissue and fetal neural precursor cells, has been tested in several clinical trials since the late 1980s [109, 110]. However, the outcomes are not encouraging and some patients even developed dyskinesias, suggesting the complexity of attempting cell replacement and circuit repair. The transplantation of xenogeneic tissues, mostly porcine tissues, has also been tested with limited success in clinical trials because of vigorous immune responses. It is therefore suggested that a combination of strategies aiming to avoid immunological reaction, modify the PD microenvironment, support cell survival, and guide synaptogenesis may be necessary [111]. Moreover, the use of fetal tissues/cells yields intense ethic controversy.

Current research efforts are focusing on seeking new cell sources. Among these, ESCs are differentiated readily into tyrosine hydroxylase positive (TH^+) cells, representing a desirable and reproducible source of defined dopaminergic neurons [112]. Again, researchers are working to obtain purified neurological cells for cell transplantation in order to avoid any contamination by undifferentiated cells as a result of the high propensity of tumorigenicity of ESCs [113]. Additionally, iPSCs offer the possibility of generating autologous neurons for transplantation. In one report, motor neurons and astroglia were derived successfully from iPSCs originating from an 82-year-old female with familial (carrying a SOD-1 mutation) amyotrophic lateral sclerosis

(ALS) [114]. Alternatively, NSCs represent an ideal cell candidate as neuroregenerative medicine with a more restricted differentiation potential, thus being easier to derive an explicitly striatal phenotype in comparison with ESCs and iPSCs [115]. In a primate PD model, transplanted NSCs could survive, migrate, and differentiate into dopamine-producing neurons and glial phenotypes and ultimately led to behavioral improvements [116]. Stimulating endogenous NSCs through infusing growth factors or using gene therapy can be a possible choice to recruit NSCs at the injured sites for circuit reconstruction and eventually behavioral improvements [117]. MSCs from different sources also can transdifferentiate into neural lineage, and the transplantation of both differentiated and undifferentiated cells has been demonstrated to produce neuroprotective effects and result in behavioral improvements in rat PD models [118, 119]. Recently, several phase I/II clinical trials have been initiated to test the safety and efficacy of stem cell-based therapies, the results of which should shed light on future development into therapeutics [120].

22.5.6 Human Immunodeficiency Virus Disease

HIV attacks the human immune system by infecting helper T cells (specifically $CD4^+$ T cells), macrophages, and dendritic cells. In general, HIV infection leads to low levels of $CD4^+$ T cells and eventually to the loss of cell-mediated immunity. Current combination antiretroviral regimens for treating HIV disease have intrinsic limits because HIV DNA persists as an integrated genome in long-lived cellular reservoirs, leading to noncurative treatments and lifelong adherence for patients [121]. In addition, many HIV-infected patients can no longer be treated with regular regimens of antiretroviral therapy. In this regard, cell-based therapy, representing a fundamentally different approach, may provide new promises. HSCs have been exploited intensely in treating HIV diseases because of their capability of reconstituting bone marrow on the one hand and being amenable to genetic manipulations on the other hand. The idea is that through the introduction of HIV resistance genes into HSCs, a long-term repopulation of the host with progeny cells would provide patients with immunization to HIV [122]. As a matter of fact, HSC-based therapy for HIV was evolved before the emergence of antiretroviral therapy in the late 1980s; however, because of the constraints in technologies and limited understanding of HIV pathogenesis, its development had been significantly halted [123].

It is now known that HIV must bind to either CCR5 or CXCR4, chemokine receptors present on many immune cells to enter cells, and *CCR5* Δ32 have been implicated to be associated with the progression of HIV disease [124]. In a clinical trial reported in 2009, when HSCs from an HLA-matched, homozygous *CCR5* Δ32 donor were implanted in an HIV-infected 42-year-old man, well known as the "Berlin patient," who developed acute myeloid leukemia and went through chemotherapy and radiation therapy to destroy the immune system cells, HIV was eradicated from the patient 20 months later at the absence of combination antiretroviral therapy [125]. This finding spikes new hope in using stem-cell-based therapy to treat HIV. Subsequently, in a very recent report, Holt et al. obtained HSCs from human umbilical cord blood and expanded them *in vitro* by treating with TPO and Flt-3L, followed by nucleofection with plasmids expressing *CCR5*-specific zinc-finger nucleases, which can induce a permanent gene disruption that is passed to daughter cells in the absence of persistent transgene expression [126]. In comparison with unmodified HSCs, when these *CCR5*-disrupted HSCs were transplanted into nonobese diabetic/severe combined immunodeficient/interleukin $2r\gamma^{null}$ (NOD/SCID/IL$2r\gamma^{null}$ or NOG) mice, a model known to support multilineage human hematopoiesis, the virus levels were lower and $CD4^+$ T cells were not depleted after being challenged with CCR5-tropic HIV [126]. However, it is unclear yet whether this technique would become a clinical reality for HIV disease because X4 variants of HIV may outgrow under this selective pressure.

22.5.7 Cartilage Tissue Regeneration

Articular cartilage in adults is an avascular, alymphatic, and aneural tissue. When damaged, only limited spontaneous repair occurs. Currently, there are no satisfactory clinical techniques for repairing articular cartilage defects. Surgical procedures such as bone marrow stimulation technique, abrasions, and microfractures generally result in the repair of cartilage defects with a fibrous tissue to fibrocartilage at best, which is known to be biochemically and biomechanically different from normal hyaline cartilage and undergo degeneration eventually [127]. Cell-based therapy promises cartilage tissue regeneration, and autologous chondrocyte implantation (ACI) has become the first biological product (Caricel) approved by the FDA on the market in the United States. ACI involves the isolation of autologous chondrocytes, *in vitro* expansion, and implantation back to the defects as illustrated in Figure 22.3 [128]. However, the long-term effectiveness of ACI still awaits to be confirmed [129]. In addition, the requirement of *in vitro* expansion of chondrocytes during the ACI procedure, which generally induces the dedifferentiation resulting in the loss of chondrocytic phenotype of chondrocytes, compromises the efficacy of ACI. Instead, because of the abundant availability through *in vitro* expansion and potent chondrogenesis of MSCs, these cells are expected to be ideal in cartilage tissue regeneration. In fact, with the limited number of reported clinical trials, the usefulness of MSCs in cartilage repair has been confirmed [130]. Nejadnik et al. reported on bone-marrow–derived MSCs transplantation into 36 patients with articular cartilage defects, and they followed up for

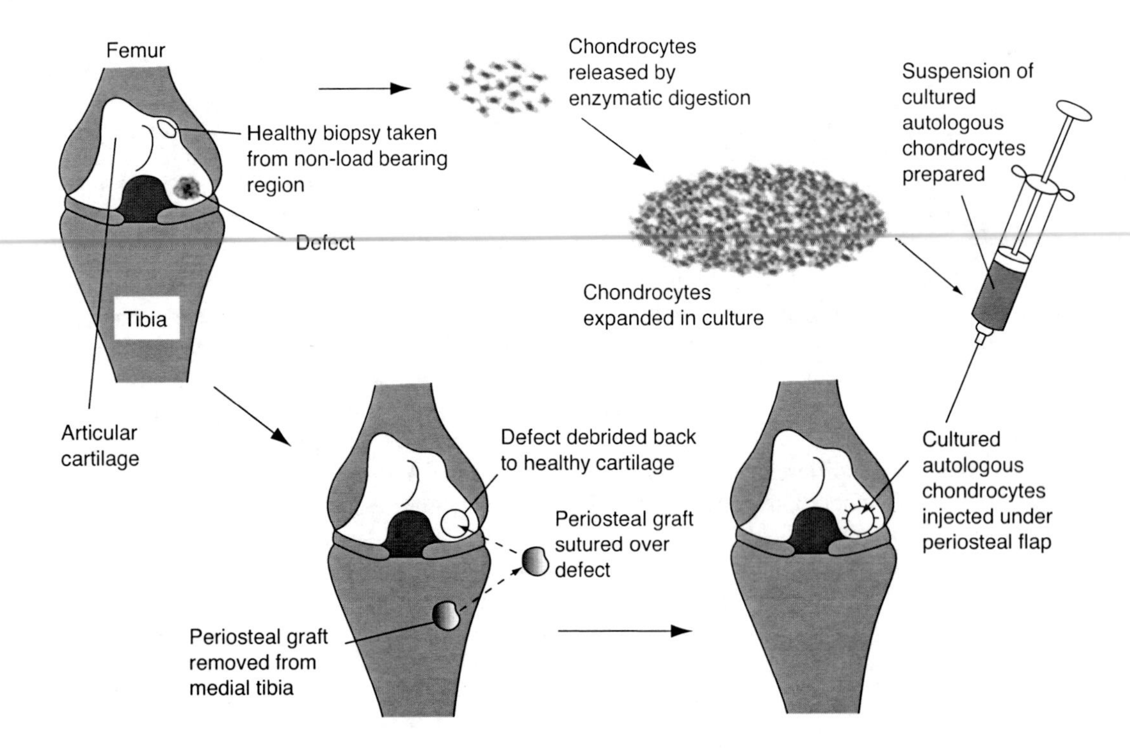

FIGURE 22.3 Procedures of autologous chondrocyte implantation. Reproduced with permission from Ref. 128.

24 months [131]. They compared the results with those undergoing the ACI procedure and concluded that MSC transplantation showed comparable benefits with ACI. Moreover, in comparison with ACI, MSC-based therapy requires one step less of surgery, thus, reducing costs for patients and minimizing donor site morbidity. Other cell types such as ESCs and iPSCs have also been explored for cartilage tissue regeneration; however, their application is limited because of ethical controversy and tumorigenicity.

22.6 BRIEF OVERVIEW ON HUMAN CASE STUDIES

The advancement of clinical development for different diseases varies. For example, bone marrow transplantation has occurred in clinical settings for decades. As such, for those diseases that can be treated potentially with bone marrow cells (containing EPCs, MSCs, and HSCs), such as myocardial infarction, clinical trials have been initiated quickly. In a long-term clinical study, named BALANCE, a 5-year follow-up of intracoronary autologous BM mononuclear cell infusion after acute myocardial infarction was performed [132]. Several key issues have been identified from a large amount of clinical trials on cardiac cell therapy, which need to be considered carefully in future studies including cell candidates, microenvironment in the disease sites, dosing, timing and method of delivery, selection of trial end points, as well as patient population [133, 134]. However, most other current clinical trials concerning cell-based therapeutics are at the stage of exploring the safety and feasibility of the procedures (phase I/II studies). It is important to note that most clinical trials involve the use of adult stem cells, which can be derived from bone marrow, umbilical cord blood, and placenta, although other cell types including β islet cells, hepatocytes, and myoblasts have been tested in different applications. Specifically, besides HSCs, MSCs represent a very promising candidate and their uses can be in very distinct situations including bone and cartilage repair, cell types into which MSCs readily differentiate, and immune conditions such as GvHD and autoimmune conditions that use the immune suppressive properties of MSCs. Considering the clinical trials registered on the National Institutes of Health's clinical trials website (http://clinicaltrials.gov), with the keyword of "mesenchymal stem cells," there are 203 clinical trials ongoing (as of November 29, 2011), which span from bone/cartilage diseases to cancer. Using "hematopoietic stem cells" as the keyword, it gives back 3450 studies.

In the clinical trials using stem cells for treating type I diabetes first initiated in 2003 in Brazil, autologous HSCs were tested to preserve β-cell mass and beneficial effects for patients have been observed including insulin-free for some period [135]. Whereas allogenic cell therapy may cause additional adverse side effects, using gene therapy in combination with HSC therapies can be very advantageous in addressing some genetic diseases, such as β-thalassemia and Wiskott-Aldrich syndrome. In a report in 2010 in the *New England Journal of Medicine*, Boztug et al. showed that HSC-based gene therapy for Wiskott-Aldrich syndrome could be corrected by autologous genetically modified HSCs to a great extent [136]. Two patients were transplanted with autologous $CD34^+$ HSCs with corrected gene *WASP* and gained correction of the primary disease phenotype, including hemorrhagic diathesis, eczema, autoimmunity, and severe infection [136]. In another clinical trial, NSCs are applied to eradicate inoperable glioblastoma (City of Hope, CA). These cells are genetically modified to produce a prodrug-activating enzyme (cytosine deaminase) that converts a nontoxic prodrug (5-fluorocytosine [5-FC]) into a cytotoxic anticancer drug (5-fluorouracil [5-FU]), eventually causing cell death at the site of the tumor. This disease is very aggressive, and patients are under treatment in the initial phase I/II study. Besides the extensive uses of adult cells, the most exciting progress is that the FDA has recently approved three applications on clinical trials with ESCs, mainly testing the safety and tolerability of cells after transplantation. Notably, in all three cases, ESCs are differentiated into lineage-committed cells before injection, i.e., oligodendrocytes in Geron's (Menlo Park, CA) trial aimed at treating spinal cord injury (initially approved in January 2009) and retinal pigment epithelium cells in Advanced Cell Technology's (Santa Monica, CA) two trials for Stargardt macular dystrophy and age-related macular degeneration.

22.7 PHARMACEUTICAL CONSIDERATIONS ON CELL-BASED THERAPEUTICS

22.7.1 Manufacturing Process

In cell-based therapy, cells are isolated from donors and are subjected to *in vitro* manipulations including purification, expansion, stimulation, differentiation, and/or genetic modification before storage and therapeutic use. As the first step in acquiring therapeutic cells, certain criteria including characteristic surface markers for stem cells should be established for their isolation, which certainly requires a profound understanding of stem cell biology. At the current stage, the isolation protocols for each cell type can be very different among different research laboratories, especially for adult stem cells, conferring cell preparations containing different cell components, which in fact represents one of the major causes that leads to conflicting results in the literature.

In most cases, the number of cells obtained from donors, especially for stem cells, is very low, and *in vitro* expansion therefore becomes necessary considering the need of a large quantity of cells in most clinical settings. Importantly, for different cell types, expansion protocols can be very different, represented by the fact that the culture medium is developed specifically for each cell type. However, the major concern lies in that most of the culture media currently used contain animal-originated proteins (e.g., fetal bovine serum), which may cause infectious agent transmission to humans [137]. Hence, developing a fully chemical defined culture medium is of great importance in cell-based therapy [138]. In particular, a feeder cell layer is generally required for maintaining the pluripotency of ESCs, which not only complicates the expansion process but also brings a high risk of contamination by animal-derived pathogens. Hence, the development of feeder-free culture for human ESCs is under intense research [139, 140]. Furthermore, it is very critical to maintain the phenotype of cells during *in vitro* cell expansion, which is especially challenging for stem cells because of the currently limited understanding of their *in vivo* microenvironment (i.e., stem cell niche). To this end, recent studies have identified several factors including oxygen tension and concentrations of metabolites that play important roles in controlling stem cell quality [141–146]. An additional issue is the expansion efficiency. For adherent cell expansion, the two-dimensional (2D) plastic tissue culture flasks used by researchers are labor intensive and susceptible to contamination because of frequent cell passaging as a result of limited surface area and manual medium changing. Besides, the nonhomogeneous nature of 2D static culture normally generates concentration gradients (e.g., pH, dissolved oxygen, and metabolites), which can be very detrimental to the quality of cells. An emerging technology is the microcarrier-based cell expansion in bioreactors, which offers a more homogeneous culture environment, a tighter control of culture parameters, and a higher productivity [147–150]. To date, several different cell types including chondrocytes, ESCs, and MSCs have been expanded successfully using this system [151–154]. Particularly, for MSCs, large-scale manufacturing processes have been developed in compliance with formal regulatory guidelines issued by international agencies [155, 156].

Generally, *in vitro* treatment to improve cell functioning is required such as priming DCs with antigens and lineage-specific differentiating stem cells. Studies have demonstrated that when $Sca\text{-}1^+$ stem cells were preconditioned with IGF-1, both cell survival and engraftment were enhanced, leading to a better improvement in myocardial function in a rat model of acute myocardial infarction [157]. Moreover, depending on the specific purpose, cells can be enforced to express proteins through genetic modification to improve cell engraftment *in vivo*, to modulate the microenvironment of diseased sites, or to deliver therapeutic modalities [22, 77, 158].

22.7.2 Administration Routes

Cells can be administered either systemically or locally. In one study, Gao et al. reported the delivery of rat bone-marrow MSCs in rats via intra-artery (i.a.), intravenous (i.v.), or intraperitoneal cavity (i.p.) infusions [159]. The most convenient method is i.v. infusion, which has been extensively applied in implantation of HSCs for bone marrow reconstitution. Following administration into the peripheral blood circulation, cells home to target tissues such as bone marrow and ischemic heart. In some cases, the i.v. infusion of cells may not be sufficient to obtain clinical benefits where a large number of cells is needed, and local administration is therefore preferred to achieve better therapeutic benefits. For example, intramyocardial injection at the per-infarct regions has been suggested to be optimal for the induction of heart repair [160].

Cells can also be encapsulated in biomaterials, which not only enables future removal of cells and prevents them from spreading in the patient's body, but also may improve their functionality by protecting them from immune attack as well as harsh inflammatory environment [161]. Among different biomaterials, hydrogels, as a result of their injectability and biocompatible properties, are very promising in facilitating cell delivery [59]. One study has demonstrated that cell/fibrin gel suspension is amenable to catheter-based delivery, which can be translated easily into clinical settings [162].

A relevant important issue is the timing of cell administration, which represents an important factor to be considered because the efficacy of cell-based therapy can be largely dependent on the status of diseases. The administration of cells at an early time point may be preferred before the establishment of pathogenesis [163]; however, the early pathogenesis normally is accompanied by strong inflammatory reactions, which is detrimental to the survival of implanted cells. As an example, an early administration of EPCs in monocrotaline-induced PH has been demonstrated to be favorable to achieve a better abrogation on the increase in right ventricular systolic pressure and hypertrophy [163, 164].

22.7.3 *In Vivo* Fates of Therapeutic Cells

Unlike conventional therapeutics, cells are "live" drugs, which can mobilize and/or reside in the body by integrating into tissues for long time and can turn over via a completely different mechanism. The biodistribution of cells can be very complicated and may relate to cell localization, migration, and survival and differentiation status. Unfortunately, currently, a satisfactory detection method on administrated cells is unavailable, although labeling cells with superparamagnetic iron oxide nanoparticles [165] or reporter gene-based imaging technology [166] has been applied in monitoring cells *in vivo*. Another challenge in studying the *in vivo* fates of cells is the immunological issue of testing human cells in animal models. Immunosuppression or immune-deficient animal models are likely to be employed, but this approach may mask immune-modulatory or immunotoxicological aspects of cells and/or may eventually change biodistribution of cells.

At the current stage, very little information is available on the biodistribution of therapeutic cells, which poses a major hurdle on the assessment of pharmacokinetics/pharmacodynamics [38]. Studies have shown that the majority of systemically administered MSCs (>80%) accumulated immediately in the lungs and was cleared with a half-life of 24 h [34, 167, 168]. Generally, only a small fraction of the original administered cell mass is capable of engrafting, and of those that do engraft, only a small percentage has been shown to differentiate into a functional replacement tissue [91, 92, 166]. However, cells have intrinsic homing properties and show responses to an injury in tissues. For example, MSCs can be recruited to injury sites [169, 170] and tumors [158] in response to chemokines, growth factors, and other soluble mediators. It is important to note that the biodistribution of cells can be affected by many biological mechanisms. For example, studies have demonstrated that co-infusion of HSCs with MSCs can promote the engraftment of HSCs in bone marrow [171].

22.7.4 Biosafety Issues

Cell-based therapeutics are emerging as a new entity in pharmaceutical science and, hence, present new biosafety issues not encountered for low-molecular-weight drugs or other biopharmaceuticals, which should be paid great attention to. However, biosafety is largely relative for cellular-based therapy and it is better to be discussed in terms of biosafety risk. Such a risk/benefit ratio can be assessed only after considering numerous factors, including the source of the cells or tissues, cell preparation methods, the intended recipients, where in the body the cell-based therapeutics will be implanted, and the method of delivery.

Tumorigenicity is one of the most concerned issues for cell-based therapeutics. A dramatic example is that a young boy developed a multifocal brain tumor after intracerebellar and intrathecal injection of human fetal NSCs for ataxia telangiectasia [172]. First, undifferentiated ESCs and iPSCs are known to form teratomas in immunocompromised animals, which sets a risk and should be assessed when using them in humans [173]. Notably, although in some cases more differentiated, lineage-committed cells are used, current differentiation protocols do not guarantee the absence of undifferentiated cells. As a matter of fact, even though ESCs were differentiated pretransplantation, teratoma formation was observed in as many as 60% of transplanted animals [174]. Second, MSCs [175], ESCs [176], and iPSCs [177] have been demonstrated to acquire chromosomal aberrations during expansion *in vitro*, which is a hallmark of cancer [178]. Evidence shows that an increased passage number of cells correlates with a higher potential for chromosomal aberrations [179]. Therefore, minimizing the culture time might be required to decrease the chance for *in vitro* genetic aberrations. Additionally, in MSC-based therapeutics, especially for those aiming at tumor targeted drug delivery, the immunoprivilege of these cells might have the potential to support tumor progression [180]. Finally, there is concern that genetically modified cells may be more prone to form tumors if the transfected gene inserts into an inappropriate place (insertional mutagenesis) and either disrupts the expression of a tumor-suppressor gene or activates an oncogene [181]. As discussed, monitoring the biodistribution of implanted cells may be extremely difficult. However, the ability to track therapeutic cells is the key to an objective assessment of risk with respect to inappropriate ectopic tissue formation or tumorigenicity. In this regard, one encouraging method is to perform direct genetic modification of cells prior to implantation with genes that can prevent the adverse events and/or eliminate the transplanted cells and their progeny when necessary, thus providing control of stem cell fates *in vivo* [182].

A unique safety issue associated with cell-based therapeutics is the immunogenicity. Although immunoprivilege of stem cells including ESCs and MSCs has been suggested, *in vitro* manipulation of cells can introduce uncertainties. A typical example comes from a report by Zhao et al. that iPSCs, initially considered to be very promising in reducing this risk of immunogenicity because of the autologous nature, induced T cell-dependent immune response in syngeneic recipients [183]. However, one complication for addressing immunotoxicity of cell products is related to the fact that typically studies are carried out in immune-compromised or immune-suppressed animals. Immunosuppression can be applied in animals but may not be medically acceptable or necessary in clinical trials. Nevertheless, supportive information may be obtained using *in vitro* assessments such as NK cell assays, serum cytotoxicity assays, mixed lymphocyte assays, Fluorescence-activated cell sorting analysis of cell-surface expression, and cytokine assay [184].

22.7.5 Regulations on Cell-Based Therapeutics

The unique properties of live cells make current regulations on drugs impractical for cell-based therapeutics, especially for stem cell products, because many physiochemical techniques such as viral inactivation, filtration, and terminal sterilization are not compatible with therapeutics of live cells any more. Clearly, conventional preclinical absorption, distribution, metabolism, excretion, and toxicity (ADMET) studies cannot be applied to cell-based products in a straightforward way.

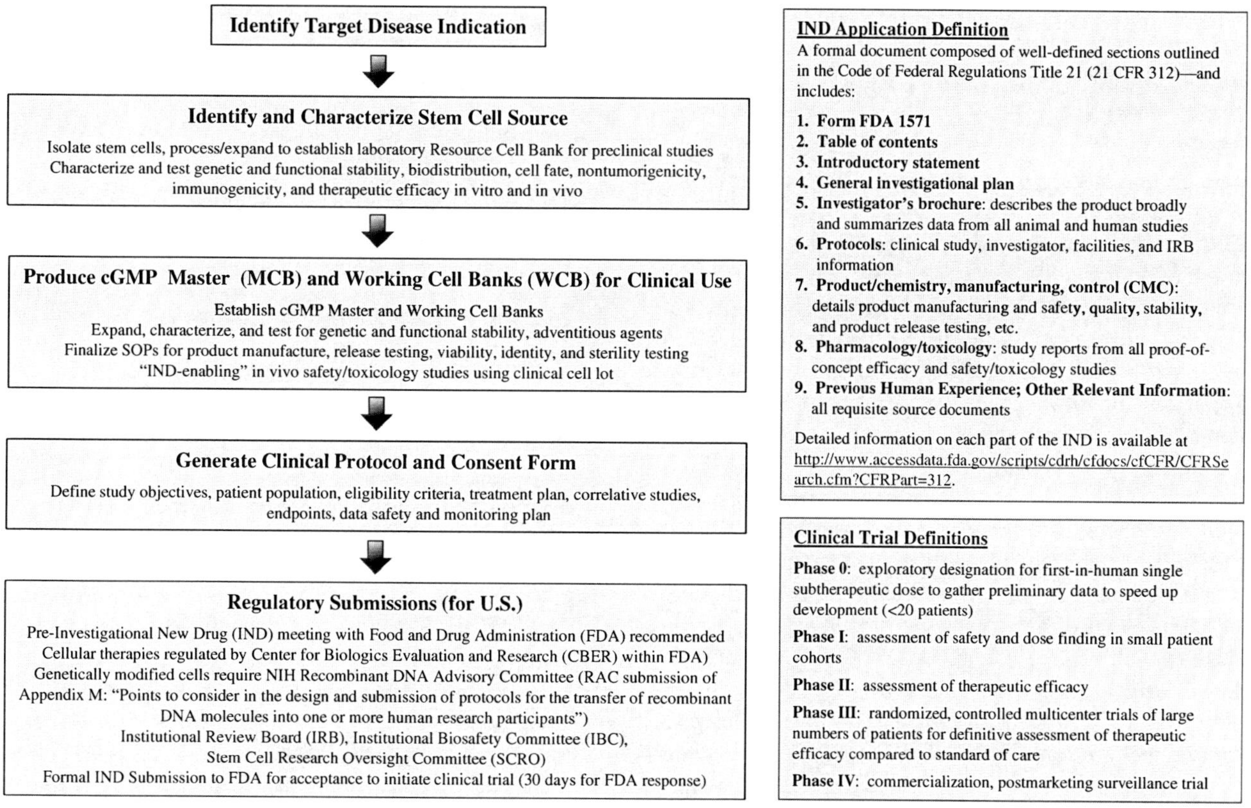

Identify Target Disease Indication

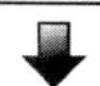

Identify and Characterize Stem Cell Source

Isolate stem cells, process/expand to establish laboratory Resource Cell Bank for preclinical studies
Characterize and test genetic and functional stability, biodistribution, cell fate, nontumorigenicity, immunogenicity, and therapeutic efficacy in vitro and in vivo

Produce cGMP Master (MCB) and Working Cell Banks (WCB) for Clinical Use

Establish cGMP Master and Working Cell Banks
Expand, characterize, and test for genetic and functional stability, adventitious agents
Finalize SOPs for product manufacture, release testing, viability, identity, and sterility testing
"IND-enabling" in vivo safety/toxicology studies using clinical cell lot

Generate Clinical Protocol and Consent Form

Define study objectives, patient population, eligibility criteria, treatment plan, correlative studies, endpoints, data safety and monitoring plan

Regulatory Submissions (for U.S.)

Pre-Investigational New Drug (IND) meeting with Food and Drug Administration (FDA) recommended
Cellular therapies regulated by Center for Biologics Evaluation and Research (CBER) within FDA)
Genetically modified cells require NIH Recombinant DNA Advisory Committee (RAC submission of Appendix M: "Points to consider in the design and submission of protocols for the transfer of recombinant DNA molecules into one or more human research participants")
Institutional Review Board (IRB), Institutional Biosafety Committee (IBC), Stem Cell Research Oversight Committee (SCRO)
Formal IND Submission to FDA for acceptance to initiate clinical trial (30 days for FDA response)

IND Application Definition

A formal document composed of well-defined sections outlined in the Code of Federal Regulations Title 21 (21 CFR 312)—and includes:

1. **Form FDA 1571**
2. **Table of contents**
3. **Introductory statement**
4. **General investigational plan**
5. **Investigator's brochure**: describes the product broadly and summarizes data from all animal and human studies
6. **Protocols**: clinical study, investigator, facilities, and IRB information
7. **Product/chemistry, manufacturing, control (CMC)**: details product manufacturing and safety, quality, stability, and product release testing, etc.
8. **Pharmacology/toxicology**: study reports from all proof-of-concept efficacy and safety/toxicology studies
9. **Previous Human Experience; Other Relevant Information**: all requisite source documents

Detailed information on each part of the IND is available at http://www.accessdata.fda.gov/scripts/cdrh/cfdocs/cfCFR/CFRSearch.cfm?CFRPart=312.

Clinical Trial Definitions

Phase 0: exploratory designation for first-in-human single subtherapeutic dose to gather preliminary data to speed up development (<20 patients)

Phase I: assessment of safety and dose finding in small patient cohorts

Phase II: assessment of therapeutic efficacy

Phase III: randomized, controlled multicenter trials of large numbers of patients for definitive assessment of therapeutic efficacy compared to standard of care

Phase IV: commercialization, postmarketing surveillance trial

FIGURE 22.4 Regulatory information for clinical trials of stem cell therapies. Reproduced with permission from Ref. 120.

Considering that many clinical trials are underway around the world, urgent attention should be given to regulatory guidelines in cell-based therapy to avoid any unscrupulous, dishonest, and unethical practices by health professionals and to prevent disappointment, unwanted side effects, and unnecessary expense on patients [185]. At the current stage, cell-based therapeutics are considered as therapeutic agents and therefore meet the definitions of several different kinds of regulated products by the FDA, including biologic products, drugs, devices, xenotransplantation products, and human cells, tissues, and cellular and tissue-based products [186]. A submission of an investigational new drug application to the FDA before studies involving humans are initiated is required according to the Public Health Safety Act, Section 351 [187]. In addition, as discussed, a genetic modification of cells before transplantation is applied in many cases, and such treatment would also be considered to be gene therapy, thus, subjecting to FDA regulations pertaining to this issue [187]. Although it is still under intensive development, in 2008, the International Society for Stem Cell Research published Guidelines for the Clinical Translation of Stem Cells (available at http://www.isscr.org/clinical_trans), which "provides a framework for the responsible and timely development of clinically useful stem-cell-based therapies" [188]. Furthermore, a roadmap for the development of the stem-cell-based therapy from bench to bedside has been proposed as shown in Figure 22.4 [120].

22.8 CONCLUSION AND FUTURE PERSPECTIVES

Although clinical uses of many forms of cell therapeutics have been available, cell-based therapy is still in its infant stage. It is noted that currently, commercial success has yet to be achieved, mostly as a result of the mixed clinical results and high specificity of each technology [189]. The evolution of a second generation of cell-based therapeutics involves many stages, but the first important issue is to make it work. Hence, many important questions remain to be seriously addressed for each form of cell therapeutics. For example, the identification of those patients who benefit most from certain cell therapy, the optimal cell type and number for patient with acute and chronic diseases, the best time and way for cell delivery, and the mechanisms of action by which cells exhibit beneficial effects need to be further evaluated. The establishment of new protocols for safety and efficacy studies as well as the manufacture of cell products is urgently needed. As the demand grows for stem cells in both drug discovery and therapeutic applications, effectively translating their promise into reality will require large-scale "industrialized" production under tightly controlled conditions. Achieving that while meeting rigorous quality and regulatory standards will depend on further research efforts in cell culture and scale-up, characterization, enrichment, purification, and process control to deliver a consistent and reproducible supply of cells safely and cost-effectively. Knowledge of the purity of the product must be known because extraneous phenotypes may either influence efficacy or contribute to a significant safety risk. This is exemplified by the temporary hold placed by the FDA on Geron's first-in-human trial of an ESCs-derived treatment for spinal cord injury (GRNOPC1), whereby one concern was surety that the manufactured cell product was fully characterized and that the mixtures of cells were predictable and free from contamination. In addition, the development of novel technologies for cell tracking and addressing the puzzle of using immunodeficient preclinical animal models because of the issue of immunogenicity should be greatly acknowledged. The use of immunocompromised animals in most studies (athymic nude mice) can complicate the interpretation of therapeutic cell function, as these animals are not totally devoid of immune cells nor are their immune systems reflective of human subjects. Finally, a strong interaction among regulatory agencies, therapy developers, and drug safety scientists is highly encouraged in this ever evolving field because clear regulatory guidelines would expedite the process of product development.

ASSESSMENT QUESTIONS

22.1. What are the dendritic cells and how can they be modulated to treat cancer?

22.2. What are the stem cells and how can they be identified generally?

22.3. What are the potential mechanisms for MSC-based therapeutics?

22.4. What is the primary concern for cell-based therapeutics?

22.5. Are there any regulatory guidelines for developing cell-based therapeutics?

REFERENCES

1. Orlando, G., Wood, K.J., Stratta, R.J., et al. (2011). Regenerative medicine and organ transplantation: Past, present, and future. *Transplantation, 91(12)*, 1310–1317.
2. Korbling, M., Estrov, Z. (2003). Adult stem cells for tissue repair—a new therapeutic concept? *New England Journal of Medicine, 349*, 570–582.
3. Orlic, D., Hill, J.M., Arai, A.E. (2002). Stem cells for myocardial regeneration. *Circulation Research 91*, 1092–1102.
4. Thomas, E.D., Lochte, H.L., Jr., Lu, W.C., et al. (1957). Intravenous infusion of bone marrow in patients receiving radiation and chemotherapy. *New England Journal of Medicine, 257*, 491–496.

5. Kurnick, N.B., Montano, A., Gerdes, J.C., et al. (1958). Preliminary observations on the treatment of postirradiation hematopoietic depression in man by the infusion of stored autogenous bone marrow. *Annals of Internal Medicine*, *49*, 973–986.
6. Mathe, G., Jammet, H., Pendic, B., et al. (1959). [Transfusions and grafts of homologous bone marrow in humans after accidental high dosage irradiation]. *Revue Française d'Études Cliniques et Biologiques*, *4*, 226–238.
7. Thomas, E.D., Lochte, H.L., Jr., Cannon, J.H., et al. (1959). Supralethal whole body irradiation and isologous marrow transplantation in man. *Journal of Clinical Investigation*, *38*, 1709–1716.
8. Mathe, G., Amiel, J.L., Schwarzenberg, L., et al. (1963). Haematopoietic chimera in man after allogenic (homologous) bone-marrow transplantation. (Control of the secondary syndrome. Specific tolerance due to the chimerism). *British Medical Journal*, *2*, 1633–1635.
9. Meuwissen, H.J., Bortin, M.M., Bach, F.H., et al. (1984). Long-term survival after bone marrow transplantation: A 15-year follow-up report of a patient with Wiskott-Aldrich syndrome. *Journal of Pediatrics*, *105*, 365–369.
10. Bach, F.H., Albertini, R.J., Joo, P., et al. (1968). Bone-marrow transplantation in a patient with the Wiskott-Aldrich syndrome. *Lancet*, *2*, 1364–1366.
11. De Koning, J., Van Bekkum, D.W., Dicke, K.A., et al. (1969). Transplantation of bone-marrow cells and fetal thymus in an infant with lymphopenic immunological deficiency. *Lancet*, *1*, 1223–1227.
12. Gatti, R.A., Meuwissen, H.J., Allen, H.D., et al. (1968). Immunological reconstitution of sex-linked lymphopenic immunological deficiency. *Lancet*, *2*, 1366–1369.
13. McCredie, K.B., Hersh, E.M., Freireich, E.J. (1971). Cells capable of colony formation in the peripheral blood of man. *Science*, *171*, 293–294.
14. Ende, M., Ende, N. (1972). Hematopoietic transplantation by means of fetal (cord) blood. A new method. *Virginia Medical Monthly*, *(1918) 99*, 276–280.
15. Baumann, I., Testa, N.G., Lange, C., et al. (1993). Haemopoietic cells mobilised into the circulation by lenograstim as alternative to bone marrow for allogeneic transplants. *Lancet*, *341*, 369.
16. Dreger, P., Haferlach, T., Eckstein, V., et al. (1994). G-CSF-mobilized peripheral blood progenitor cells for allogeneic transplantation: Safety, kinetics of mobilization, and composition of the graft. *British Journal of Haematology*, *87*, 609–613.
17. Jansen, J., Thompson, J.M., Dugan, M.J., et al. (2002). Peripheral blood progenitor cell transplantation. *Therapeutic Apheresis*, *6*, 5–14.
18. Banchereau, J., Briere, F., Caux, C., et al. (2000). Immunobiology of dendritic cells. *Annual Review of Immunology*, *18*, 767–811.
19. Steinman, R.M., Hawiger, D., Nussenzweig, M.C. (2003). Tolerogenic dendritic cells. *Annual Review of Immunology*, *21*, 685–711.
20. Blanco, P., Palucka, A.K., Gill, M., et al. (2001). Induction of dendritic cell differentiation by IFN-alpha in systemic lupus erythematosus. *Science*, *294*, 1540–1543.
21. Phillips, B., Giannoukakis, N., Trucco, M. (2009). Dendritic cell-based therapy in Type 1 diabetes mellitus. *Expert Review of Clinical Immunology*, *5*, 325–339.
22. Wu, H., Ye, Z., Mahato, R.I. (2011). Genetically modified mesenchymal stem cells for improved islet transplantation. *Molecular Pharmacology*, *8*, 1458–1470.
23. Bottino, R., Lemarchand, P., Trucco, M., et al. (2003). Gene- and cell-based therapeutics for type I diabetes mellitus. *Gene Therapy*, *10*, 875–889.
24. Staveley-O'Carroll, K., Sotomayor, E., Montgomery, J., et al. (1998). Induction of antigen-specific T cell anergy: An early event in the course of tumor progression. *Proceedings of the National Academy of Sciences USA 95*, 1178–1183.
25. Hsu, F.J., Benike, C., Fagnoni, F., et al. (1996). Vaccination of patients with B-cell lymphoma using autologous antigen-pulsed dendritic cells. *Nature Medicine*, *2*, 52–58.
26. Syme, R.M., Bryan, T.L., Gluck, S. (2001). Dendritic cell-based therapy: A review focusing on antigenic selection. *Journal of Hematotherapy and Stem Cell Research*, *10*, 601–608.
27. Asahara, T., Masuda, H., Takahashi, T., et al. (1999). Bone marrow origin of endothelial progenitor cells responsible for postnatal vasculogenesis in physiological and pathological neovascularization. *Circulation Research*, *85*, 221–228.
28. Urbich, C., Dimmeler, S. (2004). Endothelial progenitor cells: Characterization and role in vascular biology. *Circulation Research*, *95*, 343–353.
29. Leone, A.M., Rutella, S., Bonanno, G., et al. (2005). Mobilization of bone marrow-derived stem cells after myocardial infarction and left ventricular function. *European Heart Journal*, *26*, 1196–1204.
30. Hristov, M., Weber, C. (2004). Endothelial progenitor cells: Characterization, pathophysiology, and possible clinical relevance. *Journal of Cellular and Molecular Medicine*, *8*, 498–508.
31. Khakoo, A.Y., Finkel, T. (2005). Endothelial progenitor cells. *Annual Review of Medicine*, *56*, 79–101.
32. Janic, B., Guo, A.M., Iskander, A.S., et al. (2010). Human cord blood-derived AC133+ progenitor cells preserve endothelial progenitor characteristics after long term in vitro expansion. *PloS One*, *5*, e9173.
33. Friedenstein, A.J., Gorskaja, J.F., Kulagina, N.N. (1976). Fibroblast precursors in normal and irradiated mouse hematopoietic organs. *Experimental Hematology*, *4*, 267–274.
34. Beyer Nardi, N., da Silva Meirelles, L. (2006). Mesenchymal stem cells: isolation, in vitro expansion and characterization. *Handbook of Experimental Pharmacology*, 249–282.
35. Jones, E., McGonagle, D. (2008). Human bone marrow mesenchymal stem cells in vivo. *Rheumatology (Oxford)*, *47*, 126–131.
36. Le Blanc, K., Tammik, C., Rosendahl, K., et al. (2003). HLA expression and immunologic properties of differentiated and undifferentiated mesenchymal stem cells. *Experimental Hematology*, *31*, 890–896.

37. Caplan, A.I., Dennis, J.E. (2006). Mesenchymal stem cells as trophic mediators. *Journal of Cellular Biochemistry*, *98*, 1076–1084.
38. Parekkadan, B., Milwid, J.M. (2010). Mesenchymal stem cells as therapeutics. *Annual Review of Biomedical Engineering*, *12*, 87–117.
39. Dwyer, R.M., Khan, S., Barry, F.P., et al. (2011). Advances in mesenchymal stem cell-mediated gene therapy for cancer. *Stem Cell Research & Therapy*, *1*, 25.
40. Gallacher, L., Murdoch, B., Wu, D.M., et al. (2000). Isolation and characterization of human CD34(−)Lin(−) and CD34 (+)Lin(−) hematopoietic stem cells using cell surface markers AC133 and CD7. *Blood*, *95*, 2813–2820.
41. Miller, C.L., Eaves, C.J. (1997). Expansion in vitro of adult murine hematopoietic stem cells with transplantable lympho-myeloid reconstituting ability. *Proceedings of the National Academy of Sciences USA*, *94*, 13648–13653.
42. Bhatia, M., Bonnet, D., Kapp, U., et al. (1997). Quantitative analysis reveals expansion of human hematopoietic repopulating cells after short-term ex vivo culture. *Journal of Experimental Medicine*, *186*, 619–624.
43. Conneally, E., Cashman, J., Petzer, A., et al. (1997). Expansion in vitro of transplantable human cord blood stem cells demonstrated using a quantitative assay of their lympho-myeloid repopulating activity in nonobese diabetic-scid/scid mice. *Proceedings of the National Academy of Sciences USA*, *94*, 9836–9841.
44. Cartier, N., Hacein-Bey-Abina, S., Bartholomae, C.C., et al. (2009). Hematopoietic stem cell gene therapy with a lentiviral vector in X-linked adrenoleukodystrophy. *Science*, *326*, 818–823.
45. Thomson, J.A., Kalishman, J., Golos, T.G., et al. (1995). Isolation of a primate embryonic stem cell line. *Proceedings of the National Academy of Sciences USA*, *92*, 7844–7848.
46. Thomson, J.A., Itskovitz-Eldor, J., Shapiro, S.S., et al. (1998). Embryonic stem cell lines derived from human blastocysts. *Science*, *282*, 1145–1147.
47. Gepstein, L. (2002). Derivation and potential applications of human embryonic stem cells. *Circulation Research*, *91*, 866–876.
48. Takahashi, K., Yamanaka, S. (2006). Induction of pluripotent stem cells from mouse embryonic and adult fibroblast cultures by defined factors. *Cell*, *126*, 663–676.
49. Takahashi, K., Tanabe, K., Ohnuki, M., et al. (2007). Induction of pluripotent stem cells from adult human fibroblasts by defined factors. *Cell*, *131*, 861–872.
50. Yu, J., Vodyanik, M.A., Smuga-Otto, K., et al. (2007). Induced pluripotent stem cell lines derived from human somatic cells. *Science*, *318*, 1917–1920.
51. Nakagawa, M., Koyanagi, M., Tanabe, K., et al. (2008). Generation of induced pluripotent stem cells without Myc from mouse and human fibroblasts. *Nature Biotechnology*, *26*, 101–106.
52. Stadtfeld, M., Nagaya, M., Utikal, J., et al. (2008). Induced pluripotent stem cells generated without viral integration. *Science*, *322*, 945–949.
53. Okita, K., Nakagawa, M., Hyenjong, H., et al. (2008). Generation of mouse induced pluripotent stem cells without viral vectors. *Science*, *322*, 949–953.
54. Falco, M. (2009). FDA approves human embryonic stem cell study (CNN Medical News).
55. Gage, F.H. (2000). Mammalian neural stem cells. *Science*, *287*, 1433–1438.
56. Morrison, S.J., White, P.M., Zock, C., et al. (1999). Prospective identification, isolation by flow cytometry, and in vivo self-renewal of multipotent mammalian neural crest stem cells. *Cell*, *96*, 737–749.
57. Brown, A.B., Yang, W., Schmidt, N.O., et al. (2003). Intravascular delivery of neural stem cell lines to target intracranial and extracranial tumors of neural and non-neural origin. *Human Gene Therapy*, *14*, 1777–1785.
58. Hierlihy, A.M., Seale, P., Lobe, C.G., et al. (2002). The postnatal heart contains a myocardial stem cell population. *FEBS Letters*, *530*, 239–243.
59. Ye, Z., Zhou, Y., Cai, H., et al. (2011). Myocardial regeneration: Roles of stem cells and hydrogels. *Advanced Drug Delivery Reviews*, *63*, 688–697.
60. Messina, E., De Angelis, L., Frati, G., et al. (2004). Isolation and expansion of adult cardiac stem cells from human and murine heart. *Circulation Research*, *95*, 911–921.
61. Johnston, P.V., Sasano, T., Mills, K., et al. (2009). Engraftment, differentiation, and functional benefits of autologous cardiosphere-derived cells in porcine ischemic cardiomyopathy. *Circulation*, *120*, 1075-1083, 7 p following 1083.
62. Bearzi, C., Rota, M., Hosoda, T., et al. (2007). Human cardiac stem cells. *Proceedings of the National Academy of Sciences USA*, *104*, 14068–14073.
63. Budhiraja, R., Tuder, R.M., Hassoun, P.M. (2004). Endothelial dysfunction in pulmonary hypertension. *Circulation*, *109*, 159–165.
64. Raoul, W., Wagner-Ballon, O., Saber, G., et al. (2007). Effects of bone marrow-derived cells on monocrotaline- and hypoxia induced pulmonary hypertension in mice. *Respiratory Research*, *8*, 8.
65. Zhao, Y.D., Courtman, D.W., Deng, Y., et al. (2005). Rescue of monocrotaline-induced pulmonary arterial hypertension using bone marrow-derived endothelial-like progenitor cells: Efficacy of combined cell and eNOS gene therapy in established disease. *Circulation Research*, *96*, 442–450.
66. Burnham, E.L., Mealer, M., Gaydos, J., et al. (2010). Acute lung injury but not sepsis is associated with increased colony formation by peripheral blood mononuclear cells. *American Journal of Respiratory Cell and Molecular Biology*, *43*, 326–333.
67. Jarajapu, Y.P., Grant, M.B. (2010). The promise of cell-based therapies for diabetic complications: Challenges and solutions. *Circulation Research*, *106*, 854–869.
68. Tepper, O.M., Galiano, R.D., Capla, J.M., et al. (2002). Human endothelial progenitor cells from type II diabetics exhibit impaired proliferation, adhesion, and incorporation into vascular structures. *Circulation*, *106*, 2781–2786.

69. Loomans, C.J., de Koning, E.J., Staal, F.J., et al. (2004). Endothelial progenitor cell dysfunction: A novel concept in the pathogenesis of vascular complications of type 1 diabetes. *Diabetes, 53*, 195–199.
70. Fadini, G.P., Sartore, S., Schiavon, M., et al. (2006). Diabetes impairs progenitor cell mobilisation after hindlimb ischaemia-reperfusion injury in rats. *Diabetologia, 49*, 3075–3084.
71. Comerota, A.J., Link, A., Douville, J., et al. (2010). Upper extremity ischemia treated with tissue repair cells from adult bone marrow. *Journal of Vascular Surgery, 52*, 723–729.
72. Lee, R.H., Seo, M.J., Reger, R.L., et al. (2006). Multipotent stromal cells from human marrow home to and promote repair of pancreatic islets and renal glomeruli in diabetic NOD/scid mice. *American Journal of Respiratory Cell and Molecular Biology USA, 103*, 17438–17443.
73. Wu, Y., Chen, L., Scott, P.G., et al. (2007). Mesenchymal stem cells enhance wound healing through differentiation and angiogenesis. *Stem Cells, 25*, 2648–2659.
74. Kwon, D.S., Gao, X., Liu, Y.B., et al. (2008). Treatment with bone marrow-derived stromal cells accelerates wound healing in diabetic rats. *International Wound Journal, 5*, 453–463.
75. Wu, Y., Zhao, R.C., Tredget, E.E. (2010). Concise review: Bone marrow-derived stem/progenitor cells in cutaneous repair and regeneration. *Stem Cells, 28*, 905–915.
76. Gilboa, E. (2007). DC-based cancer vaccines. *Journal of Clinical Investigation, 117*, 1195–1203.
77. Smits, E.L., Anguille, S., Cools, N., et al. (2009). Dendritic cell-based cancer gene therapy. *Human Gene Therapy, 20*, 1106–1118.
78. Zielske, S.P., Livant, D.L., Lawrence, T.S. (2009). Radiation increases invasion of gene-modified mesenchymal stem cells into tumors. *International Journal of Radiation Oncology*Biology*Physics, 75*, 843–853.
79. Kidd, S., Caldwell, L., Dietrich, M., et al. (2010). Mesenchymal stromal cells alone or expressing interferon-beta suppress pancreatic tumors in vivo, an effect countered by anti-inflammatory treatment. *Cytotherapy, 12*, 615–625.
80. Sato, H., Kuwashima, N., Sakaida, T., et al. (2005). Epidermal growth factor receptor-transfected bone marrow stromal cells exhibit enhanced migratory response and therapeutic potential against murine brain tumors. *Cancer Gene Therapy, 12*, 757–768.
81. Sonabend, A.M., Ulasov, I.V., Tyler, M.A., et al. (2008). Mesenchymal stem cells effectively deliver an oncolytic adenovirus to intracranial glioma. *Stem Cells, 26*, 831–841.
82. Dembinski, J.L., Spaeth, E.L., Fueyo, J., et al. (2010). Reduction of nontarget infection and systemic toxicity by targeted delivery of conditionally replicating viruses transported in mesenchymal stem cells. *Cancer Gene Therapy, 17*, 289–297.
83. Uchibori, R., Okada, T., Ito, T., et al. (2009). Retroviral vector-producing mesenchymal stem cells for targeted suicide cancer gene therapy. *Journal of Gene Medicine, 11*, 373–381.
84. Matuskova, M., Hlubinova, K., Pastorakova, A., et al. (2010). HSV-tk expressing mesenchymal stem cells exert bystander effect on human glioblastoma cells. *Cancer Letters, 290*, 58–67.
85. Kim, S.U. (2011). Neural stem cell-based gene therapy for brain tumors. *Stem Cell Reviews, 7*, 130–140.
86. Herrmann, J.L., Abarbanell, A.M., Weil, B.R., et al. (2009). Cell-based therapy for ischemic heart disease: A clinical update. *The Annals of Thoracic Surgery, 88*, 1714–1722.
87. Perin, E.C., Silva, G.V. (2011). Cell-based therapy for chronic ischemic heart disease–a clinical perspective. *Cardiovascular Therapy, 29*, 211–217.
88. Tongers, J., Losordo, D.W., Landmesser, U. (2011). Stem and progenitor cell-based therapy in ischaemic heart disease: Promise, uncertainties, and challenges. *European Heart Journal, 32*, 1197–1206.
89. Hagege, A.A., Marolleau, J.P., Vilquin, J.T., et al. (2006). Skeletal myoblast transplantation in ischemic heart failure: Long-term follow-up of the first phase I cohort of patients. *Circulation, 114*, I108–113.
90. Abdel-Latif, A., Bolli, R., Tleyjeh, I.M., et al. (2007). Adult bone marrow-derived cells for cardiac repair: A systematic review and meta-analysis. *Archives of Internal Medicine, 167*, 989–997.
91. Hofmann, M., Wollert, K.C., Meyer, G.P., et al. (2005). Monitoring of bone marrow cell homing into the infarcted human myocardium. *Circulation, 111*, 2198–2202.
92. Freyman, T., Polin, G., Osman, H., et al. (2006). A quantitative, randomized study evaluating three methods of mesenchymal stem cell delivery following myocardial infarction. *European Heart Journal, 27*, 1114–1122.
93. Laflamme, M.A., Chen, K.Y., Naumova, A.V., et al. (2007). Cardiomyocytes derived from human embryonic stem cells in pro-survival factors enhance function of infarcted rat hearts. *Nature Biotechnology, 25*, 1015–1024.
94. Caspi, O., Huber, I., Kehat, I., et al. (2007). Transplantation of human embryonic stem cell-derived cardiomyocytes improves myocardial performance in infarcted rat hearts. *Journal of the American College of Cardiology, 50*, 1884–1893.
95. Beltrami, A.P., Barlucchi, L., Torella, D., et al. (2003). Adult cardiac stem cells are multipotent and support myocardial regeneration. *Cell, 114*, 763–776.
96. Tillmanns, J., Rota, M., Hosoda, T., et al. (2008). Formation of large coronary arteries by cardiac progenitor cells. *Proceedings of the National Academy of Sciences USA, 105*, 1668–1673.
97. Dawn, B., Stein, A.B., Urbanek, K., et al. (2005). Cardiac stem cells delivered intravascularly traverse the vessel barrier, regenerate infarcted myocardium, and improve cardiac function. *Proc Natl Acad Sci USA, 102*, 3766–3771.
98. Tarbell, K.V., Yamazaki, S., Olson, K., et al. (2004). CD25+ CD4+ T cells, expanded with dendritic cells presenting a single autoantigenic peptide, suppress autoimmune diabetes. *Journal of Experimental Medicine, 199*, 1467–1477.
99. Ma, L., Qian, S., Liang, X., et al. (2003). Prevention of diabetes in NOD mice by administration of dendritic cells deficient in nuclear transcription factor-kappaB activity. *Diabetes, 52*, 1976–1985.

100. Machen, J., Harnaha, J., Lakomy, R., et al. (2004). Antisense oligonucleotides down-regulating costimulation confer diabetes-preventive properties to nonobese diabetic mouse dendritic cells. *Journal of Immunology*, *173*, 4331–4341.

101. Phillips, B., Nylander, K., Harnaha, J., et al. (2008). A microsphere-based vaccine prevents and reverses new-onset autoimmune diabetes. *Diabetes*, *57*, 1544–1555.

102. Assady, S., Maor, G., Amit, M., et al. (2001). Insulin production by human embryonic stem cells. *Diabetes*, *50*, 1691–1697.

103. Wu, Y., Persaud, S.J., Jones, P.M. (2011). Stem cells and the endocrine pancreas. *British Medical Bulletin*, *100*, 123–135.

104. Maehr, R., Chen, S., Snitow, M., et al. (2009). Generation of pluripotent stem cells from patients with type 1 diabetes. *Proceedings of the National Academy of Sciences USA*, *106*, 15768–15773.

105. Xie, Q.P., Huang, H., Xu, B., et al. (2009). Human bone marrow mesenchymal stem cells differentiate into insulin-producing cells upon microenvironmental manipulation in vitro. *Differentiation*, *77*, 483–491.

106. Dong, Q.Y., Chen, L., Gao, G.Q., et al. (2008). Allogeneic diabetic mesenchymal stem cells transplantation in streptozotocin-induced diabetic rat. *Clinical & Investigative Medicine*, *31*, E328–337.

107. Madec, A.M., Mallone, R., Afonso, G., et al. (2009). Mesenchymal stem cells protect NOD mice from diabetes by inducing regulatory T cells. *Diabetologia*, *52*, 1391–1399.

108. Hasegawa, Y., Ogihara, T., Yamada, T., et al. (2007). Bone marrow (BM) transplantation promotes beta-cell regeneration after acute injury through BM cell mobilization. *Endocrinology*, *148*, 2006–2015.

109. Freed, C.R., Greene, P.E., Breeze, R.E., et al. (2001). Transplantation of embryonic dopamine neurons for severe Parkinson's disease. *New England Journal of Medicine*, *344*, 710–719.

110. Olanow, C.W., Goetz, C.G., Kordower, J.H., et al. (2003). A double-blind controlled trial of bilateral fetal nigral transplantation in Parkinson's disease. *Annals of Neurology*, *54*, 403–414.

111. Fitzpatrick, K.M., Raschke, J., Emborg, M.E. (2009). Cell-based therapies for Parkinson's disease: Past, present, and future. *Antioxidants & Redox Signaling*, *11*, 2189–2208.

112. Li, J.Y., Christophersen, N.S., Hall, V., et al. (2008). Critical issues of clinical human embryonic stem cell therapy for brain repair. *Trends in Neurosciences*, *31*, 146–153.

113. Hedlund, E., Pruszak, J., Lardaro, T., et al. (2008). Embryonic stem cell-derived Pitx3-enhanced green fluorescent protein midbrain dopamine neurons survive enrichment by fluorescence-activated cell sorting and function in an animal model of Parkinson's disease. *Stem Cells*, *26*, 1526–1536.

114. Dimos, J.T., Rodolfa, K.T., Niakan, K.K., et al. (2008). Induced pluripotent stem cells generated from patients with ALS can be differentiated into motor neurons. *Science*, *321*, 1218–1221.

115. Uchida, N., Buck, D.W., He, D., et al. (2000). Direct isolation of human central nervous system stem cells. *Proceedings of the National Academy of Sciences USA*, *97*, 14720–14725.

116. Redmond, D.E., Jr., Bjugstad, K.B., Teng, Y.D., et al. (2007). Behavioral improvement in a primate Parkinson's model is associated with multiple homeostatic effects of human neural stem cells. *Proceedings of the National Academy of Sciences USA*, *104*, 12175–12180.

117. Lazic, S.E., Barker, R.A. (2005). Cell-based therapies for disorders of the CNS. *Expert Opinion on Therapeutic Patents*, *15*, 1361–1376.

118. Levy, Y.S., Bahat-Stroomza, M., Barzilay, R., et al. (2008). Regenerative effect of neural-induced human mesenchymal stromal cells in rat models of Parkinson's disease. *Cytotherapy*, *10*, 340–352.

119. McCoy, M.K., Martinez, T.N., Ruhn, K.A., et al. (2008). Autologous transplants of adipose-derived adult stromal (ADAS) cells afford dopaminergic neuroprotection in a model of Parkinson's disease. *Experimental Neurology*, *210*, 14–29.

120. Aboody, K., Capela, A., Niazi, N., et al. (2011). Translating stem cell studies to the clinic for CNS repair: Current state of the art and the need for a rosetta stone. *Neuron*, *70*, 597–613.

121. Siliciano, J.D., Kajdas, J., Finzi, D., et al. (2003). Long-term follow-up studies confirm the stability of the latent reservoir for HIV-1 in resting CD4+ T cells. *Nature Medicine*, *9*, 727–728.

122. Baltimore, D. (1988). Gene therapy. Intracellular immunization. *Nature*, *335*, 395–396.

123. Deeks, S.G., McCune, J.M. (2010). Can HIV be cured with stem cell therapy? *Nature Biotechnology*, *28*, 807–810.

124. Moore, J.P., Kitchen, S.G., Pugach, P., et al. (2004). The CCR5 and CXCR4 coreceptors–central to understanding the transmission and pathogenesis of human immunodeficiency virus type 1 infection. *AIDS Research and Human Retroviruses*, *20*, 111–126.

125. Hutter, G., Nowak, D., Mossner, M., et al. (2009). Long-term control of HIV by CCR5 Delta32/Delta32 stem-cell transplantation. *New England Journal of Medicine*, *360*, 692–698.

126. Holt, N., Wang, J., Kim, K., et al. (2010). Human hematopoietic stem/progenitor cells modified by zinc-finger nucleases targeted to CCR5 control HIV-1 in vivo. *Nature Biotechnology*, *28*, 839–847.

127. Kessler, M.W., Ackerman, G., Dines, J.S., et al. (2008). Emerging technologies and fourth generation issues in cartilage repair. *Sports Medicine and Arthroscopy*, *16*, 246–254.

128. Redman, S.N., Oldfield, S.F., Archer, C.W. (2005). Current strategies for articular cartilage repair. *European Cells & Materials*, *9*, 23–32; discussion 23–32.

129. Nakamura, N., Miyama, T., Engebretsen, L., et al. (2009). Cell-based therapy in articular cartilage lesions of the knee. *Arthroscopy*, *25*, 531–552.

130. Matsumoto, T., Okabe, T., Ikawa, T., et al. (2010). Articular cartilage repair with autologous bone marrow mesenchymal cells. *Journal of Cellular Physiology*, *225*, 291–295.

131. Nejadnik, H., Hui, J.H., Feng Choong, E.P., et al. (2010). Autologous bone marrow-derived mesenchymal stem cells

versus autologous chondrocyte implantation: An observational cohort study. *American Journal of Sports Medicine*, *38*, 1110–1116.

132. Yousef, M., Schannwell, C.M., Kostering, M., et al. (2009). The BALANCE Study: Clinical benefit and long-term outcome after intracoronary autologous bone marrow cell transplantation in patients with acute myocardial infarction. *Journal of the American College of Cardiology*, *53*, 2262–2269.
133. Forrester, J.S., Makkar, R.R., Marban, E. (2009). Long-term outcome of stem cell therapy for acute myocardial infarction: Right results, wrong reasons. *Journal of the American College of Cardiology*, *53*, 2270–2272.
134. Menasche, P. (2011). Cardiac cell therapy: Lessons from clinical trials. *Journal of Molecular and Cellular Cardiology*, *50*, 258–265.
135. Couri, C.E., Voltarelli, J.C. (2009). Stem cell therapy for type 1 diabetes mellitus: A review of recent clinical trials. *Diabetology & Metabolic Syndrome*, *1*, 19.
136. Boztug, K., Schmidt, M., Schwarzer, A., et al. (2010). Stem-cell gene therapy for the Wiskott-Aldrich syndrome. *New England Journal of Medicine*, *363*, 1918–1927.
137. Spees, J.L., Gregory, C.A., Singh, H., et al. (2004). Internalized antigens must be removed to prepare hypoimmunogenic mesenchymal stem cells for cell and gene therapy. *Molecular Therapy*, *9*, 747–756.
138. Shin, S., Mitalipova, M., Noggle, S., et al. (2006). Long-term proliferation of human embryonic stem cell-derived neuroepithelial cells using defined adherent culture conditions. *Stem Cells*, *24*, 125–138.
139. Xu, C., Inokuma, M.S., Denham, J., et al. (2001). Feeder-free growth of undifferentiated human embryonic stem cells. *Nature Biotechnology*, *19*, 971–974.
140. Amit, M., Margulets, V., Segev, H., et al. (2003). Human feeder layers for human embryonic stem cells. *Biology of Reproduction*, *68*, 2150–2156.
141. Yu, B.P., Chung, H.Y. (2006). Adaptive mechanisms to oxidative stress during aging. *Mechanisms of Ageing and Development*, *127*, 436–443.
142. Fan, J., Cai, H., Tan, W.S. (2007). Role of the plasma membrane ROS-generating NADPH oxidase in CD34(+) progenitor cells preservation by hypoxia. *Journal of Biotechnology*, *130*, 455–462.
143. Fan, J.L., Cai, H.B., Yang, S., et al. (2008). Comparison between the effects of normoxia and hypoxia on antioxidant enzymes and glutathione redox state in ex vivo culture of CD34(+) cells. *Comparative Biochemistry and Physiology B-Biochemistry & Molecular Biology*, *151*, 153–158.
144. Salim, A., Nacamuli, R.P., Morgan, E.F., et al. (2004). Transient changes in oxygen tension inhibit osteogenic differentiation and Runx2 expression in osteoblasts. *The Journal of Biological Chemistry*, *279*, 40007–40016.
145. Chen, T., Zhou, Y., Tan, W.S. (2009). Influence of lactic acid on the proliferation, metabolism, and differentiation of rabbit mesenchymal stem cells. *Cell Biology and Toxicology*, *25*, 573–586.
146. Chen, T., Zhou, Y., Tan, W.S. (2009). Effects of low temperature and lactate on osteogenic differentiation of human amniotic mesenchymal stem cells. *Biotechnology and Bioprocess Engineering*, *14*, 708–715.
147. Fernandes, A.M., Fernandes, T.G., Diogo, M.M., et al. (2007). Mouse embryonic stem cell expansion in a microcarrier-based stirred culture system. *Journal of Biotechnology*, *132*, 227–236.
148. Abranches, E., Bekman, E., Henrique, D., et al. (2007). Expansion of mouse embryonic stem cells on microcarriers. *Biotechnology and Bioengineering*, *96*, 1211–1221.
149. Sart, S., Schneider, Y.J., Agathos, S.N. (2010). Influence of culture parameters on ear mesenchymal stem cells expanded on microcarriers. *Journal of Biotechnology*, *150*, 149–160.
150. Schop, D., Janssen, F.W., Borgart, E., et al. (2008). Expansion of mesenchymal stem cells using a microcarrier-based cultivation system: Growth and metabolism. *Journal of Tissue Engineering and Regenerative Medicine*, *2*, 126–135.
151. Malda, J., Kreijveld, E., Temenoff, J.S., et al. (2003). Expansion of human nasal chondrocytes on macroporous microcarriers enhances redifferentiation. *Biomaterials*, *24*, 5153–5161.
152. Eibes, G., dos Santos, F., Andrade, P.Z., et al. (2010). Maximizing the ex vivo expansion of human mesenchymal stem cells using a microcarrier-based stirred culture system. *Journal of Biotechnology*, *146*, 194–197.
153. Oh, S.K., Chen, A.K., Mok, Y., et al. (2009). Long-term microcarrier suspension cultures of human embryonic stem cells. *Stem Cell Research*, *2*, 219–230.
154. Alfred, R., Radford, J., Fan, J., et al. (2011). Efficient suspension bioreactor expansion of murine embryonic stem cells on microcarriers in serum-free medium. *Biotechnology Progress*, *27*, 811–823.
155. Brooke, G., Rossetti, T., Pelekanos, R., et al. (2009). Manufacturing of human placenta-derived mesenchymal stem cells for clinical trials. *British Journal of Haematology*, *144*, 571–579.
156. Gastens, M.H., Goltry, K., Prohaska, W., et al. (2007). Good manufacturing practice-compliant expansion of marrow-derived stem and progenitor cells for cell therapy. *Cell Transplantation*, *16*, 685–696.
157. Lu, G., Haider, H.K., Jiang, S., et al. (2009). Sca-1+ stem cell survival and engraftment in the infarcted heart: Dual role for preconditioning-induced connexin-43. *Circulation*, *119*, 2587–2596.
158. Ciavarella, S., Dominici, M., Dammacco, F., et al. (2011). Mesenchymal stem cells: A new promise in anticancer therapy. *Stem Cells and Development*, *20*, 1–10.
159. Gao, J., Dennis, J.E., Muzic, R.F., et al. (2001). The dynamic in vivo distribution of bone marrow-derived mesenchymal stem cells after infusion. *Cells Tissues Organs*, *169*, 12–20.
160. Mangi, A.A., Noiseux, N., Kong, D., et al. (2003). Mesenchymal stem cells modified with Akt prevent remodeling and restore performance of infarcted hearts. *Nature Medicine*, *9*, 1195–1201.

161. Krishna, K.A., Rao, G.V., Rao, K.S. (2007). Stem cell-based therapy for the treatment of Type 1 diabetes mellitus. *Regenerative Medicine*, *2*, 171–177.

162. Martens, T.P., Godier, A.F., Parks, J.J., et al. (2009). Percutaneous cell delivery into the heart using hydrogels polymerizing in situ. *Cell Transplantation*, *18*, 297–304.

163. Mirsky, R., Jahn, S., Koskenvuo, J.W., et al. (2011). Treatment of pulmonary arterial hypertension with circulating angiogenic cells. *American Journal of Physiology - Lung Cellular and Molecular Physiology*, *301*, L12–19.

164. Ormiston, M.L., Deng, Y., Stewart, D.J., et al. (2010). Innate immunity in the therapeutic actions of endothelial progenitor cells in pulmonary hypertension. *American Journal of Respiratory Cell and Molecular Biology*, *43*, 546–554.

165. Zhu, J., Zhou, L., XingWu, F. (2006). Tracking neural stem cells in patients with brain trauma. *New England Journal of Medicine*, *355*, 2376–2378.

166. Sallam, K., Wu, J.C. (2010). Embryonic stem cell biology: Insights from molecular imaging. *Methods in Molecular Biology*, *660*, 185–199.

167. Lee, R.H., Pulin, A.A., Seo, M.J., et al. (2009). Intravenous hMSCs improve myocardial infarction in mice because cells embolized in lung are activated to secrete the anti-inflammatory protein TSG-6. *Cell Stem Cell 5*, 54–63.

168. Schrepfer, S., Deuse, T., Reichenspurner, H., et al. (2007). Stem cell transplantation: The lung barrier. *Transplant Proceedings*, *39*, 573–576.

169. Toma, C., Pittenger, M.F., Cahill, K.S., et al. (2002). Human mesenchymal stem cells differentiate to a cardiomyocyte phenotype in the adult murine heart. *Circulation*, *105*, 93–98.

170. Morigi, M., Imberti, B., Zoja, C., et al. (2004). Mesenchymal stem cells are renotropic, helping to repair the kidney and improve function in acute renal failure. *Journal of the American Society of Nephrology*, *15*, 1794–1804.

171. Noort, W.A., Kruisselbrink, A.B., in't Anker, P.S., et al. (2002). Mesenchymal stem cells promote engraftment of human umbilical cord blood-derived CD34(+) cells in NOD/SCID mice. *Experimental Hematology*, *30*, 870–878.

172. Amariglio, N., Hirshberg, A., Scheithauer, B.W., et al. (2009). Donor-derived brain tumor following neural stem cell transplantation in an ataxia telangiectasia patient. *PLoS Med*, *6*, e1000029.

173. Ben-David, U., Benvenisty, N. (2011). The tumorigenicity of human embryonic and induced pluripotent stem cells. *Nature Reviews Cancer*, *11*, 268–277.

174. Darabi, R., Gehlbach, K., Bachoo, R.M., et al. (2008). Functional skeletal muscle regeneration from differentiating embryonic stem cells. *Nature Medicine*, *14*, 134–143.

175. Ueyama, H., Horibe, T., Hinotsu, S., et al. (2012). Chromosomal variability of human mesenchymal stem cells cultured under hypoxic conditions. *Journal of Cellular and Molecular Medicine*, *16(1)*, 72–82.

176. Baker, D.E., Harrison, N.J., Maltby, E., et al. (2007). Adaptation to culture of human embryonic stem cells and oncogenesis in vivo. *Nature Biotechnology*, *25*, 207–215.

177. Mayshar, Y., Ben-David, U., Lavon, N., et al. (2010). Identification and classification of chromosomal aberrations in human induced pluripotent stem cells. *Cell Stem Cell*, *7*, 521–531.

178. Hanahan, D., Weinberg, R.A. (2011). Hallmarks of cancer: The next generation. *Cell*, *144*, 646–674.

179. Hovatta, O., Jaconi, M., Tohonen, V., et al. (2010). A teratocarcinoma-like human embryonic stem cell (hESC) line and four hESC lines reveal potentially oncogenic genomic changes. *Plos One*, *5*, e10263.

180. Golfinopoulos, V., Pentheroudakis, G., Kamakari, S., et al. (2009). Donor-derived breast cancer in a bone marrow transplantation recipient. *Breast Cancer Research and Treatment*, *113*, 211–213.

181. Glover, D.J., Lipps, H.J., Jans, D.A. (2005). Towards safe, non-viral therapeutic gene expression in humans. *Nature Reviews Genetics*, *6*, 299–U229.

182. Kiuru, M., Boyer, J.L., O'Connor, T.P., et al. (2009). Genetic control of wayward pluripotent stem cells and their progeny after transplantation. *Cell Stem Cell*, *4*, 289–300.

183. Zhao, T., Zhang, Z.N., Rong, Z., et al. (2011). Immunogenicity of induced pluripotent stem cells. *Nature*, *474*, 212–215.

184. Okamura, R.M., Lebkowski, J., Au, M., et al. (2007). Immunological properties of human embryonic stem cell-derived oligodendrocyte progenitor cells. *Journal of Neuroimmunology*, *192*, 134–144.

185. Pepper, M.S. (2010). Cell-based therapy - navigating troubled waters. *South African Medical Journal*, *100*, 286, 288.

186. Halme, D.G., Kessler, D.A. (2006). FDA regulation of stem-cell-based therapies. *New England Journal of Medicine*, *355*, 1730–1735.

187. [Anon]. (2001). Guidance for human somatic cell therapy and gene therapy. *Human Gene Therapy*, *12*, 303–314.

188. Hyun, I., Lindvall, O., Ahrlund-Richter, L., et al. (2008). New ISSCR guidelines underscore major principles for responsible translational stem cell research. *Cell Stem Cell*, *3*, 607–609.

189. McAllister, T.N., Dusserre, N., Maruszewski, M., et al. (2008). Cell-based therapeutics from an economic perspective: Primed for a commercial success or a research sinkhole? *Regenerative Medicine*, *3*, 925–937.

23

BIOMEDICAL APPLICATIONS AND TISSUE ENGINEERING OF COLLAGEN

CHI H. LEE AND YUGYUNG LEE

23.1 CHAPTER OBJECTIVES

- To summarize the types and characteristics as well as the biomedical applications of collagen.
- To review such properties as stability, targetability, intracellular interaction, immune responses, and physiological sensitivity/biocompatibility of collagen.
- To find out the advantages and disadvantages of each collagen-based system.

23.2 INTRODUCTION

Collagen is considered one of the most useful biomaterials. As a result of its excellent biocompatibility and safety, the use of collagen in biomedical application has been rapidly growing and widely expanding to bioengineering areas. Numerous natural polymers and their synthetic analogs are used as biomaterials, but the characteristics of collagen as a biomaterial are distinctively different from those of synthetic polymers mainly in its mode of interaction in the body [1]. Collagen is a good surface-active agent and demonstrates its ability to penetrate a lipid-free interface [2]. Collagen plays an important role in the formation of tissues and organs and is involved in various functional expressions of cells.

The use of collagen as a drug delivery system is very comprehensive and diverse. Collagen can be extracted into an aqueous solution, molded into various forms of delivery systems, and exhibit biodegradability. The main applications of collagen as drug delivery systems are collagen shields in ophthalmology [3], sponges for burns/wounds [4], minipellets and tablets for protein delivery [5], gel formulation in combination with liposomes for sustained drug delivery [2], as controlling material for transdermal delivery [6], and nanoparticles for gene delivery [7].

Collagen has also been used in the tissue engineering field, including for skin replacement and bone substitutes. In addition, its uses as surgical suture [8], hemostatic agents [9, 10], and tissue engineering including basic matrices for cell culture systems [11] and replacement/substitutes for artificial blood vessels and heart valves [12–14] were reported earlier.

The main purpose of this chapter is to review biomedical applications of collagen including the collagen film, which was developed as a prototype matrix system for evaluation of tissue calcification and tumorigenic study via embedding of a single cell suspension. The advantages and disadvantages of each system are also discussed.

23.3 CHARACTERIZATION OF COLLAGEN AS A BIOMATERIAL

a. *The molecular structures of collagen:* Collagen is the primary structural material of vertebrates and is the most abundant mammalian protein accounting for

Advanced Drug Delivery, First Edition. Edited by Ashim K. Mitra, Chi H. Lee, and Kun Cheng.

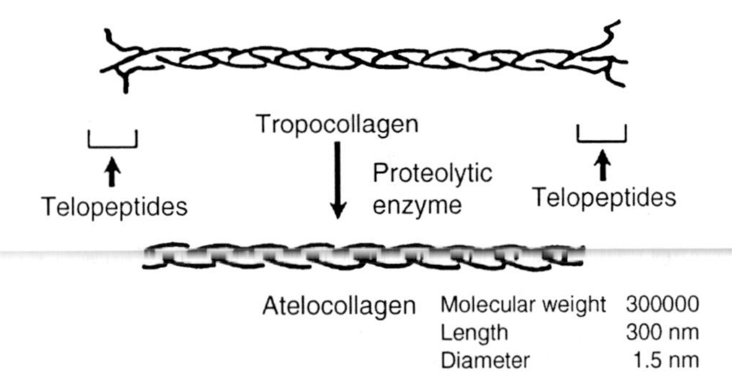

FIGURE 23.1 Schematic of collagen molecule. Reproduced from Ref. 36.

about 25% of total body proteins [15]. It is present in tissues of primarily a mechanical function. About one half of the total body collagen is in the skin and about 70% of the material other than water present in dermis of skin and tendon is collagen. Collagen made its appearance at the early stage of evolution in such primitive animals as jellyfish, coral, and sea anemones [16]. Collagen is synthesized by fibroblasts, which usually originate from pluripotential adventitial cells or reticulum cells.

The molecular structures of collagen established on the evidence from earlier studies are homo- or hetero-trimers, in which three collagen polypeptides, called chains, align in parallel and fold in the opposite directions into a unique triple-helical structure (Figure 23.1) [17–21]. The principal feature that affects a helix formation is the repeating Gly–X–Y amino acid sequence of the chains [22]. The strands are held together primarily by hydrogen bonds between adjacent —CO and —NH groups but also by covalent bonds [23]. The basic collagen molecule is stranded rod-shaped with a length and a width of about 3000 and 15 Å, respectively, and has an approximate molecular weight of 300 kDa [24, 25]. The orderly arrangement of triple helix tropocollagen molecules results in a formation of fibrils having a distinct periodicity. Nonhelical telopeptides are attached to both ends of the molecule and serve as the major source of antigenecity. Atelocollagen, which is produced by elimination of the telopeptide moieties using pepsin, has demonstrated its potential as a drug carrier, especially for gene delivery [26, 27].

To date, 28 vertebrate collagen types, I–XXVIII, encoded by 45 distinct genes have been reported [28]. Collagen XXVIII is the most recently discovered collagen exclusively expressed in the peripheral nervous system [29, 30]. The collagens are divided into two major groups: fibrillar collagens that form characteristic cross-striated fibrils and nonfibrillar collagens that do not form cross-striated fibers. I, II, and III collagen as well as types V and XI are fibril-forming collagens built up of three chains, and all are composed of the continuous triple-helical structure [31]. In type IV collagen (basement membrane), the regions with the triple helix conformation are interrupted with large nonhelical domains as well as with the short nonhelical peptide interruption. Type VI is microfibrilla collagen, and type VII is anchoring fibril collagens [32]. Fibril-associated collagens (Type IX, XI, XII, and XIV) have small chains, which contain some nonhelical domains.

b. *Functional property of collagen as a biomaterial:* The primary reason for the usefulness of collagen in biomedical application is that collagen can form fibers with extra strength and stability through its self-aggregation and cross-linking. It has high tensile strength and high affinity for water. It is easily absorbable in the body, nontoxic, biocompatible, and biodegradable [33, 34]. The major characteristics of collagen exploited for medical applications are summarized in Table 23.1 [4, 33–36].

Collagen is liable to collagenolytic degradation by enzymes, such as collagenase and telopeptide-cleaving enzymes [37]. Collagenase binds tightly to triple helices and degrades collagen starting from the surface. The melting profile of the pepsin-solubilized

TABLE 23.1 Advantages and Disadvantages of Collagen as a Biomaterial

Advantages
Available in abundance and easily purified from living organisms (constitutes more than 30% of vertebrate tissues)
Nonantigenic
Biodegradable and bioreabsorbable
Nontoxic and biocompatible
Synergic with bioactive components
Biological plastic as a result of high *tensile* strength and minimal expressibility
Hemostatic—promotes blood coagulation
Formulated in a number of different forms
Biodegradability can be regulated by crosslinking
Easily modifiable to produce materials as desired by using its functional groups
Compatible with synthetic polymers
Disadvantages
High cost of pine type I collagen
Variability of isolated collagen (e.g., crosslink density, fiber size, trace impurities, etc.)
Hydrophilicity that leads to swelling and more rapid release
Variability in enzymatic degradation rate as compared with hydrolytic degradation
Complex handling properties
Side effects, such as bovine sponge-form encephalopathy (BSF) and mineralization

collagen showed a biphasic transition, indicating that an age-related decrease in thermal stability has implications for the mechanical strength and turnover of the bone collagen [38].

In most drug delivery systems made of collagen, *in vivo* absorption of collagen is controlled by the use of crosslinking agents, such as glutaraldehyde [39], chromium tanning [40], formaldehyde [41], polyepoxy compounds [42], acyl azide [43], carbodiimides [44], and hexamethylenediisocyanate [12]. Physical and dehydrothermal treatments, such as ultraviolet and gamma-ray irradiation, have been efficiently used for introduction of crosslinks to the collagen matrix [23, 45, 46]. The thiolation process of denatured collagen allowed precise amounts of SH groups to be attached onto the protein backbone and produced oxidized and denatured thiolated collagen films that were more resistant and rigid than glutaraldehyde-treated ones under optimized conditions [47].

c. *Advantages and disadvantages of collagen-based systems:* The attractiveness of collagen in drug-incorporated particles lies in its recognition by the body as a natural constituent rather than as a foreign body, causing low immunogenicity and superior biocompatibility as compared with other natural polymers, such as albumin and gelatin [34]. Collagen can be solubilized into an aqueous solution, particularly in acidic aqueous media, engineered to exhibit tailor-made properties and converted into a number of different forms including strips, sheets, sponges, and beads, making it an ideal material for drug delivery.

Some disadvantages of collagen-based systems arose from the difficulty of assuring adequate supplies, their poor mechanical strength, and ineffectiveness in the management of infected sites [33]. There are some limitations of collagen as a drug-incorporated carrier, like the high viscosity of an aqueous phase, nondissolution in neutral pH buffers, thermal instability (denaturation), and biodegradability [48]. These limitations could be overcome by making collagen conjugates with other biomaterials or chemically modifying a collagen monomer without affecting its triple helical conformation and maintaining its native properties.

Improvement of the physical, chemical, and biological properties will be necessary to address some drawbacks in collagen-based applications. Advanced collagen delivery systems with a target release rate can be achieved by adjusting the structure of the collagen matrix or adding other proteins, such as elastin, fibronectin, or glycosaminoglycans [49–51]. A combination of collagen with other polymers, such as liposome [2, 52] and silicone [53], has been proposed to enhance the stability of a system and achieve the controlled release profiles of incorporated compounds.

d. *Adverse reactions to collagen and thrombosis:* Reports of adverse reactions to collagen have been restricted to localized redness and swelling after plastic surgery using collagen implants and wound breakdown with the use of catgut suture material [54]. Clinical reactions to collagen were rare, but two cases of allergic (IgE-mediated) reactions to bovine collagen were reported [55]. Patients in both cases developed conjunctive edema in response to the topical application of highly purified bovine collagen to the eye during ophthalmic surgery. When irritant effects and cytotoxicity of various products developed from collagen were evaluated, a cell response to exogenous collagen started shortly after the product was in contact with tissues, evoking a local and fast inflammatory response [56].

Current limitation in the preparation of collagen-based biomedical formulations and use of collagen as a coating agent for biomedical devices including a cardiovascular stent is thrombosis. Collagen shows hemostatic properties that promote blood coagulation and play an integral role in tissue generation and the repair process. Collagen sponge or gel initiates adhesion and aggregation of platelets that lead to a thrombus formation [45]. Monomeric collagen does not activate platelet aggregation, while polymeric collagen having a regular arrangement of the molecules with a length of around 1 μm does activate it, as arginine side chains of collagen are responsible for its interaction with platelets [57].

In vivo mouse models previously indicated that the intrinsic coagulation pathway, initiated by factor XII, contributes to thrombus formation in response to major vascular damage. On collagen type I, both the activation of blood coagulation proteins and the presence of other factors contribute significantly to the platelet–platelet interactions necessary for thrombus formation [58]. A recent study pointed to a dual role of collagen in thrombus formation: stimulation of glycoprotein VI signaling to form procoagulant platelets; and activation of factor XII to stimulate thrombin generation and potentiate the formation of platelet-fibrin thrombi [59].

Genetic factors that affect the interaction of platelets with collagens could represent risk factors for either thrombosis or excessive hemorrhage. The platelet levels of integrin alpha(2)beta(1), one of the major platelet collagen receptors, vary up to 10-fold in normal healthy individuals and the higher level phenotype is associated with allele 1 (807 T) of the integrin alpha(2) gene [60]. It was also found that there is roughly a 5-fold range in platelet glycoprotein VI content among normal individuals, which may also influence the risk for thromboembolism, suggesting that the level or function of platelet collagen receptors needs to be considered genetic risk factors for thrombotic onset.

Collagen-induced thrombosis can be overcome in several ways. Among them, modification of composition and purity of commercial type I as well as better standardization of the collagen coating method could be the primary strategies [61]. Other approaches include the addition of a variety of antithrombotic drugs in collagen-based systems, such as antiplatelet, anticoagulant, and thrombolytic agents [62]. Even though adverse effects including thrombosis may be discovered in the future application of collagen for gene delivery or tissue engineering, because collagen can help to avoid side effects originated from incorporated drugs or proteins, the continuous effort in development and evaluation of collagen-based systems seems to be worthwhile.

23.4 COLLAGEN-BASED DRUG DELIVERY SYSTEMS

23.4.1 Film/Sheet/Disc

Collagen film/sheet/disc has been used for the treatment of tissue infection, such as infected corneal tissue or liver cancer. The main application of collagen films is as a barrier membrane. Films with the thickness of 0.01–0.5 mm and made of biodegradable materials, such as prepared from telopeptide-free reconstituted collagen, demonstrated a slow release profile of incorporated drugs [63]. The drugs can be loaded into collagen membranes by hydrogen bonding, covalent bonding, or simple entrapment. They can be sterilized and become pliable upon hydrolyzation, while retaining adequate strength to resist manipulation.

A soluble ophthalmic insert in the form of a wafer or a film was introduced as a drug delivery system for the treatment of infected corneal tissue using a high dose of antibiotic agents, such as gentamicin [64] and tetracycline [65]. When collagen film was applied to the eye, it was completely hydrolyzed after 5–6 h [64], adding to evidence that collagen-based systems are suitable for resembling current liquid and ointment vehicles. Tetracycline released from the collagen film was detected in the plasma for more than 7 days after implantation into rabbits, and the duration of therapeutic effect was significantly lengthened [66]. The microfibrous collagen sheets developed as a local delivery carrier for ectopocide (VP-16), an anticancer agent, displayed a relatively long maintenance of drug concentrations at the target site, which in this case is the liver [67].

Some modifications on collagen film/sheet/disc have been made with a combination of crosslinkers or attaching another membrane to control the release rate of incorporated drugs. Collagen films crosslinked with chromium tanning, formaldehyde, or a combination of both have been successfully used as an implantable delivery system in achieving the sustained release of medroxyprogesterone acetate [40]. A transdermal delivery of nifedipine, from the collagen-based film, was controlled by an attached chitosan membrane, accomplishing the greatly enhanced therapeutic efficacy in the treatment of tissue infection [6].

The development of mesoporous hybrid collagen offers new possibilities for incorporating biological agents into silica structures and for controlling the release kinetics from the matrix as a result of its well-arranged pore architecture [68]. Significant differences were observed between the release patterns from the different materials (i.e., silica structures with or without collagen) and the release rate of atenolol as a model drug was influenced by the presence of collagen in the hybrid mesopores.

Although collagen films seem to offer adequate cell survival, the concerns about the long-term biocompatibility of nondegradable materials are also present. In animal models, a long-term expression of a foreign gene after implantation of transfected cells has not been successful [69]. A combination of collagen and other polymers, such as an atelocollagen matrix added onto the surface of polyurethane films, enhanced attachment and proliferation of fibroblasts and supported growth of cells [70]. Transplantation of cells embedded in a lattice of poly-tetrafluoroethylene fibers coated with rat collagen followed by a mixing with matrigel as well as a basic fibroblast growth factor revealed that a long-term expression of human β-glucuronidase by retroviral-transduced murine or canine fibroblasts was attainable through a collagen matrix approach [71–73]. Therefore, it is essential that collagen-based film/disc systems should be combined with extra matrices that could improve conditions for a long-term cell survival and therapeutic efficacy.

23.4.2 Collagen Shields

As the collagen shield was originally proposed for bandage contact lenses, collagen shields belong to the class of soluble ophthalmic inserts [74]. The idea of using a shield or hydrogel lens gradually dissolved in the cornea as a delivery device has led to the development of various drug delivery systems for ophthalmic applications.

Collagen shields are currently manufactured from porcine scleral tissue or bovine corium (dermis) collagen and contain mainly type I collagen and some type III collagen that closely resemble collagen molecules of the human eye [75]. Once in the eye, shields are hydrated by tear fluids and then soften and form a clear, pliable, thin film approximately 0.1 mm in thickness with a diameter of 14.5 mm and a base curve of 9 mm. Drug delivery by collagen shields depends on the loading conditions of medication including the solubility in the shield [76]. The collagen matrix acts as a reservoir and drugs are entrapped in the interstices of the collagen matrix in a solution for water-soluble drugs or incorporated into the shield for water-insoluble drugs. As tears flush through the shield and the shield dissolves, it provides a layer of biologically compatible collagen solution that seems to lubricate the surface of the eye, minimize rubbing of the lids on the cornea, increase the contact time between the drug and the cornea, and foster epithelial healing [3, 52]. A bolus release of drug from the lenses greatly contributed to the enhanced drug activity [77, 78]. This system allows for the higher corneal concentrations of drug and for sustained drug delivery into the cornea and the aqueous humor, conforming to the corneal surface up to 12, 24, or 72 h [79].

As shown in Table 23.2, collagen shields were used for the treatment of various local infections. The collagen shields supplemented by frequent topical applications of antibiotics has been clinically useful for preoperative and postoperative antibiotic prophylaxis, the initial treatment of bacterial keratitis, and the treatment of corneal abrasions [84, 105]. Several studies showed that shields provided equal or enhanced drug delivery of fluorescein [102], prednisolone acetate [85, 86], cyclosporine [102], and ofloxacin [99] to the anterior segment. The pharmacokinetic studies demonstrated that the collagen shield can achieve higher aqueous concentrations of topically administered moxifloxacin (0.5%) than other formulations [106] and can promote epithelial healing after corneal transplantation and radial keratomy [77, 84, 87, 107–109]. The mechanical properties of the shield proved to be effective in protecting the healing corneal epithelium from the blinking action of the eyelids [110], validating its usefulness as a potential sustained ocular delivery system [76, 111, 112].

Modifications of collagen were made to facilitate the application, to meet the highest compliance, to reduce blurring of vision, and to enhance the drug concentration and bioavailability of drugs in the cornea and aqueous humor [113]. The crosslinked collagen using glutaraldehyde or chromium tanning can serve as a drug reservoir and provide more desirable drug delivery than non-crosslinked collagen shields by increasing the contact time between the drug and the cornea. Collasomes, in the form of collagen pieces, were developed by adding long hydrocarbon side chains to the collagen [3]. Collasomes increase not only the hydrophobicity of the collagen but also the total surface area, resulting in a decrease in the diffusion rate of hydrophilic drug molecules from the collagen matrix. Collasomes can be formulated with various constituents and chemically

TABLE 23.2 Application of Collagen Shields for Various Topical Agents

Drugs Agent	References
Antibiotics	
Gentamicin	Bloomfield et al., 1978; Baziuk et al., 1992; Liang et al., 1992; Milani et al., 1993 [64, 80–82]
Vancomycin	Phinney et al., 1988 [83]
Tobramycin	O'Brien et al., 1988; Poland and Kaufman, 1988; Unnternan et al., 1988; Aquavella et al., 1988; Hobden et al., 1988; Sawusch et al., 1988a,b; Assil et al., 1992; Willoughby et al., 2002; Eshar et al., 2011 [84–92]
Netilimycin	Dorigo et al., 1995 [93]
Polymyxin B sulfate	Palmer and McDonald, 1995 [94]
Trimethoprim	Palmer and McDonald, 1995 [94]
AmphotericinB	Schwartz et al., 1990; Mendiute et al., 1995 [95, 96]
Trifluorothymidine	Gussler et al., 1990 [97]
Acyclovir	Willey et al., 1991 [98]
Ofloxacin	Taravella et al., 1999 [99]
Steroids	Aquavella et al., 1988; Sawusch et al., 1988a,b; Hwang et al., 1989; Milan et al., 1993; Palmer and McDonald, 1995 [82, 85, 86, 89, 94, 98]
Cholinergic	
Pilocarpine	Aquavella et al., 1988 [89]
Antineoplastic	
5-Fluoruuracil	Finkelstein et al., 1991 [100]
Anticoagulant	
Heparin	Murray et al., 1990 [101]
Immunodepressant	
Cyclosporin	Chen et al., 1990; Reidy et al., 1990; Sato et al., 1996; Gebhardt and Kaufman, 1995 [67, 102, 103, 104]
Gene therapy	
Plasmid DNA	Angella et al., 2000 [159]

alternated with the addition of lipid (called lacrisomes) for the delivery of water-soluble drugs like fluorescein in the treatment of dry eyes [3].

Collagen shields as a drug carrier for topical agents have numerous advantages. One of the merits of the collagen-based drug delivery systems is the ease with which the formulation can be applied to the ocular surface and their potential for clinical efficacy [105, 114]. The delivery of drugs through the impregnated collagen shield was faster, more complete, and more reliable than frequent application of other conventional treatments, such as drops, ointment, or daily subconjunctive injection [105, 109]. There was less stromal edema at the wound sites in collagen-treated corneas. The collagen shield protected keratocytes adjacent to the wound sites and diminished the inflammatory reaction of keratocyte. Moreover, the surface epithelial bonding seemed to be normal with the use of the collagen shield. A recent study shows that simple apatite coating of a collagen scaffold results in a BMP-2 carrier that renders long-term release of BMP-2 and dramatically enhances osteogenic efficacy [100].

The application of collagen shields for drug delivery is limited by several disadvantages, such as reducing visual activity, causing slight discomfort and a short duration at the inserted site [33]. Some side effects of collagen shields were also reported. Shields were implanted into rabbit and guinea pig eyes, and a potential toxic response was tested to determine whether collagen shields produce histological evidence of inflammation when implanted subconjunctively [115]. The inflammatory response in rabbits was noticeable after a 7-day implantation and was much severe than in guinea pigs, indicating that the inflammatory response in rabbits to collagen shields and their usefulness as a drug delivery system for antifibroblast drugs are species specific.

23.4.3 Collagen Sponges

Human collagen membrane has been a major resource of a collagen sponge used as a biological dressing since the 1930s [4]. Collagen sponges have the ability to absorb easily large quantities of tissue exudate and smooth adherence to the wet wound bed with preservation of a low, moist climate as well as its shielding against mechanical harm and secondary bacterial infection [116]. Collagen sponges have been useful in the treatment of severe burns and as a dressing for various types of wounds, such as pressure sores, donor sites, leg ulcers, and decubitus ulcers as well as for *in vitro* test systems [117]. Experiments using sponge implantation demonstrated a rapid recovery of skin from burn wounds by an intense infiltration of neutrophils into the sponge [118]. Coating of a collagen sponge with growth factor further facilitates dermal and epidermal wound healing [119, 120]. The sponges made from pure collagen isolated from bovine skin were swollen at pH 3.0 and were stabilized into the physical form of a sponge layer.

Collagen sponges were found suitable for short-term delivery (3–7 days) of antibiotics, such as gentamicin [121], attaining a high concentration of gentamicin at the septic focus in the abdomen and reducing local infection, while attaining a low concentration in serum without producing any systemic effects [122, 123]. Collagen sponges containing antibiotics did not show any side effects, and the collagen was reabsorbed after a few days [124].

Collagen sponges were also used for delivery of steroids through topical applications, such as intravaginal delivery of lipophilic compounds including retinoic acid [125, 126]. A collagen-based sponge was inserted into a cervical cap made of hydrogel hypan, which in contact with wet tissue surfaces adheres to them by the force of differential osmotic pressure [127]. This novel system produced high local concentrations of drugs without producing any systemic symptoms, and thus, it has been very useful for local drug delivery.

For highly resilient activity and fluid-building capacity, collagen sponges have been combined with other materials like elastin, fibronectin, or glycosaminoglycan [49–51]. The starting material can be crosslinked with glutaraldehyde and subsequently graft-co-polymerized with other polymers, such as polyhydroxyethyl methacrylate (PHEMA) [128]. The grafted PHEMA chains, which are hydrophilic, keep the membranes wet and increase their tensile strength, further affecting the efficiency in the management of infected wounds and burns. The physiological loading of fibroblasts in three-dimensional collagen lattices elicited complex and substantial changes in protease activities, suggesting the importance of matrix compliance to mechanical responses [129].

A collagen sponge as a drug carrier or a vaginal contraceptive barrier showed numerous advantages over the rubber diaphragm, such as achieving the controlled release of spermicidal agents and reducing the tissue-irritation activity. The main drawbacks of sponges seem to be the difficulty of assuring adequate supplies and their preservation. Other problems arose from their poor mechanical strength and ineffectiveness in the management of infected wounds and burns.

23.4.4 Gels/Hydrogels

Hydrogels made of collagen have been widely used as a drug carrier as a result of its ease in manufacturing and self-application. The production of a large and steady surface area is one of the major merits of collagen-based hydrogels to be suited for clinical and fundamental applications. The light scattering properties of 3D collagen hydrogels formed at two initial collagen concentrations and under several incubation temperatures were evaluated using imaging techniques and turbidity assessments [130]. The 3D collagen hydrogels could not display a unified relationship between second harmonic generation (SHG) signal directionality and fibril morphology and/or sizes, but microstructural details obtained by the multiphoton microscopy (MPM) images revealed that the dependence of SHG signals on the number of interfaces created upon assembly of 3D collagen hydrogels was accounted for the strength of the detected backscattered signals.

One well-documented application of collagen is collagen-based gel as the controlled delivery system for injectable aqueous formulations. An injectable gel formulation based on a mixture of collagen and epinephrine was developed for delivery of 5-FU in cancer therapy [131]. The disappearance of 5-FU via diffusion after intratumoral injection in mice was sustained, and its therapeutic effects were significantly improved. The subcutaneous injection of soluble collagen was efficient in the repair of dermatological defects, such as vocal fold immobility [132] and urinary incontinence [133].

Hydrogel formulations made of various combinations of natural and synthetic polymers provided advanced mechanical stability and biological acceptability stemmed from synergistic properties of both materials. Hydrogels made of a combination of collagen and polyhydroxyethyl methacrylate (PHEMA) were found stable and resilient and did not show any adverse effects or calcification after 6 months of subcutaneous implantation in rats. This system was found be very efficient in delivery of anticancer drugs including 5-FU [134].

Hybrid co-polymers of collagen with polyethylene glycol-6000 and polyvinyl pyrrolidone were prepared for the controlled delivery of contraceptive steroids [135]. Two synthetic polymers, poly(vinyl alcohol) (PVA) and poly(acrylic acid) (PAA), were blended with two biological polymers, collagen and hyaluronic acid (HA), to enhance the mechanical strength of natural polymers and to overcome the biological drawbacks of synthetic polymers. The blend of collagen-PVA hydrogel was applied to the delivery of a growth hormone (GH) [136], which was released in a controlled manner and whose release rate and quantity were dependent on the collagen content in the system.

23.4.5 A Coupling of Liposomes to Hydrogels

Liposomes are spherical lipid bilayers of phospholipids, which may form spontaneously in aqueous media [137]. The size (i.e., from 50 nm to 1000 nm in diameter) and the shape of the liposomes can be modified by altering the mixture of phospholipids, the degree of saturation of the fatty acid side chains, and the formation conditions. Liposomes are widely used as a drug carrier as a result of their biodegradability and removable versatility in terms of composition and size. The aqueous drug can be loaded into the aqueous core region, whereas hydrophobic drug can be loaded into liposomes for drug delivery.

To achieve both formulation stability and controlled release rates of entrapped materials from collagen-based hydrogels, a system consisted of liposome and collagen was introduced [21]. It was found that a coupling of liposomes to the gel-matrices enhanced the stability of the system as a result of the antioxidant effect of collagen molecules under an immobilized status [138–140]. Crosslinking the functional liposomes to a collagen gel matrix further sustained the release rate of the entrapped marker [4], thus, significantly manipulating the release rates of loaded drugs from the gel-matrix.

The formulation, in which liposome is sequestered in collagen gel, seems to have several advantages over other liposome formulations or gel formulations. This technology seems to have a potential applied for topical treatment of surgical or nonsurgical wounds and burns. As the release kinetics of hydrophilic and lipophilic substances encapsulated in liposome were similar to those of a nonencapsulated drug, the combination of liposomes with collagen seems very useful for drugs that do not penetrate the ocular surface as well as systems in need of prolonged corneal contact time [141], yielding significantly higher levels of immunosuppressive agent cyclosporin A to the cornea, anterior sclera, aqueous humor and vitreous in rabbit eyes than collagen shields without liposomes [142].

An inclusion of antimicrobials or cell growth agents, such as insulin and growth hormone, within the liposomes could facilitate enhanced cell growth and prevention of infection, while a base collagen provided a substrate for cell attachment and proliferation [138]. Moreover, as coated vesicles were more stable than control liposomes, the permeation rates of incorporated drugs from small unilamellar liposomes coated by collagen into systemic circulation were much greater [2]. Blood elimination and liver uptake of collagen-containing vesicles were about 2-fold faster and 1.5–2-fold higher than those of control liposomes, respectively. Liposome encapsulated formulations did not show any toxicity associated with liposome itself.

23.4.6 Pellet/Tablet

Minipellets made of collagen have been used for the delivery of various protein drugs [34, 36, 143–145]. A rod with a diameter and a length of 1 mm and 1 cm, respectively, is a useful shape as a drug delivery device because this rod (minipellet) is small enough to be injected into the subcutaneous space through a syringe needle and still spacious enough to contain large-molecular-weight protein drugs, such as interferon [45] and interleukin-2 [145]. A single subcutaneous injection of a minipellet produced a prolonged retention of interleukin-2 and decreased its maximal concentration in the serum. This pellet-type carrier was efficient for site-specific delivery of minocycline and lysozyme for the treatment of periodontitis symptoms.

A pellet type controlled-release delivery vehicle made of purified type I collagen for water-soluble osteogenic proteins induced cartilage and bone with a success rate of 76% [5], proving the feasibility of collagen-based pellets for soluble bioactive factors. Micropellet-containing ibuprofen was prepared with gelatin whose hydrolysis rate in the gastrointestinal tract depends on the degree of hardening by a crosslinking agent [146]. It was also shown that the physical properties of the pellets and the drug release rates from them were closely correlated with the amount of drug entrapped in the pellets as well as the degree of crosslinking of the gelatin.

Drugs are released from minipellets by means of drug dissolution and diffusion within the carrier. The affinity of drugs for collagen and the amounts of the drug included are the major determining factors for defining the release profiles of drugs from the minipellet. In some cases, it is difficult to control adequately the release rate of loaded drugs from a minipellet prepared by conventional methods as a result of initial burst release. A new double-layer minipellet, in which the lateral side of a conventional single-layer minipellet was coated with high-density collagen, was designed to overcome this problem, effectively inhibiting the initial burst of bovine serum albumin compared with the single-layer minipellet [147]. Moreover, the addition of additives such as chondroitin sulfate permitted the control of the release rate and achieved sustained-release of loaded drugs through double layers.

A collagen minipellet was also used as a vaccine delivery system and sometimes superior to biodegradable polymer microspheres that occasionally showed the risk of antigen degradation [148, 149]. A collagen minipellet as an antigen delivery vehicle was able to induce immune responses equivalent to or greater than those induced by conventional immunization with antigen in alum adjuvant [149]. A collagen minpellet for tetanus and diphtheria toxoid elicited higher antibody responses than those obtained with individual antigens or antigens adsorbed to alum and maintained the enhanced antibody levels over 48 weeks [148]. The minipellet did not induce any adverse reaction and was completely degraded after implantation in sheep for 35 days.

23.4.7 Nanoparticles/Microparticles

A property, in which the crystallites in the gel aggregates appear as multiple chain segments in the collagen-fold configuration, has been used to prepare colloidal drug delivery carriers [150]. The biodegradable collagen-based nanoparticles or nanospheres are thermally stable, readily achieving their sterilization [151]. The molecular weight profile in collagen solution was affected by pH and temperature, both of which further influenced the noncovalent interactions responsible for the molecular structure of collagen [152]. The molecular weight of collagen or gelatin has an enormous impact on the stability of the manufactured gelatin nanoparticles [153]. As a result of its small size, a large surface area, high adsorptive capacity, and ability to disperse in water to form a clear colloidal solution, collagen-based nanoparticles have demonstrated their potential to be used as a sustained-release formulation for antimicrobial agents or steroids [154].

Nanoparticles or microspheres were used as a parenteral carrier for cancer and cytoxic agents, such as campthocin [155], hydrocortisone [156], and methotrexate [157]. The gelatin microspheres showed zero-order kinetics in the release profiles of incorporated drugs, accomplishing prolonged action against rat fibrosarcoma and improved antitumor activity. Delivery of hydrocortisone, a lipophilic steroid, was not affected by the pH of the receptor medium or its binding affinity to the particles. Collagen-based nanoparticles were also used to enhance dermal delivery of retinol [151], which was very stable in the system and achieved a faster and higher transportation through the skin than the freshly precipitated retinol.

Nanoparticles can be taken up by the reticuloendothelial system [158] and enable an enhanced uptake of exogenous compounds, such as anti-HIV drugs, into a number of cells, especially macrophages [159], which serves as an additional advantage of collagen-based nanoparticles in systemic drug delivery. Attachment of collagen to silica nanoparticles by a disulfide linker, followed by the introduction of lactobionic acid (LA, a cell-specific targeting moiety), results in forming a redox-responsive system that was used for cell-specific intracellular drug delivery and efficient endocytosis [160]. The controlled release of a model drug (fluorescein isothiocyanate, FITC) was attained through cleavage of the disulfide bonds from the system.

23.5 COLLAGEN-BASED SYSTEMS FOR GENE DELIVERY

As DNA molecules are large and hydrophilic, they do not have the ability to permeate through the lipid barriers. As the delivery of the gene to cytoplasm is the first step, the DNA molecules should find their way to the nucleus. The use of biomaterials for gene delivery can potentially avoid the safety concerns involved with viral gene delivery [161]. A major concern in gene delivery strategies through bioiomaterial-based carriers is that the interior and exterior composition of polymeric gene delivery nanoparticles are often coupled with a single polymer backbone governing all functions from biophysical properties of the polymer/DNA particle to DNA condensation and release. Although cationic lipophilic compounds like liposome molecules facilitate DNA penetration into the cells, they may also prevent DNA from being transferred into the nucleus. Moreover, the efficacy of polymeric gene delivery methods is low, especially *in vivo*.

Collagen has broad application as a promising carrier for gene delivery, being capable of delivering large quantities of DNA in a direct, site-specific manner. Collagen contains reactive sites amenable for ligand conjugation, crosslinking, and other modifications that can offer the polymer tailored for a range of clinical applications. Modified collagen, such as atelocollagen, which is obtained after removal of telopeptides, has been investigated for a wide range of drug and gene delivery methods [162]. Gelatin, the industrial product of a denatured and partly amorphous form of collagen, has also been a viable gene delivery vehicle [163, 164].

It was found that formulations based on or modified by collagen were excellent candidates in achieving sustained release with site-adherent characteristics and that collagen-modified formulations were able to remain at the target sites even after reaching the equilibrium. This finding is vital, as collagen-based formulations could offer enhanced gene delivery at the targeted drug delivery site.

23.5.1 Collagen Film/Matrix

A collagen film and matrix were used as a gene delivery carrier for promoting bone formation. A composite of recombinant human bone morphogenetic protein 2 (rhBMP-2) and collagen was developed to monitor bone development and absorbent change of carrier collagen [165, 166]. The onlay implant of the mixture of rhBMP-2 and collagen resulted in active bone formation, whereas the collagen alone resulted in no bone formation. Collagen provides an anchorage for cell differentiation and remains an artificial matrix in woven bone. In a similar study, a collagen matrix loaded with BMP was placed in close contact with osteogenic cells, displaying direct osteoinduction without causing a cartilage formation [167]. These results indicated that a collagen-based film or matrix system is efficient as a biological onlay implant for gene delivery.

A collagen film and disc have numerous advantages as gene delivery systems. Systems that isolate transplanted cells from the host immune system were beneficial and economically attractive because they allowed for the utility of allogenic or even xenogenic cells in numerous patients [168–171]. The use of genetically modified cells for a long-term delivery of a therapeutic transgene product has been an attractive option for the treatment of monogenetic hereditary as well as various multifactorial nongenetic diseases [172–174]. Biodegradable collagen films or matrices have also served as a scaffold for a survival of transfected fibroblasts [175].

The feasibility of immobilizing plasmid DNA incorporated into the collagen matrix through a covalently coupled anti-DNA antibody was evaluated to achieve long-lasting and site-specific DNA delivery [176]. In cell line studies, the significant amount of green fluorescent protein (GFP)-transduced cells were detected only on the matrix loaded surface. Moreover, the overall GFP transduction efficiency in treated rabbit coronary arteries increased, validating that an anti-DNA, antibody-modified collagen-based matrix was effective as a plasmid gene delivery system. This technique thus represents an efficient and highly localized gene delivery system both *in vitro* and *in vivo*.

23.5.2 Collagen Shield

A collagen shield was further applied to the gene delivery area. Delivery of plasmid DNA into the bleb through a collagen shield enhanced chloramphenicol acetyltransferase, the reporter gene, 30-fold over injection of plasmid DNA through saline vehicle [177]. Gene therapy using naked plasmid DNA loaded in a simple collagen shield delivery was very efficient in regulating wound healing after glaucoma surgery.

23.5.3 Collagen Sponges

Like a collagen film, collagen sponges were also used as a gene delivery carrier for osteoinduction. An absorbable collagen sponge containing bacterially expressed bone morphogenetic protein 2 (rhBMP-2) was osteogenic *in vivo*, promoting bone healing in the rat model [178]. An absorbable collagen sponge containing bone morphogenetic protein 2 (rhBMP-2) stabilized endosseous dental implants in bony areas and restored normal bone formation without complication [179].

It was reported that lipoplex- and polyplex-loaded collagen sponges developed as co-polymer-protected gene vectors for therapeutic assistance of wound healing or tissue engineering were superior to naked DNA-loaded sponges in mediating sustained gene delivery *in vitro* and local transfection *in vivo* [180]. Protective co-polymers were particularly advantageous in promoting the tranfection capacity of polyplex-loaded sponges upon subcutaneous implantation, probably resulting from their stabilizing and opsonization-inhibiting properties.

23.5.4 Hydrogels

As a result of their low antigenecity, the bovine and equine collagen gel matrices were used as a gene-transfect base and well tolerated in clinical applications. Human tracheal epithelial cells grown on plastic, a condition that downregulated the expression of the receptor, failed to express the reporter gene, whereas cells from the same trachea preserved on collagen gels were transfected [181]. G-CSF transfected clonal murine fibroblast lines can survive with grafts and continue to synthesize the transgene as well as collagen *in vivo* [175].

Gels made of atelocollagen have been used as a carrier for chondrocytes to repair cartilage defects [182, 183].

Chondrocytes embedded in the atelocollagen gel gradually proliferated and maintained the chondrocyte phenotype. The grafted type I atelocollagen provided a favorable matrix for cell migration in relation to collagenase expression and modulated cell behavior [184].

23.5.5 Pellet

A collagen minipellet was studied as a delivery carrier mainly for bioactive proteins and gene vectors. Collagen with positive electric charge nucleic acid electrostatically formed a DNA/collagen complex [185]. When plasmid DNA encoded with green fluorescent protein was introduced into 293 cells, the efficiency of green florescent protein expression in the cell was dependent on the shape or size of the complex, and the efficiency of the gene expression was higher with a smaller complex. In addition, it was observed that plasmid DNA was released from minipellets in various forms of the DNA/collagen complex. The cell recognizes and effectively takes up certain shapes of complexes, indicating that collagen plays not only an integral role as a carrier in protection from degradation and performing sustained release of plasmid DNA, but also as a positive transporter of plasmid DNA into cells.

The solid nature of atelocollagen, a biocompatible polymer, *in vivo* seems to have a great potential for site- or tissue-specific transportation of target genes. A minipellet based on atelocollagen and in the form of a cylindrical shape (0.6 mm in diameter and 10 mm in length) containing 50 μg of plasmid DNA and human HST-1/FGF-4 cDNA allowed for a sustained release and expression of plasmid DNA in normal adult animals [27]. The controlled gene transfer using an atelocollagen-based pellet allowed for a prolonged systemic circulation of target products and facilitated a long-term use of naked plasmid vectors for somatic gene therapy [27]. An atecollagen-based minipellet accelerated the mRNA expression and facial nerve regeneration in the rat model, ultimately achieving facial nerve transaction and immediate repair [26].

The ultrastructural study on the mechanism involved with the bone morphogenetic protein (BMP)–collagen complex proved that direct bone formation was ectopically induced by BMPs without cartilage formation when an atelocollagen type I collagen pellet was used as a carrier [167]. Complexation of pDNA and atelocollagen in an implanted pellet produced physiologically significant levels of gene-encoding proteins in the local site and systemic circulation of animals, resulting in prolonged biological effects [162]. The applicability of atelocollage-based pellet systems can be further extended for the augmentation of the bioavailability of small-molecular-weight materials, such as antisense oligonucleotides and biologically active oligopeptides, or virus vectors.

The controlled release of rhBMP-2 (recombinant human BMP) from a collagen minipellet in cylindrical solid preparation was controlled by additives added into the system [186, 187]. Changing the preforming concentration of collagen before extrusion or the density of collagen with the use of additives may affect the permeability of protein drugs through the collagen membrane. The use of glutamic acid as an additive allows the rhBMP-2 release profiles from minipellets to be controlled and managed to the targeting amount around the implanted site, influencing the regulation of the rhBMP-2 concentration and bone formation rate.

23.5.6 Particles

Nanosphere formation is driven by a combination of electrostatic and electropic forces with sodium sulfate employed as a dissolving reagent to facilitate greater charge–charge interactions between plasmid DNA and collagen [158]. The relationship between electropic forces and gene factors was evaluated for the optimal gene delivery system. Polyion complexation between basic fibroblast growth factor and gelatin was studied by the turbidity change of a mixed solution and isoelectric electrophoresis [188]. It was found that an electrostatic interaction was the main driving force for the complexation between acidic gelatin and basic fibroblast growth factor.

The transfection levels achieved between native collagen and complexed methylated collagen for luciferase encoding plasmid were compared in both *in vitro* and *in vivo* studies [189]. As native collagen/DNA particles significantly aggregated and became destabilized at neutral pH, methylated collagen/DNA particles were more condensed and exhibited a higher charge density at pH 7.4 than native collagen/DNA particles at pH 3.

23.5.7 Scaffold

The use of a type II collagen-glycosaminoglycan (CG) scaffold was tested as a nonviral gene delivery vehicle. This scaffold was intended to produce an elevated, prolonged, and local expression of insulin-like growth factor (IGF)-1 for enhancement of cartilage regeneration in adult articular chondrocytes [190]. The sustained level of IGF-1 overexpression resulted in significantly higher amounts of tissue formation, chondrocyte-like cells, GAG accumulation, and type II collagen production, as compared with control scaffolds, validating that CG scaffolds can serve as nonviral gene delivery vehicles of microgram levels of IGF-1 plasmid.

23.5.8 A Coupling of Liposomes to Collagen

Liposome-collagen systems seemed to be an excellent candidate for gene therapy. In a research study, the efficient transfer of lac*Z* gene through both plasmid/liposome complexes and adenoviruses in both collagen sheet and collagen wrap were observed [191]. It was found that delivering the gene by collagen wrap as well as collagen sheet were effective in achieving proper gene therapy. Another finding in this research was that the gene transfer vector in the collagen collar reached the targeted tissue more effectively than the one in the collagen wrap, suggesting an efficient means of peri-adventitial gene therapy through liposome–collagen systems.

23.6 COLLAGEN-BASED SYSTEMS FOR TISSUE ENGINEERING

Tissue engineering is the use of a combination of cells, engineering and materials methods, and suitable biochemical and physiochemical factors to improve or replace biological functions. The term is closely associated with applications that repair or replace portions of or whole tissues (i.e., bone, cartilage, blood vessels, bladder, and skin).

Animal-derived recombinant collagens, especially type I, are considered one of the most useful biomaterials available in the market. They are now widely used in the tissue engineering field either in their native fibrillar forms or in various fabricated forms after denaturation, such as sponges, sheets, plugs, and pellets [192, 193]. Animal-derived collagen could provide insight into biomaterial–cellular interactions in such areas as scaffold fabrication, scaffold/cell composite construction, surgical operation and sampling, and development of histological and biological assays on the neotissues (Figure 23.2) [194].

23.6.1 Collagen as Skin Replacement and Skin Wounds

23.6.1.1 Collagen-Based Implants A method for generating a cellular layer of intestinal collagen from the porcine submucosa without compromising the native collagen structure facilitated the use of collagen in tissue engineering [195]. Collagen-based implants have been used as vehicles for transportation of cultured skin cells or drug carriers [1, 118, 196–198]. Cultured skin substitutes developed on collagen lattice like reconstituted type I collagen were used for skin replacement and skin wounds as a result of their mechanical strength and biocompatibility [4].

As implantable sponges were very efficient in recovering skin defects, various types of artificial skin have been developed in the form of a sponge. Collagen-based sponges as a substrate for human corneal cells exhibited a normal cell phenotype when individually cultured on the engineered collagen sponge matrix [199]. A type I collagen-based sponge was also used to engineer patellar tendons in rabbits under various culture conditions [200].

An allogenic cultured dermal substitute prepared by plating fibroblasts on to a collagen sponge matrix and subsequently freeze dried from a 1% aqueous solution of atelocollagen provided a good environment for epithelialization [201]. Chronic wounds resulting from diabetes have been successfully cured with allogenic cultured skin substitutes prepared from cryopreserved skin cells in which the contracted collagen lattice was used as a support for epithelial growth and differentiation to replace pathological skin [118, 202]. The addition of selected antimicrobial drugs

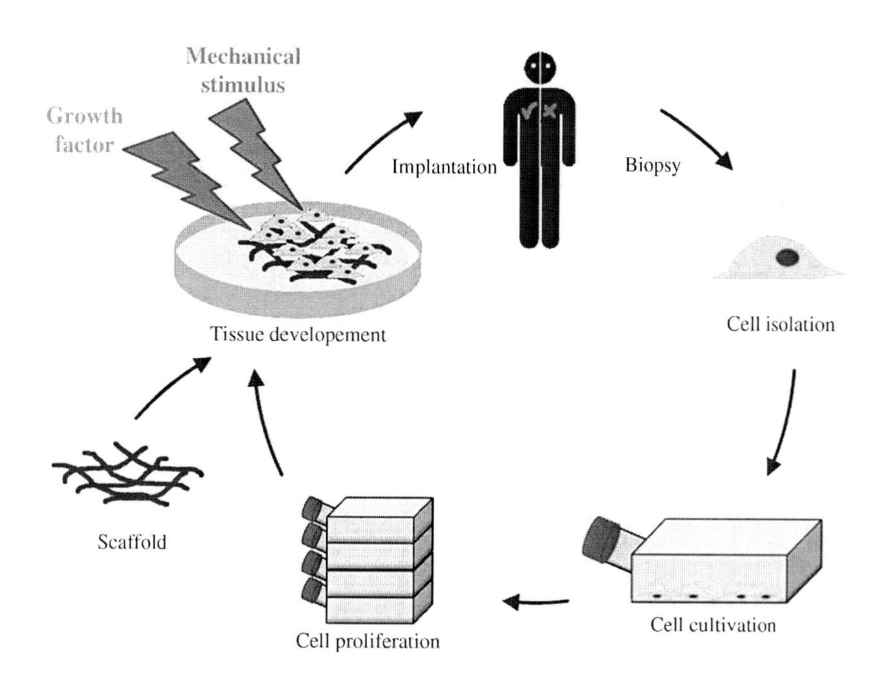

FIGURE 23.2 Tissue engineering in biomedical applications (cited from Wikipedia). (See color figure in color plate section.)

like amikacin to the bovine skin implantable collagen managed to control microbial contamination and increased therapeutic efficacy in the treatment of skin wounds [203].

23.6.1.2 The Mixture of Collagen and Other Physiological Substrates To address some limitations inherent to cultured skin substitutes, such as deficient barrier function *in vitro* and delayed keratinization after grafting in comparison with native skin autografts, several modification strategies of collagen-based systems including the combination of collagen with other proteins, such as gelatin, glycosaminoglycan, fibrin, and biotin, were proposed [204].

The modified sponge for artificial skin was developed by combining fibrillar collagen with gelatin [205]. Dehydrothermal crosslinks were used to stabilize collagen-based sponge physically and metabolically. Sponges made of gelatin by itself in a resorbable gel-foam were also used as a carrier matrix for human mesenchymal stem cells in cartilage regeneration therapy [206]. When this gelatin sponge was implanted in an osteochondral defect in the rabbit femoral condyle, gel-foam cylinders were observed to be biocompatible with no evidence of immune response or lymphatic infiltration at the site.

In the case of collagen and fibrin combination, cultured cells were best grafted directly onto the wound bed or in combination with either a thin layer of collagen or fibrin but not both [207]. It was demonstrated that the engineered neotissue based on the mixture of collagen sponge and bone-marrow-derived mesenchymal stem cells displayed enhanced collagen type I and type III expression and achieved about three fourths of the mechanical properties of normal tissue [208, 209].

The role of glycosaminoglycan and difference in its concentrations between pathological and normal tissues were reported earlier [210]. Dermal skin substitutes (membranes) made of collagen and glycosaminoglycan were found to be suitable substrates for the culture of human epidermal keratinocytes [118], reducing the rate of biodegradation and the engraftment of skin substitutes [118, 211]. Restoration of functional epidermis by cultured skin substitutes based on collagen was stimulated by incubation under reduced humidity *in vitro* [204].

Sponges in a combination of silicone and collagen were also used to address the limitations inherent to cultured skin substitutes. Acellular bilayer artificial skin composed of an outer silicone layer and an inner collagen sponge was used for a thin skin graft with split thickness, displaying superior performance in the long-term postoperative recovery of the skin graft site [53].

Biotinylation of bovine skin collagen by covalent addition of biotin has been used to attach peptide growth factors with avidin as a bridge. This technique retained the activity of peptide growth factors and demonstrated an enormous potential to be used as a modulator of the response in wound treatment [212, 213].

23.6.2 Collagen as Bone Substitutes

Among numerous tissues in the human body, bone has been considered a powerful marker for regeneration and its formation serves as a prototype model for tissue engineering based on morphogenesis. Collagen has been used as implantable carriers for bone inducing proteins, such as bone morphogenetic protein 2 (rhBMP-2) [214]. To date, collagen itself was used as bone substitutes owing to its osteoinductive activity [165]. The uses of collagen film as a gene delivery carrier for osteoinduction and collagen sponge for bone-related protein carriers were described earlier.

Type I collagen crosslinked N-telopeptide was used as a marker of bone resorption and clinically used as a marker of bone metastasis of prostate cancer and breast cancer [215, 216]. The polymorphisms of collagen type I alpha1 and vitamin D receptor were used as genetic markers for osteoporotic fracture in women [217], indicating that interlocus interaction is an integral component of osteoporotic fracture risks.

Collagen in a combination with other polymers or chemicals was also used for orthopedic defects and as a bone substitute [218]. Self-assembly of mineralized collagen composites was used as a bone graft material for the treatment of acquired and congenital orthopedic defects either by itself or in a combination with hydroxyapatite [219]. The result of this study proved that grafted demineralized bone collagen in a combination with hydroxyapatite was an excellent osteoinductive material. It was also demonstrated that the addition of 500 IU of retinoic acid to collagen at a site of a bone defect enhanced regeneration of new bone, achieving union across the defect and its complete repair [220].

23.6.3 Collagen as Bioengineered Tissues

The generation of 3D collagen scaffolds that closely mimic the structure of physiological tissue required for normal cell function has been a major challenge in the bioengineering field. Autologous tissue engineering provides an alternative for allogenic tissue transplantation. Bovine collagen type I has been evaluated as 3D scaffolds for reestablishing the collagen fibrillar structure of the skin, and some of them were already commercialized (i.e., Apligraf from Organogenesis, Inc., Canton, MA, and OrCel from Ortec Inc., Easley, SC). Corneal stroma reconstruction necessitated the creation of a stroma-like scaffold consisting of a stack of orthogonally disposed lamellae sheets of aligned collagen fibrils that were built up transforming magnetic alignment of neutralized acid-soluble type I collagen into gel through a series of gelation-rotation-gelation cycles in a horizontal magnetic field [221].

A highly porous scaffold based on a layer-by-layer collagen scaffold coated with an alginate polymer showed improved mechanical properties and controllable drug release without loss of the original biological function of the collagen scaffold [222]. In particular, the scaffold (75 vol % alginate in a collagen scaffold with a porosity of 88%) attained a Young's modulus of 30 MPa, which is approximately 9 times the value for the pure collagen scaffold (porosity – 98%). Although the scaffolds are highly porous, the drug release and initial burst were well controlled with an appropriate volume fraction of alginate. Osteoblast-like cells (MG63) readily proliferated and migrated into the interior of the scaffolds, and calcium and phosphate on the cell surfaces were well formed, similarly on pure collagen and alginate/collagen scaffolds, within only 7 days of culture. The alginate/collagen scaffolds with a drug delivery function seem to have huge potential as biomedical scaffolds for clinical use in soft and hard tissue regeneration.

Natural collagenous materials were used for surgical and abdominal wall repair as a result of their inherent low antigenecity and ability to integrate with surrounding tissues [223]. Moreover, new generations of collagen-based biological tissue are practical and reproducible resulting from the versatile properties of collagen including simple membranous configuration, relative uniformity, and abundant availability [224]. One biomedical device was surgical adhesive made of porcine collagen and polyglutamic acid, which was used for sealing air leaking from the lung that takes a relatively long period for recovery [225]. The absorption rate of collagen-based adhesive was dependent on collagen concentrations in the system.

Collagen gel or matrix as human skin substitutes have demonstrated its usefulness in tissue engineering and have led to the development of bioengineered tissues, such as blood vessels, heart valves, and ligaments [13]. A provisional extracellular support was provided from type I collagen lattice to organize the cells into a three-dimensional structure *in vitro* [11]. A small-diameter (4 mm) graft constructed from type I bovine collagen was earlier used to integrate into the host tissue and provided a scaffold for remodeling into a functional blood vessel [14]. Three-dimensional collagen scaffolds are biodegradable *in vivo*, have a large surface area for cell attachment, supported the vascularization processes, and can be used as artificial blood vessels, heart valves, or cell transplant devices [226, 227]. The use of collagen as a coated material for permeation filters made of culture endothelial cell monolayers demonstrated its effectiveness in evaluating *in vitro* vascular permeability of a drug to contrast media [228].

23.6.4 Collagen Constructs and Synthetic Collagenous Peptide Polymers

Recent progress in tissue engineering and advanced technology has led to well-characterized and reproducible collagen constructs from natural collagenous materials [229]. Biological tissue grafts in the form of a collagen-based matrix have been derived from the bladder, ureter, or small intestine [230, 231]. These collagen constructs were similar to synthetic polymer prostheses in retaining persistence. The structure-mechanical behavior relationship of biomaterials acquired from intestine submucosa displayed mechanical anisotropy and stiffer direction preferred in biomaterials [232]. The approach with a phenomenological constitutive model revealed that glycan increased the tensile stiffness and ultimate tensile strength of collagen-based matrix, further potentiating their resistance to collagen degradation [233].

Artificial collagen-like material is another important approach for collagen tissue engineering. Even though the biomaterial usage of collagen in engineering tendon and skin can be highly feasible, the use of animal-derived collagens in human sometimes caused allergic reactions and pathogen transmission. Moreover, the use of recombinant collagens may suffer from less biologic activities than native tissue as a result of a lack of undergoing significant posttranslational modifications [234].

Synthetic peptide units spontaneously polymerize in aqueous solutions through a native chemical ligation process [235]. Poly(Xaa-Yaa-Gly)$_n$ are collagenous peptide polymers with a molecular weight of about 1000 kDa [236]. The triple-helical polymers can form a nanofiber-like structure with a length in micrometers. The presence of Cys residues on the polymers also enables further crosslinking with and modification by functional moieties, producing varying structures with a limited chain length.

A novel peptide system based on self-complementary trimers of Pro-Hyp-Gly repeats was developed as collagen-like triple-helical supra-molecules through the spontaneous self-assembly process [237]. Peptide strands are tethered together by two disulphide bridges in a staggered arrangement in the trimer, which allowed for the intermolecular folding to form elongated triple-helical supra-molecules [238].

For the new form of collagen, two thirds of the protein's regular amino acids were substituted with less-flexible versions that stiffened the overall structure of the protein and helped it hold its form [239]. The breakthrough of this approach was the use of rigid analogs that have shapes similar to those the natural amino acids take in the folded, functional form of the protein. The obtained collagen holds together at temperatures far above what it takes for natural collagen to fall apart, and its three-dimensional structure is indistinguishable from that of natural collagen.

23.6.5 Computational Model for Collagen in Tissue Engineering

Tissue engineering uses the principles of biology and engineering to investigate the fundamental question of how amino acid sequences of peptides change to functional tertiary or quaternary structures and subsequently to develop biological substitutes that restore or maintain tissue function [240, 241]. Various computational models and image analysis techniques have been designed to elucidate the structural functionality of collagen and its relationship with host cell/organs or candidate compounds. The concepts of high binding affinity and specificity play a critical role in targeting delivery of drugs. By understanding the nature of collagen as drug delivery carriers and their durability in the body, the essential parameters for designing effective ligands, which interact with the systems, can be identified. It will further provide a new guide for tissue growth and organization and lead to bioactive signals for tissue-specific gene expression.

An investigation on the native collagen has led to an establishment of a structure function relationship between loaded drugs and collagen. A 3D model of fibril-forming human type II collagen was developed as synthetic collagen tissues to study the structural and functional aspects of collagen [242]. This system also allowed for the studies of the stereochemistry of all the side chain groups and specific atomic interactions as well as for further evaluation of its therapeutic effects on collagen-related diseases.

A mathematical modeling was designed for elastic scattering and light propagation approaches for three-dimensional collagen gel constructs, which can be used to obtain the scattering coefficient, the index of refraction, and the distribution of the collagen fibrils in a gel [243]. As a gel is composed of fibrils with different diameters, it was feasible to compute a best-fitting simulated spectrum as a weighted sum of the spectra corresponding to several fibril diameters, obtaining the percentages of fibrils of each diameter in the gel.

The computational model of type I collagen fibrils of the extracellular matrix (ECM) was generated to predict the structure and physical chemistry of the elements that make up the ECM [244]. It was primarily intended that, given the unit structure of the collagen molecules, the alignment of the ECM can be theoretically calculated to achieve the energy-minimum configuration among molecules. In the modeling process, a type I collagen-like triple helix backbone was computationally constructed and boundary spheres were added based on the known chemical and physical properties of the amino acid sequences. By resolving the energy-minimum state, large complex components of the extracellular space as well as other structures can be determined to provide three-dimensional structure of molecules, molecular interactions, and the tissues that they form. Along with basic knowledge of the principles of the structure of the collagen-based extracellular matrix (ECM) acquired from X-ray crystallography and nuclear magnetic resonance (NMR) spectroscopy, three-dimensional models of the ECM can define the mechanical properties of fibers and thereby characterize the functionality of the structure as a whole.

Recently, the profound understanding of the molecular structure of collagen through the computational models has led to the development of biological substitutes that improve collagen functionality in tissue. Previous studies of the structure of collagen had focused only on crystals of small fragments of the protein, so there was no information available on how it looked within intact tissue. Diffraction studies on intact collagen fibrils inside the tendons of rat tails was performed using a BioCAT beamline provided by the Advanced Photon Source (APS) to understand how the protein functioned within unbroken tissue and to transform a very basic understanding of molecular structure of tissue into a much more tangible form [245]. As the tendon tissue was kept intact, it was feasible to see how the collagen molecule binds to collagenases, a class of enzymes that when working properly help to regulate the normal growth and development of animals but when malfunctioning can lead to the metastasis of cancerous tumors or rheumatoid arthritis. The visualization of this interaction could help pharmaceutical scientists to create an inhibitor to prevent the pathological action of the enzyme.

The amount and status of collagen was used for pathological scoring of disease stage without measuring the amount of biomarker endogens. Collagen, the major component of fibrous tissue, was quantified as histopathological scoring of the fibrosis stage by computer-assisted digital image analysis (DIA). The collagen proportionate area (CPA) expressed for liver collagen showed a better histological correlationship with a hepatic venous pressure gradient (HVPG) [246]. The CPA at 1-year biopsy after liver transplantation was highly predictive of clinical outcome in patients infected with hepatitis C virus who underwent transplantation and better than HVPG [247].

23.7 COLLAGEN FILM AS A CALCIFIABLE MATRIX SYSTEM: AN EXAMPLE OF THE FORMULATION DEVELOPMENT

One of the major problems with implanted biomaterial applications is calcification, which is influenced by the structure of the implantable system and decides its *in vivo* therapeutic efficiency and clinical fate [248]. In bioprosthetic heart valves (BHVs), the aortic wall and leaflet have mainly served as calcifiable matrices. Recently, the calcification of the bioprosthetic aortic wall has been intensively studied as a result of a growing use of the stentless BHV [249]. The stentless BHV has a relatively large segment of exposed aortic wall compared with the stent valve, in which virtually no aortic wall is exposed outside the stent. Thus, bioprosthetic aortic wall calcification has a potential to cause the clinical failure of the stentless BHV.

Calcification of tissues or systems depends on chemical factors that operate at the cellular level around various tissues or biomaterials [250]. Both collagen and elastin are major components of connective tissues, which possess a structure that compromises collagen fibers intimately associated with a remarkably stable elastin network. The aortic wall in BHV is composed of 90% collagen and 10% elastin, while the leaflet is mainly composed of collagen (99%). As a result of their differences in composition, the calcification rates of the aortic wall and leaflet and their response to anticalcification agents are different. For example, ethanol pretreatment completely inhibited calcification of the porcine leaflet, while only partially (about 50%) inhibited calcification of the porcine aortic wall [251], indicating that elastin is more susceptible to tissue calcification than collagen. This finding has led to the investigation of the effects of elastin concentration on the calcification rate of implantable biomaterials.

The matrix films, which are composed of various combinations of collagen and elastin, have been developed to simulate the calcification process of implantable biomaterials and serve as a controlled delivery device for cardiovascular drugs [252, 253]. The suitability of collagen and elastin in numerous potential medical applications in reconstructive and plastic surgery including controlled delivery of bone morphogenetic protein was previously reported [214, 254]. Biomaterials should also possess mechanical properties capable of withstanding the forces and motions experienced by the normal tissues and have sufficient fatigue strength to ensure a long life of the implant *in vivo* [255]. Tensile strength can be used for evaluation of mechanical strength, resilient activity, endurance, and biocompatibility of the systems.

Collagen film has a size of 6 × 10 mm and a thickness of 1 mm. Its tensile strength was determined using the following equation:

$$\text{Tensile strength } (\sigma) = \frac{\text{Force or load } (F)}{\text{MA}}$$

where F is the maximum load (in Newtons) and MA is the minimum cross-sectional area of the film specimen (in square meters) [256]. A Chatillon DFM-10 Gauge equipped with LTC Manual Test Stand and GF-1 Grips (Ametek Test & Calibration Instruments Division, Largo, FL) was used. The tensile strength was almost constant irrespective of a loading ratio of collagen and elastin and within a durable range as shown in Table 23.3. There was no sign of swelling of the system, which is a sensitive marker of collagen deterioration [257]. This matrix system was endurable after subcutaneous implantation in the rat for up to three weeks and exhibited no side effect or infection. As the concentration of elastin in a system increased from 10% to 90%, the total amount of accumulated calcium upon implantation in the rat subcutaneous model also increased (Figure 23.3), indicating that elastin has a more intimate role in tissue calcification than collagen. Therefore, this system can be used as a calcifiable matrix simulating the calcification process of implantable tissues, such as BHV, as well as a drug carrier for local and systemic delivery of various anticalcification agents, cardiovascular drugs, and antibiotics in the treatment of heart diseases.

TABLE 23.3 The Tensile Strength of the Collagen Elastin Matrix (CEM) Containing Various Combinations of Collagen and Elastin [235]

CEM Composition (Collagen:Elastin)	Tensile Strength (MPa ± S.D.)
90:10	2.9 ± 0.2
50:50	3.0 ± 0.3
20:80	3.1 ± 0.4

The collagen-based matrix can also be used as a lattice for tissue culture systems, which provides the substrate for the embedding of a single cell suspension or a small tumor specimen. Three-dimensional aggregates can be kept viable and proliferating for weeks, yielding higher degrees of resemblance compared with the *in vivo* tumors from which they were derived [200, 258–260]. The matrix remained stable in shape and size during the cell culture process. The

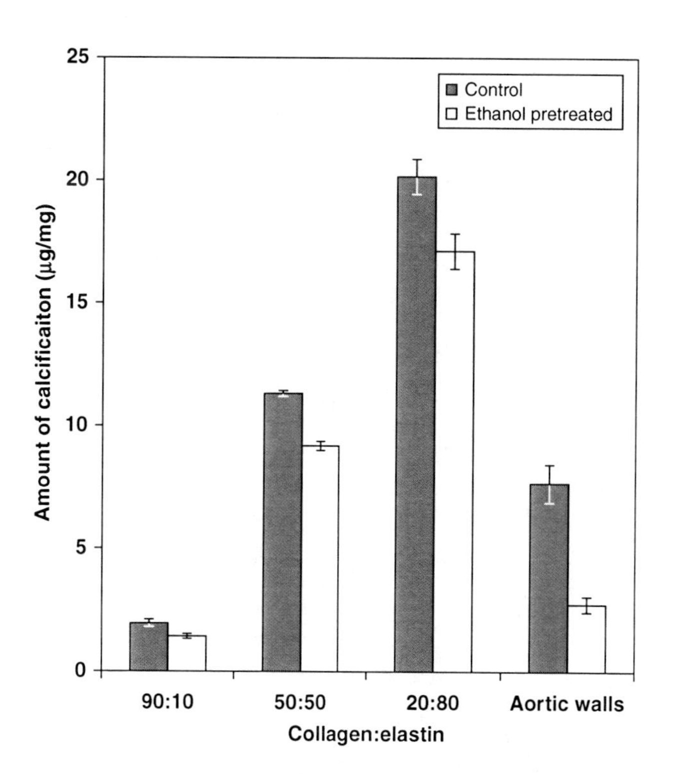

FIGURE 23.3 The effect of elastin and ethanol (80%) pretreatment on the calcification rate of CEM and porcine aortic walls implanted in the rat subcutaneous model for 7 days ($N = 6$) [235].

three-dimensional model showed more resistance to anticancer drugs than cells growing as monolayers, serving as an advanced model for the characterization of the biological and biochemical aspects of human solid tumors. Collagen-based matrix cultures could offer an efficient tool for the study of the mechanisms behind human tumor progress.

23.8 CONCLUSION

Collagen has various advantages as a biomaterial and is widely used as a carrier system for delivery of drugs, proteins, and genes. The examples described in this chapter represent selected applications of collagen in the biomedical field. The successful demonstration of usefulness of human skin substitutes made of collagen has led to the development of bioengineering tissues, such as blood vessels and ligaments. The investigation on native collagen for drug delivery systems and tissue engineering may lead to a better understanding of pathological diseases. Collagen-based biomaterials are expected to become a useful matrix substance for various biomedical applications in the future.

ASSESMENT QUESTIONS

23.1. What are the major properties of collagen as a biomaterial?

23.2. What are the advantages and disadvantages of collagen-based biomaterials or systems?

23.3. Define or briefly describe the following terms: Tropocollagen and Collasomes.

23.4. What is the major drawback in biomedical application of collagen?

23.5. For blood-contacting implants, there should be instances when thrombus formation is desirable and when it is detrimental. Please give an example of each, and explain your reasoning.

REFERENCES

1. McPherson, J.M., Sawamura, S., Amstrong, R. (1986). An examination of the biologic response to injectable, glutaraldehyde cross-linked collagen implants. *Journal of Biomedical Materials Research*, *20*, 93–107.
2. Fonseca, M.J., Alsina, M.A., Reig, F. (1999). Coating liposomes with collagen (Mr 50 000) increases uptake into liver. *Biochimica et Biophysica Acta*, *1279*(2), 259–265.
3. Kaufman, H.E., et al. (1994). Collagen-based drug delivery and artificial tears. *Journal of Ocular Pharmacology*, *10*, 17–27.
4. Rao, K.P. (1995). Recent developments of collagen-based materials for medical applications and drug delivery systems. *Journal of Biomaterials Science*, *7*(*7*), 623–645.
5. Lucas, P.A., et al. (1989). Ectopic induction of cartilage and bone by water soluble proteins from bovine bone using a collagenous delivery vehicle. *Journal of Biomedical Materials Research*, *23*, 23–39.
6. Thacharodi, D., Rao, K.P. (1996). Rate-controlling biopolymer membranes as transdermal delivery systems for nifedipine: Development and in vitro evaluations. *Biomaterials*, *17*, 1307–1311.
7. Rossler, B., Kreuter, J., Scherer, D. (1995). Collagen microparticles: Preparation and properties. *Journal of Microencapsulation*, *12*, 49–57.
8. Miller, J.M., Zoll, D.R., Brown, E.O. (1964). Clinical observation on use of an extrude collagen suture. *Archives of Surgery*, *88*, 167–174.
9. Cameron, W.J. (1978). A new topical hemostatic agent in gynecological surgery. *Obstetrics & Gynecology*, *51*, 118–122.
10. Browder, I.W., Litwin, M.S. (1986). Use of absorbable collagen for hemostasis in general surgical patients. *The American Surgeon*, *52*, 492–494.
11. Kemp, P.D. Tissue engineering and cell populated collagen matrices, in C. Streuli and M. Grant (eds.), *Methods in Molecular Biology*, Springer, New York, NY, 2000, pp. 287–293.
12. Chvapil, M., et al. (1993). Collagen fibers as a temporary scaffold for replacement of ACL in goats. *Journal of Biomedical Materials Research*, *27*(*3*), 313–325.
13. Auger, F.A., et al. (1998). Tissue-engineered human skin substitutes developed from collagen populated hydrated gels: Clinical and fundamental applications. *Medical & Biological Engineering & Computing*, *36*, 801–812.
14. Huynh, T., et al. (1999). Remodeling of an acellular collagen graft into a physiologically responsive neovessel. *Nature Biotechnology*, *17*, 1083–1086.
15. Harkness, R.D. (1961). Biological functions of collagen. *Biological Reviews*, *36*, 399–463.
16. Bergeon, M.T. (1967). Collagen: A review. *Journal - Oklahoma State Medical Association*, *60*(*6*), 330–332.
17. Gross, J. *Comparative Biochemistry 5*, Academic Press, New York, NY, 1963, pp. 307–345.
18. Ramachandran, G.N., Sasisekharan, V. (1965). Refinement of the structure of collagen. *Biochimica et Biophysica Acta*, *109* (*27*), *1*, 314–316.
19. Burge, R.E. The structure and function of connective and skeletal tissue, in *Proceedings of NATO Advanced Study Group*, Butterworth, St. Andrews, 1964, pp. 2–7.
20. Miyata, T., Taira, T., Noishiki, Y. (1992). Collagen engineering for biomaterial use. *Clinical Materials*, *9*(*3–4*), 139–148.
21. Rao, K.P., Alamelu, S. (1992). Effect of crosslinking agent on the release of an aqueous marker from liposomes sequestered in collagen and chitosan gels. *Journal of Membrane Science*, *71*, 161.

22. Piez, K.A. (1984). Molecular and aggregate structures of the collagens, in K.A. Piez and A.H. Reddi (eds.), *Extracellular Matrix Biochemistry*, Elsevier, New York, NY, pp. 1–40.
23. Harkness, R.D. (1966). Collagen. *Science Progress Oxford*, *54*, 257–274.
24. Traub, W., Piez, K.A. The chemistry and structure of collagen, in C.B. Anfinsen, J.T. Edsalla and F.M. Richards (eds.), *Advances in Protein Chemistry*, Academic Press, New York, NY, 1971, p. 245.
25. Nimni, M.E., Harkness, R.D. Molecular structures and functions of collagen, in Nimni ME (ed.), *Collagen-Biochemistry I*, CRC Press, Boca Raton, FL, 1988, pp. 1–79.
26. Kohmura, E., et al. (1999). BNDF atelocollagen mini-pellet accelerates facial nerve regeneration. *Brain Research*, *849*, 235–238.
27. Ochiya, T., et al. (1999). New Delivery system for plasmid DNA in vivo using atelocollagen as a carrier material: The Minipellet. *Nature Medicine*, *5(6)*, 707–710.
28. Chu, Mon Li. Structural proteins: Genes for collagen, in *eLS*, Wiley, Chichester, U.K., 2011.
29. Veit, G., et al. (2006). Collagen XXVIII, a novel von Willebrand factor A domain-containing protein with many imperfections in the collagenous domain. *Journal of Biological Chemistry*, *281*, 3494–3504.
30. Grimal, S., et al. (2010). Collagen XXVIII is a distinctive component of the peripheral nervous system nodes of ranvier and surrounds nonmyelinating glial cells. *Glia*, *58(16)*, 1977–1987.
31. Timpl, R. Immunology of the collagens, in K.A. Piez and A. H. Reddi (eds.), *Extracellular Matrix Biochemistry*, Elsevier, New York, NY, 1984, pp. 159–190.
32. Samuel, C.S., Coghlan, J.P., Bateman, J.F. (1998). Effects of relaxin, pregnancy and parturition on collagen metabolism in the rat public symphysis. *Journal of Endocrinology*, *159*, 117–125.
33. Friess, W. (1998). Collagen-biomaterial for drug delivery. *European Journal of Pharmaceutics and Biopharmaceutics*, *45*, 113–136.
34. Maeda, M., et al. (1999). Microstructure and release characteristics of the minipellet, a collagen based drug delivery system for controlled release of protein drugs. *Journal of Controlled Release*, *62*, 313–324.
35. Jerome, A., Ramshaw, J.A. (1992). Editorial: Collagen-based. *Biomaterials*, *9*, 137–138.
36. Fujioka, K., Maeda M., Hojo T., Sato, A. (1998). Protein release from collagen matrices. *Advanced Drug Delivery Reviews*, *31(3)*, 247–266.
37. Woolley, D.E. (1984). Mammalian collagenases, in K.A. Piez and A.H. Reddi (eds.), *Extracellular matrix Biochemistry*, Elsevier, New York, NY, pp. 119–158.
38. Danielsen, C.C. (1990). Age-related thermal stability and susceptibility to proteolysis of rat bone collagen. *Biochemical Journal*, *272*, 697–701.
39. Barbani, N., et al. (1995). Bioartificial materials based on collagen: 1. Collagen cross-linking with gaseous glutaraldehyde. *Journal of Biomaterials Science*, *7*, 461–469.
40. Bradley, W.G., Wilkes, G.L. (1977). Some mechanical property considerations of reconstituted collagen for drug release supports. *Biomaterials, Medical Devices & Artificial Organs*, *5*, 159–175.
41. Ruderman, R.J., et al. (1973). Prolonged resorption of collagen sponges: Vapor-phase treatment with formaldehyde. *Journal of Biomedical Materials Research*, *7*, 263–265.
42. Tu, R., et al. (1993). Kinetic study of collagen fixation with polyepoxy fixatives. *Journal of Biomedical Materials Research*, *27*, 3–9.
43. Petite, H., et al. (1990). Use of the acyl azide method for crosslinking collagen rich tissues such as pericardium. *Journal of Biomedical Materials Research*, *24*, 179–187.
44. Nimni, M.E., et al. Bioprosthesis derived from crosslinked and chemically modified collagenous tissue, in Nimni ME, (ed.), *Collagen Biotechnology III*, CRC Press, Boca Raton, FL, 1988, pp. 1–38.
45. Miyata, T., et al. (1971). Effects of ultraviolet irradiation on native and telopeptide-poor collagen. *Biochimica et Biophysica Acta*, *229*, 672–680.
46. Gorham, S.D., et al. (1992). Effect of chemical modifications on the susceptibility of collagen to proteolysis. II. Dehydrothermal crosslinking. *International Journal of Biological Macromolecules*, *14*, 129–138.
47. Nicholas, F.L., Gagnieu, C.H. (1997). Denatured thiolated collagen. II. Crosslinking by oxidation. *Biomaterials*, *18*, 815–821.
48. Sehgal, P.K., Srinivasan, A. (2006). Collagen-coated microparticles in drug delivery. *Journal of Non-Crystalline Solids*, *352(32–35)*, 15.
49. Doillon, C.J., Silver, F.H. (1986). Collagen- based wound dressing effects of hyaluronic acid and fibronectin on wound healing. *Biomaterials*, *7*, 3–8.
50. Lefebvre, F., et al. (1992). New artificial connective matrix-like structure made of elastin solubilized peptides and collagens: Elaboration, biochemical and structural properties. *Biomaterials*, *13*, 28–33.
51. Lefebvre, F., et al. (1996). New preparation and microstructure of the EndoPatch elastin–collagen containing glycosaminoglycans. *Biomaterials*, *17*, 1813–1818.
52. Kaufman, H.E. (1988). Collagen shield symposium. *Journal of Cataract & Refractive Surgery*, *14(5)*, 487–488.
53. Suzuki, S., et al. (2000). Long-term follow-up study of artificial dermis composed of outer silicone layer and inner collagen sponge. *British Journal of Plastic Surgery*, *53(8)*, 659–666.
54. Webster, R.C., Kattner, M.D., Smith, R.C. (1984). Injectable collagen for augmentation of facial areas. *Archives of Otolaryngology*, *110*, 652–656.
55. Mullins, R.J., Richards, C., Walker, T., (1996). Allergic reactions to oral, surgical and topical bovine collagen.

Anaphylactic risk for surgeons. *Australian and New Zealand Journal of Ophthalmology*, *24(3)*, 257–260.

56. Trasciatti, S., et al. (1998). In vitro effects of different formulations of bovine collagen on cultured human skin. *Biomaterials*, *19*, 897–903.
57. Wang, C.L., et al. (1978). Collagen-induced platelet aggregation and release. *Biochimica et Biophysica Acta*, *544*, 555–567.
58. Badimon, L., et al. (1988). Platelet thrombus formation on collagen type I. A model of deep vessel injury. Influence of blood rheology, von Willebrand factor, and blood coagulation. *Circulation*, *78(6)*, 1431–1442.
59. Van der Meijden, P.E.J., et al. (2009). Dual role of collagen in factor XII–dependent thrombus formation. *Blood*, *114(4)*, 881–890.
60. Furihata, K., Nugent, D.J., Kunicki, T.J. (2002). Influence of platelet collagen receptor polymorphisms on risk for arterial thrombosis. *Archives of Pathology & Laboratory Medicine*, *126(3)*, 305–309.
61. Heemsker, J.W.M., et al. (2011). Collagen surfaces to measure thrombus formation under flow: Possibilities for standardization. *Journal of Thrombosis and Haemostasis*, *9(4)*, 856–858.
62. Collins, B., Hollidge, C. (2003). Antithrombotic drug market, *Nature Reviews Drug Discovery*, *2*, 11–12.
63. Rubin, A.L., et al. (1973). Collagen as a vehicle for drug delivery. *Journal of Clinical Pharmacology*, 309–312.
64. Bloomfield, S.E., et al. (1978). Soluble gentamycin ophthalmic inserts as a drug delivery system. *Archives of Ophthalmology*, *96*, 885–887.
65. Minabe, M., et al. (1989a). Subgingival administration of tetracycline on a collagen film. *Journal of Periodontology*, *60*, 552–556.
66. Minabe, M., et al. (1989b). Application of a local drug delivery system to periodontal therapy: I. Development of collagen preparations with immmobilized tetracycline. *Journal of Periodontology*, *60*, 113–117.
67. Sato, H., et al. (1996). Microdialysis assessment of microfibrous collagen containing a p-glycoprotein-mediated transport inhibitor, cyclosporine A, for local delivery of etoposide. *Research in Pharmacy*, *13*, 1565–1569.
68. Fagundes, L.B., et al. (2009). SBA-15-collagen hybrid material for drug delivery applications. *Expert Opinion on Drug Delivery*, *6(7)*, 687–695.
69. Aebischer, P., et al. (1996). Intrathecal delivery of CNTF using encapsulated genetically modified xenogenic cells in amyotrophic lateral sclerosis. *Nature Medicine*, *2*, 696–699.
70. Park, J.C., et al. (2000). Type I atelocollagen grafting onto ozone-treated polyurethane films: Cell attachment, proliferation, and collagen synthesis. *Journal of Biomedical Materials Research*, *52(4)*, 669–677.
71. Moullier, P., et al. (1993a). Correction of lysosomal storage in the liver and spleen of MPS VII mice by implantation of genetically modified skin fibroblasts. *Nature Genetics*, *4*, 154–159.
72. Moullier, P., et al. (1993b). Continuous systemic secretion of lysosomal enzyme by genetically-modified mouse skin fibroblasts. *Transplantation*, *56*, 427–432.
73. Moullier, P., et al. (1995). Long-term delivery of a lysosomal enzyme by genetically modified fibroblasts in dogs. *Nature Medicine*, *1*, 353–357.
74. Wedge, C.I., Rootman, D.S. (1992). Collagen shields: Efficacy, safety and comfort in the treatment of human traumatic corneal abrasion and effect on vision in healthy eyes. *Canadian Journal of Ophthalmology*, *27(6)*, 295–298.
75. Harrison, K.W. (1989). Collagen corneal shields—an important therapeutic modality. *Journal of Ophthalmic Nursing and Technology*, *8(3)*, 97–98.
76. Willoughby, C.E., Batterbury, M., Kaye, S.B., (2002). Collagen corneal shields. *Survey of Ophthalmology*, *47*, 174–182.
77. Waltman, S.R., Kaufman, H.E. (1970). Use of hydrophilic soft lenses to increase ocular penetration of topical drugs. Investigative Ophthalmology, *9*, 250–255.
78. Podos, S.M., et al. (1972). Pilocarpine therapy with soft contact lenses. *American Journal of Ophthalmology*, *73*, 336–341.
79. Leaders, F.E., et al. (1973). New polymers in drug delivery. *Annals of Ophthalmology*, *5*, 513–522.
80. Baziuk, N., et al. (1992). Collagen shields and intraocular drug delivery: Concentration of gentamicin in the aqueous and vitreous of a rabbit eye after lensectomy and vitrectomy. *International Ophthalmology*, *16*, 101–107.
81. Liang, F.G., et al. (1992). Noncross-linked collagen discs and cross-linked collagen shields in the delivery of gentamicin to rabbit eyes. *Investigative Ophthalmology & Visual Science*, *33*, 2194–2198.
82. Milani, J.K., et al. (1993). Collagen shields impregnated with gentamicin-dexamethasone as a potential drug delivery device. *American Journal of Opthamology*, *116*, 622–627.
83. Phinney, R.B., et al. (1988). Collagen shield delivery of gentamycin and vancomycin. *Archives of Opthalmology*, *106*, 1599–1604.
84. Poland, D.E., Kaufman, H.E. (1988). Clinical uses of collagen shields. *Journal of Cataract and Refractive Surgery*, *14*, 489–491.
85. Sawusch, M.R., et al. (1988). Use of collagen corneal shields in the treatment of bacterial keritis. *American Journal of Opthalmology*, *106*, 279–281.
86. Sawusch, M.R., O'brien, T.P., Updegraff, S.A. (1989). Collagen corneal shields enhance penetration of topical prednisolon acetate. *Journal of Cataract and Refractive Surgery*, *15*, 625–628.
87. Unterman, S.R., et al. (1888). Collagen shield drug delivery: Therapeutic concentrations of tobramycin in the rabbit cornea and aqueous humor. *Journal of Cataract and Refractive Surgery*, *14*, 500–504.
88. O'brien, T.P., et al. (1988). Use of collagen corneal shields soft contact lenses to enhance penetration of topical tobramycin. *Journal of Cataract and Refractive Surgery*, *14*, 505–507.

89. Aquavella, J.V., Ruffini, J.J., LoCascio, J.A. (1988). Use of collagen shields as a surgical adjunct. *Journal of Cataract and Refractive Surgery*, *14*, 492–495.

90. Hobden, J.A., et al. (1988). Treatment of experimental Pseudomonas keratitis using collagen shields containing tobramycin. *Archives of Opthalmology*, *106*, 1605–1607.

91. Assil, K.K., et al. (1992). Efficacy of tobramycin-soaked collagen shield vs. tobramycin eyedrop loaden dose for sustained experimental Pseudomonas aeruginosa induced keratitis in rabbits. *American Journal of Ophthalmology*, *113*, 418–423.

92. Willoughby, C.E., Batterbury, M., Kaye, S.B. (2002). Collagen corneal shields. *Survey of Ophthalmology*, *47*, 174–182.

93. Dorigo, M.T., De Natale, R., Miglioli, P.A. (1995). Collagen shields delivery of netilmicin: A study of ocular pharmacokinetics. *Chemotherapy*, *41*, 1–4.

94. Palmer, R.M., McDonald, M.B. (1995). A corneal lens/shield system to promote postoperative corneal epithelial healing. *Journal of Cataract and Refractive Surgery*, *21*, 125–126.

95. Schwartz, S.D., et al. (1990). Collagen shield delivery of amphotericin B. *American Journal of Opthalmology*, *109*, 701–704.

96. Mendicute, J., et al. (1995). The use of collagen shields impregnated with amphotericin B to treat aspergillus keratomycosis. *Contact Lens Association of Ophthalmologists Journal*, *21*, 252–255.

97. Gussler, J.R., et al. (1990). Collagen shield delivery of trifluorothymidine. *Journal of Cataract and Refractive Surgery*, *16*, 719–722.

98. Willey, D.E., et al. (1991). Ocular acyclovir delivery by collagen discs: A mouse model to screen anti-viral agents. *Current Eye Research*, *10*, 167–169.

99. Taravella, M.J., et al. (1999). Collagen shield delivery of ofloxacin to the human eye. *Journal of Cataract and Refractive Surgery*, *25(4)*, 562–565.

100. Yang HS, et al. (2011). Apatite-coated collagen scaffold for bone morphogenetic protein-2 delivery. *Tissue Engineering Part A*, *17(17–18)*, 2153–2164.

101. Hwang, D.G., et al. (1989). Collagen shield enhancement of topical dexamethasone penetration. *Archives of Ophthalmology*, *107*, 1375–1380.

102. Reidy, J.J., Gebhardt, B.M., Kaufman, H.E. (1990). The collagen shield: A new vehicle for delivery of cyclosporine A to the eye. *Cornea*, *9*, 196–199.

103. Murray, T.G., et al. (1990). Collagen shield heparin delivery for prevention of postoperative fibrin. *Archives of Opthalmology*, *108*, 104–106.

104. Chen, Y. F., et al. (1990). Cyclosporin-containing collagen shields suppress corneal allograftrejection. *American Journal of Ophtalmology*, *109*, 132–137.

105. Friedberg, M.L., Pleyer, U., Mondino, B.J. (1991). Device drug delivery to the eye. *Ophthalmology*, *98*, 725–732.

106. Hariprasad, S.M., et al. (2004). Human intraocular penetration pharmacokinetics of moxifloxacin 0.5% via topical and collagen shield routes of administration. *Transactions of the American Ophthalmological Society*, *102*, 149–155.

107. Robin, J.B., et al. (1990). The effect of collagen shields on rabbit corneal re-epithelization after chemical debridement. *Investigative Ophthalmology & Visual Science*. *31*, 1294–1300.

108. Shaker, G.J., et al. (1989). Effect of collagen shield on cat corneal epithelial wound healing. *Investigative Ophthalmology & Visual Science*, *30*, 1565–1568.

109. Marmer, H. (1988). Therapeutic and protective properties of the corneal shield. *Journal of Cataract & Refractive Surgery*, *14*, 496–499.

110. Mondino, B.J., (1991). Collagen shields. *American Journal of Ophthalmology*, *112(5)*, 587–590.

111. Bourlais, C.L., et al. (1998). Ophthalmic drug delivery systems—recent advances. *Progress in Retinal and Eye Research*, *17*, 33–58.

112. Kaur, I.P., Kanwar, M., (2002). Ocular preparations: The formulation approach. *Drug Development and Industrial Pharmacy*, *28*, 473–493.

113. Kuwano, M., Horibe, Y., Kawashima, Y. (1997). Effect of collagen cross-linking in collagen corneal shields on occular drug delivery. *Journal of Pharmacology Therapeutics*, *13*, 31–40.

114. Lee, V.H. (1990). New directions in the optimization of ocular drug delivery. *Journal of Ocular Pharmacology*, *6*, 157–164.

115. Finkelstein, I., et al. (1991). Further evaluation of collagen shields as a delivery sytem for 5-fluoruracil: Histopathological observations. *Canadian Journal of Ophthalmology*, *26*, 129–132.

116. Pachence, J.M., Berg, R.A., Silver, F.H. (2000). Collagen: Its place in the medical device industry. *Medical Device and Diagnostic Industry*, *9*, 49–55.

117. Geesin, J.C., et al. (1996). Development of a skin model based on insoluble fibrillar collagen. *Journal of Biomedical Materials Research*, *33*, 1–8.

118. Boyce, S.T., Christanson, D., Hansbrough, J.F. (1988). Structure of a collagen-GAG dermal skin substitute optimized for cultured human epidermal keratinocytes. *Journal of Biomedical Materials Research*, *22*, 939–957.

119. Marks, M.G., Doillon, C., Silver, F.H. (1991). Effects of fibroblasts and basic fibroblast growth factor on facilitation of dermal wound healing by type I collagen matrices. *Journal of Biomedical Materials Research*, *25*, 683–696.

120. Royce, P.M., et al. (1995). The enhancement of cellular infiltration and vascularization of a collagenous dermal implant in the rat by platelet-derived growth factor BB. *Journal of Dermatology Science*, *10*, 42–52.

121. Wachol-Drewek, Z., Zpfeiffer, M., Scholl, E. (1996). Comparative investigation of drug delivery of collagen implants saturated in antibiotic solutions and a sponge containing gentamycin. *Biomaterials*, *17*, 1733–1738.

122. Vaneerdeweg, W., et al. (1988). Comparison between plain and gentamicin containing collagen sponges in infected peritoneal cavity in rats. *European Journal of Surgery*, *164* (8), 617–621.

123. Vaneerdeweg, W., et al. (2000). Effect of gentamicin-containing sponges on the healing of colonic anastomoses in a rat model of peritonitis. *European Journal of Surgery*, *166*(*12*), 959–962.
124. Stemberger, A., et al. (1997). Local treatment of bone and soft tissue infections with the collagen gentamicin sponge. *European Journal of Surgery*, *578*(*163*), 17–26.
125. Dorr, R.T., et al. (1982). In vitro retinoid binding and release from a collagen sponge material in a simulated intravaginal environment. *Journal of Biomedical Materials Research*, *16*, 839–850.
126. Chvapil, M., et al. (1985). Collagen sponge as vaginal contraceptive barrier: Critical summary of seven years of research. *American Journal of Obstetrics and Gynecology*, *151*, 325–329.
127. Peng, Y.-M., et al. (1986). Cervical tissue uptake of all-trans-retinoic acid delivered via a collagen sponge-cervical cap delivery device in patients with cervical dysplasia. *Investigational New Drugs*, *4*, 245–249.
128. Sastry, T.O., Rao, P.K. High performance biomaterials, in M. Szycher (ed.), *A Comprehensive Guide to Medical/Pharmaceutical Application*, Technomic, Lancaster, PA, 1991, p. 171.
129. Prajapati, R.T., et al. (2000). Mechanical loading regulates protease production by fibroblasts in three dimensional collagen substrates. *Wound Repair and Regeneration*, *8*, 226–237.
130. Hwang, Y.J., Lyubovitsky, J.G. (2011). Collagen hydrogel characterization: Multi-scale and multi-modality approach. *Analytical Methods*, *3*, 529–536.
131. Sahai, A., et al. (1995). An injectable sustained release drug delivery system markedly enhances intratumoral retention of C14-fluorouracil in murine fibro sarcomas. *Research in Pharmacy*. *12*, S227.
132. Remacle, M., Dujardin, J.M., Lawson, G. (1995). Treatment of vocal fold immobility by glutaraldehyde-crosslinked collagen injection: Long term results. *Annals of Otology, Rhinology & Laryngology*, *104*, 437–441.
133. Shortliffe, L.M.D., et al. (1989). Treatment of urinary incontinence by the periurethal implantation of glutaraldehyde crosslinked collagen. *Journal of Urology*, *141*, 538–541.
134. Jeyanthi, J., Nagarajan, B., Rao, K.P. (1991). Solid tumour chemotherapy using implantable collagen-poly (HEMA) hydrogel containing 5-fluorouracil. *Journal of Pharmacy and Pharmacology*, *43*(*1*), 60–62.
135. Shantha, K.L., Rao, K.P. (1993). Hybrid Copolymers for controlled release of contraceptive steroids. *Journal of Bioactive and Compatible Polymers*, *8*(2), 142–157.
136. Cascone, M.G., Sim, B., Downes, S. (1995). Blends of synthetic and natural polymers as drug delivery systems for growth hormone. *Biomaterials*, *16*, 569–574.
137. Banerjee, R. (2001). Liposomes: Applications in medicine. *Journal of Biomaterials Applications*, *16*(*1*), 3–21.
138. Weiner, A.L., et al. (1985). Liposome-collagen gel matrix: A novel sustained drug delivery system. *Journal of Pharmacy & Pharmaceutical Sciences*, *74*, 922–925.
139. Pajean, M., Herbage, D. (1993). Effect of collagen on liposome permeability. *International Journal of Pharmacy*, *91*, 209.
140. Shi, X., et al. (2001). The aggregation behavior of collagen in aqueous solution and its property of stabilizing liposomes in vitro. *Biomaterial*, *22*, 1627–1634.
141. Grammer, J.B., et al. (1996). Impregnation of collagen corneal shields with liposomes: Uptake and release of hydrophilic and lipophilic marker substances. *Current Eye Research*, *15*(*8*), 815–823.
142. Pleyer, U., et al. (1994). Ocular absorption of cyclosporine A from liposomes incorporated into collagen shields. *Current Eye Research*, *13*(*3*), 177–181.
143. Takenaka, H., Fujioka, K., Takada, Y. (1986). New formulations of bioactive materials. *Pharmaceutical Technology of Japan*, *2*, 1083–1091.
144. Yamahira, Y., et al. (1991). Sustained release injections. European Patent. 84112313.6.
145. Matsuoka, J., et al. (1988). Development of an interleukin-2 slow delivery system. *Asio Transcations*, *34*, 729–731.
146. Tayade, P.T., Kale, R.D. (2004). Encapsulation of water-insoluble drug by a cross-linking technique: Effect of process and formulation variables on encapsulation efficiency, particle size, and in vitro dissolution rate. *Journal of American Association of Pharmaceutical Scientists*, *6*, E12.
147. Maeda, H., et al. (2003). Design of long-acting formulation of protein drugs with a double-layer structure and its application to rhG-CSF. *Journal of Controlled Release*, *91*, 281–297.
148. Higaki, M., et al. (2001). Collagen minipellet as a controlled release delivery system for tetanus and diphtheria toxoid. *Vaccine*, *19*, 3091–3096.
149. Lofthouse, S., et al. (2001). The application of biodegradable collagen minipellets as vaccine delivery vehicles in mice and sheep. *Vaccine*, *19*, 4318–4327.
150. Muller, R.H., Mader, K., Gohla, S. (2000). Solid lipid nanoparticles for controlled drug delivery-a review of the state of the art. *European Journal of Pharmaceutics and Biopharmaceutics*, *50*, 161–177.
151. Rossler, B., Kreuter, J., Scherer, D. (1994). Effect of collagen microparticles on the stability of retinol and its absorption into hairless mouse skin in vitro. *Pharmazie*, *49*, 175–179.
152. Farrugia, C.A., Groves, M.J. (1999). Gelatin behavior in dilute aqueous solution: Designing a nanoparticulate formulation. *Journal of Pharmacy and Pharmacology*, *51*, 643–649.
153. Coester, C.J., et al. (2000). Gelatin nanoparticles by two step desolvation, a new preparation method, surface modifications and cell uptake. *Journal of Microencapsulation*, *17*, 187–193.
154. El-Samaligy, M.S., Rohdewald, P. (1983). Reconstituted collagen nanoparticles, a novel drug carrier delivery system. *Journal of Pharmacy and Pharmacology*, *35*, 537–539.
155. Yang, C., et al. (1999). Body distribution in mice of intravenously injected camptothecin solid lipid nanoparticles and targeting effect on brain. *Journal of Controlled Release*, *59*, 299–307.

156. Berthold, A., Cremer, K., Kreuter, J., (1998). Collagen microparticles: Carriers for glucocorticosteroids. *European Journal of Pharmaceutics and Biopharmaceutics*, *45*, 23–29.

157. Narayani, R., Rao, K.P. (1994). Controlled release of anticancer drug methotrexate from biodegradable gelatin microspheres. *Journal of Microencapsulation*, *11(1)*, 69–77.

158. Marty, J.J., Openheim, R.C., Speiser, P. (1978). Nanoparticles-a new colloidal drug delivery system. *Pharmaceutica Acta Helvetiae*, *53*, 17–23.

159. Bender, A., et al. (1996). Efficiency of nanoparticles as a carrier system for antiviral agents in human monocytes/macrophages in vitro. *Antimicrobial Agents and Chemotherapy*, *40*, 1467–1471.

160. Luo, Z., et al. (2011). Mesoporous silica nanoparticles end-capped with collagen: Redox-responsive nanoreservoirs for targeted drug delivery. *Angewandte Chemie International Edition*, *50(3)*, 640–643.

161. Posadas, I., Guerra, F.J., Ceña, V. (2010). Nonviral vectors for the delivery of small interfering RNAs to the CNS. *Nanomedicine*, *5(8)*, 1219–1236.

162. Sano, A., et al. (2003). Collagen in drug delivery and tissue engineering; Atelocollagen for protein and gene delivery. *Advanced Drug Delivery Reviews*, *55(12)*, 1651–1677.

163. Zwiorek, K., et al. (2004). Gelatin nanoparticles as a new and simple gene delivery system. *Journal of Pharmacy & Pharmaceutical Sciences*, *7(4)*, 22–28.

164. Kaul, G., Amiji, M. (2005). Tumor-targeted gene delivery using poly(ethylene glycol)-modified gelatin nanoparticles: In vitro and in vivo studies. *Pharmaceutical Research*, *22(6)*, 951–961.

165. Murata, M., et al. (1999). Bone augmentation by recombinant human BMP-2 and collagen on adult rat parietal bone. *International Journal of Oral and Maxillofacial Surgery*, *28(3)*, 232–237.

166. Murata, M., et al. (2000). Bone augmentation by onlay implant using recombinant human BMP-2 and collagen on adult rat skull without periosteum. *Clinical Oral Implants Research*, *11(4)*, 289–295.

167. Nakagawa, T., Tagawa, T., (2000). Ultrastructural study of direct bone formation induced by BMPs-collagen complex implanted into an ectopic site. *Oral Diseases*, *6(3)*, 172–179.

168. Liu, H.W., Ofosu, F.A., Chang, P.L. (1993). Expression of human factor IX by microencapsulated recombinant fibroblasts. *Human Gene Therapy*, *4*, 291–301.

169. Al-Hendy, A., et al. (1995). Correction of the growth defect in dwarf mice with nonautologous microencapsulated myoblasts—an alternative approach to somatic gene therapy. *Human Gene Therapy*, *6(2)*, 165–175.

170. Tani, K., et al. (1989). Implantation of fibroblasts transfected with human granulocyte colony-stimulating factor cDNA into mice as a model of cytokine supplement gene therapy. *Blood*, *74*, 1274–1280.

171. Brauker, J. S., et al. (1995). Immunoisolation in somatic cell gene therapy. *Journal of Cellular Biochemistry*, *21B*, D1–D15.

172. Barr, E., Leiden, J.M. (1991). Systemic delivery of recombinant proteins by genetically modified myoblasts. *Science*, *254*, 1507–1509.

173. Scharfmann, R., Axelord, J.H., Verma, I.M. (1991). Long-term in vivo expression of retrovirus-mediated gene transfer in mouse fibroblast implants. *Proceedings of the National Academy of Science of the USA*, *88*, 4626–4630.

174. Heartlein, M.W., et al. (1994). Long-term production and delivery of human growth hormone in vivo. *Proceedings of the National Academy of Science of the USA*, *91*, 10967–10971.

175. Rosenthal, F.M., Kohler, G. (1997). Collagen as matrix for neo-organ formation by gene-transfected fibroblasts. *Anticancer Research*, *17*, 1179–1186.

176. Jin, X., et al. (2008). Antibody modified collagen matrix for site-specific gene delivery. *ACS Symposium Series*, *992(13)*, 243–261.

177. Angella, G.J., et al. (2000). Enhanced short-term plasmid transfection of filtration surgery tissues. *Investigative Ophthalmology & Visual Science*, *41(13)*, 4158–4162.

178. Kimura, M., et al. (2000). Bone-inductive efficacy of recombinant human bone morphogenetic protein-2 expressed in Escherichia coli: An experimental study in rat mandibular defects. *Scandinavian Journal of Plastic and Reconstructive Surgery and Hand Surgery*, *34(4)*, 289–299.

179. Cochran, D.L., et al. (2000). Evaluation of recombinant human bone morphogenetic protein-2 in oral applications including the use of endosseous implants: 3-year results of a pilot study in humans. *Journal of Periodontology*, *71(8)*, 1241–1257.

180. Scherer, F., et al. (2002). Nonviral vector loaded collagen sponges for sustained gene delivery in vitro and in vivo. *Journal of Gene Medicine*, *4(6)*, 634–643.

181. Ferkol, T., Kaetzel, C.S., Davis, P.B. (1993). Gene transfer into respiratory epithelial cells by targetting the polymeric immunoglobulin receptor. *Journal of Clinical Investigation*, *92*, 2394–2400.

182. Uchio, Y., et al. (2000). Human chondrocyte proliferation and matrix synthesis cultured in Atelocollagen gel. *Journal of Biomedical Materials Research*, *50(2)*, 138–143.

183. Katsube, K., et al. (2000). Repair of articular cartilage defects with cultured chondrocytes in Atelocollagen gel. Comparison with cultured chondrocytes in suspension. *Archives of Orthopaedic and Trauma Surgery*, *120(3–4)*, 121–127.

184. Suh, H., et al. (2001). Behavior of osteoblasts on a type I atelocollagen grafted ozone oxidized poly L-lactic acid membrane. *Biomaterials*, *22(3)*, 219–230.

185. Honma, K., et al. (2001). Atelocollagen-based gene transfer in cells allows high-throughput screening of gene functions. *Biochemical and Biophysical Research Communications*, *289*, 1075–1081.

186. Maeda, H., Sano, A., Fujioka, K. (2004a). Controlled release of rhBMP-2 from collagen minipellet and the relationship between release profile and ectopic bone formation. *International Journal of Pharmacy*, *275*, 109–122.

187. Maeda, H., Sano, A., Fujioka, K. (2004b). Profile of rhBMP-2 release from collagen minipellet and induction of ectopic bone formation. *Drug Development and Industrial Pharmacy*, *30*, 473–480.

188. Muniruzzaman, T., Tabata, Y., Ikada, Y. (1998). Complexation of basic fibroblast growth factor with gelatin. *Journal of Biomaterials Science, Polymer Edition*, *9*, 459–473.

189. Wang, Lee, L., et al. (2004). Evaluation of collagen and methylated collagen as gene carriers. *International Journal of Pharmaceutics*, *279*, 115–126.

190. Capito, R.M., Spector, M. (2007). Collagen scaffolds for nonviral IGF-1 gene delivery in articular cartilage tissue engineering. *Gene Therapy*, *14*, 721.

191. Pakkanen, T.M., et al. (2000). Periadventitial LacZ gene transfer to pig carotid arteries using a biodegradable collagen collar or a wrap of collagen sheet with adenoviruses and plasmid-liposome complexes. *Journal of Gene Medicine*, *2*, 52–60.

192. Canty, E.G., Kadler, K.E. (2005). Procollagen trafficking, processing and fibrillogenesis. *Journal of Cellular Science*, *118*, 1341–1353.

193. Metcalfe, A.D., Ferguson, M.W. (2007). Tissue engineering of replacement skin: The crossroads of biomaterials, wound healing, embryonic development, stem cells and regeneration. *Journal of The Royal Society Interface*, *4*, 413–437.

194. Cen, L., et al. (2008). Collagen tissue engineering: Development of novel biomaterials and applications. *Pediatric Research*, *63(5)*, 492–496.

195. Abraham, A., et al. (2000). Evaluation of the porcine intestinal collagen layer as a biomaterial. *Journal of Biomedical Materials Research*, *51*, 442–452.

196. Leipziger, L.S., et al. (1985). Dermal wound repair: Role of collagen matrix implants and sysnthetic polymer dressings. *Journal of the American Academy of Dermatology*, *12*, 409–419.

197. Deatherage, J.R., Miller, E.J. (1987). Packaging and delivery of bone induction factors in a collagenous implant. *Collagen Release Research*, *7*, 225–231.

198. Harriger, M.D., et al. (1997). Glutaraldehyde crosslinking of collagen substrates inhibits degradation in skin substitutes grafted to athymic mice. *Journal of Biomedical Materials Research*, *35*, 137–145.

199. Orwin, E.J., Hubel, A. (2000). In vitro culture characteristics of corneal epithelial, endothelial, and keratocyte cells in a native collagen matrix. *Tissue Engineering*, *6(4)*, 307–319.

200. Awad, H.A., et al. (2003). Repair of patellar tendon injuries using a cell-collagen composite. *Journal of Orthopaedic Research*, *21*, 420–431.

201. Yamada, N., Uchinuma, E., Kuroyanagi, Y. (1999). Clinical evaluation of an allogeneic cultured dermal substitute composed of fibroblasts within a spongy collagen matrix. *Scandinavian Journal of Plastic and Reconstructive Surgery and Hand Surgery*, *33(2)*, 147–154.

202. Yannas, I.V., et al. (1989). Synthesis and characterization of a model extracellular matrix that induces partial regeneration of adult mammalian skin. *Proceedings of the National Academy of Science of the USA*, *86*, 933–937.

203. Boyce, S.T., et al. (1993). Attachment of an aminoglycoside, amikacin, to implantable collagen for local delivery in wounds. *Antimicrobial Agents and Chemotherapy*, *37*, 1890–1895.

204. Supp, A.P., et al. (1999). Incubation of cultured skin substitutes in reduced humidity promotes cornification in vitro and stable engraftment in athymic mice. *Wound Repair Regeneration*, *7*, 226–237.

205. Koide, M., et al. (1993). A new type of biomaterial for artificial skin: Dehydrothermally cross-linked composites of fibrillar and denatured collagens. *Journal of Biomedical Materials Research*, *27*, 79–87.

206. Ponticiello, M.S., et al. (2000). Gelatin-based resorbable sponge as a carrier matrix for human mesenchymal stem cells in cartilage regeneration therapy. *Journal of Biomedical Materials Research*, *52(2)*, 246–255.

207. Lam, P.K., et al. (1999). The efficacy of collagen dermis membrane and fibrin on cultured epidermal graft using an athymic mouse model. *Annals of Plastic Surgery*, *43*, 523–528.

208. Juncosa-Melvin, et al. (2006). Effects of mechanical stimulation on the biomechanics and histology of stem cell-collagen sponge constructs for rabbit patellar tendon repair. *Tissue Engineering*, *1*, 2291–2300.

209. Juncosa-Melvin, N., et al. (2007). Mechanical stimulation increases collagen type I and collagen type III gene expression of stem cell-collagen sponge constructs for patellar tendon repair. *Tissue Engineering*, *13*, 1219–1226.

210. Sobolewski, K., et al. (1995). Collagen, elastin and glycosaminoglycans in aortic aneurysms. Acta Biochimica. *Polonica*, *42*, 301–308.

211. Boyce S.T., et al. (1995). Comparative assessment of cultured skin substitutes and native skin autograft for treatment of full-thickness burns. *Annals of Surgery*, *222*, 743–752.

212. Boyce, S.T., Stompro, B.E., Hansbrough, J.F. (1992). Biotinylation of implantable collagen for drug delivery. *Journal of Biomedical Materials Research*, *26*, 547–553.

213. Stompro, B.E., Hansbrough, J.F., Boyce, S.T. (1989). Attachment of peptide growth factors to implantable collagen. *Journal of Surgical Research*, *46*, 413–421.

214. Reddi, A.H. (2000). Morphogenesis and tissue engineering of bone and cartilage: Inductive signals, stem cells, and biomimetic biomaterials. *Tissue Engineering*, *6(4)*, 351–359.

215. Kobayashi, Y., Ochi, M., Tokue, A. (2000). Clinical usefulness of crosslinked N-telopeptide of type I collagen as a bone metastatic marker in patients with prostate cancer: Comparison with serum PICP, PINP and ICTP. *Hinyokika*, *46*, 869–872.

216. Ulrich, U., et al. (2001). Cross linked type I collagen C- and N-telopeptides in women with bone metastases from breast cancer. *Archives of Gynecology and Obstetrics*, *264*, 186–190.

217. Uitterlinden, A.G., et al. (2001). Interaction between the vitamin D receptor gene and collagen type Ialpha 1 gene

in susceptibility for fracture. *Journal of Bone and Mineral Research*, *15*, 379–385.

218. Cui, F.Z., Li, Y., Ge, J. (2007). Self-assembly of mineralized collagen composites. *Materials Science and Engineering: R: Reports*, *57*, 1–27.
219. Takaoka, K., et al. (1988). Ectopic bone induction on and in porous hydroxyapatite combined with collagen and bone morphogenetic protein. *Clinical Orthopaedics*, *234*, 250–254.
220. Sela, J., et al. (2000). Retinoic acid enhances the effect of collagen on bone union, following induced non-union defect in guinea pig ulna. *Inflammation Research*, *49*, 679–683.
221. Torbet, J., et al. (2007). Orthogonal scaffold of magnetically aligned collagen lamellae for corneal stroma reconstruction. *Biomaterials*. *28*, 4268–4276.
222. Lee, H.J., Ahn, S.H., Kim, G.H. (2012). Three-dimensional collagen/alginate hybrid scaffolds functionalized with a drug delivery system (DDS) for bone tissue regeneration. *Chemistry of Materials*, *24(5)*, 881–891.
223. Van der Laan, J.S., et al. (1991). Tee-plasma polymerized dermal sheep collagen for the repair of abdominal wall defects. *International Journal of Artificial Organs*, *14*, 661–666.
224. Grant, M.E. (2007). From collagen chemistry towards cell therapy-a personal journey. *International Journal of Experimental Pathology*, *88*, 203–214.
225. Sekine, T., et al. (2001). A new type of surgical adhesive made from porcine collagen and polyglutamic acid. *Journal of Biomedical Materials Research*, *54*, 305–310.
226. Kuzuya, M., Kinsell, J.L. (1994). Induction of endothelial cell differentiation in vitro by fibroblast-derived soluble factors. *Experimental Cell Research*, *215*, 310–318.
227. Chevallay, B., Herbage, D. (2000). Collagen-based biomaterials as 3D scaffold for cell cultures: Applications for tissue engineering and gene therapy. *Medical, & Biological Engineering & Computing*, *38(2)*, 211–218.
228. Matin-Chouly, C.A., et al. (1999). In vitro evaluation of vascular permeability to contrast media using cultured endothelial cell monolayers. *Investigative Radiology*, *34*, 663–668.
229. Sanchez, C., Arribart, H., Guille, M.M. (2005). Biomimetism and bioinspiration as tools for the design of innovative materials and systems. *Nature Materials*, *4*, 277–288.
230. Clarke, K.M., et al. (1996). Intestine submucosa and polypropylene mesh for abdominal wall repair in dogs. *Journal of Surgery Research*, *60*, 107–114.
231. Desgrandchamps, F. (2000). Biomaterials in functional reconstruction. *Current Opinion in Urology*, *10(3)*, 201–206.
232. Gloeckner, D.C., et al. (2000). Mechanical evaluation and design of a multilayered collagenous repair. *Biomaterial*. *52*, 365–373.
233. Girton, T.S., et al. (1990). Mechanisms of stiffening and strengthening in media equivalents fabricated using glycation. *Journal of Biomechanical Engineering*, *122*, 216–223.
234. Koide, T. (2007). Designed triple-helical peptides as tools for collagen biochemistry and matrix engineering. *Philosophical Transactions of the Royal Society of London - Series B: Biological Sciences*, *362*, 1281–1291.
235. Smith, K., Rennie M.J. (2007). New approaches and recent results concerning human-tissue collagen synthesis. *Current Opinion in Clinical Nutrition and Metabolic Care*, *10*, 582–590.
236. Paramonov, S.E., Gauba, V., Hartgerink, J.D. (2005). Synthesis of collagen-like peptide polymers by native chemical ligation. *Macromolecules*, *38*, 7555–7561.
237. Koide, T., et al. (2005). Self-complementary peptides for the formation of collagen-like triple helical supramolecules. *Bioorganic & Medicinal Chemistry Letters*, *15*, 5230–5233.
238. Kotch, F.W., Raines, R.T. (2006). Self-assembly of synthetic collagen triple helices. *Proceedings of the National Academy of Science of the USA*, *103*, 3028–3033.
239. University of Wisconsin-Madison. (2010, January 13). Scientists create super-strong *collagen*. Retrieved July 3, 2011, from http://www.sciencedaily.com.
240. Langer, R., Vacanti, J.P. (1993). Tissue engineering. *Science*, *260*, 920–926.
241. Langer, R. (2000). Tissue engineering. *Molecular Therapy*, *1*, 12–15.
242. Chen, J.M., Sheldon, A., Pincus, M.R., (1995). Three dimensional energy-minimized model of human type II smith collagen microfibrill. *Journal of Biomolecular Structure & Dynamics*, *12*, 1129–1156.
243. Caria, A., et al. (2004). Elastic scattering and light transport in three-dimensional collagen gel constructs: A mathematical model and computer Simulation approach. *NanoBioscience*, *3* (2), 85–89.
244. Israelowitz, M., et al. (2005). Computational modeling of type I collagen fibers to determine the extracellular matrix structure of connective tissues. *Protein Engineering, Design and Selection*, *18(7)*, 329–335.
245. Perumal, S., Anti pova, O., Orgel, J.P.R. (2008). Collagen fibril architecture, domain organization, and triple-helical conformation govern its proteolysis. *Proceedings of the National Academy of Sciences of the USA*, *105(8)*, 2824–2829.
246. Calvaruso, V., et al. (2009). Computer-assisted image analysis of liver collagen: Relationship to Ishak scoring and hepatic venous pressure gradient. *Hepatology*, *49(4)*, 1236–1244.
247. Manousou, P., et al. (2011). Digital image analysis of liver collagen predicts clinical outcome of recurrent hepatitis C virus 1 year after liver transplantation. *Liver Transplants*, *17(2)*, 178–188.
248. Schoen, F.J., et al. (1992). Antimineralization treatments for bioprosthetic heart valves: Assessment of efficacy and safety. *Journal of Thoracic Cardiovascular Surgery*, *104(5)*, 1285–1288.
249. Wright, G.A., Faught, J.M., Olin, J.M. (2009). Assessing anticalcification treatments in bioprosthetic tissue by using the New Zealand rabbit intramuscular model. *Comparative Medicine*, *59(3)*, 266–271.
250. Wada, T., et al. (1999). Calcification of vascular smooth muscle cell cultures: Inhibition by osteopontin. *Circulation Research*, *84*, 166–178.
251. Lee, C.H., et al. (1998). Inhibition of aortic wall calcification in bioprosthetic heart valves by ethanol pretreatment:

Biochemical and biophysical mechanisms. *Journal of Biomedical Materials Research*, *42(1)*, 30–37.

252. Singla, A., Lee, C.H. (2003). Inhibition of CEM calcification by the sequential pretreatment with Ethanol and EDTA. *Journal of Biomedical Materials Research*, *64(4)*, 706–713.
253. Singla, A., Lee, C.H. (2002). Effect of elastin on the calcification rate of collagen-elastin matrix systems. *Journal of Biomedical Materials Research*, *60(3)*, 368–374.
254. Vardaxis, N.J., Boon, M.E., Ruijgrok, J.M. (1996). Calcification of cross-linked collagen-elastin membrane implants in vivo and their proposed use in bone regeneration. *Biomaterials*, *17*, 1489–1497.
255. Meaney, D.F. (1995). Mechanical properties of implantable biomaterials. *Clinics in Podiatric Medicine and Surgery*, *12(3)*, 363–384.
256. Fell, J.T., Newton, J.M. (1970). Determination of tablet strength by diametrical compression test. *Journal of Pharmacy & Pharmaceutical Sciences*, *69*, 688–691.
257. Bank, R.A., et al. (2000). The increased swelling and instantaneous deformation of osteoarthritic cartilage is highly correlated with collagen degradation. *Arthritis & Rheumatism*, *43*, 2202–2210.
258. Boyce, S.T. (1998). Skin substitutes from cultured cells and collagen-GAG polymers. *Medical, & Biological Engineering & Computing*, *36*, 791–800.
259. Lee, C.H., Singla, A., Lee, Y. (2001). Biomedical application of Collagen. *International Journal of Pharmaceutics*, *221(1–2)*, 1–22.
260. Eshar, D., Wyre, D.R., Schoster, J.V. (2011). Use of collagen shields for treatment of chronic bilateral corneal ulcers in a pet rabbit. *Journal of Small Animal Practice*, *53(7)*, 380–383.
261. Gebhardt, B.M., Kaufman, H.E. (1995). Collagen as a delivery system for hydrophobic drugs: Studies with cyclosporinee. *Journal of Ocular Pharmacology and Therapeutics*, *11*, 319–327.

24

MOLECULAR IMAGING OF DRUG DELIVERY

ZHENG-RONG LU

24.1 CHAPTER OBJECTIVES

- To enlist the commonly used imaging modalities that can be used in the development of drug delivery systems.
- To learn the fundamental concepts and principles of the imaging modalities.
- To understand the applications of the imaging modalities in the development of drug delivery systems.

24.2 INTRODUCTION

Molecular imaging allows for noninvasive visualization and measurement of molecular markers along with biological, metabolic, and physiological processes in living organisms [1–4]. Various imaging modalities have been developed using the electromagnetic spectrum to visualize objects normally invisible to the human eye. From low-frequency to high-frequency wavelengths in the electromagnetic spectrum, ultrasound imaging, magnetic resonance imaging (MRI), optical imaging, X-ray computerized tomography (CT), γ-ray scintigraphy, single-photon emission computed tomography (SPECT), and positron emission tomography (PET) are commonly used imaging modalities in biomedical research and clinical practice. Imaging probes or contrast agents are often needed for these imaging modalities for functional and molecular imaging [5–8]. The concept of drug delivery can be applied in molecular imaging for the design of effective and target-specific imaging agents and probes. Molecular imaging provides a noninvasive tool for investigating the drug delivery efficiency and therapeutic efficacy of drug delivery systems. The combination of drug delivery and molecular imaging has resulted in the development of new diagnostic and therapeutic regimens, including image-guided therapies, theranostics, or personalized medicine. These new regimens have a potential to provide earlier and more accurate disease diagnosis, efficacious treatment, rapid and noninvasive assessment of therapeutic efficacy, and the best possible therapeutic outcomes [5–7]. The characteristics of the commonly used imaging modalities and their applications in drug delivery are summarized in Table 24.1.

24.3 IMAGING MODALITIES

24.3.1 Ultrasound Imaging

Ultrasound imaging measures the interaction of high-frequency sound waves (1–10 MHz) with the tissue of interest [8–10]. Sound waves travel fast in solids and liquids, and slow in gas. When sound waves are applied to a subject through a transducer, they are reflected at the interface of tissues or organs of different densities and recorded in the transducer. High-resolution morphological images can be constructed based on the echoes, attenuation of the sound, and sound speed. Real-time two-dimensional (2D) and

Advanced Drug Delivery, First Edition. Edited by Ashim K. Mitra, Chi H. Lee, and Kun Cheng.

TABLE 24.1 Characteristics and Applications of Commonly Used Imaging Modalities

	Ultrasound	MRI	Optical Imaging	X-Ray CT	SPECT	PET
Energy (eV)	$<10^{-5}$	$<10^{-5}$	2–3	3–150 K	100–200 K	511 K
Tissue penetration	Unlimited	Unlimited	Limited	Unlimited	Unlimited	Unlimited
Sensitivity for molecular imaging (mol/kg)	10^{-4}	10^{-4}	10^{-6}	10^{-2}	10^{-10}	10^{-10}
Imaging agents	Microbubbles	Gd(III), Mn(II) chelates, iron oxide particles	Fluorophores	Iodine, heavy elements	γ-emitters ^{111}In, ^{99m}Tc	Positron emitters, ^{18}F, ^{11}C
Anatomic imaging	Good	Good	Fair	Good	Poor	Poor
Pharmacokinetics	Quantitative	Semiquantitative	Quantitative	Quantitative	Quantitative	Quantitative
Pharmacodynamics	Quantitative	Quantitative	Qualitative	Quantitative	Quantitative	Quantitative

three-dimensional images can be obtained with advanced ultrasound imaging technologies, e.g., Doppler imaging technology [11, 12]. Microbubbles ($<10\,\mu m$) generate strong echoes, enhance echo differences between tissue types, and are effective contrast agents for accurate ultrasonic diagnostic imaging [13]. Microbubbles are composed of a shell of biocompatible materials, including denatured proteins, lipids or polymers, filled with inert gas with low water solubility, such as air, nitrogen, SF_6 or C_3F_8, or other low-density perfluorocarbons. Ultrasound imaging is highly sensitive in detecting the microbubbles developed for diagnostic imaging and molecular imaging [14–18]. Microbubbles have also been used as carriers for the delivery of chemotherapeutics, proteins, and nucleic acids [8, 18]. Ultrasonic imaging can provide real-time tracking of *in vivo* drug delivery processes and tissue interactions of a single microbubble. It can also guide and specifically activate the burst and release of the drug from drug loading microbubbles [19–21].

24.3.2 Magnetic Resonance Imaging

MRI measures the longitudinal (T_1) and transverse (T_2) relaxation rates of protons (mainly water protons) in the body [22]. Water forms approximately 60% of the body weight of a normal human adult. Different tissues have different proton density and different T_1 and T_2 relaxation rates, thereby generating different MR signals. The longitudinal (T_1) relaxation or spin-lattice relaxation involves the return of magnetized protons from a high-energy state to an equilibrium state by dissipating their excess energy to their surroundings. The transverse (T_2) relaxation or spin-spin relaxation involves energy transfer from proton to proton. High-resolution three-dimensional anatomic images are constructed from the signals of the proton relaxations in different tissues. Paramagnetic materials, including paramagnetic metal chelates and nanoparticles, are used as MRI contrast agents to enhance the image contrast between the tissue of interest and its surrounding tissues [23, 24]. The paramagnetic materials increase the relaxation rates of surrounding water protons, resulting in enhanced MR signal contrast. Stable paramagnetic chelates, e.g., Gd(III) chelates and Mn(II) chelates, are commonly used as T_1-weighted contrast agents, which increase T_1 relaxation rate and MR signal, resulting in positive or bright image enhancement [25]. Paramagnetic nanoparticles, e.g., iron oxide nanoparticles, are used mainly as T_2-weighted contrast agents, which increase T_2 relaxation and reduce the MR signal, resulting in negative or dark image enhancement [26]. Paramagnetic chelates have been incorporated into various drug delivery systems, including polymers, liposomes, and nanoparticles, to modify their pharmacokinetics and to achieve more effective contrast enhancement for vascular imaging and cancer imaging [27–30]. Targeting agents have been conjugated to the delivery systems of the contrast agents for molecular imaging with MRI [31, 32]. Paramagnetic nanoparticles have also been modified with biocompatible polymers and targeting agents to design targeted nanoparticular MRI contrast agents [33, 34].

24.3.3 Optical Imaging

Optical imaging mainly uses visible and infrared lights to visualize the morphology, biomarkers, and biological processes of the subject of interest. Fluorescence and luminescence imaging techniques are the popular optical imaging modalities in biological and biomedical research [35, 36]. Fluorescence imaging measures the fluorescence emitted from a fluorophore after excitation with an external light source. Luminescence imaging detects the light emission from a chemical or biochemical reaction with no external excitation. Both fluorescence and bioluminescence imaging have been routinely used for *in vitro* and *in vivo* evaluation of drug delivery systems [37–39]. The drug delivery systems are often labeled with a fluorophore to allow for visualization of the delivery process at both cellular and tissue levels. Microscopic fluorescence imaging and confocal fluorescence microscopy are commonly used for visualizing the cellular interaction and intracellular trafficking of drug delivery systems with high resolution and sensitivity [40, 41]. Bioluminescence imaging is effective for *in vitro* and *in vivo* study gene expression with a reporter gene and is commonly used for evaluating the efficiency of delivery systems for nucleic acids [42, 43]. Near infrared (NIR) lights (650–900 nm), having relatively low tissue absorption, is commonly used for *in vivo* fluorescence imaging [44, 45]. Optical imaging for *in vivo* study of drug delivery is often limited by the depth of light penetration into tissues.

24.3.4 X-Ray Computed Tomography

X-ray radiography measures the attenuation of X-rays by the tissues through which they pass. When an X-ray beam passes through the body, it can be scattered or absorbed by the tissues based on their density, resulting in loss of X-ray intensity, known as attenuation. An image of the body is constructed from the attenuated X-rays recorded on X-ray sensitive cameras. X-ray attenuation is strong in dense tissue (such as bone) and weak in soft tissues. CT provides three-dimensional anatomic images of the body with high spatial resolution [46, 47] but has a low sensitivity for molecular imaging. Biologically inert substances containing heavy elements, e.g., iodine and barium, are effective for attenuating X-rays and are used as contrast agents for CT [48]. Biocompatible iodinated benzene derivatives, required in high doses, are commonly used as the CT contrast agents. The principle of drug delivery has also been applied to improve the *in vivo* properties of CT contrast agents. Various drug delivery systems have been used to modify the pharmacokinetics and biodistribution of iodinated contrast agents [49, 50]. Recently, nanoparticles, including gold nanoparticles, have been prepared as CT contrast agents [51, 52].

24.3.5 Single-Photon Emission Computed Tomography

SPECT detects the γ-rays emitted by radioactive isotopes [53]. SPECT requires the administration of radiopharmaceuticals or radiotracers. Each decay of the radioisotope emits one γ-ray, which is detected by a rotating camera and processed by a computer to generate three-dimensional images. SPECT has a high sensitivity for detecting radiopharmaceuticals and is effective for molecular imaging. Although SPECT provides quantitative information about their distribution in the body, it is not effective for high-resolution anatomical imaging. Radiopharmaceuticals or radiotracers for SPECT are composed of the radionuclides decaying by γ-ray emission [54]. The γ-rays with energy greater than 30 keV have minimal absorption by the body and are preferable for SPECT. The commonly used SPECT tracers are the complexes of radioactive transition metal chelates (e.g., In-111 and Tc-99m) that have relatively short half-lives [55–58]. Targeted imaging probes have been developed by conjugating the radioactive complexes to targeting agents for molecular imaging of biomarkers [58]. Organic compounds labeled with radioactive iodine are also used as SPECT imaging agents [59]. SPECT is effective for noninvasive investigation of the *in vivo* drug delivery process. It can be used for quantitative measurement of pharmacokinetics and delivery efficiency of drug delivery systems and noninvasive evaluation of therapeutic response [60–62]. Drug delivery systems can be labeled with radioactive isotopes through chemical conjugation or modification allowing for pharmacokinetics and biodistribution of the labeled delivery systems to be quantitatively measured [63].

24.3.6 Positron Emission Tomography

PET also detects γ-rays from the body after administration of radiopharmaceuticals containing radionuclides that emit positrons [53, 64]. Each decay of PET radionuclides or probes emits one positron, which then annihilates with an electron in the tissue to give a pair of γ-rays with energy of 511 KeV at almost 180°. The γ-rays are recorded by detectors and processed by a computer to produce three-dimensional images. PET is highly sensitive for detecting its probes and generally is used for functional and molecular imaging. The commonly used PET isotopes are the derivatives of C-11, N-13, O-15, and F-18 isotopes [65]. Biologically active molecules are often labeled with these isotopes by replacing one or more atoms in their chemical structures while still maintaining their biological activity [66, 67]. PET is useful for noninvasive evaluation of the biological and pharmaceutical properties of a drug or drug candidate after labeling with a positron emitter [68]. The half-lives of C-11, N-13, O-15, and F-18 are 20.4, 9.96, 2.07, and 109.7 min. An on-site cyclotron is required for the production of positron emitters before imaging. Positron emitters with a relatively long half-life, e.g., ^{64}Cu(II), have been used to label drug delivery systems [69–73]. The probes with a longer half-life allow for continuous tracking *in vivo* drug delivery for several days.

24.4 MOLECULAR IMAGING OF DRUG DELIVERY

Drug delivery is a process of transporting therapeutics to diseased tissues and cells to achieve enhanced therapeutic efficacy. Molecular imaging provides a noninvasive tool for investigating the mechanism and process of drug delivery. Intracellular and *in vivo* delivery processes can be visualized continuously by molecular imaging by labeling drug delivery systems with imaging probes. The drug delivery efficiency can also be determined quantitatively by molecular imaging modalities, such as SPECT and PET. Molecular imaging provides more accurate assessment of whole-body pharmaceutical properties, including pharmacokinetics, biodistribution, targeting efficiency, and pharmacodynamics, of drug delivery systems than conventional methods in both preclinical and clinical development. Accurate determination of the delivery process of drug delivery systems using molecular imaging will assist the optimization, design, and development of more effective drug delivery systems.

24.4.1 Molecular Imaging of Intracellular Drug Delivery

Intracellular drug delivery is a critical step for many therapeutic agents, including chemotherapeutics, proteins, and nucleic acids, to achieve efficacious treatment. Confocal microscopic fluorescence imaging is used routinely for investigating intracellular delivery, including target binding, cellular interaction, intracellular trafficking, and drug release, of drug delivery systems. Targeting agents and delivery systems can be labeled readily with a fluorophore to allow for imaging cellular binding of the targeting agents and delivery systems, and the intracellular behavior of the systems. Some drug compounds have intrinsic fluorescence and their drug delivery systems can be evaluated directly with fluorescence imaging to track the intracellular fate of the drug [74]. Drug carriers can also be labeled with a fluorophore with a different emission wavelength to study the intracellular fate of both the drug and the carrier.

Monoclonal antibodies bind to their targets specifically and are often used as targeting agents for targeted drug delivery. The binding of antibodies to their targets on cell surface can be visualized by confocal fluorescence imaging after they are labeled with a fluorophore. Figure 24.1 shows the confocal fluorescence images of OVCAR-3 cancer cells after incubation with an OV-TL 16 antibody labeled with rhodamine isothiocyanate (RITC) at 0 °C [75]. Confocal fluorescence imaging clearly revealed the recognition and binding of the antibody to its receptor on OVCAR-3 cell surface. The strong fluorescence signal on the cell surface indicated the binding of the antibody to the cancer cells. Because the cells were incubated with the labeled antibody at the low temperature, the bound antibody remained on the cell surface with minimal internalization [75].

Confocal fluorescence microscopy is effective to visualize the intracellular properties of drug delivery systems. Figure 24.2 shows the intracellular fate of *N*-(2-hydroxypropyl)methacrylamide (HPMA) co-polymers revealed by confocal fluorescence microscope [76]. HPMA co-polymers are biocompatible water-soluble drug carriers and have been used for preparing drug conjugates for the delivery of anticancer drugs. Dynamic confocal fluorescence images clearly showed the nuclear localization of the fluorescence-labeled co-polymers after cytoplasmic injection. The labeled polymers entered the nucleus as early as 15 min and substantially localized in the nucleus by 60 min postinjection. The strong presence of the conjugate in the nucleus was maintained for at least 24 h, indicating the preferential nuclear partition of the polymers [76].

Figure 24.3 shows the confocal fluorescence images of the intracellular uptake of an antibody fragment Fab′ targeted HPMA co-polymer Mce_6 conjugate in OVCAR-3 human ovarian carcinoma cells [41]. Mesochlorin e_6 (Mce_6) is a photosensitizer for photodynamic therapy and has intrinsic fluorescence. OV-TL 16 antibody Fab′ fragment targeted HPMA co-polymer Mce_6 conjugate was prepared for targeted delivery of Mce_6 for photodynamic therapy of ovarian cancer. The targeted Mce_6 conjugate demonstrated cytotoxicity two orders of magnitude higher than a nontargeted HPMA co-polymer Mce_6 conjugate. Confocal fluorescence imaging based on the fluorescence of Mce_6 revealed high cellular uptake of the targeted polymer Mce_6 conjugate in OVCAR-3 cancer cells 6 h after the incubation, whereas little uptake was observed with the nontargeted conjugate. High

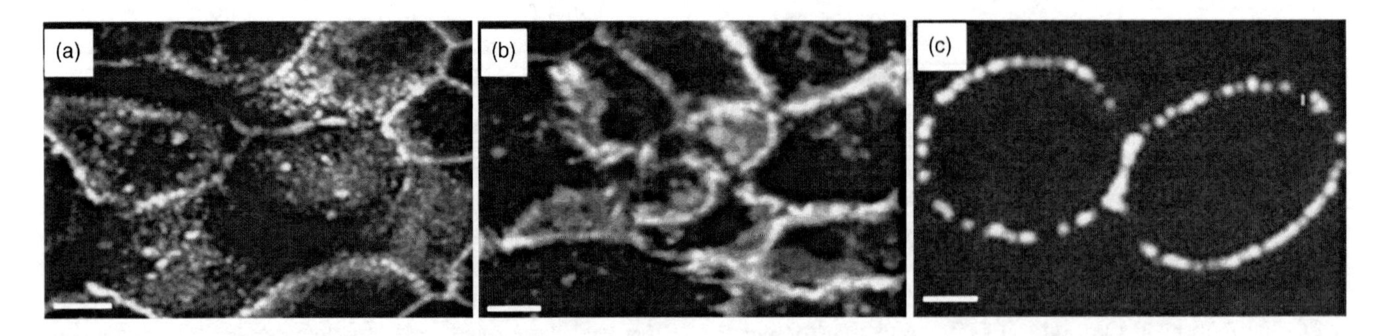

FIGURE 24.1 The binding of the OV-TL16 antibody to the cell surface of human ovarian carcinoma OVCAR-3 cells. Fluorescence images show the upper cell surface (a) and an optical section through the bottom part (b) of a cluster of cells, and an optical section through the lower middle region of mitotic cells (c). Bar: 5 μm. Adapted from Ref. 75.

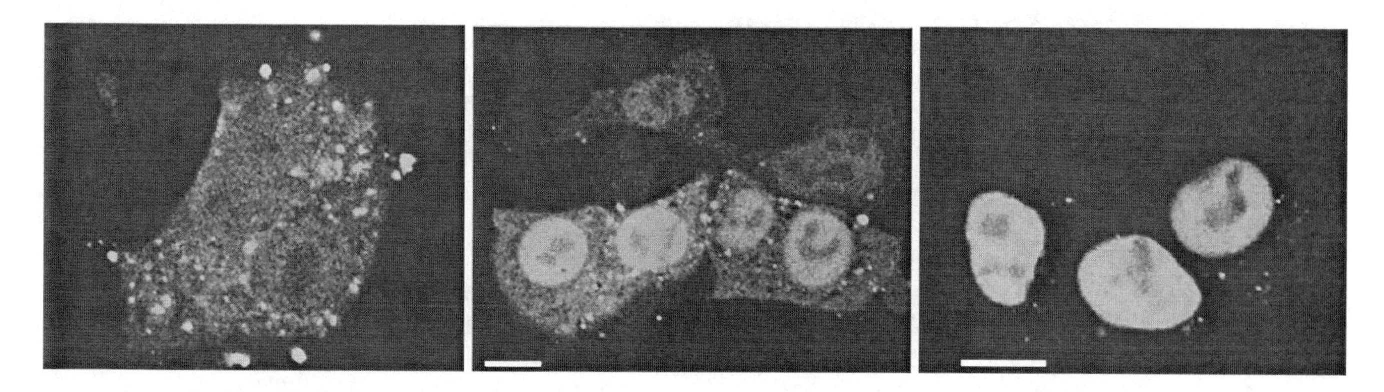

FIGURE 24.2 Confocal images of Hep G2 cells at 15 min (left), 60 (middle) min, and 24 h (right) after cytoplasmic injection of fluorescein-labeled HPMA co-polymers. Adapted from Ref. 76. (See color figure in color plate section.)

intracellular uptake of the targeted conjugate correlated very well with its high cytotoxicity. Fluorescence imaging also showed punctuated intracellular distribution of the targeted conjugate, indicating the presence of the drug conjugate in the endosomal-lysosomal compartments. The results obtained from *in vitro* imaging study can be predictive of the therapeutic efficacy of the drug delivery systems in their early development stage [77].

24.4.2 Molecular Imaging of *In Vivo* Drug Delivery

The pharmacokinetics, biodistribution, and *in vivo* drug delivery efficiency of drug delivery systems are evaluated traditionally by blood and urine sampling and surgery-based methods. These methods are typically invasive and require a large number of animals in preclinical studies. Furthermore, the pharmacokinetic data obtained with surgical methods cannot reflect accurately the true biodistribution in tissues. Molecular imaging allows for noninvasive longitudinal visualization of pharmacokinetics of drug delivery systems in a small number of experimental subjects after they are labeled with imaging probes or contrast agents. Fluorescence imaging, MRI, SPECT, PET, and ultrasound imaging can be used for noninvasive evaluation of drug delivery systems. Fluorescence imaging is suitable for the study of the drug delivery into superficial tissues because of shallow light penetration [37]. Contrast-enhanced MRI provides high-resolution and whole-body visualization of the pharmacokinetics and biodistribution of drug delivery systems after being labeled with an MRI contrast agent [27]. SPECT and PET can provide sensitive and quantitative measurement of radioactively labeled drug delivery systems [53, 72]. Ultrasound imaging is effective for evaluation of microbubble based delivery systems [38].

HPMA co-polymers were labeled with an MRI contrast agent Gd-DOTA for investigating their *in vivo* properties by MRI in animal models [27, 78]. pHPMA-GFLG-(Gd-DOTA) conjugates of 28, 60, and 121 kDa were prepared

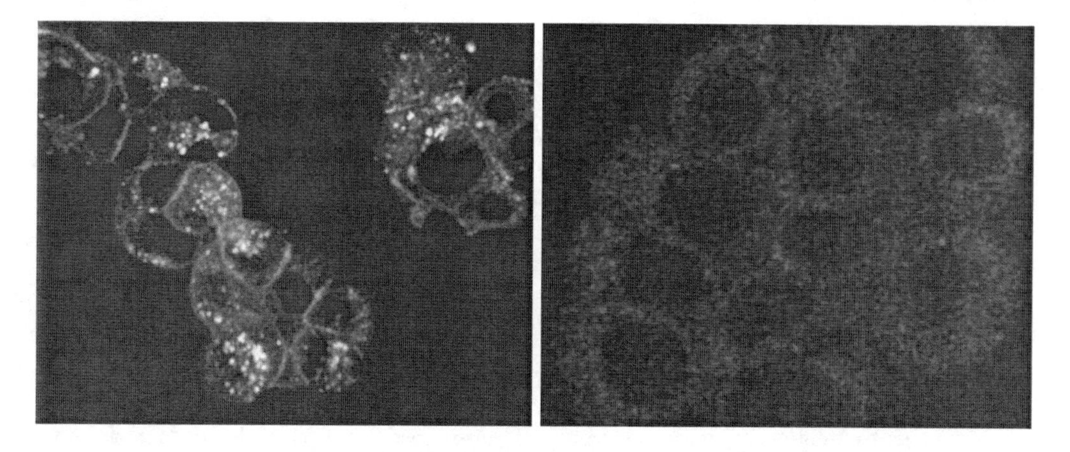

FIGURE 24.3 Confocal fluorescence images of OVCAR-3 human ovarian cancer cells after 6 h of incubation at 37 °C with the OV-TL16 antibody Fab′ fragment targeted pHPMA-Mce_6 conjugate (left) and pHPMA-Mce_6 conjugate (right) based on the intrinsic fluorescence of Mce_6.

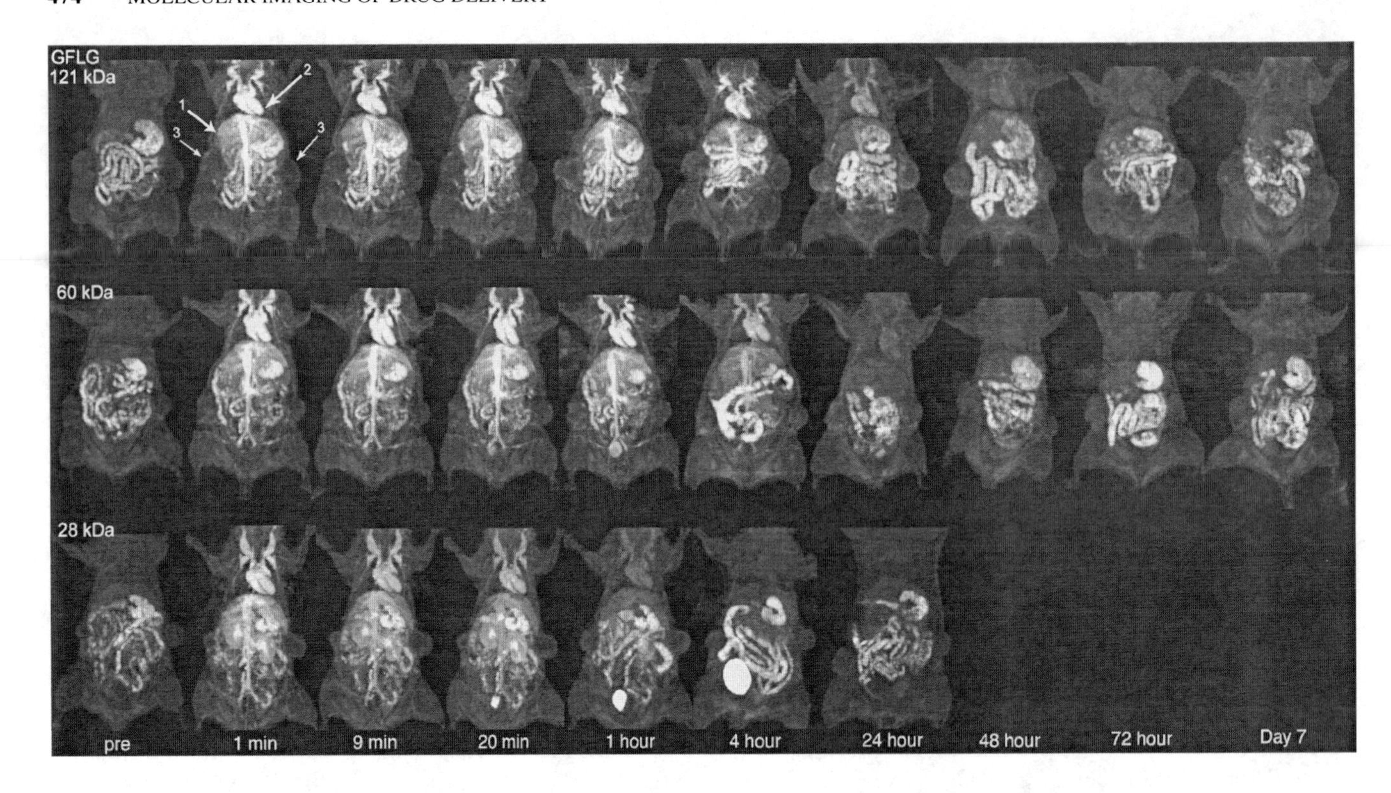

FIGURE 24.4 Three-dimensional MIP MR images of mice bearing MDA-MB-231 human breast carcinoma xenografts injected with pHPMA-GFLG-(Gd-DOTA monoamide) conjugates with molecular weights of 28, 60, and 121 kDa before contrast and at various time points after the injection of the conjugates at a dose of 0.03 mmol-Gd/kg. Arrows are pointing to the liver (1), heart (2), and tumor (3). Bright signal in the blood and the fluid of the urinary bladder indicates a high concentration of the conjugate. The bright signal from the stomach and intestine is from the food and fluid. Adapted from Ref. 27.

by co-polymerization of HPMA with a monomer containing Gd-DOTA and by fractionation with size exclusion chromatography. Figure 24.4 shows the representative three-dimensional T_1-weighted dynamic MR images of mice bearing MDA-MB-231 human breast carcinoma xenografts before and after the injection of the pHPMA-GFLG-(Gd-DO3A) conjugates at a dose of 0.03 mmol-Gd/kg [27]. The three-dimensional MR images clearly revealed the whole-body distribution of the conjugates of different molecular weights. The brightness of images in the organs and tissues indirectly reflected the biodistribution of the conjugates in the body. The bright signals indicated high concentration in the tissues, with the exception of the intestines and stomach, in which the bright signal was from the food in the gastrointestinal tract. The size-dependent pharmacokinetics and biodistribution of the conjugates in the blood, liver, and kidneys were shown clearly in the dynamic MR images. The high-molecular-weight HPMA conjugates had more prolonged blood circulation than the low-molecular-weight conjugates. The low-molecular-weight conjugates cleared more rapidly from the blood circulation via renal filtration than the high-molecular-weight conjugates, resulting in a strong MR signal in the urinary bladder.

Prolonged blood circulation of the high-molecular-weight conjugates resulted in high and prolonged tumor accumulation of the polymers. Figure 24.5 shows the color-coded 2D T_1-weighted spin-echo high-resolution images of tumor tissues before and after the injection of the labeled HPMA co-polymers [27]. MR images revealed the size-dependent gradual tumor accumulation and heterogeneous distribution of the conjugates. The color intensity reflects the concentration of the conjugates in tumor tissue. The dynamic MRI data showed that the high-molecular-weight polymer drug conjugates were more effective for tumor drug delivery than the low-molecular-weight conjugates.

The effectiveness of SPECT for visualizing biodistribution of drug delivery systems labeled with radioactive isotopes was demonstrated with a radioactively labeled HPMA co-polymer drug conjugate. Galactosamine targeted pHPMA-GlyPhe-LeuGly-Dox (PK2, Mw = 31 kDa) was developed for targeted delivery of an anticancer drug doxorubicin to treat liver cancer. The biodistribution of the liver-targeting drug conjugate in human patients was evaluated noninvasively with SPECT [79]. The conjugate was labeled with a γ-emitter ^{123}I and the whole-body biodistribution of the labeled conjugate was visualized by SPECT. Figure 24.6 shows the whole-body

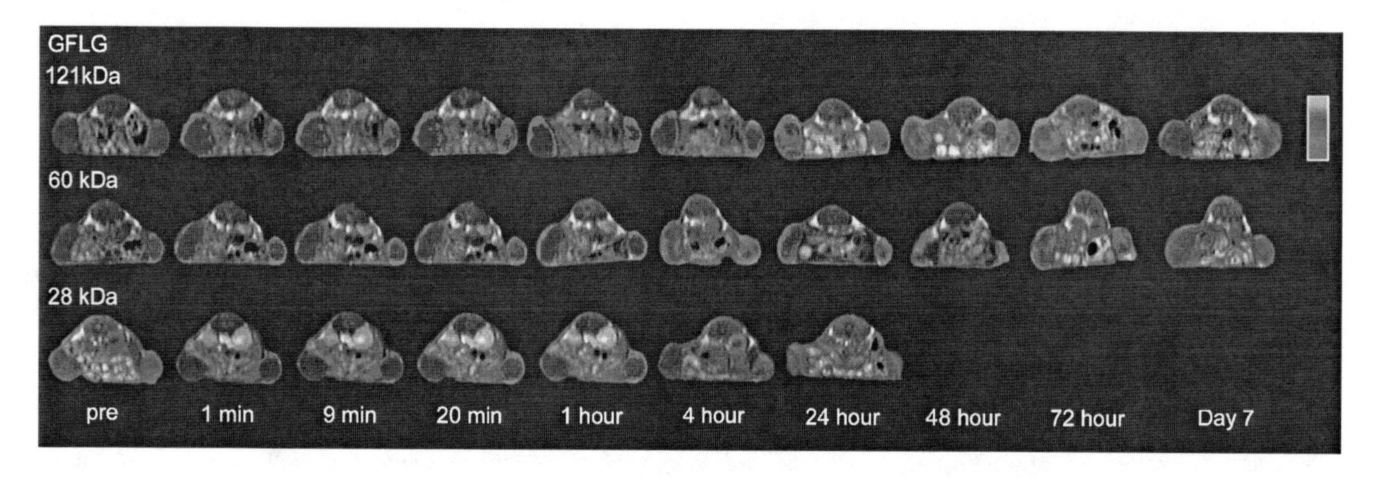

FIGURE 24.5 Color-coded 2D axial spin-echo MR images of mice injected with pHPMA-GFLG-(Gd-DOTA monoamide) conjugates with molecular weights of 28, 60, and 121 kDa before contrast and at various time points after the injection of the conjugates at a dose of 0.03 mmol-Gd/kg. The color distribution represents the accumulation and distribution of the conjugates. Adapted from Ref. 27.

images of the biodistribution of the labeled PK2 in a patient at different time points after the infusion [79]. Strong signal intensity in the liver was shown at 4 h and maintained at 48 h postinjection, indicating strong liver accumulation of the targeted conjugate. SPECT allows noninvasive evaluation of the whole-body biodistribution in human patients, which is not possible with conventional methods.

Liposomes are nanosized delivery systems for chemotherapeutics, biologics, and nucleic acids and have been approved for clinical use [80, 81]. Imaging agents or probes can be encapsulated readily inside liposomes or incorporated

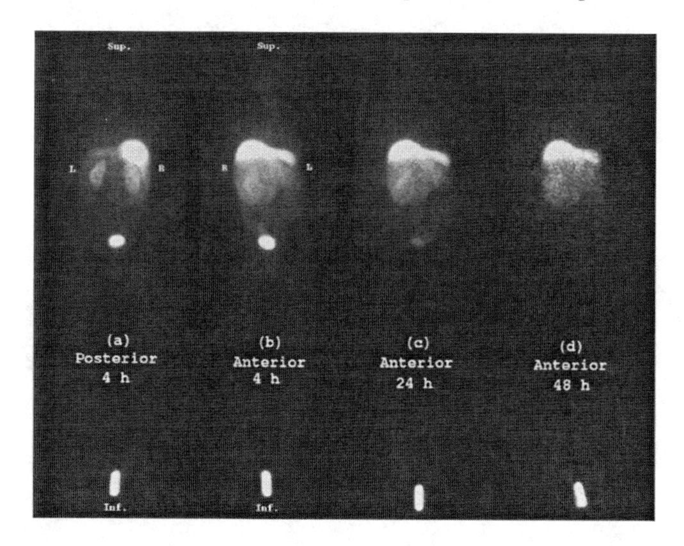

FIGURE 24.6 Whole body SPECT images of ^{123}I-labeled galactosamine targeted pHPMA-DOX conjugate (PK2) of a patient acquired at 4 h (posterior view) and 4, 24, and 48 h (anterior view) after the end of infusion. The bright signal indicates the concentration of the conjugate. Adapted from Ref. 79.

in the lipid bilayers for noninvasive evaluation of the liposomes in both preclinical and clinical development [28, 60, 63]. Multiple imaging agents can also be incorporated into liposomes to allow for multimodality imaging of the delivery systems [63]. The *in vivo* properties, including pharmacokinetics and biodistribution, of labeled liposomes can be evaluated continuously and noninvasively by molecular imaging in both preclinical and clinical development. For example, liposomal drug delivery systems are often PEGylated to minimize nonspecific tissue interactions, prolong blood circulation, and enhance tumor drug accumulation [82–84]. The *in vivo* drug delivery efficiency and whole-body biodistribution of a PEGylated liposomal drug delivery system in patients was evaluated continuously by γ-scintigraphy and SPECT after it was labeled by a (In-111)-DTPA chelate [85]. The serial γ-scintigraphic images after administration of the PEGylated liposomes labeled with (In-111)-DTPA for up to a week clearly revealed the dynamic whole-body biodistribution, gradual clearance from the blood circulation, and prolonged tumor accumulation of the labeled liposomes. Detailed three-dimensional information on tumor accumulation of liposomes can be obtained by SPECT [85].

Microbubbles have been used for the delivery of therapeutic agents, including anticancer drugs and plasmid DNA [15, 86–90]. The combination of ultrasound imaging and drug delivery allows for tracking the localization of the drug loading microbubbles in the body. The microbubbles can then be destroyed specifically in the target tissues by focused ultrasound under imaging guidance to release the drug payloads. For example, doxorubicin was loaded to perfluoropentane microbubbles coated with block co-polymers for both ultrasonic cancer imaging and targeted cancer therapy [91]. Tumor accumulation of the drug-loading microbubbles was visualized by ultrasound imaging. The microbubbles were then activated with tumor-targeted ultrasound to facilitate the intratumoral drug release. The combination approach resulted in significant tumor regression in a mouse tumor model [91]. The microbubbles have also been used for ultrasound guided delivery and release of proteins and nucleic acids [90, 92, 93].

24.5 IMAGING THERAPEUTIC EFFICACY OF DRUG DELIVERY SYSTEMS

Early and accurate evaluation of the effectiveness and therapeutic efficacy of drug delivery systems is crucial for accurate identification of promising drug delivery systems for further development. Molecular imaging is an effective tool for rapid and accurate assessment of therapeutic efficacy of drug delivery systems in both preclinical and clinical studies. Traditionally, biomedical imaging is used to evaluate therapeutic efficacy based on the morphological changes of a target tissue in response to a treatment. However, visible morphological change may take a long time to develop after the treatment if there is any change at all. Molecular imaging provides a timely assessment of therapeutic efficacy based on accurate measurements of molecular, metabolic, and physiological properties before any significant morphological change of the target tissues [94]. Bioluminescence imaging with reporter genes is an effective tool for noninvasive determination of transfection efficiency of gene delivery systems and gene silencing efficiency of small interfering RNA (siRNA) delivery systems in animal models. Nuclear medicine is used commonly for the assessment of the molecular and metabolic changes [95–98]. Molecular changes can also be determined by magnetic resonance spectroscopy (MRS) [99, 100]. The physiological responses based on vascular and tissue permeability and perfusion can be determined by dynamic contrast-enhanced MRI [101–104].

24.5.1 Bioluminescence Imaging of *In Vivo* Transfection Efficiency of Nucleic Acids

Gene therapy has a potential to treat various human diseases. Effective gene therapy requires efficient delivery and transfection of therapeutic nucleic acids, including both DNA and RNA, into the cells in target tissues [105–107]. Bioluminescence imaging is an effective modality to determine noninvasively the real-time transfection efficiency of a delivery system with a reporter gene [108, 109]. Firefly luciferase is used commonly as a reporter gene for determining the delivery and transfection efficiency of gene delivery systems in animal models. D-Luciferin is required for bioluminescence imaging with firefly luciferase. The biochemical reaction of luciferase with D-luciferin emits luminescence light with a wavelength about 560 nm. Luciferase activity can be determined quantitatively based on luminescence intensity recorded by an imaging system and used for assessing the transfection efficiency of the delivery system.

Plasmid DNA expressing firefly luciferase is often used for evaluating *in vitro* and *in vivo* transfection of gene delivery systems. The plasmid DNA can be incorporated readily into various delivery systems, including both viral and nonviral delivery systems [43, 110–114]. Transfection efficiency of the delivery systems can be determined readily based on the luciferase activity in the target tissue measured by a bioluminescence imaging system. For example, cationic PAMAM dendrimers are used as the carriers for gene delivery [115, 116]. The tumor gene transfection efficiency of a generation-5 PAMAM dendrimer in a mouse tumor model after systemic administration was revealed clearly by bioluminescence imaging with a CpG free hEF1 alpha-driven plasmid DNA encoding firefly luciferase. Figure 24.7 shows the dynamic bioluminescence images in the tumor of an A/J mouse bearing Neuro2a tumor xenograft after transfection luciferase gene with G5 dendrimer [115]. The dendrimer resulted in strong luciferase activity in tumor up to 3 days after injection. Significant luciferase activity could be

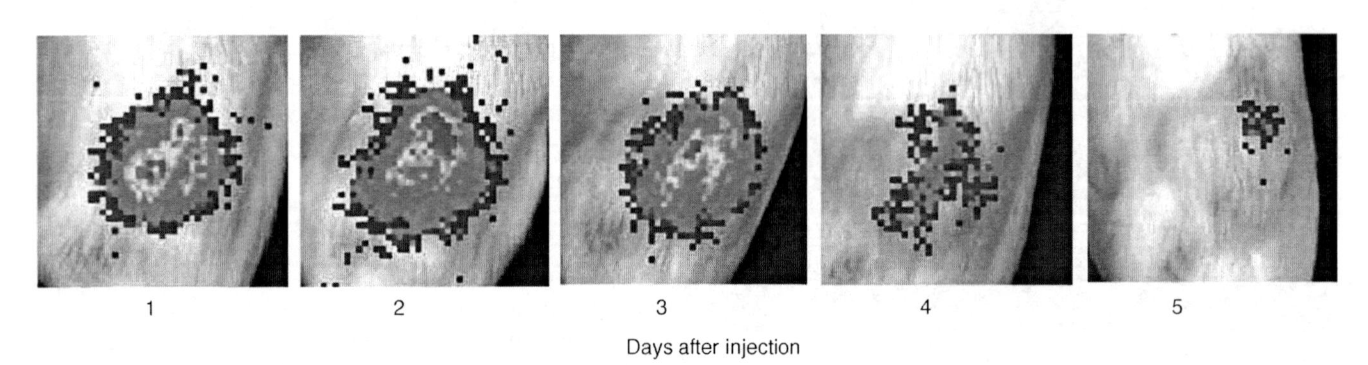

FIGURE 24.7 Dynamic bioluminescence images of an A/J mouse bearing Neuro2a tumor xenograft at different days after intravenous injection of pCpG-hCMV-Luc/PAMAM G5 polyplexes. Blue color represents the lowest intensity and red for the highest intensity. Adapted from Ref. 115. (See color figure in color plate section.)

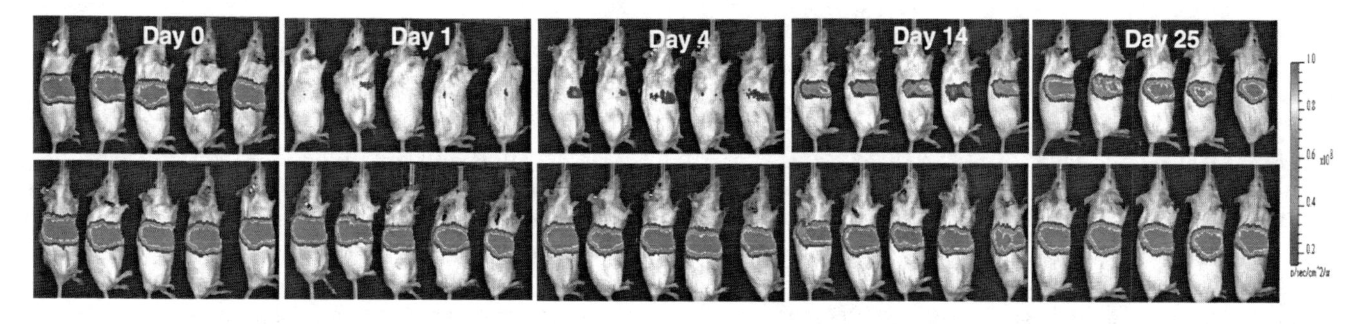

FIGURE 24.8 Color-coded bioluminescence images of a group of mice with constitutive expression of luciferase in the liver before and after the treatment with a lipid nanoparticle of antiluciferase siRNA at 3 mg/kg. Blue color represents the lowest intensity and red for the highest intensity. Adapted from Ref. 123. (See color figure in color plate section.)

still observed on day 5. The bioluminescence study revealed that the G5 PAMAM dendrimer could result in transient gene expression in the tumor up to 5 days in the tested animal model.

RNA interference (RNAi) is a natural biological process using siRNA to control gene expression [117–120]. RNAi with siRNA has a potential to treat human diseases by regulating disease-related genes. Bioluminescence imaging with firefly luciferase reporter gene is also effective for noninvasive real-time evaluation of the *in vitro* and *in vivo* gene silencing efficiency of siRNA delivery systems [121, 122]. Transfection efficiency or pharmacodynamics of siRNA delivery systems can be determined quantitatively by silencing luciferase activity in target cells or tissues with an antiluciferase siRNA. When the siRNA is transfected in target cells with constitutive expression of luciferase reporter gene, it induces the RNAi machinery to destroy luciferase messenger RNA (mRNA) and blocks luciferase expression, resulting in a decrease of luciferase activity. Figure 24.8 shows the bioluminescence images of a group of mice with luciferase expression in the liver before and after the treatment with a lipid siRNA nanoparticle [123]. It was observed that luciferase mRNA could be correlated linearly to bioluminescence [123, 124]. As revealed by bioluminescence imaging, the lipid siRNA nanoparticle resulted in the maximum silencing efficiency in the liver 3 days after the treatment. It took about 25 days for bioluminescence to recover to the pretreatment level after a single dose of 3 or 6 mg/kg. The pharmacodynamic properties determined by noninvasive bioluminescence imaging are valuable for the identification of suitable delivery systems for further development.

24.5.2 Therapeutic Efficacy Evaluation with PET

PET with ^{18}F-FDG is a commonly used method for noninvasive imaging of tissue metabolism in response to therapies in preclinical and clinical studies [125]. It measures metabolic activities of the tissue of interest based on quantification of ^{18}F-FDG uptake. ^{18}F-FDG is a glucose derivative and is taken by cells via glucose membrane transporters. ^{18}F-FDG is trapped in the cells of high glucose uptake and metabolic activities after it converts to ^{18}F-FDG-6-phosphate, which cannot be metabolized further. ^{18}F-FDG-PET can thereby differentiate tissues of high metabolic activities from less active tissues. Proliferative tumor tissues are highly metabolic active and have higher accumulation of ^{18}F-FDG than normal tissues, generating a stronger PET signal. ^{18}F-FDG-PET is used routinely in clinical practice for evaluating the efficacy of anticancer therapies and predicting therapeutic outcomes [126, 127]. Dual imaging modalities, e.g., PET/CT and PET/MRI, are available to correlate PET imaging with high-resolution anatomic images from CT and MRI [128–130].

FDG-PET is an effective tool for assessing the therapeutic efficacy of drug delivery systems in preclinical and clinical development [131–133]. If an anticancer drug delivery system can prevent tumor growth and kill cancer cells effectively, then a significant signal reduction can be observed in PET images compared with the pretreatment level before any morphological changes can be observed. High-resolution small-animal PET and PET/CT are available for the evaluation of drug delivery systems in small animal models. The tumor response to a delivery system can be detected by FDG-PET as early as 1 h after the treatment [134]. Significant signal reduction and decrease of ^{18}F-FDG uptake in the treated tumor was observed at 1 h after the initiation of photodynamic therapy, whereas little change was observed in the untreated control tumor.

24.5.3 Therapeutic Efficacy Evaluation with Dynamic Contrast Enhanced (DCE) MRI

DCE MRI measures the uptake kinetics of an MRI contrast agent in the tissue of interest [101]. Vascular parameters, including blood volume and vascular permeability, can be readily calculated from the uptake kinetics of the contrast agent [135–137]. The vascular parameters measured by DCE-MRI are feasible quantitative biomarkers for noninvasive evaluation of the therapeutic efficacy of drug delivery systems. In oncology, malignant tumors are highly angiogenic and have high vascular permeability. Effective cancer treatment generally results in the reduction of tumor angiogenesis and decreased vascular permeability. DCE-MRI can measure the accurate changes of the tumor vascular parameters as early as a few hours after the initiation of the treatment [138]. The size of MRI contrast agents has a significant impact on the accurate characterization of tumor vascular parameters with DCE-MRI. Preclinical studies have shown that macromolecular MRI contrast agents are more effective for quantitative measurement of tumor vascular parameters than low-molecular-weight contrast agents in DCE-MRI because of their preferential permeation through angiogenic blood vessels [138–141].

Figure 24.9 shows the representative signal enhancement (ΔSI)–time curves in the tumor periphery of a biodegradable macromolecular MRI contrast agent GDCC-40 and a low-molecular-weight agent Gd(DTPA-BMA) before and after the treatment with the antiangiogenic drug Avastin® in a mouse colon cancer model [102]. GDCC-40, Gd-DTPA cystamine co-polymers with a molecular weight of 40 kDa, is a biodegradable macromolecular contrast agent designed to facilitate the excretion of the contrast agent and to minimize the retention of toxic Gd(III) ions [142]. The signal-time curves measured by DCE-MRI represent the tumor uptake kinetics of the contrast agents. An approximately 50% decrease of uptake of GDCC-40 was observed in the tumor periphery at 36 h after the initial treatment compared with the uptake before the treatment. The uptake of GDCC-40 increased slightly at 7 days after the treatment with Avastin compared with that measured at 36 h after the first injection. DCE-MRI with Gd(DTPA-BMA) did not show significant changes of Gd(DTPA-BMA) uptake in tumor before and after the treatment with Avastin.

The vascular parameters of tumor tissues can be calculated by suitable pharmacokinetic models from the DCE-MRI data. A two-compartment bidirectional exchange kinetic model $C_T(t) = K^{trans} \int_0^t C_p(\theta) e^{-k_{ep}(t-\theta)} d\theta + f^{PV} C_p(t)$ is used to calculate the vascular parameters K^{trans} and f^{PV} from the signal enhancement (ΔSI)–time data in Figure 24.9 [102, 143]. $C_p(t)$ and $C_T(t)$ are the contrast agent concentrations in plasma and in the tumor. K^{trans} is the endothelial transfer coefficient, k_{ep} is the rate constant of reflux from the extravascular and extracellular space (EES) back to blood, θ is a Laplace operator, and f^{PV} is the fractional plasma volume. At low-contrast-agent concentrations in DCE-MRI studies, the assumption of the linear correlation of MRI signal to the concentration of a contrast agent is often used in fitting the DCE-MRI data. The calculated K^{trans} and f^{PV} parameters from the DCE-MRI data with the agents GDCC-40 and Gd(DTPA-BMA) before and after the treatments with Avastin are plotted in Figure 24.10. Both K^{trans} and f^{PV} values in tumor periphery obtained from DCE-MRI with GDCC-40 significantly decreased at 36 h after the treatment compared with the pretreatment values ($p < 0.05$). The values increased at 7 days after three treatments and were similar to the

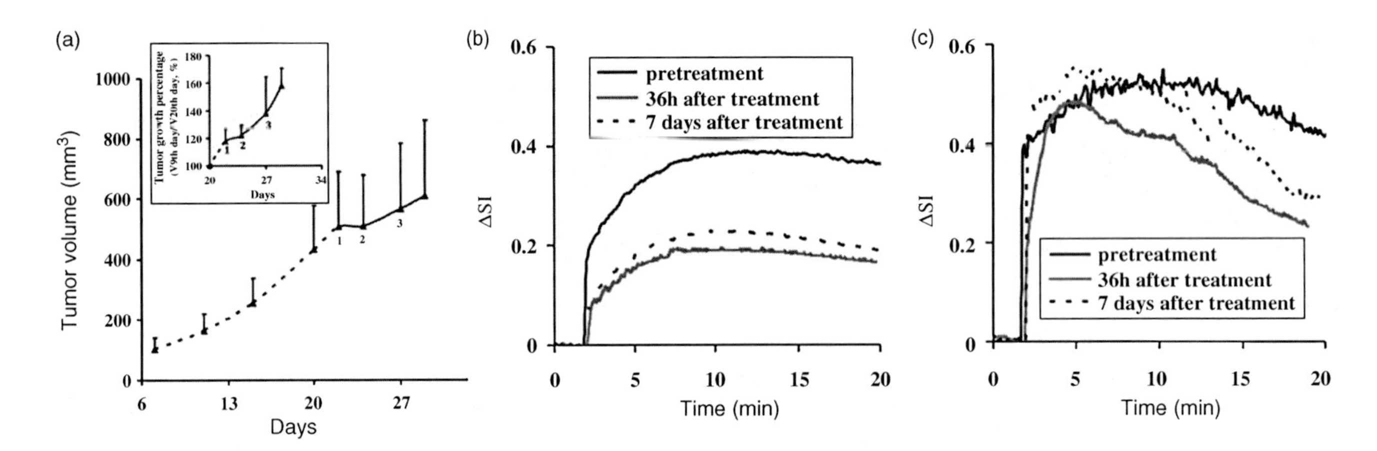

FIGURE 24.9 Tumor volume and normalized tumor growth percentage relative to the tumor size of the day 20 (inset) before and after treatment with Avastin (a) and dynamic signal changes in the tumor before and after the treatment measured by DCE-MRI with (Gd-DTPA)-cystamine co-polymers (40 kDa, b) and Gd(DTPA-BMA) (c). Treatment was started on the day 22 by intraperitoneal administration of Avastin at a dose of 200 μg/mouse every 2 days in 6 days. 1: First treatment; 2: second treatment; 3: third treatment. Tumor growth was temporarily arrested by initial administration of Avastin and then resumed at a slower rate even after the second and third administrations. Adapted from Ref. 102.

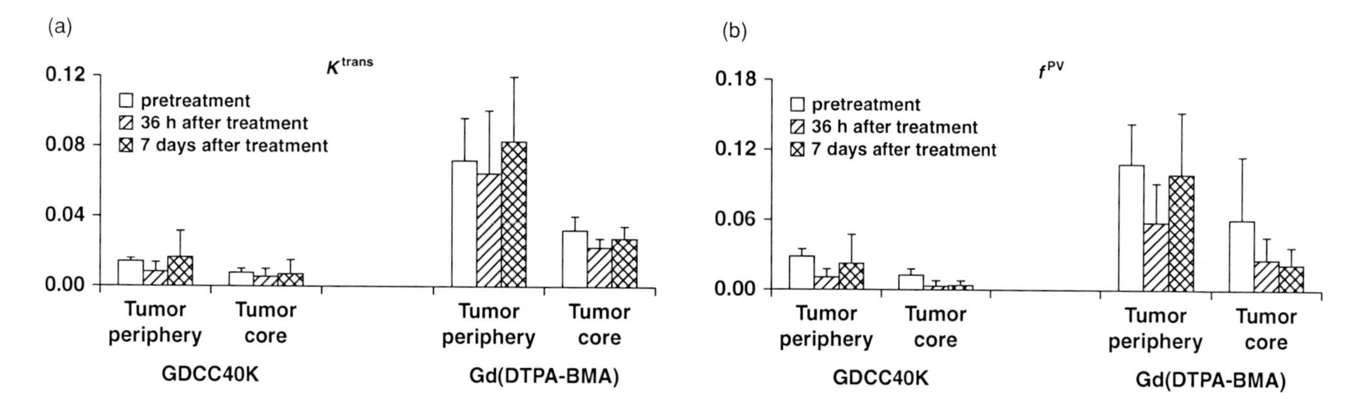

FIGURE 24.10 The vascular parameters K^{trans} (a) and f^{PV} (b) for GDCC-40 and Gd(DTPA-BMA) before and after Avastin administration calculated from the DCE-MRI data in Figure 24.9b and c. $^{*}p < 0.05$. K^{trans} = endothelial transfer coefficient (mL of plasma/mL of tissue/min), f^{PV} = fractional vascular volume (mL of plasma/mL of tissue). Adapted from Ref. 102.

pretreatment values ($p > 0.05$). The data correlated well to the tumor volume changes in response to the treatment. In comparison, the K^{trans} and f^{PV} in both tumor periphery and tumor core estimated from DCE-MRI with Gd(DTPA-BMA) after treatments were not significantly different from the pretreatment values ($p > 0.05$).

DCE-MRI with macromolecular contrast agents provides more accurate assessment of the therapeutic efficacy of cancer therapies than low-molecular MRI contrast agents. Currently, no macromolecular MRI contrast agent has been approved for clinical use. Nevertheless, DCE-MRI with macromolecular agents is an effective tool for noninvasive evaluation of therapeutic efficacy of drug delivery systems in preclinical development.

24.6 THERANOSTICS

Theranostics is the combination of therapeutics and diagnostics for achieving individualized pharmacotherapy. It measures a diverse set of biomarkers, including genomic, proteomic, metabolic, and physiological biomarkers; predicts patients' response to therapies; and determines the best treatment to achieve the best possible therapeutic outcomes. The combination of drug delivery and molecular imaging produces a novel class of theranostics [144, 145]. Various theranostics have been reported by the incorporation of therapeutics and diagnostics on the same polymer or nanoparticle drug delivery platform [146–148]. Theranostics allow for noninvasive tracking of drug delivery with molecular imaging, delivery of both imaging agent and therapeutics to the target site for diagnosis and therapy, and rapid assessment of responses to the therapies. The concept of drug delivery based theranostics can be illustrated with a recent study of a bifunctional polymeric drug conjugate for image-guided photodynamic therapy.

Photodynamic therapy (PDT) is a minimally invasive therapeutic modality for cancer treatment [149–151]. It involves the delivery of photosensitizers to tumor tissues followed by activation with a laser of a specific wavelength. Accurate localization of tumor tissue is necessary for directing laser light to activate the photosensitizer in the tumor tissue. Poly(L-glutamic acid)-Mce$_6$-(Gd-DOTA) conjugate and its PEGylated conjugate were prepared for delivering an MRI contrast agent and a photosensitizer for tumor localization with MRI, noninvasive determination of tumor drug delivery and accumulation, and image-guided photodynamic therapy [152, 153]. The structures of the bifunctional conjugates are shown in Figure 24.11. Whole-body high-resolution MR images revealed the biodistribution of the bifunctional conjugates and the structural effect of the conjugates on their biodistribution in mice bearing a human breast cancer xenograft [153]. Figure 24.12 shows the representative three-dimensional maximum intensity projection (MIP) images of the mice before and at different time points after injection of PEG-PGA-(Gd-DOTA)-Mce$_6$, PGA-(Gd-DOTA)-Mce$_6$, and PGA-(Gd-DOTA) conjugates at a dose of 0.05 mmol-Gd/kg. The PEGylated conjugate had more prolonged vascular enhancement and less liver enhancement than the non-PEGylated conjugate and the control. PEGylation of the bifunctional conjugate significantly reduced nonspecific liver uptake and increased blood circulation.

The prolonged blood circulation of the PEGylated conjugate resulted in a higher tumor accumulation than the non-PEGylated PGA-(Gd-DO3A)-Mce$_6$. Figure 24.13 shows the dynamic signal-to-noise ratios (SNRs) of different conjugates in tumor. High SNR reflects high tumor accumulation of the PEGylated conjugate [153]. The PEGylated conjugate resulted in more effective tumor growth inhibition after photodynamic therapy than the non-PEGylated conjugate. Figure 24.14a shows the percentage of tumor size change

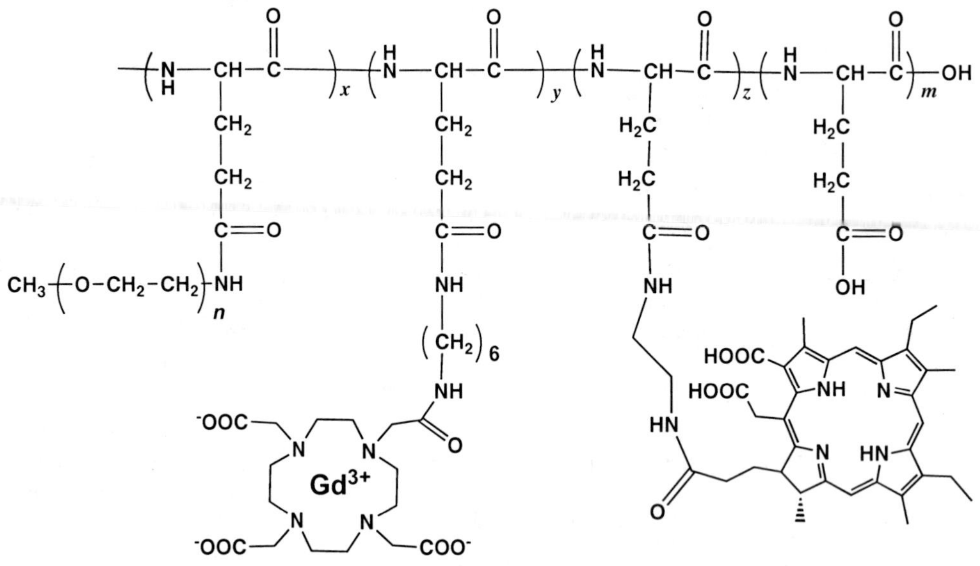

FIGURE 24.11 Structure of PEG-PGA-(Gd-DOTA monoamide)-Mce_6 conjugate.

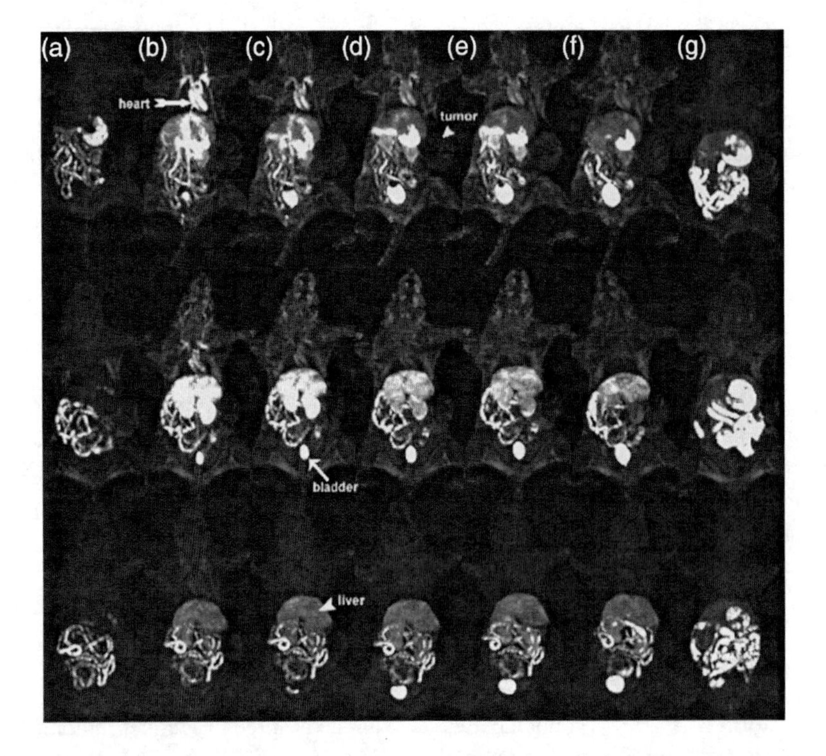

FIGURE 24.12 Three-dimensional MIP MR images of the mice bearing MDA-MB-231 breast tumor xenografts showing the biodistribution of PEG-PGA-(Gd-DO3A)-Mce_6 (top panel), PGA-(Gd-DO3A)-Mce_6 (middle panel), and PGA-(Gd-DO3A) (bottom panel) before (a) and at 2 min (b), 5 min (c), 15 min (d), 30 min (e), 2 h (f), and 18 h (g) postinjection at a dose of 0.05 mmol-Gd/kg. Bright signal in the blood and the fluid of the urinary bladder indicates a high concentration of the conjugate. The bright signal from the stomach and intestine is from the food and fluid. Adapted from Ref. 153.

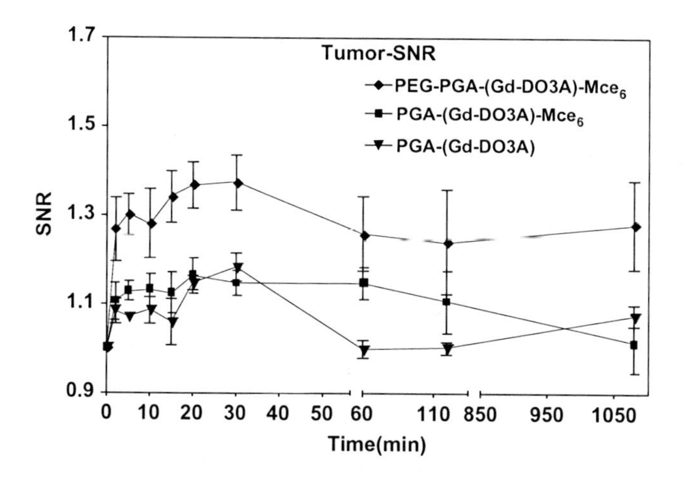

FIGURE 24.13 The signal-to-noise ratio (SNR) in the tumor of the mice bearing MDA-MB-231 breast tumor xenografts indicating the tumor concentration of PEG-PGA-(Gd-DO3A)-Mce_6, PGA-(Gd-DO3A)-Mce_6, and PGA-(Gd-DO3A) after the IV injection of the conjugates at a dose of 0.05 mmol-Gd/kg. Adapted from Ref. 153.

after the treatment with the PEGylated, non-PEGylated and control conjugates compared with that before the treatment. The therapeutic efficacy of different conjugates was also assessed noninvasively by dynamic contrast-enhanced MRI with a biodegradable macromolecular MRI contrast agent (Gd-DTPA)-cystine co-polymers. Figure 24.14b shows the dynamic change of relative signal intensity in the peripheral tumor tissues, representing tumor uptake kinetics of the contrast agent. Tumor uptake kinetics of the contrast agent could be correlated to tumor response to therapies or therapeutic efficacy. Generally, effective tumor treatment resulted in a decrease of tumor angiogenesis and reduced tumor vascular permeability to macromolecules, and consequently low tumor uptake kinetics measured by DCE-MRI. The tumor treated with the PEGylated PGA-(Gd-DOTA) conjugate had lower uptake kinetics than those treated with the non-PEGylated Mce_6 conjugate and control, indicating more significantly reduced vascular permeability of the tumors treated with the PEGylated conjugate and higher therapeutic efficacy. The tumor uptake kinetics of the contrast agent determined by DCE-MRI correlated well with the tumor growth after the treatment with different conjugates.

24.7 SUMMARY

Molecular imaging provides noninvasive methods for evaluating drug delivery systems in both preclinical and clinical development. The combination of molecular imaging and drug delivery allows for the design and development of more effective imaging agents and drug delivery systems. New drug delivery systems and therapeutic modalities with improved drug delivery efficiency and therapeutic efficacy can be developed with the assistance of molecular imaging. Personalized patient care can be tailored using the combination of molecular imaging and efficient drug delivery to achieve the maximum therapeutic outcome. Until now, molecular imaging had not yet reached its full potential for its application in drug delivery. Therefore, the continuous advancement of the integration of molecular imaging and

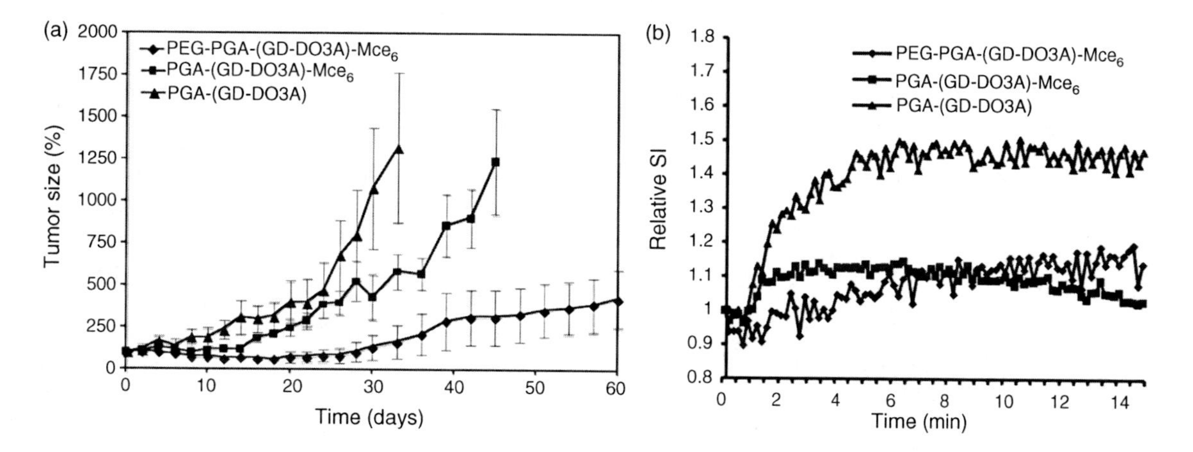

FIGURE 24.14 (a) Tumor growth curve, the percentage increase in relative tumor size, for the mice bearing MDA-MB-231 breast tumor xenografts after photodynamic treatments at 18 and 24 h postinjection of PEG-PGA-(Gd-DO3A)-Mce_6, PGA-(Gd-DO3A)-Mce_6 at a Mce_6 equivalent dose of 6.0 mg/kg, and PGA-(Gd-DO3A), at a dose of 0.045 mmol-Gd/kg. (b) Relative signal intensity plots of the DCE-MRI data showing the dynamic uptake of (Gd-DTPA)-cystine co-polymers in tumor periphery, which is rich of angiogenic blood vessels, of tumor bearing mice after PDT with the conjugates. Adapted from Ref. 153.

drug delivery will have a revolutionary impact on personalized patient care.

ASSESSMENT QUESTIONS

24.1. What are the characteristics of ultrasound imaging, optical imaging, magnetic resonance imaging, X-ray CT, SPECT, and PET, respectively?

24.2. What are the roles of molecular imaging in drug delivery?

24.3. What imaging modalities can be used for quantitative determination of a drug delivery system?

24.4. What are the differences between contrast-enhanced MRI and SPECT for determination of the biodistribution of the drug delivery systems?

24.5. What imaging agents can be used for labeling drug delivery systems for noninvasive visualization of their biodistribution?

24.6. What is the mechanism for (^{18}F)-FGD PET measuring the therapeutic efficacy of an anticancer drug delivery system?

24.7. How do you quantitatively determine the *in vivo* transfection efficiency of a cationic nonviral gene delivery system?

24.8. How do you measure *in vivo* gene silencing efficiency noninvasively in the tumor tissue of a siRNA delivery system in an animal tumor model?

24.9. How does dynamic contrast-enhanced MRI measure the therapeutic efficacy of a targeted liposomal drug delivery system containing an anticancer drug?

24.10. How does ultrasound technology work for image-guided drug delivery in cancer therapy?

24.11. What is theranostics? How does it work?

REFERENCES

1. Gross, S., Piwnica-Worms, D. (2006). Molecular imaging strategies for drug discovery and development. *Current Opinion in Chemical Biology*, *10*, 334–342.
2. Rudin, M., Weissleder, R. (2003). Molecular imaging in drug discovery and development. *Nature Reviews Drug Discovery*, *2*, 123–131.
3. Kelloff, G.J., Krohn, K.A., Larson, S.M., Weissleder, R., Mankoff, D.A., Hoffman, J.M., Link, J.M., Guyton, K.Z., Eckelman, W.C., Scher, H.I., O'Shaughnessy, J., Cheson, B. D., Sigman, C.C., Tatum, J.L., Mills, G.Q., Sullivan, D.C., Woodcock, J. (2005). The progress and promise of molecular imaging probes in oncologic drug development. *Clinical Cancer Research*, *11*, 7967–7985.
4. Willmann, J.K., van Bruggen, N., Dinkelborg, L.M., Gambhir, S.S. (2008). Molecular imaging in drug development. *Nature Reviews Drug Discovery*, *7*, 591–607.
5. Melancon, M.P., Elliott, A., Ji, X., Shetty, A., Yang, Z., Tian, M., Taylor, B., Stafford, R.J., Li, C. (2011). Theranostics with multifunctional magnetic gold nanoshells: Photothermal therapy and t2* magnetic resonance imaging. *Investigative Radiology*, *46*, 132–140.
6. Ng, K.K., Lovell, J.F., Zheng, G. (2011). Lipoprotein-inspired nanoparticles for cancer theranostics. *Accounts of Chemical Research*, *44(10)*, 1105–1113.
7. Sajja, H.K., East, M.P., Mao, H., Wang, Y.A., Nie, S., Yang, L. (2009). Development of multifunctional nanoparticles for targeted drug delivery and noninvasive imaging of therapeutic effect. *Current Drug Discovery Technologies*, *6*, 43–51.
8. Qin, S., Caskey, C.F., Ferrara, K.W. (2009). Ultrasound contrast microbubbles in imaging and therapy: Physical principles and engineering. *Physics in Medicine and Biology*, *54*, R27–57.
9. Deshpande, N., Needles, A., Willmann, J.K. (2010). Molecular ultrasound imaging: Current status and future directions. *Clinical Radiology*, *65*, 567–581.
10. Gessner, R., Dayton, P.A. (2010). Advances in molecular imaging with ultrasound. *Molecular Imaging*, *9*, 117–127.
11. Fayssoil, A. (2009). Tissue Doppler characterization of cardiac phenotype in mouse. *European Journal of Radiology*, *72*, 82–84.
12. Tsivgoulis, G., Alexandrov, A.V., Sloan, M.A. (2009). Advances in transcranial Doppler ultrasonography. *Current Neurology and Neuroscience Reports*, *9*, 46–54.
13. Klibanov, A.L. (2007). Ultrasound molecular imaging with targeted microbubble contrast agents. *Journal of Nuclear Cardiology*, *14*, 876–884.
14. Schneider, M. (2008). Molecular imaging and ultrasound-assisted drug delivery. *Journal of Endourology*, *22*, 795–802.
15. Klibanov, A.L. (2006). Microbubble contrast agents: Targeted ultrasound imaging and ultrasound-assisted drug-delivery applications. *Investigative Radiology*, *41*, 354–362.
16. Cosgrove, D., Harvey, C. (2009). Clinical uses of microbubbles in diagnosis and treatment. *Medical & Biological Engineering & Computing*, *47*, 813–826.
17. Klibanov, A.L. (2009). Preparation of targeted microbubbles: Ultrasound contrast agents for molecular imaging. *Medical & Biological Engineering & Computing*, *47*, 875–882.
18. Stride, E. (2009). Physical principles of microbubbles for ultrasound imaging and therapy. *Cerebrovascular Disease*, *27 Suppl 2*, 1–13.
19. Bohmer, M.R., Klibanov, A.L., Tiemann, K., Hall, C.S., Gruell, H., Steinbach, O.C. (2009). Ultrasound triggered image-guided drug delivery. *European Journal of Radiology*, *70*, 242–253.
20. Husseini, G.A., Pitt, W.G. (2009). Ultrasonic-activated micellar drug delivery for cancer treatment. *Journal of Pharmaceutical Sciences*, *98*, 795–811.

21. Pua, E.C., Zhong, P. (2009). Ultrasound-mediated drug delivery. *IEEE Engineering in Medicine and Biology Magazine*, *28*, 64–75.
22. Liang, Z.P., Lauterbur, P.C. *Principles of Magnetic Resonance Imaging: A Signal Processing Perspective*. IEEE Inc., New York, 2000.
23. Waters, E.A., Wickline, S.A. (2008). Contrast agents for MRI. *Basic Research in Cardiology*, *103*, 114–121.
24. Strijkers, G.J., Mulder, W.J., van Tilborg, G.A., Nicolay, K. (2007). MRI contrast agents: Current status and future perspectives. *Anticancer Agents in Medicinal Chemistry*, *7*, 291–305.
25. Caravan, P., Ellison, J.J., McMurry, T.J., Lauffer, R.B. (1999). Gadolinium(III). Chelates as MRI contrast agents: Structure, dynamics, and applications. *Chemical Reviews*, *99*, 2293–2352.
26. White, D.L. (1991). Paramagnetic iron (III) MRI contrast agents. *Magnetic Resonance in Medicine*, *22*, 309–312.
27. Wang, Y., Ye, F., Jeong, E.K., Sun, Y., Parker, D.L., Lu, Z.R. (2007). Noninvasive visualization of pharmacokinetics, biodistribution and tumor targeting of poly[*N*-(2-hydroxypropyl) methacrylamide] in mice using contrast enhanced MRI. *Pharmaceutical Research*, *24*, 1208–1216.
28. Mikhaylova, M., Stasinopoulos, I., Kato, Y., Artemov, D., Bhujwalla, Z.M. (2009). Imaging of cationic multifunctional liposome-mediated delivery of COX-2 siRNA. *Cancer Gene Therapy*, *16*, 217–226.
29. Erdogan, S., Medarova, Z.O., Roby, A., Moore, A., Torchilin, V.P. (2008). Enhanced tumor MR imaging with gadolinium-loaded polychelating polymer-containing tumor-targeted liposomes. *Journal of Magnetic Resonance Imaging*, *27*, 574–580.
30. Rowe, M.D., Thamm, D.H., Kraft, S.L., Boyes, S.G. (2009). Polymer-modified gadolinium metal-organic framework nanoparticles used as multifunctional nanomedicines for the targeted imaging and treatment of cancer. *Biomacromolecules*, *10*, 983–993.
31. Tan, M., Wu, X., Jeong, E.K., Chen, Q., Parker, D.L., Lu, Z.R. (2010). An effective targeted nanoglobular manganese(II) chelate conjugate for magnetic resonance molecular imaging of tumor extracellular matrix. *Molecular Pharmacology*, *7*, 936–943.
32. Erdogan, S., Torchilin, V.P. (2010). Gadolinium-loaded polychelating polymer-containing tumor-targeted liposomes. *Methods in Molecular Biology*, *605*, 321–334.
33. Chen, K., Xie, J., Xu, H., Behera, D., Michalski, M.H., Biswal, S., Wang, A., Chen, X. (2009). Triblock copolymer coated iron oxide nanoparticle conjugate for tumor integrin targeting. *Biomaterials*, *30*, 6912–6919.
34. Kiessling, F., Huppert, J., Zhang, C., Jayapaul, J., Zwick, S., Woenne, E.C., Mueller, M.M., Zentgraf, H., Eisenhut, M., Addadi, Y., Neeman, M., Semmler, W. (2009). RGD-labeled USPIO inhibits adhesion and endocytotic activity of alpha v beta3-integrin-expressing glioma cells and only accumulates in the vascular tumor compartment. *Radiology*, *253*, 462–469.
35. Weissleder, R., Ntziachristos, V. (2003). Shedding light onto live molecular targets. *Nature Medicine*, *9*, 123–128.
36. Wang, G., Cong, W., Shen, H., Qian, X., Henry, M., Wang, Y. (2008). Overview of bioluminescence tomography–a new molecular imaging modality. *Frontiers in Bioscience*, *13*, 1281–1293.
37. Feng, B., Tomizawa, K., Michiue, H., Han, X.J., Miyatake, S., Matsui, H. (2010). Development of a bifunctional immunoliposome system for combined drug delivery and imaging in vivo. *Biomaterials*, *31*, 4139–4145.
38. Mohan, P., Rapoport, N. (2010). Doxorubicin as a molecular nanotheranostic agent: Effect of doxorubicin encapsulation in micelles or nanoemulsions on the ultrasound-mediated intracellular delivery and nuclear trafficking. *Molecular Pharmacology*, *7*, 1959–1973.
39. McCann, T.E., Kosaka, N., Mitsunaga, M., Choyke, P.L., Gildersleeve, J.C., Kobayashi, H. (2010). Biodistribution and excretion of monosaccharide-albumin conjugates measured with in vivo near-infrared fluorescence imaging. *Bioconjugate Chemistry*, *21*, 1925–1932.
40. Bothun, G.D., Rabideau, A.E., Stoner, M.A. (2009). Hepatoma cell uptake of cationic multifluorescent quantum dot liposomes. *Journal of Physical Chemistry B*, *113*, 7725–7728.
41. Lu, Z. R., Kopeckova, P., Kopecek, J. (1999). Polymerizable Fab′ antibody fragments for targeting of anticancer drugs. *Nature Biotechnology*, *17*, 1101–1104.
42. Takeshita, F., Hokaiwado, N., Honma, K., Banas, A., Ochiya, T. (2009). Local and systemic delivery of siRNAs for oligonucleotide therapy. *Methods in Molecular Biology*, *487*, 83–92.
43. Hauck, E.S., Zou, S., Scarfo, K., Nantz, M.H., Hecker, J.G. (2008). Whole animal in vivo imaging after transient, nonviral gene delivery to the rat central nervous system. *Molecular Therapy*, *16*, 1857–1864.
44. Ghoroghchian, P.P., Therien, M.J., Hammer, D.A. (2009). In vivo fluorescence imaging: A personal perspective. *Wiley Interdisciplinary Reviews: Nanomedicine and Nanobiotechnology*, *1*, 156–167.
45. Volodkin, D.V., Skirtach, A.G., Mohwald, H. (2009). Near-IR remote release from assemblies of liposomes and nanoparticles. *Angewandte Chemie International Edition England*, *48*, 1807–1809.
46. Seeram, E. *Computed Tomography: Physics Principles, Clinical Applications, and Quality Control*, 2nd ed. W.B. Saunders Company, Philadelphia, PA, 2001.
47. Henwood, S. *Clinical CT: Techniques and Practice*. Greenwich Medical Media Ltd., London, U.K., 1999.
48. Dawson, P., Cosgrove, D.O., Grainger, R.G. *Textbook of Contrast Media*. Isis Medical Media Ltd., Oxford, U.K., 1999.
49. Hallouard, F., Anton, N., Choquet, P., Constantinesco, A., Vandamme, T. (2010). Iodinated blood pool contrast media for preclinical X-ray imaging applications–a review. *Biomaterials*, *31*, 6249–6268.
50. Elrod, D.B., Partha, R., Danila, D., Casscells, S.W., Conyers, J.L. (2009). An iodinated liposomal computed tomographic contrast agent prepared from a diiodophosphatidylcholine lipid. *Nanomedicine*, *5*, 42–45.

51. Jackson, P.A., Rahman, W.N., Wong, C.J., Ackerly, T., Geso, M. (2010). Potential dependent superiority of gold nanoparticles in comparison to iodinated contrast agents. *European Journal of Radiology*, *75*, 104–109.
52. Popovtzer, R., Agrawal, A., Kotov, N.A., Popovtzer, A., Balter, J., Carey, T.E., Kopelman, R. (2008). Targeted gold nanoparticles enable molecular CT imaging of cancer. *Nano Letters*, *8*, 4593–4596.
53. Wernick, M.N., Aarsvold, J.N. *Emission Tomography: The Fundamentals of PET and SPECT*. Elsevier Academic Press, San Diego, CA, 2004.
54. Saha, G.B. *Fundamentals of Nuclear Pharmacy*, 5th ed. Springer, New York, 2004.
55. Agdeppa, E.D., Spilker, M.E. (2009). A review of imaging agent development. *AAPS Journal*, *11*, 286–299.
56. Bowen, M.L., Orvig, C. (2008). 99m-Technetium carbohydrate conjugates as potential agents in molecular imaging. *Chemical Communications (Cambridge)*, 5077–5091.
57. Ozker, K. (2000). Current developments in single photon radiopharmaceuticals for tumor imaging. *Current Pharmaceutical Design*, *6*, 1123–1126.
58. Schillaci, O., Corleto, V.D., Annibale, B., Scopinaro, F., Delle Fave, G. (1999). Single photon emission computed tomography procedure improves accuracy of somatostatin receptor scintigraphy in gastro-entero pancreatic tumours. *Italian Journal of Gastroenterology and Hepatology*, *31 Suppl 2*, S186–S189.
59. Ross, S.A., Seibyl, J.P. (2004). Research applications of selected 123I-labeled neuroreceptor SPECT imaging ligands. *Journal of Nuclear Medicine Technology*, *32*, 209–214.
60. Phillips, W.T., Goins, B.A., Bao, A. (2009). Radioactive liposomes. *Wiley Interdisciplinary Reviews: Nanomedicine and Nanobiotechnology*, *1*, 69–83.
61. Chen, M.C., Wong, H.S., Lin, K.J., Chen, H.L., Wey, S.P., Sonaje, K., Lin, Y.H., Chu, C.Y., Sung, H.W. (2009). The characteristics, biodistribution and bioavailability of a chitosan-based nanoparticulate system for the oral delivery of heparin. *Biomaterials*, *30*, 6629–6637.
62. Merkel, O. M., Beyerle, A., Librizzi, D., Pfestroff, A., Behr, T. M., Sproat, B., Barth, P. J., Kissel, T. (2009). Nonviral siRNA delivery to the lung: Investigation of PEG-PEI polyplexes and their in vivo performance. *Molecular Pharmacology*, *6*, 1246–1260.
63. Chen, L.C., Chang, C.H., Yu, C.Y., Chang, Y.J., Wu, Y.H., Lee, W.C., Yeh, C.H., Lee, T.W., Ting, G. (2008). Pharmacokinetics, micro-SPECT/CT imaging and therapeutic efficacy of (188) Re-DXR-liposome in C26 colon carcinoma ascites mice model. *Nuclear Medicine and Biology*, *35*, 883–893.
64. Phelps, M.E. *PET: Molecular Imaging and Its Biological Applications*. Springer, New York, 2004.
65. Welch, M.J., Redvanly, C.S. *Handbook of Radiopharmaceuticals*. John Wiley & Sons, Ltd., New York, 2003.
66. Serdons, K., Verbruggen, A., Bormans, G.M. (2009). Developing new molecular imaging probes for PET. *Methods*, *48*, 104–111.
67. Kopka, K., Schober, O., Wagner, S. (2008). (18)F-labelled cardiac PET tracers: Selected probes for the molecular imaging of transporters, receptors and proteases. *Basic Research in Cardiology*, *103*, 131–143.
68. Gupta, N., Price, P.M., Aboagye, E.O. (2002). PET for in vivo pharmacokinetic and pharmacodynamic measurements. *European Journal of Cancer*, *38*, 2094–2107.
69. Shokeen, M., Fettig, N.M., Rossin, R. (2008). Synthesis, in vitro and in vivo evaluation of radiolabeled nanoparticles. *Quarterly Journal of Nuclear Medicine and Molecular Imaging*, *52*, 267–277.
70. Yang, X., Hong, H., Grailer, J.J., Rowland, I.J., Javadi, A., Hurley, S.A., Xiao, Y., Yang, Y., Zhang, Y., Nickles, R.J., Cai, W., Steeber, D.A., Gong, S. (2011). cRGD-functionalized, DOX-conjugated, and ^{64}Cu-labeled superparamagnetic iron oxide nanoparticles for targeted anticancer drug delivery and PET/MR imaging. *Biomaterials*, *32*, 4151–4160.
71. Rygh, C.B., Qin, S., Seo, J.W., Mahakian, L.M., Zhang, H., Adamson, R., Chen, J.Q., Borowsky, A.D., Cardiff, R.D., Reed, R.K., Curry, F.R., Ferrara, K.W. (2011). Longitudinal investigation of permeability and distribution of macromolecules in mouse malignant transformation using PET. *Clinical Cancer Research*, *17*, 550–559.
72. Schluep, T., Hwang, J., Hildebrandt, I.J., Czernin, J., Choi, C. H., Alabi, C.A., Mack, B.C., Davis, M. E. (2009). Pharmacokinetics and tumor dynamics of the nanoparticle IT-101 from PET imaging and tumor histological measurements. *Proceedings of the National Academy of Sciences USA*, *106*, 11394–11399.
73. Bartlett, D.W., Su, H., Hildebrandt, I.J., Weber, W.A., Davis, M.E. (2007). Impact of tumor-specific targeting on the biodistribution and efficacy of siRNA nanoparticles measured by multimodality in vivo imaging. *Proceedings of the National Academy of Sciences USA*, *104*, 15549–15554.
74. Omelyanenko, V., Kopeckova, P., Gentry, C., Kopecek, J. (1998). Targetable HPMA copolymer-adriamycin conjugates. Recognition, internalization, and subcellular fate. *Journal of Controlled Release*, *53*, 25–37.
75. Omelyanenko, V., Gentry, C., Kopeckova, P., Kopecek, J. (1998). HPMA copolymer-anticancer drug-OV-TL16 antibody conjugates. II. Processing in epithelial ovarian carcinoma cells in vitro. *International Journal of Cancer*, *75*, 600–608.
76. Jensen, K.D., Kopeckova, P., Bridge, J.H., Kopecek, J. (2001). The cytoplasmic escape and nuclear accumulation of endocytosed and microinjected HPMA copolymers and a basic kinetic study in Hep G2 cells. *AAPS PharmSciTech*, *3*, E32.
77. Lu, Z.R., Shiah, J.G., Kopeckova, P., Kopecek, J. (2001). Preparation and biological evaluation of polymerizable antibody Fab′ fragment targeted polymeric drug delivery system. *Journal of Controlled Release*, *74*, 263–268.
78. Wang, D., Miller, S.C., Sima, M., Parker, D., Buswell, H., Goodrich, K.C., Kopeckova, P., Kopecek, J. (2004). The arthrotropism of macromolecules in adjuvant-induced arthritis rat model: A preliminary study. *Pharmaceutical Research*, *21*, 1741–1749.

79. Julyan, P.J., Seymour, L.W., Ferry, D.R., Daryani, S., Boivin, C.M., Doran, J., David, M., erson, D., Christodoulou, C., Young, A.M., Hesslewood, S., Kerr, D.J. (1999). Preliminary clinical study of the distribution of HPMA copolymers bearing doxorubicin and galactosamine. *Journal of Controlled Release*, *57*, 281–290.

80. Moreau, P. (2009). Combination regimens using doxorubicin and pegylated liposomal doxorubicin prior to autologous transplantation in multiple myeloma. *Expert Review of Anticancer Therapy*, *9*, 885–890.

81. Visani, G., Isidori, A. (2009). Nonpegylated liposomal doxorubicin in the treatment of B-cell non-Hodgkin's lymphoma: Where we stand. *Expert Review of Anticancer Therapy*, *9*, 357–363.

82. Minisini, A.M., Andreetta, C., Fasola, G., Puglisi, F. (2008). Pegylated liposomal doxorubicin in elderly patients with metastatic breast cancer. *Expert Review of Anticancer Therapy*, *8*, 331–342.

83. Huwyler, J., Drewe, J., Krahenbuhl, S. (2008). Tumor targeting using liposomal antineoplastic drugs. *International Journal of Nanomedicine*, *3*, 21–9.

84. Harrington, K.J., Lewanski, C., Northcote, A.D., Whittaker, J., Peters, A.M., Vile, R.G., Stewart, J.S. (2001). Phase II study of pegylated liposomal doxorubicin (Caelyx) as induction chemotherapy for patients with squamous cell cancer of the head and neck. *European Journal of Cancer*, *37*, 2015–2022.

85. Harrington, K.J., Mohammadtaghi, S., Uster, P.S., Glass, D., Peters, A.M., Vile, R.G., Stewart, J.S. (2001). Effective targeting of solid tumors in patients with locally advanced cancers by radiolabeled pegylated liposomes. *Clinical Cancer Research*, *7*, 243–254.

86. Deelman, L.E., Decleves, A.E., Rychak, J.J., Sharma, K. (2010). Targeted renal therapies through microbubbles and ultrasound. *Advanced Drug Delivery Reviews*, *62*, 1369–1377.

87. Mayer, C.R., Geis, N.A., Katus, H.A., Bekeredjian, R. (2008). Ultrasound targeted microbubble destruction for drug and gene delivery. *Expert Opinion on Drug Delivery*, *5*, 1121–1138.

88. Mayer, C.R., Bekeredjian, R. (2008). Ultrasonic gene and drug delivery to the cardiovascular system. *Advanced Drug Delivery Reviews*, *60*, 1177–1192.

89. Ferrara, K., Pollard, R., Borden, M. (2007). Ultrasound microbubble contrast agents: Fundamentals and application to gene and drug delivery. *Annual Review of Biomedical Engineering*, *9*, 415–947.

90. Bekeredjian, R., Kuecherer, H.F., Kroll, R.D., Katus, H.A., Hardt, S.E. (2007). Ultrasound-targeted microbubble destruction augments protein delivery into testes. *Urology*, *69*, 386–389.

91. Rapoport, N., Gao, Z., Kennedy, A. (2007). Multifunctional nanoparticles for combining ultrasonic tumor imaging and targeted chemotherapy. *Journal of the National Cancer Institute*, *99*, 1095–1106.

92. Vandenbroucke, R.E., Lentacker, I., Demeester, J., De Smedt, S.C., Sanders, N.N. (2008). Ultrasound assisted siRNA delivery using PEG-siPlex loaded microbubbles. *Journal of Controlled Release*, *126*, 265–273.

93. Duvshani-Eshet, M., Adam, D., Machluf, M. (2006). The effects of albumin-coated microbubbles in DNA delivery mediated by therapeutic ultrasound. *Journal of Controlled Release*, *112*, 156–166.

94. Vriens, D., van Laarhoven, H.W., van Asten, J.J., Krabbe, P. F., Visser, E.P., Heerschap, A., Punt, C.J., de Geus-Oei, L.F., Oyen, W.J. (2009). Chemotherapy response monitoring of colorectal liver metastases by dynamic Gd-DTPA-enhanced MRI perfusion parameters and 18F-FDG PET metabolic rate. *Journal of Nuclear Medicine*, *50*, 1777–1784.

95. Dierckx, R., Maes, A., Peeters, M., Van De Wiele, C. (2009). FDG PET for monitoring response to local and locoregional therapy in HCC and liver metastases. *Quarterly Journal of Nuclear Medicine and Molecular Imaging*, *53*, 336–342.

96. Niu, G., Li, Z., Cao, Q., Chen, X. (2009). Monitoring therapeutic response of human ovarian cancer to 17-DMAG by noninvasive PET imaging with (64)Cu-DOTA-trastuzumab. *European Journal of Nuclear Medicine and Molecular Imaging*, *36*, 1510–159.

97. Decoster, L., Schallier, D., Everaert, H., Nieboer, K., Meysman, M., Neyns, B., De Mey, J., De Greve, J. (2008). Complete metabolic tumour response, assessed by 18-fluorodeoxyglucose positron emission tomography (18FDG-PET), after induction chemotherapy predicts a favourable outcome in patients with locally advanced non-small cell lung cancer (NSCLC). *Lung Cancer*, *62*, 55–61.

98. Sciagra, R., Parodi, G., Pupi, A., Migliorini, A., Valenti, R., Moschi, G., Santoro, G.M., Memisha, G., Antoniucci, D. (2005). Gated SPECT evaluation of outcome after abciximab-supported primary infarct artery stenting for acute myocardial infarction: The scintigraphic data of the abciximab and carbostent evaluation (ACE) randomized trial. *Journal of Nuclear Medicine*, *46*, 722–727.

99. Tozaki, M., Oyama, Y., Fukuma, E. (2010). Preliminary study of early response to neoadjuvant chemotherapy after the first cycle in breast cancer: Comparison of 1H magnetic resonance spectroscopy with diffusion magnetic resonance imaging. *Japanese Journal of Radiology*, *28*, 101–109.

100. Morvan, D., Demidem, A. (2007). Metabolomics by proton nuclear magnetic resonance spectroscopy of the response to chloroethylnitrosourea reveals drug efficacy and tumor adaptive metabolic pathways. *Cancer Research*, *67*, 2150–2159.

101. Craciunescu, O.I., Blackwell, K.L., Jones, E.L., Macfall, J.R., Yu, D., Vujaskovic, Z., Wong, T.Z., Liotcheva, V., Rosen, E. L., Prosnitz, L.R., Samulski, T.V., Dewhirst, M.W. (2009). DCE-MRI parameters have potential to predict response of locally advanced breast cancer patients to neoadjuvant chemotherapy and hyperthermia: A pilot study. *International Journal of Hyperthermia*, *25*, 405–415.

102. Wu, X., Jeong, E.K., Emerson, L., Hoffman, J., Parker, D.L., Lu, Z.R. (2010). Noninvasive evaluation of antiangiogenic effect in a mouse tumor model by DCE-MRI with Gd-DTPA cystamine copolymers. *Molecular Pharmacology*, *7*, 41–48.

103. Jarnagin, W.R., Schwartz, L.H., Gultekin, D.H., Gonen, M., Haviland, D., Shia, J., D'Angelica, M., Fong, Y., Dematteo, R., Tse, A., Blumgart, L.H., Kemeny, N. (2009). Regional chemotherapy for unresectable primary liver cancer: Results

of a phase II clinical trial and assessment of DCE-MRI as a biomarker of survival. *Annals of Oncology*, *20*, 1589–1595.

104. Dafni, H., Kim, S.J., Bankson, J.A., Sankaranarayanapillai, M., Ronen, S.M. (2008). Macromolecular dynamic contrast-enhanced (DCE)-MRI detects reduced vascular permeability in a prostate cancer bone metastasis model following anti-platelet-derived growth factor receptor (PDGFR) therapy, indicating a drop in vascular endothelial growth factor receptor (VEGFR) activation. *Magnetic Resonance in Medicine*, *60*, 822–833.
105. Mahato, R.I. (1999). Non-viral peptide-based approaches to gene delivery. *Journal of Drug Targeting*, *7*, 249–268.
106. Gao, K., Huang, L. (2009). Nonviral methods for siRNA delivery. *Molecular Pharmacology*, *6*, 651–658.
107. Oh, Y.K., Park, T.G. (2009). siRNA delivery systems for cancer treatment. *Advanced Drug Delivery Reviews*, *61*, 850–862.
108. Moore, A., Medarova, Z. (2009). Imaging of siRNA delivery and silencing. *Methods in Molecular Biology*, *487*, 93–110.
109. Raty, J.K., Liimatainen, T., Unelma Kaikkonen, M., Grohn, O., Airenne, K.J., Yla-Herttuala, S. (2007). Non-invasive imaging in gene therapy. *Molecular Therapy*, *15*, 1579–1586.
110. Iyer, M., Salazar, F.B., Wu, L., Carey, M., Gambhir, S.S. (2006). Bioluminescence imaging of systemic tumor targeting using a prostate-specific lentiviral vector. *Human Gene Therapy*, *17*, 125–132.
111. Mizuno, T., Mohri, K., Nasu, S., Danjo, K., Okamoto, H. (2009). Dual imaging of pulmonary delivery and gene expression of dry powder inhalant by fluorescence and bioluminescence. *Journal of Controlled Release*, *134*, 149–154.
112. Peterson, J.R., Infanger, D.W., Braga, V.A., Zhang, Y., Sharma, R.V., Engelhardt, J.F., Davisson, R.L. (2008). Longitudinal noninvasive monitoring of transcription factor activation in cardiovascular regulatory nuclei using bioluminescence imaging. *Physiological Genomics*, *33*, 292–299.
113. Centelles, M.N., Qian, C., Campanero, M.A., Irache, J.M. (2008). New methodologies to characterize the effectiveness of the gene transfer mediated by DNA-chitosan nanoparticles. *International Journal of Nanomedicine*, *3*, 451–460.
114. Niu, G., Xiong, Z., Cheng, Z., Cai, W., Gambhir, S.S., Xing, L., Chen, X. (2007). In vivo bioluminescence tumor imaging of RGD peptide-modified adenoviral vector encoding firefly luciferase reporter gene. *Molecular Imaging and Biology*, *9*, 126–134.
115. Navarro, G., Maiwald, G., Haase, R., Rogach, A.L., Wagner, E., de Ilarduya, C.T., Ogris, M. (2010). Low generation PAMAM dendrimer and CpG free plasmids allow targeted and extended transgene expression in tumors after systemic delivery. *Journal of Controlled Release*, *146*, 99–105.
116. Gao, Y., Gao, G., He, Y., Liu, T., Qi, R. (2008). Recent advances of dendrimers in delivery of genes and drugs. *Mini Reviews in Medicinal Chemistry*, *8*, 889–900.
117. Kurreck, J. (2009). RNA interference: From basic research to therapeutic applications. *Angewandte Chemie International Edition England*, *48*, 1378–1398.
118. Fire, A.Z. (2007). Gene silencing by double-stranded RNA. *Cell Death and Differentiation*, *14*, 1998–2012.
119. Hannon, G.J. (2002). RNA interference. *Nature*, *418*, 244–51.
120. Meister, G., Tuschl, T. (2004). Mechanisms of gene silencing by double-stranded RNA. *Nature*, *431*, 343–349.
121. Wang, Q., Ilves, H., Chu, P., Contag, C.H., Leake, D., Johnston, B.H., Kaspar, R.L. (2007). Delivery and inhibition of reporter genes by small interfering RNAs in a mouse skin model. *Journal of Investigative Dermatology*, *127*, 2577–2584.
122. McAnuff, M.A., Rettig, G.R., Rice, K.G. (2007). Potency of siRNA versus shRNA mediated knockdown in vivo. *Journal of Pharmaceutical Sciences*, *96*, 2922–2930.
123. Wei, J., Jones, J., Kang, J., Card, A., Krimm, M., Hancock, P., Pei, Y., Ason, B., Payson, E., Dubinina, N., Cancilla, M., Stroh, M., Burchard, J., Sachs, A.B., Hochman, J.H., Flanagan, W.M., Kuklin, N.A. (2011). RNA-induced silencing complex-bound small interfering RNA is a determinant of RNA interference-mediated gene silencing in mice. *Molecular Pharmacology*, *79*, 953–963.
124. Tao, W., Davide, J.P., Cai, M., Zhang, G.J., South, V.J., Matter, A., Ng, B., Zhang, Y., Sepp-Lorenzino, L. (2010). Noninvasive imaging of lipid nanoparticle-mediated systemic delivery of small-interfering RNA to the liver. *Molecular Therapy*, *18*, 1657–1666.
125. Juweid, M.E., Cheson, B.D. (2006). Positron-emission tomography and assessment of cancer therapy. *New England Journal of Medicine*, *354*, 496–507.
126. Inohara, H., Enomoto, K., Tomiyama, Y., Higuchi, I., Inoue, T., Hatazawa, J. (2010). Impact of FDG-PET on prediction of clinical outcome after concurrent chemoradiotherapy in hypopharyngeal carcinoma. *Molecular Imaging and Biology*, *12*, 89–97.
127. Subedi, N., Scarsbrook, A., Darby, M., Korde, K., Mc Shane, P., Muers, M.F. (2009). The clinical impact of integrated FDG PET-CT on management decisions in patients with lung cancer. *Lung Cancer*, *64*, 301–307.
128. Pichler, B.J., Judenhofer, M.S., Pfannenberg, C. (2008). Multimodal imaging approaches: PET/CT and PET/MRI. *Handbook of Experimental Pharmacology*, 109–132.
129. Grigsby, P.W. (2009). PET/CT imaging to guide cervical cancer therapy. *Future Oncology*, *5*, 953–958.
130. Zaidi, H., Vees, H., Wissmeyer, M. (2009). Molecular PET/CT imaging-guided radiation therapy treatment planning. *Academic Radiology*, *16*, 1108–1133.
131. Li, X., Li, R., Qian, X., Ding, Y., Tu, Y., Guo, R., Hu, Y., Jiang, X., Guo, W., Liu, B. (2008). Superior antitumor efficiency of cisplatin-loaded nanoparticles by intratumoral delivery with decreased tumor metabolism rate. *European Journal of Pharmaceutics and Biopharmaceutics*, *70*, 726–734.
132. Medina, O.P., Pillarsetty, N., Glekas, A., Punzalan, B., Longo, V., Gonen, M., Zanzonico, P., Smith-Jones, P., Larson, S.M. (2011). Optimizing tumor targeting of the lipophilic EGFR-binding radiotracer SKI 243 using a liposomal nanoparticle delivery system. *Journal of Controlled Release*, *149*, 292–298.

133. Groot-Wassink, T., Aboagye, E.O., Wang, Y., Lemoine, N.R., Reader, A.J., Vassaux, G. (2004). Quantitative imaging of Na/I symporter transgene expression using positron emission tomography in the living animal. *Molecular Therapy*, *9*, 436–442.

134. Berard, V., Rousseau, J.A., Cadorette, J., Hubert, L., Bentourkia, M., van Lier, J.E., Lecomte, R. (2006). Dynamic imaging of transient metabolic processes by small-animal PET for the evaluation of photosensitizers in photodynamic therapy of cancer. *Journal of Nuclear Medicine*, *47*, 1119–1126.

135. Padhani, A.R. (2003). MRI for assessing antivascular cancer treatments. *British Journal of Radiology*, *76 Spec No 1*, S60–S80.

136. O'Connor, J.P., Jackson, A., Parker, G.J., Jayson, G.C. (2007). DCE-MRI biomarkers in the clinical evaluation of antiangiogenic and vascular disrupting agents. *British Journal of Cancer*, *96*, 189–195.

137. Cheng, H.L. (2007). Dynamic contrast-enhanced MRI in oncology drug development. *Current Clinical Pharmacology*, *2*, 111–122.

138. Feng, Y., Emerson, L., Jeong, E.K., Parker, D.L., Lu, Z.R. (2009). Application of a biodegradable macromolecular contrast agent in dynamic contrast-enhanced MRI for assessing the efficacy of indocyanine green-enhanced photothermal cancer therapy. *Journal of Magnetic Resonance Imaging*, *30*, 401–406.

139. Preda, A., van Vliet, M., Krestin, G.P., Brasch, R.C., van Dijke, C.F. (2006). Magnetic resonance macromolecular agents for monitoring tumor microvessels and angiogenesis inhibition. *Investigative Radiology*, *41*, 325–331.

140. Feng, Y., Jeong, E.K., Mohs, A.M., Emerson, L., Lu, Z.R. (2008). Characterization of tumor angiogenesis with dynamic contrast-enhanced MRI and biodegradable macromolecular contrast agents in mice. *Magnetic Resonance in Medicine*, *60*, 1347–1352.

141. Barrett, T., Kobayashi, H., Brechbiel, M., Choyke, P.L. (2006). Macromolecular MRI contrast agents for imaging tumor angiogenesis. *European Journal of Radiology*, *60*, 353–366.

142. Lu, Z.R., Parker, D.L., Goodrich, K.C., Wang, X., Dalle, J.G., Buswell, H.R. (2004). Extracellular biodegradable macromolecular gadolinium(III) complexes for MRI. *Magnetic Resonance in Medicine*, *51*, 27–34.

143. Weidensteiner, C., Rausch, M., McSheehy, P.M., Allegrini, P.R. (2006). Quantitative dynamic contrast-enhanced MRI in tumor-bearing rats and mice with inversion recovery True-FISP and two contrast agents at 4.7 T. *Journal of Magnetic Resonance Imaging*, *24*, 646–656.

144. Janib, S.M., Moses, A.S., MacKay, J.A. (2010). Imaging and drug delivery using theranostic nanoparticles. *Advanced Drug Delivery Reviews*, *62*, 1052–1063.

145. Kelkar, S.S., Reineke, T.M. (2011). Theranostics: Combining imaging and therapy. *Bioconjugate Chemistry*, *22*, 1879–1903.

146. Al-Jamal, W.T., Kostarelos, K. (2011). Liposomes: From a clinically established drug delivery system to a nanoparticle platform for theranostic nanomedicine. *Accounts of Chemical Research*, *44*, 1094–1104.

147. Tan, M., Lu, Z.R. (2011). Integrin targeted MR imaging. *Theranostics*, *1*, 83–101.

148. Xie, J., Lee, S., Chen, X. (2010). Nanoparticle-based theranostic agents. *Advanced Drug Delivery Reviews*, *62*, 1064–1079.

149. Choudhary, S., Nouri, K., Elsaie, M.L. (2009). Photodynamic therapy in dermatology: A review. *Lasers in Medical Science*, *24*, 971–980.

150. Dai, T., Huang, Y.Y., Hamblin, M.R. (2009). Photodynamic therapy for localized infections–state of the art. *Photodiagnosis and Photodynamics Therapy*, *6*, 170–188.

151. Moore, C. M., Pendse, D., Emberton, M. (2009). Photodynamic therapy for prostate cancer–a review of current status and future promise. *Nature Clinical Practice Urology*, *6*, 18–30.

152. Vaidya, A., Sun, Y., Ke, T., Jeong, E.K., Lu, Z.R. (2006). Contrast enhanced MRI-guided photodynamic therapy for site-specific cancer treatment. *Magnetic Resonance in Medicine*, *56*, 761–767.

153. Vaidya, A., Sun, Y., Feng, Y., Emerson, L., Jeong, E.K., Lu, Z. R. (2008). Contrast-enhanced MRI-guided photodynamic cancer therapy with a pegylated bifunctional polymer conjugate. *Pharmaceutical Research*, *25*, 2002–2011.

ANSWERS

CHAPTER 1

1.1. b.

1.2. Absorption rate constant (ka). Most drugs have faster absorption rate constants compared with their elimination rate constants. By changing the release rate from a modified formulation, the terminal elimination rate will be governed by a slower absorption rate (flip-flop absorption phenomenon).

1.3. The physicochemical properties of the drug, nature of the drug product, and anatomy and physiology at the absorption site.

1.4. Basic drugs can be absorbed better at pH 7 compared with acidic drugs. Intestinal absorption in the rat at pH 7 were reported to be 41%, 35%, NA, and 30%, respectively (Florence and Attwood [73, p. 341]).

1.5. Barriers to protein delivery include epithelia, metabolism/instability, clearance, immunology, and size/nature of the molecules.

1.6. Transcytosis by enterocytes or M cells will be major mechanisms for nanoparticle delivery of a vaccine. Paracellular transport and passive diffusion may contribute much less.

1.7. The most important transporters include P-gp (MDR1), BCRP, MRP2, MCT1, ASBT, PEPT1, and OATP.

1.8. As Fick's law stated as in Equation (1.1), the formulation improving a larger surface area for the particles, higher solubility, greater sink concentration in the systemic circulation near absorptive sites, bigger diffusivity of a drug, better lipophilicity, and thinner absorptive distance will increase the oral absorption of the drug product.

1.9. **a.** *Passive Diffusion:* Passive diffusion is the movement of a solute across a membrane down the electrochemical gradient without the assistance of a transport protein. It does not require any biological energy, but it does follow Fick's law.

b. *Unstirred Water Layer:* The unstirred or stagnant water layer is an additional barrier to drug transport that exists in parallel with the luminal surface of the intestinal membrane. The unstirred layer, whose thickness ranges from 0.01 to 1 mm, reduces the absorption rate and shifts the inflection point in the pH—absorption profile to the right for an acid and to the left for a basic compound.

c. *Tight Junction:* Tight junctions are closely associated areas of two cells whose membranes join together, forming a virtually impermeable barrier to fluid. Tight junctions are composed of the structural proteins, the scaffold proteins, and the actin cytoskeleton. Occludin and claudins are structural proteins of the tight junctions. The scaffold proteins consist of zonula occluden-1 (ZO-1), ZO-2, fodrin, cingulin, symplekin, 7H6, and p130. Paracellular transport of drugs mostly occurs via tight junctions.

d. *Luminal pH:* The luminal pH is the pH in the lumen of the gastrointestinal tract. The pH at the absorption site is an integral factor in drug absorption because many drugs are either weak organic acids or bases. The luminal pH in the stomach and small intestines are

Advanced Drug Delivery, First Edition. Edited by Ashim K. Mitra, Chi H. Lee, and Kun Cheng.

about 1 and 6 to 7, respectively, with high variability when food is present.

1.10. Three key functions of the gastrointestinal tract: barrier to bioavailability, barrier to immunity, and barrier to microorganisms. Various nutrients and exogenous compounds can be selectively absorbed via sequential events such as dissolution, precipitation, enzymatic or chemical degradation, membrane permeation, and first-pass metabolism. The intestinal epithelium serves as an efficient barrier to immunity between the external environment and the body to deal with continuous exposures of antigen loads from ingested food, resident bacteria, and invading viruses. In addition, the GI tract provides an effective barrier to micro-organisms by maintaining the acidic pH of the stomach and the antibacterial activity of pancreatic enzymes, biles, and other intestinal secretions.

1.11. First-pass or presystemic metabolism refers to the loss of drug through biotransformation by eliminating organs (GI tract and liver) during its passage to systemic circulation after oral administration. The low drug concentration or complete absence of the drug in plasma after oral administration is indicative of first-pass effects.

CHAPTER 2

2.1. Solubility is an intrinsic material characteristic for a specific molecule that can be qualitatively defined as the spontaneous interaction of two or more substances to form a homogenous molecular dispersion. Solubility depends on the physical and chemical properties of the solute and the solvent as well as on such factors as temperature, pressure, the pH of the solution, and to a lesser extent, the state of subdivision of the solute.

2.2. About 30–40% of the lead substances available today have an aqueous solubility less than 10 μM or 5 mg/mL at pH 7. Hence, much effort is placed on enhancement of the solubility of poorly soluble compounds. The candidate molecules with optimum solubility are crucial to achieving their target bioavailability and therapeutic responses.

2.3. Several examples in the literature demonstrate the effects of changing crystal morphology on an *in vivo* dissolution rate with potential for improving bioavailability. The habit modification of dipyridamole by crystallization showed that dissolution of rod-shaped particles was faster than rectangular needle-shaped crystals. Similarly, phenytoin can be crystallized into a needle-like rhombic shape with different dissolution properties, which is ascribed to changes in surface area rather than to improvements in the wetting of more polar surface moieties. However, it was also noted that the crystal habit of doped crystals played an integral role in the enhancement of the intrinsic dissolution rate of phenytoin as a result of increased abundance in polar groups.

2.4. As a result of the unique characteristics of surfactants, their low concentrations added to water will form a stable monolayer. As the amount of surfactant added increases, a monolayer becomes a bilayer. If the concentration of surfactant is sufficiently high, the bilayer becomes unstable and micelles are formed. An important property of micelles particularly in pharmaceutical application is their ability to increase the aqueous solubility of sparingly soluble substances. At surfactant concentrations above the critical micelle concentration, the solubility of a drug increases linearly with the concentration of surfactant. As the solubilization is the partitioning process of the drug between the micelle and the aqueous phase, the standard free energy of solubilization (ΔG_s^0) can be expressed by the following equation: $\Delta G_s^0 = -RT \ln P$, where R is the universal gas constant, T is the absolute temperature, and P is the partition coefficient between the micelle and the aqueous phase.

2.5. Microemulsions are thermodynamically stable, isotropically clear dispersions of two immiscible liquids, such as oil and water, which are stabilized by an interfacial film of surfactant molecules. As a result of their superior properties in solubilization and stability, microemulsions offer distinct advantages over unstable dispersions like emulsions and suspensions. Oil-soluble drugs can be formulated in oil-in-water microemulsion, whereas water-soluble ones are better suited for water-in-oil systems.

2.6. Enhancement in solubility and dissolution of hydrophobic drug from solid dispersion is brought on by the following mechanisms:

i. *Reduction in particle size:* A drug may exist molecularly, as amorphous clusters, or as size-reduced crystals in the matrix in solid dispersion. When a drug exists molecularly or as amorphous clusters, no energy is required to break the crystal lattice, thereby leading to enhancement in solubility. An increase in surface area by reduction in drug crystal size leads to enhancement in both solubility and dissolution.

ii. *Improved wettability of drug particles:* In a solid dispersion system, a drug is thoroughly dispersed in a hydrophilic carrier. Hence, drug wettability is enhanced in solid dispersions by the hydrophilic carriers even in the absence of surface active agents.

iii. *Particles with higher porosity:* Particles in solid dispersions have been found to have a higher degree of porosity. The increased porosity of solid dispersion particles improves water penetration and hence causes rapid dissolution.

2.7. The most common degradation pathways involve hydrolysis, dehydration, oxidation, intramolecular cyclization, photolysis, and racemization.

2.8. For light-sensitive materials, sunlight or artificial light could lead to photodegradation of the active principle as well as change the physicochemical properties of the product. For example, as the product becomes discolored or cloudy in appearance, a loss in viscosity, a change in dissolution rate, or a precipitation is observed. The drug molecule may be affected directly or indirectly by irradiation, depending on how the radiant energy is transferred to the substance. Direct photochemical reactions occur when the drug molecule itself absorbs energy. In an indirect reaction, the energy may be absorbed by nondrug molecules (e.g., excipient, impurity, and degradation product) in the formulation. The energy is shared by the active ingredient, which is subjected to subsequent degradation.

2.9. The Arrhenius equation (given below) could be applied to predict the stability of various pharmaceuticals:

$$\ln k = \ln A - \frac{E_a}{RT}$$

where R is the gas constant, E_a is the activation energy, and A is the frequency factor, which is an indication of the entropy of activation for the process. Arrhenius kinetics is a linear dependence of the natural logarithm of the reaction rate, k, versus the reciprocal of the absolute temperature, T.

2.10. Co-crystal formation involves complexation of neutral molecules rather than ions, and thus, it has been potentially employed with all APIs, including acidic, basic, and nonionizable molecules. There is also a large number of nontoxic "counter-molecules" that may be considered to be potential co-crystal candidates, possibly broadening the scope of pharmaceutical co-crystallization.

2.11. The impurities present in the excipient can promote oxidation reactions, such as nucleophilic/electrophilic addition with drugs. Excipients may also exert catalyzing effects toward drug degradation. They can affect drug stability by providing moisture. Excipients having strong water-entrapping abilities that tend to lower the drug degradation rates, as was seen from colloidal silica. They can also affect drug stability by altering the microclimate pH. The surface acidity of excipients resulting from the presence of carboxylic acid groups has been reported to be a factor contributing to drug degradation.

2.12. Cyclodexterins have a "donut" shape, with the interior portion of the molecule being relatively hydrophobic and the exterior being relatively hydrophilic. As a result of their unique chemical structure, they are capable of forming "inclusion" complexes with various drug molecules to protect them from the chemical degradation.

CHAPTER 3

3.1. Two major superfamilies of membrane-drug transporters are (i) ABC (ATP binding cassette) and (ii) SLC (solute carrier) transporters. The ABCs, as active transporters, operate by ATP hydrolysis to expel their substrate out of the cell across the lipid bilayer. The ABC proteins are encoded by 49 genes and are categorized into seven subclasses. The P-glycoprotein (P-gp) is the most well-documented transporter in the ABC superfamily and is encoded by the MDR1 (ABCB1) gene. Lipophilic drugs, substrates for efflux transporters, diffuse through cellular lipid bilayers, but efflux transporters present in the membrane of some vital tissues (intestine, liver, BBB, kidney) extrude them out of cells lowering drug concentrations in the tissue. Again, these efflux transporters overexpress in tumor cells and in other tissues in response to many drugs. Such overexpression may cause subtherapeutic concentrations of drugs that may lead to drug resistance and therapeutic failure. The influx transporters belong to the SLC (solute carrier) transporter family. The SLC superfamily consists of 43 families that participate in drug absorption. These include carriers for peptides, vitamins, organic anions, organic cations, glucose, and other nutrients. These transporters are involved in the pharmacokinetic and pharmacodynamic pathways of drug molecules. Drug molecules are modified chemically to achieve desired lipophilicity and solubility targeting various influx transporters that will ultimately improve drug bioavailability. For example, beta lactam antibiotics use a peptide transporter for absorption. The prodrug of ACV (val-val ACV) can be absorbed more than ACV by using PEPT. The influx transporters can be used as molecular targets for tissue-selective drug delivery and for reducing systemic toxicity. For example, folic acid conjugated cancer drugs can be targeted to tumor cells that overexpress the folate transporter.

3.2. c.

3.3. c.

3.4. g.

3.5. a.

3.6. f.

3.7. The sodium-dependent multivitamin transporter (SMVT) and the sodium-dependent vitamin C transporter (SVCT1 and SVCT2).

3.8. a.

3.9. Ascorbic acid (AA, vitamin C) is an essential nutrient required for cellular growth, function, wound healing, and immunity. Sodium-dependent vitamin C transporters (SVCT1 and SVCT2) were cloned recently from human and rat DNA libraries. Both isoforms have a similar function and can mediate L-AA transport. This transporter is present in many tissues such as the intestine, kidney, brain, eye, bone, and skin. SVCT1 expresses mainly on the apical membrane, and SVCT2 is present on both the apical and the basolateral membrane of MDCK cells. Various inter- and intracellular stimuli (hormones, paracrine factors, signaling molecules, etc.) are engaged in the regulation of expression of SVCT.

3.10. Nanotechnology provides an alternative strategy to circumvent MDR by offering a means to encapsulate drugs to lipids, gelatin, and polymers producing nanoparticles that are resistant to drug efflux. These nanoparticles take advantage of the endocytosis process simultaneously evading MDR proteins on cell membranes. Moreover, these nanoparticles can be surface decorated with folic acid, biotin, and so on for receptor-mediated targeted delivery. Figure 3.6 demonstrates the mechanism of efflux evasion via endocytosis after encapsulation of the substrate drug molecule in nanoparticles. Inclusion of targeting ligands on the surface of nanoparticles has the potential of affecting tumor-specific drug delivery and retention, thus, minimizing systemic toxicity.

CHAPTER 4

4.1. A biomaterial is a nonviable material used in a medical device intended to assess, treat, augment, or replace any nonfunctional part of a living system or to function in intimate contact with living tissues or biological systems. Biomaterial has been categorized based on:

a. Mechanism of tissue interaction to the material surface:

1. Bioinert biomaterial
2. Bioactive (biointeractive) biomaterial
3. Bioresorbable (viable) biomaterial
4. Replant biomaterial

b. Material selection

1. Composites
2. Metals
3. Ceramics
4. Polymer

4.2. The fundamental requirement to be qualified as a biomaterial is that material must be biocompatible, safe, cost-effective, and not generate any toxic, allergic, or carcinogenic responses. The selection of material for biomedical application is mainly based on material compatibility within a biological system.

4.3. The three major considerations are as follows:

1. Biocompatibility may not be exclusively dependent on the material characteristics but also on the location in which the material is used. It is highly likely that material response may vary from one application site to another.
2. It is sometimes required that material should interact rather than being inert in nature with the tissue to generate its effects (e.g., blood contacting materials designed to develop a neointima).
3. In some cases, it is required for material to degrade over time rather than remaining intact for an indefinite period (e.g., resorbable materials: sutures and biodegradable drug delivery systems).

4.4. Biomaterial exhibits four different types of interactions within the biological system depending on the material properties.

1. *Chemical Interaction:* The ultimate outcomes of chemical (metal) interactions include corrosion, degradation, and protein deposition. In addition to immunogenic responses, metal degradation products may also generate other responses, such as metabolic changes, initiation of lymphocyte toxins, variations in host–parasite interactions, and development of chemical carcinogenesis.
2. *Mechanical Interaction:* The development of a fibrous encapsulation, thrombus formation, and calcification are the ultimate outcomes of mechanical interaction between biomaterial and the host system. The outcomes of foreign body reaction and fibrous encapsulation serve as a biological restriction of integration and *in vivo* performance of biomaterial implants.
3. *Pharmacological Interaction:* Toxic leaching, embrittlement, and cell lysis are the major consequences of pharmacological biomaterial interactions.
4. *Surface Interaction:* Biomaterial-mediated surface interactions with the host system will trigger a series of host reactions including blood–material interactions, complement activation on biomaterial surfaces, and macrophage adhesion followed by fusion or capsulation. The ultimate outcome of the above events would be acute or chronic inflammation, granulation, foreign body reaction, and fibrosis.

4.5. Blood compatibility of the implanted devise depends on properties of biomaterial, design of device, and patient state. However, biological properties of biomaterial (surface roughness and surface charge) are the only regulating factor to control blood compatibility.

4.6. **d.** All of the above.

4.7. **d.** All of the above.

4.8. **a.** Graft polymer.

4.9. Biodegradable polymers are materials that are designed to undergo gradual degradation in physiological conditions into nontoxic products. Examples of commonly used biodegradable–bioresorbable polymers in tissue engineering include polylactide, polycaprolactone, polyglycolic acid, polyester-ether such as polydioxanone, and others.

4.10. The potential advantages of biodegradable polymers over non-biodegradable polymers and metallic systems are as follows:

1. Gradual degradation of the polymer into nontoxic products
2. Eliminates requirement of second surgery for removal of implants
3. Eliminates problems such as corrosion, difficulties in magnetic resonance imaging, and release of metallic particles unlike metallic implants
4. Transferring loads to the healing soft tissue and bone fracture
5. Improved drug release profiles by modifying polymeric block ratio

4.11. An ideal biodegradable polymer should not produce an inflammatory response upon implantation, should have degradation time similar to the regeneration or healing of the targeted tissue, and should produce nontoxic products on degradation that can be easily excreted from the body.

4.12. Blood coagulation, hemolysis, and release of proinflammatory cytokines are a few biocompatibility issues associated with several biodegradable polymers.

4.13. Diffusion.

4.14. Its pore size. High porosity and pore microstructure could be achieved through controlling manufacture parameters. Macromolecules such as bone regenerating growth factors or antibodies could be incorporated into hydroxyapatite granules to enhance its therapeutic efficacy.

4.15. Delivery vehicles. Spherical hydroxyapatite fabricated by various methods could be used as drug carriers, especially for the bone-inducing agents, as well as anti-inflammatory drugs or antibacterial agents.

4.16. **d.** All of the above.

4.17. Arterial blood is corrosive to trigger nickel ion release from Nitinol alloy surface, causing potential adverse inflammation. In this case, the surface property of Nitinol medical devices needs to be modified to enhance resistance to peeling.

4.18. **b.** Biodegradability.

4.19. Compared with titanium and stainless steel, CoCr has a greater fatigue life with regard to their sensitivity to intraoperative contouring, thus, being more suitable as arthrodesis constructs.

4.20. **a.** Osteoconductivity.

4.21. **d.** All of the above.

4.22. Composite materials are strong, tailor-made solids containing two or more distinct constituent materials or phases.

4.23. The advantages of composite materials over homogeneous materials include 1) high strength;

2) light weight; 3) corrosion resistance; 4) durability; and 5) design flexibility.

4.24. Natural composites often exhibit particulate, porous, and fibrous structural features on different microscales. Natural composites include bone, wood, dentin, cartilage, and skin. Natural foams include lung, cancellous bone, and wood.

4.25. Composite materials can be categorized into 1) macrofiller composite (>10 μm); 2) hybrid composite and homogenic microfiller composite (0.01–0.1 μm); and 3) inhomogenic microfiller composite (0.01–0.1 μm). The use of nanofillers and nanoclusters in hybrid composites can help microfiller composites to enhance the long-term stability and can obtain the polishing properties. When superficial filler particles are disoriented due to abrasion, nanoclusters of the nanocomposites are broken down into nanoparticles.

4.26. **e.**

4.27. The nanotubes are "smart" because they could be designed to encapsulate and then open up to deliver a drug or gene in a particular location in the body. The smart bio-nanotubes have a trilayered structure consisting of a microtubular protein called tubulin, coated with a bilayer of lipid, followed by coating of tubulin protein in the form of rings or spirals where proteins had either open ends (negatively overcharged) or closed ends (positively overcharged with lipid caps). The integral variable for smart bio-nanotubes that regulates the release profile of loaded drug is the comparative thickness of protein lipid versus protein coats.

4.28. The first-generation biomaterials are bioinert materials including stainless steel and polyethylene. The second-generation biomaterials aim to beneficially interact with the body, which include hydroxyapatitie-reinforced polyethylene (HAPEX), bioglass, and so on. The bioresorbable and bioactive materials are classified as "third-generation" biomaterials, as a result of their ability of closely mimicking the natural function and helping the body to heal itself.

4.29. Several biodegradable and bioabsorbable biomaterials composed of co-polymers like polyglycolic acid (PGA), polylactic acid (PLA), and polyglycolide lactide (PGLA) have been used by researchers for would healing. Examples:

1. Bioglass®-poly(D,L-lactide) (PDLLA) composite exhibits improved microstructural homogeneity and uniformity along the suture length through an additional PDLLA coating.
2. Composite polyglactin 910, a synthetic absorbable monofilament surgical suture material, shows good mechanical properties, minimal tissue reactions, and easy and reproducible fabrication.

4.30. Stimuli responsive materials are referred to as materials whose properties can be considerably altered by external stimuli, such as changes of temperature, mechanical stress, pH, moisture, or electric or magnetic fields.

4.31. Electro-conductive hydrogels (ECHs) are polymeric blends or co-networks that combine inherently conductive electro-active polymers with highly hydrated hydrogels.

4.32. When a crack occurs in the epoxy composite material, the microcapsules near the creak are broken and release the resin. The resin subsequently fills the crack and reacts with a Grubbs catalyst dispersed in the epoxy composite, leading to the polymerization of the resin and repair of the crack.

4.33. PEG molecules are strongly hydrophilic and form a surface-bound hydrated layer around the nanoparticles, which limit the interactions with cell surface proteins and elimination by the immune system.

4.34. **b.** Composite interpenetrating network of poly (dimethyl siloxane) and poly(*N*-isopropyl acrylamide).

CHAPTER 5

5.1. **c.**

5.2. **c.**

5.3. Physical targeting, active targeting, and passive targeting.

5.4. Peptides, monoclonal antibody, folic acid, and aptamers.

5.5. 1-C; 2-F; 3-E; 4-B; 5-D, and 6-A.

CHAPTER 6

6.1. **d.**

6.2. **e.**

6.3. **d.**

6.4. Solubility can be increased by two ways: 1) formulation strategies including the formation of stable salts, use of surfactants, co-solvents, solubilizing agents, or complexing agents; and 2) prodrug strategies including derivatization of a drug molecule using either a neutral (polyethylene glycol, PEG) or a charged (phosphate or succinate esters) promoiety.

6.5. **d.**

6.6. The ultimate goal in drug delivery is to deliver the drug at the specific site without any adverse reactions. This selectivity can be accomplished by targeting specific transporters/receptors, antigens, and enzymes. The localization of these transporters, receptors, and antigens in various tissues has been well characterized, studied, and exploited to design prodrugs to treat various diseases. By chemical modification or coupling to a ligand for a known transporter, the parent drug can be transported. Such transporter-targeted prodrugs also increase the bioavailability, resulting in enhanced therapeutic activity.

6.7. The most important biochemical barrier to absorption of drugs is the presence of efflux transporters. Efflux transporters like P-glycoprotein (P-gp), multidrug resistance protein (MRP), and breast cancer resistant protein (BCRP) secrete drugs back into the lumen, thus, lowering their intracellular concentration. During translocation across cell membranes, the transporter-targeted prodrug is not accessible to bind with efflux transporters. Hence, these site-specific prodrugs offer dual advantage by increasing the absorption and evading efflux proteins simultaneously.

6.8. **d.**

6.9. Formulation of prodrugs helps in providing controlled and sustained prodrug delivery. Furthermore, these nanosystems can also protect the prodrug from rapid metabolism, simultaneously evading efflux transporters.

CHAPTER 7

7.1. **1.**

7.2. Nanoparticles from preformed polymer can be prepared by the following methods:

1. Salting out method
2. Single emulsion-solvent evaporation method
3. Double emulsion-solvent evaporation method
4. Emulsification/solvent diffusion

7.3. Nanoparticles are colloidal solid particles with the size range of 10 to 1000 nm. Depending on the type of fabrication material, nanoparticles can be allocated into three major categories:

1. Polymeric nanoparticles
2. Solid lipid nanoparticles
3. Inorganic nanoparticles

7.4. Chitosan, sodium alginate, poly(lactide-co-glycolide), polycaprolactone, and polylactide are the examples of most commonly employed polymers for fabrication of polymeric nanoparticles.

7.5.

1. It can be employed for drug administration via any route, e.g., oral, intravenous and intraocular.
2. Site-specific drug delivery can be achieved by surface decoration with targeting ligand.
3. It can employed for delivering small hydrophilic and hydrophobic drugs as well as macromolecules.
4. Controlled and sustained drug delivery.
5. It protects entrapped drug from enzymatic or acidic degradation.

7.6. *Advantages:* Simple, easy, and reproducible large-scale manufacturing. Feasibility of conjugating targeting moiety on the surface of micelles for active targeting. Ability to develop clear aqueous solutions with hydrophilic corona that helps in preventing opsonization.

Disadvantages: Structure of micelles is fragile in nature. Subjected to extreme dilution upon administration. Premature drug release with no sustained/controlled release profiles.

7.7. Critical micellar concentration (CMC) is defined as the concentration of monomers in the solvent system at which aggregation of monomers is initiated.

7.8. There are two major methods of micelle preparations: (1) direct dissolution or simple equilibration and (2) organic solvent method. The organic solvent method includes 1) dialysis, 2) oil-in-water method, 3) solvent casting, and 4) freeze drying.

7.9. **1.**

7.10. **3.**

7.11. True.

7.12. Based on the structural morphology, liposomes can be classified as small or large unilamellar vesicles (SUVs, LUVs), multilamellar vesicles (MLVs), giant unilamellar or multilamellar vesicles (GUVs, GMVs), and multivesicular vesicles (MVVs).

CHAPTER 8

8.1. The efficient delivery of the drug to the target tissue depends on the chemical and physical properties of the conjugate as well as on the pathological conditions of the tissue environment.

8.2. Physiological impairment includes a decrease in nutrients and O_2 supply and accumulation of cellular metabolites. Pathological abnormalities like hypoxia, lower pH, and depletion of nutrients are the utilized strategies for enhancement of the pharmacological efficacy through modulating the physical affinity of the carrier systems.

8.3. Physiological-based approaches involve variables such as pH, temperature, and magnetism, whereas target ligands include monoclonal antibodies, peptides, polysaccharides, and transporters.

CHAPTER 9

9.1. Implants are single-unit drug delivery systems designed to deliver drug molecules at a therapeutically desired rate over a prolonged period of time and offer sustained drug release.

9.2. **d.**

9.3. Polymeric implantable systems are a type of implant that exploits the application of polymer and polymeric membranes for achieving controlled drug release in biological systems. Depending on the property of the polymer used, polymeric implantable drug delivery systems are subclassified into two categories: 1) non-biodegradable implant systems and 2) biodegradable implant systems.

9.4. **d.**

9.5. Polyglycolic acid (PGA), polylactic acid (PGA), polyaspartic acid (PAA) and poly (ε-caprolactone) (PCL) are the examples of most commonly employed polymers for fabrication of biodegradable implant systems.

9.6. Non-biodegradable implants are mainly fabricated from silicone, polyvinyl alcohol, and ethylene vinyl acetate polymers.

9.7. In the reservoir system, drug solution is surrounded by a polymeric membrane, while in matrix systems, the drug is uniformly dispersed into a polymeric matrix.

9.8. The ideal characteristics of implantable pumps are: 1) The pump should be capable of delivering the drug at controlled, sustained rates for prolonged periods of time; 2) the pump should provide a wide range of drug delivery rate (accuracy and precision of drug delivery should be preferably less than ±5% based on *in vitro* measurements); 3) it should offer protection against physical, chemical, and biological degradation of the drug; 4) it should be safe, noninflammatory, nontoxic, nonallergic, nonmutagenic, noncarcinogenic, and nonthrombogenic; 5) it should be leak free, offer overdose protection, and be convenient to use; 6) it should possess a sufficient drug reservoir, whose life is evaluated by drug requirement and the maximum drug concentration; 7) it should also possess a long battery life, be easily monitored, have ease of programmability, and be capable of adjusting the parameters as and when required; 8) it should be preferably implanted under local anesthesia rather than under general anesthesia because of frequent and regular complications by the latter; and 9) it should be easily sterilized to reduce the exposure of microorganisms after implantation.

9.9. **c.**

9.10. The desirable criteria for biological evaluation of biomaterials include the following: 1) The biomaterial should be compatible with various drugs and should not alter the pharmacological activity of the respective drug; 2) the biomaterial should be easily sterilizable without altering its physical, chemical, and mechanical properties; 3) the biomaterial should be molded into different shapes depending on the need (upon implantation, it should not lose it shape and be stable enough because these delivery systems are placed for a long period of time); 4) biodegradable biomaterials should be capable of degrading in a controlled fashion when exposed to the tissue environment; 5) the biomaterial should be chemically inert and not be altered by any physical or chemical stresses caused by local tissues (it should not interact with tissues surrounding the implanted tissues); (f) the biomaterial should be devoid of any toxicity and must not elicit allergic or hypersensitivity reactions or inflammatory and immunogenic responses (the biomaterial itself or the breakdown products should not be carcinogenic and not cause any thrombogenicity); and (g) most importantly, the biomaterial should be easily removed from the implanted site after its use or easily replaced in case of nonbioerodible materials.

CHAPTER 10

10.1. Aptamer targets show a great degree of diversity spanning from small molecules to amino acids, peptides, proteins, and whole cells. Aptamers can be selected from large pools of random oligonucleotide libraries by virtue of selective binding to purified molecules, whole living cells, and animals with high specificity and affinity. However, there are some drawbacks to consider for each target species. For example, relative to peptides and proteins, small molecules provide fewer sites for aptamer binding, and thus, it may not be easy to produce large numbers of aptamers that recognize a wide range of small molecules of interest. On the other hand, protein targets are structurally much larger and therefore provide multiple binding sites for aptamers. Most aptamers currently available for targeting applications have been developed against well-characterized purified proteins. However, selections against purified proteins are hampered by the limited number of purified receptors available, especially when the protein targets are insoluble or the targets are functionally part of multiprotein complexes. Although in many cases the recombinant production and purification of extracellular domains is possible, it is not guaranteed that the domain will still adopt a native conformation. To overcome these limitations, selection protocols based on living cells such as Cell-SELEX have been developed as alternative methods. In contrast to the selection processes against purified proteins, cell-based selections can be performed without prior knowledge of targets or multiprotein complexes expressed on the cell surface. Furthermore, intact living cells with many native receptor proteins can be used as targets during the selection procedure. This allows for a variety of ligands targeting several proteins on the same cell to be isolated from such screenings. As this strategy relies on the differences between the target cell population and the control cell population used for counter-selection (e.g. defined phenotype, protein expression levels, different protein conformations, etc.), multiple ligands recognizing only the target cell population and not the control/normal cells can be identified. Both conventional SELEX and cell-SELEX isolate aptamers under *in vitro* conditions by using either biologically purified proteins or whole living cells as targets. However, aptamer binding depends on the conformation of its target, which in turn is largely influenced by the target's physiological environment. Therefore, conventional SELEX and cell-SELEX may not generate the most relevant aptamers capable of localizing to specific tissues *in vivo*. In an effort to target the *in vivo* context of disease-specific moieties, an *in vivo* selection process was developed by using an animal model as the target [45]. Mi et al. designed an "*in vivo* selection" approach to screen a library of nuclease-resistant RNA oligonucleotides in tumor-bearing mice in order to identify candidates with the ability to localize to hepatic colon cancer metastases. One of the selected molecules was an RNA Apt that binds to p68, an RNA helicase that has been shown to be upregulated in colorectal cancer. For *in vivo* selection processes of aptamer targets, problems may arise, however, as a result of degradation and clearance of aptamers prior to binding events. For the purpose of improving the circulation half-life of aptamers, PEGylation of aptamers has been carried out. PEG molecules of high molecular weights have been conjugated to aptamers without affecting their binding ability to targets.

Using conventional SELEX, cell SELEX, and *in vivo* SELEX, researchers now can search aptamers with their binding targets under a wide range of environments. Despite the differences in practice, the SELEX technique allows for aptamer discovery unrestrained by the complexity of nucleic-acid–target interactions and thus can generate aptamers with unpredictable and unimaginable molecular configurations and targeted functions.

10.2. Aptamers have advantageous features to small-molecule ligands in that they can bind to their targets with high affinities, which is akin to that of antibody binding affinities. Unlike antibodies, aptamers can easily be chemically modified as a result of their high stability. Additionally, antibodies are far less immunogenic than antibodies. The preparation of antibodies relies on the induction of an immune response in animals; however, SELEX processes have much more versatility and can be fabricated for a range of nonimmunogenic targets. Furthermore, aptamers are capable of differentiating different cell types including normal and cancer cells and even between different varieties of cancer cells. Aptamers have substantial potential for drug delivery applications as they can either activate or inhibit extracellular targets or they can be conjugated to drugs themselves. One key characteristic that endows Apts with high specificity against targets is their secondary structure that arises from their specific nucleotide sequence. However, this secondary structure may be affected by heat, exonuclease or endonuclease degradation, and other environmental factors that could limit the stability of Apts and their binding properties. As a single aptamer is capable of delivering many drug molecules at the same time and could be more effective than using aptamers as drugs themselves, aptamer-mediated drug delivery can be an attractive option in drug delivery applications. In contrast to the *in vivo* production of other targeting molecules such as antibodies, the chemical production process of aptamers is not prone to viral or bacterial contamination. In addition, the stability of nucleic acid backbones allows aptamers to adapt to diverse chemical environments and engineering processes; show tolerance to heat, pH, and organic solvents; and be denatured and renatured multiples times without significant loss of activity. In addition, aptamers can be easily conjugated to various delivery platforms. The ability to attach fluorescent dyes or chemical groups allows aptamers to bring rich functionalities and integrate with advanced drug delivery systems. Aptamers show further potential because further efforts are now underway to use SELEX selection processes for identifying ligands capable of specific cellular internalization and transcytosis (transport across the cell interior).

10.3. In choosing a targeting ligand for specific drug delivery, a number of practical challenges should be considered, which include 1) the use of targeting ligands that are biocompatible, biodegradable/bioeliminable materials; 2) the use of simple, robust, and reproducible bioconjugation chemistries for the attachment of precursors and targeting ligands to drug delivery vehicles; 3) facile target ligand-drug assemblies that avoid multistep preparation and purification steps; 4) optimization of targeted drug delivery system biophysicochemical properties (e.g., size, charge, hydrophilicity, etc.) to achieve optimal drug attachment, long circulation half-life, suitable biodistribution, differential target tissue accumulation, efficacious target tissue drug concentration, and drug exposure kinetics; 5) validation of target ligand-drug delivery vehicle stability and predictable shelf-life; and 6) development or adaptation of scalable processes and units of operations amenable to the manufacturing of large quantities of ligand targeted-drug delivery systems for clinical development and commercialization.

Ligand targeted-drug delivery systems can lead to therapeutics being specifically retained in tissues and/or cells, resulting in a higher dose and duration of drug exposure within the target tissue. However, ultimately the question remains as to whether targeted therapies demonstrate dramatic improvements in clinical outcomes, which need to be demonstrated through well-executed larger clinical trials. Beyond the regulatory requirements of demonstrating safety, efficacy, quality, and cost-effectiveness, further challenges of each targeted technology need to be investigated on a case-by-case basis, and these challenges must be met in order to harness their tremendous potential as a new class of targeted therapeutics.

CHAPTER 11

11.1. Nanofibers are biocompatible and biodegradable polymeric fibers having a diameter of less than 100 nanometers. Nanofibers offers unique benefits such as higher catalytic efficiency, controlled pore size, enhanced cellular interactions, and the ability to modulate aqueous solubility, biocompatibility, and bio-recognition of therapeutic agents.

11.2. 1) synthetic polymer blends, 2) natural polymer blends, 3) natural–synthetic polymer blends, and 4) hydrophilic and hydrophobic polymer blends.

11.3. Polymeric nanofibers can be processed using several techniques such as electrospinning, self-assembly, phase separation, and template synthesis.

11.4. Three major parameters affect the electrospinning process during nanofiber preparation:

- **i.** System parameters (polymer molecular weight, distribution, and architecture)
- **ii.** Process parameters (orifice diameter, flow rate of polymer, and electric potential)
- **iii.** Ambient parameters (solution temperature, humidity, air velocity, and static electricity)

11.5. **d.**

11.6. Some drugs have an unfavorable pharmacokinetic (PK) profile. Therefore, use of nanofibers might be able to improve the PK, which would enhance the efficacy of the drug *in vivo*.

11.7. **a.**

11.8. **c.**

11.9. **b.**

CHAPTER 12

12.1. The number of junctions within one facet gives the triangulation number. Hence, $T = 1$, 4, and 16 for a), b), and c), respectively. There can be placed three building blocks at a junction giving rise to 3, 12, and 48 building blocks for a), b), and c), respectively.

12.2. In a), each triangular facet hosts three protein blocks giving in total 60 blocks; hence, $T=1$. In b), each triangular facet hosts one hexamer giving in total 20 hexamers of 120 blocks. Twelve pentamers account for the remaining 60 blocks. A total of 180 blocks is characteristic of $T=3$. Alternatively, $10(T-1)$ hexamers $= 20$; hence, $T=3$.

12.3. The least common multiple defines the number of the blocks and is 15. One variant of their arrangement is shown in Figure 12.8.

12.4. All native nanoparticles assemble from proteins or peptides from the bottom up. Proteins are sequence-defined polymers that employ a limited number of structurally rigid folding motifs that in turn have exact and predictable measures. For example, the distances between successive residues in a β-sheet and α-helix are always 0.33 nm and 0.15 nm, respectively, which means that one β-sheet or one α-helix of 20 residues would always span 6.6 nm and 3 nm. These folding motifs are therefore the main determinants of protein shapes and forms used for nanoparticle construction.

CHAPTER 13

13.1. Oral, intravenous, buccal, sublingual, nasal, and pulmonary are few major routes used for peptide and protein drug delivery.

13.2. Large molecular size, hydrophilicity, and susceptibility to enzymatic degradation can reduce oral absorption of proteins.

13.3. **d.**

13.4. Peptidases, papain, proteases, trypsin-like activity enzymes, and cathespin are a few enzymes capable of degrading peptides or proteins.

13.5. **e.**

13.6. Prodrugs are chemical derivatives that are required to undergo biotransformation to generate parent drug molecules.

13.7. Lipidation, PEGylation, and cyclic prodrug derivatization are a few approaches explored to increase protein absorption.

13.8. Proteins are highly hydrophilic in nature. This hydrophilicity reduces the membrane interaction of proteins as cell membrane is lipophilic in nature. Lipidation involves conjugation of lipids to protein molecules. Hence, the addition of lipids lowers the hydrophilicity of proteins that in turn enhances the interaction with cell membrane.

13.9. Peptide transporters such as PepT1 and PepT2 can transport di- and tripeptides.

13.10. **e.**

13.11. Drug delivery systems (mostly a polymer) with the ability of adhesion with a biological system (gastrointestinal mucosa) are referred to as bioadhesive systems. Bioadhesive systems are mainly designed:

- **i.** To increase the residence time and interaction of delivery system at the absorption site
- **ii.** To increase the concentration gradient and instant absorption of the therapeutic agent
- **iii.** To prevent active drug dilution or biodegradation in the luminal fluids
- **iv.** To enhance drug/delivery system localization at a target site

13.12. Hydroxyethyl methacrylate (HEMA), chitosan, alginate, gelatin, and dextran.

13.13. **1.** To encapsulate the therapeutic protein or peptide in a micelle's core; 2) to ensure the chemical and physical stability of the protein during and after processing of final formulation; 3) to encapsulate a small amount of proteins over wide batch sizes in a reproducible manner; and 4) to offer narrow size distribution of final formulation.

13.14. **1.** Immunoliposomes (conjugated to antibodies or antibody fragments), 2) stealth liposomes (conjugated with a protective layer of PEG to prevent opsonin recognition and rapid clearance), 3) long circulating immune-liposomes (conjugated with both a protective polymer and an antibody), and 4) surface-modified liposomes (surface modification using stimuli-responsive lipids, cell penetrating peptides, and diagnostic agents).

CHAPTER 14

14.1. The main types of nucleic acids therapeutics include plasmids, small interfering RNAs, oligonucleotides, aptamers, and ribozymes. Plasmids are circular, double-stranded DNA molecules, which need to enter the nucleus to express a particular therapeutic gene. Oligonucleotides can be classified into antisense ODNs and antigene ODNs. Antisense ODNs are single-stranded DNA oligonucleotides that inhibit gene expression at the posttranscription level. Antisense

ODNs can be designed to be complimentary to either mRNA or pre-mRNA to sterically block translation machinery or sterically inhibit pre-mRNA splicing or trigger the mRNA degradation at the ODN binding site by endogenous RNase H. By contrast, antigene ODNs work at the transcription level. Antigene ODN blocks gene transcription by forming a triplex with genomic DNA in a sequence-specific manner on the polypurine-polypyrimidine tract. Synthetic siRNA is double-stranded RNA of 21–23 nucleotides in length that can specifically silence its target gene in eukaryotic cells. Once inside the cells, the siRNA is unwound by an ATP-dependent helicase, and its antisense strand is incorporated into the RNA induced silencing complex (RISC). Subsequently, the antisense strand guides the RISC to its complementary mRNA, and Argonaute protein (AGO), a catalytic component in the RISC, triggers the degradation of the mRNA. Aptamers are artificial, short, single-stranded DNA or RNA oligonucleotides that can bind to macromolecules and small molecules with a high affinity. Ribozymes are catalytically active RNA molecules that can catalyze a chemical reaction of their substrate, most of which are an RNA molecule. Ribozymes bind to substrate RNAs via Watson-Crick base pairing and cleave the target RNA in a nonhydrolytic reaction.

14.2. Compared with small-molecule drugs, nucleic acids are promising therapeutics because a great variety of human diseases are caused by aberrant gene expressions. Through introducing therapeutic nucleic acids, defective genes can be corrected, replaced, or silenced. In addition, some of the nucleic acids therapeutics can regulate a variety of targets that are "undruggable" by conventional small molecular and monoclonal antibody drugs. Moreover, as developing traditional small-molecule drugs become more and more costly and time-consuming for the pharmaceutical industry, nucleic acids therapeutics is the new hope to solve these difficulties since theoretically it just needs to change the sequence of the nucleic acids once a successful delivery system has been developed.

14.3. Generally, nucleic acids have a relatively large molecular weight with negative charge, which prevent them from passing through biological membrane and increase the potential of triggering unwanted side effects. Also the biological properties of nucleic acids also prevent its potential application as therapeutics, including their instability and susceptibility to being degraded by nucleases. There are a series of either physical or biological barriers standing between the initiate site of injection and the final site of action. These barriers mainly include the difficulties in escaping the fate of degradation by various nucleases, clearance by the reticuloendothelial system, and excretion by the kidney; and in passing through various biological membranes, escaping from the endosome, and entering the nucleus.

14.4. First, chemical modification is usually regarded as a very effective way to increase its stability and reduce the toxicity of nucleic acids. All three basic structural units of nucleic acids including the sugar group, the phosphate group, and the nucleobase have been extensively explored for a great variety of modifications. Local administration is another strategy that is widely employed in many clinical studies to bypass the biological barriers associated with systemic administration. Also other common strategies include using viral or nonviral vectors to protect nucleic acids from degradation and enhance the biodistribution and therapeutic effect.

14.5. There are many nonviral materials used in nucleic acids delivery. The most common materials can be classified into a lipid-based, polymer-based, and peptide/protein-based delivery system or their combination. Liposomes are globular vesicles with a phospholipid bilayer and an aqueous core. They are formed by the mixture of cationic lipids, cholesterol, and neutral helper lipids at various ratios. As a result of their amphipthic nature, a wide variety of hydrophobic and hydrophilic agents can be loaded into liposomes. One problem associated with the lipid-based system is the short circulation time in the blood as a result of the excessive surface charge, which can lead to interaction with plasma proteins and elimination from the RES. To circumvent RES clearance and increase the circulation time of lipoplexes, polyethylene glycol (PEG) has been successfully employed to shield the positive charge of the system and prolong the circulation half-life of lipoplexes. Cationic polymers are another class of carriers that have been widely exploited for the delivery of nucleic acids. Among them, PEI, cationic dentrimer, and chitosan are the three most commonly used carriers. Similar to cationic lipids, these cationic polymers can condense nucleic acids to form nanoscale polyplexes. Cell-penetrating peptides (CPPs), also known as protein transduction domains (PTDs), are a class of peptides composed of basic amino acids that carry a net positive charge at physiological pH. Cationic peptides with repeated lysine and/or argentine are capable of condensing nucleic acids into small and compact particle efficiently. The net positive charge of the particles is able to interact with a negative charged biological membrane and facilitate the delivery of nucleic acids.

CHAPTER 15

15.1. c. Immune protection acquired by an animal/human through transfer from another animal/human, respectively, is termed passive immunity. This is the type of immunity an infant receives from his/her mother. Immunoglobulins and hyperimmune globulins are used to induce passive immunity. Active immunity is produced by an individual's own immunity, and it is acquired either by disease or vaccination.

15.2. b. Most micro-organisms are detected and destroyed within minutes or hours by short-lasting, nonspecific, and limited number of germline encoded innate immune receptors, whereas an adaptive immune response is carried by somatic receptors, and displays immunological memory against heterogeneous and mutating pathogens imparting long-lasting protection, but it is a delayed immune response.

15.3. b. IgG has a serum half-life of 25–35 days, although mast-cell bound IgE has the longest half-life. IgG immune complexes are opsonized for phagocytosis through binding to the IgG receptors on neutrophils and macrophages and through a complement system.

15.4. d. A primary immune response is characterized by the appearance of IgM antibodies during 3–4 days of viral antigen exposure. The peak primary immune response occurs 10 days after the antigen is encountered, and the serum contains both IgM and IgG antibodies.

15.5. d. Patients with an uncertain history of vaccination and Tetanus-prone injuries require both active and passive vaccination. Tetanus immunoglobulins provide immediate protection, while Tetanus toxoid administration leads to the establishment of a memory immune response. An individual with active vaccination requires no treatment if the last vaccination was administered less than 5 years earlier.

15.6. b. $CD8^+$ or cytotoxic T cells recognize the antigen-peptide fragments (epitopes) bound to MHC class I molecules on the surface of antigen presenting cells (e.g., macrophages or dendritic cells), while $CD4^+$ T cells recognize the antigen-peptide fragments bound to MHC class II molecules.

15.7. b. B cells secrete antibodies and bind to toxins. Secreted antibodies cause opsonization of antibody-toxin complexes. Antibodies play an important role in conferring extracellular immune protection. An effector CTL kills a virus infected cell when it recognizes peptide fragments of an internal viral protein bound to class I MHC proteins on the surface of an infected cell (e.g., DC or macrophage). Interferons are proteins secreted from viral infected cells, and they induce the appearance of antiviral proteins in other cells.

15.8. b. Live attenuated vaccines replicate and produce long-lasting immune response. Live attenuated vaccines require low doses compared with inactivated or killed vaccines. Inactivated or killed vaccines are not competent for replication and require high doses.

15.9. b. A live attenuated influenza vaccine is available in injectable (IM) and intranasal forms. A yellow fever vaccine is administered subcutaneously; an inactivated polio vaccine is available for IM administration; and a live attenuated MMR vaccine is approved for SC administration.

15.10. b. An inactivated polio vaccine is approved in the United States.

15.11. b. Pneumococcal and meningococcal vaccines are available as polysaccharide and conjugate forms; a hemophilus b influenza vaccine is available as a meningococcal protein and tetanus toxoid conjugates; a polio vaccine is available as an inactivated protein vaccine and small pox vaccine containing a live attenuated virus; and Japanese encephalitis and anthrax vaccines contain respective inactivated proteins.

15.12. c. The hepatitis B vaccine is produced by insertion of a segment of the respective viral gene into the gene of yeast, *Saccharomyces cerevisiae*. The modified yeast cell produces a pure hepatitis B surface antigen.

15.13. b. Inactivated vaccines produce pain, swelling, and redness at the site of injection. Vaccine adjuvants may contribute to local adverse reactions, while live vaccines produce fever and myalgia.

15.14. d. The Bacillus of Calmette and Guerrin vaccine contains a live attenuated culture preparation of Bacillus of Calmette and Guerrin strain of *Mycobacterium bovis*; the varicella vaccine contains a live attenuated virus; and DTaP contains diphtheria, tetanus toxoids, and an inactivated pertussis protein.

15.15. c. The minimal interval between doses of most vaccines is 4 weeks. The last dose of the series is separated from the previous dose by 4–6 months. Decreasing the interval compromises immune response, while increasing the interval does not affect the immune response.

15.16. c. The hepatitis B vaccine is recommended at birth to decrease the incidence of hepatitis B in infants of hepatitis B infected mothers.

15.17. b. cDNAs is the DNA synthesized from mRNA. In this process, RNA is used as the template and mRNA uses a reverse transcriptase enzyme for DNA synthesis. This phenomenon is the reversal of the transcription where mRNA is synthesized from DNA.

15.18. Affinity between T-cell receptor and MHC (II)-antigen-peptide complex, density of the complex, nature of DC subsets (myeloid DC vs lymphoid DC), types of co-stimulatory molecules expressed on naïve $CD4^+$ T cells, and types of cytokines secreted by dendritic cells, naïve $CD4^+$ T cells differentiate first into T_H0 cells, and then either into T_H1 or T_H2 or T_H17 helper cells. Adjuvants have no preservative action.

15.19. d.

15.20. b. Particle size plays a key role in particle-based adjuvant systems. Particles in the size range 0.1–1 μm are taken up by dendritic cells, and they initiate adaptive immune responses.

15.21. Mucosal tolerance eliminates oral and nasal routes of administration. In the case of alum adjuvanted vaccines (e.g., hepatitis, diphtheria, tetanus, and pertussis vaccines), the intramuscular route is strongly preferred because subcutaneous administration leads to an increased incidence of local reactions such as irritation, inflammation, granuloma formation, and necrosis.

15.22. Langerhans cells are key antigen presenting cells in the epidermis.

15.23. Liquid suspensions also cause aqueous degradation. Both dry powder and lyophilized powder exist in a solid state condition, and they improve the stability of vaccines. In both approaches, vaccine antigens are mixed with bulking excipients to improve the content uniformity or assist in processing (lyophilization). Dry powder or lyophilized powder is mixed with appropriate diluents before administration.

15.24. d.

CHAPTER 16

16.1. b.

16.2. c.

16.3. c.

16.4. d.

16.5. d.

16.6. b.

16.7. b.

16.8. e.

16.9. e.

16.10. The U.S. FDA uses an "aggregate weight of evidence" approach to evaluate the bioequivalence of metered nasal and inhalation products. This approach uses the following criteria for documentation of bioequivalence: 1) *in vitro* studies between test and reference products to support equivalent performance of the metering device, 2) pharmacokinetic studies to establish equivalence in systemic exposure, and 3) pharmacodynamic or clinical endpoint studies to demonstrate equivalence in local action.

16.11. Characterization tests for nanomaterial-containing drug products may include 1) particle size and size distribution, 2) particle shape or architecture, 3) surface chemistry (such as charge, coating, and density), and 4) aggregation or agglomeration state. See the text in this chapter for the reasons why the tests are particularly important for these products.

CHAPTER 17

17.1. Tumor angiogenesis, tumor hypoxia, acidic pH, interstitial hypertension, and metastasis.

17.2. The EPR effect is a phenomenon that nanoparticles or macromolecules ranging from 20 to 200 nm tend to extravasate and accumulate inside the interstitial space in tumor tissues. The tumor vasculature is structurally and functionally abnormal compared with normal vessels in healthy tissues. Tumor vessels are unevenly distributed, heterogeneous, chaotic, irregularly branched, tortuous, leaky, thin-walled, and pericyte-depleted.

Generally, the tumor microenvironment is characterized by large fenestration, lack of smooth muscle layers, and ineffective lymphatic drainage, and therefore, it helps to accumulate nanoscale particles and macromolecules in tumor tissues rather than in normal tissues.

17.3. Based on its composition and structure, the liposome can be classified into three types: conventional liposome, stealth liposome, and targeted liposome. The conventional liposome is the first generation of liposomes to be used in therapeutic applications. Generally, the conventional liposome is only composed of neutral and/or charged lipids plus co-lipids. It is also the most popular liposome formulation in translational research. The stealth liposome is a second-generation liposome, and its surface is modified with PEG. Compared with the conventional liposome, the stealth liposome escapes uptake by the mononuclear phagocyte system and avoids the lysis of the complement system, which dramatically prolongs blood circulation time and improves biodistribution. Moreover, the PEGylated liposome exhibits stability with minimal vesicle aggregation. Targeted liposomes are prepared by coupling targeting ligands to the PEG-end of stealth liposomes via a stable or cleavable linker. Targeted liposomes cannot increase the drug accumulation in tumors compared with stealth liposomes, but they exhibit more selectivity and higher uptake. The targeting ligands include monoclonal antibodies or their fragments, peptides, aptamers, small molecules, and natural receptor ligands.

17.4. Antibody–drug conjugates are constructed by covalently conjugating a recombinant antibody to a cytotoxic chemical via a synthetic linker. Cytotoxic chemicals provide the pharmacological potency, while highly specific antibodies serve as the targeting agent, which also includes a carrier that increases the half-life and biocompatibility of the conjugate. The antibody–drug conjugates are generally taken up by tumor cells via receptor-mediated endocytosis. Theoretically, the number of antigens/targets per tumor cell is limited (10^3–10^6). Only thousands of antibody–drug molecules can be internalized to release the active parent drugs. The drug payload of antibody–drug conjugates is generally low, and each antibody molecule only conjugates with one to three cytotoxic molecules. Therefore, the chemical toxin must be highly potent and able to kill tumor cells at a very low dose.

17.5. ANG1005 is composed of Angiopep-2 linked to three molecules of paclitaxel with a cleavable succinyl ester linkage. After conjugation, Angiopep-2 dramatically increases the capacity of uptake of paclitaxel into the brain. The peptide Angiopep-2 is a ligand that binds to the low-density lipoprotein receptor-related protein (LRP) receptor at the BBB. The binding of Angiopep-2 with the LRP receptor results in crossing the BBB by receptor-mediated transport. The *in vivo* uptake of ANG1005 into the brain and brain tumors is 4–54-fold higher than that of paclitaxel. Moreover, ANG1005 bypasses P-gp and resides in the brain much longer even after capillary deletion and vascular washout.

CHAPTER 18

18.1. Some of the main cardiovascular diseases are as follows: atherosclerosis (hyperlipidemia/hypercholesterolemia), coronary artery diseases, angina pectoris, myocardial infarction (heart attack), congestive heart failure, and hypertension.

18.2. Some of the main cardiovascular drug classes are as follows: diuretics, α blockers, β blockers, angiotensin converting enzyme (ACE), angiotensin II receptor blockers (ARBs), nitrovasodilators, Ca^{2+} channel blockers, and statins.

18.3. Renin converts angiotensinogen into angiotensin-I, which is converted into angiotensin-II by ACE. Angiotensin-II binds to the AT1 receptor causing blood vessels to constrict and an increase in blood pressure.

18.4. The characteristic sequence of chemical bonds present in all nitrovasodilator drugs is the nitrate ester/C–O–NO_2/carbon–oxygen–nitrogen bond.

18.5. Statins inhibit HMG-CoA reductase.

18.6. The calcium channel blockers/antagonists inhibit the L-type calcium channel.

18.7. Angiotensin II binds to the AT1 receptor to control arterial blood pressure.

18.8. Organic nitrates or nitric oxide cause relaxation of vascular smooth muscle leading to vasodilation.

18.9. The low-molecular-mass organic nitrates such as nitroglycerin are administered with an inert carrier such as lactose because they are volatile and an oily liquid.

18.10. The most effective drugs for the reduction of LDL levels are statins.

18.11. Statins are competitive inhibitors of 3-hydroxy-3-methylglutaryl coenzyme A (HMG-CoA) reductase, which catalyzes an early, rate-limiting step in cholesterol biosynthesis.

18.12. Some statins like lovastatin and simvastatin are less water soluble than other statins because they are lactone prodrugs.

18.13. The ACE converts angiotensin I into angiotensin II.

18.14. The first clinically used angiotensin II receptor blocker (ARB) developed was losartan.

18.15. The heart and the circulation system are the two main components of the cardiovascular system.

18.16. A fully developed and mature heart consists of four compartments or chambers.

18.17. Two major circulation systems constitute the cardiovascular system: the systemic and pulmonary circulation systems.

18.18. In systemic circulation, arteries carry oxygenated blood away from the heart, while veins carry deoxygenated blood back to the heart. However, the roles are reversed in the pulmonary circulation, in which the pulmonary artery carries deoxygenated blood into the lungs while the pulmonary vein transports oxygenated blood back to the heart from the lungs.

18.19. A mammalian heart has four valves: two atrioventricular valves and two semilunar valves.

a. The mitral valve and tricuspid valve are the atrioventricular valves, located between the atria and ventricles. They prevent backflow of blood from the ventricle to the atria.

b. The aortic valve and pulmonary valve are the semilunar valves, located between the artery and the ventricle. They pump blood into the artery and prevent backflow.

18.20. Structural differences between type I and type II valves are based on location, function, and valve hemodynamics.

a. Leaflets of type I valves are thinner and lack chordae tendinae, as they function in a rhythmic pattern in response to pressure gradient from aorta/artery to prevent backflow of blood.

b. Leaflets of type II valves are thicker as a result of spongiosa and atrialis layers at the leaflet edges. During ventricular systole, thick and vascular walls of ventricles apply large force (compared with a pressure gradient in the aorta) to pump blood to the lungs or the body. Type II valves regulate blood flow from the ventricle to the atria. To prevent prolapse in this process, leaflets are anchored to the ventricle wall with chordae tendinae, which become tense holding flaps together.

18.21. **a.** The conditions and constraints required for a new artificial valve graft are as follows:

1. *Biological requirements:* biocompatible, biodegradable, nontoxic, and nonimmunogenic.

2. *Mechanical requirements:* Mechanical strength, durability, and long-term stability.

3. *Material requirements:* Porosity, ability to deliver bioactive molecules, and ease of processability.

Material of choice: Scaffolds prepared from naturally or synthetically obtained extracellular matrix proteins like collagen, elastin, and hyaluronic acid.

b. We would perform the following testes to assess biocompatibility:

1. *In vitro* assessment

i. *Biological reactivity test:* Biological compatibility of mammalian cells to artificial graft surface

2. *In vivo* animal studies using shunt method

i. *Immunohistochemistry:* Immunological reactions

ii. *Calcification study:* Formation of calcium deposits triggered as a result of inflammation

iii. *Surface characterization:* Changes in surface morphology on contact with blood.

c. From the above tests, long-term durability and biocompatibility assessment under valve failure conditions cannot be performed. Accelerated wear testing, dynamic failure mode testing, and cavitation study are a few of the FDA recommended studies to replicate heart hemodynamics and disease conditions. These experiments are performed using specially designed chambers equipped with high-performance pressure transducers, stroboscopes, still/video cameras, and valve testers. These studies provide accelerated testing information, which cannot be obtained using conventional *in vitro* or *in vivo* studies.

18.22.
- Autograft—from recipient, no concern regarding compatibility
- Allograft—from the same species, tissue typing necessary
- Isograft—from identical twins, no concern regarding compatibility
- Xenograft—from different species, most probability of incompatibility
  - ✓ Xenograph—has natural valve action, so there is less chance of hemolysis and coagulation; quiet; cannot be reconnected to chordae tendinae

✓ Disk—possibility of hemolysis as a result of structure; low coagulation as a result of use of pyrolitic carbon; noisy; low aspect ratio; may leak

✓ Poppet—ball must be chosen carefully to avoid swelling/sticking; high aspect ratio; possible hemolysis as a result of cage

18.23.
- Allograft—tissue or organ from a donor of the same species; example: cadaveric donation
- Xenograft—tissue or organ from a donor of a different species; example: baboon heart transplant for infants
- Testing required—ABO (blood) typing, T-cell crossmatch, HLA testing
- Xenografts are less likely to be accepted as a result of the foreign proteins located on the cells; these will have a greater difference from the recipient than will those of a donor of the same species

18.24. Porcine xenograft:

Advantages
- Biocompatible functional properties (e.g., hemodynamics).
- Anticoagulants (resistance to thrombosis) therapy is not required.
- Valves do not make clicking noise.

Disadvantages
- Prone to calcification.
- Pig valves last between 10 and 15 years, while cow valves can last beyond 20 years in some cases.
- Immune rejection.

Metallic valves:

Advantages
- Durability and lower risk of valve replacement or re-operations.

Disadvantages
- Anticoagulant therapy is required.
- Clicking noise in patients.

18.25. Testing required: ABO (blood) typing, T-cell crossmatch, HLA testing. Histocompatibility—presence of antigens on cell surfaces, which are recognized as foreign by the recipient's immune system.

18.26. Major causes of bioprosthetic heart valve failure are as follows:
- Congenital bicuspid aortic valve disease
- Infective endocarditis
- Rheumatic fever
- Myxomatous degeneration
- Aortic aneurysm

18.27. The major steps for tissue calcification are as follows:

a. Initiation

b. Nucleation

c. Proliferation

18.28. Application of tissue engineering in synthetic heart valves:

a. Can improve material biocompatibility

b. Enhance cell adhesion and migration

c. Increase matrix biomechanical properties

d. Reduce immunogenic reactions

e. Reduce the need for allografts and xenografts

18.29. Factors involved:
- Degree of thrombogeneity
- Degree of hemolysis effects

Properties that influence these factors:
- Surface roughness—smooth reduces coagulation and hemolysis
- Surface tension—low minimizes adhesion and prevents coagulation; high builds up hemolysis-resistant layer
- Surface charge—negative repels blood cells and prevents coagulation

18.30.
- Least likely to be carcinogenic
  - Any material that is inert
  - No chemical pathway for carcinogenesis from ceramics has been identified to date
- Types of testing
  - Ames test in tissue culture to determine mutagenic potential
  - *In vivo* animal test to determine tumor incidence
- Limitations
  - Mutagenicity does not indicate carcinogenicity: lack of mutagenicity implies lack of carcinogenicity
  - *In vivo* tests do not generally exceed latency period for carcinogenic materials
  - Tumor generation in a small number of animals is often not statistically significant, especially as a result of spontaneous tumor generation

CHAPTER 19

19.1. b.

19.2. d.

19.3. d.

19.4. e.

19.5. Implants control the release kinetics of drugs from polymeric delivery systems by using various polymer and polymeric membranes. This is an invasive technique in which implants are placed at the pars plana of the eye.

Classification of implants:

a. Non-biodegradable solid implants

b. Biodegradable solid implants

19.6. The different types of stem cells are as follows:

a. Retinal progenitor cell (RPC)

b. Embryonic stem cell (ESC)

c. Induced pluripotent stem cell (iPS)

d. Mesenchymal stem cell (MSC)

e. Bone marrow (BM)

19.7. Upon repetitive dosing through the intravitreal route, damage to the eye may occur in the form of retinal detachment, cataract, hyperemia, and endophthalmitis.

19.8. Membrane transporters are the membrane-bound proteins that help in translocation of nutrients across the biological membranes. Transporter systems are classified into two categories: 1) efflux transporters and 2) influx transporters. These efflux and influx transporters belong to the ATP binding cassette superfamily and solute carrier (SLC) superfamily, respectively. An efflux transporter (depending on its polarization) acts as a hindrance for entry of the drug molecule into the cell, whereas an influx transporter (depending on their polarization) facilitates entry of the drug molecule into the cell.

19.9. An ideal drug delivery system must provide 1) controlled release of drugs, 2) drug targeting through a systemic route, and 3) enhancement of drug permeation through a barrier. The two approaches, i.e., 1) and 2) are used to overcome the difficulties in delivering the drug to the posterior segment of the eye by topical administration. Approach 2 is used for the drugs that are administered systemically for ocular tissues. This approach is used not only to facilitate drug efficacy but also to rarefy adverse effects.

CHAPTER 20

20.1. True.

20.2. True.

20.3. An increase in viscosity leads to a prolongation of a system's contact time on the delivery site (Barry, 1974; Dolz et al., 1997). To remain in the cervix, the formulation must be thick enough not to run out of the vagina or flow down the back of cervix. As gelation is reversible, removal is facilitated by immersion into or turning back to the original pH.

20.4. Thixotropy is the property exhibited by the pseudo-plastic systems that exhibit the time-dependent change in the viscosity.

The properties suitable for vaginal delivery systems provide a response to environmental changes (pH change from 4.4 to 7.4), such that the liquid formulation after instillation undergoes a phase transition in the cavity upon exposure to male semen to form a visco-elastic gel, withstanding *in vivo* shearing action of fluid movements and achieving a longer residence in the cervical mucosa.

20.5. Clearly specify your rationale behind the equations, and define and identify all the necessary variables.

CHAPTER 21

21.1. Expression of tight junctions between brain capillary endothelial cells prevents passive diffusion of hydrophilic therapeutic agents from systemic circulation. Moreover, efflux proteins expressed on the luminal side of brain capillary cells also extrudes therapeutic agents to systemic circulation. These two factors play an important role in reducing the brain permeability of therapeutic agents.

21.2. Intravenous, intra-arterial, and transnasal delivery approaches have been employed for delivery of drugs to the brain. Intravenous delivery is the common route for brain drug delivery. Drugs administered by intravenous route bypass first-pass metabolism. Moreover, the brain is highly perfused with blood capillaries and the large surface area of the brain is connected with a capillary network. Hence, this route is more suitable for brain drug targeting. Intra-arterial delivery involves direct injection into blood, which allows the drug to reach brain capillaries before the drug enters peripheral circulation. Intra-arterial delivery has similar advantages to intravenous delivery. However, for drugs administered by both routes, the BBB is the rate-limiting barrier. Transnasal delivery allows for the drug to diffuse into systemic circulation from the respiratory region and/or the drug may reach the brain directly via olfactory and trigeminal neuronal pathways.

21.3. Nasal cavities are divided into three regions, nasal vestibular, respiratory, and olfactory regions. The nasal vestibular region is responsible for filtering out airborne particles and has no significant role in drug absorption. The respiratory region is the largest part of the nasal cavity and is highly vascularized. The respiratory region is responsible for drug absorption into systemic circulation. The drug absorption pathways include paracellular and transcellular pathways, transcytosis, and carrier-mediated transport. The olfactory region (next to the respiratory region) is the major portal for drug absorption into the brain. Drug absorption pathways from the olfactory region include paracellular, transcellular, olfactory and trigeminal neuronal, perivascular, and CSF pathways.

21.4. Intracerebral (intraparenchymal), intraventricular (transcranial), and intrathecal (intra-CSF) delivery approaches have been employed for direct brain delivery of drugs. All these approaches are invasive. Drugs have to diffuse to target tissue from the site of injection. Drug diffusion decreases exponentially with the distance between injection and target sites. Therefore, these approaches are combined with convection enhanced delivery that involves site-specific administration. Intrathecal delivery involves administration of the drug directly into CSF at the cistern magna of the brain. This is less invasive compared with intracerebral and intraventricular injections. A major limitation with the intrathecal route is rapid drug clearance from CSF to blood. Therefore, drugs cannot reach the deep parenchymal tissue. Hence, this rote is mainly employed for spinal diseases.

21.5. Efflux proteins such as P-glycoprotein (P-gp), multidrug resistance associated protein (MRP2), and breast cancer resistance protein (BCRP) are expressed on brain capillary endothelial cells.

21.6. Efflux proteins require energy to efflux therapeutic agents. This energy is supplied from ATP hydrolysis.

21.7. Modulation of efflux proteins with use of inhibitors, a prodrug approach, and use of a novel drug delivery system such as nanoparticles and liposomes have been explored to enhance the brain permeability of therapeutic agents.

21.8. Nutrient transporters such as amino acid, biotin, riboflavin, glucose, and ascorbic acid transporters are reported to be expressed on brain capillary endothelial cells.

21.9. **d.**

21.10. **d.**

21.11. The lipidation approach involves conjugation of fatty acids or lipids to therapeutic agents that are highly hydrophilic in nature. Such conjugation decreases the hydrophilic characteristics of therapeutic agents, thereby increasing interaction with the absorbing cell membrane.

CHAPTER 22

22.1. Dendritic cells are primarily antigen presenting cells in the body. Their main function is to process antigen material and present it on the surface to other cells, e.g., T cells, of the immune system, which then specifically recognize and ultimately eliminate the antigen source. Dendritic cells can not only induce innate and adaptive immune responses, but also they can maintain immunological tolerance in the steady state. For cancer therapy, dendritic cells can be *in vitro* challenged with tumor-associated antigens such as cancer extracts, cancer antigens, RNA of cancer tissues, and cancer cells to present a potent antigenic stimulus to T cells and induce tumor-specific immune reactions.

22.2. Stem cells are defined by their self-renewal capacity and the pluri/multipotency in differentiation into different lineages. Based on their origin, stem cells can be embryonic stem cells, which are isolated from the inner cell mass of blastocysts, and adult stem cells, which are resident in postnatal tissues, such as bone marrow, brain, and heart. Although embryonic stem cells can differentiate into all derivatives of the three primary germ layers, ectoderm, endoderm, and mesoderm, adult stem cells are responsible for maintaining cellular homeostasis of tissues by replenishing cells that are lost through maturation and senescence or through injury and have only multipotency, giving rise to progeny of several distinct cell types. In general, adult stem cells can be isolated based on their specific surface antigen markers, which are distinct for different adult stem cells.

22.3. MSCs are extremely versatile and are very promising as cell-based therapeutics. They can not only differentiate into mesodermal lineages, but also they can transdifferentiate into myoblasts, neural precursors, cardiomyocytes, and other cell types. In addition, MSCs are considered immunoprivileged as a result of the lack of HLA class II surface antigens and thus can be used as allogeneic products. Most importantly, MSCs secrete multiple anti-inflammatory, angiogenic, neurotrophic, immunomodulatory, and antifibrotic factors. The immunosuppressive ability of MSCs makes them very promising in treating immune-related diseases, such as acute graft-versus-host disease, liver disease, diabetic foot ulcers, cutaneous wounds, neurological disease, and bone marrow transplantation, among others. Furthermore, the homing property of MSCs to injured sites as well as tumors makes them an ideal vehicle for delivery of therapeutic agents, for example, cancer gene therapy.

22.4. Tumorigenicity is one of the most concerned issues for cell-based therapeutics. First of all, undifferentiated ESCs and iPSCs can form teratomas in immunocompromised animals, which sets another risk and should be assessed when using them in humans. Although in some cases more differentiated, lineage-committed cells are used, current differentiation protocols do not guarantee cell preparations free of undifferentiated cells. Second, MSCs, ESCs, and iPSCs have been demonstrated to acquire chromosomal aberrations during expansion in culture, which is a hallmark of human cancer. Minimizing the culture time might be required in order to decrease the chance for *in vitro* genetic aberrations. Additionally, immunoprivilege of MSCs may present a risk of supporting tumor progression. Finally, there is the concern that genetically modified cells may be more prone to form tumors if the transfected gene inserts into an inappropriate place (insertional mutagenesis) and either disrupts the expression of a tumor-suppressor gene or activates an oncogene.

22.5. For cell-based therapeutics, the unique properties of living cells make the current regulations on drugs impractical, especially for stem-cell products and there is an urgent need to draft regulatory guidelines for developing cell-based therapeutics. At the current stage, cell-based therapeutics are considered therapeutic agents and therefore meet the definitions of several different kinds of regulated products by the FDA including biologic products, drugs, devices, xenotransplantation products, and human cells, tissues, and cellular and tissue-based products. A submission of an investigational new drug application to the FDA before studies involving humans are initiated is required according to the Public Health Safety Act, Section 351. In addition, in many cases, a genetic modification of cells before transplantation is applied and such treatment would also be considered to be gene therapy, thus, subjecting to FDA regulations pertaining to this issue. Although it is still under intensive development, in 2008, the International Society for Stem Cell Research published Guidelines for the Clinical Translation of Stem Cells (available at http://www.isscr.org/clinical_trans), which "provides a framework for the responsible and timely development of clinically useful stem-cell-based therapies." In addition, a roadmap for the development of the stem-cell-based therapy from bench to bedside has been proposed.

CHAPTER 23

23.1. As a result of its excellent biocompatibility and safety, the use of collagen in biomedical application has been rapidly growing and widely expanding to bioengineering areas.

23.2. The attractiveness of collagen in drug-incorporated particles lies in its recognition by the body as a natural constituent rather than as a foreign body, causing low immunogenicity and superior biocompatibility as compared with other natural polymers, such as albumin and gelatin. Collagen can be solubilized into an aqueous solution, particularly in acidic aqueous media, engineered to exhibit tailor-made properties and converted into a number of different forms including strips, sheets, sponges, and beads, making it an ideal material for drug delivery.

Some disadvantages of collagen-based systems arose from the difficulty of assuring adequate supplies, their poor mechanical strength, and ineffectiveness in the management of infected sites. There are some limitations of collagen as a drug-incorporated carrier, like the high viscosity of an aqueous phase, nondissolution in neutral pH buffers, thermal instability (denaturation), and biodegradability. These limitations could be overcome by making collagen conjugates with other biomaterials or chemically modifying a collagen monomer without affecting its triple helical conformation and maintaining its native properties.

23.3. *Tropocollagen:* The orderly arrangement of triple helix tropocollagen molecules results in a formation of fibrils having a distinct periodicity. Nonhelical telopeptides are attached to both ends of the molecule and serve as the major source of antigenecity. Atelocollagen, which is produced by elimination of the telopeptide moieties using pepsin, has demonstrated its potential as a drug carrier, especially for gene delivery.

Collasomes: Collasomes were developed by adding long hydrocarbon side chains to the collagen. Collasomes can be formulated with various constituents and chemically alternated with the addition of lipid (called lacrisomes) for the delivery of water-soluble drugs. Collasomes increase not only the hydrophobicity of the collagen but also the total surface area, resulting in a decrease in the diffusion rate of hydrophilic drug molecules from the collagen matrix.

23.4. One of the major problems with implanted biomaterial applications is calcification, which is influenced by the structure of the implantable system that decides its *in vivo* therapeutic efficiency and clinical fate. In bioprosthetic heart valves (BHVs), the aortic wall and leaflet have mainly served as calcifiable matrices. Thus, bioprosthetic aortic wall calcification mainly resulting from collagen has a potential to cause the clinical failure of the BHV or other collagen-based formulations.

23.5. Desirable—vessel grafts: a clot seals the fabric and provides a biocompatible surface. Undesirable—heart valves: a clot interferes with the action of the valve, which may cause an embolus.

CHAPTER 24

24.1. *Ultrasound imaging* measures the interaction of high-frequency sound waves (1–10 MHz) with the tissue of interest. Sound waves travel fast in solids and liquids and slow in gas. When sound waves are applied to a subject through a transducer, they are reflected at the interface of tissues or organs of different densities and recorded in the transducer. High-resolution morphological images can be constructed based on the echoes, attenuation of the sound, and sound speed.

Magnetic resonance imaging (MRI) measures the longitudinal (T_1) and transverse (T_2) relaxation rates of protons (mainly water protons) in the body. Water forms approximately 60% of the body weight of a normal human adult. Different tissues have different proton density and different T_1 and T_2 relaxation rates thereby generating different MR signals. High-resolution, three-dimensional anatomic images are constructed from the signals of the proton relaxations in different tissues.

Optical imaging mainly uses visible and infrared lights to visualize the morphology, biomarkers, and biological processes of the subject of interest. Fluorescence and luminescence imaging techniques are the popular optical imaging modalities in biological and biomedical research. Fluorescence imaging measures the fluorescence emitted from a fluorophore after excitation with an external light source. Luminescence imaging detects the light emission from a chemical or biochemical reaction with no external excitation.

X-ray radiography measures the attenuation of X-rays by the tissues through which they pass. When an X-ray beam passes through the body, it can be scattered or absorbed by the tissues based on their densities, resulting in loss of X-ray intensity, known as attenuation. An image of the body is constructed from the attenuated X-rays recorded on X-ray sensitive cameras. X-Ray attenuation is strong in dense tissue (such as bone) and weak in soft tissues.

Single-photon emission computed tomography (SPECT) detects the γ-rays emitted by radioactive isotopes. SPECT requires the administration of radiopharmaceuticals or radiotracers. Each decay of the radioisotopes emits one γ-ray, which is detected by a rotating camera and processed by a computer to generate three-dimensional images. SPECT has a high sensitivity for detecting radiopharmaceuticals and is effective for molecular imaging. Although SPECT provides quantitative information about their distribution in the body, it is not effective for high-resolution anatomical imaging.

Positron emission tomography (PET) also detects γ-rays from the body after administration of radiopharmaceuticals containing radionuclides that emit positrons. Each decay of PET radionuclides or probes emits one positron, which then annihilates with an electron in the tissue to give a pair of γ-rays with energy of 511 KeV at almost 180. The γ-rays are recorded by detectors and processed by a computer to produce three-dimensional images. PET is highly sensitive for detecting its probes and generally used for functional and molecular imaging.

24.2. Drug delivery is a process of transporting therapeutics to diseased tissues and cells to achieve enhanced therapeutic efficacy. Molecular imaging provides a noninvasive tool for investigating the mechanism and process of drug delivery. Intracellular and *in vivo* delivery processes can be continuously visualized by molecular imaging by labeling drug delivery systems with imaging probes. The drug delivery efficiency can also be quantitatively determined by molecular imaging modalities, such as SPECT and PET. Molecular imaging provides a more accurate assessment of whole-body pharmaceutical properties, including pharmacokinetics, biodistribution, and targeting efficiency, of drug delivery systems than conventional methods in both preclinical and clinical development. Accurate determination of the delivery process of drug delivery systems using molecular imaging will assist the optimization, design, and development of more effective drug delivery systems.

24.3. SPECT and PET can provide sensitive and quantitative measurement of radioactively labeled drug delivery systems.

24.4. Contrast-enhanced MRI provides high-resolution and whole-body visualization of the pharmacokinetics and biodistribution of drug delivery systems. SPECT provides sensitive and quantitative measurement of radioactively labeled drug delivery systems.

24.5. Fluorescence imaging, MRI, SPECT, PET, and ultrasound imaging can be used for noninvasive evaluation of drug delivery systems.

24.6. PET with ^{18}F-FDG is a commonly used method for noninvasive imaging of tissue metabolism in response to therapies in preclinical and clinical studies. It measures metabolic activities of the tissue of interest based on quantification of ^{18}F-FDG uptake. ^{18}F-FDG is a glucose derivative that is taken by cells via glucose membrane transporters. ^{18}F-FDG is trapped in the cells of high glucose uptake and metabolic activities after it converts to ^{18}F-FDG-6-phosphate, which cannot be metabolized further. ^{18}F-FDG-PET can thereby differentiate tissues of high metabolic activities from less active tissues. Proliferative tumor tissues are highly metabolic active and have higher accumulation of ^{18}F-FDG than normal tissues, generating a stronger PET signal. ^{18}F-FDG-PET is routinely used in clinical practice for evaluating the efficacy of anticancer therapies and predicting therapeutic outcomes.

24.7. Bioluminescence imaging is an effective modality to determine noninvasively the real-time transfection efficiency of a nonviral gene delivery system with a reporter gene, such as the plasmid DNA expressing firefly luciferase.

24.8. Bioluminescence imaging with a firefly luciferase reporter gene is effective for noninvasive real-time evaluation of the *in vitro* and *in vivo* gene silencing efficiency of siRNA delivery systems. Transfection efficiency or pharmacodynamics of siRNA delivery systems can be quantitatively determined by silencing luciferase activity in tumor tissues with an anti-luciferase siRNA. When the siRNA is transfected in the tumor cells expressing the luciferase reporter gene, it induces the RNAi machinery to destroy luciferase mRNA and blocks luciferase expression, resulting in a decrease of luciferase activity.

24.9. DCE-MRI can quantitatively measure the tumor vascular properties, which can be correlated to tumor angiogenesis. The anticancer efficacy of the delivery system can be determined by the changes of the vascular properties measured by DCE-MRI. A positive response of the tumor to the therapy should be the decrease of tumor angiogenesis.

24.10. Microbubbles loaded with therapeutics can be visualized and localized by ultrasound imaging. The bubbles can then be destroyed by a different ultrasound frequency to release the therapeutics.

24.11. Theranostics is the combination of therapeutics and diagnostics for achieving individualized pharmacotherapy. It measures a diverse set of biomarkers, including genomic, proteomic, metabolic, and physiological biomarkers; predicts patients' responses to therapies; and determines the best treatment to achieve the best possible therapeutic outcomes.

INDEX

Advanced Drug Delivery, First Edition. Edited by Ashim K. Mitra, Chi H. Lee, and Kun Cheng.